a LANGE medical book

Smith's
General Urology

Sixteenth edition

Edited by

Emil A. Tanagho, MD
Professor of Urology
University of California School of Medicine
San Francisco

Jack W. McAninch, MD, FACS
Professor of Urology
University of California School of Medicine
Chief, Department of Urology
San Francisco General Hospital
San Francisco

Lange Medical Books/McGraw-Hill
Medical Publishing Division

New York   San Francisco   Lisbon   London   Madrid   Mexico City
Milan   New Delhi   San Juan   Seoul   Singapore   Sydney   Toronto

Smith's General Urology, Sixteenth Edition

Copyright © 2004, 2000 by The McGraw-Hill Companies, Inc. All Rights Reserved. Printed in the United States of America. Except as permitted under the United States Copyright Act of 1976, no part of this publication may be reproduced or distributed in any form or by any means, or stored in a data base or retrieval system, without the prior written permission of the publisher.

Previous edition copyright © 1995 Appleton & Lange.

2 3 4 5 6 7 8 9 0   DOC/DOC   0 9 8 7 6 5 4

ISBN: 0-07-139648-9
ISSN: 0892-1245

Notice

Medicine is an ever-changing science. As new research and clinical experience broaden our knowledge, changes in treatment and drug therapy are required. The authors and the publisher of this work have checked with sources believed to be reliable in their efforts to provide information that is complete and generally in accord with the standards accepted at the time of publication. However, in view of the possibility of human error or changes in medical sciences, neither the editors nor the publisher nor any other party who has been involved in the preparation or publication of this work warrants that the information contained herein is in every respect accurate or complete, and they disclaim all responsibility for any errors or omissions or for the results obtained from use of the information contained in this work. Readers are encouraged to confirm the information contained herein with other sources. For example and in particular, readers are advised to check the product information sheet included in the package of each drug they plan to administer to be certain that the information contained in this work is accurate and that changes have not been made in the recommended dose or in the contraindications for administration. This recommendation is of particular importance in connection with new or infrequently used drugs.

This book was set in Times Roman by Pine Tree Composition.
The editors were Janet Foltin, Janene Matragano Oransky, and Karen G. Edmonson.
The production manager was Phil Galea.
The cover designer was Mary McKeon.
The art director was Charissa Baker.
The index was prepared by Kathi Unger.
RR Donnelley was printer and binder.

This book is printed on acid-free paper.

INTERNATIONAL EDITION ISBN: 0-07-121969-2

Copyright © 2004. Exclusive rights by **The McGraw-Hill Companies, Inc.,** for manufacture and export. This book cannot be reexported from the country to which it is consigned by McGraw-Hill. The International Edition is not available in North America.

Contents

Authors

William J.C. Amend, Jr., MD
Professor of Clinical Medicine and Surgery, Division Chief, Department of Nephrology, University of California School of Medicine, San Francisco

Susan Barbour, RN, FNP, WOCN
Clinical Nurse Specialist, University of California San Francisco Medical Center, San Francisco

Laurence S. Baskin, MD
Chief of Pediatric Urology, UCSF Children's Hospital, San Francisco; Atending Urologist, Children's Hospital Oakland, Oakland

Timothy G. Berger, MD
Executive Vice Chair and Director of Clinics, Department of Dermatology; Clinical Professor of Dermatology, University of California School of Medicine, San Francisco

Allan I. Bloom, MD
Lecturer, Vascular and Interventional Radiology, Department of Radiology, Hadassah University Hospital, Jerusalem, Israel

Peter N. Bretan, Jr., MD, FACS
Clinical Associate Professor of Urology, University of California School of Medicine, San Francisco; Chief, Northern California Renal Transplant Program, Santa Rosa Memorial Hospital, San Francisco

Peter R. Carroll, MD
Professor and Chair, Department of Urology, Ken and Donna Derr-Chevron Endowed Chair in Prostate Cancer, University of California School of Medicine, San Francisco

Robert Dreicer, MD, FACP
Director, Genitourinary Medical Oncology, Associate Director, Experimental Therapeutics, Department of Hematology/Oncology, The Urologic Institute Cleveland Clinic Foundation, Cleveland

Steven C. Eberhardt, MD
Clinical Assistant Radiologist, Memorial Sloan-Kettering Cancer Center; Assistant Professor of Radiology, Weill Medical College, Cornell University, New York

Christian Gilfrich, MD
Department of Urology, Johannes Gutenberg University Medical School, Mainz, Germany

Roy L. Gordon, MD
Professor of Radiology, Chief of Interventional Radiology, Department of Radiology, University of California School of Medicine, San Francisco

Gary D. Grossfeld, MD
Private Practice, Greenbrae, California

Hedvig Hricak, MD
Chairman, Department of Radiology, Memorial Sloan-Kettering Cancer Center; Professor of Radiology, Cornell University, New York

Christopher J. Kane, MD, FACS
Associate Professor of Urology, University of California School of Medicine, San Francisco; Chief, Department of Urology, Veterans Affairs Medical Center, San Francisco

Barry A. Kogan, MD
Professor of Urology and Pediatrics; Chief, Division of Urology, Albany Medical College, Albany, New York

Badrinath R. Konety, MD, MBA
Assistant Professor of Urology and Epidemiology, University of Iowa, Iowa City

Karl J. Kreder, MD
Professor and Clinical Vice Chair, Director of Urodynamics and Reconstructive Urology, Department of Urology, University of Iowa, Iowa City

John N. Krieger, MD
Professor of Urology, University of Washington; Chief, Section of Urology, VA Puget Sound Health Care System, Seattle

Marcus A. Krupp, MD, FACP
Clinical Professor of Medicine, Emeritus, Stanford University Medical School, Stanford

Tom F. Lue, MD
Professor of Urology, University of California School of Medicine, San Francisco

Jack W. McAninch, MD, FACS
Professor of Urology, University of California School of Medicine, San Francisco; Chief, Department of Urology, San Francisco General Hospital, San Francisco

Hiep-Thieu Nguyen, MD
Assistant Professor of Urology and Pediatrics, University of California School of Medicine, San Francisco; UCSF Children's Hospital, San Francisco

Joseph C. Presti, Jr., MD
Associate Professor of Urology, Director, Genitourinary Oncology Program, Stanford University School of Medicine, Stanford

Mack Roach, III, MD
Professor of Radiation Oncology and Urology, University of California School of Medicine, San Francisco; San Francisco Comprehensive Cancer Center, San Francisco

Eric J. Small, MD
Professor of Medicine and Urology, University of California School of Medicine, San Franicsco; Program Member, UCSFComprehensive Cancer Center, San Francisco

R. Ernest Sosa, MD
Associate Professor of Urology, New York Presbyterian Hospital, Weill Medical College of Cornell University, New York

Joycelyn L. Speight, MD, PhD
Clinical Instructor of Radiation Oncology, University of California School of Medicine, San Francisco; Member, UCSFComprehensive Cancer Center, San Francisco

Marshall L. Stoller, MD
Professor of Urology, University of California School of Medicine, San Francisco

Emil A. Tanagho, MD
Professor of Urology, University of California School of Medicine, San Francisco

Joachim W. Thüroff, MD
Professor Department of Urology, and Chairman Johannes Gutenberg University Medical School, Mainz, Germany

Paul J. Turek, MD
Associate Professor of Urology and Obstetrics-Gynecology and Reproductive Science; Director, Male Reproductive Center and Laboratory, University of California School of Medicine, San Francisco

E. Darracott Vaughn, MD
James J. Colt Professor of Urology, Weill Medical College of Cornell University, New York-Presbyterian Hospital, New York

Flavio G. Vincenti, MD
Clinical Professor of Medicine and Nephrology, Department of Medicine, University of California School of Medicine, San Francisco

Richard D. Williams, MD
Rubin H. Flocks Chair, Professor and Head, Department of Urology, University of Iowa, Iowa City

J. Stuart Wolf, MD
Director, Michigan Center for Minimally Invasive Urology; Associate Professor of Urology, University of Michigan, Ann Arbor

Preface

Smith's General Urology, 16th Edition, provides in a concise format the information necessary for the understanding, diagnosis, and treatment of diseases managed by urologic surgeons. Our goal has been to keep the book current, to the point, and readable.

Medical students will find this book useful because of its concise, easy-to-follow format and organization and its breadth of information. Interns and residents, as well as practicing physicians in urology or general medicine, will find it an efficient and current reference, particularly because of its emphasis on diagnosis and treatment.

The 16th edition is a thorough revision of the book. No new chapters have been added. However, three chapters were completely rewritten by new authors: Chapter 13: Bacterial Infections of the Genitourinary Tract, Hiep T. Nguyen, MD; Chapter 29: Disorders of the Adrenal Glands, Christopher J. Kane, MD; and Chapter 41: Abnormalities of Sexual Determination & Differentiation, Laurence S. Baskin, MD. The total number of chapters has been reduced to 43, as we eliminated one chapter (Urologic Laser Surgery) and incorporated six others in related chapters. To these, and to all our ongoing contributors, we are deeply indebted.

The book has been reviewed and updated throughout, with emphasis on current references. The several hundred illustrations have been further modernized and improved, including many fine anatomic drawings and the latest imaging techniques. Since the 11th Edition, the following translations have been published: Chinese, French, Greek, Italian, Japanese, Korean, Portuguese, Russian, Spanish, and Turkish.

We greatly appreciate the assistance of our sponsoring editor, Janet Foltin, and Development Editor, Janene Matragrano Oransky, whose expertise and patience have been instrumental in bringing this edition to completion.

Emil A. Tanagho, MD
Jack W. McAninch, MD

San Francisco
October 2003

Anatomy of the Genitourinary Tract 1

Emil A. Tanagho, MD

Urology deals with diseases and disorders of the male genitourinary tract and the female urinary tract. Surgical diseases of the adrenal gland are also included. These systems are illustrated in Figures 1–1 and 1–2.

ADRENALS

Gross Appearance

A. ANATOMY

Each kidney is capped by an adrenal gland, and both organs are enclosed within Gerota's (perirenal) fascia. Each adrenal weighs about 5 g. The right adrenal is triangular in shape; the left is more rounded and crescentic. Each gland is composed of a cortex, chiefly influenced by the pituitary gland, and a medulla derived from chromaffin tissue.

B. RELATIONS

Figure 1–2 shows the relation of the adrenals to other organs. The right adrenal lies between the liver and the vena cava. The left adrenal lies close to the aorta and is covered on its lower surface by the pancreas; superiorly and laterally, it is related to the spleen.

Histology

The adrenal cortex is composed of 3 distinct layers: the outer zona glomerulosa, the middle zona fasciculata, and the inner zona reticularis. The medulla lies centrally and is made up of polyhedral cells containing eosinophilic granular cytoplasm. These chromaffin cells are accompanied by ganglion and small round cells.

Blood Supply

A. ARTERIAL

Each adrenal receives 3 arteries: one from the inferior phrenic artery, one from the aorta, and one from the renal artery.

B. VENOUS

Blood from the right adrenal is drained by a very short vein that empties into the vena cava; the left adrenal vein terminates in the left renal vein.

Lymphatics

The lymphatic vessels accompany the suprarenal vein and drain into the lumbar lymph nodes.

KIDNEYS

Gross Appearance

A. ANATOMY

The kidneys lie along the borders of the psoas muscles and are therefore obliquely placed. The position of the liver causes the right kidney to be lower than the left (Figures 1–2 and 1–3). The adult kidney weighs about 150 g.

The kidneys are supported by the perirenal fat (which is enclosed in the perirenal fascia), the renal vascular pedicle, abdominal muscle tone, and the general bulk of the abdominal viscera. Variations in these factors permit variations in the degree of renal mobility. The average descent on inspiration or on assuming the upright position is 4–5 cm. Lack of mobility suggests abnormal fixation (eg, perinephritis), but extreme mobility is not necessarily pathologic.

On longitudinal section (Figure 1–4), the kidney is seen to be made up of an outer cortex, a central medulla, and the internal calices and pelvis. The cortex is homogeneous in appearance. Portions of it project toward the pelvis between the papillae and fornices and are called the columns of Bertin. The medulla consists of numerous pyramids formed by the converging collecting renal tubules, which drain into the minor calices at the tip of the papillae.

B. RELATIONS

Figures 1–2 and 1–3 show the relations of the kidneys to adjacent organs and structures. Their intimacy with intraperitoneal organs and the autonomic innervation they share with these organs explain, in part, some of the gastrointestinal symptoms that accompany genitourinary disease.

Histology

A. NEPHRON

The functioning unit of the kidney is the nephron, which is composed of a tubule that has both secretory

Upper tract
Kidneys
Ureters

Adrenal

Adrenal

Renal vascular
pedicle

Spermatic or
ovarian artery

Spermatic or
ovarian artery

Spermatic or
ovarian vein

Spermatic or
ovarian vein

Psoas muscle

Mid tract
Bladder

Trigone

Lower tract
Vas deferens
Seminal vesicles
Verumontanum
Prostate
Urethra

Corpus cavernosum

Testicle

Figure 1–1. Anatomy of the male genitourinary tract. The upper and mid tracts have urologic function only. The lower tract has both genital and urinary functions.

Figure 1–2. Relations of kidney, ureters, and bladder (anterior aspect).

and excretory functions (Figure 1–4). The secretory portion is contained largely within the cortex and consists of a renal corpuscle and the secretory part of the renal tubule. The excretory portion of this duct lies in the medulla. The renal corpuscle is composed of the vascular glomerulus, which projects into Bowman's capsule, which, in turn, is continuous with the epithelium of the proximal convoluted tubule. The secretory portion of the renal tubule is made up of the proximal convoluted tubule, the loop of Henle, and the distal convoluted tubule.

The excretory portion of the nephron is the collecting tubule, which is continuous with the distal end of the ascending limb of the convoluted tubule. It empties its contents through the tip (papilla) of a pyramid into a minor calyx.

B. Supporting Tissue

The renal stroma is composed of loose connective tissue and contains blood vessels, capillaries, nerves, and lymphatics.

Blood Supply (Figures 1–2, 1–4, and 1–5)

A. Arterial

Usually there is one renal artery, a branch of the aorta, that enters the hilum of the kidney between the pelvis, which normally lies posteriorly, and the renal vein. It

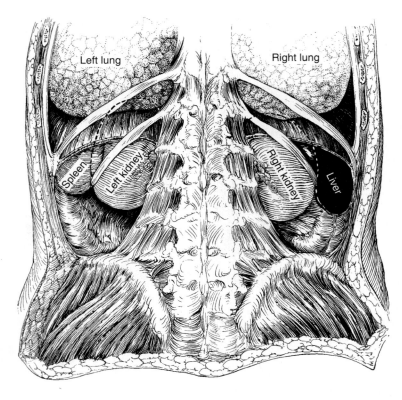

Figure 1–3. Relations of kidneys (posterior aspect). The dashed lines represent the outline of the kidneys where they are obscured by overlying structures.

may branch before it reaches the kidney, and 2 or more separate arteries may be noted. In duplication of the pelvis and ureter, it is usual for each renal segment to have its own arterial supply.

The renal artery divides into anterior and posterior branches. The posterior branch supplies the mid segment of the posterior surface. The anterior branch supplies both upper and lower poles as well as the entire anterior surface. The renal arteries are all end arteries.

The renal artery further divides into interlobar arteries, which ascend in the columns of Bertin (between the pyramids) and then arch along the base of the pyramids (arcuate arteries). The renal artery then ascends as interlobular arteries. From these vessels, smaller (afferent) branches pass to the glomeruli. From the glomerular tuft, efferent arterioles pass to the tubules in the stroma.

B. VENOUS

The renal veins are paired with the arteries, but any of them will drain the entire kidney if the others are tied off.

Although the renal artery and vein are usually the sole blood vessels of the kidney, accessory renal vessels are common and may be of clinical importance if they are so placed to compress the ureter, in which case hydronephrosis may result.

Nerve Supply

The renal nerves derived from the renal plexus accompany the renal vessels throughout the renal parenchyma.

Lymphatics

The lymphatics of the kidney drain into the lumbar lymph nodes.

CALICES, RENAL PELVIS, & URETER

Gross Appearance

A. ANATOMY

1. Calices—The tips of the minor calices (8–12 in number) are indented by the projecting pyramids (Figure 1–4). These calices unite to form 2 or 3 major calices, which join to form the renal pelvis.

2. Renal pelvis—The pelvis may be entirely intrarenal or partly intrarenal and partly extrarenal. Inferomedially, it tapers to form the ureter.

3. Ureter—The adult ureter is about 30 cm long, varying in direct relation to the height of the individual. It follows a rather smooth S curve. Areas of relative narrowing are found (1) at the ureteropelvic junction, (2)

Figure 1–4. Anatomy and histology of the kidney and ureter. **Upper left:** Diagram of the nephron and its blood supply (Courtesy of Merck, Sharp, & Dohme: Seminar: 1947;9[3].) **Upper right:** Cast of the pelvic caliceal system and the arterial supply of the kidney. **Middle:** Renal calices, pelvis, and ureter (posterior aspect). **Lower left:** Histology of the ureter. The smooth-muscle bundles are arranged in both a spiral and a longitudinal manner. **Lower right:** Longitudinal section of kidney showing calices, pelvis, ureter, and renal blood supply (posterior aspect).

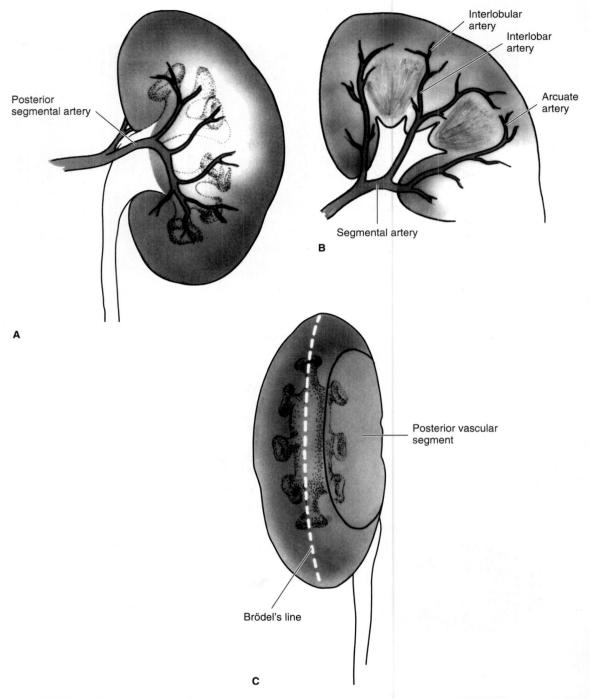

Figure 1–5. **A:** The posterior branch of the renal artery and its distribution to the central segment of the posterior surface of the kidney. **B:** Branches of the anterior division of the renal artery supplying the entire anterior surface of the kidney as well as the upper and lower poles at both surfaces. The segmental branches lead to interlobar, arcuate, and interlobular arteries. **C:** The lateral convex margin of the kidney. Brödel's line, which is 1 cm from the convex margin, is the bloodless plane demarcated by the distribution of the posterior branch of the renal artery.

where the ureter crosses over the iliac vessels, and (3) where it courses through the bladder wall.

B. RELATIONS

1. Calices—The calices are intrarenal and are intimately related to the renal parenchyma.

2. Renal pelvis—If the pelvis is partly extrarenal, it lies along the lateral border of the psoas muscle and on the quadratus lumborum muscle; the renal vascular pedicle is placed just anterior to it. The left renal pelvis lies at the level of the first or second lumbar vertebra; the right pelvis is a little lower.

3. Ureter—As followed from above downward, the ureters lie on the psoas muscles, pass medially to the sacroiliac joints, and then swing laterally near the ischial spines before passing medially to penetrate the base of the bladder (Figure 1–2). In females, the uterine arteries are closely related to the juxtavesical portion of the ureters. The ureters are covered by the posterior peritoneum; their lowermost portions are closely attached to it, while the juxtavesical portions are embedded in vascular retroperitoneal fat.

The vasa deferentia, as they leave the internal inguinal rings, sweep over the lateral pelvic walls anterior to the ureters (Figure 1–6). They lie medial to the latter before joining the seminal vesicle and penetrating the base of the prostate to become the ejaculatory ducts.

Histology (Figure 1–4)

The walls of the calices, pelvis, and ureters are composed of transitional cell epithelium under which lies

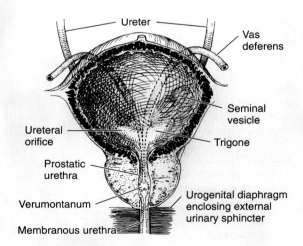

Figure 1–6. Anatomy and relations of the ureters, bladder, prostate, seminal vesicles, and vasa deferentia (anterior view).

loose connective and elastic tissue (lamina propria). External to these are a mixture of helical and longitudinal smooth muscle fibers. They are not arranged in definite layers. The outermost adventitial coat is composed of fibrous connective tissue.

Blood Supply

A. ARTERIAL

The renal calices, pelvis, and upper ureters derive their blood supply from the renal arteries; the mid ureter is fed by the internal spermatic (or ovarian) arteries. The lowermost portion of the ureter is served by branches from the common iliac, internal iliac (hypogastric), and vesical arteries.

B. VENOUS

The veins of the renal calices, pelvis, and ureters are paired with the arteries.

Lymphatics

The lymphatics of the upper portions of the ureters as well as those from the pelvis and calices enter the lumbar lymph nodes. The lymphatics of the mid ureter pass to the internal iliac (hypogastric) and common iliac lymph nodes; the lower ureteral lymphatics empty into the vesical and hypogastric lymph nodes.

BLADDER

Gross Appearance

The bladder is a hollow muscular organ that serves as a reservoir for urine. In women, its posterior wall and dome are invaginated by the uterus. The adult bladder normally has a capacity of 400–500 mL.

A. ANATOMY

When empty, the adult bladder lies behind the pubic symphysis and is largely a pelvic organ. In infants and children, it is situated higher. When it is full, it rises well above the symphysis and can readily be palpated or percussed. When overdistended, as in acute or chronic urinary retention, it may cause the lower abdomen to bulge visibly.

Extending from the dome of the bladder to the umbilicus is a fibrous cord, the median umbilical ligament, which represents the obliterated urachus. The ureters enter the bladder posteroinferiorly in an oblique manner and at these points are about 5 cm apart (Figure 1–6). The orifices, situated at the extremities of the crescent-shaped interureteric ridge that forms the proximal border of the trigone, are about 2.5 cm apart. The

Figure 1–7. **Left:** Histology of the prostate. Epithelial glands embedded in a mixture of connective and elastic tissue and smooth muscle. **Right:** Histology of the bladder. The mucosa is transitional cell in type and lies on a well-developed submucosal layer of connective tissue. The detrusor muscle is composed of interlacing longitudinal, circular, and spiral smooth-muscle bundles.

trigone occupies the area between the ridge and the bladder neck.

The internal sphincter, or bladder neck, is not a true circular sphincter but a thickening formed by interlaced and converging muscle fibers of the detrusor as they pass distally to become the smooth musculature of the urethra.

B. Relations

In males, the bladder is related posteriorly to the seminal vesicles, vasa deferentia, ureters, and rectum (Figures 1–8 and 1–9). In females, the uterus and vagina are interposed between the bladder and rectum (Figure 1–10). The dome and posterior surfaces are covered by peritoneum; hence, in this area the bladder is closely related to the small intestine and sigmoid colon. In both males and females, the bladder is related to the posterior surface of the pubic symphysis, and, when distended, it is in contact with the lower abdominal wall.

Histology (Figure 1–7)

The mucosa of the bladder is composed of transitional epithelium. Beneath it is a well-developed submucosal layer formed largely of connective and elastic tissues. External to the submucosa is the detrusor muscle, which is made up of a mixture of smooth muscle fibers

arranged at random in a longitudinal, circular, and spiral manner without any layer formation or specific orientation except close to the internal meatus, where the detrusor muscle assumes 3 definite layers: inner longitudinal, middle circular, and outer longitudinal.

Blood Supply

A. Arterial

The bladder is supplied with blood by the superior, middle, and inferior vesical arteries, which arise from the anterior trunk of the internal iliac (hypogastric) artery, and by smaller branches from the obturator and inferior gluteal arteries. In females, the uterine and vaginal arteries also send branches to the bladder.

B. Venous

Surrounding the bladder is a rich plexus of veins that ultimately empties into the internal iliac (hypogastric) veins.

Lymphatics

The lymphatics of the bladder drain into the vesical, external iliac, internal iliac (hypogastric), and common iliac lymph nodes.

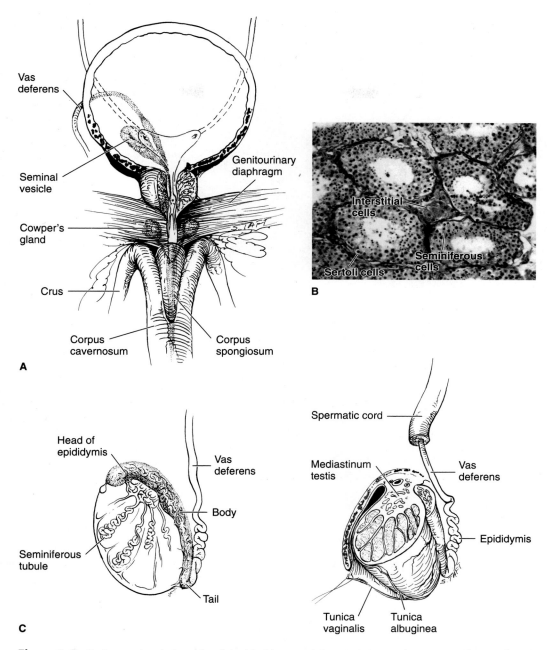

Figure 1–8. **A:** Anatomic relationship of the bladder, prostate, prostatomembranous urethra, and root of the penis. **B:** Histology of the testis. Seminiferous tubules lined by supporting basement membrane for the Sertoli and spermatogenic cells. The latter are in various stages of development. **C:** Cross sections of the testis and epididymis. (**A** and **C** are reproduced, with permission, from Tanagho EA: Anatomy of the lower urinary tract. In: Walsh PC et al [editors]: *Campbell's Urology*, 6th ed., vol. 1. Saunders, 1992.)

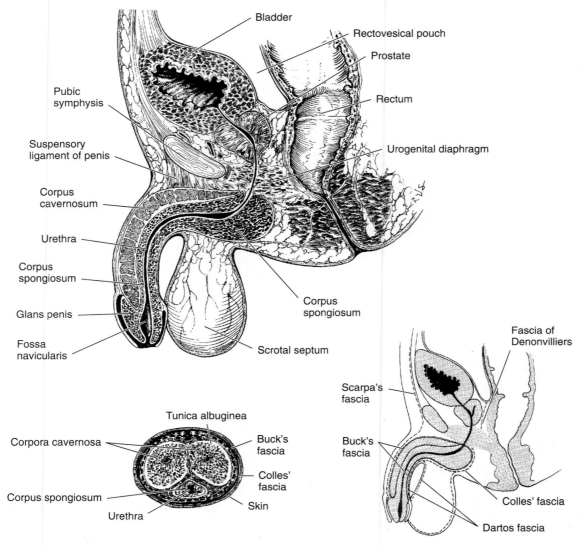

Figure 1–9. **Top:** Relations of the bladder, prostate, seminal vesicles, penis, urethra, and scrotal contents. **Lower left:** Transverse section through the penis. The paired upper structures are the corpora cavernosa. The single lower body surrounding the urethra is the corpus spongiosum. **Lower right:** Fascial planes of the lower genitourinary tract. (After Wesson.)

PROSTATE GLAND

Gross Appearance

A. ANATOMY

The prostate is a fibromuscular and glandular organ lying just inferior to the bladder (Figures 1–6 and 1–8). The normal prostate weighs about 20 g and contains the posterior urethra, which is about 2.5 cm in length.

It is supported anteriorly by the puboprostatic ligaments and inferiorly by the urogenital diaphragm (Figure 1–6). The prostate is perforated posteriorly by the ejaculatory ducts, which pass obliquely to empty through the verumontanum on the floor of the prostatic urethra just proximal to the striated external urinary sphincter (Figure 1–11).

According to the classification of Lowsley, the prostate consists of 5 lobes: anterior, posterior, median,

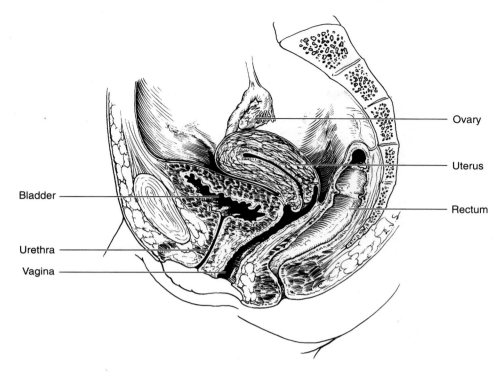

Bladder

Urethra

Vagina

Ovary

Uterus

Rectum

Figure 1–10. Anatomy and relations of the bladder, urethra, uterus and ovary, vagina, and rectum.

right lateral, and left lateral. According to McNeal (1972), the prostate has a peripheral zone, a central zone, and a transitional zone; an anterior segment; and a preprostatic sphincteric zone (Figure 1–12). The segment of urethra that traverses the prostate gland is the prostatic urethra. It is lined by an inner longitudinal layer of muscle (continuous with a similar layer of the vesical wall). Incorporated within the prostate gland is an abundant amount of smooth musculature derived primarily from the external longitudinal bladder musculature. This musculature represents the true smooth involuntary sphincter of the posterior urethra in males.

Prostatic adenoma develops from the periurethral glands at the site of the median or lateral lobes. The posterior lobe, however, is prone to cancerous degeneration.

B. Relations

The prostate gland lies behind the pubic symphysis. Located closely to the posterosuperior surface are the vasa deferentia and seminal vesicles (Figure 1–8). Posteriorly, the prostate is separated from the rectum by the 2 layers of Denonvilliers' fascia, serosal rudiments of the pouch of Douglas, which once extended to the urogenital diaphragm (Figure 1–9).

Histology (Figure 1–7)

The prostate consists of a thin fibrous capsule under which are circularly oriented smooth muscle fibers and collagenous tissue that surrounds the urethra (involuntary sphincter). Deep to this layer lies the prostatic stroma, composed of connective and elastic tissues and smooth muscle fibers in which are embedded the epithelial glands. These glands drain into the major excretory ducts (about 25 in number), which open chiefly on the floor of the urethra between the verumontanum and the vesical neck. Just beneath the transitional epithelium of the prostatic urethra lie the periurethral glands.

Blood Supply

A. Arterial

The arterial supply to the prostate is derived from the inferior vesical, internal pudendal, and middle rectal (hemorrhoidal) arteries.

B. Venous

The veins from the prostate drain into the periprostatic plexus, which has connections with the deep dorsal vein of the penis and the internal iliac (hypogastric) veins.

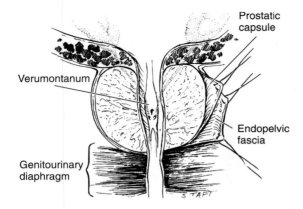

Figure 1–11. Section of the prostate gland shows the prostatic urethra, verumontanum, and crista urethralis, in addition to the opening of the prostatic utricle and the 2 ejaculatory ducts in the midline. Note that the prostate is surrounded by the prostatic capsule, which is covered by another prostatic sheath derived from the endopelvic fascia. The prostate is resting on the genitourinary diaphragm. (Reproduced, with permission, from Tanagho EA: Anatomy of the lower urinary tract. In: Walsh PC et al [editors]: *Campbell's Urology*, 6th ed., vol. 1. Saunders, 1992.)

Nerve Supply

The prostate gland receives a rich nerve supply from the sympathetic and parasympathetic nerve plexuses.

Lymphatics

The lymphatics from the prostate drain into the internal iliac (hypogastric), sacral, vesical, and external iliac lymph nodes.

SEMINAL VESICLES

Gross Appearance

The seminal vesicles lie just cephalic to the prostate under the base of the bladder (Figures 1–6 and 1–8). They are about 6 cm long and quite soft. Each vesicle joins its corresponding vas deferens to form the ejaculatory duct. The ureters lie medial to each, and the rectum is contiguous with their posterior surfaces.

Histology

The mucous membrane is pseudostratified. The submucosa consists of dense connective tissue covered by a thin layer of muscle that in turn is encapsulated by connective tissue.

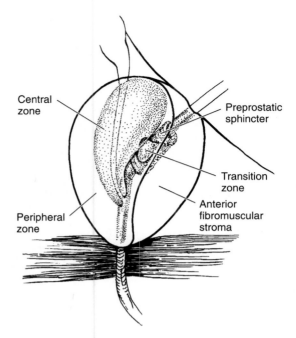

Figure 1–12. Anatomy of the prostate gland (adapted from McNeal). (Reproduced, with permission, from Tanagho EA: Anatomy of the lower urinary tract. In: Walsh PC et al [editors]: *Campbell's Urology*, 6th ed., vol. 1. Saunders, 1992.)

Blood Supply

The blood supply is similar to that of the prostate gland.

Nerve Supply

The nerve supply is mainly from the sympathetic nerve plexus.

Lymphatics

The lymphatics of the seminal vesicles are those that serve the prostate.

SPERMATIC CORD

Gross Appearance

The 2 spermatic cords extend from the internal inguinal rings through the inguinal canals to the testicles (Figure 1–8). Each cord contains the vas deferens, the internal and external spermatic arteries, the artery of the vas, the venous pampiniform plexus (which forms the spermatic vein superiorly), lymph vessels, and nerves. All of the preceding are enclosed in investing layers of thin fascia. A few fibers of the cremaster muscle insert on the cords in the inguinal canal.

Histology

The fascia covering the cord is formed of loose connective tissue that supports arteries, veins, and lymphatics. The vas deferens is a small, thick-walled tube consisting of an internal mucosa and submucosa surrounded by 3 well-defined layers of smooth muscle encased in a covering of fibrous tissue. Above the testes, this tube is straight. Its proximal 4 cm tends to be convoluted.

Blood Supply

A. ARTERIAL

The external spermatic artery, a branch of the inferior epigastric, supplies the fascial coverings of the cord. The internal spermatic artery passes through the cord on its way to the testis. The deferential artery is close to the vas.

B. VENOUS

The veins from the testis and the coverings of the spermatic cord form the pampiniform plexus, which, at the internal inguinal ring, unites to form the spermatic vein.

Lymphatics

The lymphatics from the spermatic cord empty into the external iliac lymph nodes.

EPIDIDYMIS

Gross Appearance

A. ANATOMY

The upper portion of the epididymis (globus major) is connected to the testis by numerous efferent ducts from the testis (Figure 1–8). The epididymis consists of a markedly coiled duct that, at its lower pole (globus minor), is continuous with the vas deferens. An appendix of the epididymis is often seen on its upper pole; this is a cystic body that in some cases is pedunculated but in others is sessile.

B. RELATIONS

The epididymis lies posterolateral to the testis and is nearest to the testis at its upper pole. Its lower pole is connected to the testis by fibrous tissue. The vas lies posteromedial to the epididymis.

Histology

The epididymis is covered by serosa. The ductus epididymidis is lined by pseudostratified columnar epithelium throughout its length.

Blood Supply

A. ARTERIAL

The arterial supply to the epididymis comes from the internal spermatic artery and the artery of the vas (deferential artery).

B. VENOUS

The venous blood drains into the pampiniform plexus, which becomes the spermatic vein.

Lymphatics

The lymphatics drain into the external iliac and internal iliac (hypogastric) lymph nodes.

TESTIS

Gross Appearance

A. ANATOMY

The average testicle measures about 4 × 3 × 2.5 cm (Figure 1–8). It has a dense fascial covering called the tunica albuginea testis, which, posteriorly, is invaginated somewhat into the body of the testis to form the mediastinum testis. This fibrous mediastinum sends fibrous septa into the testis, thus separating it into about 250 lobules.

The testis is covered anteriorly and laterally by the visceral layer of the serous tunica vaginalis, which is continuous with the parietal layer that separates the testis from the scrotal wall.

At the upper pole of the testis is the appendix testis, a small pedunculated or sessile body similar in appearance to the appendix of the epididymis.

B. RELATIONS

The testis is closely attached posterolaterally to the epididymis, particularly at its upper and lower poles.

Histology (Figure 1–8)

Each lobule contains 1–4 markedly convoluted seminiferous tubules, each of which is about 60 cm long. These ducts converge at the mediastinum testis, where they connect with the efferent ducts that drain into the epididymis.

The seminiferous tubule has a basement membrane containing connective and elastic tissue. This supports the seminiferous cells, which are of 2 types: (1) Sertoli (supporting) cells and (2) spermatogenic cells. The stroma between the seminiferous tubules contains connective tissue in which the interstitial Leydig cells are located.

Blood Supply

The blood supply to the testes is closely associated with that to the kidneys because of the common embryologic origin of the two organs.

A. ARTERIAL

The arteries to the testes (internal spermatics) arise from the aorta just below the renal arteries and course through the spermatic cords to the testes, where they anastomose with the arteries of the vasa deferentia that branch off from the internal iliac (hypogastric) artery.

B. VENOUS

The blood from the testis returns in the pampiniform plexus of the spermatic cord. At the internal inguinal ring, the pampiniform plexus forms the spermatic vein.

The right spermatic vein enters the vena cava just below the right renal vein; the left spermatic vein empties into the left renal vein.

Lymphatics

The lymphatic vessels from the testes pass to the lumbar lymph nodes, which in turn are connected to the mediastinal nodes.

SCROTUM

Gross Appearance

Beneath the corrugated skin of the scrotum lies the dartos muscle. Deep to this are the 3 fascial layers derived from the abdominal wall at the time of testicular descent. Beneath these is the parietal layer of the tunica vaginalis.

The scrotum is divided into 2 sacs by a septum of connective tissue. The scrotum not only supports the testes but, by relaxation or contraction of its muscular layer, helps to regulate their environmental temperature.

Histology

The dartos muscle, under the skin of the scrotum, is unstriated. The deeper layer is made up of connective tissue.

Blood Supply

A. ARTERIAL

The arteries to the scrotum arise from the femoral, internal pudendal, and inferior epigastric arteries.

B. VENOUS

The veins are paired with the arteries.

Lymphatics

The lymphatics drain into the superficial inguinal and subinguinal lymph nodes.

PENIS & MALE URETHRA

Gross Appearance

The penis is composed of 2 corpora cavernosa and the corpus spongiosum, which contains the urethra, whose diameter is 8–9 mm. These corpora are capped distally by the glans. Each corpus is enclosed in a fascial sheath (tunica albuginea), and all are surrounded by a thick fibrous envelope known as Buck's fascia. A covering of skin, devoid of fat, is loosely applied about these bodies. The prepuce forms a hood over the glans.

Beneath the skin of the penis (and scrotum) and extending from the base of the glans to the urogenital diaphragm is Colles' fascia, which is continuous with Scarpa's fascia of the lower abdominal wall (Figure 1–9).

The proximal ends of the corpora cavernosa are attached to the pelvic bones just anterior to the ischial tuberosities. Occupying a depression of their ventral surface in the midline is the corpus spongiosum, which is connected proximally to the undersurface of the urogenital diaphragm, through which emerges the membranous urethra. This portion of the corpus spongiosum is surrounded by the bulbospongiosus muscle. Its distal end expands to form the glans penis.

The suspensory ligament of the penis arises from the linea alba and pubic symphysis and inserts into the fascial covering of the corpora cavernosa.

Histology

A. CORPORA AND GLANS PENIS

The corpora cavernosa, the corpus spongiosum, and the glans penis are composed of septa of smooth muscle and erectile tissue that enclose vascular cavities.

B. URETHRA

The urethral mucosa that traverses the glans penis is formed of squamous epithelium. Proximal to this, the mucosa is transitional in type. Underneath the mucosa is the submucosa, which contains connective and elastic tissue and smooth muscle. In the submucosa are the numerous glands of Littre, whose ducts connect with the urethral lumen. The urethra is surrounded by the vascular corpus spongiosum and the glans penis.

Blood Supply

A. ARTERIAL

The penis and urethra are supplied by the internal pudendal arteries. Each artery divides into a deep artery of the penis (which supplies the corpora cavernosa), a dorsal artery of the penis, and the bulbourethral artery. These branches supply the corpus spongiosum, the glans penis, and the urethra.

B. VENOUS

The superficial dorsal vein lies external to Buck's fascia. The deep dorsal vein is placed beneath Buck's fascia and lies between the dorsal arteries. These veins connect with the pudendal plexus, which drains into the internal pudendal vein.

Lymphatics

Lymphatic drainage from the skin of the penis is to the superficial inguinal and subinguinal lymph nodes. The lymphatics from the glans penis pass to the subinguinal and external iliac nodes. The lymphatics from the deep urethra drain into the internal iliac (hypogastric) and common iliac lymph nodes.

FEMALE URETHRA

The adult female urethra is about 4 cm long and 8 mm in diameter. It is slightly curved and lies beneath the pubic symphysis just anterior to the vagina.

The epithelial lining of the female urethra is squamous in its distal portion and pseudostratified or transitional in the remainder. The submucosa is made up of connective and elastic tissues and spongy venous spaces. Embedded in it are many periurethral glands, which are most numerous distally; the largest of these are the periurethral glands of Skene, which open on the floor of the urethra just inside the meatus.

External to the submucosa is a longitudinal layer of smooth muscle continuous with the inner longitudinal layer of the bladder wall. Surrounding this is a heavy layer of circular smooth muscle fibers extending from the external vesical muscular layer. They constitute the true involuntary urethral sphincter. External to this is the circular striated (voluntary) sphincter surrounding the middle third of the urethra; this constitutes an intensive element in the musculature of the urethra.

The arterial supply to the female urethra is derived from the inferior vesical, vaginal, and internal pudendal arteries. Blood from the urethra drains into the internal pudendal veins.

Lymphatic drainage from the external portion of the urethra is to the inguinal and subinguinal lymph nodes. Drainage from the deep urethra is into the internal iliac (hypogastric) lymph nodes.

Nerve Supply to the Genitourinary Organs

See Figures 3–2 and 3–3.

REFERENCES

Adrenals

Avisse C et al: Surgical anatomy and embryology of the adrenal glands. Surg Clin North Am 2000;80:403.

Edmonds DK: Congenital malformations of the genital tract. Obstet Gynecol Clin North Am 2000;27:49.

Peppercorn PD, Reznek RH: State-of-the-art C and MRI of the adrenal gland. Eur Radiol 1997;7:822.

Rosol TJ et al: Adrenal gland: Structure, function, and mechanisms of toxicity. Toxicol Pathol 2001;29:41.

Kidneys

Aizenstein RI et al: The perinephric space and renal fascia: Review of normal anatomy, pathology, and pathways of disease spread. J Magn Reson Imaging 1998;8:517.

Amis ES Jr, Cronan JJ: The renal sinus: An imaging review and proposed nomenclature for sinus cysts. J Urol 1988;139:1151.

Chestbrough RM et al: Gerota versus Zuckerkandl: The renal fascia revisited. Radiology 1989;173:845.

Cockett ATK: Lymphatic network of kidney. 1. Anatomic and physiologic considerations. Urology 1977;9:125.

Emamian SA et al: Kidney dimensions at sonography: Correlation with age, sex, and habitus in 655 adult volunteers. AJR 1993;160:83.

Hoeltl W, Hruby W, Aharinejad S: Renal vein anatomy and its implications for retroperitoneal surgery. J Urol 1990;143:1108.

Kikinis R et al: Normal and hydronephrotic kidney: Evaluation of renal function with contrast-enhanced MR imaging. Radiology 1987;165:837.

Mandell J et al: Structural genitourinary defects detected in utero. Radiology 1991;178:193.

Nolte-Ernsting CC, Adam GB, Gunther RW: MR urography: Examination techniques and clinical applications. Eur Radiol 2001;11:355.

Ohlson L: Normal collecting ducts: Visualization at urography. Radiology 1989;170:33.

Patten RM et al: The fetal genitourinary tract. Radiol Clin North Am 1990;28:115.

Potter EL: Development of the human glomerulus. Arch Pathol 1965;80:241.

Prince MR: Renal MR angiography: A comprehensive approach. J Magn Reson Imaging 1998;8:511.

Resnick MI, Pounds DM, Boyce WH: Surgical anatomy of the human kidney and its applications. Urology 1981;17:367.

Sampaio FJ: Anatomical background for nephron-sparing surgery in renal cell carcinoma. J Urol 1992;147:999.

Sampaio FJ, Aragao AH: Anatomical relationship between the intrarenal arteries and the kidney collecting system. J Urol 1990;143:679.

Sampaio FJ et al: Intrarenal access: 3-dimensional anatomical study. J Urol 1992;148:1769.

Calices, Renal Pelvis, & Ureters

el-Galley RE, Keane TE: Embryology, anatomy, and surgical applications of the kidney and ureter. Surg Clin North Am 2000; 80:381.

Koff SA et al: Pathophysiology of ureteropelvic junction obstruction: Experimental and clinical observations. J Urol 1986; 136:336.

Osathanondh V, Potter EL: Development of human kidney shown by microdissection. 2. Renal pelvis, calyces, and papillae. 3. Formation and interrelationships of collecting tubules and nephrons. 4. Formation of tubular portions of nephrons. 5. Development of vascular pattern of glomerulus. Arch Pathol 1963;76:277, 290 and 1966;82:391, 403.

Tanagho EA: The ureterovesical junction: Anatomy and physiology. In: Chisholm GD, Williams DI (editors): *Scientific Foundations of Urology*. Heinemann, 1982.

Bladder & Urethra

Andersson KE: Neurotransmitters and neuroreceptors in the lower urinary tract. Curr Opin Obstet Gynecol 1996;8:361.

Banson ML: Normal MR anatomy and techniques for imaging of the male pelvis. Magn Reson Imaging Clin North Am 1996;4:481.

Bernhardt TM, Rapp-Bernhardt U: Virtual cystoscopy of the bladder based on CT and MRI data. Abdom Imaging 2001; 26:325.

Chai TC, Steers WD: Neurophysiology of micturition and continence. Urol Clin North Am 1996;23:221.

Creed KE, Van der Werf BA: The innervation and properties of the urethral striated muscle. Scand J Urol Nephrol Suppl 2001; 207:8.

Dorschner W, Stolzenburg JU, Neuhaus J: Structure and function of the bladder neck. Adv Anat Embryol Cell Biol 2001; 159:III–XII, 1–109.

Elbadawi A: Functional anatomy of the organs of micturition. Urol Clin North Am 1996;23:177.

Elbadawi A: Ultrastructure of vesicourethral innervation. 1. Neuroeffector and cell junctions in male internal sphincter. J Urol 1982;128:180.

Gosling JA, Dixon DS: The structure and innervation of smooth muscle in the wall of the bladder neck and proximal urethra. Br J Urol 1975;47:549.

Hutch JA: *Anatomy and Physiology of the Bladder, Trigone and Urethra*. Appleton-Century-Crofts, 1972.

Hutch JA: The internal urinary sphincter: A double loop system. J Urol 1971;105:375.

Juenemann KP et al: Clinical significance of sacral and pudendal nerve anatomy. J Urol 1988;139:74.

Lewis SA: Everything you wanted to know about the bladder epithelium but were afraid to ask. Am J Physiol Renal Physiol 2000;278:F867.

Sandler CM, Corriere JN Jr: Urethrography in the diagnosis of acute urethral injuries. Urol Clin North Am 1989;16:283.

Schlegel PN, Walsh PC: Neuroanatomical approach to radical cystoprostatectomy with preservation of sexual function. J Urol 1987;138:1402.

Tanagho EA: Anatomy of the lower urinary tract. In: Walsh PC et al (editors): *Campbell's Urology*, 6th ed., vol. 1, p. 40. Saunders, 1992.

Tanagho EA, Miller ER: Functional considerations of urethral sphincteric dynamics. J Urol 1973;109:273.

Tanagho EA, Pugh RCB: The anatomy and function of the ureterovesical junction. Br J Urol 1963;35:151.

Tanagho EA, Schmidt RA, de Araujo CG: Urinary striated sphincter: What is its nerve supply? Urology 1982;20:415.

Tanagho EA, Smith DR: The anatomy and function of the bladder neck. Br J Urol 1966;38:54.

Prostate

Allen KS et al: Age-related changes of the prostate: Evaluation by MR imaging. AJR 1989;152:77.

Greene DR, Fitzpatrick JM, Scardino PT: Anatomy of the prostate and distribution of early prostate cancer. Semin Surg Oncol 1995;11:9.

Hricak H et al: MR imaging of the prostate gland: Normal anatomy. AJR 1987;148:51.

McNeal JE: The prostate and prostatic urethra: A morphologic study. J Urol 1972;107:1008.

Myers RP: Male urethral sphincteric anatomy and radical prostatectomy. Urol Clin North Am 1991;18:211.

Myers RP, Goellner JR, Cahill DR: Prostate shape, external striated urethral sphincter and radical prostatectomy: The apical dissection. J Urol 1987;138:543.

Older RA, Watson LR: Ultrasound anatomy of the normal male reproductive tract. J Clin Ultrasound 1996;24:389.

Wein AJ, Benson Gs, Jacobowitz D: Lack of evidence for adrenergic innervation of external urethral sphincter. J Urol 1979; 121:324.

Wheeler TM: Anatomic considerations in carcinoma of the prostate. Urol Clin North Am 1989;16:623.

Spermatic Cord

Baker LL et al: MR imaging of the scrotum: Normal anatomy. Radiology 1987;163:89.

Wishahi MM: Anatomy of spermatic venous plexus (pampiniform plexus) in men with and without varicocele: Intraoperative venographic study. J Urol 1992;147:1285.

Testis

Busch FM, Sayegh ES: Roentgenographic visualization of human testicular lymphatics: A preliminary report. J Urol 1963;89: 106.

Oyen RH: Scrotal ultrasound. Eur Radiol 2002;12:19.

Takihara H et al: Significance of testicular size measurement in andrology: 2. Correlation of testicular size with testicular function. J Urol 1987;137:416.

Female Urethra

DeLancey JO: Structural aspects of the extrinsic continence mechanism. Obstet Gynecol 1988;72:296.

Mostwin JL: Current concepts of female pelvic anatomy and physiology. Urol Clin North Am 1991;18:175.

Ulmsten U: Some reflections and hypotheses on the pathophysiology of female urinary incontinence. Acta Obstet Gynecol Scand Suppl 1997;166:3.

Embryology of the Genitourinary System

Emil A. Tanagho, MD

At birth, the genital and urinary systems are related only in the sense that they share certain common passages. Embryologically, however, they are intimately related. Because of the complex interrelationships of the embryonic phases of the 2 systems, they are discussed here as 5 subdivisions: the nephric system, the vesicourethral unit, the gonads, the genital duct system, and the external genitalia.

■ NEPHRIC SYSTEM

The nephric system develops progressively as 3 distinct entities: pronephros, mesonephros, and metanephros.

Pronephros

The pronephros is the earliest nephric stage in humans, and it corresponds to the mature structure of the most primitive vertebrate. It extends from the fourth to the 14th somites and consists of 6–10 pairs of tubules. These open into a pair of primary ducts that are formed at the same level, extend caudally, and eventually reach and open into the cloaca. The pronephros is a vestigial structure that disappears completely by the fourth week of embryonic life (Figure 2–1).

Mesonephros

The mature excretory organ of the higher fish and amphibians corresponds to the embryonic mesonephros. It is the principal excretory organ during early embryonic life (4–8 weeks). It, too, gradually degenerates, although parts of its duct system become associated with the male reproductive organs. The mesonephric tubules develop from the intermediate mesoderm caudal to the pronephros shortly before pronephric degeneration. The mesonephric tubules differ from those of the pronephros in that they develop a cuplike outgrowth into which a knot of capillaries is pushed. This is called Bowman's capsule, and the tuft of capillaries is called a glomerulus. In their growth, the mesonephric tubules extend toward and establish a connection with the nearby primary nephric duct as it grows caudally to join the cloaca (Figure 2–1). This primary nephric duct is now called the mesonephric duct. After establishing their connection with the nephric duct, the primordial tubules elongate and become S-shaped. As the tubules elongate, a series of secondary branchings increase their surface exposure, thereby enhancing their capacity for interchanging material with the blood in adjacent capillaries. Leaving the glomerulus, the blood is carried by one or more efferent vessels that soon break up into a rich capillary plexus closely related to the mesonephric tubules. The mesonephros, which forms early in the fourth week, reaches its maximum size by the end of the second month.

Metanephros

The metanephros, the final phase of development of the nephric system, originates from both the intermediate mesoderm and the mesonephric duct. Development begins in the 5- to 6-mm embryo with a budlike outgrowth from the mesonephric duct as it bends to join the cloaca. This ureteral bud grows cephalad and collects mesoderm from the nephrogenic cord of the intermediate mesoderm around its tip. This mesoderm with the metanephric cap moves, with the growing ureteral bud, more and more cephalad from its point of origin. During this cephalic migration, the metanephric cap becomes progressively larger, and rapid internal differentiation takes place. Meanwhile, the cephalic end of the ureteral bud expands within the growing mass of metanephrogenic tissue to form the renal pelvis (Figure 2–1). Numerous outgrowths from the renal pelvic dilatation push radially into this growing mass and form hollow ducts that branch and rebranch as they push toward the periphery. These form the primary collecting ducts of the kidney. Mesodermal cells become arranged in small vesicular masses that lie close to the blind end of the collecting ducts. Each of these vesicular masses will form a uriniferous tubule draining into the duct nearest to its point of origin.

As the kidney grows, increasing numbers of tubules are formed in its peripheral zone. These vesicular masses develop a central cavity and become S-shaped.

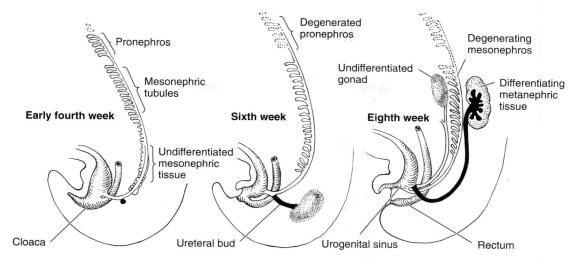

Figure 2–1. Schematic representation of the development of the nephric system. Only a few of the tubules of the pronephros are seen early in the fourth week, while the mesonephric tissue differentiates into mesonephric tubules that progressively join the mesonephric duct. The first sign of the ureteral bud from the mesonephric duct is seen. At 6 weeks, the pronephros has completely degenerated and the mesonephric tubules start to do so. The ureteral bud grows dorsocranially and has met the metanephrogenic cap. At the eighth week, there is cranial migration of the differentiating metanephros. The cranial end of the ureteric bud expands and starts to show multiple successive outgrowths. (Adapted from several sources.)

One end of the S coalesces with the terminal portion of the collecting tubules, resulting in a continuous canal. The proximal portion of the S develops into the distal and proximal convoluted tubules and into Henle's loop; the distal end becomes the glomerulus and Bowman's capsule. At this stage, the undifferentiated mesoderm and the immature glomeruli are readily visible on microscopic examination (Figure 2–2). The glomeruli are fully developed by the 36th week or when the fetus weighs 2500 g (Osathanondh and Potter, 1964a and b). The metanephros arises opposite the 28th somite (fourth lumbar segment). At term, it has ascended to the level of the first lumbar or even the 12th thoracic vertebra. This ascent of the kidney is due not only to actual cephalic migration but also to differential growth in the caudal part of the body. During the early period of ascent (seventh to ninth weeks), the kidney slides above the arterial bifurcation and rotates 90 degrees. Its convex border is now directed laterally, not dorsally. Ascent proceeds more slowly until the kidney reaches its final position.

Certain features of these 3 phases of development must be emphasized: (1) The 3 successive units of the system develop from the intermediate mesoderm. (2) The tubules at all levels appear as independent primordia and only secondarily unite with the duct system. (3) The nephric duct is laid down as the duct of the

pronephros and develops from the union of the ends of the anterior pronephric tubules. (4) This pronephric duct serves subsequently as the mesonephric duct and as such gives rise to the ureter. (5) The nephric duct reaches the cloaca by independent caudal growth. (6) The embryonic ureter is an outgrowth of the nephric duct, yet the kidney tubules differentiate from adjacent metanephric blastema.

ANOMALIES OF THE NEPHRIC SYSTEM

Failure of the metanephros to ascend leads to **ectopic kidney.** An ectopic kidney may be on the proper side but low (simple ectopy) or on the opposite side (crossed ectopy) with or without fusion. Failure to rotate during ascent causes a **malrotated kidney.**

Fusion of the paired metanephric masses leads to various anomalies—most commonly **horseshoe kidney.**

The ureteral bud from the mesonephric duct may bifurcate, causing a **bifid ureter** at various levels depending on the time of the bud's subdivision. An accessory ureteral bud may develop from the mesonephric duct, thereby forming a **duplicated ureter,** usually meeting the same metanephric mass. Rarely, each bud has a separate metanephric mass, resulting in **supernumerary kidneys.**

Figure 2–2. Progressive stages in the differentiation of the nephrons and their linkage with the branching collecting tubules. A small lump of metanephric tissue is associated with each terminal collecting tubule. These are then arranged in vesicular masses that later differentiate into a uriniferous tubule draining into the duct near which it arises. At one end, Bowman's capsule and the glomerulus differentiate; the other end establishes communication with the nearby collecting tubules.

If the double ureteral buds are close together on the mesonephric duct, they open near each other in the bladder. In this case, the main ureteral bud, which is the first to appear and the most caudal on the mesonephric ducts, reaches the bladder first. It then starts to move upward and laterally and is followed later by the second accessory bud as it reaches the urogenital sinus. The main ureteral bud (now more cranial on the urogenital sinus) drains the lower portion of the kidney. The 2 ureteral buds re-verse their relationship as they move from the mesonephric duct to the urogenital sinus. This is why double ureters always cross (Weigert-Meyer law). If the 2 ureteral buds are widely separated on the mesonephric duct, the accessory bud appears more proximal and ends in the bladder with an ectopic orifice lower than the normal one. This ectopic orifice could still be in the bladder close to its outlet, in the urethra, or even in the genital duct system (Figure 2–3). A single ureteral bud that

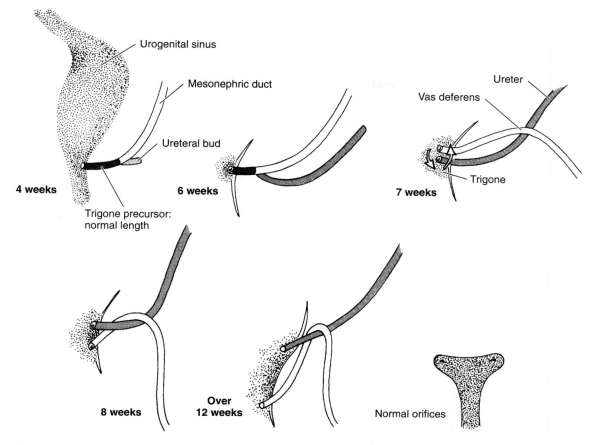

Figure 2–3. The development of the ureteral bud from the mesonephric duct and the relationship of both to the urogenital sinus. The ureteral bud appears at the fourth week. The mesonephric duct distal to this ureteral bud is gradually absorbed into the urogenital sinus, resulting in separate endings for the ureter and the mesonephric duct. The mesonephric tissue that is incorporated into the urogenital sinus expands and forms the trigonal tissue.

arises higher than normal on the mesonephric duct can also end in a similar ectopic location.

Lack of development of a ureteral bud results in a **solitary kidney** and a hemitrigone.

■ VESICOURETHRAL UNIT

The blind end of the hindgut caudal to the point of origin of the allantois expands to form the cloaca, which is separated from the outside by a thin plate of tissue (the cloacal membrane) lying in an ectodermal depression (the proctodeum) under the root of the tail. At the 4-mm stage, starting at the cephalic portion of the cloaca where the allantois and gut meet, the cloaca progressively divides into 2 compartments by the caudal growth of a crescentic fold, the urorectal fold. The 2 limbs of the fold bulge into the lumen of the cloaca from either side, eventually meeting and fusing. The division of the cloaca into a ventral portion (urogenital sinus) and a dorsal portion (rectum) is completed during the seventh week. During the development of the urorectal septum, the cloacal membrane undergoes a reverse rotation, so that the ectodermal surface is no longer directed toward the developing anterior abdominal wall but gradually is turned to face caudally and slightly posteriorly. This change facilitates the subdivision of the cloaca and is brought about mainly by development of the infraumbilical portion of the anterior abdominal wall and regression of the tail. The mesoderm that passes around the cloacal membrane to the caudal attachment of the umbilical cord proliferates and grows, forming a surface elevation, the genital tubercle. Further growth of the infraumbilical part of the abdominal wall progressively separates the umbilical cord from the genital tubercle. The division of the cloaca is completed before the cloacal membrane ruptures, and its 2 parts therefore have separate openings. The ventral part is the primitive urogenital sinus, which has the shape of an elongated cylinder and is continuous cranially with the allantois; its external opening is the urogenital ostium. The dorsal part is the rectum, and its external opening is the anus.

The urogenital sinus receives the mesonephric ducts. The caudal end of the mesonephric duct distal to the ureteral bud is progressively absorbed into the urogenital sinus. By the seventh week, the mesonephric duct and the ureteral bud have independent opening sites. This introduces an island of mesodermal tissue amid the surrounding endoderm of the urogenital sinus. As development progresses, the opening of the mesonephric duct (which will become the ejaculatory duct) migrates downward and medially. The opening of the ureteral bud (which will become the ureteral orifice) migrates upward and laterally. The absorbed mesoderm of the mesonephric duct expands with this migration to occupy the area limited by the final position of these tubes (Figure 2–3). This will later be differentiated as the trigonal structure, which is the only mesodermal inclusion in the endodermal vesicourethral unit.

The urogenital sinus can be divided into 2 main segments; the dividing line, the junction of the combined müllerian ducts with the dorsal wall of the urogenital sinus, is an elevation called Müller's tubercle, which is the most fixed reference point in the whole structure and which is discussed in a subsequent section. The segments are as follows:

(1) The ventral and pelvic portion forms the bladder, part of the urethra in males, and the whole urethra in females. This portion receives the ureter.

(2) The urethral, or phallic, portion receives the mesonephric and the fused müllerian ducts. This will be part of the urethra in males and forms the lower fifth of the vagina and the vaginal vestibule in females.

During the third month, the ventral part of the urogenital sinus starts to expand and forms an epithelial sac whose apex tapers into an elongated, narrowed urachus. The pelvic portion remains narrow and tubular; it forms the whole urethra in females and the supramontanal portion of the prostatic urethra in males. The splanchnic mesoderm surrounding the ventral and pelvic portion of the urogenital sinus begins to differentiate into interlacing bands of smooth muscle fibers and an outer fibrous connective tissue coat. By the 12th week, the layers characteristic of the adult urethra and bladder are recognizable (Figure 2–4).

The part of the urogenital sinus caudal to the opening of the müllerian duct forms the vaginal vestibule and contributes to the lower fifth of the vagina in females (Figure 2–5). In males, it forms the inframontanal part of the prostatic urethra and the membranous urethra. The penile urethra is formed by the fusion of the urethral folds on the ventral surface of the genital tubercle. In females, the urethral folds remain separate and form the labia minora. The glandular urethra in males is formed by canalization of the urethral plate. The bladder originally extends up to the umbilicus, where it is connected to the allantois that extends into the umbilical cord. The allantois usually is obliterated at the level of the umbilicus by the 15th week. The bladder then starts to descend by the 18th week. As it descends, its apex becomes stretched and narrowed, and it pulls on the already obliterated allantois, now called the urachus. By the 20th week, the bladder is well separated from the umbilicus, and the stretched urachus becomes the middle umbilical ligament.

PROSTATE

The prostate develops as multiple solid outgrowths of the urethral epithelium both above and below the entrance of the mesonephric duct. These simple, tubular outgrowths begin to develop in 5 distinct groups at the end of the 11th week and are complete by the 16th week (112-mm stage). They branch and rebranch, ending in a complex duct system that encounters the differentiating mesenchymal cells around this segment of the urogenital sinus. These mesenchymal cells start to develop around the tubules by the 16th week and become denser at the periphery to form the prostatic capsule. By the 22nd week, the muscular stroma is considerably developed, and it continues to increase progressively until birth.

From the 5 groups of epithelial buds, 5 lobes are eventually formed: anterior, posterior, median, and 2 lateral lobes. Initially, these lobes are widely separated, but later they meet, with no definite septa dividing them. Tubules of each lobe do not intermingle with each other but simply lie side by side.

The anterior lobe tubules begin to develop simultaneously with those of the other lobes. Although in the early stages the anterior lobe tubules are large and show multiple branches, gradually they contract and lose most of the branches. They continue to shrink, so that at birth they show no lumen and appear as small, solid embryonic epithelial outgrowths. In contrast, the tubules of the posterior lobe are fewer in number yet larger, with extensive branching. These tubules, as they grow, extend posterior to the developing median and

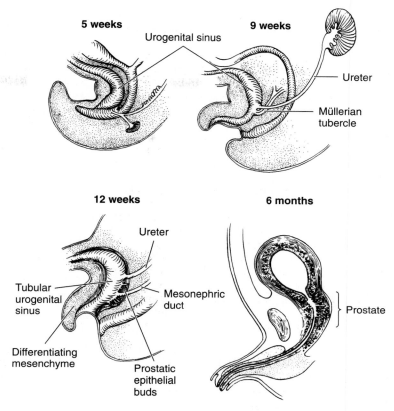

Figure 2–4. Differentiation of the urogenital sinus in males. At the fifth week, the progressively growing urorectal septum is separating the urogenital sinus from the rectum. The former receives the mesonephric duct and the ureteral bud. It retains its tubular structure until the 12th week, when the surrounding mesenchyme starts to differentiate into the muscle fibers around the whole structure. The prostate gland develops as multiple epithelial outgrowths just above and below the mesonephric duct. During the third month, the ventral part of the urogenital sinus expands to form the bladder proper; the pelvic part remains narrow and tubular, forming part of the urethra. (Reproduced, with permission, from Tanagho EA, Smith DR: Mechanisms of urinary continence. 1. Embryologic, anatomic, and pathologic considerations. J Urol 1969;100:640.)

lateral lobes and form the posterior aspect of the gland, which may be felt rectally.

ANOMALIES OF THE VESICOURETHRAL UNIT

Failure of the cloaca to subdivide is rare and results in a **persistent cloaca.** Incomplete subdivision is more frequent, ending with **rectovesical, rectourethral,** or **rectovestibular fistulas** (usually with **imperforate anus** or **anal atresia**).

Failure of descent or incomplete descent of the bladder leads to a **urinary umbilical fistula** (**urachal fistula**), **urachal cyst,** or **urachal diverticulum** depending on the stage and degree of maldescent.

Development of the genital primordia in an area more caudal than normal can result in formation of the corpora cavernosa just caudal to the urogenital sinus outlet, with the urethral groove on its dorsal surface. This defect results in complete or incomplete **epispadias** depending on its degree. A more extensive defect results in **vesical exstrophy.** Failure of fusion of urethral folds leads to various grades of **hypospadias.** This

defect, because of its mechanism, never extends proximal to the bulbous urethra. This is in contrast to epispadias, which usually involves the entire urethra up to the internal meatus.

■ GONADS

Most of the structures that make up the embryonic genital system have been taken over from other systems, and their readaptation to genital function is a secondary and relatively late phase in their development. The early differentiation of such structures is therefore independent of sexuality. Furthermore, each embryo is at first morphologically bisexual, possessing all the necessary structures for either sex. The development of one set of sex primordia and the gradual involution of the other are determined by the sex of the gonad.

The sexually undifferentiated gonad is a composite structure. Male and female potentials are represented by specific histologic elements (medulla and cortex) that

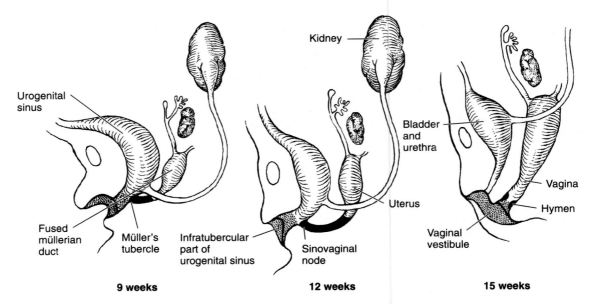

Figure 2–5. Differentiation of the urogenital sinus and the müllerian ducts in the female embryo. At 9 weeks, the urogenital sinus receives the fused müllerian ducts at Müller's tubercle (sinovaginal node), which is solidly packed with cells. As the urogenital sinus distal to Müller's tubercle becomes wider and shallower (15 weeks), the urethra and fused müllerian duct will have separate openings. The distal part of the urogenital sinus forms the vaginal vestibule and the lower fifth of the vagina (shaded area), and that part above Müller's tubercle forms the urinary bladder and the entire female urethra. The fused müllerian ducts form the uterus and the upper four-fifths of the vagina. The hymen is formed at the junction of the sinovaginal node and the urogenital sinus.

have alternative roles in gonadogenesis. Normal differentiation involves the gradual predominance of one component.

The primitive sex glands make their appearance during the fifth and sixth weeks within a localized region of the thickening known as the urogenital ridge (this contains both the nephric and the genital primordia). At the sixth week, the gonad consists of a superficial germinal epithelium and an internal blastema. The blastemal mass is derived mainly from proliferative ingrowth from the superficial epithelium, which comes loose from its basement membrane.

During the seventh week, the gonad begins to assume the characteristics of a testis or ovary. Differentiation of the ovary usually occurs somewhat later than differentiation of the testis.

If the gonad develops into a testis, the gland increases in size and shortens into a more compact organ while achieving a more caudal location. Its broad attachment to the mesonephros is converted into a gonadal mesentery known as the mesorchium. The cells of the germinal epithelium grow into the underlying mesenchyme and form cordlike masses. These are radi-

ally arranged and converge toward the mesorchium, where a dense portion of the blastemal mass is also emerging as the primordium of the rete testis. A network of strands soon forms that is continuous with the testis cords. The latter also split into 3–4 daughter cords. These eventually become differentiated into the seminiferous tubules by which the spermatozoa are produced. The rete testis unites with the mesonephric components that will form the male genital ducts, as discussed in a subsequent section (Figure 2–6).

If the gonad develops into an ovary, it (like the testis) gains a mesentery (mesovarium) and settles in a more caudal position. The internal blastema differentiates in the ninth week into a primary cortex beneath the germinal epithelium and a loose primary medulla. A compact cellular mass bulges from the medulla into the mesovarium and establishes the primitive rete ovarii. At 3–4 months of age, the internal cell mass becomes young ova. A new definitive cortex is formed from the germinal epithelium as well as from the blastema in the form of distinct cellular cords (Pflüger's tubes), and a permanent medulla is formed. The cortex differentiates into ovarian follicles containing ova.

Figure 2–6. Transformation of the undifferentiated genital system into the definitive male and female systems.

Descent of the Gonads

A. Testis

In addition to its early caudal migration, the testis later leaves the abdominal cavity and descends into the scrotum. By the third month of fetal life, the testis is located retroperitoneally in the false pelvis. A fibromuscular band (the gubernaculum) extends from the lower pole of the testis through the developing muscular layers of the anterior abdominal wall to terminate in the subcutaneous tissue of the scrotal swelling. The gubernaculum also has several other subsidiary strands that extend to adjacent regions. Just below the lower pole of the testis, the peritoneum herniates as a diverticulum along the anterior aspect of the gubernaculum, eventually reaching the scrotal sac through the anterior abdominal muscles (the processus vaginalis). The testis remains at the abdominal end of the inguinal canal until the seventh month. It then passes through the inguinal canal behind (but invaginating) the processus vaginalis. Normally, it reaches the scrotal sac by the end of the eighth month.

B. Ovary

In addition to undergoing an early internal descent, the ovary becomes attached through the gubernaculum to the tissues of the genital fold and then attaches itself to the developing uterovaginal canal at its junction with the uterine (fallopian) tubes. This part of the gubernaculum between the ovary and uterus becomes the ovarian ligament; the part between the uterus and the labia majora becomes the round ligament of the uterus. These ligaments prevent extra-abdominal descent, and the ovary enters the true pelvis. It eventually lies posterior to the uterine tubes on the superior surface of the urogenital mesentery, which has descended with the ovary and now forms the broad ligament. A small processus vaginalis forms and passes toward the labial swelling, but it is usually obliterated at full term.

GONADAL ANOMALIES

Lack of development of the gonads is called **gonadal agenesis.** Incomplete development with arrest at a certain phase is called **hypogenesis. Supernumerary gonads** are rare. The commonest anomaly involves descent of the gonads, especially the testis. Retention of the testis in the abdomen or arrest of its descent at any point along its natural pathway is called **cryptorchidism,** which may be either unilateral or bilateral. If the testis does not follow the main gubernacular structure but follows one of its subsidiary strands, it will end in an abnormal position, resulting in **ectopic testis.**

Failure of union between the rete testis and mesonephros results in a testis separate from the male genital ducts (the epididymis) and azoospermia.

■ GENITAL DUCT SYSTEM

Alongside the indifferent gonads, there are, early in embryonic life, 2 different yet closely related ducts. One is primarily a nephric duct (wolffian duct), yet it also serves as a genital duct if the embryo develops into a male. The other (müllerian duct) is primarily a genital structure from the start.

Both ducts grow caudally to join the primitive urogenital sinus. The wolffian duct (known as the pronephric duct at the 4-mm stage) joins the ventral part of the cloaca, which will be the urogenital sinus. This duct gives rise to the ureteral bud close to its caudal end. The ureteral bud grows cranially and meets metanephrogenic tissue. The part of each mesonephric duct caudal to the origin of the ureteric bud becomes absorbed into the wall of the primitive urogenital sinus, so that the mesonephric duct and ureter open independently. This is achieved at the 15-mm stage (seventh week). During this period, starting at the 10-mm stage, the müllerian ducts start to develop. They reach the urogenital sinus relatively late—at the 30-mm stage (ninth week)—their partially fused blind ends producing the elevation called Müller's tubercle. Müller's tubercle is the most constant and reliable point of reference in the whole system.

If the gonad starts to develop into a testis (17-mm stage, seventh week), the wolffian duct will start to differentiate into the male duct system, forming the epididymis, vas deferens, seminal vesicles, and ejaculatory ducts. At this time, the müllerian duct proceeds toward its junction with the urogenital sinus and immediately starts to degenerate. Only its upper and lower ends persist, the former as the appendix testis and the latter as part of the prostatic utricle.

If the gonad starts to differentiate into an ovary (22-mm stage, eighth week), the müllerian duct system forms the uterine (fallopian) tubes, uterus, and most of the vagina. The wolffian ducts, aside from their contribution to the urogenital sinus, remain rudimentary.

MALE DUCT SYSTEM

Epididymis

Because of the proximity of the differentiating gonads and the nephric duct, some of the mesonephric tubules are retained as the efferent ductules, and their lumens become continuous with those of the rete testis. These tubules, together with the part of the mesonephric duct into which they empty, will form the epididymis. Each coiled ductule makes a conical mass known as the lobule of the epididymis. The cranial end of the mesonephric duct becomes highly convoluted, completing the formation of the epididymis. This is an example of direct inclusion of a nephric structure into the genital system. Additional mesonephric tubules, both cephalad and caudal to those that were included in the formation of the epididymis, remain as rudimentary structures, that is, the appendix of the epididymis and the paradidymis.

Vas Deferens, Seminal Vesicles, & Ejaculatory Ducts

The mesonephric duct caudal to the portion forming the epididymis forms the vas deferens. Shortly before this duct joins the urethra (urogenital sinus), a localized dilatation (ampulla) develops, and the saccular convoluted structure that will form the seminal vesicle is evaginated from its wall. The mesonephric duct between the origin of the seminal vesicle and the urethra forms the ejaculatory duct. The whole mesonephric duct now achieves its characteristic thick investment of smooth muscle, with a narrow lumen along most of its length.

Both above and below the point of entrance of the mesonephric duct into the urethra, multiple outgrowths of urethral epithelium mark the beginning of the development of the prostate. As these epithelial buds grow, they meet the developing muscular fibers around the urogenital sinus, and some of these fibers become entangled in the branching tubules of the growing prostate and become incorporated into it, forming its muscular stroma (Figure 2–4).

FEMALE DUCT SYSTEM

The müllerian ducts, which are a paired system, are seen alongside the mesonephric duct. It is not known whether they arise directly from the mesonephric ducts or separately as an invagination of the celomic epithelium into the parenchyma lateral to the cranial extremity of the mesonephric duct, but the latter theory is favored. The müllerian duct develops and runs lateral to the mesonephric duct. Its opening into the celomic cavity persists as the peritoneal ostium of the uterine tube (later it develops fimbriae). The other end grows caudally as a solid tip and then crosses in front of the mesonephric duct at the caudal extremity of the mesonephros. It continues its growth in a caudomedial direction until it meets and fuses with the müllerian duct of the opposite side. The fusion is partial at first, so there is a temporary septum between the 2 lumens.

This later disappears, leaving one cavity that will form the uterovaginal canal. The potential lumen of the vaginal canal is completely packed with cells. The solid tip of this cord pushes the epithelium of the urogenital sinus outward, where it becomes Müller's tubercle (33-mm stage, ninth week). The müllerian ducts actually fuse at the 63-mm stage (13th week), forming the sinovaginal node, which receives a limited contribution from the urogenital sinus. (This contribution forms the lower fifth of the vagina.)

The urogenital sinus distal to Müller's tubercle, originally narrow and deep, shortens, widens, and opens to form the floor of the pudendal or vulval cleft. This results in separate openings for the vagina and urethra and also brings the vaginal orifice to its final position nearer the surface. At the same time, the vaginal segment increases appreciably in length. The vaginal vestibule is derived from the infratubercular segment of the urogenital sinus (in males, the same segment will form the inframontanal part of the prostatic urethra and the membranous urethra). The labia minora are formed from the urethral folds (in males they form the pendulous urethra). The hymen is the remnant of the müllerian tubercle. The lower fifth of the vagina is derived from the portion of the urogenital sinus that combines with the sinovaginal node. The remainder of the vagina and the uterus are formed from the lower (fused) third of the müllerian ducts. The uterine tubes (fallopian tubes, oviducts) are the cephalic two-thirds of the müllerian ducts (Figure 2–6).

ANOMALIES OF THE GONADAL DUCT SYSTEM

Nonunion of the rete testis and the efferent ductules can occur and, if bilateral, causes **azoospermia** and **sterility.** Failure of the müllerian ducts to approximate or to fuse completely can lead to various degrees of **duplication** in the genital ducts. **Congenital absence** of one or both uterine tubes or of the uterus or vagina occurs rarely.

Arrested development of the infratubercular segment of the urogenital sinus leads to its persistence, with the urethra and vagina having a common duct to the outside (**urogenital sinus**).

■ EXTERNAL GENITALIA

During the eighth week, external sexual differentiation begins to occur. Not until 3 months, however, do the progressively developing external genitalia attain characteristics that can be recognized as distinctively male or female. During the indifferent stage of sexual development, 3 small protuberances appear on the external aspect of the cloacal membrane. In front is the genital tubercle, and on either side of the membrane are the genital swellings.

With the breakdown of the urogenital membrane (17-mm stage, seventh week), the primitive urogenital sinus achieves a separate opening on the undersurface of the genital tubercle.

MALE EXTERNAL GENITALIA

The urogenital sinus opening extends on the ventral aspect of the genital tubercle as the urethral groove. The primitive urogenital orifice and the urethral groove are bounded on either side by the urethral folds. The genital tubercle becomes elongated to form the phallus. The corpora cavernosa are indicated in the seventh week as paired mesenchymal columns within the shaft of the penis. By the 10th week, the urethral folds start to fuse from the urogenital sinus orifice toward the tip of the phallus. At the 14th week, the fusion is complete and results in the formation of the penile urethra. The corpus spongiosum results from the differentiation of the mesenchymal masses around the formed penile urethra.

The glans penis becomes defined by the development of a circular coronary sulcus around the distal part of the phallus. The urethral groove and the fusing folds do not extend beyond the coronary sulcus. The glandular urethra develops as a result of canalization of an ectodermal epithelial cord that has grown through the glans. This canalization reaches and communicates with the distal end of the previously formed penile urethra. During the third month, a fold of skin at the base of the glans begins growing distally and, 2 months later, surrounds the glans. This forms the prepuce. Meanwhile, the genital swellings shift caudally and are recognizable as scrotal swellings. They meet and fuse, resulting in the formation of the scrotum, with 2 compartments partially separated by a median septum and a median raphe, indicating their line of fusion.

FEMALE EXTERNAL GENITALIA

Until the eighth week, the appearance of the female external genitalia closely resembles that of the male genitalia except that the urethral groove is shorter. The genital tubercle, which becomes bent caudally and lags in development, becomes the clitoris. As in males (though on a minor scale), mesenchymal columns differentiate into corpora cavernosa, and a coronary sulcus identifies the glans clitoridis. The most caudal part of the urogenital sinus shortens and widens, forming the vaginal vestibule. The urethral folds do not fuse but remain separate as the labia minora. The genital swellings meet in front of the anus, forming the posterior commissure, while the swellings as a whole enlarge and remain separated on either side of the vestibule and form the labia majora.

ANOMALIES OF THE EXTERNAL GENITALIA

Absence or duplication of the penis or clitoris is very rare. More commonly, the penis remains rudimentary or the clitoris shows hypertrophy. These anomalies may be seen alone or, more frequently, in association with **pseudohermaphroditism.** Concealed penis and transposition of penis and scrotum are relatively rare anomalies.

Failure or incomplete fusion of the urethral folds results in **hypospadias** (see preceding discussion). Penile development is also anomalous in cases of **epispadias** and **exstrophy** (see preceding discussion).

REFERENCES

General

Arey LB: *Developmental Anatomy: A Textbook and Laboratory Manual of Embryology,* 7th ed. Saunders, 1974.

Carlson BM: *Patten's Foundations of Embryology,* 6th ed. McGraw-Hill, 1996.

Fine RN: Diagnosis and treatment of fetal urinary tract abnormalities. J Pediatr 1992;121:333.

FitzGerald MJT: *Human Embryology: A Regional Approach.* Harper & Row, 1978.

Gilbert SG: *Pictorial Human Embryology.* University of Washington Press, 1989.

Marshall FF: Embryology of the lower genitourinary tract. Urol Clin North Am 1978;5:3.

Reddy PP, Mandell J: Prenatal diagnosis. Therapeutic implications. Urol Clin North Am 1998;25:171.

Stephens FD: *Congenital Malformations of the Urinary Tract.* Praeger, 1983.

Stephens FD: Embryopathy of malformations. J Urol 1982;127:13.

Tanagho EA: Developmental anatomy and urogenital abnormalities. In: Raz S (editor): *Female Urology,* 2nd ed. Saunders, 1986.

Tanagho EA: Embryologic development of the urinary tract. In: Ball TP (editor): *AUA Update Series.* American Urological Association, 1982.

Vaughan ED Jr, Middleton GW: Pertinent genitourinary embryology: Review for practicing urologist. Urology 1975;6:139.

Anomalies of the Nephric System

Avni EF et al: Multicystic dysplastic kidney: Natural history from in utero diagnosis and postnatal followup. J Urol 1987; 138:1420.

Bomalaski MD, Hirschl RB, Bloom DA: Vesicoureteral reflux and ureteropelvic junction obstruction: Association, treatment options and outcome. J Urol 1997;157:969.

Chevalier RL: Effects of ureteral obstruction on renal growth. Pediatr Nephrol 1995;9:594.

Churchill BM, Abara EO, McLorie GA: Ureteral duplication, ectopy and ureteroceles. Pediatr Clin North Am 1987;34:1273.

Corrales JG, Elder JS: Segmental multicystic kidney and ipsilateral duplication anomalies. J Urol 1996;155:1398.

Cox R, Strachan JR, Woodhouse CR: Twenty-year follow-up of primary megaureter. Eur Urol 1990;17:43.

Decter RM: Renal duplication and fusion anomalies. Pediatr Clin North Am 1997;44:1323.

El-Galley RE, Keane TE: Embryology, anatomy, and surgical applications of the kidney and ureter. Surg Clin North Am 2000;80:381.

Glassberg KI: Normal and abnormal development of the kidney: A clinician's interpretation of current knowledge. J Urol 2002; 167:2339.

Higashihara E et al: Medullary sponge kidney and hyperparathyroidism. Urology 1988;31:155.

Keating MA et al: Changing concepts in management of primary obstructive megaureter. J Urol 1989;142:636.

MacDermot KD et al: Prenatal diagnosis of autosomal dominant polycystic kidney disease (PKD1) presenting in utero and prognosis for very early onset disease. J Med Genet 1998; 35:13.

Magee MC: Ureteroceles and duplicated systems: Embryologic hypothesis. J Urol 1980;123:605.

Maher ER, Kaelin WG Jr: Von Hippel-Lindau disease. Medicine (Baltimore) 1997;76:381.

Mesrobian HG, Rushton HG, Bulas D: Unilateral renal agenesis may result from in utero regression of multicystic renal dysplasia. J Urol 1993;150:793.

Murcia NS, Sweeney WE Jr, Avner ED: New insights into the molecular pathophysiology of polycystic kidney disease. Kidney Int 1999;55:1187.

Nguyen HT, Kogan BA: Upper urinary tract obstruction: Experimental and clinical aspects. Br J Urol 1998;81(Suppl 2):13.

Osathanondh V, Potter EL: Pathogenesis of polycystic kidneys: Survey of results of microdissection. Arch Pathol 1964a; 77:510.

Osathanondh V, Potter EL: Pathogenesis of polycystic kidneys: Type 4 due to urethral obstruction. Arch Pathol 1964b; 77:502.

Pope JC IV et al: How they begin and how they end: Classic and new theories for the development and deterioration of congenital anomalies of the kidney and urinary tract, CAKUT. J Am Soc Nephrol 1999;10:2018.

Prasad PV, Priatna A: Functional imaging of the kidneys with fast MRI techniques. Eur J Radiol 1999;29:133.

Robson WL, Leung AK, Rogers RC: Unilateral renal agenesis. Adv Pediatr 1995;42:575.

Ross JH, Kay R: Ureteropelvic junction obstruction in anomalous kidneys. Urol Clin North Am 1998;25:219.

Scherz HC et al: Ectopic ureteroceles: Surgical management with preservation of continence. Review of 60 cases. J Urol 1989; 142:538.

Soderdahl DW, Shiraki IW, Schamber DT: Bilateral ureteral quadruplication. J Urol 1976;116:255.

Somlo S, Markowitz GS: The pathogenesis of autosomal dominant polycystic kidney disease: An update. Curr Opin Nephrol Hypertens 2000;9:385.

Tanagho EA: Development of the ureter. In: Bergman H (editor): The Ureter, 2nd ed. Springer-Verlag, 1981.

Tanagho EA: Ureteroceles: Embryogenesis, pathogenesis and management. J Cont Educ Urol (Feb) 1979;18:13.

Thomsen HS et al: Renal cystic diseases. Eur Radiol 1997;7:1267.

Tokunaka S et al: Morphological study of ureterocele: Possible clue to its embryogenesis as evidenced by locally arrested myogenesis. J Urol 1981;126:726.

Zerres K et al: Autosomal recessive polycystic kidney disease. Contrib Nephrol 1997;122:10.

Anomalies of the Vesicourethral Unit

Asopa HS: Newer concepts in the management of hypospadias and its complications. Ann R Coll Surg Engl 1998;80:161.

Austin PF et al: The prenatal diagnosis of cloacal exstrophy. J Urol 1998;160(3 Pt 2):1179.

Baskin LS: Hypospadias and urethral development. J Urol 2000; 163:951.

Begg RC: The urachus, its anatomy, histology and development. J Anat 1930;64:170.

Belman AB: Hypospadias update. Urology 1997;49:166.

Burbige KA et al: Prune belly syndrome: 35 years of experience. J Urol 1987;137:86.

Churchill BM et al: Emergency treatment and long-term follow-up of posterior urethral valves. Urol Clin North Am 1990; 17:343.

Chwalle R: The process of formation of cystic dilatations of the vesical end of the ureter and of diverticula at the ureteral ostium. Urol Cutan Rev 1927;31:499.

Connor JP et al: Long-term follow-up of 207 patients with bladder exstrophy: An evolution in treatment. J Urol 1989; 142:793.

Dinneen MD, Duffy PG: Posterior urethral valves. Br J Urol 1996;78:275.

Duckett JW: The current hype in hypospadiology. Br J Urol 1995; 76 (Suppl 3):1.

Eagle JR Jr, Barrett GS: Congenital deficiency of abdominal musculature with associated genitourinary abnormalities: A syndrome. Report of nine cases. Pediatrics 1950;6:721.

Elmassalme FN et al: Duplication of urethra—case report and review of literature. Eur J Pediatr Surg 1997;7:313.

Escham W, Holt HA: Complete duplication of bladder and urethra. J Urol 1980;123:773.

Goh DW, Davey RB, Dewan PA: Bladder, urethral, and vaginal duplication. J Pediatr Surg 1995;30:125.

Greskovich FJ III, Nyberg LM Jr: The prune belly syndrome: A review of its etiology, defects, treatment and prognosis. J Urol 1988;140:707.

Hinman F Jr: Surgical disorders of the bladder and umbilicus of urachal origin. Surg Gynecol Obstet 1961;113:605.

Jaramillo D, Lebowitz RL, Hendren WH: The cloacal malformation: Radiologic findings and imaging recommendations. Radiology 1990;177:441.

Jeffs RD: Exstrophy, epispadias, and cloacal and urogenital sinus abnormalities. Pediatr Clin North Am 1987;34:1233.

Landes RR, Melnick I, Klein R: Vesical exstrophy with epispadias: Twenty-year follow-up. Urology 1977;9:53.

Mackie GG: Abnormalities of the ureteral bud. Urol Clin North Am 1978;5:161.

Manzoni GA, Ransley PG, Hurwitz RS: Cloacal exstrophy and cloacal exstrophy variants: A proposed system of classification. J Urol 1987;138:1065.

Massad CA et al: Morphology and histochemistry of infant testes in the prune belly syndrome. J Urol 1991;146:1598.

Mesrobian HG, Kelalis PP, Kramer SA: Long-term followup of 103 patients with bladder exstrophy. J Urol 1988;139:719.

Mouriquand PD, Persad R, Sharma S: Hypospadias repair: Current principles and procedures. Br J Urol 1995;76(Suppl 3):9.

Nguyen HT, Kogan BA: Fetal bladder physiology. Adv Exp Med Biol 1999;462:121.

Orvis BR, Bottles K, Kogan BA: Testicular histology in fetuses with the prune belly syndrome and posterior urethral valves. J Urol 1988;139:335.

Randall A, Campbell EW: Anomalous relationship of the right ureter to the vena cava. J Urol 1935;34:565.

Rosenfeld B et al: Type III posterior urethral valves: Presentation and management. J Pediatr Surg 1994;29:81.

Shapiro E: Embryologic development of the prostate: Insights into the etiology and treatment of benign prostatic hyperplasia. Urol Clin North Am 1990;17:487.

Silver RI: What is the etiology of hypospadias? A review of recent research. Del Med J 2000;72:343.

Stein R, Thuroff JW: Hypospadias and bladder exstrophy. Curr Opin Urol 2002;12:195.

Stephens FD: The female anus, perineum and vestibule: Embryogenesis and deformities. J Obstet Gynaecol Br Commonw 1968;8:55.

Tanagho EA: Embryologic basis for lower ureteral anomalies: A hypothesis. Urology 1976;7:451.

Uehling DT: Posterior urethral valves: Functional classification. Urology 1980;15:27.

Van Savage JG et al: An algorithm for the management of anterior urethral valves. J Urol 1997;158(3 Pt 2):1030.

Wakhlu AK et al: Congenital megalourethra. J Pediatr Surg 1996;31:441.

Workman SJ, Kogan BA: Fetal bladder histology in posterior urethral valves and the prune belly syndrome. J Urol 1990; 144:337.

Gonadal Anomalies

Barteczko KJ, Jacob MI: The testicular descent in humans: Origin, development and fate of the gubernaculum Hunteri, processus vaginalis peritonei, and gonadal ligaments. Adv Anat Embryol Cell Biol 2000;156:III–X, 1.

Belville C, Josso N, Picard JY: Persistence of müllerian derivatives in males. Am J Med Genet 1999;89:218.

Ben-Chaim J, Gearhart JP: Current management of bladder exstrophy. Scand J Urol Nephrol 1997;31:103.

Borzi PA, Thomas DF: Cantwell-Ransley epispadias repair in male epispadias and bladder exstrophy. J Urol 1994;151:457.

Crankson SJ, Ahmed S: Female bladder exstrophy. Int Urogynecol J Pelvic Floor Dysfunct 1997;8:98.

DePalma L, Carter D, Weiss RM: Epididymal and vas deferens immaturity in cryptorchidism. J Urol 1988;140:1166.

Diez Garcia R et al: Peno-scrotal transposition. Eur J Pediatr Surg 1995;5:222.

Elder JS, Isaacs JT, Walsh PC: Androgenic sensitivity of gubernaculum testis: Evidence for hormonal/mechanical interactions in testicular descent. J Urol 1982;127:170.

Gad YZ et al: 5 alpha-reductase deficiency in patients with micropenis. J Inherited Metab Dis 1997;20:95.

Hadziselimovic F et al: The significance of postnatal gonadotropin surge for testicular development in normal and cryptorchid testes. J Urol 1986;136:274.

Honoré LH: Unilateral anorchism: Report of 11 cases with discussion of etiology and pathogenesis. Urology 1978;11:251.

Johnson P et al: Inferior vesical fissure. J Urol 1995;154:1478.

Kaplan LM et al: Association between abdominal wall defects and cryptorchidism. J Urol 1986;136:645.

Koff WJ, Scaletscky R: Malformations of the epididymis in undescended testis. J Urol 1990;143:340.

Mollard P, Basset T, Mure PY: Female epispadias. J Urol 1997; 158:1543.

Nef S, Parada LF: Hormones in male sexual development. Genes Dev 2000;14:3075.

Newman K, Randolph J, Anderson K: The surgical management of infants and children with ambiguous genitalia: Lessons learned from 25 years. Ann Surg 1992;215:644.

Pagon RA: Diagnostic approach to the newborn with ambiguous genitalia. Pediatr Clin North Am 1987;34:1019.

Parker KL, Schedl A, Schimmer BP: Gene interactions in gonadal development. Annu Rev Physiol 1999;61:417.

Pujol A et al: The value of bilateral biopsy in unilateral cryptorchidism. Eur Urol 1978;4:85.

Rajfer J, Walsh PC: Testicular descent: Normal and abnormal. Urol Clin North Am 1978;5:223.

Rajfer J et al: Hormonal therapy of cryptorchidism: A randomized, double-blind study comparing human chorionic gonadotropin and gonadotropin-releasing hormone. N Engl J Med 1986;314:466.

Toppari J, Kaleva M: Maldescendus testis. Horm Res 1999;51:261.

Zaontz MR, Packer MG: Abnormalities of the external genitalia. Pediatr Clin North Am 1997;44:1267.

Symptoms of Disorders of the Genitourinary Tract

3

Jack W. McAninch, MD

In the workup of any patient, the history is of paramount importance; this is particularly true in urology. It is necessary to discuss here only those urologic symptoms that are apt to be brought to the physician's attention by the patient. It is important to know not only whether the disease is acute or chronic but also whether it is recurrent, since recurring symptoms may represent acute exacerbations of chronic disease.

Obtaining the history is an art that depends on the skill and methods used to elicit information. The history is only as accurate as the patient's ability to describe the symptoms. This subjective information is important in establishing an accurate diagnosis.

SYSTEMIC MANIFESTATIONS

Symptoms of fever and weight loss should be sought. The presence of fever associated with other symptoms of urinary tract infection may be helpful in evaluating the site of the infection. Simple acute cystitis is essentially an afebrile disease. Acute pyelonephritis or prostatitis is apt to cause high temperatures (to 40 °C [104 °F]), often accompanied by violent chills. Infants and children who have acute pyelonephritis may have high temperatures without other localizing symptoms or signs. Such a clinical picture, therefore, *invariably* requires bacteriologic study of the urine.

A history of unexplained attacks of fever occurring even years before may represent otherwise asymptomatic pyelonephritis. Renal carcinoma sometimes causes fever that may reach 39 °C (102.2 °F) or more. The absence of fever does not by any means rule out renal infection, for it is the rule that chronic pyelonephritis does not cause fever.

Weight loss is to be expected in the advanced stages of cancer, but it may be noticed also when renal insufficiency due to obstruction or infection supervenes. In children who have "failure to thrive" (low weight and less than average height for age), chronic obstruction, urinary tract infection, or both should be suspected.

General malaise may be noted with tumors, chronic pyelonephritis, or renal failure.

The presence of many of these symptoms may be compatible with human immunodeficiency virus (HIV; see Chapter 15).

LOCAL & REFERRED PAIN

Two types of pain have their origins in the genitourinary organs: local and referred. The latter is especially common.

Local pain is felt in or near the involved organ. Thus, the pain from a diseased kidney (T10–12, L1) is felt in the costovertebral angle and in the flank in the region of and below the 12th rib. Pain from an inflamed testicle is felt in the gonad itself.

Referred pain originates in a diseased organ but is felt at some distance from that organ. The ureteral colic (Figure 3–1) caused by a stone in the upper ureter may be associated with severe pain in the ipsilateral testicle; this is explained by the common innervation of these 2 structures (T11–12). A stone in the lower ureter may cause pain referred to the scrotal wall; in this instance, the testis itself is not hyperesthetic. The burning pain with voiding that accompanies acute cystitis is felt in the distal urethra in females and in the glandular urethra in males (S2–3).

Abnormalities of a urologic organ can also cause pain in any other organ (eg, gastrointestinal, gynecologic) that has a sensory nerve supply common to both (Figures 3–2 and 3–3).

Kidney Pain (Figure 3–1)

Typical renal pain is felt as a dull and constant ache in the costovertebral angle just lateral to the sacrospinalis muscle and just below the 12th rib. This pain often spreads along the subcostal area toward the umbilicus or lower abdominal quadrant. It may be expected in the renal diseases that cause sudden distention of the renal capsule. Acute pyelonephritis (with its sudden edema) and acute ureteral obstruction (with its sudden renal back pressure) both cause this typical pain. It should be pointed out, however, that many urologic renal diseases are painless because their progression is so slow that

Figure 3–1. Referred pain from kidney (dotted areas) and ureter (shaded areas).

sudden capsular distention does not occur. Such diseases include cancer, chronic pyelonephritis, staghorn calculus, tuberculosis, polycystic kidney, and hydronephrosis due to chronic ureteral obstruction.

Ureteral Pain (Figure 3–1)

Ureteral pain is typically stimulated by acute obstruction (passage of a stone or a blood clot). In this instance, there is back pain from renal capsular distention combined with severe colicky pain (due to renal pelvic and ureteral muscle spasm) that radiates from the costovertebral angle down toward the lower anterior abdominal quadrant, along the course of the ureter. In men, it may also be felt in the bladder, scrotum, or testicle. In women, it may radiate into the vulva. The severity and colicky nature of this pain are caused by the hyperperistalsis and spasm of this smooth muscle

organ as it attempts to rid itself of a foreign body or to overcome obstruction.

The physician may be able to judge the position of a ureteral stone by the history of pain and the site of referral. If the stone is lodged in the upper ureter, the pain radiates to the testicle, since the nerve supply of this organ is similar to that of the kidney and upper ureter (T11–12). With stones in the mid portion of the ureter on the right side, the pain is referred to McBurney's point and may therefore simulate appendicitis; on the left side, it may resemble diverticulitis or other diseases of the descending or sigmoid colon (T12, L1). As the stone approaches the bladder, inflammation and edema of the ureteral orifice ensue, and symptoms of vesical irritability such as urinary frequency and urgency may occur. It is important to realize, however, that in mild ureteral obstruction, as seen in the congenital stenoses, there is usually no pain, either renal or ureteral.

Figure 3–2. Diagrammatic representation of autonomic nerve supply to gastrointestinal and genitourinary tracts.

Figure 3–3. Diagrammatic representation of sensory nerves of gastrointestinal and genitourinary tracts.

Labels in figure:

Vagus nerve

CIII
IV
V

ThI
II
III
IV
V
VI
VII
VIII
IX
X
XI
XII

LI
II
III
IV
V

SI
II
III
IV

Esophagus
Diaphragm
Stomach
Liver
Gallbladder
Pancreas
Spleen
Renal pelvis and ureter
Colon
Small intestine
Rectum
Ureter
Bladder
Gonad
Genitalia

Lines are dotted, broken, or solid for ease of identification only; they are all sensory nerves.

Vesical Pain

The overdistended bladder of the patient in acute urinary retention causes agonizing pain in the suprapubic area. Other than this, however, constant suprapubic pain not related to the act of urination is usually not of urologic origin.

The patient in chronic urinary retention due to bladder neck obstruction or neurogenic bladder may experience little or no suprapubic discomfort even though the bladder reaches the level of the umbilicus.

The most common cause of bladder pain is infection; the pain is usually not felt over the bladder but is referred to the distal urethra and is related to the act of urination. Terminal dysuria may be a major complaint in severe cystitis.

Prostatic Pain

Direct pain from the prostate gland is not common. Occasionally, when the prostate is acutely inflamed, the patient may feel a vague discomfort or fullness in the perineal or rectal area (S2–4). Lumbosacral backache is occasionally experienced as referred pain from the prostate but is not a common symptom of prostatitis. Inflammation of the gland may cause dysuria, frequency, and urgency.

Testicular Pain

Testicular pain due to trauma, infection, or torsion of the spermatic cord is very severe and is felt locally, although there may be some radiation of the discomfort along the spermatic cord into the lower abdomen. Uninfected hydrocele, spermatocele, and tumor of the testis do not commonly cause pain. A varicocele may cause a dull ache in the testicle that is increased after heavy exercise. At times, the first symptom of an early indirect inguinal hernia may be testicular pain (referred). Pain from a stone in the upper ureter may be referred to the testicle.

Epididymal Pain

Acute infection of the epididymis is the only painful disease of this organ and is quite common. The pain begins in the scrotum, and some degree of neighborhood inflammatory reaction involves the adjacent testis as well, further aggravating the discomfort. In the early stages of epididymitis, pain may first be felt in the groin or lower abdominal quadrant. (If on the right side, it may simulate appendicitis.) This may be a referred type of pain but can be secondary to associated inflammation of the vas deferens.

GASTROINTESTINAL SYMPTOMS OF UROLOGIC DISEASES

Whether renal or ureteral disease is painful or not, gastrointestinal symptoms are often present. The patient with acute pyelonephritis not only has localized back pain, symptoms of vesical irritability, chills, and fever but also generalized abdominal pain and distention. A patient who is passing a stone down the ureter has typical renal and ureteral colic and, usually, hematuria and may experience severe nausea and vomiting as well as abdominal distention. However, the urinary symptoms so far overshadow the gastrointestinal symptoms that the latter are usually ignored. Inadvertent overdistention of the renal pelvis (eg, with opaque material in order to obtain adequate retrograde urograms) may cause the patient to become nauseated, to vomit, and to complain of cramplike pain in the abdomen. This clinical experiment demonstrates the renointestinal reflex, which may lead to confusing symptoms. In the very common "silent" urologic diseases, some degree of gastrointestinal symptomatology may be present, which could mislead the clinician into seeking the diagnosis in the intraperitoneal zone.

Cause of the Mimicry

A. Renointestinal Reflexes

Renointestinal reflexes account for most of the confusion. They arise because of the common autonomic and sensory innervations of the two systems (Figures 3–2 and 3–3). Afferent stimuli from the renal capsule or musculature of the pelvis may, by reflex action, cause pylorospasm (symptoms of peptic ulcer) or other changes in tone of the smooth muscles of the enteric tract and its adnexa.

B. Organ Relationships

The right kidney is closely related to the hepatic flexure of the colon, the duodenum, the head of the pancreas, the common bile duct, the liver, and the gallbladder (Figure 1–3). The left kidney lies just behind the splenic flexure of the colon and is closely related to the stomach, pancreas, and spleen. Inflammations or tumors in the retroperitoneum thus may extend into or displace intraperitoneal organs, causing them to produce symptoms.

C. Peritoneal Irritation

The anterior surfaces of the kidneys are covered by peritoneum. Renal inflammation, therefore, causes peritoneal irritation, which can lead to muscle rigidity and rebound tenderness.

The symptoms arising from chronic renal disease (eg, noninfected hydronephrosis, staghorn calculus, cancer, chronic pyelonephritis) may be entirely gastrointestinal and may simulate in every way the syndromes of peptic ulcer, gallbladder disease, or appendicitis, or other, less specific gastrointestinal complaints. If a thorough survey of the gastrointestinal tract fails to demonstrate suspected disease processes, the physician should give every consideration to study of the urinary tract.

SYMPTOMS RELATED TO THE ACT OF URINATION

Many conditions cause symptoms of "cystitis." These include infections of the bladder, vesical inflammation due to chemical or x-radiation reactions, interstitial cystitis, prostatitis, psychoneurosis, torsion or rupture of an ovarian cyst, and foreign bodies in the bladder. Often, however, the patient with chronic cystitis notices no symptoms of vesical irritability. Irritating chemicals or soap on the urethral meatus may cause cystitislike symptoms of dysuria, frequency, and urgency. This has been specifically noted in young girls taking frequent bubble baths.

Frequency, Nocturia, & Urgency

The normal capacity of the bladder is about 400 mL. Frequency may be caused by residual urine, which decreases the functional capacity of the organ. When the mucosa, submucosa, and even the muscularis become inflamed (eg, infection, foreign body, stones, tumor), the capacity of the bladder decreases sharply. This decrease is due to 2 factors: the pain resulting from even mild stretching of the bladder and the loss of bladder compliance resulting from inflammatory edema. When the bladder is normal, urination can be delayed if circumstances require it, but this is not so in acute cystitis. Once the diminished bladder capacity is reached, any further distention may be agonizing, and the patient may urinate involuntarily if voiding does not occur immediately. During very severe acute infections, the desire to urinate may be constant, and each voiding may produce only a few milliliters of urine. Day frequency without nocturia and acute or chronic frequency lasting only a few hours suggest nervous tension.

Diseases that cause fibrosis of the bladder are accompanied by frequency of urination. Examples of such diseases are tuberculosis, radiation cystitis, interstitial cystitis, and schistosomiasis. The presence of stones or foreign bodies causes vesical irritability, but secondary infection is almost always present.

Nocturia may be a symptom of renal disease related to a decrease in the functioning renal parenchyma with loss of concentrating power. Nocturia can occur in the absence of disease in persons who drink excessive amounts of fluid in the late evening. Coffee and alcoholic beverages, because of their specific diuretic effect, often produce nocturia if consumed just before bedtime. In older people who are ambulatory, some fluid retention may develop secondary to mild heart failure or varicose veins. With recumbency at night, this fluid is mobilized, leading to nocturia in these patients.

A very low or very high urine pH can irritate the bladder and cause frequency of urination.

Dysuria

Painful urination is usually related to acute inflammation of the bladder, urethra, or prostate. At times, the pain is described as "burning" on urination and is usually located in the distal urethra in men. Women usually localize the pain to the urethra. The pain is present only with voiding and disappears soon after micturition is completed. More severe pain sometimes occurs in the bladder just at the end of voiding, suggesting that inflammation of the bladder is the likely cause. Pain also may be more marked at the beginning of or throughout the act of urination. Dysuria often is the first symptom suggesting urinary infection and is often associated with urinary frequency and urgency.

Enuresis

Strictly speaking, enuresis means bedwetting at night. It is physiologic during the first 2 or 3 years of life but becomes troublesome, particularly to parents, after that age. It may be functional or secondary to delayed neuromuscular maturation of the urethrovesical component, but it may present as a symptom of organic disease (eg, infection, distal urethral stenosis in girls, posterior urethral valves in boys, neurogenic bladder). If wetting occurs also during the daytime, however, or if there are other urinary symptoms, urologic investigation is essential. In adult life, enuresis may be replaced by nocturia for which no organic basis can be found.

Symptoms of Bladder Outlet Obstruction

A. HESITANCY

Hesitancy in initiating the urinary stream is one of the early symptoms of bladder outlet obstruction. As the degree of obstruction increases, hesitancy is prolonged and the patient often strains to force urine through the obstruction. Prostate obstruction and urethral stricture are common causes of this symptom.

B. LOSS OF FORCE AND DECREASE OF CALIBER OF THE STREAM

Progressive loss of force and caliber of the urinary stream is noted as urethral resistance increases despite the generation of increased intravesical pressure. This can be evaluated by measuring urinary flow rates; in normal circumstances with a full bladder a maximal flow of 20 mL/s should be achieved.

C. TERMINAL DRIBBLING

Terminal dribbling becomes more and more noticeable as obstruction progresses and is a most distressing symptom.

D. URGENCY

A strong, sudden desire to urinate is caused by hyperactivity and irritability of the bladder, resulting from obstruction, inflammation, or neuropathic bladder disease. In most circumstances, the patient is able to control temporarily the sudden need to void, but loss of small amounts of urine may occur (urgency incontinence).

E. ACUTE URINARY RETENTION

Sudden inability to urinate may supervene. The patient experiences increasingly agonizing suprapubic pain associated with severe urgency and may dribble only small amounts of urine.

F. CHRONIC URINARY RETENTION

Chronic urinary retention may cause little discomfort to the patient even though there is great hesitancy in starting the stream and marked reduction of its force and caliber. Constant dribbling of urine (paradoxic incontinence) may be experienced; it may be likened to water pouring over a dam.

G. INTERRUPTION OF THE URINARY STREAM

Interruption may be abrupt and accompanied by severe pain radiating down the urethra. This type of reaction strongly suggests the complication of vesical calculus.

H. SENSE OF RESIDUAL URINE

The patient often feels that urine is still in the bladder even after urination has been completed.

I. CYSTITIS

Recurring episodes of acute cystitis suggest the presence of residual urine.

Incontinence (See also Chapter 27.)

There are many reasons for incontinence. The history often gives a clue to its cause.

A. TRUE INCONTINENCE

The patient may lose urine without warning; this may be a constant or periodic symptom. The more obvious causes include exstrophy of the bladder, epispadias, vesicovaginal fistula, and ectopic ureteral orifice. Injury to the urethral smooth muscle sphincters may occur during prostatectomy or childbirth. Congenital or acquired neurogenic diseases may lead to dysfunction of the bladder and incontinence.

B. STRESS INCONTINENCE

When slight weakness of the sphincteric mechanisms is present, urine may be lost in association with physical strain (eg, coughing, laughing, rising from a chair). This is common in multiparous women who have weakened muscle support of the bladder neck and urethra. Occasionally, neuropathic bladder dysfunction can cause stress incontinence. The patient stays dry while lying in bed.

C. URGE INCONTINENCE

Urgency may be so precipitate and severe that there is involuntary loss of urine. Urge incontinence not infrequently occurs with acute cystitis, particularly in women, since women seem to have relatively poor anatomic sphincters. Urge incontinence is a common symptom of an upper motor neuron lesion.

D. OVERFLOW INCONTINENCE

Paradoxic incontinence is loss of urine due to chronic urinary retention or secondary to a flaccid bladder. The intravesical pressure finally equals the urethral resistance; urine then constantly dribbles forth.

Oliguria & Anuria

Oliguria and anuria may be caused by acute renal failure (due to shock or dehydration), fluid-ion imbalance, or bilateral ureteral obstruction.

Pneumaturia

The passage of gas in the urine strongly suggests a fistula between the urinary tract and the bowel. This occurs most commonly in the bladder or urethra but may be seen also in the ureter or renal pelvis. Carcinoma of the sigmoid colon, diverticulitis with abscess formation, regional enteritis, and trauma cause most vesical fistulas. Congenital anomalies account for most urethroenteric fistulas. Certain bacteria, by the process of fermentation, may liberate gas on rare occasions.

Cloudy Urine

Patients often complain of cloudy urine, but it is most often cloudy merely because it is alkaline; this causes precipitation of phosphate. Infection can also cause urine to be cloudy and malodorous. A properly performed urinalysis will reveal the cause of cloudiness.

Chyluria

The passage of lymphatic fluid or chyle is noted by the patient as passage of milky white urine. This represents a lymphatic–urinary system fistula. Most often, the cause is obstruction of the renal lymphatics, which results in forniceal rupture and leakage. Filariasis, trauma, tuberculosis, and retroperitoneal tumors have caused the problem.

Bloody Urine

Hematuria is a danger signal that cannot be ignored. Carcinoma of the kidney or bladder, calculi, and infection are a few of the conditions in which hematuria is typically demonstrable at the time of presentation. It is important to know whether urination is painful or not, whether the hematuria is associated with symptoms of vesical irritability, and whether blood is seen in all or only a portion of the urinary stream. The hemoglobinuria that occurs as a feature of the hemolytic syndromes may also cause the urine to be red.

A. Bloody Urine in Relation to Symptoms and Diseases

Hematuria associated with renal colic suggests a ureteral stone, although a clot from a bleeding renal tumor can cause the same type of pain.

Hematuria is not uncommonly associated with nonspecific, tuberculous, or schistosomal infection of the bladder. The bleeding is often terminal (bladder neck or prostate), although it may be present throughout urination (vesical or upper tract). Stone in the bladder often causes hematuria, but infection is usually present, and there are symptoms of bladder neck obstruction, neurogenic bladder, or cystocele.

Dilated veins may develop at the bladder neck secondary to enlargement of the prostate. These may rupture when the patient strains to urinate, resulting in gross or microscopic hematuria.

Hematuria without other symptoms (silent hematuria) must be regarded as a symptom of tumor of the bladder or kidney until proved otherwise. It is usually intermittent; bleeding may not recur for months. Complacency because the bleeding stops spontaneously must be condemned. Less common causes of silent hematuria are staghorn calculus, polycystic kidneys, benign prostatic hyperplasia, solitary renal cyst, sickle cell disease, and hydronephrosis. Painless bleeding is common with acute glomerulonephritis. Recurrent bleeding is occasionally seen in children suffering from focal glomerulitis. Joggers and people who engage in participatory sports frequently develop transient proteinuria and gross or microscopic hematuria.

B. Time of Hematuria

Learning whether the hematuria is partial (initial, terminal) or total (present throughout urination) is often of help in identifying the site of bleeding. Initial hematuria suggests an anterior urethral lesion (eg, urethritis, stricture, meatal stenosis in young boys). Terminal hematuria usually arises from the posterior urethra, bladder neck, or trigone. Among the common causes are posterior urethritis and polyps and tumors of the vesical neck.

Total hematuria has its source at or above the level of the bladder (eg, stone, tumor, tuberculosis, nephritis).

OTHER OBJECTIVE MANIFESTATIONS

Urethral Discharge

Urethral discharge in men is one of the most common urologic complaints. The causative organism is usually *Neisseria gonorrhoeae* or *Chlamydia trachomatis*. The discharge is often accompanied by local burning on urination or an itching sensation in the urethra (see Chapter 15).

Skin Lesions of the External Genitalia (See Chapters 15 and 40.)

An ulceration of the glans penis or its shaft may represent syphilitic chancre, chancroid, herpes simplex, or squamous cell carcinoma. Venereal warts of the penis are common.

Visible or Palpable Masses

The patient may notice a visible or palpable mass in the upper abdomen that may represent renal tumor, hydronephrosis, or polycystic kidney. Enlarged lymph nodes in the neck may contain metastatic tumor from the prostate or testis. Lumps in the groin may represent spread of tumor of the penis or lymphadenitis from chancroid, syphilis, or lymphogranuloma venereum. Painless masses in the scrotal contents are common and include hydrocele, varicocele, spermatocele, chronic epididymitis, hernia, and testicular tumor.

Edema

Edema of the legs may result from compression of the iliac veins by lymphatic metastases from prostatic cancer. Edema of the genitalia suggests filariasis, chronic ascites, or lymphatic blockage from radiotherapy for pelvic malignancies.

Bloody Ejaculation

Inflammation of the prostate or seminal vesicles can cause hematospermia.

Gynecomastia

Often idiopathic, gynecomastia is common in elderly men, particularly those taking estrogens for control of prostatic cancer. It is also seen in association with choriocarcinoma and interstitial cell and Sertoli cell tumors of the testis. Certain endocrinologic diseases, for example, Klinefelter syndrome, may also cause gynecomastia.

COMPLAINTS RELATED TO SEXUAL PROBLEMS

Many people have genitourinary complaints on a purely psychological or emotional basis. In others, organic symptoms may be increased in severity because of tension states. It is important, therefore, to seek clues that might give evidence of emotional stress.

In women, the relationship of the menses to ureteral pain or vesical complaints should be determined, although menstruation may exacerbate both organic and functional vesical and renal difficulties.

Many patients recognize that the state of their "nerves" has a direct effect on their symptoms. They often realize that their "cystitis" develops after a tension-producing or anxiety-producing episode in their personal or occupational environment.

Sexual Difficulties in Men

Men may complain directly of sexual difficulty. However, they are often so ashamed of loss of sexual power that they cannot admit it even to a physician. In such cases, they may ask for "prostate treatment" and hope that the physician will understand that they have sexual complaints and that they will be treated accordingly. The main sexual symptoms include impaired quality of erection, premature loss of erection, absence of ejaculate with orgasm, premature ejaculation, and even loss of desire.

Sexual Difficulties in Women

Women who have the psychosomatic cystitis syndrome almost always admit to an unhappy sex life. They notice that frequency or vaginal-urethral pain often occurs on the day following the incomplete sexual act. Many of them recognize the inadequacy of their sexual experiences as one of the underlying causes of urologic complaints; too frequently, however, the physician either does not ask them pertinent questions or, if patients volunteer this information, ignores it.

REFERENCES

Ahn JH, Morey AF, McAninch JW: Workup and management of traumatic hematuria. Emerg Med Clin North Am 1998; 16:145.

Andreoli SP: Renal manifestations of systemic diseases. Semin Nephrol 1998;18:270.

Bird VG et al: A comparison of unenhanced helical computerized tomography findings and renal obstruction determined by furosemide 99m-technetium mercaptoacetyltriglycine diuretic scintirenography for patients with acute renal colic. J Urol 2002;167:1597.

Bower WF, Moore KH, Adams RD: A novel clinical evaluation of childhood incontinence and urinary urgency. J Urol 2001; 166:2411.

Clark AJ, Norman RW: "Mirror pain" as an unusual presentation of renal colic. Urology 1998;51:116.

Collins MM et al: Prevalence and correlates of prostatitis in the health professionals' follow-up study cohort. J Urol 2002; 167:1363.

Cummings JM et al: Adult testicular torsion. J Urol 2002;167: 2109.

Feld LG et al: Hematuria: An integrated medical and surgical approach. Pediatr Clin North Am 1997;44:1191.

Fredell L et al: Heredity of hypospadias and the significance of low birth weight. J Urol 2002;167:1423.

Gatti JM et al: Acute urinary retention in children. J Urol 2001; 165:918.

Glassberg KI: Normal and abnormal development of the kidney: A clinician's interpretation of current knowledge. J Urol 2002; 167:2339.

Hamm M et al: Low dose unenhanced helical computerized tomography for the evaluation of acute flank pain. J Urol 2002; 167:1687.

Hjalmas K: Nocturnal enuresis: Basic facts and new horizons. Eur Urol 1998;33(Suppl 3):53.

Homma Y et al: Significance of nocturia in the international prostate symptom score for benign prostatic hyperplasia. J Urol 2002;167:172.

Kershen RT, Azadzoi KM, Siroky MB: Blood flow, pressure and compliance in the male human bladder. J Urol 2002; 168:121.

Khadra MH et al: A prospective analysis of 1930 patients with hematuria to evaluate current diagnostic practice. J Urol 2000;163:524.

Konety BR, Getzenberg RH: Urine based markers of urological malignancy. J Urol 2001;165:600.

Kotsis SV et al: Early onset prostate cancer: Predictors of clinical grade. J Urol 2002;167:1659.

Kurowski K: The women with dysuria. Am Fam Physician 1998; 57(9):2155.

Lang EK et al: Computerized tomography tailored for the assessment of microscopic hematuria. J Urol 2002;167:547.

Leissner J et al: The pelvic plexus and antireflux surgery: Topographical findings and clinical consequences. J Urol 2001; 165:1652.

Li J et al: Absent hematuria and expensive computerized tomography: Case characteristics of emergency urolithiasis. J Urol 2001;165:782.

McCarthy JJ: Outpatient evaluation of hematuria: Locating the source of bleeding. Postgrad Med 1997;101(Feb 2):125, 131.

Niall O et al: A comparison of noncontrast computerized tomography with excretory urography in the assessment of acute flank pain. J Urol 1999;161:534.

Nickel JC et al: Predictors of patient response to antibiotic therapy for the chronic prostatitis/chronic pelvic pain syndrome: A prospective multicenter clinical trial. J Urol 2001;165:1539.

Nickel JC et al: The patient with chronic epididymitis: Characterization of an enigmatic syndrome. J Urol 2002;167:1701.

Nitti VW et al: Lower urinary tract symptoms in young men: Videourodynamic findings and correlation with noninvasive measures. J Urol 2002;168:135.

Paajanen H, Tainio H, Laato M: A chance of misdiagnosis between acute appendicitis and renal colic. Scand J Urol Nephrol 1996;30:363.

Parulkar BG et al: Renal colic during pregnancy: A case for conservative treatment. J Urol 1998;159:365.

Roberts RO et al: Longitudinal changes in peak urinary flow rates in a community based cohort. J Urol 2000;163:107.

Schulz MW et al: A comparison of techniques for eliciting patient preferences in patients with benign prostatic hyperplasia. J Urol 2002;168:155.

Shekarriz B, Lu H-F, Stoller ML: Correlation of unilateral urolithiasis with sleep posture. J Urol 2001;165:1085.

Swinn MJ et al: The cause and natural history of isolated urinary retention in young women. J Urol 2002;167:151.

Van der Weide MJA et al: Lower urinary tract symptoms after renal transplantation. J Urol 2001;166:1237.

Weiss JP, Blaivas JG: Nocturia. J Urol 2000;163:5.

Physical Examination of the Genitourinary Tract

4

Emil A. Tanagho, MD

The history will suggest whether a complete or partial examination is indicated. The symptom of urethral discharge usually does not require a thorough physical examination; on the other hand, painless hematuria certainly requires a careful examination of the genitourinary tract. In this chapter the urologic aspects of the physical examination are discussed.

■ EXAMINATION OF THE KIDNEYS

Inspection

On occasion, a mass that is visible in the upper abdominal area if soft (eg, as in hydronephrosis), may be difficult to palpate. Fullness in the costovertebral angle may be consistent with cancer (eg, neuroblastoma in children) or perinephric infection. The presence and persistence of indentations in the skin from lying on wrinkled sheets suggest edema of the skin secondary to perinephric abscess. If this disease is suspected, one should have the patient lie on a rough towel and observe for indentations.

Palpation

The kidneys lie rather high under the diaphragm and lower ribs and are therefore well protected from injury. Because of the position of the liver, the right kidney is lower than the left. The kidneys are difficult to palpate in men because of the resistance of abdominal muscle tone and because the kidneys in men are more fixed than those in women and move only slightly with change of posture or respiration. The lower part of the right kidney can sometimes be felt, especially in thin patients, but the left kidney usually cannot be felt unless it is enlarged or displaced.

The most successful method of renal palpation is carried out with the patient lying in the supine position on a hard surface (Figure 4–1). The kidney is lifted by one hand in the costovertebral angle. On deep inspiration, the kidney moves downward; when it is lowest, the other hand is pushed firmly and deeply beneath the costal margin in an effort to trap the kidney below that point. If this is successful, the anterior hand can palpate the size, shape, and consistency of the organ as it slips back into its normal position.

The kidney sometimes can be palpated best with the examiner standing behind the seated patient. At other times, if the patient is lying on one side, the uppermost kidney drops downward and medially, thereby making it more accessible to palpation.

Perlman and Williams (1976) described a very effective method of identifying renal anomalies in newborns. The fingers are placed in the costovertebral angle, with the thumb anterior. The thumb does the feeling. With this technique, the kidneys can be palpated 95% of the time. Anomalies were found in 0.5% of 11,000 newborns.

An enlarged renal mass suggests compensatory hypertrophy (if the other kidney is absent or atrophic), hydronephrosis, tumor, cyst, or polycystic disease. A mass in this area, however, may be a retroperitoneal tumor, the spleen, a lesion of the bowel (eg, tumor, abscess), a lesion of the gallbladder, or a pancreatic cyst. Tumors may have the consistency of normal tissue; they may also be nodular. Hydronephroses may be firm or soft. Polycystic kidneys are usually nodular and firm.

An acutely infected kidney is tender, but this is difficult to elicit, since marked muscle spasm is usually present. Because normal kidneys are often tender also, this sign is not always helpful.

Although renal pain may be diffusely felt in the back, tenderness is usually well localized just lateral to the sacrospinalis muscle and just below the twelfth rib (costovertebral angle [CVA]). This may be elicited by palpation or, more sharply, by percussion over that area.

Percussion

At times, a greatly enlarged kidney cannot be felt on palpation, particularly if it is soft. This can be true of hydronephrosis. Such masses may be readily outlined by percussion, however, both anteriorly and posteriorly; this part of the examination should never be omitted.

Figure 4–1. Method of palpation of the kidney. The posterior hand lifts the kidney upward. The anterior hand feels for the kidney. The patient then takes a deep breath; this causes the kidney to descend. As the patient inhales, the fingers of the anterior hand are plunged inward at the costal margin. If the kidney is mobile or enlarged, it can be felt between the two hands.

Percussion is of particular value in outlining an enlarging mass in the flank following renal trauma (progressive hemorrhage), when tenderness and muscle spasm prevent proper palpation.

Transillumination

Transillumination may prove quite helpful in children under age 1 year who present with a suprapubic or flank mass. A 2- or 3-cell flashlight with an opaque flange protruding beyond the lens is an adequate instrument. The flashlight is applied at right angles to the abdomen. The fiberoptic light cord, used to illuminate various optical instruments, is an excellent source of cold light. A dark room is required. A distended bladder or cystic mass will transilluminate; a solid mass will not. Flank masses also may be tested by applying the light posteriorly.

Differentiation of Renal & Radicular Pain

Radicular pain is commonly felt in the costovertebral and subcostal areas. It may spread along the course of the ureter as well and is the most common cause of so-called kidney pain. Every patient who complains of flank pain should be examined for evidence of nerve root irritation. Frequent causes are poor posture (scoliosis, kyphosis), arthritic changes in the costovertebral or costotransverse joints, impingement of a rib spur on a subcostal nerve, hypertrophy of costovertebral ligaments pressing on a nerve, and intervertebral disk disease (Smith and Raney, 1976). Radicular pain may be noted as an aftermath of a flank incision wherein a rib may become dislocated, causing the costal nerve to impinge on the edge of a ligament. Pain experienced during the preeruptive phase of herpes zoster involving any of the segments between T11 and L2 also may simulate pain of renal origin.

Radiculitis usually causes hyperesthesia of the area of skin served by the irritated peripheral nerve. This hypersensitivity can be elicited by means of the pinwheel or by grasping and pinching both skin and fat of the abdomen and flanks. Pressure exerted by the thumb over the costovertebral joints reveals local tenderness at the point of emergence of the involved peripheral nerve.

Auscultation

Auscultation of the costovertebral areas and upper abdominal quadrants may reveal a systolic bruit, which is often associated with stenosis or aneurysm of the renal artery. Bruits over the femoral arteries may be found in association with Leriche syndrome, which may be a cause of impotence.

■ EXAMINATION OF THE BLADDER

The bladder cannot be felt unless it is moderately distended. In adults, if it is percussible, it contains at least 150 mL of urine. In acute or (more commonly) chronic urinary retention, the bladder may reach or even rise above the umbilicus, in which case its outline may be seen and usually felt. (In chronic retention, in which the bladder wall is flabby, the bladder may be difficult to palpate. In this instance, percussion is of great value.)

In male infants or young boys, palpation of a hard mass deep in the center of the pelvis is compatible with a thickened hypertrophied bladder secondary to obstruction caused by posterior urethral valves.

A sliding inguinal hernia containing some bladder wall can be diagnosed (when the bladder is full) by compression of the scrotal mass. The bladder will be found to distend additionally.

A few instances have been reported wherein marked edema of the legs has developed secondary to compression of the iliac vessels by a distended bladder. Bimanual (abdominorectal or abdominovaginal) palpation may reveal the extent of a vesical tumor. To be successful, it must be done under anesthesia.

■ EXAMINATION OF THE EXTERNAL MALE GENITALIA

PENIS

Inspection

If the patient has not been circumcised, the foreskin should be retracted. This may reveal tumor or balanitis as the cause of a foul discharge. If retraction is not possible in phimosis, surgical correction (dorsal slit or circumcision) is indicated.

The observation of a poor urinary stream is significant. In newborns, neurogenic (neuropathic) bladder or the presence of posterior urethral valves should be considered. In men, such a finding suggests urethral stricture or prostatic obstruction.

The scars of healed syphilis may be an important clue. An active ulcer requires bacteriologic or pathologic study (eg, syphilitic chancre, epithelioma). Superficial ulcers or vesicles are compatible with herpes simplex; they are often interpreted by the patient as a serious sexually transmitted disease, possibly syphilis. Venereal warts may be observed.

Meatal stenosis is a common cause of bloody spotting in male infants. On rare occasions, it may be of such degree as to cause advanced bilateral hydronephrosis. It is easily corrected by meatotomy.

The position of the meatus should be noted. It may be located proximal to the tip of the glans on either the dorsum (epispadias) or the ventral surface (hypospadias). In either instance, there is apt to be abnormal curvature of the penis—dorsally with epispadias, ventrally with hypospadias. The urethral orifice is often stenotic in the latter.

Micropenis or macropenis may be observed.

Palpation

Palpation of the dorsal surface of the shaft may reveal a fibrous plaque involving the fascial covering of the corpora cavernosa. This is typical of Peyronie disease. Tender areas of induration felt along the urethra may signify periurethritis secondary to urethral stricture.

Urethral Discharge

Urethral discharge is the most common complaint referable to the male sex organ. Gonococcal pus is usually profuse, thick, and yellow or gray-brown. Nongonorrheal discharges may be similar in appearance but are often thin, mucoid, and scanty. Although gonorrhea must be ruled out as the cause of a urethral discharge, a significant percentage of such cases are found to be caused by chlamydiae. Patients with urethral discharge should be examined also for other sexually transmitted diseases; multiple infection is not uncommon.

Bloody discharge should suggest the possibility of a foreign body in the urethra (male or female), urethral stricture, or tumor.

Urethral discharge must always be sought before the patient is asked to void.

SCROTUM

Angioneurotic edema and infections and inflammations of the skin of the scrotum are not common. Small sebaceous cysts are occasionally seen. Malignant tumors are rare. The scrotum is bifid when midscrotal or perineal hypospadias is present.

Elephantiasis of the scrotum is caused by obstruction to lymphatic drainage. It is endemic in the tropics and is due to filariasis. Elephantiasis may result from radical resection of the lymph nodes of the inguinal and femoral areas, in which case the skin of the penis is also involved. Small hemangiomas of the skin are common and may bleed spontaneously.

Scrotal ultrasound is helpful in evaluating scrotal contents.

TESTIS

The testes should be carefully palpated with the fingers of both hands. A hard area in the testis proper must be regarded as a malignant tumor until proved otherwise. Transillumination of all scrotal masses should be done routinely. With the patient in a dark room, a strong flashlight or fiberoptic light is placed against the scrotal sac posteriorly. A hydrocele will cause the intrascrotal mass to glow red. Light is not transmitted through a solid tumor. Tumors are often smooth but may be nodular. Testes seem abnormally heavy. A testis replaced by tumor or damaged by gumma is insensitive to pressure, and the usual sickening sensation is absent. About 10% of tumors are associated with a secondary hydrocele that may have to be aspirated before definitive palpation can be done.

The testis may be absent from the scrotum. This may represent transient (physiologic retractile testis) or true cryptorchidism. Palpation of the groins may reveal the presence of the organ.

The atrophic testis (following postoperative orchiopexy, mumps orchitis, or torsion of the spermatic cord) may be flabby and at times hypersensitive but is usually firm and hyposensitive. Although spermatogenesis may be lost, androgen function is occasionally maintained.

EPIDIDYMIS

The epididymis is sometimes rather closely attached to the posterior surface of the testis, and at other times it is quite free of it. The epididymis should be carefully palpated for size and induration. Induration implies infection (primary tumors are exceedingly rare).

In the acute stage of epididymitis, the testis and epididymis are indistinguishable by palpation; the testicle and epididymis may be adherent to the scrotum, which is usually quite red. Tenderness is exquisite. With few exceptions, the infecting organism is *Neisseria gonorrhoeae, Chlamydia trachomatis,* or *Escherichia coli.*

Chronic painless induration should suggest tuberculosis or schistosomiasis, although nonspecific chronic epididymitis is also a possibility. Other signs of tuberculosis of the genitourinary tract usually present include "sterile" pyuria, a thickened seminal vesicle, a nodular prostate, and "beading" of the vas deferens.

SPERMATIC CORD & VAS DEFERENS

A swelling in the spermatic cord may be cystic (eg, hydrocele or hernia) or solid (eg, connective tissue tumor). The latter is rare. Lipoma in the investing fascia of the cord may simulate hernia. Diffuse swelling and induration of the cord are seen with filarial funiculitis.

Careful palpation of the vas deferens may reveal thickening (eg, chronic infection), fusiform enlargements (the "beading" caused by tuberculosis), or even absence of the vas. The latter finding is of importance in infertile males; it is rare.

When a male patient stands, a mass of dilated veins (varicocele) may be noted behind and above the testis. The degree of dilatation decreases with recumbency and can be increased by the Valsalva maneuver. The major sequel of varicocele is infertility (see Chapter 42).

TESTICULAR TUNICS & ADNEXA

Hydroceles are usually cystic but on occasion are so tense that they simulate solid tumors. Transillumination makes the differential diagnosis. They may develop secondary to nonspecific acute or tuberculous epididymitis, trauma, or tumor of the testis. The latter is a distinct possibility if hydrocele appears spontaneously between the ages of 18 and 35. It should be aspirated to permit careful palpation of underlying structures.

Hydrocele usually surrounds the testis completely. Cystic masses that are separate from but in the region of the upper pole of the testis are probably spermatoceles. Aspiration reveals the typical thin, milky fluid, which contains sperm.

■ EXAMINATION OF THE FEMALE GENITALIA

VAGINAL EXAMINATION

Diseases of the female genital tract may involve the urinary organs secondarily, thereby making a thorough gynecologic examination essential. Commonly associated are urethrocystitis secondary to urethral diverticulitis or cervicitis, pyelonephritis during pregnancy, and ureteral obstruction from metastatic nodes or direct extension in cancer of the cervix.

Inspection

In newborns and children especially, the vaginal vestibule should be inspected for a single opening (common urogenital sinus), labial fusion, split clitoris and lack of fusion of the anterior fourchette (epispadias), or hypertrophied clitoris and scrotalization of the labia majora (adrenogenital syndrome).

The urinary meatus may reveal a reddened, tender, friable lesion (urethral caruncle) or a reddened, everted posterior lip, which is often seen with senile urethritis and vaginitis. Biopsy is indicated if a malignant tumor cannot be ruled out. The diagnosis of senile vaginitis (and urethritis) is established by staining a smear of the vaginal epithelium with Lugol's solution. It should be examined immediately after rinsing, because the brown dye in the cells fades quickly. Cells lacking glycogen (hypoestrogenism) do not take up the stain, whereas normal cells do.

Multiple painful small ulcers or blisterlike lesions may be noted; these probably represent herpes virus type 2 infection, which may have serious sequels.

Smears and cultures of urethral or vaginal discharge should be made. Gonococci are relatively easy to identify; culture of chlamydiae requires techniques seldom available to the physician.

The presence of skenitis and bartholinitis may reveal the source of persistent urethritis or cystitis. The condition of the vaginal wall should be observed. Bacteriologic study of the secretions may be helpful. Urethrocele and cystocele may cause residual urine and lead to persistent infection of the bladder. They are often found in association with stress incontinence. A bulge in the anterior vaginal wall may represent a urethral diverticulum. The cervix should be inspected to detect cancer or infection. Taking biopsy specimens or making Papanicolaou smears may be indicated.

Palpation

At times, the urethra, the base of the bladder, and the lower ureters may be tender on palpation, but little can be deduced from this. Induration of the urethra or trigonal area or a mass involving either may be a clue to an existing tumor. A soft mass found in this area could be a urethral diverticulum. Pressure on such a lesion may cause pus to extrude from the urethra. A stone in the lower ureter may be palpable. Evidence of enlargement of the uterus (eg, pregnancy, myomas) or diseases or inflammations of the colon or adnexa may afford a clue to the cause of urinary symptoms (eg, compression of a ureter by a malignant ovarian tumor, endometriosis, or diverticulitis of the sigmoid colon adherent to the bladder).

Carcinoma of the cervix may invade the base of the bladder, causing vesical irritability or hematuria; its metastases to iliac lymph nodes may compress the ureters.

Rectal examination may afford further information and is the obvious route of examination in children and virgins.

■ RECTAL EXAMINATION IN MALES

SPHINCTER & LOWER RECTUM

The estimation of sphincter tone is of great importance. Laxity of the muscle strongly suggests similar changes in the urinary sphincters and detrusor and may be a clue to the diagnosis of neurogenic disease. The same is true for a spastic anal sphincter. In addition to the digital prostatic examination, the examiner should palpate the entire lower rectum to rule out stenosis, internal hemorrhoids, cryptitis, rectal fistulas, mucosal polyps, and rectal cancer and should use bidigital palpation for Cowper's glands. Testing perianal sensation is mandatory.

PROSTATE

A specimen of urine for routine analysis should be collected before the rectal examination is made. This is of the utmost importance, since prostatic massage (or even palpation at times) forces prostatic secretion into the posterior urethra. If this secretion contains pus, a specimen of urine voided after the rectal examination will be contaminated by it.

Size

The average prostate is about 4 cm in length and width. It is widest superiorly at the bladder neck. As the gland enlarges, the lateral sulci become relatively deeper and the median furrow becomes obliterated. The prostate may also elongate. The clinical importance of prostatic hyperplasia is measured by the severity of symptoms and the amount of residual urine rather than by the size of the gland. On rectal examination, the prostate may be of normal size and consistency in a patient with acute urinary retention.

Consistency

Normally, the consistency of the gland is similar to that of the contracted thenar eminence of the thumb (with the thumb completely opposed to the little finger). It is rather rubbery. It may be mushy if congested (due to lack of intercourse or to chronic infection with impaired drainage), indurated (due to chronic infection with or without calculi), or stony-hard (due to advanced carcinoma).

The difficulty lies in differentiating firm areas in the prostate: fibrosis from nonspecific infection, granulomatous prostatitis, nodulation from tuberculosis, or firm areas due to prostatic calculi or early cancer. Generally speaking, nodules caused by infection are raised above the surface of the gland. At their edges, the induration gradually fades to the normal softness of surrounding tissue. In cancer, conversely, the suspicious lesion is usually not raised; it is hard and has a sharp edge (ie, there is an abrupt change in consistency on the same plane). It tends to arise in the lateral sulcus (Figure 4–2).

Even the most experienced clinicians sometimes have trouble making this differentiation. In the absence of other signs of tuberculosis and in the absence of pus in the prostatic secretion, cancer is likely, particularly if an x-ray fails to show prostatic calculi (which are seen just behind or above the symphysis). Serum acid phosphatase determinations and radiograms of bones are of no help in diagnosing early carcinoma of the prostate. The prostate-specific antigen (PSA) level can be helpful if elevated. Transrectal ultrasound-guided biopsy can be diagnostic.

Mobility

The mobility of the gland varies. Occasionally, it has great mobility; at other times, very little. With advanced carcinoma, it is fixed because of local extension through the capsule. The prostate should be routinely massaged in adults and its secretion examined microscopically. It should not be massaged, however, in the

Figure 4–2. Differential diagnosis of prostatic nodules. **A:** Inflammatory area is raised above the surface of the gland; induration decreases gradually at its periphery. **B:** Cancerous nodule is not raised; there is an abrupt change in consistency at its edges.

presence of an acute urethral discharge, acute prostatitis, or acute prostatocystitis; in men near the stage of complete urinary retention (because it may precipitate complete retention); or in men suffering from obvious cancer of the gland. Even without symptoms, massage is necessary, for prostatitis is commonly asymptomatic. Diagnosis and treatment of such silent disease is important in preventing cystitis and epididymitis.

Massage & Prostatic Smear

Copious amounts of secretion may be obtained from some prostate glands and little or none from others. The amount obtained depends to some extent on the vigor with which the massage is carried out. If no secretion is obtained, the patient should be asked to void even a few drops of urine; these will contain adequate secretion for examination. Microscopic examination of the secretion is done under low-power magnification. Normal secretion contains numerous lecithin bodies, which are refractile, like red cells, but much smaller than red cells. Only an occasional white cell is present. A few epithelial cells and, rarely, corpora amylacea are seen. Sperm may be present, but its absence is of no significance.

The presence of large numbers of pus cells is pathologic and suggests the diagnosis of prostatitis. Stained smears are usually impractical. It is difficult to fix this material on the slide, and even when this is successful, pyogenic bacteria are usually not found. Acid-fast organisms can often be found by appropriate staining methods.

On occasion, it may be necessary to obtain cultures of prostatic secretion in order to demonstrate nonspecific organisms, tubercle bacilli, gonococci, or chlamydiae. After thorough cleansing of the glans and emptying of the bladder (to mechanically cleanse the urethra), massage is done. Drops of secretion are collected in a sterile tube of appropriate culture medium.

SEMINAL VESICLES

Palpation of the seminal vesicles should be attempted. The vesicles are situated under the base of the bladder and diverge from below upward (Figure 1–8). Normal seminal vesicles are usually not palpable, but when the vesicles are overdistended they may feel quite cystic. In the presence of chronic infection (particularly tuberculosis or schistosomiasis) or in association with advanced carcinoma of the prostate, they may be markedly indurated. Stripping of the seminal vesicles should be done in association with prostatic massage, for the vesicles are usually infected when prostatitis is present. Primary tumors of the vesicles are very rare. A cystic mass may rarely be felt over the prostate or just above it. This probably represents a cyst of the müllerian duct or the utricle. The latter is occasionally associated with severe hypospadias.

LYMPH NODES

It should be remembered that generalized lymphadenopathy usually occurs early in human immunodeficiency syndrome (HIV) (see Chapter 15).

Inguinal & Subinguinal Lymph Nodes

With inflammatory lesions of the skin of the penis and scrotum or vulva, the inguinal and subinguinal lymph nodes may be involved. Such diseases include chancroid, syphilitic chancre, lymphogranuloma venereum, and, on occasion, gonorrhea.

Malignant tumors (squamous cell carcinoma) involving the penis, glans, scrotal skin, or distal urethra in women metastasize to the inguinal and subinguinal nodes. Testicular tumors do not spread to these nodes unless they have invaded the scrotal skin or the patient has previously undergone orchiopexy.

Other Lymph Nodes

Tumors of the testis and prostate may involve the left supraclavicular nodes. Tumors of the bladder and prostate typically metastasize to the internal iliac, external iliac, and preaortic nodes, although only occasionally are they so large as to be palpable. Upper abdominal masses near the midline in a young man should suggest metastases from cancer of the testis; the primary growth may be minute and completely hidden in the substance of what appears to be a normal testicle.

NEUROLOGIC EXAMINATION

A careful neurologic survey may uncover sensory or motor impairment that will account for residual urine (neuropathic bladder) or incontinence. Since the bladder and its sphincter are innervated by the second to fourth sacral segments, much information can be gained by testing anal sphincter tone and the sensation of the perianal skin and by eliciting the Achilles tendon and bulbocavernosus reflexes. The bulbocavernosus reflex is elicited by placing a finger in the patient's rectum and squeezing the glans penis or clitoris or by jerking on an indwelling Foley catheter. The normal reflex is contraction of the anal sphincter and bulbocavernosus muscles in response to these maneuvers.

It is wise, particularly in children, to seek a dimple over the lumbosacral area. One should palpate the sacrum to be sure it is present and normally formed. Sacral agenesis or partial development is compatible with deficits of S2–4. If findings seem abnormal, x-ray examination is indicated.

REFERENCES

General

Daniels IR, Layer GT: Gynaecomastia. Eur J Surg 2001;167:885.

Examination of the Kidneys

Acino S, Resnick MI: Office urologic ultrasound. Urol Clin North Am 1988;15:577.

Ahn JH, Morey AF, McAninch JW: Workup and management of traumatic hematuria. Emerg Med Clin North Am 1998; 16:145.

Bagley DH, Rivas D: Upper urinary tract filling defects: Flexible ureteroscopic diagnosis. J Urol 1990;143:1196.

Dockery WD, Stolpen AH: State-of-the-art magnetic resonance imaging of the kidneys and upper urinary tract. J Endourol 1999;13:417.

Gross GW, Boal DK: Sonographic assessment of normal renal size in children with myelodysplasia. J Urol 1988;140:784.

Lowe LH et al: Pediatric renal masses: Wilms tumor and beyond. Radiographics 2000;20:1585.

Mofenson HC, Greensher J: Transillumination of the abdomen in infants. Am J Dis Child 1968;115:428.

Perlman M, Williams J: Detection of renal anomalies by abdominal palpation in newborn infants. Br Med J 1976;3:347.

Pretorius ES, Wickstrom ML, Siegelman ES: MR imaging of renal neoplasms. Magn Reson Imaging Clin N Am 2000;8:813.

Restrepo NC, Carey PO: Evaluating hematuria in adults. Am Fam Physician 1989;40(2):149.

Ross JH: Pheochromocytoma: Special considerations in children. Urol Clin North Am 2000;27:393.

Smith DR, Raney FL Jr: Radiculitis distress as a mimic of renal pain. J Urol 1976;116:269.

Walther MM, Keiser HR, Linehan WM: Pheochromocytoma: Evaluation, diagnosis, and treatment. World J Urol 1999;17:35.

External Genitalia in Males

Andersen B, Mitchell M: Recent advances in hypospadias: Current surgical technique and research in incidence and etiology. Curr Urol Rep 2001;2:122.

Bemelmans BL et al: Penile sensory disorders in erectile dysfunction: Results of a comprehensive neuro-urophysiological diagnostic evaluation in 123 patients. J Urol 1991;146:777.

Conway GS et al: Importance of scrotal ultrasonography in gynaecomastia. Br Med J 1988;297:1176.

Dubinsky TJ, Chen P, Maklad N: Color-flow and power Doppler imaging of the testes. World J Urol 1998;16:35.

Galejs LE: Diagnosis and treatment of the acute scrotum. Am Fam Physician 1999;59:817.

Hall S, Oates RD: Unilateral absence of the scrotal vas deferens associated with contralateral mesonephric duct anomalies resulting in infertility: Laboratory, physical and radiographic findings, and therapeutic alternatives. J Urol 1993;150:1161.

Hanson P et al: Sacral reflex latencies in tethered cord syndrome. Am J Phys Med Rehab 1993;72(1):39.

Horstman WG: Scrotal imaging. Urol Clin North Am 1997; 24:653.

Lavoipierre AM: Ultrasound of the prostate and testicles. World J Surg 2000;24:198.

Lavoisier P et al: Bulbocavernosus reflex: Its validity as a diagnostic test of neurogenic impotence. J Urol 1989;141:311.

Leissner J et al: The undescended testis: Considerations and impact on fertility. BJU Int 1999;83:885.

Marcozzi D, Suner S: The nontraumatic, acute scrotum. Emerg Med Clin North Am 2001;19:547.

Oyen RH: Scrotal ultrasound. Eur Radiol 2002;12:19.

Pavlica P, Barozzi L: Imaging of the acute scrotum. Eur Radiol 2001;11:220.

Rivkees SA et al: Accuracy and reproducibility of clinical measures of testicular volume. J Pediatr 1987;110:914.

Sherrard J, Barlow D: Gonorrhoea in men: Clinical and diagnostic aspects. Genitourin Med 1996;72:422.

Wolf CK, Maizels M, Furness PD 3rd: The undescended testicle. Compr Ther 2001;27:11.

External Genitalia in Females

Edmonds DK: Congenital malformations of the genital tract. Obstet Gynecol Clin North Am 2000;27:49.

Redman JF: Techniques of genital examination and bladder catheterization in female children. Urol Clin North Am 1990;17:1.

Prostate

Carroll P et al: Prostate-specific antigen best practice policy—part II: Prostate cancer staging and post-treatment follow-up. Urology 2001;57:225.

Clarke HS Jr: Benign prostatic hyperplasia. Am J Med Sci 1997; 314:239.

Goldstein MM, Messing EM: Prostate and bladder cancer screening. J Am Coll Surg 1998;186:63.

Grossfeld GD, Coakley FV: Benign prostatic hyperplasia: Clinical overview and value of diagnostic imaging. Radiol Clin North Am 2000;38:31.

Kirby RS: The clinical assessment of benign prostatic hyperplasia. Cancer 1992;70(1 Suppl):284.

Kubik-Huch RA, Hailemariam S, Hamm B: CT and MRI of the male genital tract: Radiologic-pathologic correlation. Eur Radiol 1999;9:16.

Lummus WE, Thompson I: Prostatitis. Emerg Med Clin North Am 2001;19:691.

Nickel JC: The Pre and Post Massage Test (PPMT): A simple screen for prostatitis. Tech Urol 1997;3:38.

Obek C et al: Comparison of digital rectal examination and biopsy results with the radical prostatectomy specimen. J Urol 1999; 161:494.

Neurologic Examination

Cardenas DD, Mayo ME, Turner LR: Lower urinary changes over time in suprasacral spinal cord injury. Paraplegia 1995; 33:326.

Vodusek DB: Electromyogram, evoked sensory and motor potentials in neurourology. Neurophysiol Clin 1997;27:204.

Zermann DH et al: The male chronic pelvic pain syndrome. World J Urol 2001;19:173.

Urologic Laboratory Examination

Karl J. Kreder, Jr, MD, & Richard D. Williams, MD

Examination of specimens of urine, blood, and genitourinary secretions or exudates commonly directs the subsequent urologic workup and frequently establishes a diagnosis. Since approximately 20% of patients who visit a primary physician's office have a urologic problem, it is important for the physician to have a broad knowledge of the laboratory methods available to test appropriate specimens. Judicious use of such tests permits rapid, accurate, and cost-effective determination of the probable diagnosis and directs the management of patients with urologic disease.

EXAMINATION OF URINE

Urinalysis is one of the most important and useful urologic tests available, yet all too often the necessary details are neglected and significant information is overlooked or misinterpreted. Reasons for inadequate urinalyses include (1) improper collection, (2) failure to examine the specimen immediately, (3) incomplete examination (eg, most laboratories do not perform a microscopic analysis unless it is specifically requested by the provider), (4) inexperience of the examiner, and (5) inadequate appreciation of the significance of the findings.

The necessity of routine urinalysis as a screen in asymptomatic individuals, those admitted to hospitals, or those undergoing elective surgery continues to be debated. Numerous studies indicate that in these situations urinalysis is not cost-effective, that is, does not uncover more than 2.5% of conditions requiring treatment and thus is not routinely necessary. Patients presenting with urinary tract symptoms or signs, however, should undergo urinalysis. Studies also indicate that if macroscopic urinalysis (dip-strip) is normal, microscopic analysis is not necessary. If the patient has signs or symptoms suggestive of urologic disease, or the dipstick is positive for protein, heme, leukocyte esterase, or nitrite, a complete urinalysis, including microscopic examination of the sediment, should be completed.

Urine Collection

A. TIMING OF COLLECTION

It is best to examine urine that has been properly obtained in the office. First-voided morning specimens are helpful for qualitative protein testing in patients with possible orthostatic proteinuria and for specific gravity assessment as a presumptive test of renal function in patients with minimal renal disease due to diabetes mellitus or sickle cell anemia or in those with suspected diabetes insipidus. Evaluation of multiple morning specimens may be required to obviate the variability often encountered. Urine specimens that are obtained immediately after the patient has eaten or that have been left standing for a few hours become alkaline and thus may contain lysed red cells, disintegrated casts, or rapidly multiplying bacteria; therefore, a freshly voided specimen obtained a few hours after the patient has eaten and examined within 1 h of voiding is most reliable. The patient's state of hydration may alter the concentration of urinary constituents. Timed urine collections may be required for definitive assessment of renal function or proteinuria.

B. METHOD OF COLLECTION

Proper collection of the specimen is particularly important when patients have hematuria or proteinuria or are being evaluated for urinary tract infection. Examination of a urine specimen collected sequentially during voiding in several containers may help to identify the site of origin of hematuria or urinary tract infection. To gather consistent and meaningful urinalysis data, urine must be collected by a uniform method in the physician's office or laboratory. The specimen should be obtained before a genital or rectal examination in order to prevent contamination from the introitus or expressed prostatic secretions. Urine obtained from a condom, chronic catheter, or intestinal conduit drainage bag is *not* a proper specimen for urinalysis.

1. Men—It is usually simple to collect a clean-voided midstream urine sample from men. Routine instructions may be printed on a sheet given to the patient or placed on the lavatory wall. The procedure should include (1) retraction of the foreskin (a common source of contamination of the specimen) and cleansing of the meatus with benzalkonium chloride or hexachlorophene; (2) passing the first part of the stream (15–30 mL) without collection; (3) collecting the next or midstream portion (approximately 50–100 mL) in a sterile specimen container, which is capped immediately afterward; and (4) completely emptying the bladder into the toilet. A portion of the specimen is prepared immediately for both macroscopic and microscopic examination, and the rest is saved in the sterile container for subsequent culture if this proves necessary.

With this midstream clean-catch method, the likelihood that the specimen will be contaminated by meatal or urethral secretions is markedly decreased, although not completely eliminated. In adult males, it is rarely necessary to collect urine by catheterization unless urinary retention is present.

2. Women—The best method for collecting a clean-voided midstream specimen from a woman is as follows: (1) The patient is placed on the examining table in the lithotomy position. (2) The vulva and urethral meatus are cleansed with benzalkonium chloride or hexachlorophene. (3) The labia are separated. (4) The patient is instructed to initiate voiding into a container held close to the vulva. After she has passed the first 10–20 mL of urine, the next 50–100 mL is collected in a sterile container that is immediately capped. (5) The patient is allowed to complete emptying of the bladder. Because this technique requires considerable effort, it is acceptable to have the patient provide an initial specimen in a nonsterile container in the office lavatory. If results of urinalysis are normal, no further study is indicated; if abnormal, a urine specimen must be obtained by the more exacting technique. In either case, the specimen should be prepared for immediate examination.

If a satisfactory specimen cannot be obtained by the method described, one should not hesitate to obtain a specimen by catheterization. Catheterization may be necessary to determine whether residual urine is present or to eliminate nonvaginal sources of hematuria. The possibility of introducing bladder infection by catheter is minimal when catheterization is performed.

3. Children—Urine for analysis, other than bacterial cultures, can be obtained from males or females by covering the cleansed urethral meatus with a plastic bag; a urine specimen for culture may require catheterization or suprapubic needle aspiration. In girls, catheterization with a small catheter attached to a centrifuge tube is appropriate, but boys should *not* be routinely catheterized. It is often preferable in either sex to proceed with suprapubic needle aspiration. This is easier if the patient has been previously hydrated, so that the bladder is full. Suprapubic needle aspiration is performed as follows: (1) Cleanse the suprapubic area by sponging with alcohol. (2) With a small amount of local anesthetic, raise an intradermal wheal on the midline 1–2 cm above the pubis (the bladder lies just above the pubis in

young children). (3) Attach a 10-mL syringe to a 22-gauge needle. Insert the needle perpendicularly through the abdominal wheal into the bladder wall, maintaining gentle suction with the syringe so that urine will be aspirated as soon as the bladder is entered.

Macroscopic Examination

Macroscopic examination of urine often provides a clue when diagnosis is difficult.

A. Color and Appearance

Urine is often colored owing to drugs: phenazopyridine (Pyridium) will turn the urine orange; rifampin will turn it yellow-orange; nitrofurantoin will turn it brown; and L-dopa, α-methyldopa, and metronidazole will turn it reddish-brown. Red urine does not always signify hematuria. A red discoloration unassociated with intact erythrocytes in the urine can result from beta-cyanin excretion after beet ingestion, phenolphthalein in laxatives, ingestion of vegetable dyes, concentrated urate excretion, myoglobinuria due to significant muscle trauma, or hemoglobinuria following hemolysis. In addition, *Serratia marcescens* bacteria can cause the "red diaper" syndrome. However, whenever red urine is seen, hematuria must be ruled out by microscopic analysis. Cloudy urine is commonly thought to represent pyuria, but more often the cloudiness is due to large amounts of amorphous phosphates, which disappear with the addition of acid, or urates, which dissolve with the use of alkali. The odor of urine is rarely clinically significant.

B. Specific Gravity

The specific gravity of urine (normal, 1.003–1.030) is often important for diagnostic purposes: that of patients with significant intracranial trauma may be low owing to a lack of antidiuretic hormone (vasopressin); that of patients with primary diabetes insipidus is less than 1.010 even after overnight dehydration; that of patients with extensive acute renal tubular damage is consistently 1.010 (similar to the specific gravity of plasma); and a low specific gravity can be an early sign of renal damage from conditions such as sickle cell anemia. Urine specific gravity is the simplest time-honored test for evaluating hydration in postoperative patients. The specific gravity of urine may affect the results of other urine tests: in dilute urine, a pregnancy test may be falsely negative; in concentrated urine, protein may be falsely positive on dip-strips yet unconfirmed on quantitative tests. The specific gravity of urine may be falsely elevated by the presence of glucose, protein, artificial plasma expanders, or intravenous contrast agents.

Studies of specific-gravity reagent strips (method based on ionic alteration of a polyelectrolyte solution) have shown the method to be rapid, reliable, and unaffected by elevated amounts of glucose or contrast medium; however, alkaline pH may falsely lower the result (0.005/pH unit > 7.0). In the routine office setting, these strips are as reliable as either the hydrometer or refractometer methods.

C. CHEMICAL TESTS

Chemically impregnated reagent strips are accurate and have simplified routine urinalysis greatly. However, they must be monitored routinely by appropriate standardized quality-control reagents. The dip-strips are reliable only when not outdated and when used with *room temperature* urine.

1. pH—The pH of urine is important in a few specific clinical situations. Patients with uric acid stones rarely have a urinary pH over 6.5 (uric acid is soluble in alkaline urine). Patients with calcium stones, nephrocalcinosis, or both may have renal tubular acidosis and will be unable to acidify urine below pH 6.0. With urinary tract infections caused by urea-splitting organisms (most commonly *Proteus* species), the urinary pH tends to be over 7.0. It should be reemphasized that urine obtained within 2 h of a large meal or left standing at room temperature for several hours tends to be alkaline. The indicator paper in most dip-strips is quite accurate; however, confirmation by a pH meter is occasionally required.

2. Protein—Dip-strips containing bromphenol blue can be used to determine the presence of > 10 mg/dL protein in urine, but persistent proteinuria detected in this manner requires quantitative protein testing for confirmation. The dip-strip measures primarily albumin and is not sensitive to Bence-Jones proteins (immunoglobulins). Concentrated urine may give a false-positive result, as will urine containing numerous white blood cells (leukocytes) or vaginal secretions replete with epithelial cells. Orthostatic proteinuria can be demonstrated by detecting elevated protein levels in a urine specimen obtained after the patient has been in the upright position for several hours, whereas normal levels are found before ambulation. Prolonged fever and excessive physical exertion are also common causes of transient proteinuria.

Persistently elevated protein levels in the urine (> 150 mg/24 h) may indicate significant disease. Therefore, specific quantitative protein tests, electrophoretic studies of the urine, or both may be required to determine the specific type of protein that is present.

3. Glucose—The glucose oxidase-peroxidase tests used in dip-strips are quite accurate and specific for urinary glucose. False-positive results may be obtained when patients have ingested large doses of aspirin, ascorbic acid, or cephalosporins. An occasional patient has a blood glucose level below 180 mg/dL and yet has significant glucosuria; this indicates a low renal threshold of glucose excretion. However, most patients with a positive reading have diabetes mellitus.

4. Hemoglobin—The dip-strip test for hemoglobin is not specific for erythrocytes and should be used only to *screen* for hematuria, with microscopic analysis of the urinary sediment used for confirmation. Free hemoglobin or myoglobin in the urine may give a positive reading; ascorbic acid in the urine can inhibit the dip-strip reaction and give a false-negative result. Note that dilute urine (< 1.008) will lyse erythrocytes and thus provide a positive dip-strip reading for hemoglobin but no visible erythrocytes on microscopic analysis.

5. Bacteria and leukocytes—Test strips to determine the number of bacteria (nitrite) or leukocytes (leukocyte esterase) as predictors of bacteriuria are as accurate as microscopic sediment analysis in studies using quantitative urine cultures as the standard. The nitrite reductase test depends on the conversion of nitrate to nitrite. Many of the bacteria responsible for urinary tract infections, particularly enterobacteria, are capable of reducing nitrate to nitrite and therefore detectable by this test. When the nitrite test is positive, it suggests the presence of greater than 100,000 organisms per milliliter; however, several factors can lead to false-negative results. The nitrite test is positive only for coagulase-splitting bacteria and thus when used alone is only 40–60% accurate. Urine must be in the bladder for a sufficient time before sampling for the reduction of nitrate to occur (> 4 h); therefore, this test is most likely to be positive when first-voided morning urine is tested. A false-negative test will also result if the bacteria present do not contain nitrate reductase or if dietary nitrate is absent. A false-negative nitrite study may occur in a patient taking vitamin C. The leukocyte esterase test is a widely used chemical test that depends on the presence of esterase in granulocytic leukocytes. The leukocyte esterase test is an indication of pyuria and will remain positive even after the leukocytes have degenerated. The test accurately identifies patients with 10–12 leukocytes per high-power field in a centrifuged specimen. Although this test is a good indicator of pyuria, it does not detect bacteriuria. Therefore, it is often combined with the nitrite test to detect both bacteriuria and inflammation to maximize the chances of predicting urinary tract infection. Used together, the 2 tests are as predictive as the microscopic analysis but not as accurate as a urine culture. A false-negative leukocyte esterase study can be caused by glucosuria, or by phenazopyridine hydrochloride (Pyridium), nitrofurantoin, vitamin C, or rifampin in the urine.

Microscopic Examination

To be most accurate, the microscopic sediment examination should be done personally by an experienced physician or technician. Early-morning urine is the best specimen if it can be examined within a few minutes of collection. In most cases, the sediment can be prepared as follows: (1) Centrifuge a 10-mL specimen at 2000 rpm for 5 min. (2) Decant the supernatant. (3) Resuspend the sediment in the remaining 1 mL of urine by tapping the tube gently against a countertop. (4) Place 1 drop of the mixture on a microscope slide, cover with a coverslip, and examine first under a low-power ($\times$ 10) and then under a high-power ($\times$ 40) lens. For maximal contrast of the elements in the sediment, the microscope diaphragm should be nearly closed to prevent overillumination. Significant elements (particularly bacteria) are more easily seen if the slide is stained with methylene blue, but staining is not essential. Figure 5–1 shows typical findings in the urinary sediment.

A. STAINING

Staining with methylene blue (available commercially) may be helpful in microscopic examination of urinary sediment.

The urinary sediment is prepared as follows: (1) Place a drop of the centrifuged sediment on a glass slide and let it air dry. (2) Add a few drops of methylene blue for 10–20 s. (3) Rinse with tap water and let air dry. Do not blot. (4) Examine the slide under oil immersion (with $\times$ 100 lens) without a coverslip.

The slide can be stained with Gram's stain (Table 5–1) instead of methylene blue, but this is more complex and time-consuming to perform, and the only advantage over staining with methylene blue is that

Figure 5–1. Microscopic examination of urine sediment. (Redrawn after Todd-Sanford-Davidson.)

Table 5–1. Gram's staining method (Hucker modification).

1. Fix smear by heat.
2. Cover with crystal violet for 1 min.
3. Wash with water. Do not blot.
4. Cover with Gram's iodine for 1 min.
5. Wash with water. Do not blot.
6. Decolorize for 10–30 s with gentle agitation in acetone (30 mL) and alcohol (70 mL).
7. Wash with water. Do not blot.
8. Cover for 10–30 s with safranin (2.5% solution in 95% alcohol).
9. Wash with water and let dry.

Neisseria gonorrhoeae (gram-negative intracellular diplococci) can be more readily identified.

B. INTERPRETATION

1. Bacteria—The significance of bacteria in the urinary sediment is discussed in the section that follows on bacteriuria.

2. Leukocytes—Just as the presence of bacteria in the sediment is not an absolute indication of infection, neither is the finding of pyuria. In the sediment from clean-voided midstream specimens from men and those obtained by suprapubic aspiration or catheterization in women, a finding of more than 5 leukocytes per high-power field is generally considered abnormal (pyuria). If the patient has symptoms of a urinary tract infection as well as pyuria and bacteriuria, one is justified in making a diagnosis of infection and initiating empiric therapy. However, in a study of female patients with symptoms of urinary tract infection (Komaroff, 1984), 61% of those with pyuria had no bacterial growth from bladder urine obtained by catheterization or suprapubic aspiration. This underscores the unreliability of urinalysis alone for diagnosing urinary tract infections and further emphasizes the need for confirmation by bacterial cultures.

Renal tuberculosis can cause "sterile" acid-pyuria and should be considered in any patient with persistent pyuria and negative results on routine bacterial cultures. Specific staining of the urinary sediment for acid-fast bacteria (Ziehl-Neelsen stain) can be diagnostic; however, results will be positive from the sediment of spot specimens in only approximately 50% of patients with renal tuberculosis, whereas they are positive in the sediment of 24-h specimens in 70–80% of such cases. *Mycobacterium smegmatis,* a commensal organism, may be present in the urine (particularly in uncircumcised men) and can give false-positive results on acid-fast stains.

Urolithiasis can also cause pyuria. In patients with persistent pyuria, the physician should consider obtaining at least a plain x-ray of the abdomen and possibly an intravenous urogram to determine whether urolithiasis is present. Similarly, a retained foreign body such as a self-induced bladder object or a forgotten internal ureteral stent can cause pyuria. A plain x-ray (KUB film) of the abdomen should reveal the offender.

3. Erythrocytes—The presence of even a few erythrocytes in the urine (hematuria) is abnormal and requires further investigation. Although gross hematuria is more alarming to the patient, microscopic hematuria is no less significant. Infrequent causes of hematuria include strenuous exercise (long-distance running), vaginal bleeding, and inflammation of organs near or directly adjoining the urinary tract, for example, diverticulitis or appendicitis. Hematuria associated with cystitis or urethritis generally clears after treatment. Persistent hematuria in an otherwise asymptomatic patient of either sex and any age signifies disease and is an indication for further testing.

In patients with microscopic hematuria, a 3-container method for collection of urine can provide information on the site of origin of erythrocytes: (1) Give the patient 3 containers, labeled 1, 2, and 3 (or initial, mid, and terminal). (2) Instruct the patient to urinate and to collect the initial portion of the urine stream (10–15 mL) in the first container, the middle portion (30–40 mL) in the second, and the final portion (5–10 mL) in the third. (3) Using methods described previously, centrifuge the 3 specimens individually, prepare slides of the urinary sediment (with or without staining), and examine the slides microscopically. If erythrocytes predominate in the initial portion of the specimen, they are usually from the anterior urethra; those in the terminal portion are generally from the bladder neck or posterior urethra; and the presence of equal numbers of erythrocytes in all 3 containers usually indicates a source above the bladder neck (bladder, ureters, or kidneys). It is important to collect the urine before physical examination (particularly before rectal examination in men) to avoid misleading results.

The 3-container test may not be necessary in patients with gross hematuria, since the patients (men in particular) can usually tell the physician which portion of the stream contains the darkest urine (ie, the most erythrocytes). A specific dysmorphic erythrocyte configuration that can be detected with phase-contrast microscopy or by particle analyzer study of the urinary sediment and is highly indicative of active glomerular disease (Figure 5–2) has been described by Stamey and Kindrachuk (1985). This dysmorphism is thought to be a result of extreme changes in osmolality and the high concentration of urinary chemical constituents affecting erythrocytes during passage through the kidney tubules. An automated system for measuring electrical

Figure 5–2. **Left:** Dysmorphic erythrocytes in urine (arrows), viewed under light microscopy (magnification × 400). **Right:** Dysmorphic erythrocytes in urine (identical field), viewed under phase-contrast microscopy. (Reproduced, with permission, from Stamey TA, Kindrachuk RW: *Urinary Sediment and Urinalysis: A Practical Guide for the Health Science Professional.* Saunders, 1985.)

flow impedance has been shown to accurately detect, enumerate, and size erythrocytes in urine and is highly accurate in distinguishing glomerular from neonglomerular red cells (Kore, Dow, and Desai, 1999).

4. Epithelial cells—Squamous epithelial cells in the urinary sediment indicate contamination of the specimen from the distal urethra in males and from the introitus in females; no other significance should be placed on them. It is not uncommon to find transitional epithelial cells in the normal urinary sediment; however, if they are present in large numbers or clumps and are abnormal histologically (including large nuclei, multiple nucleoli, and an increased ratio of nucleus to cytoplasm), they are indicative of a malignant process affecting the urothelium (Figure 5–3).

5. Casts—Casts are formed in the distal tubules and collecting ducts and, for the most part, are not seen in normal urinary sediment; therefore, they commonly signify intrinsic renal disease.

Although **leukocyte casts** have been considered suggestive of pyelonephritis, they are not an absolute indicator and should not be used as the sole criterion for diagnosis. Leukocyte casts must be distinguished from **epithelial cell casts,** because the latter have little significance when present in small numbers. The distinction can be made easily if a small amount of acetic acid is added under the coverslip to enhance nuclear detail. (Note that casts tend to congregate near the edges of the coverslip.) Epithelial cell or leukocyte casts in large numbers signify underlying intrinsic renal disease requiring further diagnostic workup. In renal transplant recipients, an increase in the number of epithelial cells or casts from the renal tubules may be an early indication of acute graft rejection.

Erythrocyte casts are pathognomonic of underlying glomerulitis or vasculitis.

Hyaline casts probably represent a mixture of mucus and globulin congealed in the tubules; in small numbers, they are not significant. Hyaline casts are commonly seen in urine specimens taken after exercise and in concentrated or highly acidic urine specimens. Casts are rarely seen in alkaline urine and are therefore not usually present in urine specimens that have been left standing or in specimens from patients unable to acidify.

A

B

C

Figure 5–3. Papanicolaou-stained bladder cytology specimens. **A:** Normal cells (left) and malignant cells (right). **B:** High-power view of malignant cells. **C:** Papillary cluster of malignant cells. (Courtesy of Larry Kluskens, MD, Cytopathology Laboratory, University of Iowa.)

Granular casts most commonly represent disintegrated epithelial cells, leukocytes, or protein; they usually indicate intrinsic renal tubular disease.

6. Other findings—The finding of crystals in urine can be helpful in some instances, but the mere presence of crystals does not indicate disease. Crystals form in normal urine below room temperature. Cystine, leucine, tyrosine, cholesterol, bilirubin, hematoidin, and sulfonamide crystals are abnormal findings of varying importance. Several types of crystals that may be found on microscopic examination of urinary sediment are shown in Figure 5–1.

The use of protease inhibitors for treatment of human immunodeficiency virus (HIV) has resulted in urolithiasis due to indinavir crystal formation in urine. The characteristic crystals are flat, rectangular plates, often in a fan or star-burst pattern (Gagnon, Tsoukas, and Watters, 1998; Kopp et al, 1997).

The presence of trichomonads or yeast cells in the stained or unstained smear of sediment from a properly obtained urine specimen establishes a diagnosis and the need for treatment.

Artifacts present in the urine sediment can be difficult to differentiate from real abnormalities. Dirt and small pieces of vegetable fiber or hair are frequently found, but the most common artifacts are starch granules from examination gloves.

Bacteriuria

A. MICROSCOPIC EXAMINATION

A presumptive diagnosis of bacterial infection may be made on the basis of results of microscopic examination of the urinary sediment. If several bacteria per high-power field are found in a urine specimen obtained by suprapubic aspiration or catheterization in a woman or in a properly obtained clean-voided midstream specimen from a man, a provisional diagnosis of bacterial infection can be made and empiric treatment started. The findings should be confirmed by bacterial culture.

Finding several bacteria per high-power field in a voided specimen from a woman is of little significance. It is easier to distinguish and count bacteria and to differentiate leukocytes from transitional epithelial cells when slides are stained with methylene blue (see earlier section). Newer methods using flow cytometry–based urine analysis (UF-50) can detect bacteria with nearly 80% accuracy.

B. BACTERIAL CULTURES

The presumptive diagnosis of bacterial infection based on microscopic examination of the urinary sediment should be confirmed by culture.

1. Indications and interpretation—Cultures can be used to estimate the number of bacteria in the urine (quantitative cultures), to identify the exact organism present, and to predict which drugs will be effective in treating the infection. Cultures are particularly important in patients with recurrent or persistent infections, renal insufficiency, or drug allergies.

The number of bacteria present in the urine (colony count) is influenced by the method used to collect the urine specimen, the patient's hydration status, and whether the patient has been taking antimicrobial drugs. The concept that urinary tract infection is present only when the urine specimen contains 10^5 or more bacteria per milliliter is not an absolute rule; a lower count does not exclude the possibility of an infection, particularly in a symptomatic patient. Cultures with growth of multiple organisms usually signify contamination. The presence of a few organisms in a specimen with a low specific gravity is more significant than the same finding in a specimen with a high specific gravity, because the former is more dilute.

Identifying the drugs to which the bacteria are sensitive may or may not be necessary. *Escherichia coli,* which causes 85% of "routine" urinary tract infections, is known to be sensitive to numerous oral antimicrobial drugs. However, in patients with septicemia, renal insufficiency, diabetes mellitus, or suspected enterococcal, *Proteus,* or *Pseudomonas* infections, it is important to determine the antibiotic sensitivity of the organism and the drug concentration necessary for efficacious treatment. Monitoring antibiotic levels in blood and urine during treatment may be indicated, especially in severely ill patients and those receiving highly toxic drugs. These measurements can be done by most hospital laboratories.

2. Rapid tests for bacteriuria—In general, seriously ill or hospitalized patients with urinary tract infections should have cultures processed by an accredited bacteriology laboratory. However, for "routine" infections encountered in office practice, there are many satisfactory, cost-effective testing methods.

Rapid methods to screen for bacteria include growth-independent systems and growth-dependent systems. Several growth-dependent systems are available. One measures the turbidity of urine incubated in a broth medium for several hours. Positive results can be determined in as short a time period as 4 h; however, 12 h of growth is required before a test sample can be regarded as negative. Another growth-dependent system is based on the measurement of electrical conductance; however, this test has a high false-positive rate. A single screening test uses the leukocyte esterase test and the nitrite test. One growth-independent screening test is an automated system of microscopy with acridine-orange staining. This system is very sensitive and predictive for a urinary tract infection, but it has a high false-negative rate and is costly. Another test traps leukocytes and bacteria in a filter. A dye is then applied to the filter, and a color change is indicative of a urinary tract infection. This system is very rapid; however, the filter is prone to clogging, and pigmented urine may interfere with the colorimetric end point. Particles in the urine (both bacteria and leukocytes) can be counted by measuring electrical impedance, although the test is less accurate when counting bacteria.

Reliable culture methods involve use of small strips or glass slides coated with eosin–methylene blue agar on one side and nutrient agar on the other. The strips or slides are dipped in the urine specimen and then incubated for 24 h. Although these methods are easy to use, their disadvantages are that (1) not all bacteria will grow under these conditions, and (2) the accuracy of colony counts is debatable.

Perhaps preferable for the physician's office (but still subject to some of the same limitations) is use of a divided plastic culture plate with blood agar on one side and deoxycholate agar on the other. A known amount of urine is inoculated onto the agar on each side of the plate, and colony counts are determined at 24–48 h. The numbers of bacteria in 1 mL of the original urine specimen can be determined by multiplying the number of colonies by the volume (in milliliters) and dilution (if any) of the inoculum. If antibiotic sensitivity testing is also desired, an additional culture plate can be inoculated and small antibiotic-impregnated disks placed on the agar. Zones of growth inhibition seen around the disks at 12–24 h indicate sensitivity.

3. Cultures for tuberculosis—Urine smears stained for acid-fast bacilli (Ziehl-Neelsen stain performed by the laboratory) may provide evidence to support the diagnosis of renal tuberculosis. However, regardless of the result of the smear, multiple urine cultures should be performed if renal tuberculosis is suspected, both to confirm the presence of *Mycobacterium* and to determine its species. Numerous atypical mycobacteria have been found to cause renal tuberculosis. Since they are not always sensitive to the commonly used antituberculous drugs, sensitivity testing may also be indicated. Because the procedures for urine culture for mycobacteria vary from one laboratory to another, the physician should consult the laboratory beforehand. Mycobacteria grow slowly; thus, culture results may require 6–8 weeks or longer.

Other Urine Tests

Many other tests of urine can be helpful in determining the presence of urologic disease.

A. UROTHELIAL CANCER TESTS

1. Urine cytology—The evaluation of voided or bladder wash (barbotage) urine for bladder urothelial cancer cells has been quite successful for higher-grade (2–3) transitional cell cancers. Lower-grade tumors less commonly shed abnormal cells. Cystoscopy remains the standard diagnostic test for initial diagnosis and surveillance of bladder cancer.

2. Bladder tumor antigen test—The bladder tumor antigen test (BTA; Bard Diagnostic Sciences, Inc, Redmond, WA) is a latex agglutination assay for the qualitative detection of bladder tumor antigen in the urine.

3. Bladder tumor antigen stat test—The BTA *stat* test (Bard Diagnostic Sciences) is a single-step immunochromatographic assay that detects a human complement factor that is similar to human complement factor H (hCFH).

4. Nuclear matrix protein 22—The nuclear matrix protein 22 test (NMP22; Matritech, Inc, Newton, MA) is an immunoassay. Normal subjects will have low levels of NMP22 in the urine, whereas patients with active transitional cell carcinoma may have high levels of urinary NMP22.

5. FDP—Bladder tumor cells normally produce vascular endothelial growth factor leading to leakage of plasminogen, fibrinogen, and other clotting factors, which convert fibrinogen into fibrin and fibrinogen degradation products. The AuraTek FDP test (PerImmune, Inc, Rockville, MD) is an immunoassay that measures fibrin/fibrinogen degradation products (FDP) in the urine.

6. QUANTICYT System—The QUANTICYT System is a computer-based cytologic image analysis system. This system evaluates 50 randomly selected images containing 100–500 nuclei for DNA content and nuclear shape (van der Poel et al, 1996).

The characteristics of these bladder cancer tests are compared in Table 5–2.

Table 5–2. Comparison of different urine tests for bladder transitional cell carcinoma.

Test	Sensitivity (%)	Specificity (%)
NMP22	71	75
BTA	52	85
BTA *stat*	66	67
FDP	68	78
Telomerase	74	79
QUANTICYT	52	82
FISH	73	100
Flow cytometry	59	84
BLCA-4	96	100
Lewis X	80	86
Hyaluronidase	100	89
Hyaluronic acid	92	93
Survivin	100	95
Cytology	49	96

BTA, bladder tumor antigen; FDP, fibrin/fibrinogen degradation products; NMP22, nuclear matrix protein 22.
Source: Konety BR, Getzenberg RH: Urine based markers of urological malignancy. J Urol 2001;165:600.

7. Other tests—Other tests in development that require further clinical studies include fluorescent studies, flow cytometry, Lewis X antigen, hyaluronidase/hyaluronic acid, telomerase, BLCA-4, and survivin (Table 5–2).

B. HORMONAL STUDIES

Tests for abnormalities in adrenal hormone secretion are important in the workup of patients with suspected adrenal tumors. Pheochromocytoma and neuroblastoma can be detected by measuring the excretion of vanillylmandelic acid. However, urinary levels of metanephrine, epinephrine, and norepinephrine are more sensitive indicators, particularly in cases of pheochromocytoma. Although high levels of aldosterone in urine usually indicate an aldosterone-secreting tumor, drug interference may cause false-positive or false-negative results. Other adrenocortical tumors may be detected by their production of elevated levels of urinary 17-ketosteroids, although more specific urinary steroid tests are now available.

C. STUDIES OF STONE CONSTITUENTS

Patients with recurrent urolithiasis may have an underlying abnormality of excretion of calcium, uric acid, oxalate, magnesium, or citrate. Samples of 24-h urine collections can be tested to determine abnormally high levels of each. A few patients may have elevated cystine levels in urine. The nitroprusside test, a simple *qualitative* screening test for cystine, may indicate the need for quantifying cystine levels in timed urine collections. Whenever a stone is recovered, a formal stone analysis is recommended.

D. Miscellaneous Studies

In patients with suspected fistulas of the urinary tract and bowel (eg, cancer of the colon, diverticulitis, regional ileitis), discoloration of the urine after ingestion of a poorly absorbed dye such as phenol red will confirm the diagnosis. In an equally satisfactory test for fistulas, the patient is instructed to ingest gelatin capsules filled with granulated charcoal and to submit a urine sample several days later. Examination of the centrifuged urinary sediment will reveal the typical black granules if a fistula is present.

EXAMINATION OF URETHRAL DISCHARGE & VAGINAL EXUDATE

Urethral Discharge

Examination of urethral discharge in males can be particularly helpful in establishing a diagnosis. The following procedure, although exacting, provides proper specimens for determining the site of origin of bacteriuria or pyuria. Four sterile containers are labeled VB_1, VB_2, EPS, and VB_3 (VB = voided bladder urine; EPS = expressed prostatic secretions). The patient is instructed to retract the foreskin and cleanse the meatus with benzalkonium chloride or hexachlorophene and to collect the urine specimens, capping the containers immediately afterward. The initial 10–15 mL of urine is collected in container VB_1 and the subsequent 15–30 mL in container VB_2. The prostate is then massaged, and secretions are collected in container EPS. The patient voids a final time, collecting the specimen in container VB_3. An aliquot of each specimen is tested for nitrite and leukocyte esterase and then centrifuged, and the sediment is prepared for microscopic examination as described previously. A separate aliquot of each VB specimen and the EPS specimen are saved for subsequent culture if necessary. The presence of leukocytes or bacteria (or both) only in VB_1 indicates anterior urethritis; if present in all 3 VB specimens, they may indicate cystitis or upper urinary tract infection; if present in EPS or VB_3 only, they indicate a prostatic source of infection. Quantitative cultures can be similarly interpreted. Patients with positive results should be treated with appropriate antimicrobial drugs.

If the patient presents with the thick yellowish discharge typical of *N gonorrhoeae* infection, the discharge should be stained with Gram's stain and examined for gram-negative intracellular diplococci. It is important to remember that commensal bacteria in smegma may produce false-positive results.

If the patient presents with clear or whitish urethral discharge, a smear of the discharge obtained by milking the urethra or from VB_1 should be stained with methylene blue or Gram's stain and examined microscopically. The presence of trichomonads, yeast cells, or bacteria in properly collected specimens indicates disease requiring treatment.

In cases of acute epididymitis, urinalysis and urine culture are often helpful in establishing the cause. Epididymitis is most commonly caused by *Chlamydia* species in young men and by *E coli* in men over 35 years of age. Culturing chlamydiae is time-consuming and expensive. Although a rapid immunofluorescence method of identifying *Chlamydia* is available, it is usually best to proceed with therapy based on the age of the patient and guided by clinical results.

The diagnosis of any sexually transmitted disease should raise the question of acquired immunodeficiency syndrome (AIDS). A study by Hart (1991) demonstrated that many patients who presented to a sexually transmitted disease clinic did not request to be tested for HIV infection. Had the clinical staff not provided education and urged HIV testing for all patients, 44% of patients diagnosed with HIV would have been missed.

Vaginal Exudate

The underlying cause of vaginitis is often a viral, yeast, or protozoal infection or the presence of a foreign body (eg, retained tampon), and a simple physical examination may be all that is required for diagnosis.

Vaginal secretions obtained by use of a swab can be examined either stained or unstained. A drop of saline is added to a drop of specimen on a glass slide, mixed thoroughly, and covered with a coverslip. Examination under a low- or high-power lens may reveal yeast cells or trichomonads, thus suggesting appropriate therapy. Since bacteria are always present in the vagina, they generally are not significant findings in a wet smear.

RENAL FUNCTION TESTS

Urine Specific Gravity

With diminished renal function, the ability of the kidneys to concentrate urine lessens progressively until the specific gravity of urine reaches 1.006–1.010. However, the ability to dilute urine tends to be maintained until renal damage is extreme. Even in uremia, although the concentrating power of the kidneys is limited to a specific gravity of 1.010, dilution power in the specific gravity range of 1.002–1.004 may still be found. Determination of urine osmolality is undoubtedly a more meaningful measurement of renal function, but determination of specific gravity lends itself to office diagnosis.

Serum Creatinine

Creatinine, the end product of the metabolism of creatine in skeletal muscle, is normally excreted by the kidneys. Because individual daily creatinine production is constant, the serum level is a direct reflection of renal function. Serum creatinine levels remain within the normal range (0.8–1.2 mg/dL in adults; 0.4–0.8 mg/dL in young children) until approximately 50% of renal function has been lost. Unlike most other excretory products, the serum creatinine level generally is not influenced by dietary intake or hydration status.

Endogenous Creatinine Clearance

Because creatinine production is stable and creatinine is filtered through the glomerulus (although a small amount is probably secreted), its renal clearance is essentially equal to the glomerular filtration rate. The endogenous creatinine clearance test has thus become the most accurate and reliable measure of renal function available without resorting to infusion of exogenous substances such as inulin or radionuclides. Determination of creatinine clearance requires only the collection of a timed (usually 24-h) urine specimen and a serum specimen. The clearance is calculated as follows:

$$Clearance = UV/P$$

where: U = creatinine in urine (in mg/dL)

P = creatinine in plasma (in mg/dL)

V = mL of urine excreted (per minute
or 24 h)

The resulting clearance is expressed in milliliters per minute, with 90–110 mL/min considered normal.

Because muscle mass differs among individuals, further standardization has been achieved by using the following formula:

$$UV/P = 1.73 \ m^2 / Estimated \ surface \ area$$

$$= Corrected \ clearance$$

A corrected clearance level of 70–140 mL/min is considered normal.

Although creatinine is highly reliable as an estimate of renal function, values may be falsely low, particularly if only part of the urine is collected over the timed period or if a serum specimen is not collected concurrently.

Blood Urea Nitrogen

Urea is the primary metabolite of protein catabolism and is excreted entirely by the kidneys. The blood urea nitrogen (BUN) level is therefore related to the glomerular filtration rate. Unlike creatinine, however, BUN is influenced by dietary protein intake, hydration status, and gastrointestinal bleeding. Approximately two-thirds of renal function must be lost before a significant rise in BUN level becomes evident. For these reasons, an elevated BUN level is less specific for renal insufficiency than an elevated serum creatinine level. However, the BUN-creatinine (BUN-Cr) ratio can provide specific diagnostic information. It is normally 10:1; in dehydrated patients and those with bilateral urinary obstruction or urinary extravasation, the ratio may range from 20:1 to 40:1; patients with advanced hepatic insufficiency and overhydrated patients may exhibit a lower than normal BUN level and BUN-Cr ratio. In patients with renal insufficiency, extremely high BUN levels may develop that can be partially controlled by a decrease in dietary protein.

EXAMINATION OF BLOOD, SERUM, & PLASMA

Complete Blood Count

Normochromic normocytic anemia is often seen with chronic renal insufficiency. Chronic blood loss from microscopic hematuria is usually not sufficient to cause anemia, although gross hematuria certainly can be. A specific increase in the number of erythrocytes, as manifested by elevated hemoglobin and hematocrit levels (erythrocytosis, not polycythemia), may be indicative of a paraneoplastic syndrome associated with renal cell cancer. The leukocyte count is usually nonspecific, although marked elevations may indicate an underlying leukemia that may be the cause of urologic symptoms.

Blood Clotting Studies

Clotting studies are generally not necessary unless an insidious disorder such as von Willebrand disease, hepatic disease, or a sensitivity to ingested salicylates is suspected in a patient with unexplained hematuria. The determination of prothrombin time and bleeding time (and perhaps partial thromboplastin time) is usually sufficient. A platelet count is important in patients receiving chemotherapy and those who have received extensive radiation therapy.

Electrolyte Studies

Serum sodium and potassium determinations may be indicated in patients taking diuretics or digitalis preparations and in patients who have just undergone transurethral prostatectomy. Serum calcium determinations are useful in patients with calcium urolithiasis. Elevated calcium levels are occasionally indicative of a paraneoplastic syndrome in patients with renal cell cancer. Serum albumin levels should be measured simultaneously with calcium levels to adequately assess the significance of the latter.

Prostate Cancer Markers

Prostate-specific antigen (PSA) is an extremely important prostate cancer marker. PSA is prostate-specific but not cancer-specific. Serum elevation greater than 4.0 ng/mL is correlated with prostatic cancer; however, serum levels vary with prostate volume, inflammation, and amount of cancer within the gland. PSA has become useful as a screening tool and is most useful as a marker of effective treatment (falls to zero following removal of organ-confined cancer) and early recurrence (antedates other clinical evidence of tumor by 6 months or more). The percentage of free PSA (ratio of unbound to total PSA) in the serum has been approved for use in diagnosing prostate cancer. Studies show that when the percentage of free PSA is < 10%, approximately 60% of men will have prostate cancer, whereas if the percentage of free PSA is > 25%, only 8% will have it (Catalona et al, 1995).

Table 5–3. Laboratory values that *do not* change with age.

Hepatic function tests
Serum bilirubin
AST
ALT
GGTP
Coagulation tests
Biochemical tests
Serum electrolytes
Total protein
Calcium
Phosphorus
Serum folate
Arterial blood tests
pH
$Paco_2$
Renal function tests
Serum creatinine
Thyroid function tests
T_4
Complete blood count
Hematocrit
Hemoglobin
Erythrocyte indices
Platelet count

AST, aspartate aminotransferase; ALT, alanine aminotransferase; GGTP, gamma-glutamyltransferase.

Hormonal Studies

Serum parathyroid hormone studies are useful in determining the presence of a parathyroid adenoma in patients with urolithiasis and an elevated serum calcium level. Measurement of parathyroid hormone is not reliable, however, as a sole screening test for parathyroid adenoma and should not be used routinely in all patients with urolithiasis. Serum renin levels may be elevated in patients with renal hypertension, although many conditions can cause false-positive results. Studies of adrenal steroid hormones (eg, aldosterone, cortisol, epinephrine, norepinephrine) are useful in determining adrenal function or the presence of adrenal tumors. Determinations of serum levels of the beta-subunit of hCG and of alpha-fetoprotein are indispensable in staging and in treatment follow-up for testicular tumors. One of these tumor markers is usually elevated in up to

Table 5–4. Laboratory values that *do* change with age.

Value	Degree of Change
Alkaline phosphatase	Increases by 20% between third and eighth decades
Biochemical tests	
Serum albumin	Slight decline
Uric acid	Slight increase
Total cholesterol	Increases by 30–40 mg/dL by age 55 in women and age 60 in men
HDL cholesterol	Increases by 30% in men; decreases 50% in women
Triglycerides	Increases by 30% in men and 50% in women
Serum B_{12}	Slight decrease
Serum magnesium	Decreases by 15% between third and eighth decades
Pao_2	Decreases by 25% between third and eighth decades
Creatinine clearance	Decreases by 10 mL/min/1.73 sq m/decade
Thyroid function tests	
T_3	Possible slight decrease
TSH	Possible slight increase
Glucose tolerance tests	
Fasting blood sugar	Minimal increase (within normal range)
1-Hour postprandial blood sugar	Increases by 10 mg/dL/decade after age 30
2-Hour postprandial blood sugar	Increases up to 100 plus age after age 40
Leukocyte count	Decreases

HDL, high-density lipoprotein; TSH, thyroid-stimulating hormone.

85% of patients with nonseminomatous testicular tumors and can predict the recrudescence of tumor several months before disease is clinically evident. Serum testosterone studies can help to establish the cause of impotence or infertility.

Other Studies

The finding of elevated fasting plasma glucose levels in patients with urologic disease can establish the diagnosis of diabetes mellitus and thus indicate a possible cause of renal insufficiency, neurovesical dysfunction, impotence, or recurrent urinary tract infection. Serum uric acid levels are often elevated in patients with uric acid stones. Elevated serum complement levels may be diagnostic of underlying glomerulopathies.

LABORATORY VALUES IN ELDERLY PATIENTS

Clearly, some laboratory values change as patients age, others stay the same, and the effects of aging on some are as yet unknown. Laboratory values that do not change with increasing age include complete blood count, serum electrolytes, and hepatic function tests, among others (Table 5–3). Laboratory values that change as patients age include creatinine clearance, alkaline phosphatase, uric acid, and cholesterol (Table 5–4).

Other factors that may make laboratory interpretation more difficult include atypical disease presentation, multiple concurrent diseases, and prescription and nonprescription drug use.

REFERENCES

Berger RE et al: *Chlamydia trachomatis* as a cause of acute "idiopathic" epididymitis. N Engl J Med 1978;298:301.

Bolann BJ, Sandberg S, Digranes A: Implications of probability analysis for interpreting results of leukocyte esterase and nitrite test strips. Clin Chem 1989;35:1663.

Catalona WJ et al: Evaluation of percentage of free serum PSA to improve specificity of prostate cancer screening. JAMA 1995; 274:1214.

Cavalieri TA, Chopra A, Bryman PN: When outside the norm is normal: Interpreting lab data in the aged. Geriatrics 1992; 47:66.

Gagnon RF, Tsoukas CM, Watters AK: Light microscopy of indinavir urinary crystals. Ann Intern Med 1998;128:321.

Hart G: Factors associated with requesting and refusing human immunodeficiency virus antibody testing. Med J Aust 1991; 155:586.

Khanna OP, Son DL: Screening for urinary tract infection using Bac-T-Screen bacteriuria device. Urology 1986;27:424.

Komaroff AL: Acute dysuria in women. N Engl J Med 1984; 310:368.

Konety BR, Getzenberg RH: Urine based markers of urological malignancy. J Urol 2001;165:600.

Kopp JB et al: Crystalluria and urinary tract abnormalities associated with indinavir. Ann Intern Med 1997;127:119.

Kore R, Dow C, Desai K: A new automated system for urine analysis: A simple, cost-effective and reliable method for distinguishing between glomerular and nonglomerular sources of haematuria. BJU Int 1999;84:454.

Lawrence VA, Gafni A, Gross M: The unproven utility of the preoperative urinalysis: Economic evaluation. J Clin Epidemiol 1989;42:1185.

Lohr JA et al: Making a presumptive diagnosis of urinary tract infection by using a urinalysis performed in an on-site laboratory. J Pediatr 1993;122:22.

Lotan Y, Roehrborn C: Cost-effectiveness of a modified care protocol substituting bladder tumor markers for cystoscopy for the followup of patients with transitional cell carcinoma of the bladder: A decision analytical approach. J Urol 2002;167:75.

Messing EM et al: Urinary tract cancers found by homescreening with hematuria dipsticks in healthy men over 50 years of age. Cancer 1989;64:2361.

Morgan MG, McKenzie H: Controversies in the laboratory diagnosis of community-acquired urinary tract infection. Eur J Clin Microbiol Infect Dis 1993;12:491.

Okada H et al: Automated urinalysis: Evaluation of the Sysmex UF-50. Am J Clin Pathol 2001;115(4):605.

Okada H et al: Detection of significant bacteriuria by automated urinalysis using flow cytometry. J Clin Microbiol 2000;38: 2870.

Pels RJ et al: Dipstick urinalysis screening of asymptomatic adults for urinary tract disorders. 2. Bacteriuria. JAMA 1989;262: 1221.

Saad A et al: A study comparing various noninvasive methods of detecting bladder cancer in urine. BJU Int 2002;89(4):369.

Sarosdy MF et al: Improved detection of recurrent bladder cancer using the Bard BTA *stat* test. Urology 1997;50:349.

Schmetter BS et al: A multicenter trial evaluation of the fibrin/fibrinogen degradation products test for detection and monitoring of bladder cancer. J Urol 1997;158:801.

Smith SD et al: Urine detection of survivin and diagnosis of bladder cancer. JAMA 2001;285:324.

Soloway MS et al: Use of a new tumor marker, urinary NMP22, in the detection of occult or rapidly recurring transitional cell carcinoma of the urinary tract following surgical treatment. J Urol 1996;156:363.

Stamey TA, Kindrachuk RW: *Urinary Sediment and Urinalysis: A Practical Guide for the Health Science Professional.* Saunders, 1985.

van der Poel HG et al: QUANTICYT: Karyometric analysis of bladder washing for patients with superficial bladder cancer. Urology 1996;48:357.

Van Nostrand J, Junkins A, Bartholdi R: Poor predictive ability of urinalysis and microscopic examination to detect urinary tract infection. Am J Clin Pathol 2000;113(5):709.

Radiology of the Urinary Tract

Steven C. Eberhardt, MD, & Hedvig Hricak, MD, PhD

6

The field of diagnostic radiology continues to evolve, most noticeably in refinements to cross-sectional techniques. Imaging of the urinary tract, as a result, has become more precise, with new procedures offering a great selection of options, and new imaging algorithms are being implemented. Ultrasonography, computed tomography (CT), and magnetic resonance imaging (MRI) provide higher soft-tissue contrast resolution than conventional radiography, as well as multiplanar imaging capability, resulting in significant advances in almost all areas of uroradiology. Although such advances have produced new algorithms for how to best proceed with diagnostic imaging evaluation, the approach in any particular case also depends greatly on the equipment and professional talent available. In summary, ever-changing uroradiology remains indispensable in the diagnosis and treatment of patients with urologic disorders. This chapter will discuss the imaging techniques used in uroradiology, with summaries of the advantages and disadvantages of the various techniques, and will end with a brief discussion comparing imaging methods.

RADIOGRAPHY

X-rays are electromagnetic waves with photon energies that typically fall between those of gamma rays and ultraviolet radiation. Radiography is possible because tissues differ in their ability to absorb x-rays. A radiopaque contrast medium is frequently employed to enhance soft-tissue contrast.

Newer imaging techniques are replacing conventional radiography for diagnosis of many urologic problems; however, radiography remains in use for some urologic disorders. Therefore, the urologist should be familiar with x-ray equipment and uroradiologic techniques. The basic types of uroradiologic studies are plain (conventional) abdominal films (also known as KUB, which stands for kidney, ureter, bladder); intravenous urograms (IVU); cystourethrograms; urethrograms; and angiograms. These studies are described separately in sections that follow.

Basic Equipment & Techniques

A. RADIOGRAPHY FLUOROSCOPY

Many conventional x-ray units contain both radiographic and fluoroscopic capabilities. These require a high-voltage power supply, an x-ray tube, a collimating device, and an x-ray detector or film. Fluoroscopic units also use an electronic image intensifier and an image display system. Today, more radiology departments are becoming completely "filmless" as digital recording, displaying, and archiving of images are replacing film-based techniques.

B. IMAGE INTENSIFICATION

Image intensifiers, coupled to video cameras, electronically augment the ordinary dim fluoroscopic image. Acquired images can be recorded and simultaneously viewed on monitors, usually in the x-ray room.

C. IMAGE RECORDING

Conventional recording of an x-ray image uses film and intensifying screens. The image intensifier and camera can be used to capture dynamic and static images. Real-time images may be recorded using photographic cine cameras, though this has been largely replaced by conventional or digital video. Conventional spot images may be acquired on x-ray film, or on modern equipment digitally recorded, including rapid-sequence images at up to 8 per second.

D. CONTRAST MEDIA

Radiographic contrast media used in uroradiology are water-soluble iodinated compounds that are radiopaque. Similar compounds are used for basic radiographic techniques and computed tomography, though iodine concentrations will differ depending on preference and route of administration. In general, intravenous administration for CT or IVU is performed with 200 mg iodine per pound body weight in adults, and direct instillation to the collecting system or bladders uses the same media diluted to 15–45% concentration. The extracellular distribution of these agents results in improved contrast resolution and conspicuity of various structures.

Significant advances in water-soluble contrast media occurred with the introduction of low-osmolality (nonionic) organic iodine-containing compounds. When compared with conventional high-osmolality agents, these nonionic agents significantly improve patient tolerance and decrease the incidence of adverse reactions. Whether they reduce the mortality associated with the use of contrast media has not been proved. The major obstacle to the universal use of nonionic agents is higher cost.

E. ADVERSE REACTIONS

All procedures using intravascular contrast media carry a small but definite risk of adverse reactions. The overall incidence of adverse reactions is about 5%. Reactions in nonintravenous use (ie, cystograms) are extremely rare but have been reported.

Most reactions are minor; for example, nausea, vomiting, hives, rash, or flushing, and usually require no treatment other than reassurance. Cardiopulmonary and anaphylactoid reactions can occur with little warning and can be life-threatening or fatal. In a large meta-analysis, the incidence of death due to intravascular injection of contrast media was 0.9 deaths per 100,000 injections. There are no reliable methods for pretesting patients for possible adverse reactions; therefore, the risks and benefits of contrast use should be carefully evaluated for each patient before the procedure is initiated.

Nonionic contrast media have produced fewer adverse reactions than the higher-osmolality ionic contrast agents and are being used increasingly, particularly in patients with previous reactions or in patients with a history of allergies. In many departments, they are used exclusively.

Treatment of adverse reactions involves the use of antihistamines, epinephrine, vascular volume expanders, and cardiopulmonary drugs as well as ancillary procedures indicated by the nature and severity of the reaction.

In some cases a radiographic examination using intravascular contrast media is critical even if the patient has had a prior moderate or severe reaction. Such patients are given nonionic contrast agents and are pretreated with corticosteroids, sometimes in combination with antihistamines, in an effort to prevent recurrence. This preventive treatment is not always successful, so any decision to administer contrast media under these circumstances should be carefully weighed against the risks.

Nephrotoxicity caused by intravascular contrast agents is another concern. The pathogenesis of contrast nephropathy likely involves medullary ischemia due to contrast-induced vasoconstriction and direct tubular injury. Patients at higher risk are those with preexisting renal insufficiency, diabetes, or dehydration or patients who receive higher volumes of contrast material. Alternative procedures can be selected in high-risk patients. If contrast use is deemed necessary in a high-risk individual, contrast nephropathy can be minimized through attention to proper hydration, discontinuation of drugs that may exacerbate toxic effects (ie, metformin, nonsteroidal anti-inflammatory drugs), and reduction of contrast volume.

Advantages & Disadvantages

Radiography produces anatomic images of almost any body part. Costs are moderate compared with cross-sectional imaging systems. Space requirements are modest, and portable equipment is available for use in hospital wards, operating rooms, and intensive care units. Because a great many specialists are trained in radiography, the use of radiography is not confined to large medical centers. The major disadvantage of radiographic imaging is the use of ionizing radiation and relatively poor soft-tissue contrast. The evaluation of the urinary tract almost always requires opacification by iodine contrast media.

1. Plain Film of the Abdomen (Figures 6–1 through 6–3)

A plain film of the abdomen, frequently called a KUB (kidney-ureter-bladder) film, is the simplest uroradiologic examination. It is generally the preliminary radiograph in extended radiologic examinations, such as intravenous urography, and is usually taken with the patient supine. It may demonstrate osseous abnormalities, abnormal calcifications, or large soft-tissue masses.

Kidney outlines usually can be seen on the plain film, so that their size, number, shape, and position can be assessed. The size of normal adult kidneys varies widely. The long diameter (the length) of the kidney is the most widely used and most convenient radiographic measurement. The average adult kidney is about 12–14 cm long. In children older than 2 years of age, the length of a normal kidney is approximately equal to the distance from the top of the first to the bottom of the fourth lumbar vertebral body. Patterns of calcification in the urinary tract (Figures 6–1 and 6–2) may help to identify specific diseases.

Figure 6–1. Plain films of the abdomen with abnormal radiopacities. **Upper left:** Bilateral nephrocalcinosis. Young adult male with renal tubular acidosis. **Upper right:** Bilateral staghorn calculi. 37-year-old woman with chronic pyelonephritis and history of previous right staghorn pyelolithotomy. **Lower left:** Renal tuberculosis. Shrunken, autonephrectomized, and calcified right tuberculous kidney (arrows). 74-year-old man with history of renal and thoracolumbar spinal tuberculosis. **Lower right:** Papillary adenocarcinoma of the right kidney. Remarkable tumor surface calcifications. Multiple pulmonary metastases (arrows) from the renal cancer. 22-year-old woman with painless soft-tissue mass in the neck.

2. Urography (Figures 6–4 through 6–8)

The collecting structures of the kidneys, ureters, and bladder can be demonstrated radiologically with contrast media by the following methods:

Intravenous Urography

The IVU, also known as excretory urography (EU) (Figure 6–4), or intravenous pyelography (IVP), can demonstrate a wide variety of urinary tract lesions (Figures 6–4 and 6–5), is simple to perform, and is well tolerated by most patients.

Sonography, CT, and MRI have replaced urography in many cases. Nevertheless, urography is still occasionally used and is useful for demonstrating small lesions in the urinary tract (eg, papillary necrosis, medullary sponge kidney, uroepithelial tumors, pyeloureteritis cystica).

A. PATIENT PREPARATION

At one time dehydration was advocated as optimal preparation for intravenous urography (EU). This is no longer required. Furthermore, dehydration is to be avoided in infants, debilitated and elderly patients, and patients with diabetes mellitus, renal failure, multiple myeloma, or hyperuricemia.

It is controversial whether preliminary bowel cleansing is beneficial. The choice may be made according to individual preference.

Figure 6–2. Plain films of the abdomen with abnormal radiopacities. **Left:** Schistosomiasis calcification (arrows) in bladder and left ureter. 19-year-old male native of Aden with weight loss and hematuria. **Right:** Large vaginolith (open arrow) and small, barely visible bladder calculus (solid arrow). 4-year-old girl with common urogenital sinus.

B. Standard Technique

Following a preliminary plain film of the abdomen, additional radiographs are taken at timed intervals after the intravenous injection of iodine-containing contrast medium. Normal kidneys promptly excrete contrast agents, almost entirely by glomerular filtration.

The volume and speed of injection of the radiographic contrast medium (rapid bolus, slow infusion, etc) as well as the number and type of films taken vary by preference, patient tolerance, and clinical problem.

C. Technique Modifications

Radiographic tomography, x-ray imaging of a selected plane in the body, permits recognition of kidney structures that otherwise are obscured on standard radiograms by extrarenal shadows; for example, those due to bone or feces (Figure 6–6). **Image-intensified fluoroscopy** permits study of urinary tract dynamics. **"Immediate" films,** which are taken immediately after the rapid (bolus) injection of contrast, typically show a dense nephrogram and permit better visualization of renal outlines. **Abdominal (ureteral) compression devices** temporarily obstruct the upper urinary tract during excretory urography and improve the filling of renal collecting structures. **"Delayed" films,** taken hours later or on the following day, can contribute useful information. **"Upright" films,** taken with the patient standing or partially erect, reveal the degree of mobility and drainage of the kidneys and, if taken immediately after the patient has voided (**"postvoiding" film**), show any residual urine in the bladder.

Retrograde Urograms

Retrograde urography is a minimally invasive procedure that requires cystoscopy and the placement of catheters in the ureters. A radiopaque contrast medium is introduced into the ureters or renal collecting structures through the ureteral catheters (Figures 6–7 through 6–8), and radiographs of the abdomen are taken. This study must be performed by a urologist or experienced interventional uroradiologist. Some type of local or general anesthesia should be used, and the procedure occasionally causes later morbidity or urinary tract infection.

Retrograde urograms may be necessary if excretory urograms or CT urogram (CTU) are unsatisfactory, if

Figure 6–3. Plain films of the abdomen with abnormal radiolucencies. **Upper left:** Emphysematous pyelonephritis. Interstitial striated pattern of radiolucent gas (arrows) throughout the entire left kidney. Similar changes were present in the right kidney. 58-year-old diabetic man with pyuria and septic shock. **Upper right:** Gas pyelogram. No interstitial gas, but gas fills dilated left kidney calices, pelvis, and ureter. 50-year-old diabetic woman with sepsis and left upper urinary tract infection due to gas-forming microorganisms. **Lower left:** Renal angiomyolipoma. Plain film tomogram shows left kidney mass containing radiolucent fat (arrows). 69-year-old woman with weight loss and left flank pain. **Lower right:** Calcified renal *Echinococcus* cysts. Retroperitoneal gas insufflation study, tomogram, adult male. Note how radiolucent gas (arrows) has dissected in the retroperitoneum about the minimally calcified cysts in the upper pole of the kidney.

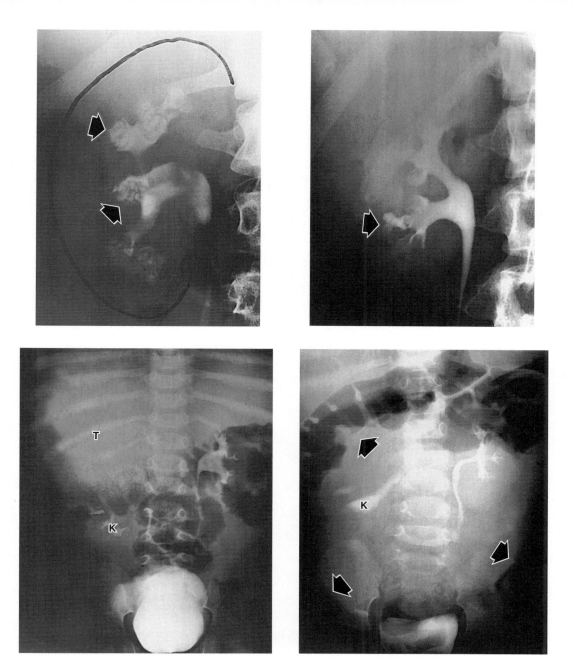

Figure 6–4. Abnormal excretory urograms. **Upper left:** Medullary sponge kidney. Pronounced medullary tubular ectasia (arrows) of entire right kidney. Similar findings were present in upper pole pyramids of left kidney, and small medullary calculi were present in some areas of tubular ectasia in both kidneys. 34-year-old woman with repeated bouts of chills, fever, and left flank pain. **Upper right:** Renal tuberculosis. Irregular cavitation of lower pole pyramid (arrow). 22-year-old woman with positive urine culture for tuberculosis. **Lower left:** Adrenal neuroblastoma. Diffuse small calcifications in a large right upper quadrant mass (T) depressing the right kidney (K). 12-year-old girl with proptosis of the right eye and an abdominal tumor. **Lower right:** Wilms tumor. Huge tumor of right kidney filling the entire abdomen (arrows), displacing bowel, and deforming collecting structures of the right kidney (K). Left kidney normal. 21-month-old girl with large abdominal mass.

Figure 6–5. Abnormal excretory urograms. **Upper left:** Crossed fused ectopia. Composite of 2 films from an excretory urogram shows ectopic right kidney (R) fused to left kidney (L). Right ureter (arrows) crosses midline and enters normally into right side of bladder. Healthy 31-year-old female potential kidney donor. **Upper right:** Renal artery aneurysm. Right kidney collecting structures draped around a central mass. 41-year-old woman with hypertension and right abdominal bruit. **Lower left:** Infantile polycystic kidney disease. Very large kidneys with radiopaque spoke pattern radiating out to cortex. 26 h after administration of intravenous contrast medium. 4-month-old female with bilateral abdominal masses. **Lower right:** Renal cell carcinoma. Unusual circular and curvilinear eggshell calcifications (arrows) in the tumor, which is compressing the infundibulum to deform upper pole calices. 39-year-old man with history of unroofing of left kidney cyst 3 years earlier.

Figure 6–6. Radiographic tomography. Tomography is used to image a plane in the body. The technique was widely used in uroradiology, often permitting demonstration of lesions otherwise hidden by overlying soft tissues or obscuring bowel shadows. However, CT is rapidly replacing conventional excretory urograms, and thus tomography is declining in its use as well. **Left:** Transitional cell carcinoma. The tumor in the pelvis (arrow) is clearly shown free of obscuring gas shadows present on the nontomographic films. 56-year-old man with history of renal calculi. **Right:** Renal cell carcinoma (T). Displacement of mid-kidney collecting structures and a nephrogram defect are seen free of obscuring splenic flexure fecal shadows that were present on the nontomographic films. 44-year-old woman with fever, weight loss, anemia, and history of contralateral nephrectomy for carcinoma 15 years earlier.

the patient has a history of adverse reaction to intravenous contrast media, or if other methods of imaging are unavailable or inappropriate.

Percutaneous Urograms

Outlining the renal collecting structures and ureters by percutaneous catheter is occasionally done when excretory or retrograde urography has failed or is contraindicated, or when there is a nephrostomy tube in place and delineation of the collecting system is desired. For antegrade studies, contrast medium is introduced either through nephrostomy tubes (nephrostogram) or by direct injection into the renal collecting structures via a percutaneous puncture through the patient's back. Percutaneous retrograde urograms of the upper urinary tract are made by retrograde injection of contrast medium through the opening of a skin ureterostomy or pyelostomy (skin ureterogram, skin urogram) or through the ostium of an interposed conduit, usually a segment of small bowel (loopogram).

3. Cystography & Voiding Cystourethrography (Figures 6–9 through 6–12)

Direct instillation of contrast media into the urinary bladder (cystography) is preferred over excretory urography for a more thorough examination of the bladder. Contrast is usually instilled via a transurethral catheter, but when necessary can be administered via percutaneous suprapubic bladder puncture. Radiographs can be taken using standard overhead x-rays, or during

Figure 6–7. Retrograde urograms and nephrostograms; lower ureters not all shown. **Upper left:** Normal retrograde urogram. Intrarenal collecting structures, pelvis, and ureter are normal. Adult male with microscopic hematuria and previous technically unsatisfactory excretory urogram. **Upper right:** Squamous cell carcinoma. Marked irregular filling defects involving calices, pelvis, and proximal ureter, with communicating abscess cavity in upper pole (arrow). Kidney also showed squamous metaplasia and contained calculi. 51-year-old woman with 2-week history of left flank cellulitis and tenderness. **Lower left:** Transitional cell carcinoma. Severe deformity with filling defects in right upper pole calices (curved arrow) and blood clots in lower calices and at ureteropelvic junction (straight arrow). 65-year-old man with gross hematuria and right flank pain. **Lower right:** Fungus balls. Nephrostogram revealing 2 filling defects (arrows) in renal pelvis. Copious fungal matter aspirated through nephrostomy catheter. 65-year-old diabetic woman who had undergone left nephrectomy, with percutaneous nephrostomy catheter (white arrow) for obstruction of right kidney.

Figure 6–8. Abnormal retrograde urograms. **Upper left:** Idiopathic retroperitoneal fibrosis. Smooth narrowing of both mid ureters (arrows), with bilateral proximal ureterectasis and hydronephrosis. 51-year-old woman with no urinary tract symptoms. **Upper right:** Functional ureteral obstruction. Obstruction was due to congenitally abnormal muscle arrangements in the affected very distal ureter (curved arrow). Pronounced hydronephrosis and dilatation of ureter (U) proximal to the short segment of abnormal ureter. 13-year-old boy with repeated urinary tract infections. **Lower left:** Transitional cell carcinoma of the ureter. No contrast medium has passed beyond the large, bulky, right ureteral tumor (arrow). The ureteral widening below the tumor is distinctive and is sometimes referred to as the "champagne glass" sign (in this instance, the glass is tipped on its side). 76-year-old man with nonfunctioning right kidney. **Lower right:** Ureteral constrictions secondary to extension of carcinoma of the colon. Bilateral distal ureteral narrowings (arrows) with upper tract obstruction. Composite of separate retrograde urograms. E, unintended extravasation about tip of left ureteral catheter. 76-year-old man with cancer of the sigmoid colon.

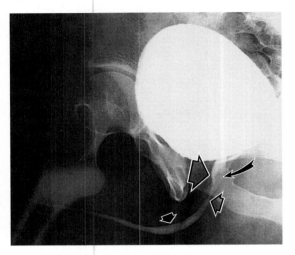

Figure 6–9. Normal voiding cystourethrograms. **Left:** Normal female bladder and urethra. Arrow indicates urethral meatus. 22-year-old woman with voiding symptoms. **Right:** Normal male penile urethra. Large open arrow, prostatic urethra; small open arrow, membranous urethra; closed arrow, penile urethra; curved arrow, verumontanum. 27-year-old man with vague right lower abdominal and testicular pain.

fluoroscopy. Voiding cystourethrograms are radiographs of the bladder and urethra obtained during micturition. Cystography and cystourethrography are important radiologic techniques for detecting vesicoureteral reflux and may be used in the workup of patients with urinary stress incontinence. CT cystography (CT of the pelvis after the instillation of dilute contrast medium into the bladder) has been shown useful in the evaluation of traumatic bladder rupture.

4. Urethrography (Figures 6–13 through 6–15)

The urethra can be imaged radiographically by retrograde injection of radiopaque fluid or in antegrade fashion with voiding cystourethrography or with voiding following excretory urography. The antegrade technique is required when lesions of the posterior urethra (for example, posterior urethral valves) are suspected; the retrograde technique is more useful for examining the anterior (penile) urethra.

5. Vasography (Figure 6–16)

Vasoseminal vesiculography is most often used in the investigation of male sterility. The radiopaque contrast medium is introduced into the ductal system by direct injection into an ejaculatory duct following panendoscopy or, more commonly, by injection into the vas deferens after it has been surgically exposed through a small incision in the scrotal neck.

6. Lymphangiography (Figure 6–17)

Lymphangiography is performed by injecting an oily contrast medium through a cannula into a lymphatic vessel in the foot to produce radiopacification of the inguinal, pelvic, and retroperitoneal lymphatic system. This procedure has been largely abandoned and replaced by CT and MRI.

7. Angiography

Nearly 50 years after Seldinger described techniques for percutaneous arteriography, catheter angiography maintains a role in treatment of some urologic disorders but is being replaced by CT or MRI for diagnostic examinations. Although an established imaging technique with proven value and an acceptable incidence of complications and morbidity, angiography is moderately invasive and relatively expensive.

Figure 6–10. Abnormal cystograms: retrograde cystograms or "cystograms" as part of excretory urogram studies. **Upper left:** Ectopic ureterocele. Giant ureterocele (straight arrows) to hydronephrotic, nonfunctioning upper portion (curved arrow) of duplex right kidney. 9-month-old female with urinary tract infections. **Upper right:** Pelvic lipomatosis. Pear-shaped bladder and increased radiolucency of the pelvic soft tissues secondary to pelvic lipomatosis is of severity sufficient to produce obstructive dilatation of the upper urinary tracts. Filling defects (arrows) at bladder base are due to cystitis glandularis. 62-year-old man with intermittent left flank pain. **Lower left:** Rupture of the membranous urethra. Pear-shaped bladder secondary to extraperitoneal extravasation (E) and perivesical hematoma. Arrow, inflated balloon of Foley catheter. 41-year-old man with renal transplant, after a motor vehicle accident that resulted in pelvic bone fractures, separation of the sacroiliac joints, and dislocation of the left (L) but not the right hip prosthesis (patient has bilateral hip prostheses). **Lower right:** Bladder hernia. Bilateral obstructive ureterectasis (small arrows) secondary to remarkable herniation of the entire bladder (large arrow, B) into the inguinal region, 5'5", 225-pound, 53-year-old man with panniculus reaching to mid thigh, complaining of difficulty voiding.

Figure 6–11. Abnormal cystograms: retrograde cystograms or "cystograms" as part of excretory urogram studies. **Upper left:** Neurogenic bladder. This neurogenic bladder has a "Christmas-tree" shape, with gross trabeculation and many diverticula. Residual myelographic contrast medium in spinal canal (straight arrow). Right vesicoureteral reflux (curved arrow). 70-year-old man with urinary incontinence. **Upper right:** Congenital "hourglass" bladder. Transverse concentric muscular band (arrows) separates upper and lower bladder segments, both of which contracted and emptied simultaneously and completely with voiding. 66-year-old woman with urinary stress incontinence. **Lower left:** Hodgkin's disease of bladder. Global thickening of the bladder wall (arrows), more apparent on the left. 54-year-old man with generalized Hodgkin's disease. **Lower right:** Papillary transitional cell bladder carcinoma. Huge (12 cm) cauliflowerlike bladder mass (arrows) filling almost the entire bladder. "Cystogram" film of an excretory urogram in a 40-year-old man with recurrent bladder tumor.

Figure 6–12. Abnormal prostate and posterior urethra: cystograms and urethrograms. **Upper left:** Benign prostatic hyperplasia. Gross enlargement of prostate gland producing marked elevation (arrows) of the bladder base. The bladder shows small diverticula and slight trabeculation. Excretory urogram (cystogram) in a 65-year-old man with history of obstructive voiding symptoms. **Upper right:** Foreign body (eyeliner pencil cover) lodged in bladder and prostatic urethra, with urethrorectal fistula. Radiopaque medium enters rectum and sigmoid colon (S) through fistula (arrow) from prostatic urethra. Retrograde urethrogram in a 43-year-old transsexual man. **Lower left:** Rhabdomyosarcoma of prostate. Lobulated filling defects (large arrow) encroaching on widened prostatic urethra. Voiding cystourethrogram in a 5-year-old boy with voiding difficulties. Small arrow, penile urethra. **Lower right:** Posterior urethral valves. Marked dilatation and elongation of prostatic urethra (P), with reflux into prostatic ducts (straight arrow) secondary to posterior urethral valves (curved arrow) with bilateral vesicoureteral reflux into dilated ureters (U). Voiding cystourethrogram in a 10-day-old male.

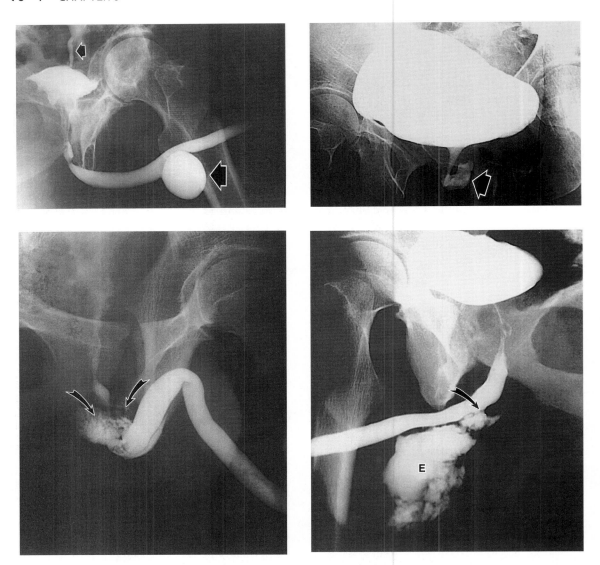

Figure 6–13. Abnormal anterior urethras: voiding cystourethrograms and retrograde urethrograms. **Upper left:** Voiding cystourethrogram in a 78-year-old man with a history of urethral diverticulum of unknown etiology. 4-cm anterior urethral diverticulum (large arrow) and left vesicoureteral reflux (small arrow). **Upper right:** Urethral diverticulum in a woman. Large irregular diverticulum (arrow). Voiding cystourethrogram in a 51-year-old woman with voiding difficulties and suspected urethral stricture. **Lower left:** Ruptured urethra. Extravasation of contrast medium around the bulbous urethra (arrows). Retrograde urethrogram in a 16-year-old boy in whom blunt perineal trauma was followed by bloody urethral discharge and inability to void. **Lower right:** Urethroscrotal fistula. Extravasation (E) into extraurethral tissues from fistula in bulbous urethra (arrow). Retrograde urethrogram in a 26-year-old man after end-to-end urethroplasty for stricture.

Figure 6–14. Abnormal anterior urethras: retrograde urethrograms. **Upper left:** Urethral carcinoma. Gross irregularities with filling defects involving most of penile urethra. Poorly differentiated carcinoma of anterior urethra in a 59-year-old man with obstructive voiding symptoms and inguinal adenopathy. **Upper right:** Urethral carcinoma. Filling of irregular sinus tracts and channels in a large epidermoid carcinoma of the bulbocavernous urethra (straight arrow). There are multiple thin transverse strictures of the penile urethra (curved arrow). 75-year-old man with obstructive voiding symptoms and 30-year history of urethral strictures requiring dilatations. **Lower left:** Focal urethral stricture (arrow). Middle-aged man with obstructive voiding symptoms who denied any previous urethritis. **Lower right:** Urethral strictures. Multiple strictures in the bulbocavernous urethra (lower arrow) with reflux into Cowper's gland (middle arrow) and prostatic ducts (upper arrow). B, bladder; D, bladder diverticulum. 62-year-old man with 25-year history of urethral strictures requiring frequent dilatations.

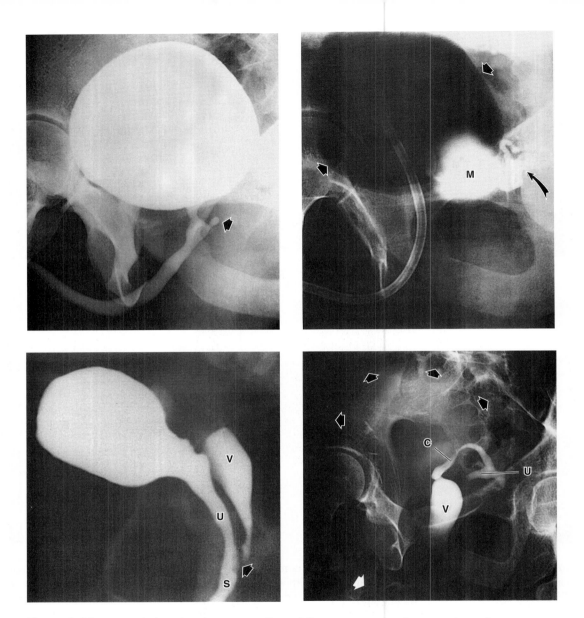

Figure 6–15. Congenital genitourinary anomalies: voiding cystograms and retrograde urethrograms. **Upper left:** Utricle. Midline outpouching (arrow) from verumontanum between orifices of ejaculatory ducts, representing müllerian duct cyst. **Upper right:** Gas cystogram combined with injection of utricle, oblique view. M, grossly dilated utricle (müllerian duct cyst); straight arrows, bladder distended with air; curved arrow, coincident partial filling of left seminal vesicle and vas deferens. 34-year-old man with urgency, frequency, and suspected retrograde ejaculation. **Lower left:** Common urogenital sinus. Vagina (V) and urethra (U) join (at arrow) into a common urogenital sinus (S). Voiding cystourethrogram in a 3-week-old female pseudohermaphrodite with ambiguous genitalia and congenital adrenal hyperplasia. **Lower right:** Male pseudohermaphrodite. Bladder is distended with urine (black arrows). Retrograde urethrogram via hypospadiac meatus has fortuitously and selectively filled with contrast medium an extensive müllerian duct remnant consisting of vagina (V), cervix and cervical canal (C), and retroverted uterus (U). Residual contrast medium in hypoplastic anterior urethra (white arrow). 27-year-old man with small external genitalia, hypospadias, and perineal pain.

Figure 6–16. Vasoseminal vesiculography (vasography). **Left:** Normal left vasoseminal vesiculogram. V, vas deferens; S, seminal vesicle; E, ejaculatory duct. 40-year-old man with hypospermia. **Right:** Seminal vesiculitis. Bilateral vasogram. Mass (M) produced by the swollen, nonfilling right seminal vesicle has displaced both ejaculatory ducts (E) toward the left and indented the medial aspect of the proximal left seminal vesicle and vas deferens (V). 33-year-old man with painful ejaculations after repair of right varicocele.

Aortorenal & Selective Renal Arteriography (Figure 6–18)

Arteriographic studies are performed almost exclusively by percutaneous needle puncture and catheterization of the common femoral arteries. Rapid-sequence images are obtained during catheter injection of nonionic contrast. Aortograms at the level of the renal vessels using multi-hole "flush" catheters demonstrate renal arteries, including anomalies. Selective catheterization of renal arteries follows.

Indications for renal arteriography include suspected renal artery stenosis (renovascular hypertension), vascular malformations, tumor embolization to minimize surgical blood loss or treat bleeding tumors, and trauma. Diagnostic renal angiography to demonstrate renal vascular anatomy is uncommon today, because this information may usually be obtained noninvasively. Complications from catheter angiography include bleeding at the puncture site, contrast allergy or nephrotoxicity, and renal or distal emboli.

Inferior Venacavography & Selective Venography (Figures 6–19 and 6–20)

The common femoral veins or, less commonly, the internal jugular vein is catheterized for catheter angiography of the inferior vena cava and renal and adrenal veins. Risks of bleeding and emboli present in arterial studies are virtually eliminated. Venography is rarely used today since the information can be obtained at cross-sectional imaging (CT or MRI) in almost all cases. Adrenal and renal venography is performed occasionally in the setting of venous sampling to localize hormone secretion in patients with indeterminate noninvasive imaging studies.

Miscellaneous Urologic Angiography (Figure 6–21)

Although angiography has little or no value in examination of the ureter, bladder, adrenals, and prostate, angiograms of these structures may be indicated in

Figure 6–17. Lymphangiography. **Left:** Metastatic testicular choriocarcinoma. Enlarged thoracolumbar lymph nodes partially replaced by metastatic tumor (arrows). 26-year-old man with enlarged left supraclavicular node after orchiectomy for choriocarcinoma. **Right:** Hodgkin's disease. Kidneys and ureters displaced by grossly involved abdominal and pelvic lymph nodes. 52-year-old woman with stage IV Hodgkin's disease.

particular clinical situations, in which case the studies are usually "tailored" to the clinical problem. In this era of multiple cross-sectional methods, these procedures are rarely used.

Corpus cavernosograms are made by direct injection of suitable contrast material into the corpora cavernosa of the penis. They can be useful in examining for Peyronie's disease, impotence, priapism, and traumatic penile lesions, but these also are not commonly performed.

SONOGRAPHY
(Figures 6–22 through 6–27)

Basic Principles

Sound is the mechanical propagation of pressure changes, or waves, through a deformable medium. A wave frequency of one cycle/second (cps) is called a hertz (Hz). Sound frequencies greater than 20 kHz are beyond the range of human hearing and are called **ul-**trasound. Medical sonography uses ultrasound to produce images. The frequencies commonly used in medical sonography are between 3.5 and 10 MHz.

Ultrasound waves for imaging are generated by transducers, devices that convert electrical energy to sound energy and vice versa. These transducers are special piezoelectric crystals that emit ultrasonic waves when they are deformed by an electrical voltage and, conversely, generate an electrical potential when struck by reflected sound waves. Thus, they act as both sonic transmitters and detectors. In general concept, medical sonography resembles naval submarine sonar. Ultrasound images are reflection images formed when part of the sound that was emitted by the transducer bounces back from tissue interfaces to the transducer. The sound reflected by stationary tissues forms the data set for anatomic gray-scale images. The sound reflected by moving structures (eg, flowing blood in a vessel) has an altered frequency due to the Doppler effect. By determining the Doppler shift, vascular flow direction and velocity can be encoded graphically (spectral Doppler) or by color (color Doppler). A more sensitive method

Figure 6–18. Angiography: aortorenal arteriography. **Upper left:** Normal abdominal aortogram. The aortic catheter is hidden by the opacified normal aorta. Right (R) and left renal arteries and branches are well shown, as are the splenic (S) and hepatic (H) arteries arising from the celiac axis. The superior mesenteric artery is superimposed over the aortic silhouette and is not visible on this study. 28-year-old healthy female potential kidney donor. **Upper right:** Multiple renal arteries. Horseshoe kidney with 3 renal arteries on each side, the 2 lowermost (3) supplying the renal isthmus. 42-year-old man with recurrent calculous disease, after left pyelolithotomy. **Lower left:** Bilateral renal artery stenoses. Typical angiographic appearance and location of stenoses caused by atherosclerosis (small arrows) and fibromuscular dysplasia (large arrows). 58-year-old woman with abdominal bruits and a 16-year history of hypertension. **Lower right:** Vascular parasitism by kidney cancer. Selective inferior mesenteric arteriogram (M) demonstrating large blood supply to a hypervascular adenocarcinoma (T) of the upper pole. Asterisks, renal pelvis. 69-year-old woman with polycythemia.

Figure 6–19. Angiography: inferior venacavography. **Upper left:** Normal inferior vena cava (C). Unusual retrograde filling of morphologically normal renal veins (arrows) from antegrade injection into the inferior vena cava is probably due to reduced venous outflow from the kidneys with the patient in Valsalva maneuver. B, retained contrast material in the cecum from previous barium enema examination. Woman with arteriolar nephrosclerosis and renal failure. **Upper right:** Inferior vena cava obstruction. Complete block of the vena cava (curved arrow) by extension from right renal vein of tumor thrombus from a right renal carcinoma. Note cephalad blood return via the paralumbar veins (straight arrows). 60-year-old man with gross hematuria. **Lower left:** Double inferior vena cava (R, L). Persistent left supracardinal vein anomaly. 23-year-old man after orchiectomy for testicular teratocarcinoma. **Lower right:** Retrocaval ureter. Hydronephrosis and proximal ureterectasis secondary to congenitally abnormal course of the right ureter behind the inferior vena cava (C). Catheter is in the right ureter, with its tip (arrow) at the lower curve of the redundant, dilated proximal ureter (asterisk). 17-year-old girl with history of pyelonephritis.

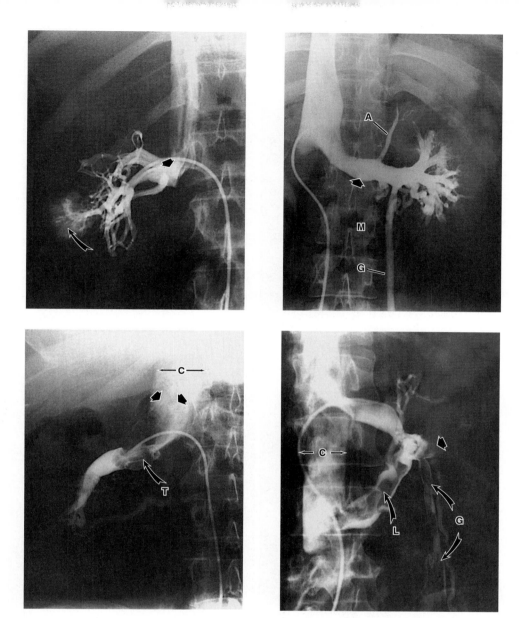

Figure 6–20. Angiography: renal venography. **Upper left:** Normal right renal vein. The right renal vein (straight arrow) is short and, unlike the left renal vein, does not receive the adrenal or gonadal vein; these veins empty directly into the inferior vena cava. Curved arrow, segmental intravasation of contrast medium from inadvertent wedging of the catheter tip in a small vein during injection. 19-year-old man with glomerulonephritis and nephrotic syndrome. **Upper right:** Normal left renal vein. On the left side, the adrenal (A) and gonadal (G) veins enter the renal vein (arrow). M, radiographic localization marker. Young woman with proteinuria. **Lower left:** Tumor thrombus. Straight arrows, upper margin of filling defect of the renal vein tumor thrombus (T) that extends into the vena cava (C). 68-year-old man with gross hematuria from adenocarcinoma of the right kidney. **Lower right:** Circumaortic left renal vein thrombosis. The catheter is in the patent upper limb of the venous anomaly. There is thrombosis of the intrarenal vein (straight arrow), with extension of thrombus into the lower limb (L) of the circumaortic renal vein and into the gonadal vein (G). C, inferior vena cava. 54-year-old man with nephrotic syndrome and edema of the legs and scrotum.

Figure 6–21. Angiography: miscellaneous urovenography. **Upper left:** Penoscrotal varices. Penile venography. Many tortuous veins in the penis (P) and scrotum (S). 14-year-old boy with long-standing penile and scrotal varicosities and numerous scrotal phleboliths. **Upper right:** Varicocele. Gonadal venography. Dilated, tortuous varicosities of the pampiniform plexus in the left scrotum. 31-year-old man with recurrence of scrotal pain after varicocele ligation. **Lower left:** Normal corpora cavernosogram. Injection of contrast medium into the left corpus (L), with normal (albeit slightly less) filling of the right corpus (R). 57-year-old man with impotence. **Lower right:** Penile fibrosis. Corpora cavernosogram. Injection of right corpus produces no filling of the proximal right corpus (arrow); there is normal filling of the left corpus (L). 33-year-old man with "crooked penis" following unsuccessful penile prosthesis operation.

Figure 6–22. Sonography of the kidney. **Upper:** Normal kidney. Renal cortex (C), normal renal sinus echoes (S). **Middle:** Moderate hydronephrosis and hydroureter; dilated renal pelvis (P). Dilated proximal ureter (prox ure). **Lower:** Severe hydronephrosis of the transplanted kidney, compound sagittal scans, dilated clubbed calices (C), dilated renal pelvis (P).

of detecting flow, called power mode Doppler, is available on modern equipment. This technique displays the integrated power of the Doppler signal rather than the mean Doppler frequency shift. Direction or velocity of flow is not displayed in the power mode.

Reflected sound received by the transducer is converted into electrical signals that are analyzed by computer algorithms and rapidly converted into video images viewed directly on a real-time display. Images are rapidly updated on the display, giving an integrated cross-sectional anatomic depiction of the site studied. Individual frames may be frozen during an examination for motion-free analysis and recording, or continuous images may be recorded as digital or conventional video.

Clinical Applications

Ultrasound is commonly used for the evaluation of the kidney, urinary bladder, prostate, testis, and penis.

Ultrasound is useful for assessing renal size and growth. It is also helpful in triage for patients with renal failure. For example, small echogenic kidneys suggest renal parenchymal (medical) disease, whereas a dilated pelvocaliceal system indicates an obstructive, and potentially reversible, cause of renal failure.

Renal ultrasound is useful in detection and characterization of renal masses. Ultrasound provides an effective method of distinguishing benign cortical cysts from potentially malignant solid renal lesions. Since the most common renal lesion is a simple cortical cyst, ultrasound is a cost-effective method to confirm this diagnosis. Ultrasound may also be used to follow up mildly complicated cysts detected on CT; for example, hyperdense cysts or cysts with thin septations.

The differential diagnosis for echogenic renal masses includes renal stones, angiomyolipomas, renal cell carcinomas, and, less commonly, abscesses and hematomas. All echogenic renal masses should be correlated with clinical history and, if necessary, confirmed with another imaging modality or follow-up ultrasound. Thin-section CT showing fat within the renal lesion characterizes it as a benign angiomyolipoma, and no further investigation is required. Echogenic lesions smaller than 1 cm are more difficult to characterize by CT owing to partial volume averaging; in the correct clinical setting, follow-up ultrasound rather than repeat CT scan may be more useful.

Doppler sonography is useful for the evaluation of renal vessels, vascularity of renal masses, and complications following renal transplant. It can detect renal vein thrombosis, renal artery stenosis, and ureteral obstruction prior to the development of hydronephrosis, arteriovenous fistulas, and pseudoaneurysms. Perinephric

Figure 6–23. Renal calculi and the consequence of obstruction as detected by sonography. Longitudinal (**upper left**) and transverse (**upper right**) scans of the right kidney showing calicectasis (C) and renal calculus (arrow). **Lower left:** Renal calculus (arrow) at the infundibulum causing dilatation of the upper pole calyx (C). **Lower right:** Acute obstruction of the right kidney (K) with spontaneous urine (U) extravasation into the perirenal space. Renal calculus (arrow).

fluid collections following renal transplantation, extracorporeal shock wave lithotripsy, or acute obstructions are reliably detected by ultrasound.

Developments in other imaging modalities have decreased the use of ultrasound in several clinical scenarios. Most patients with suspected renovascular hypertension are evaluated with CTA, MRA, or radionuclide renography rather than Doppler ultrasonography. Unenhanced helical CT is now the initial procedure of choice for the evaluation of the patient with acute flank pain and suspected urolithiasis. In addition to rapidly and sensitively detecting renal stones without the need for intravenous contrast medium, helical CT also has the potential for identifying other causes of flank pain, such as appendicitis and diverticulitis. In the past, a combination of KUB and ultrasound was advocated for the evaluation of hematuria, but recent studies indicate that IVU, CT (CTU), or both are the preferred modalities to evaluate this common clinical problem.

Applications of bladder sonography include assessment of bladder volume and bladder wall thickness and detection of bladder calculi and tumors. The suprapubic, transabdominal approach is most commonly used. The transurethral approach during cystoscopy has been recommended for tumor detection and staging.

Ultrasound examination of the testis has become an extension of the physical examination. The superficial location of the testis allows the use of a high-frequency transducer (5–10 MHz), which produces excellent spatial resolution. The addition of color Doppler sonography provides simultaneous display of morphology and blood flow. Normal intratesticular arterial blood flow is

Figure 6–24. Sonography of renal neoplasms. **Upper left:** Simple renal cyst (Cy) demonstrating sharp interfaces toward the renal parenchyma, no internal echoes, and increase through transmission. **Upper right:** Complex renal cyst (arrow) with lobulated margins and thick wall. **Lower left:** Solid tumor (T) in upper pole of left kidney with increased echogenicity relative to adjacent renal parenchyma. Pathology was oncocytoma. **Lower right:** Small renal tumor (T) in the right kidney (K) the echogenicity of which is similar to that of the remaining renal parenchyma. The diagnosis is established by localized bulge in the outline.

consistently detected with power or color Doppler. Sonography is highly accurate in differentiating intratesticular from extratesticular disease and in the detection of intratesticular pathology. Ultrasound is commonly used to evaluate acute conditions of the scrotum. It can distinguish between inflammatory processes, inguinal hernias, and acute testicular torsion. In addition, epididymitis not responding to antibiotics within 2 weeks should be investigated further with scrotal ultrasonography.

Advantages & Disadvantages

The main advantages of ultrasound are ease of use, high patient tolerance, noninvasiveness, lack of ioniz-ing radiation, low relative cost, and wide availability. Disadvantages include a relatively low signal-to-noise level, tissue nonspecificity, limited field of view, and dependence on the operator's skill and the patient's habitus.

COMPUTED TOMOGRAPHY SCANNING (Figures 6–28 through 6–34)

Basic Principles

In CT scanning, a thin, collimated beam of x-rays is passed through the patient and captured by an array of solid-state or gas detectors.

Figure 6–25. Sonography with comparative study. Film from IVP (**left**) and transabdominal ultrasound (**right**) of the urinary bladder in a patient with duplication of the left kidney, ectopic ureterocele, and a calculus (arrow) within it. Urinary bladder (B).

The interconnected x-ray source and detector system are rapidly rotated in the gantry around the recumbent patient. Computers integrate the collected x-ray transmission data to reconstruct a cross-sectional image (tomogram).

Spiral (or helical) CT uses a slip-ring gantry that rotates continuously while the patient moves constantly through the collimated x-ray beam. A helical exposure covering 30 cm of tissue can be obtained during a single 30-second breath-hold. Spiral CT technology affords the ability to image during specific phases of contrast bolus enhancement, including the ability to perform CT angiography, and allows improved image reformations. The latest major CT innovation is **multidetector (or multislice)** helical CT technology. The basis for it is an array of multiple rows of detectors in a helical scanner such that multiple scan images can be acquired per gantry rotation and, as a by-product, thinner sections and higher resolution achieved. Such systems are optimally paired with powerful computer workstations so that high-quality three-dimensional and multiplanar reformations can be quickly generated and analyzed.

Clinical Applications

Renal CT is most commonly used in the evaluation of acute flank pain, hematuria, renal infection (search for abscess), and renal trauma, and in the characterization and staging of renal neoplasm. CT evaluation of renal anatomy and pathology generally requires intravenous injection of iodinated contrast media; noncontrast scans are needed, however, when renal or perirenal calcification, hemorrhage, or urine extravasation is suspected, since scans obtained after the administration of contrast media may mask these abnormalities. Also, precontrast and postcontrast scans are required to determine whether a mass is solid or cystic.

Contrast media are usually administered as a rapid intravenous bolus for assessment of renal anatomy or measurement of aortorenal transit time. Using a bolus injection and rapid-sequence scanning, renal arterial opacification is followed immediately by enhancement of the cortex. A nephrogram phase with medullary enhancement is reached within 60 s. Excretion of contrast material into the collecting structures can be expected within 2–3 min after initiation of contrast administration.

Figure 6–26. The use of transrectal ultrasound in the evaluation of the prostatic urethra. **Upper left:** Sonographic appearance of the prostatic urethra (U) following transurethral resection as seen on transrectal ultrasound in the sagittal plane of scanning. Urinary bladder (B). The urethra (U) is dilated to the level of the verumontanum (arrow). Peripheral zone (P), rectum (R). **Upper right:** The prostatic urethra (U) is dilated to the level to the membranous urethra (arrow). Urinary bladder (B). The cursors are placed to measure the length of the prostatic urethra. **Lower left and lower right:** Examples of testicular cancer. **Lower left:** The right testis (T) is normal. There is a hypoechoic lesion within the left testis (asterisk). At surgery, it was a seminoma. **Lower right:** The lesion (asterisk) within the right testis is hypoechoic with a hyperechogenic focus (arrow). Embryonal carcinoma was present at surgery. Surrounding normal testicular tissue (T).

Figure 6–27. Gray-scale and Doppler sonography: acute rejection in a renal transplant. **Upper left:** Gray-scale ultrasound image of transplant kidney shows loss of corticomedullary differentiation. A small fluid collection is seen within the renal pelvis (arrow). Native external iliac vessels are seen as tubular hypoechoic structures (arrowheads). **Upper right and lower left:** Color Doppler images demonstrate flow within the native external iliac artery (arrowheads), the transplant renal artery (long arrow), and the interlobar arteries (short arrow). **Lower right:** Spectral Doppler analysis reveals an elevated resistive index of 0.84. These findings are compatible with but not specific for acute rejection.

Figure 6–28. CT scans: adrenal glands. **Upper left:** Normal adrenal glands (arrows) have inverted arrowhead or Y shape. 48-year-old woman with melanoma. **Upper right:** CT densitometry. Thin-section CT of incidental right adrenal mass (M) performed without intravenous contrast. Region of interest density measurement was below 10 Hounsfield units (near zero), compatible with adrenal adenoma, confirmed by pathologic findings. **Lower left:** Bilateral adrenal lymphoma. Enlarged adrenal glands (arrows) anterior to normal kidneys. L, liver. 53-year-old man with abdominal pain and histiocytic lymphoma of the central nervous system. **Lower right:** Left adrenal carcinoma. Large tumor (T) in left upper retroperitoneum with necrotic or cystic changes. Differential for CT included exophytic renal carcinoma. 52-year-old woman with pulmonary nodules (metastases).

Figure 6–29. CT scans: kidneys. **Left:** Simple renal cyst. Cyst (arrow) has a CT number close to that of water. 49-year-old man with flank pain. **Right:** New hydronephrosis, severe on left and mild on right. Dilated left renal pelvis and delayed left nephrogram (arrow). 40-year-old woman with ovarian carcinoma and peritoneal metastases.

Although CT can detect ureteral tumors, the role of CT in the evaluation of the ureters is mostly in tumor staging and diagnosis of the cause and level of obstruction. Helical CT without oral or intravenous contrast is the preferred imaging modality for patients with renal colic or suspected urolithiasis (Figure 6–33).

In the evaluation of the urinary bladder, CT is used primarily in staging bladder tumors and in diagnosing bladder rupture following trauma. Performing CT after filling the bladder with dilute contrast medium (CT cystography) improves the sensitivity of this modality for detecting tumors and bladder rupture. For prostate diseases, CT is used for detection of lymphadenopathy and to delineate prostatic abscesses. CT is used for detection of the abdominal location of suspected undescended testes, for staging of testicular tumors, and in the search for nodal or distant metastasis. CTA or MRA are replacing conventional angiography for diagnostic examinations.

Advantages & Disadvantages

The main advantages of CT include a wide field of view, the ability to detect subtle differences in the x-ray attenuation properties of various tissues, good spatial resolution, anatomic cross-sectional images, and operator independence. A considerable amount of diagnostic information available from CT scans depends on patterns of contrast enhancement, so a carefully tailored examination is essential. Reformatted helical image data in different planes and in 3-D has made renal CT imaging, with renal angiography and urography, valuable in preoperative planning, such as for partial nephrectomy. Limitations of CT include restriction to the transaxial plane for direct imaging, tissue nonspecificity, low soft-tissue contrast resolution, and the need for contrast media (both oral and intravenous). Even with careful use of contrast media, tissue contrast is sometimes unsatisfactory.

MAGNETIC RESONANCE IMAGING (Figures 6–35 through 6–42)

Basic Principles

Clinical MRI has its basis in the nuclear properties of the hydrogen atoms in the body. Hydrogen nuclei, when considered as aggregates, sometimes referred to as "protons," behave like tiny magnets, with net polarity (positive one direction, negative opposite) oriented along an axis at any given point in space. Ordinarily, the axes of the hydrogen nuclei in the body are randomly oriented. However, if the nuclei are placed in a strong magnetic field (like that produced in an MRI scanner), they precess (wobble like a spinning top) around the lines of magnetic force.

Figure 6–30. CT scans: kidneys. **Upper left:** Renal cell carcinoma. The left renal tumor (arrow) shows central necrosis. Note calcification in the arteriosclerotic abdominal aorta. 61-year-old man with previous right nephrectomy for renal carcinoma. **Upper right:** Recurrent renal adenocarcinoma. Massive recurrence in right renal fossa (T), with extensive invasion of posterior soft tissues and destruction of vertebral bodies (arrows). 51-year-old man after right nephrectomy for carcinoma. **Lower left:** Renal angiomyolipomas. Bilateral heterogeneous renal masses. The larger lesions all showed areas of macroscopic fat density (arrows). 35-year-old woman with probable lymphangioleiomyomatosis. **Lower right:** Right renal pelvic laceration. Enhanced CT scan through the kidneys shows extravasation of radiopaque material (arrow). Hemorrhage into the psoas and back muscles has enlarged their image (asterisk). 22-year-old man with laceration of the right renal pelvis due to a stab wound.

Figure 6–31. CT scans of kidneys. **Upper left:** 42-year-old woman with severe right pyelonephritis. An image through the upper pole of the right kidney shows low-density fluid collections between residual strands of enhancing renal parenchyma. Low-density inflammatory lymph nodes (arrows) displace the inferior vena cava anteriorly. **Upper right:** An image through the mid pole of the right kidney in the same patient reveals an enlarged kidney with marked destruction and striation of the renal parenchyma. Note the multiple low-density fluid collections. **Lower left:** Exophytic renal cell carcinoma. An image through the mid pole of the right kidney shows an apparent extrinsic mass (white arrowheads) displacing the kidney laterally. The renal artery (long arrows) and renal vein (short arrows) are draped over the mass anteriorly. The renal vein is free of thrombus. **Lower right:** A lower image in the same patient reveals that the mass arises from the kidney. The renal parenchyma (short arrows) and contrast-containing collecting system (long arrows) are splayed by the mass.

When hydrogen nuclei in a strong magnetic field are additionally stimulated by short, pulsed radio waves of appropriate frequency, they absorb energy and invert their orientation with respect to the magnetic field. At the termination of radiofrequency pulses, the hydrogen nuclei return at various rates to their original orientation within the magnetic field, emitting energy in the form of radio waves. This phenomenon is called **nu-clear magnetic resonance.** The emitted weak radio signals from the resonating hydrogen nuclei are received by sophisticated antenna, or coils, and transformed with various computer programs into cross-sectional images.

Different MR signal intensities reflect different hydrogen densities in body tissues, as well as differing physical, cellular, and chemical microenvironments and

Figure 6–32. 3-D CT and CTA for renal mass, performed on multidetector CT scanner. Coronal oblique reformatted image with volume rendering shows a small enhancing mass (m) in the lower pole of the left kidney. The kidney has two renal arteries (arrows). The lower one, which serves the tumor, is the primary artery. 69-year-old man with solitary kidney and indeterminate lesion on prior CT.

also flow (fluid) characteristics. The signals emitted from nuclei under MR investigation contain no innate spatial information. Spatial localization is achieved through varying the magnetic field in space (gradients), because emitted frequencies are proportional to magnetic field. Timing of precession (phase) is also controlled and varied to provide spatial localization of emitted signals.

Some biologically important nuclei other than hydrogen are MR-sensitive, including phosphorus, sodium, and potassium, but these occur in lower physiologic concentrations than hydrogen. Imaging of these nuclei for tissue typing and mapping and as biologic tracers (MR spectroscopy) is undergoing intense research and development.

Clinical Applications

MRI has been applied in imaging the kidney, retroperitoneum, urinary bladder, prostate, testis, and penis. Applications for MR in renal imaging include demonstration of congenital anomalies, diagnosis of renal vein thrombosis, and staging of renal cell carcinoma. MR angiography, which does not require intravenous contrast media, is useful in evaluating renal transplant vessels, renal vein tumor or thrombosis, and renal artery stenosis.

The use of contrast media in MRI of the kidney has broadened clinical applications. Using bolus injection of gadolinium and rapid-sequence imaging, both

Figure 6–33. Helical CT without oral or intravenous contrast in a 42-year-old man with left flank pain. **Left:** CT image through the kidneys shows enlargement of the left kidney compared with the right, left pelvicalicectasis (P), and a stone in the mid pole of the left kidney (arrow). L, liver; S, spleen. **Right:** CT image through the base of the bladder shows an 8-mm stone (arrow) at the left ureterovesical junction with associated edema involving the left hemitrigone. Posterior to the ureteral stone is a 5-mm phlebolith (open arrow) within a pelvic vein.

Figure 6–34. CT scans: retroperitoneum, bladder, prostate. **Upper left:** Perirenal hematoma. Hematoma (arrow) displaces the left kidney anteriorly. G, gallbladder. 16-year-old boy with acute glomerulonephritis; low-grade fever and left flank pain following left renal biopsy. **Upper right:** Retroperitoneal metastatic seminoma. Huge retroperitoneal mass of metastatic nodes (T) destroying vertebral body (arrow), obliterating outlines of central abdominal and retroperitoneal structures, and displacing kidneys laterally and bowel anteriorly. 46-year-old man with metastatic anaplastic testicular seminoma. **Lower left:** CT scan, transitional cell carcinoma of the urinary bladder with tumor (T) extension into the bladder diverticulum. There is tumor extension into the perivesical fat (arrows). **Lower right:** CT scan, transitional cell carcinoma of the urinary bladder with bilateral ureteral obstruction. Tumor (T), dilated ureters (U).

Figure 6–35. MRI appearance of the normal kidney. **Upper left:** T1-weighted conventional spin-echo image showing detailed anatomy of the kidney with differentiation between higher signal intensity cortex (C) and lower signal intensity medulla (M). Left renal vein (arrow), inferior vena cava (I). **Upper right:** T1-weighted spin-echo image using fat saturation technique. Because the fat signal has been suppressed, the computer automatically adjusts the gray scale of the signal intensity, rendering even better contrast between higher signal intensity cortex (C) and lower signal intensity medulla (M). Inferior vena cava (I). **Lower left and lower right:** Images of the normal kidney using GRASS (gradient recall acquisition steady state) technique. Gradient echo technique images are obtained while the patient is holding his breath. **Lower left:** Noncontrast scan. **Lower right:** Scan obtained following gadolinium-DTPA injection of the contrast medium. The scan was obtained during the nephrogram phase showing uniform enhancement of both kidneys (K). There has been enhancement of the liver (L) and spleen (S).

Figure 6–36. MR images. **Upper left and upper right:** Horseshoe kidney. Nonenhanced T1-weighted image (**upper left**); m, medulla; c, renal cortex. Gadolinium-DTPA–enhanced T1-weighted image (**upper right**). Following injection of the contrast medium, there is uniform enhancement of the renal cortex (C). The addition of the contrast enhancement shows that the part of the kidney in front of the aorta (A) and the inferior vena cava (I) is functioning renal parenchyma. **Lower left and lower right:** Chemical shift imaging, adrenal adenoma. On in-phase gradient T1-weighted image (**lower left**) there is a soft-tissue intensity 2.7-cm mass in the left adrenal gland (arrow). Opposed phase T1-weighted image (**lower right**) shows marked signal loss in the lesion consistent with intracellular lipid; and therefore, a benign adenoma. 30-year-old woman with indeterminate adrenal lesion noted on prior CT.

Figure 6–37. MRI appearance of renal cell carcinoma. The advantages of MRI are multiplanar imaging and the use of contrast media for better tumor characterization. **Upper left:** Sagittal T1-weighted image shows a large renal cell carcinoma (T) arising from the inferior pole of the right kidney (K). Tumor extension in the posterior perirenal space (arrow). Liver (L). **Upper right:** Coronal image of a large renal cell carcinoma (T) replacing almost the entire parenchyma of the left kidney (K). Superior displacement of the pancreas (arrows). Liver (L). **Lower left and lower right:** Fat saturation images before and after injection of the contrast medium. Heterogeneous tumor (T) (**lower right**) in the posterior part of the right kidney shows heterogeneous enhancement following injection of gadolinium. The tumor is extending into the renal vein (arrows) and to the inferior vena cava (I). Kidney (K).

Figure 6–38. Precontrast and postcontrast CT and MRI of a renal cell carcinoma adjacent to a cyst. **Upper left:** Precontrast CT image through the left kidney reveals a prominent posterior bulge (long arrow), which proved to be a cyst, and a subtle posterolateral convex contour deformity, which contains tiny calcifications (short arrow). **Upper right:** Postcontrast CT image reveals a nonenhancing cyst posteriorly (long arrow). The posterolateral contour deformity is caused by an enhancing renal cell carcinoma (short arrow) with a central low-density fluid collection. **Lower left:** Precontrast T1-weighted image shows similar intensities for the cyst, tumor, and normal renal parenchyma. **Lower right:** Postcontrast T1-weighted image. The cyst (long arrow) is nonenhancing. The margins of the enhancing renal cell carcinoma (short arrows) are seen. The central fluid collection does not enhance.

Figure 6–39. Gadolinium-enhanced renal MRA. A, aorta; I, inferior vena cava. A, aorta; I, inferior vena cava. **Left:** Maximum intensity projection (MIP) image from a renal MRA in a 22-year-old potential renal donor. The renal arteries are normal. **Right:** MIP image from a renal MRA in a 56-year-old man with suspected renovascular hypertension shows an atrophic left kidney with an occluded left renal artery (arrow) and a severely stenotic right renal artery (arrow). The collateral capsular renal vessels are not seen.

anatomy and function of the kidney can be assessed. Gadolinium, similar to iodine contrast media, is an extracellular contrast agent primarily excreted by glomerular filtration. Unlike iodine contrast media, however, gadolinium has good renal tolerance in patients with preexisting renal failure.

Iodinated contrast agents used in radiography and CT increase attenuation linearly with their concentration. The effect of gadolinium on MR tissue signal intensity is more complex, though in general at lower concentrations gadolinium causes an increase in signal intensity.

The use of gadolinium has extended the application of MRI to the evaluation of renal obstruction (magnetic resonance intravenous urography may be used when other studies are inconclusive) and the detection and characterization of renal tumors. Although MRI is capable of imaging blood vessels without contrast media, gadolinium bolus followed by rapid imaging can also be used for this purpose. This gadolinium-enhanced MRA is useful for assessing renal artery stenosis and for evaluating potential renal donors (Figure 6–39).

MRI is used primarily to stage bladder tumors and to differentiate between benign bladder wall hypertrophy and infiltrating malignant neoplasm. In imaging the prostate gland, MRI is principally used to stage patients with prostate cancer. MR spectroscopy increases specificity and reduces interobserver variability in this setting. MRI of the testis is appropriate when other imaging studies are inconclusive and is applicable to the evaluation of undescended testis, trauma, epididymoorchitis, and tumors.

A modification of the MRI technique, called **chemical shift** imaging, can detect microscopic amounts of fat within lesions (Figure 6–36, lower images). This technique is commonly used to characterize adrenal masses. Adrenal masses containing fat are either adrenal adenomas or myelolipomas, so the CT or MRI demonstration of fat in an adrenal lesion characterizes it as a benign lesion, even in the patient with cancer.

MR urography utilizes the sensitivity of MR imaging to demonstrate fluid (urine), producing urogram-like pictures without the need for contrast media. This technique is sensitive in the detection of ureterohydronephrosis and is particularly useful in patients in whom contrast material is contraindicated, such as patients with prior contrast reactions or renal failure.

Advantages & Disadvantages

Advantages of MRI include direct imaging in any plane desired (though transverse, sagittal, and coronal are most standard), choice of large or small field of view, excellent soft-tissue contrast, imaging without exposure to ionizing radiation, and (as compared to ultrasonography) less operator dependence. MRI can image blood vessels and the urinary tract without contrast material. MR scanning, however, is not without drawbacks. The scanning time is relatively slow, and as a result image clarity is often inferior compared with that of CT. Absolute contraindications to MRI include the presence of (1) intracranial aneurysm clips, unless the referring physician is certain that the clip is made of a nonferromagnetic material (such as titanium); (2) intra-orbital

Figure 6–40. MRI examination of the pelvis. The upper images are examples of the ability of MRI to demonstrate a bladder tumor (T) and show its extent (arrows). **Upper left:** T1-weighted. **Upper right:** T2-weighted transaxial image. The large tumor (T) at the bladder base shows perivesical extension. Also seen is a dilated right ureter (arrow). **Lower left and lower right:** Prostate cancer. Axial T2-weighted image (**lower left**) shows dominant tumor at the right prostatic base (low signal area compared to higher signal in center and left side), with extracapsular extension into the right neurovascular bundle (arrow). Coronal T2-weighted image (**lower right**) in the same patient shows the tumor in right base and mid-gland also with bilateral seminal vesicle invasion (arrows). MRI is consistent with stage T3b (American Joint Committee on Cancer). 60-year-old man with prostate cancer diagnosed on biopsy from the right base.

Figure 6–41. MRI of seminal vesicles, ductus deferens, and ejaculatory ducts. **Upper left:** T2-weighted image, normal seminal vesicles, ductus deferens, and ejaculatory ducts. The ampullae of the ductus deferens (long arrows) are normally of high signal intensity on T2-weighted images and are immediately medial to the seminal vesicles (short arrows). The seminal vesicles are also of high signal intensity and are draped over the prostate gland. **Upper right:** Seminal vesicle and ductus deferens calculi. Coronal T2-weighted images show low-signal calculi within the proximal ductus deferens and medial aspect of the seminal vesicle on the left side (arrows). The patient had a history of prostatitis, prostatic pain, and hemorrhagic ejaculate. **Lower left:** Axial T2-weighted image through the prostate. The peripheral zone is of normal high signal intensity. The normal ejaculatory ducts (arrows) are identified as two small foci of high signal intensity within the lower-signal central zone. **Lower right:** Axial T2-weighted image through the prostate reveals a low-signal-intensity calculus (arrow) within the right ejaculatory duct (same patient as in upper right image).

metal fragments; and (3) any electrically, magnetically, or mechanically activated implants (including cardiac pacemakers, biostimulators, neurostimulators, cochlear implants, and hearing aids). Relative contraindications such as pregnancy should always be viewed in the light of risk versus benefit of the examination.

COMPARISON OF IMAGING METHODS (Figures 6–43 through 6–46)

As new imaging methods have been developed, changes have occurred in patterns of use for each type of imaging. For example, increased familiarity with and

Figure 6–42. MRI appearance of scrotal contents. **Upper left:** Normal testis, T2-weighted image. The testicular tissue is of homogeneous high signal intensity. The tunica albuginea (arrows) demonstrates low signal intensity, as does the mediastinum testis (open arrowhead). A small amount of fluid—hydrocele (H). Epididymis (E) is of low signal intensity. **Upper right:** Hydrocele of the right scrotum (T2-weighted image). Hydrocele (H) demonstrates high signal intensity. Testis (T). Tunica albuginea (curved black arrows). Varicocele (asterisk). **Lower left and lower right:** Images of a testicular tumor. On the proton density image (**lower left**), the signal intensity from both testicles is similar. On the T2-weighted image (**lower right**), testicular tumor (asterisk) demonstrates lower signal intensity as compared with the higher signal intensity of the normal testicular tissue (T).

Figure 6–43. Comparison of imaging methods in the evaluation of renal cell carcinoma. **Upper left:** CT scan showing a renal cyst (Cy) in the right kidney. There is bulging (arrow) in the contour of the left kidney (K), but it is difficult to discern if the lesion represents a neoplasm. **Upper right:** Angiogram showing small vascular lesions in the inferior pole of the left kidney (arrows). **Lower left and lower right:** MRI scans. **Lower left:** T1-weighted non-contrast scan. **Lower right:** T1-weighted postcontrast scan. The renal cyst (Cy) in the right kidney does not show any enhancement. The lesion (arrow) in the left kidney (K) shows marked enhancement, indicating that it is solid in nature. In this example, the contrast-enhanced MRI is superior to CT in the detection and characterization of the left renal mass.

Figure 6–44. Comparison of imaging methods: metastatic extra-adrenal familial pheochromocytoma. 10-year-old boy with hypertension and seizures precipitated by abdominal palpation. Family history of multiple extra-adrenal pheochromocytomas in the mother. **Upper left:** Excretory urogram. The right ureter is dilated and elevated (curved arrow), with the right posterior portion of the bladder displaced toward the left (straight arrow). The urographic diagnosis is possible extra-adrenal paravesical pheochromocytoma. **Upper right:** Right femoral arteriogram. Tumor stain (arrow) in right paravesical location. The angiographic diagnosis is extra-adrenal paravesical pheochromocytoma. **Lower left:** CT scan. Transverse tomogram through bladder (B) shows the tumor (T) indenting the bladder (arrows). R, rectum. **Lower right:** CT scan. Transverse tomogram through bladder. Recurrence of symptoms following removal of the right paravesical pheochromocytoma prompted another CT study, which shows recurrent tumor (arrow) in the bladder wall. Each imaging study complemented or supplemented the previous one. None, however, diagnosed the small liver metastases discovered at surgery.

Figure 6–45. Comparison of imaging methods. **Upper left** is an example of a nonenhanced CT scan, and **upper right** is an ultrasound study in the demonstration of renal calcifications. Fine calcifications in the medullary region indicate medullary nephrocalcinosis. They are of high density on CT (arrows) and are shown as echogenic foci (arrows) on an ultrasound scan. **Lower left and lower right:** Example of images of a transitional cell carcinoma and the calcified renal cyst. Retrograde urogram (**lower left**) shows filling defects due to tumor in the renal pelvis (black arrow) at ureteropelvic junction, and also seen are the calcifications in a lower pole mass (white arrows). Note that the infundibulum and calices of the lower pole failed to opacify in this 45-year-old woman with hematuria. On the CT scan (**lower right**), the cystic nature of the calcified renal mass (curved arrow) is well demonstrated, and the CT scan shows better the extent of the tumor (T), which involves the entire lower pole of the kidney and extends into the dilated renal pelvis.

Figure 6–46. Comparison of imaging methods. **Upper left and upper right:** Psoas abscess. Excretory urogram (**upper left**) reveals abnormal orientation of the right kidney and an enlarged psoas muscle. On the CT scan (**upper right**) in the same patient, the psoas abscess (arrow) is well seen. The CT scan is exceptionally helpful for imaging retroperitoneal structures. The abscess was drained percutaneously under CT control. **Lower left and lower right:** Demonstration of an arterial venous malformation to the seminal vesicles. On the CT scan (**lower left**), the right seminal vesicle (SV) is enlarged, but the nature of the enlargement (arrow) is difficult to discern. On an MRI scan (**lower right**), the enlarged vessels (arrows) are demonstrated as the flowing blood within the vessel lacks signal intensity in contrast to the medium signal intensity of the seminal vesicles (SV). Urinary bladder (B).

confidence in sonography and CT scanning have resulted in a decrease in the use of some long-established conventional uroradiologic studies such as excretory urography.

Several factors are involved in these changes: (1) the increased effectiveness of newer imaging methods over older ones for some aspects of urodiagnosis; (2) the availability of equipment, trained technical personnel to operate it, and physicians to interpret the results; (3) increased awareness of the hazards of ionizing radiation; and (4) the desire to use noninvasive examinations if possible.

Because so many different types of imaging are available, each with different costs, risks, and areas of effectiveness, it may be difficult for the clinician to decide which method will yield the most information with the least cost and risk. A particular study may be critical in one diagnostic situation but useless in another. For example, sonography is an excellent noninvasive, relatively inexpensive method for differentiating simple cysts from other mass lesions in the kidney but is much less effective in imaging the adrenal glands and ureters than is CT scanning. Sonography also relies considerably on the skill of the operator. CT scanning produces excellent images and is currently the preferred imaging method for the examination of the retroperitoneum. MRI rivals CT scanning in imaging capability for some structures; for example, the kidney, but has surpassed CT in imaging the pelvis. With advances in equipment and techniques, the use of MRI in urology will likely grow.

The patient and the clinician both benefit from careful consultation with the radiologist to ensure that the methods of imaging chosen are of value in diagnosis and treatment planning and do not duplicate or merely confirm established findings, with loss of time and additional expense.

REFERENCES

Contrast Agents

Albrecht T, Dawson P: Gadolinium-DTPA as x-ray contrast medium in clinical studies. Br J Radiol 2000;73(872):878.

Caro JJ, Trindade E, McGregor M: The risks of death and of severe nonfatal reactions with high- vs low-osmolality contrast media: A meta-analysis. AJR 1991;156(4):825.

Cohan RH, Ellis JH: Iodinated contrast material in uroradiology: Choice of agent and management of complications. Urol Clin North Am 1997;24(3):471.

Freed KS et al: Breakthrough adverse reactions to low-osmolar contrast media after steroid premedication. AJR 2001;176(6):1389.

Stacul F: Current iodinated contrast media. Eur Radiol 2001;11(4):690.

Townsend RR et al: Safety of intravenous gadolinium (Gd-BOPTA) infusion in patients with renal insufficiency. Am J Kidney Dis 2000;36(6):1207.

Violon D: Renal failure and iodinated contrast media: A review. JBR-BTR 1999;82(2):57.

Weese DL, Greenberg HM, Zimmern PE: Contrast media reactions during voiding cystourethrography or retrograde pyelography. Urology 1993;41(1)81.

Radiography

Amis ES Jr: Epitaph for the urogram. Radiology 1999;213(3):639.

Chan DY et al: Image-guided therapy in urology. J Endourol 2001;15(1):105.

Chen MY et al: Abnormal calcification on plain radiographs of the abdomen. Crit Rev Diagn Imaging 1999;40(2–3):63.

Dalla Palma L: What is left of i.v. urography? Eur Radiol 2001;11(6):931.

Dyer RB, Chen MY, Zagoria RJ: Intravenous urography: Technique and interpretation. Radiographics 2001;21(4):799; discussion, 822.

Gallagher HJ, Tolley DA: 2000 AD: Still a role for the intravenous urogram in stone management? Curr Opin Urol 2000;10(6)551.

Hession P et al: Intravenous urography in urinary tract surveillance in carcinoma of the bladder. Clin Radiol 1999;54(7):465.

Little MA et al: The diagnostic yield of intravenous urography. Nephrol Dial Transplant 2000;15(2):200.

McFarlane JP et al: Outpatient ureteric procedures: A new method for retrograde ureteropyelography and ureteric stent placement. BJU Int 2001;87(3):172.

Miller DC, Forauer A, Faerber GJ: Successful angioembolization of renal artery pseudoaneurysms after blunt abdominal trauma. Urology 2002;59(3):444.

Morey AF et al: Bladder rupture after blunt trauma: Guidelines for diagnostic imaging. J Trauma 2001;51(4):683.

Shurrab AE et al: Increasing the diagnostic yield of renal angiography for the diagnosis of atheromatous renovascular disease. Br J Radiol 2001;74(879):213.

Spinosa DJ et al: Interventional uroradiologic procedures performed using gadodiamide as an alternative to iodinated contrast material. Cardiovasc Intervent Radiol 2000;23(1):72.

Ultrasound

Agrawal A et al: Clinical and sonographic findings in carcinoma of the penis. J Clin Ultrasound 2000;28(8):399.

Bateman GA, Cuganesan R: Renal vein Doppler sonography of obstructive uropathy. AJR 2002;178(4):921.

Baxter GM: Ultrasound of renal transplantation. Clin Radiol 2001;56(10):802.

Caoili EM et al: Evaluation of sonographically guided percutaneous core biopsy of renal masses. AJR 2002;179(2):373.

Chow L et al: Power Doppler imaging and resistance index measurement in the evaluation of acute renal transplant rejection. J Clin Ultrasound 2001;29(9):483.

Datta SN et al: Urinary tract ultrasonography in the evaluation of haematuria—A report of over 1,000 cases. Ann R Coll Surg Engl 2002;84(3):203.

Dohle GR, Schroder FH: Ultrasonographic assessment of the scrotum. Lancet 2000;11(356):1625.

Frauscher F et al: Comparison of contrast enhanced color Doppler targeted biopsy with conventional systematic biopsy: Impact on prostate cancer detection. J Urol 2002;167(4):1648.

Frauscher F et al: Laparoscopic pyeloplasty for UPJ obstruction with crossing vessels: Contrast-enhanced color Doppler findings and long-term outcome. Urology 2002;59(4):500.

Lapeyre M et al: Color-flow Doppler sonography of pseudoaneurysms in patients with bleeding renal angiomyolipoma. AJR 2002;179(1):145.

Leventis AK et al: Characteristics of normal prostate vascular anatomy as displayed by power Doppler. Prostate 2001;1 (46):281.

Morey AF, McAninch JW: Sonographic staging of anterior urethral strictures. J Urol 2000;163(4):1070.

Pavlica P, Barozzi L: Imaging of the acute scrotum. Eur Radiol 2001;11(2):220.

Ragheb D, Higgins JL Jr: Ultrasonography of the scrotum: Technique, anatomy, and pathologic entities. J Ultrasound Med 2002;21(2):171.

Varsamidis K, Varsamidou E, Mavropoulos G: Doppler ultrasonography in testicular tumors presenting with acute scrotal pain. Acta Radiol 2001;42(2):230.

Computed Tomography

Abramson S et al: Impact in the emergency department of unenhanced CT on diagnostic confidence and therapeutic efficacy in patients with suspected renal colic: A prospective survey. AJR 2000;175(6):1689.

Boridy IC et al: Acute ureterolithiasis: Nonenhanced helical CT findings of perinephric edema for prediction of degree of ureteral obstruction. Radiology 1999a;213(3):663.

Boridy IC et al: Ureterolithiasis: Value of the tail sign in differentiating phleboliths from ureteral calculi at nonenhanced helical CT. Radiology 1999b;211(3):619.

Caoili EM: Imaging of the urinary tract using multidetector computed tomography urography. Semin Urol Oncol 2002;20 (3):174.

Caoili EM et al: Urinary tract abnormalities: Initial experience with multidetector row CT urography. Radiology 2002;222 (2):353.

Chow LC, Sommer FG: Multidetector CT urography with abdominal compression and three-dimensional reconstruction. AJR 2001;177(4):849.

Curry NS, Cochran ST, Bissada NK: Cystic renal masses: Accurate Bosniak classification requires adequate renal CT. AJR 2000; 175(2):339.

Homer JA, Davies-Payne DL, Peddinti BS: Randomized prospective comparison of non-contrast enhanced helical computed tomography and intravenous urography in the diagnosis of acute ureteric colic. Australas Radiol 2001;45(3):285.

Kawashima A et al: Imaging evaluation of posttraumatic renal injuries. Abdom Imaging 2002;27(2):199.

Leder RA, Nelson RC: Three-dimensional CT of the genitourinary tract. J Endourol 2001;15(1):37.

Macari M, Bosniak MA: Delayed CT to evaluate renal masses incidentally discovered at contrast-enhanced CT: Demonstration of vascularity with enhancement. Radiology 1999;213 (3):674.

Pao DM et al: Utility of routine trauma CT in the detection of bladder rupture. Acad Radiol 2000;7(5):317.

Shokeir AA et al: Noncontrast computed tomography in obstructive anuria: A prospective study. Urology 2002;59(6):861.

Vaccaro JP, Brody JM: CT cystography in the evaluation of major bladder trauma. Radiographics 2000;20(5):1373.

Comparison of Imaging

Andrews SJ et al: Ultrasonography and abdominal radiography versus intravenous urography in investigation of urinary tract infection in men: Prospective incident cohort study. BMJ 2002;23(324):454.

Bernhardt TM, Rapp-Bernhardt U: Virtual cystoscopy of the bladder based on CT and MRI data. Abdom Imaging 2001;26 (3):325.

Bigongiari LR et al: Trauma to the bladder and urethra. Radiology 2000;215(Suppl):733.

Bluth EI et al: Obstructive voiding symptoms secondary to prostate disease. Radiology 2000;215(Suppl):693.

Brehmer M: Imaging for microscopic haematuria. Curr Opin Urol 2002;12(2):155.

Dalla Palma L, Pozzi-Mucelli R, Stacul F: Present-day imaging of patients with renal colic. Eur Radiol 2001;11(1):4.

Heidenreich A, Desgrandschamps F, Terrier F: Modern approach of diagnosis and management of acute flank pain: Review of all imaging modalities. Eur Urol 2002;41(4):351.

Heneghan JP et al: Compression CT urography: A comparison with IVU in the opacification of the collecting system and ureters. J Comput Assist Tomogr 2001;25(3):343.

Hilton S: Imaging of renal cell carcinoma. Semin Oncol 2000; 27(2):150.

Jaffe JS et al: A new diagnostic algorithm for the evaluation of microscopic hematuria. Urology 2001;57(5):889.

Jung P et al: Magnetic resonance urography enhanced by gadolinium and diuretics: A comparison with conventional urography in diagnosing the cause of ureteric obstruction. BJU Int 2000;86(9):960.

Kawashima A et al: Imaging of renal trauma: A comprehensive review. Radiographics 2001;21(3):557.

Keogan MT: Radiology of urinary diversions. Curr Opin Urol 2000;10(2):117.

Livingston L, Larsen CR: Seminal vesicle cyst with ipsilateral renal agenesis. AJR 2000;175(1):177.

Mayo-Smith WW et al: State-of-the-art adrenal imaging. Radiographics 2001;21(4):995.

Narepalem N et al: Comparison of helical computerized tomography and plain radiography for estimating urinary stone size. J Urol 2002;167(3):1235.

Sandler CM et al: Imaging in acute pyelonephritis. Radiology 2000;215(Suppl):677.

Shokeir AA, Abdulmaaboud M: Prospective comparison of nonenhanced helical computerized tomography and Doppler ultrasonography for the diagnosis of renal colic. J Urol 2001;165(4):1082.

Sourtzis S et al: Radiologic investigation of renal colic: Unenhanced helical CT compared with excretory urography. AJR 1999;172(6):1491.

Sudah M et al: Patients with acute flank pain: Comparison of MR urography with enhanced helical CT. Radiology 2002;223(1):98.

Teigen EL, Newhouse JH: Imaging renal masses. Curr Opin Urol 2000;10(5):421.

Wefer AE et al: Advances in uroradiological imaging. BJU Int 2002;89(5):477.

MRI

Blandino A et al: MR pyelography in 115 patients with a dilated renal collecting system. Acta Radiol 2001;42(5):532.

Coakley FV et al: Prostate cancer tumor volume: Measurement with endorectal MR and MR spectroscopic imaging. Radiology 2002;223(1):91.

Katzberg RW et al: Functional, dynamic, and anatomic MR urography: Feasibility and preliminary findings. Acad Radiol 2001;8(11):1083.

Koutcher JA, Zakian K, Hricak H: Magnetic resonance spectroscopic studies of the prostate. Mol Urol 2000;4(3):143; discussion, 153.

Kurhanewicz J et al: The prostate: MR imaging and spectroscopy; Present and future. Radiol Clin North Am 2000;38(1):115.

Muglia V et al: Magnetic resonance imaging of scrotal diseases: When it makes the difference. Urology 2002;59(3):419.

Neimatallah MA et al: Magnetic resonance imaging in renal transplantation. J Magn Reson Imaging 1999;10(3):357.

Nolte-Ernsting CC, Adam GB, Gunther RW: MR urography: Examination techniques and clinical applications. Euro Radiol 2001;11(3):355.

Pretorius ES et al: MR imaging of the penis. Radiographics 2001;21:S283; discussion, S298.

Ryu J, Kim B: MR imaging of the male and female urethra. Radiographics 2001;21(5):1169.

Scheidler J et al: Prostate cancer: Localization with three-dimensional proton MR spectroscopic imaging—clinicopathologic study. Radiology 1999;213(2):473.

Soulie M et al: Assessment of the risk of positive surgical margins with pelvic phased-array magnetic resonance imaging in patients with clinically localized prostate cancer: A prospective study. Urology 2001;58(2):228.

Sudah M et al: MR urography in evaluation of acute flank pain: T2-weighted sequences and gadolinium-enhanced three-dimensional FLASH compared with urography. AJR 2001;176(1):105.

Yu KK et al: Prostate cancer: Prediction of extracapsular extension with endorectal MR imaging and three dimensional proton MR spectroscopic imaging. Radiology 1999;213(2):481.

Vosshenrich R, Fisher U: Contrast-enhanced MR angiography of abdominal vessels: Is there still a role for angiography? Eur Radiol 2002;12(1):218.

Vascular Interventional Radiology* | 7

Allan I. Bloom, MD, & Roy L. Gordon, MD

Interventional uroradiologic procedures can be divided into 2 major groups: vascular and percutaneous nonvascular. Percutaneous nonvascular interventional procedures are discussed elsewhere. The intravascular route is used, as the therapy of choice, for the embolization of arteriovenous fistulas (AVFs) or malformations, and for bleeding sites. Transcatheter embolization is used for tumor embolization, for the ablation of renal function, for the treatment of testicular vein and ovarian vein varices, and for the treatment of high-flow priapism. Balloon angioplasty and stenting of stenotic renal arteries are frequently performed endovascular techniques for the treatment of ischemic nephropathy and secondary hypertension. Renal artery aneurysms may also be treated using these catheter-directed techniques. Occasionally, fibrinolytic agents are delivered via an endovascular catheter to occluded renal arteries. This chapter will review these intravascular interventions.

TRANSCATHETER EMBOLIZATION

Renal Arteriovenous Fistulas & Malformations

Transcatheter embolization is the treatment of choice for renal arteriovenous fistulas, which may be congenital, spontaneous, or acquired. Iatrogenic AVFs are the type most commonly treated by transcatheter embolization. These occur as a complication of such procedures as percutaneous renal biopsy, nephrostomy placement, and pyelolithotomy (Lovaria et al, 1999). Trauma or surgery can also result in AVFs. AVF occurring in the transplant kidney is successfully managed by embolization. The classical angiographic finding of spontaneous or acquired AVF is a feeding artery with an early draining vein. Ancillary findings include pseudoaneurysm and extravasation of contrast material. Congenital AVFs (AV malformations) consist of a group of multiple coiled communicating vessels that may be associated with enlarged feeding arteries and draining veins.

The modes of clinical presentation include hematuria; retroperitoneal or intraperitoneal hemorrhage;

and congestive heart failure, cardiomegaly, or both. Hypertension can occur as a consequence of ischemia secondary to venous shunting of blood away from the affected area. A bruit may be heard on physical examination. Duplex Doppler ultrasound is the most useful diagnostic study, performed before angiographic intervention.

Successful intervention requires the angiographic identification, selective catheterization, and embolization of the feeding artery (Figure 7–1A, B). Using a transfemoral approach, an abdominal aortogram is performed to identify the arterial supply to the bleeding kidney. In the case of a renal transplant, an initial pelvic angiogram is performed in a steep oblique projection. The artery supplying the bleeding site is selectively catheterized. A 3F coaxial microcatheter is then used for subselective catheterization and embolization of the feeding artery. The use of a microcatheter allows accurate placement of the embolic material. Microcoils are used for the occlusion of iatrogenic AVFs because they can be deployed very precisely, thereby minimizing the loss of renal parenchyma due to resultant ischemia (Figure 7–2A–C.)

The procedure is usually performed without significant complications. Very rarely, inadvertent nontarget embolization or thrombosis of the renal artery can occur.

Bleeding Sites

Transcatheter embolization plays a key role in the management of hemorrhage in the urinary tract originating in the kidney, ureter, bladder, and pelvis (Velmahos et al, 2000). Acute life-threatening hemorrhage can occur as a consequence of trauma, instrumentation, and tumors. Chronic intractable hemorrhage is associated with radiation cystitis, tumors, prostatectomy, and infiltrative disorders. Hemodynamically stable patients undergo a noninvasive diagnostic study such as contrast-enhanced computed tomography (CT), before embolization.

Pelvic fractures resulting in life-threatening hemorrhage require embolization for control if resuscitation and external pelvic fixation have been ineffective. Embolization has been shown to be very effective at arresting hemorrhage. Using a transfemoral approach, the practitioner performs a nonselective pelvic arteriogram before selective catheterization and embolization of the hypogastric arteries. Because of contralateral crossover

*The authors wish to thank Dr Anthony Verstandig, Hadassah University Hospital, Jerusalem, Israel, for providing the clinical information and images of the patient depicted in Figures 7–4A and 7–4B.

A   **B**

Figure 7–1. Transcatheter embolization of a large arteriovenous malformation (AVM) in a 64-year-old woman with hematuria. **A:** A conventional film midstream aortogram. An enlarged left renal artery is seen. There is a large serpiginous AVM arising from the lower pole renal artery branch with aneurysmal dilatation of the draining renal vein. **B:** Selective left renal digital subtraction arteriogram (DSA) after coil embolization shows cessation of flow in the AVM. Coils have been placed in the terminal portion of the lower pole artery and within the AVM. Embolization resulted in resolution of the hematuria.

blood supply, pelvic lesions are treated by bilateral embolization. Gelfoam pledgets are frequently used. They can be deployed rapidly, are immediately effective if the patient has a normal coagulation profile, and produce temporary vascular occlusion. Gelfoam sponge is easily cut into pieces appropriate to the caliber of the vessel to be embolized. Coils may be used with, or instead of, Gelfoam. However, if used, they may hamper future access to the hypogastric artery in the event of rebleeding. Small embolic materials such as Gelfoam powder or Ivalon particles are not used to treat hemorrhage from pelvic trauma. They produce very peripheral occlusion of small vessels, thereby risking ischemia of nontarget organs.

Complications specific to pelvic embolization are extremely uncommon. Nontarget embolization is rare.

Tumors

A. RENAL CELL CARCINOMA

Primary renal cell carcinoma (RCC) is treated by surgical excision. In some cases preoperative occlusive em-

bolization of the renal artery is used as an adjunct to surgery. Embolization reduces intraoperative hemorrhage and allows immediate ligation of the renal vein. It is used in patients with very large tumors and also in tumors supplied by many parasitized vessels. Embolization accentuates cleavage planes and therefore facilitates nephrectomy. The optimal time delay between embolization and surgery is probably 1 day. Embolization may also favorably impact patient survival (Zielinski, Szmigielski, and Petrovich, 2000).

Palliation of nonresectable disease that causes pain and hematuria can be achieved by transcatheter embolization. Patients with bilateral RCC, and those with RCC in a single kidney, can undergo subselective embolization as an alternative to surgery, thereby sparing normal parenchyma. Embolization of RCC metastases to bone is performed before surgical resection to decrease intraoperative blood loss (Chatziioannou et al, 2000). CT or magnetic resonance imaging may be used for tumor evaluation before and after intervention.

A transfemoral aortogram and selective arteriogram are performed to determine the blood supply to the

A   B   C

Figure 7–2. Transcatheter embolization of a postbiopsy arteriovenous fistula (AVF) in a 14-year-old boy with hypertension and prior renal transplantation. A bruit was heard on examination. **A:** Pelvic arteriogram (DSA) shows an AVF arising from a lower pole branch artery. There is aneurysmal dilatation of the draining vein. **B:** DSA shows that the renal artery has been selectively catheterized, and a 3F coaxial catheter is positioned peripherally within the lower pole branch artery supplying the AVF. Several microcoils have been placed (arrow) and no flow is seen in the AVF. **C:** Completion DSA of the main renal artery shows absent flow in the AVF (arrow) with minimal devascularization of lower pole parenchyma (curved arrow).

kidney and tumor. An occlusive balloon catheter may be placed within the vessel and inflated before embolization to prevent reflux of embolic material and inadvertent nontarget embolization. However, many physicians use a simple selective catheter. Gelfoam pledgets are used for preoperative embolization (Figure 7–3A, B). Coils are not used because they can be dislodged during surgery when the kidney is manipulated. Absolute ethanol is the preferred embolic material for ablative palliative embolization of nonresectable tumor. Bone metastases are embolized by positioning a microcatheter in the vessel(s) supplying the tumor and injecting polyvinyl alcohol until maximal obliteration of the angiographic tumor stain is achieved.

Tumor embolization is a safe procedure. Complications such as puncture-site hematoma and inadvertent nontarget embolization occur in less than 2% of patients. Almost all patients, however, experience postembolization syndrome (PES). PES consists of severe pain, nausea and vomiting, fever, and leukocytosis. It is probably caused by tissue necrosis that results from successful embolization. Transient ileus, transient hypertension, sepsis, and reversible renal failure have also been described. PES occurs within a few hours of the procedure and may last for several days. Its occurrence should not delay surgical intervention. Tissue swelling and tissue gas formation are seen on imaging studies.

The severity of PES is related to the quantity of infarcted tissue. Analgesics and antibiotics are used for treatment. Administration of steroids and antibiotics before embolization may reduce the severity of PES.

B. ANGIOMYOLIPOMA

Selective embolization has proved to be an effective method of controlling hemorrhage from benign renal lesions while preserving normal parenchyma. This technique has been used in the treatment of active bleeding from angiomyolipoma (Khaitan et al, 2001) and for the elective prevention of hemorrhage, especially if the tumors are multiple or bilateral, as in patients with tuberous sclerosis. The procedure is effective in decreasing tumor size and in preventing or treating hemorrhage in 85–90% of patients. CT can clearly identify the fat component of the tumor and is therefore used for diagnosis before intervention and for follow-up.

The technique for embolization is similar to that described for RCC. Through a transfemoral approach, angiography is used to define the arterial supply to the kidney and tumor. The feeding vessels are then selectively catheterized using a coaxial microcatheter. The tumor volume is estimated, and an equal amount of absolute ethanol admixed with iodized oil is carefully injected until the flow ceases. Ethanol is easy to handle, is inexpensive, and produces permanent occlusion of the

A B

Figure 7–3. Preoperative embolization of a large right renal cell carcinoma (RCC) in a 28-year-old woman. **A:** Digital subtraction arteriogram (DSA) of the right renal artery shows a large hypervascular mass involving most of the right kidney. There is tumor thrombus within the renal vein. **B:** Completion DSA of the right renal artery after Gelfoam embolization shows complete cessation of flow within the tumor and kidney. Contrast is seen within the main renal artery only.

vascular bed. Iodized oil is radiopaque and therefore is useful for visualizing the flow of the embolic material during the embolization. It remains within the tumor, thereby allowing measurement of tumor response on follow-up CT. An occlusion balloon is reserved for more proximal embolization in a main renal artery when the risk of nontarget embolization is greatest.

The reported complications are similar to those seen after RCC embolization. Recurrence of tumor hemorrhage occurs in approximately 10–15% of patients and is treated by repeat embolization. A short-term tapered dose of prednisone may reduce PES after the procedure (Bissler et al, 2002).

Ablation of Renal Function

Total renal infarction using transcatheter embolization may be indicated in certain circumstances: namely, abolition of urine production to assist in healing or palliation of terminal patients with urinary fistulas; prevention of excessive proteinuria; management of uncontrollable hypertension; and rarely for benign obstructive uropathy in patients who are poor surgical candidates (De Baere et al, 2000; Toussi, McConnell, and

Srinivasan, 2001). For patients with end-stage renal disease and intractable hypertension or nephrotic syndrome, the advantages of ablation must be weighed against the loss of production of vitamin D_3 and erythropoietic factors and, occasionally, the loss of the ability to eliminate some water. Total renal ablation must be achieved so that perfusion of surviving parenchyma via pericapsular branches cannot occur. The embolic agent must perfuse the entire renal substance but be safe if it passes through the kidney into the venous circulation. The technique is applicable in adults and children and in both native and allograft kidneys. Renal ablation appears to be a safe procedure, which is successful in most patients (De Baere et al, 2000).

Initially, a midstream aortogram is performed to identify the arterial supply to the kidneys. This is followed by renal artery catheterization and selective arteriography. An occlusion balloon catheter is placed in the vessel and contrast medium is injected to measure the volume of embolic agent needed to fill the vascular tree of the kidney. Absolute ethanol is the embolic agent of choice for the reasons mentioned above. An equal volume is carefully injected with the balloon inflated to prevent reflux to nontarget regions. The contents are then aspirated and an angiogram is performed to assess flow. The procedure is repeated as many times as necessary until complete cessation of blood flow is achieved.

PES of several days' duration occurs in all patients and is managed with antibiotics and analgesics. Inadvertent embolization of the adrenal artery and other visceral vessels is a rare but serious complication that can be avoided by using the occlusion balloon technique. Systemic toxicity from ethanol injection is not a clinical problem. Morbidity and mortality from the procedure is less than from surgical nephrectomy.

Embolization of Primary Varicocele

The subject of varicocele and male infertility is discussed in detail in Chapter 42. The basis for intervention is the presence of a varicocele on physical examination; most varicoceles are left-sided. Color Doppler sonography is usually performed routinely before intervention. Several reports have suggested a positive association between improvement of seminal parameters and pregnancy. Surgery and percutaneous transvenous embolization appear to be equally effective. However, advantages of the percutaneous route include greater patient comfort, ease of bilateral treatment, and reduced recovery time.

The procedure is performed with conscious intravenous sedation and local anesthesia. The transjugular venous approach is preferred by many physicians, although the procedure can be performed transfemorally. Direct ultrasound guidance is used to access the jugular vein; a catheter is then guided fluoroscopically into the left gonadal vein. The left gonadal vein usually drains into the left renal vein, whereas the right gonadal vein usually drains directly into the inferior vena cava. The patient is placed in reverse Trendelenburg position and left gonadal venography is performed. A positive venogram result demonstrates incompetence with filling of collateral vessels. Embolization is achieved by placing coils within the gonadal vein, commencing at the region of the inguinal ligament and continuing cranially toward the renal vein, until the gonadal vein and collateral vessels have been occluded. If a right-sided varicocele is also present, the right gonadal vein is then interrogated and embolized.

The recurrence rate of varicocele after embolization is approximately 4%. Minor complications include contrast extravasation from perforation of the vein, nontarget embolization, venospasm, and hematoma. Rarely, cardiac arrhythmia and contrast allergy can occur.

Embolization of Ovarian Vein Varices (Pelvic Congestion Syndrome)

Pelvic congestion syndrome is a recognized cause of chronic pelvic pain in women that has been associated with lumbo-ovarian vein varices. Dyspareunia, when present, may be a poor prognostic indicator. Symptoms are often worse with fatigue, before menstruation, and in the upright position. Occasionally, vulval and thigh varicosities are present on examination. The cause is probably multifactorial. The diagnosis of varicosed pelvic veins is confirmed by duplex Doppler ultrasound that is also used for postintervention follow-up. CT venography or magnetic resonance venography are alternative noninvasive diagnostic tests.

Transvenous embolization has produced durable relief of symptoms in most patients (> 70%). Most responses occur within 2 weeks of treatment; however, continued improvement has been reported up to 12 months after the procedure (Venbrux et al, 2002). Using either a transfemoral or a transjugular approach, the ovarian veins are individually catheterized, and embolic agents such as coils or synthetic glue are deployed in the vessel at the level of the pelvic inlet (Figure 7–4A, B). Occasionally, embolization of internal iliac vein tributaries may be necessary.

Reported complications are similar to those for varicocele embolization. The procedure does not appear to have a deleterious effect on fertility or the menstrual cycle.

Treatment of High-Flow Priapism

High-flow priapism is a fairly rare condition resulting from increased arterial flow into the lacunar spaces of the cavernous tissue. The "arteriocavernous fistula" most often results from penile or perineal trauma. In some cases the cause is unknown. Color Doppler sonography demonstrates the abnormality.

Transcatheter embolization is a minimally invasive, successful treatment for this condition (Ciampalini et al, 2002). A nonselective transfemoral pelvic angiogram is performed to demonstrate the fistula, which originates from the pudendal artery. This procedure is followed by superselective catheterization of the injured artery using a microcatheter. The fistula is then closed by accurately deploying microcoils (Figure 7–5A, B). This technique preserves blood flow to the penis, thereby allowing normal erectile function in most cases. The use of microcoils prevents possible ischemic injury to the perineum.

In the event of recurrence after embolization, repeat embolization is successful in nearly all patients. Surgery should be reserved for patients in whom embolization fails.

RENAL ARTERY ANGIOPLASTY & STENTING

Ischemic nephropathy due to atherosclerotic vascular disease and renal artery stenosis is a leading cause of progressive renal failure. Renal artery stenosis is the

A   B

Figure 7–4. Embolization of ovarian vein varices in a 30-year-old multiparous woman with pelvic congestion syndrome. She complained of increasing pelvic pain and dyspareunia. On examination there were prominent vulval varicosities. **A:** Transjugular right ovarian venography demonstrates multiple large ovarian vein varices. **B:** Radiograph taken after coil embolization of both ovarian veins and tributaries of the internal iliac veins. The varices have been occluded. The patient's symptoms resolved after the procedure.

most common cause of secondary hypertension. Surgical revascularization is an established method of treatment, with reported success rates of > 70%. In recent years, percutaneous transluminal angioplasty (PTA) and stent placement have become a viable alternative to surgery (Leertouwer et al, 2000). Percutaneous transluminal angioplasty is the treatment of choice in the management of fibromuscular dysplasia occurring in a subset of hypertensive patients. The technique involves the use of an inflatable balloon catheter that is positioned endoluminally across the stenosis and then inflated (angioplasty).

Several diagnostic imaging modalities are used for patient selection and for post-procedure follow-up, including captopril radioisotope assay, duplex Doppler ultrasound, CT angiography, magnetic resonance angiography, and arteriography. The advantages and disadvantages of these techniques are beyond the scope of this chapter.

Renal artery stenosis is described as ostial, nonostial, or branch vessel stenosis. An ostial lesion is located within 3 mm of the aortic lumen and is typical of atherosclerotic vascular disease. In fibromuscular dysplasia, nonostial and branch vessel lesions are more typically seen. The initial technical success rate of PTA varies. It may be as low as 35% for some atherosclerotic vascular disease ostial lesions, but in most series the overall rate approximates 95–100%. PTA results in stabilization or improvement of renal function in most patients with ischemic nephropathy and also leads to durable improvement or cure in most of those with hypertension. The best results after PTA have been achieved in hypertensive patients with fibromuscular dysplasia, in whom improvement or cure is achieved in approximately 90%.

Stent placement has traditionally been reserved for immediate failure or complication of PTA, such as elastic recoil or flow limiting intimal dissection, for residual stenoses of > 30%, for a > 20 mm Hg peak systolic

A

B

Figure 7–5. A 17-year-old male had normal erectile function before a skateboard straddle injury. He had a painless partial erection for 13 months and was unable to achieve full erection for intercourse. **A:** A right internal iliac arteriogram shows a cavernosal arteriosinusoidal fistula arising from the internal pudendal artery (arrow). **B:** Repeat angiography after selective microcoil embolization for the fistula shows occlusion of the fistula (arrow). After the procedure there was complete detumescence, with return of normal sexual function over the next 3 months.

pressure gradient after PTA, for early restenosis, and for ostial lesions that are difficult to treat by PTA alone. Renal artery stenting results in stabilization (38% of patients) or improvement (30% of patients) of renal function and in durable improvement (49%) or cure (20%) of hypertension (Leertouwer et al, 2000). PTA and stenting have also been used successfully to treat renal allograft artery stenosis. Primary patency rates vary after stenting. The average restenosis rate is approximately 17% after 6–12 months' follow-up. However, the rate increased to 20–30% with longer follow-up. Secondary patency may be achieved in > 90% of patients.

Usually, the transfemoral approach is used, although a transaxillary approach may be required. Initially, a midstream aortogram is performed to identify the renal arteries, followed by a selective injection to evaluate the morphology and location of the stenosis, the diameter of the vessel, and the percentage of stenosis. In the presence of altered renal function with elevated creatinine levels, alternatives to iodinated contrast agents include gadolinium and carbon dioxide gas. Indicators of a significant stenosis include a reduction of cross-sectional diameter of at least 50%, post-stenotic dilatation, collateral vessels to the affected kidney, and a transtenotic systolic pressure gradient of > 20 mm Hg across the lesion. Before intervention, an oral antiplatelet agent such as clopidogrel is administered. The patient is heparinized and a vasodilating agent (eg, nitroglycerine) is given via the arterial catheter. Initially, the lesion is

crossed with a guidewire. If a high-grade stenosis is present, predilatation with a small balloon may be necessary before definitive angioplasty or stent placement. An outer guiding catheter or sheath is used to facilitate contrast injection during the procedure and to improve catheter stability. Continuous fluoroscopic guidance and "vascular road-mapping" are also used to ensure precision. Frequently, a small tear in the vessel intima is seen after PTA. We prefer to use a balloon expandable stent because it can be very accurately deployed. The minimal recommended vessel diameter for stenting is 6 mm. A 10- to 20-mm-long stent is used, and approximately 1–2 mm should protrude into the aortic lumen when ostial lesions are treated (Figure 7–6A, B).

Success of the procedure is defined by < 30% residual stenosis and by the resolution of a significant transtenotic pressure gradient. We frequently use a percutaneous closure device to achieve hemostasis. Antiplatelet medication is continued for 6 weeks after the procedure, and the patient is carefully followed up by clinical evaluation and repeat imaging.

The reported complication rate after PTA and stenting varies considerably but ranges from 3% to 10% in experienced operators. Complications include puncture-site hematoma; femoral artery pseudoaneurysm; contrast nephropathy; cholesterol embolization; stent malpositioning; and injury to the renal artery such as dissection, thrombosis, and rupture. Rarely, procedure-related deaths have occurred.

A   B

Figure 7–6. Renal artery stenting in an 80-year-old woman with labile hypertension and right renal artery stenosis due to atherosclerotic vascular disease. Her hypertension was poorly controlled on 3 antihypertensive medications. **A:** A midstream aortogram at the level of the renal arteries demonstrates a high-grade ostial right renal artery stenosis. **B:** Repeat midstream aortogram after placement of a 20-mm-long Palmaz stent, dilated to 6 mm. A widely patent renal artery is seen. The stent protrudes slightly into the aortic lumen. The patient's hypertension improved after the procedure.

OTHER ENDOVASCULAR PROCEDURES

Renal Artery Aneurysms

Renal artery aneurysms are rare and are usually not symptomatic. They carry the risk of rupture, with associated life-threatening hemorrhage. Occasionally, they are associated with renovascular hypertension. Distal embolization may occur, leading to parenchymal infarction. The indications for treatment of renal artery aneurysms include diameter greater than 2.5 cm, interval enlargement, renovascular hypertension, pain, hematuria, intrarenal thromboemboli, and lesions in women of childbearing age. The diagnosis is made by color Doppler sonography, CT, or magnetic resonance imaging.

In the high-risk surgical patient, endovascular techniques may be well-suited to aneurysm repair, by excluding the aneurysm while preserving flow to the kidney. Depending on the location of the aneurysm, its relationship to branch vessels, and the presence or absence of a "neck," either a stent graft or transcatheter embolization are possible treatment options (Rundback et al, 2000; Karkos et al, 2000). A stent graft is a metallic stent that is covered by surgical graft material. Its deployment across the aneurysm results in internal reconstruction of the vessel, with exclusion of blood flow to the aneurysm due to the impervious graft material. The cavity of the aneurysm may then thrombose.

Selective embolization of an aneurysm that is supplied by a branch vessel is performed by occluding blood flow proximally using coils. This approach results in distal parenchymal infarction and therefore can only be safely performed if there is sufficient renal functional reserve. If there is an identifiable neck separating the aneurysm from the native vessel, coils may be used to pack the aneurysm cavity, thereby resulting in thrombosis of the aneurysm while at the same time preserving distal flow.

The risks of the procedure are similar to those reported above. Long-term results of endovascular repair are not yet available.

CATHETER-DIRECTED FIBRINOLYSIS

This procedure has been used extensively in the peripheral vasculature but with only limited success in the management of native renal artery or aortorenal bypass graft thrombosis (Rouviere et al, 2002). Small series or individual case reports have suggested a possible role in the treatment of recent renal artery occlusion before PTA and for the treatment of acute renal artery thromboembolic disease.

The diagnosis is made by noninvasive imaging such as duplex Doppler ultrasound, magnetic resonance imaging, or CT angiography and is then confirmed by angiography, at which time fibrinolytic therapy is begun. A diagnostic arteriogram is performed from a transfemoral approach, after which an infusion catheter or wire is embedded within the thrombosed segment. Tissue plasminogen activator (t-PA) is currently the most frequently used fibrinolytic agent in the United

States. Several infusion protocols exist. Our preferred technique is continuous infusion of 1–2 mg t-PA per hour. Prophylactic antibiotics are administered. The patient is monitored for puncture-site and systemic bleeding in the intensive care or step-down unit throughout the infusion therapy. A repeat arteriogram is performed 12–24 h after the initiation of therapy. When recanalization has been achieved, an underlying stenotic lesion is usually identified, at which time PTA or stenting is performed.

Complications include puncture-site and systemic hemorrhage and infection. Bleeding may be severe enough to require transfusion or to discontinue the infusion. The incidence of complications is related to the duration of therapy and to the dose administered.

REFERENCES

Bissler JJ et al: Reduction of postembolization syndrome after ablation or renal angiomyolipoma. Am J Kidney Dis 2002;39 (5):966.

Chatziioannou AN et al: Preoperative embolization of bone metastases from renal cell carcinoma. Eur Radiol 2000;10(4):593.

Ciampalini S et al: High-flow priapism: Treatment and long term follow-up. Urology 2002;59(1):110.

De Baere T et al: Transcatheter ethanol ablation in 20 patients with persistent urine leaks: An alternative to surgical nephrectomy. J Urol 2000;164(4):1148.

Karkos CD et al: Renal artery aneurysm: Endovascular treatment by coil embolization with preservation of renal blood flow. Eur J Vasc Endovasc Surg 2000;19(2):214.

Khaitan A et al: Management of renal angiomyolipoma in complex clinical situations. Urol Int 2001;67(1):28.

Leertouwer TC et al: Stent placement for renal artery stenosis: Where do we stand? A meta-analysis. Radiology 2000;216 (1):78.

Lovaria A et al: Interventional radiology in the treatment of urological vascular complications. Ann Urol (Paris) 1999;33(3):156.

Rouviere O et al: Acute thrombosis of renal transplant artery: Graft salvage by means of intra-arterial fibrinolysis. Transplantation 2002;73(3):403.

Rundback JH et al: Percutaneous stent-graft management of renal artery aneurysms. JVIR 2000;11:1189.

Toussi H, McConnell C, Srinivasan V: Renal artery embolization for benign obstructive uropathy. J Urol 2001;165(4):1162.

Velmahos GC et al: Angiographic embolization of bilateral internal iliac arteries to control life-threatening hemorrhage after blunt trauma to the pelvis. Am Surg 2000;66(9):858.

Venbrux A et al: Pelvic congestion syndrome (pelvic venous incompetence): Impact of ovarian vein and internal iliac vein embolotherapy on menstrual cycle and chronic pelvic pain. JVIR 2002;13:171.

Zielinski H, Szmigielski S, Petrovich Z: Comparison of preoperative embolization followed by radical nephrectomy with radical nephrectomy alone for renal cell carcinoma. Am J Clin Oncol 2000;23(1):6.

Percutaneous Endourology & Ureterorenoscopy

8

Joachim W. Thüroff, MD, & Christian P. Gilfrich, MD

In contrast to retrograde instrumentation such as ureterorenoscopy, which invades the urinary tract via the natural route of the urethra under endoscopic guidance, techniques of antegrade instrumentation involve access via a percutaneous puncture. This approach must respect the intrarenal anatomy just as in open surgical nephrotomy, and imaging techniques are essential to guide the procedure.

First, and most important, a puncture route must be established that will provide straightforward access to the target and safe, bloodless instrumentation. Visualization of the puncture needle and target and precise guidance to the target require the use of imaging techniques such as ultrasound, fluoroscopy, and, in selected cases, computed tomography (CT).

Contraindications to percutaneous kidney puncture are blood clotting anomalies due to coagulopathies or pharmacologic anticoagulation. Preparation and draping of the surgical field are required as for open surgery, and the same standards of asepsis must be followed. Local anesthesia only is sufficient for puncture of the kidney and small-bore tract dilation (6–12F) for antegrade insertion of a ureteral stent or nephrostomy catheter. Lidocaine hydrochloride 1% USP, 10 mL, can be given for infiltration of the skin and tissues along the intended route of puncture down to the renal capsule. During dilation of the tract, administration of a local anesthetic in lubricant (eg, lidocaine hydrochloride jelly 2%) serves the dual purpose of anesthetization and lubrication. Dilation of nephrostomy tracts up to 30F and extraction of small renal stones can be done under local anesthesia.

Percutaneous nephrolithotomy (PNL) is still indicated for treatment of staghorn calculi and stones in caliceal diverticula, but the extent of intrarenal instrumentation for stone disintegration and extraction usually requires epidural or general anesthesia. Because puncture, tract dilation, and stone disintegration and removal are preferably performed as a one-stage procedure, the use of local anesthesia in PNL is limited.

IMAGING & PUNCTURE TECHNIQUES

Percutaneous puncture of the renal collecting system may be performed for diagnostic procedures (eg, antegrade pyelography, pressure/perfusion studies) or to establish access for therapeutic interventions (Table 8–1).

Both ultrasonic scanning and fluoroscopy provide visualization and guidance for a safe, accurate percutaneous puncture, but ultrasound has definite advantages:

(1) No intravenous or retrograde administration of contrast dye.
(2) No radiation exposure.
(3) Continuous real-time control of puncture.
(4) Imaging of radiolucent, non-contrast-enhancing renal and extrarenal structures (eg, renal cyst, retroperitoneal tumor) for puncture.
(5) Imaging of all tissues along an intended nephrostomy tract (eg, bowel, lung).
(6) Imaging in numerous planes simply by shifting, tilting, and rotating the scanning head.
(7) Three-dimensional information during puncture.

Once the puncture needle has entered the renal collecting system, fluoroscopy is required for control and guidance of subsequent steps (eg, guidewire insertion, tract dilation, catheter insertion). In selected cases, insertion and placement of a nephrostomy catheter in a dilated renal system may be possible with ultrasonic control only. Fluoroscopy provides a 2-dimensional image with complete integration of all information from the third (anterior-posterior) dimension, so that the entire length of radiopaque catheter, wires, and so on can be visualized.

For percutaneous puncture of the renal collecting system, the patient should be placed on the fluoroscopy table in the prone position. Radiolucent bolsters may be placed under the abdomen to correct for lumbar lordosis and to support the kidney. A standard puncture

Table 8–1. Indications for percutaneous puncture of the renal collecting system.

Diagnostic indications
  Antegrade pyelography
  Pressure/perfusion study (Whitaker test)
Therapeutic indications
  Nephrostomy catheter drainage
  Antegrade ureteral stenting
  Dilation of ureteral strictures
  Percutaneous endopyeloplasty
  Perfusion chemolysis of renal stones
  Percutaneous nephrolithotomy (PNL)
  Percutaneous resection and coagulation of urothelial
    tumors

Figure 8–1. Renal ultrasound. **A:** The longitudinal axis of the kidney forms a 30-degree angle with the midline. **B:** The transverse axis of the kidney forms a 45-degree angle with both a horizontal and a vertical line.

site is in the posterior axillary line midway between the 12th rib and the ileal crest; this site ensures that later the patient does not lie on the nephrostomy catheter in the supine position. Ultrasonic scanning is performed below the 12th rib to obtain a median longitudinal scan through the kidney. For optimal coupling of the ultrasonic beam to the skin, sterile gel (eg, K-Y jelly) is applied to the skin at the scanning site. In the frontal view of an intravenous pyelogram, the long axis of the kidney usually follows the psoas muscle, forming about a 30-degree angle with the midline (Figure 8–1A). In the transverse view of a CT scan, the transverse axis of the kidney forms about a 45-degree angle with both a horizontal and a sagittal line (Figure 8–1B). The position and direction of the transducer should be oriented roughly to the following marks: below the 12th rib (if possible), cranial to the puncture site, with a 30-degree caudal-lateral rotation, and with a 45-degree lateral tilt of the scanning head.

Factors that may influence the choice of scanning technique and puncture site include patient size; position and rotation of the kidney; anomalies of bony structures; positions of the colon, spleen, liver, and lung relative to the kidney; and the target of puncture (upper, middle, or lower calyx; caliceal diverticulum). The scanning head can be positioned to provide the best visualization and optimum puncture site for each patient. Thus, a puncture site as high as above the 11th rib may be chosen if the lung is not visualized in the puncture route. A different puncture site must be chosen if bowel gas or the liver or spleen is visualized within the intended nephrostomy route.

The route of puncture should always aim through a pyramid into a dorsal calyx; puncture into an infundibulum may result in bleeding from segmental and interlobar vessels in the renal sinus, and direct puncture of the renal pelvis renders dilation of the nephrostomy tract and insertion of catheters and instruments diffi-

cult, with increased risk of accidental catheter dislodgment after successful entry. For large, complete staghorn calculi, when PNL is to be performed for debulking the stone volume (followed by ESWL for disintegrating retained caliceal stones), puncture is usually performed through a lower dorsal calyx, a position from which the lower caliceal group, the renal pelvis, and part of the upper caliceal group can be reached easily with rigid instruments. However, for staghorn stones that can be completely removed by PNL alone (without ESWL), another route (eg, middle or upper calyx puncture) may be chosen. Stones in caliceal diverticula are better approached by direct puncture of the diverticulum.

Once chosen, the target for access to the renal collecting system must be visualized ultrasonically. The cutaneous puncture site should be chosen in a virtual caudal extension of the perpendicular orientation (width) of the scanning plane. Skin and fascia are incised with a No. 11 blade. At this time, the scanning head may be shifted over the incision to measure the exact distance between the incision and the target. A 16- to 18-gauge puncture needle (Figure 8–2) may then

Figure 8–2. Universal nephrostomy set (Bard-Angiomed), containing (1) coaxial 17.5-gauge needle/6F catheter system with obturator; (2) fine needle (22 gauge); (3) 0.035-in stiff guidewire with floppy J-tip; (4) coaxial 10F dilator/12F introducer catheter system; and (5) 10F pigtail nephrostomy catheter.

be inserted blindly through the incision and aimed in the direction previously determined by ultrasound. However, the needle should never be advanced blindly farther than through the abdominal fascia.

The scanning head is now placed in such a way that both the target and the puncture needle are visualized in the same scanning plane, and the needle is aligned so that its tip can be clearly seen. Vibrating the needle makes the tip more visible while the position of the scanning head is being adjusted. The needle can be

safely moved back and forth down to the renal capsule as often as necessary, but the renal parenchyma ideally should be punctured only once.

A needle guide can be used to direct the needle exactly within the ultrasonic scanning plane. With some needle guides, the angle of puncture relative to the longitudinal axis of the scanning plane (depth) is also fixed and may be indicated on the monitor by an electronically generated beam. If a steeper or flatter angle of puncture is desired, the entire scanning head and attached needle guide must be tilted, and the choice of puncture site is therefore limited. Another drawback of this device is that it does not allow for independent adjustment of the puncture and scanning direction if the needle deviates from its intended direction after being advanced through the skin. This frequently occurs in patients with scars from previous operations and becomes more of a problem the farther the target is from the cutaneous puncture site. Freehand puncture with individual adjustment of puncture and scanning direction is preferable in these cases.

Movement of the kidney during respiration may complicate puncture if the target is small and is visible on the monitor only during a specific respiratory phase. If the direction of the needle and the position of the target are aligned and both are clearly seen on the monitor, the needle is advanced through the renal capsule during the appropriate phase of respiration (Figure 8–3). In this phase, the kidney is usually pushed to some extent by the puncture needle, so that visualization of needle and target may be momentarily impaired. However, as soon as the tip of the needle has penetrated the fibrous renal capsule, it is seen even

Figure 8–3. Ultrasonically guided puncture of a dorsal lower calyx. Needle must be in the scanning plane to be visualized.

more clearly. If both the tip of the needle and the target are visualized clearly at the same spot on the scanning plane, the needle is in the desired space.

Antegrade injection of a small amount of contrast dye for fluoroscopy outlines the renal collecting system after successful puncture. However, if the collecting system has not been successfully punctured at the first attempt, contrast dye may fill the interlobar veins, which form a basketlike structure around the calyx, or may extravasate. In rare cases in which contrast dye is injected into the adventitia of the renal collecting system, extravasation may assume the configuration of the collecting system, mimicking successful puncture. Care must be taken to inject the least amount of dye necessary so that further fluoroscopic and ultrasonic orientation will not be hindered. A larger amount of dye injected outside the collecting system may compress the calyx to be entered and render puncture more difficult. If the position of the needle tip on ultrasound is close to its destination (ascertained by a small vibratory movement), the needle should be retracted a few millimeters only and readvanced at the appropriate angle and tilt. Once the collecting system is entered (Figure 8–4A), fluoroscopy alone is used to guide the subsequent steps of the procedure.

If fluoroscopy is used instead of ultrasound for guiding renal puncture, a fine-needle (20–22 gauge) puncture technique may be used. Intravenous or retrograde

administration of contrast dye is needed. With retrograde injection, a ureteral balloon occlusion catheter can be inserted and blocked in the ureteropelvic junction to cause slight distention of the renal collecting system; this facilitates puncture of a nondilated system. First, a 16- to 18-gauge needle is inserted through the abdominal wall only, and a longer fine needle is inserted coaxially through the larger needle (Figure 8–4B). This technique improves control of the fine needle. As soon as the fine needle has entered the collecting system, the larger needle can be advanced over the fine needle, which serves as a guide. After withdrawal of the fine needle, a regular guidewire can be inserted through the large needle into the collecting system.

Urine aspirated from the collecting system should be cultured, especially if there is suspicion of a urinary tract infection.

ANTEGRADE PYELOGRAPHY & PRESSURE/PERFUSION STUDIES

Renal puncture is rarely indicated for diagnostic antegrade pyelography only, because less invasive radiographic techniques are available (eg, intravenous pyelography with tomograms, ultrasound, CT, magnetic resonance imaging, retrograde pyelography). However, obtaining a radiograph after antegrade injection of contrast dye should be an integral part of every percutaneous puncture for any indication. Before contrast dye is injected, urine must be aspirated to decompress an obstructed collecting system. The contrast dye should be diluted to 20–30% for better visualization of details; antegrade pyelography then provides images of the collecting system with about the same resolution of detail as retrograde pyelography.

Antegrade pyelography is also performed in conjunction with a percutaneous pressure/perfusion study (Whitaker test) to assess pyeloureteral resistance. Percutaneous urodynamic studies of the dilated upper urinary tract are indicated only in the 10–30% of cases in which noninvasive radioisotope studies (diuresis renogram) fail to differentiate an obstructed from a nonobstructed dilated system. (This is more likely in cases of ureterovesical obstruction than in pelvicureteral obstruction, in which diuresis renograms are reliable.)

The Whitaker test provides simultaneous measurements of intrapelvic and intravesical pressures during antegrade perfusion, with flow rates of 5, 10, 15, and 20 mL/min. Puncture of the renal collecting system is performed with a coaxial needle/catheter system with an outer 6F catheter for the renal pressure/perfusion study; thus, puncture and catheter insertion can be done as a one-step procedure. Perfusion is started with

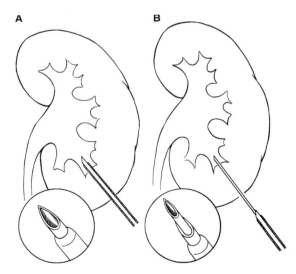

Figure 8–4. Percutaneous puncture techniques. **A:** Ultrasonically guided technique: puncture with a 16- to 18-gauge coaxial needle/catheter system. **B:** Fluoroscopically guided technique: coaxial fine-needle puncture through a larger needle/catheter system.

flow rates of 5–10 mL/min until a steady-state equilibrium of pressure readings is reached and the entire upper urinary tract is opacified (Figure 8–5). Pressure readings may be obtained intermittently, from the perfusion catheter via a 3-way stopcock, or continuously, if a double-lumen nephrostomy catheter or 2 separate catheters for perfusion and pressure measurement are used. Continuous recordings during perfusion from a single-lumen perfusion catheter via a T connection yield erroneous pressure readings (the smaller the lumen of the nephrostomy catheter and the higher the perfusion rate, the higher the pressure reading), unless the resistance of the entire system was previously calibrated for each rate of perfusion. To obtain accurate pressure readings, the positions of the intrapelvic and intravesical pressure manometers must be adjusted to the level of the renal pelvis and bladder, respectively. At a flow rate of 10 mL/min, differential pressures (renal pelvic pressure minus bladder pressure) below 13 cm water are normal, between 14 and 22 cm water suggest mild obstruction, and above 22 cm water suggest moderate to severe obstruction. At flow rates of 15 mL/min and 20 mL/min, upper limits of normal pressure are 18 cm and 21 cm water, respectively.

PERCUTANEOUS CATHETER PLACEMENT

Percutaneous nephrostomy catheter placement for drainage and decompression of the upper urinary tract is indicated if retrograde ureteral catheterization is not advisable (eg, in sepsis secondary to ureteral obstruction) or proves to be impossible (eg, impassable ureteral obstruction due to stone, tumor, or stricture). After percutaneous endourologic procedures, a nephrostomy catheter is usually left indwelling for a few days. To convert a nephrostomy catheter diversion into an internal stent drainage, antegrade ureteral stenting through the nephrostomy tract may be attempted even in cases in which previous attempts at retrograde stenting have failed. The antegrade approach to stenting can be expected to be successful if failure of retrograde stenting was not related to mere mechanical ureteral obstruction but rather to ureteral tortuosity, false passage (uretero-vaginal fistula, urinoma after open surgery), or inability to identify the orifice endoscopically (ureteroileal anastomosis).

For diagnostic procedures such as pressure/perfusion studies (Whitaker test), a 6F catheter is sufficient. Catheters of this size can be placed in a one-step procedure of puncture if coaxial needle/catheter systems are used (Figure 8–2). For therapeutic interventions such as nephrostomy drainage or antegrade ureteral stenting, softer, larger catheters must be inserted, and puncture tract dilation is necessary before catheter insertion. For dilation of a puncture tract, a 0.035- or 0.038-in guidewire must be inserted into the collecting system, either directly through the puncture needle or through the outer catheter of a coaxial needle/catheter system. Curved-tip (J) guidewires are less likely to cause damage to the mucosa of the renal pelvis than are straight guidewires. One of the most common problems of tract dilation is kinking of the guidewire during insertion of fascial dilators; therefore, guidewires with a floppy tip and a stiff proximal section (Lunderquist wire) are preferable over floppy guidewires. If the tip of the guidewire cannot be advanced into the renal pelvis because it is trapped in a dilated calyx with a narrow infundibulum or because an obstructing stone hinders passage, the outer catheter of a coaxial needle/catheter system can be used to manipulate the guidewire into the

Figure 8–5. Whitaker test in a dilated upper tract after vesicoureteral reimplantation (prune belly syndrome). Antegrade perfusion with 10 mL/min results in a vesicopelvic pressure gradient of 10 cm of water, with unobstructed flow.

collecting system (Figure 8–6A), or angiographic catheters with different curved-tip configurations may be inserted over the guidewire for this purpose. Once the guidewire is in the correct position (upper calyx, renal pelvis, upper ureter), radiopaque fascial dilators can be inserted under fluoroscopic control with rotating movement of the dilator during advancement. If flexible plastic fascial dilators are used, sequential insertion of dilators of increasing size (usually in 2F steps) is necessary. If stiff metal or Kevlar dilators are used, dilation from 6F to 10–12F is possible in a one-step procedure.

After tract dilation, relatively stiff nephrostomy catheters (eg, polyethylene catheters) can be introduced easily over the guidewire. However, if softer catheters (eg, silicone or polyurethane) are to be inserted, use of an introducer catheter is helpful. An introducer catheter is also helpful for antegrade ureteral stenting

and for insertion of nephrostomy catheters with various self-retaining configurations of the tip (eg, pigtail). These catheters can be stretched into a straight configuration while being inserted through the introducer catheter and over a guidewire; the tip resumes its original configuration due to the memory function of the material once the guidewire is withdrawn. The introducer catheter can be inserted with the last fascial dilator in a one-step procedure if a coaxial dilator/introducer catheter system is used (Figures 8–6B and C). The use of an introducer catheter provides universal access to the renal collecting system for placement of all types of catheters (nephrostomy catheters [Figure 8–6D], ureteral stents, balloon dilation catheters) and safety and working wires for different systems of large-bore nephrostomy tract dilation required for insertion of endoscopic instruments.

Figure 8–6. Small-bore tract dilation and nephrostomy catheter insertion. **A:** J-guidewire inserted through the needle-catheter system and advanced with assistance of the catheter into the renal pelvis. **B:** Insertion of a coaxial dilator/introducer catheter system over the guidewire. Stiff proximal section of the guidewire prevents extrarenal kinking. **C:** After the dilator has entered the collecting system, the introducer catheter is advanced over its tip. **D:** Pigtail nephrostomy catheter is inserted into the renal pelvis over the guidewire and through the introducer catheter.

Nephrostomy catheters should be soft to avoid discomfort and irritation of the renal pelvis and should have a self-retaining mechanism or should be placed with enough slack to prevent dislodgment from the collecting system during movement of the kidney. Standard nephrostomy catheters are Malecot catheters, pigtail catheters, and loop catheters. Loop catheters have a very effective retaining mechanism; it may cause serious complications, however, if the catheter is accidentally pulled out of the kidney.

Antegrade ureteral stenting can be done through an introducer catheter using either open- or closed-tip stents. Catheters with open-tip configuration are advanced with a pusher catheter over a guidewire, which must be inserted through the introducer sheath down the ureter and into the bladder as a first step. Catheters with closed-tip configuration are advanced by pushing the indwelling wire. In either technique, a thread should be pulled through one of the proximal side holes of the catheter so that the catheter can be pulled back into the renal pelvis if it is advanced too far. The thread must be pulled out before the guidewire is withdrawn so that the pusher catheter can still hold the double-J stent in place.

An introducer catheter may also be used for insertion of a 7F balloon dilation catheter over a guidewire into the ureter to dilate ureteral strictures to 12–18F with balloon pressures of up to 15 atm. After successful dilation, an 8–10F stent is usually left indwelling for several weeks. This technique is most successful in ureteral strictures that are a complication of recent surgery for benign disorders, except ureteropelvic obstruction. Long-standing strictures or strictures due to tumor compression of the ureter, radiation damage, or ischemic ureteral necrosis after radical pelvic surgery are not likely to respond favorably to balloon dilation. Long-term results of ureteral balloon dilation cannot be determined from published data, either because the periods of follow-up were too short or because balloon dilations were repeated periodically.

PERFUSION-CHEMOLYSIS OF RENAL STONES

Nephrostomy catheters may be used for perfusion of the renal collecting system with chemolytic agents for dissolution of renal stones. In principle, uric acid, cystine, struvite, or apatite stones are amenable to chemolysis. However, the success of ESWL and the possibility of oral chemolysis (for uric acid stones) have limited the use of percutaneous chemolysis to adjunctive treatment of residual stones after open surgery, PNL, or ESWL. Primary percutaneous chemolysis may still be indicated in patients who are poor anesthetic risks. Benefits of

percutaneous chemolysis must be weighed against disadvantages and possible risks, for example, prolonged hospitalization for dissolution of large stones (cystine, struvite, or apatite stones) and possible complications of treating infection stones (sepsis, hypermagnesemia).

To limit risks, perfusion chemolysis should always be performed with a double-catheter system for irrigation and simultaneous continuous drainage. This is achieved by using either 2 separately or coaxially inserted nephrostomy catheters (Figure 8–7A) or a ureteral catheter in conjunction with a nephrostomy catheter (Figure 8–7B). To ensure effective flow around the stone, the irrigation catheter must be placed close to the stone. Lack of continuous, complete drainage of the perfusate with increased intrapelvic pressures above 30 cm water may lead to pyelotubular and pyelovenous reflux of chemolytic agents and, possibly, infected urine, resulting in hypermagnesemia (perfusion with hemiacidrin or Suby's solution G or M) and sepsis. Irrigation should be started only in the absence of urinary tract infection or if infection is under control. Irrigation must first be tested with saline at the lowest possible height above kidney level to achieve a flow rate of 100–120 mL/h. Discomfort, pain, or leakage of perfusate may indicate inappropriate drainage of the irrigant, and patients should be instructed to interrupt the irrigation themselves in such instances.

Uric acid stones can be dissolved by sodium or potassium bicarbonate solution; cystine stones with D-penicillamine, acetylcysteine, or tromethamine-E solution; and struvite and apatite stones with Suby's solution G or M or hemiacidrin (Renacidin; not FDA-approved for renal irrigation). Patients must be monitored for developing urinary tract infection or fever, and serum creatinine, phosphorus (hemiacidrin-perfusion), and magnesium levels (perfusion with hemiacidrin, Suby's solution G or M) must be obtained every other day.

The time necessary for complete stone dissolution depends on the composition and size of the stone and may vary from a few days (uric acid stones) to several weeks (cystine or struvite stones).

ENDOSCOPIC INTRARENAL INSTRUMENTATION

Nephroscopes are endoscopic instruments with sheaths of 15–26F that are inserted percutaneously through a nephrostomy tract. Standard rigid instruments are available in sizes 24–26F; these have telescopes with offset eyepieces (Figure 8–8, left). Rigid instruments such as graspers and ultrasound probes can be inserted through a central working channel (Figure 8–8, right). Flexible fiberoptic nephroscopes may be used as well. These have a deflecting mechanism for the tip that al-

A

B

Figure 8–7. Catheter placement for perfusion chemolysis of renal stones. **A:** Perfusion and drainage of the irrigating fluid through 2 nephrostomy catheters. **B:** Perfusion through nephrostomy catheter, and drainage of the irrigant through ureteral catheter.

lows inspection of otherwise difficult-to-reach calyces. A smaller working channel allows insertion of flexible instruments such as stone baskets, wire graspers, and electrohydraulic or laser probes. However, instrumentation through flexible nephroscopes is limited by the size and flexibility of working instruments such as stone forceps, and flexible endoscopes do not offer the optical quality and durability of rigid nephroscopes.

Nephroscopy is rarely indicated for diagnostic purposes only; in most cases, it is performed for percutaneous lithotripsy and extraction of renal stones (PNL). However, ESWL has gradually replaced PNL for treatment of renal stones and is now used in more than 90% of cases. PNL is still indicated in cases for which ESWL is not the primary choice of treatment. Such cases include urinary obstruction not caused by the stone itself, large-volume stones, and stones that cannot be positioned within the focus of the shock wave apparatus. Nephroscopes also may be used for direct-vision internal incision of ureteropelvic stenosis and for palliative treatment of urothelial cancer of the upper urinary tract.

Insertion of a nephroscope into the renal collecting system requires dilation of the puncture tract to 24–30F. A safety wire should be inserted parallel to the working wire and advanced into an upper calyx or the upper ureter to guide the way back into the collecting system in case the dilator and working wire become dislodged accidentally. Insertion of an introducer catheter during small-bore tract dilation to 10–12F facilitates parallel insertion of safety and working wires. The central metal catheter of a coaxial metal dilator system (Figure 8–9, left), the central plastic catheter for insertion of sequential plastic dilators, or a balloon dilator catheter can be inserted over the working wire. Balloon dilator catheters of 9F size can dilate a nephrostomy tract to a diameter of 30F under pressure up to 10–12 atm in a one-step procedure. This may prove difficult or impossible if perirenal scar tissue from previous surgery prevents complete expansion of the balloon over its entire length. Sequential plastic dilators allow stepwise dilation of the tract under fluoroscopic control; however, on withdrawal for insertion of the next larger dilator, compression of the tract is lost intermittently and bleeding occurs into the collecting system, sometimes hindering subsequent endoscopy. Coaxial metal dilators (Figure 8–9, right) (each dilator slides over the next smaller one) allow stepwise tract dilation even in the presence of severe scarring with continuous nephrostomy tract compression for improved hemostasis.

With any dilation technique, the last step is insertion of a working sheath, which may be either the 24–26F metal working sheath of the nephroscope or a larger plastic sheath. With the balloon dilation tech-

Figure 8–8. Rigid nephroscope. **Left:** A continuous-flow sheath, telescope with offset eyepiece for central access to a straight working channel, and rigid forceps and graspers. **Right:** Graspers and forceps for percutaneous endoscopic stone extraction.

Figure 8–9. Large-bore tract dilation for nephroscopy. **Left:** Insertion of the central catheter of the Alken dilator system over a working wire through an introducer catheter (see also Figure 8–7). An introducer catheter allows parallel insertion of a safety wire into the collecting system. **Right:** Alken coaxial metal dilators for sequential tract dilation without loss of tract compression. Final step is coaxial insertion of a plastic working sheath or the metal nephroscope sheath.

nique, the working sheath must be introduced over a plastic dilator; with use of serial plastic or coaxial metal dilators, the working sheath slides over the last dilator. A 28–30F plastic working sheath is preferable to a metal nephroscope sheath in all cases in which extensive, prolonged instrumentation is anticipated (eg, staghorn stones). Larger plastic sheaths not only provide better irrigation with lower intrapelvic pressures than do continuous-flow nephroscope sheaths but also allow easier extraction of large stone fragments.

Renal Stones

In the era of ESWL, indications for PNL are limited to 4 types of stone disease:

(1) Urinary obstruction not caused by the stone itself (eg, stone in a caliceal diverticulum [Figure 8–10, left and right], stone in association with ureteropelvic stenosis). These stones could be broken up by ESWL, but gravel would not pass spontaneously.

(2) Large-volume stones (> 3 cm, stone surface > 500 mm^2) (Figure 8–11, left and right) (eg, staghorn stones). These stones can be treated by several sessions of ESWL, but only about 30% of patients become stone free. However, problems associated with passing large quantities of gravel (eg, ureteral obstruction, pain, fever, sepsis) can be prevented by first percutaneously debulking the stone and then performing ESWL for endoscopically inaccessible stones.

(3) Stones that cannot be positioned within the focus of the shock wave apparatus (eg, stones in kidneys

Figure 8–10. Stone in upper caliceal diverticulum requiring percutaneous nephrolithotomy. **Left:** Plain abdominal radiograph. **Right:** Intravenous pyelogram.

with abnormal position due to anomalies of the urinary tract or skeleton, stones in transplanted kidneys).

(4) PNL may be of benefit for lower-pole caliceal calculi even under the 2–3 cm range. The overall stone-free rate for these stones with ESWL is only about 60%.

Large-volume staghorn stones are a much more common indication for PNL than stones that can be extracted in toto. Small stones can be extracted with a variety of rigid forceps and graspers (Figure 8–8, right). Stones may be retrieved from difficult-to-reach calyces with flexible wire baskets and graspers inserted through flexible nephroscopes. Large stones must be disintegrated using mechanical, ultrasonic, electrohydraulic, or laser energy. Strong nutcracker-type forceps (visual lithotrite, stone punch; derived from instruments for transurethral

Figure 8–11. Staghorn stone requiring combined percutaneous nephrolithotomy and extracorporeal shockwave lithotripsy. **Left:** Plain abdominal radiograph. **Right:** Intravenous pyelogram.

bladder stone disintegration) can be used only in a spacious renal pelvis. Hollow ultrasonic probes allow for controllable, systematic stone disintegration under continuous suction for removal of sand and smaller fragments. Electrohydraulic probes are more powerful than ultrasonic probes and may be used through flexible nephroscopes, but they do not provide continuous suction and are associated with a higher risk of scattering stone fragments into inaccessible calyces and of damaging the mucosa of the renal pelvis. However, with electrohydraulic probes and the holmium:YAG laser, disintegration of hard or large stones is faster.

For soft stones, continuous disintegration and evacuation of fragments with ultrasound probes is most time-efficient. Hard stones should be broken up into the largest possible fragments that can be extracted through the working sheath. The ureteropelvic portion of a staghorn stone should be left in place until the procedure is nearly completed, as it will act like a plug in a drain to prevent the loss of fragments into the ureter. An antegradely or retrogradely positioned ureteral balloon occlusion catheter might serve the same purpose; however, the extra procedure of retrograde ureteral catheterization is rarely indicated.

Normal saline should be used as the irrigation fluid except in the case of electrohydraulic lithotripsy, in which 1/6 normal saline is more appropriate. However, even with the low-pressure system provided by a large plastic working sheath, considerable amounts of irrigation fluid may be absorbed if small veins are opened and intrarenal manipulation is prolonged. This may cause transurethral resection (TUR) syndrome with use of hypotonic fluids. Intraoperative administration of diuretics (eg, mannitol, 12.5 g) is advisable and also has proved effective in preventing intrarenal reflux. If there is suspicion of extravasation, contrast dye must be injected and a diagnostic radiograph obtained. On completion of the procedure, a plain film should be obtained and a nephrostomy catheter placed. A Foley catheter with a 5-mL balloon may be inserted through a fenestrated trocar or the plastic working sheath, which then is withdrawn and cut lengthwise for removal from the Foley catheter. Malecot catheters or straight polyethylene catheters (eg, chest tubes) may be used as well and should be secured to the skin with sutures. A final nephrostogram documents appropriate position of the catheter.

Nephrostomy catheters may be removed after 1–4 days. If ESWL is to be performed, it can be done 1–4 days after the percutaneous procedure. The nephrostomy catheter should be left in place during and after ESWL to provide drainage for urine and stone gravel and to allow for a second endoscopic procedure if some of the stone fragments do not pass spontaneously after ESWL.

Ureteropelvic Stenosis

With the advent of PNL and ureterorenoscopy, other endosurgical techniques have been developed that are similar to procedures used in the lower urinary tract. Direct-vision internal incision of ureteropelvic stenosis (pyelolysis, endopyelotomy, endopyeloplasty) seems to be a natural outgrowth of endoscopic techniques in the upper urinary tract. Compared with the retrograde techniques of endopyelotomy (incision with a cold knife, Acucise catheter, Greenwald electrode, or laser) and the endoballoon rupture, the antegrade technique offers the advantage of an incision under direct vision. The cold-knife incision must be extended into the perirenal fat and is stented for 4–6 weeks to allow for healing, according to the principle of Davis' intubated ureterotomy.

Success rates of antegrade endopyelotomy of up to 65–95% are reported for primary cases and up to 89% for secondary cases after failed open-surgical pyeloplasty.

The success rates for retrograde endopyelotomy with fewer patients and less follow-up than in antegrade endopyelotomy range between 79% and 94%; for the Acucise endopyelotomy, between 73% and 81%. The candidates for best endoscopic (antegrade and retrograde) outcome are those with less than grade II hydronephrosis and good renal function.

In most reports on endopyelotomy, the criteria of success differ from those of open pyeloplasty; relief of subjective symptoms is given priority over results of imaging studies such as decompression of a dilated collecting system on intravenous pyelography or renal ultrasound. Inadequate results after endopyelotomy may be related to a crossing vessel or to redundancy of the renal pelvis, which would be resected during open pyeloplasty. According to the law of Laplace, wall tension of a renal pelvis is, at the same intrapelvic pressures, higher in a more dilated collecting system with a larger diameter than in a less dilated system with a smaller diameter. A raised wall tension supposedly represents a more important pathogenetic factor for developing progressive dilatation than do elevated intrapelvic pressures due to anatomic obstruction of outflow. Secondary open pyeloplasty after failed endopyelotomy may be a more tedious operation with less satisfactory results in cases with extensive periureteral scarring due to extravasation of urine after endopyelotomy than primary open pyeloplasty.

Renal Pelvis Tumor

Another technique of endoscopic surgery in the upper urinary tract is use of electroresection, electrocoagulation, electrovaporization, and neodymium:YAG laser coagulation for treatment of urothelial tumors of the renal pelvis. However, with the limited reports of treatment of upper urinary tract urothelial cancer endoscopically, recurrence rates are yet to be compared with those of standard surgical treatment.

Ensuring a strict follow-up, percutaneous management of transitional cell carcinoma of the collecting system may be an alternative to nephroureterectomy for patients with grade I disease and for palliative treatment.

PERCUTANEOUS ASPIRATION & BIOPSY

Percutaneous puncture of cystic or solid lesions of the kidney and the adjacent retroperitoneum is usually performed for diagnostic purposes, in some cases in combination with therapeutic intentions such as drainage of fluid collections or obliteration of renal cysts (Tables 8–2 and 8–3). Because most of these lesions are radiolucent and are not enhanced with intravenously administered contrast dye, they cannot be visualized by fluoroscopy. Thus, ultrasound or CT is the imaging technique of choice to depict these lesions and guide percutaneous puncture. The technique of ultrasonically guided puncture is the same whether the target is the renal collecting system or a cystic or solid renal or extrarenal lesion. For cytologic aspiration, a fine-needle (20–22 gauge) aspiration technique is used that is comparable to fine-needle aspiration biopsy of the prostate. There is no evidence that one type of needle is preferable to the others. For aspiration and evacuation of renal cysts or extrarenal fluid collections (urinoma, lymphocele), the same coaxial needle/catheter system can be used as for percutaneous puncture of the renal collecting system. A small catheter (6–10F) is placed for a few days to ensure complete drainage of fluid. When fluids of high viscosity (abscess, hematoma) are to be

Table 8–2. Indications for puncture of renal and retroperitoneal lesions.

Diagnostic indications
Fluid aspiration
Fluid chemistry
Bacteriology and sensitivity
Cytology
Radiography with percutaneously injected contrast dye
Histology (core biopsy)
Therapeutic indications
Catheter drainage
Urinoma, lymphocele
Abscess, hematoma
Fluid evacuation and injection of sclerosing agent
Simple renal cyst

Table 8–3. Differential diagnosis of renal and retroperitoneal lesions.

Renal cystic lesion
Benign cyst
Hydrocalix
Abscess
Hematoma
Cystic tumor
Tumor in cyst
Retroperitoneal fluid collection
Urinoma
Lymphocele
Hematoma
Abscess
Cystic tumor
Solid renal and retroperitoneal lesions
Benign tumor
Malignant primary tumor
Metastatic tumor

drained, large-bore catheters (14–20F) must be inserted, necessitating dilation of the percutaneous tract. Percutaneous renal biopsy for histologic diagnosis and classification of renal disease is performed with 14- to 16-gauge needles (eg, Franklin-Silverman, Tru-Cut) at the lower pole of the kidney.

Renal Cysts

Renal cysts are found in about 50% of autopsy specimens in persons over the age of 50 years and are a frequent accidental finding on ultrasound or CT studies. Only a few cases require diagnostic percutaneous puncture. Indications for diagnostic puncture of a cystic lesion are an irregular, thick wall and internal echoes on ultrasound examination, density numbers on CT higher than those of serous fluid, and hematuria. Puncture for therapeutic procedures (evacuation of fluid and instillation of a sclerosing agent) is indicated only if, due to its size or location, the cyst causes compression and urinary obstruction of a caliceal infundibulum or the ureter, or discomfort and pain.

Various tests may be performed on aspirated fluid. No one test is pathognomonic except cytologic findings of malignant cells. However, neoplasms within a cyst are exceedingly rare, and cystic degeneration of a renal neoplasm can usually be easily identified by ultrasound and CT. Benign cysts contain clear, straw-colored fluid with low fat and protein content and lactic acid dehydrogenase levels of less than 250 mIU/mL. Cancer is suspected if the fluid is bloody or murky and has a high content of fat, protein, and lactic acid dehydrogenase. After aspiration of 20–30% of the cystic fluid, the same amount of 60% contrast dye is injected, and diagnostic radiographs are obtained in the prone, supine, upright, decubitus, and Trendelenburg positions. If necessary, another 20–30% of the cystic fluid may be replaced by air for obtaining double-contrast radiographs.

For therapeutic obliteration of cysts, sclerosing agents such as Pantopaque or 95% ethanol can be injected after complete evacuation of the cystic fluid. A volume of 10–100 mL of 95% ethanol, approximating 10–20% of the original volume of cystic fluid, is injected into the cyst and should be drained after 30 min.

Retroperitoneal Fluid Collections

Low-viscosity retroperitoneal fluid collections (urinoma, lymphocele) are usually a complication of surgical procedures. However, urinoma may also be caused by exogenous trauma or by fornix rupture due to acute ureteral obstruction. Percutaneous techniques of catheter drainage eliminate the need for open surgical revision in most cases.

Insertion of a small (6–10F) catheter (with numerous side holes) is usually sufficient. Adjunctive procedures are performed to ensure sealing of the fluid leak and obliteration of the cystic lesion. In cases of urinoma, the upper urinary tract must also be drained by a ureteral catheter or percutaneous nephrostomy catheter until drainage from the urinoma stops. Lymphoceles that develop following pelvic or retroperitoneal lymphadenectomy or renal transplantation often undergo spontaneous regression and usually do not require puncture and drainage. However, large lymphoceles developing after retroperitoneal lymphadenectomy may cause pain and even ureteral obstruction (Figure 8–12). Patients should be treated with parenteral nutrition and abdominal compression by bandaging, but if lymph drainage after percutaneous puncture and catheter placement persists for more than 1 week, surgical intervention with intraperitoneal marsupialization of the lymphocele and ligation or electrocoagulation of lymphatic vessels is indicated.

High-viscosity fluid collections (hematoma, abscess) usually require large-bore (14–20F) percutaneous catheters for sufficient drainage. Perirenal hematomas are most frequently caused by surgical or exogenous trauma and rarely develop spontaneously in the presence of a bleeding disorder or due to rupture of a renal tumor. Indications for percutaneous drainage are rare, as most small hematomas resolve spontaneously and should be followed by ultrasound or CT only. A hematoma that increases in size requires surgical intervention rather than percutaneous drainage. Secondary infection of a hematoma may be an indication for percutaneous drainage.

A perirenal abscess is mostly a complication of open surgery; hematogenic renal abscess (renal carbuncle) is

Figure 8–12. Percutaneous drainage of a lymphocele causing ureteral displacement and compression.

less frequent. Indications for puncture and drainage should be based on CT finding of a unifocal process that can be effectively and safely drained percutaneously. Multifocal renal abscess formation is not amenable to percutaneous drainage.

Renal & Retroperitoneal Tumors

Percutaneous aspiration biopsy of renal and retroperitoneal tumors is indicated if less invasive radiographic studies are inconclusive and if cytologic findings may have an impact on further medical or surgical therapy (Figure 8–13). If curative treatment by open surgery seems to be feasible, aspiration biopsy is generally not indicated. If the identity of a renal lesion is questionable or if conservative, organ-sparing surgery is technically feasible, surgical excision of the lesion with intraoperative frozen sections is preferable over percutaneous aspiration biopsy. However, aspiration biopsy may be indicated to avoid radical nephrectomy of a possibly benign lesion. In multifocal or possibly metastatic lesions, cytologic evaluation can be crucial for planning surgical or medical therapy, and in these cases, aspiration biopsy is usually indicated. Interpretation of cytologic findings is limited by a 10–25% incidence of false-negative findings and the difficulty in discriminating normal renal tubular cells from low-grade renal cell cancer. As a rare complication, tumor seeding in the puncture tract has been described. The aspirate is immediately spread on glass slides. For standard Papanicolaou stains, alcohol fixation must be used.

Renal Biopsy

Renal biopsy for diagnosis and classification of medical renal disease can be performed percutaneously or by open surgery. Because specimens, rather than aspirates, are needed for diagnostic histologic study, large-bore (14–16 gauge) Franklin-Silverman or Tru-Cut needles are used. Ultrasonic or fluoroscopic guidance is preferable to blind renal puncture. However, even with puncture aimed precisely at the dorsal aspect of the lower pole of the kidney, where accidental injury to large vessels is less likely, bleeding is to be expected because of the vascularity of the parenchyma and is the major complication of this procedure (about 5% of cases, with a mortality rate of 0.1%). Hematoma can usually be followed conservatively by ultrasound or CT, but transvascular embolization, open surgical revision, and even nephrectomy have been required following diagnostic renal biopsy. Therefore, open surgical biopsy rather than percutaneous biopsy is indicated in patients with solitary kidneys or uncontrolled hypertension.

URETERORENOSCOPY

Ureterorenoscopy is endoscopy of the ureter up to the renal pelvis for both diagnostic evaluation and therapeutic intervention (Table 8–4).

Ureterorenoscopes (Figure 8–14) are endoscopes for retrograde insertion into the ureter; however, they also may be used in an antegrade fashion via a percutaneously established nephrostomy tract. Rigid ureterorenoscopes are available in sizes 6.9–12.6F, and semirigid fiberoptic ureterorenoscopes and flexible ureterorenoscopes may be found in sizes 6.2–9.3F. The smallest instruments are for diagnostic procedures only. Larger instruments, with a 3–6F working channel, can accept stone baskets, wire graspers, stone forceps, biopsy forceps, and ultrasonic, electrohydraulic, or laser probes for stone disintegration. Flexible ureterorenoscopes follow the topographic anatomy of the ureter more easily and facilitate inspection of middle and lower renal calyces if a deflecting mechanism for the tip

Figure 8–13. Percutaneous fine-needle biopsy. **Left:** Aspiration biopsy of a renal lesion. **Right:** Guidance with computed tomography scanning for fine-needle aspiration biopsy of an exophytic renal cell carcinoma.

of the instrument is provided. However, the use of instrumentation through flexible nephroscopes is limited by the size and flexibility of working instruments such as stone forceps, and flexible ureterorenoscopes do not offer the optical quality and durability of rigid instruments.

Insertion of a ureterorenoscope into the ureteral orifice may be facilitated by dilation of the intramural

Table 8–4. Indications for ureterorenoscopy.

Diagnostic indications
    Lesions of ureter or renal pelvis
    Hematuria from upper tract
Therapeutic indications
    Ureteral stone treatment
    Direct vision internal ureterotomy of ureteral strictures
    Endoscopic resection and coagulation of ureteral tumors

---

ureter, either with sequential plastic dilators of increasing size, which are slid over a guidewire, or with a balloon dilator catheter (Figure 8–15). Dilation of the ureter is often unnecessary if a small (3–5F) ureteral catheter is inserted through the working channel of the ureterorenoscope into the ureter as a guide, and the ureterorenoscope is then rotated 180 degrees and introduced in an upside-down orientation (Figure 8–16). In this position, the ureteral catheter will spread the roof of the intramural ureter like a tent and the nose of the instrument will slide flat on the trigone into the orifice. The orifice and intramural ureter will thus be dilated only to the extent necessary for insertion of the instrument.

Diagnostic Ureterorenoscopy

Indications for diagnostic ureterorenoscopy are those rare lesions of the ureter or renal pelvis whose nature

Figure 8–14. Ureterorenoscopes: Telescopes with center and offset eyepieces for use through a 12.5F working sheath. 10.5F ureterorenoscope with integrated sheath (asterisk).

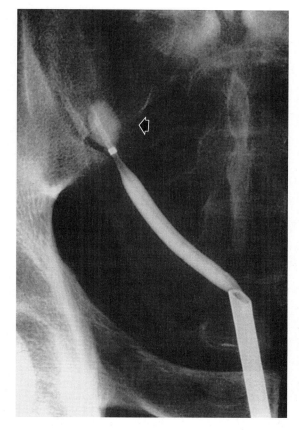

Figure 8–15. Ureteral dilation with balloon catheter before ureterorenoscopic removal of a distal ureteral stone (arrow).

cannot be determined with less invasive diagnostic procedures such as retrograde pyelography, selective urinary cytology, CT, or magnetic resonance imaging. If a small ureterorenoscope without a working channel is used for a diagnostic procedure, a biopsy of a lesion cannot be obtained. If ureterorenoscopy is performed for evaluation of hematuria from the upper tract, the source of bleeding can rarely be identified during gross hematuria because of limited irrigation through ureterorenoscopes, resulting in poor visibility. If the urine has cleared, the chances of identifying a lesion that could not be detected on radiographic studies are small as well.

Ureteral Stones

Ureterorenoscopy is most frequently performed for treatment of ureteral stones, although more than 90% of ureteral stones can be treated by ESWL either in situ or after dislodgment of the ureteral stone into the renal pelvis using a ureteral catheter (push-back or flush-back procedures). For the remaining indications of ureteral stone treatment, ureterorenoscopy is used for extraction of stones, dislodgment of stones into the renal pelvis for subsequent ESWL, and intraureteral stone disintegration.

For extraction of distal ureteral stones that are unresponsive to ESWL, short rigid ureterorenoscopes and alligator forceps or Dormia baskets are most helpful. Impacted proximal ureteral stones that did not respond to in situ ESWL and could not be dislodged with a ureteral catheter usually can be repositioned into the renal pelvis under direct vision for subsequent ESWL using a small semirigid or rigid ureterorenoscope. If the stones are too large or impacted, intraureteral lithotripsy for stone disintegration may be necessary in a few cases.

To prevent the pushing back of stones or fragments into the renal pelvis during lithotripsy, a 3F wire basket can be used to hold the stone during disintegration or a 3F balloon catheter can be passed alongside the stone and be blocked proximally. Ultrasound probes allow safe stone disintegration under continuous suction, but they are not as effective as electrohydraulic and laser probes and can be used through rigid ureterorenoscopes only. Both electrohydraulic and laser probes can be used through rigid or flexible ureterorenoscopes. Laser probes for intraureteral lithotripsy have the smallest diameter (< 11F) and do not injure the mucosa of the ureter if used under direct vision. Several pulsed lasers such as the holmium:YAG laser, pulsed-dye laser, and

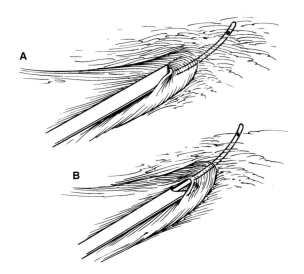

Figure 8–16. Ureterorenoscopy. **A:** Straightforward advancement of the instrument over a thin ureteral catheter can catch the mucosa of the orifice. **B:** With 180-degree upside-down rotation of the instrument, the ureteral catheter holds the orifice open like a tent.

Alexandrite laser are available for intraureteral lithotripsy. Electrohydraulic probes, which are available in sizes 1.6–5F, require less expensive equipment, but they bear the risk of ureteral damage if used inappropriately.

If ureteral perforation occurs as a complication of intraureteral instrumentation, ureteral stenting using a 6–8F double-J stent for 2–6 weeks usually allows healing without late sequelae. Stents should be used for a few days even after uncomplicated ureterorenoscopy to prevent pain from urinary stasis because of edema of the intramural ureter after instrumentation. If there is ureteral perforation and a stent has been placed, the bladder should be on continuous drainage for a few days using a transurethral Foley catheter or a suprapubic cystotomy catheter to prevent urinoma formation from vesicoureteral reflux via the double-J stent.

Ureteral Strictures

Direct-vision internal ureterotomy of ureteral strictures is the ureterorenoscopic variant of percutaneous endopyeloplasty for ureteropelvic stenosis (see the section: Endoscopic Intrarenal Instrumentation, Ureteropelvic Stenosis). Cold-knife incision of the stenosis into the periureteral fat and stenting of the ureter for 4–6 weeks are the principles of Davis' intubated ureterotomy.

Best results are obtained in ureteral strictures that are a complication of surgery for benign disorders if treatment is established early. However, long-term results of this technique as compared with open surgical repair remain to be determined. Long-standing strictures or strictures due to external ureteral compression, radiation damage, or ischemic ureteral necrosis after surgery are not satisfactorily treated by internal ureterotomy.

Ureteral Tumors

Endoscopic electroresection and laser coagulation of ureteral tumors are the ureterorenoscopic variants of percutaneous endoscopic treatment of renal pelvis tumors (see the section: Endoscopic Intrarenal Instrumentation, Renal Pelvis Tumor). Although rare, benign fibroepithelioma of the ureter is sufficiently treated by ureterorenoscopic techniques, the same precautions and limitations apply for endoscopic treatment of urothelial cancer of the ureter as listed previously for percutaneous endoscopic treatment of renal pelvis tumors.

REFERENCES

Percutaneous Puncture & Catheter Placement

Dyer RB, Assimos DG, Regan JD: Update on interventional uroradiology. Urol Clin North Am 1997;24:623.

Goodwin WE, Casey WC, Woolf W: Percutaneous trocar (needle) nephrostomy in hydronephrosis. JAMA 1955;157:891.

Kaye KW, Goldberg ME: Applied anatomy of the kidney and ureter. Urol Clin North Am 1982;9:3.

Lau MWM et al: Urinary tract obstruction and nephrostomy drainage in pelvic malignant disease. Br J Urol 1995;76:565.

Pedersen JF: Percutaneous nephrostomy guided by ultrasound. J Urol 1974;112:157.

See WA: Continuous antegrade infusion of Adriamycin as adjuvant therapy for upper tract urothelial malignancies. Urology 2000;56(2):216.

Seldinger SI: Catheter replacement of the needle in percutaneous arteriography. Acta Radiol 1953;39:368.

Smith AD, Badlani GH: Special use of retrograde percutaneous nephrostomy. J Endourol 1987;1:23.

Tekin MI et al: Practical approach to terminate urinary extravasation: Percutaneous fistula tract embolization with N-butyl cyanoacrylate in a case with partial nephrectomy. Tech Urol 2001;7(1):67.

Thüroff JW, Alken P: Ultrasound for renal puncture and fluoroscopy for tract dilatation and catheter placement: A combined approach. Endourology 1987;2:1.

Thüroff JW, Becht E: Urologist's ultrasound. In: Lytton B et al (editors): *Advances in Urology,* vol. 1. Year Book Medical Publishers, 1988.

Antegrade Pressure/Perfusion Studies

Ahlawat R, Basarge N: Objective evaluation of the outcome of endopyelotomy using Whitaker's test and diuretic renography. Br J Urol 1995;76:686.

Jones A et al: Compliance studies, pressure flow measurements and renal function assessment in patients with upper urinary tract dilatation. J Urol 1987;138:571.

Kashi SH, Irving HC, Sadek SA: Does the Whitaker test add to antegrade pyelography in the investigation of collecting system dilatation in renal allografts? Br J Radiol 1993;66:877.

Pagne S, Ramsay J: The effect of double-J-stents on renal pelvic dynamics in the pig. J Urol 1988;140:637.

Whitaker RH: Methods of assessing obstruction in dilated ureters. Br J Urol 1973;45:15.

Whitaker RH, Buxton-Thomas MS: A comparison of pressure flow studies and renography in equivocal upper urinary tract obstruction. J Urol 1984;131:446.

Woodburg P et al: Constant pressure perfusion: A method to determine obstruction in the upper urinary tract. J Urol 1989; 142:632.

Percutaneous Renal Stone Treatment

Albala DM et al: Lower pole I: A prospective randomized trial of extracorporeal shock wave lithotripsy and percutaneous nephrostolithotomy for lower pole nephrolithiasis: Initial results. J Urol 2001;166(6):2072.

Alken P, Günther R, Thüroff J: Percutaneous nephrolithotomy: A routine procedure? Br J Urol [Suppl] 1983;51:1.

Cato AR, Tulloch AGS: Hypermagnesemia in a uremic patient during renal pelvis irrigation with renacidin. J Urol 1974; 111:313.

Chatham JR et al: Effect of percutaneous nephrolithotomy on differential renal function as measured by mercaptoacetyl triglycine nuclear renography. Urology 2002;59(4):522, discussion 525.

el-Damanhoury H, Burger R, Hohenfellner R: Surgical aspects of urolithiasis in children. Pediatr Nephrol 1991;5:339.

Feng MI et al: Prospective randomized study of various techniques of percutaneous nephrolithotomy. Urology 2001;58(3):345.

Fernström I, Johansson B: Percutaneous pyelolithotomy: A new extraction technique. Scand J Urol Nephrol 1976;10:257.

Heimbach D et al: Percutaneous chemolysis: An important tool in the treatment of urolithiasis. Int Urol Nephrol 1998;30 (6):655.

Holman E et al: Simultaneous bilateral compared with unilateral percutaneous nephrolithotomy. BJU Int 2002;89(4):334.

Lahme S et al: Minimally invasive PCNL in patients with renal pelvic and calyceal stones. Eur Urol 2001;40(6):619.

Limb J, Bellman GC: Tubeless percutaneous renal surgery: Review of first 112 patients. Urology 2002;59(4):527, discussion 531.

Minon Cifuentes J et al: Percutaneous nephrolithotomy in transplanted kidney. Urology 1991;38:232.

Ramakumar S, Segura JW: Renal calculi: Percutaneous management [review]. Urol Clin North Am 2000;27(4):617.

Rao PN et al: Prediction of septicemia following endourological manipulation for stones in the upper urinary tract. J Urol 1991;146:955.

Schwartz BF, Stoller M: Percutaneous management of caliceal diverticula [review]. Urol Clin North Am 2000;27(4):635.

Segura JW: Role of percutaneous procedures in the management of renal calculi. Urol Clin North Am 1990;17:207.

Segura JW et al: Percutaneous removal of kidney stones: Review of 1000 cases. J Urol 1985;134:1077.

Suby HI, Albright F: Dissolution of phosphatic urinary calculi by the retrograde introduction of citrate solution containing magnesium. N Engl J Med 1943;228:81.

Thüroff JW, Alken P: Stones in caliceal diverticula: Removal by percutaneous nephrolithotomy. In: Jonas U, Dabhoiwala NF, Debruyne FMJ (editors): *Endourology: New and Approved Techniques.* Springer-Verlag, 1988.

Wong MY: An update on percutaneous nephrolithotomy in the management of urinary calculi [review]. Curr Opin Urol 2001;11(4):367.

Percutaneous Endoscopic Surgery

Aslan P, Preminger GM: Retrograde balloon cautery incision of ureteropelvic junction obstruction. Urol Clin North Am 1998;25:295.

Bernardo NO, Smith AD: Percutaneous endopyelotomy. Urology 2000;56:322.

Danuser H et al: Endopyelotomy for primary ureteropelvic junction obstruction: Risk factors determine the success rate. J Urol 1998;159(1):56.

Danuser H et al: Influence of stent size on the success of antegrade endopyelotomy for primary ureteropelvic junction obstruction: Results of 2 consecutive series. J Urol 2001;166(3):902.

Davis DM: Intubated ureterotomy: A new operation for ureteral and ureteropelvic strictures. Surg Gynecol Obstet 1943;76: 513.

Delakas D et al: Long-term results after percutaneous minimally invasive procedure treatment of symptomatic simple renal cysts. Int Urol Nephrol 2001;32(3):321.

Delvecchio FC et al: Combined antegrade and retrograde endoscopic approach for the management of urinary diversion-associated pathology. J Endourol 2000;14(3):251.

Figenshau RS, Clayman RV: Endourologic options for management of ureteropelvic junction obstruction in the pediatric patient. Urol Clin North Am 1998;25:199.

Goldfischer ER, Smith AD: Endopyelotomy revisited. Urology 1998;51:855.

Hauser S, Studer UE: Therapy of carcinoma of the kidney pelvis. Urologe A 2001;40(6):452.

Hibi H et al: Retrograde ureteroscopic endopyelotomy using the holmium:YAG laser. Int J Urol 2002;9(2):77.

Hulbert JC et al: Percutaneous intrarenal marsupialization of a perirenal cystic collection: Endocystolysis. J Urol 1988;139: 1039.

Hvarness H, Krarup T, Eldrup J: Long-term remission of transitional cell carcinoma after Bacillus Calmette-Guérin instillation in the renal pelvis. J Urol 2001;166(5):1829.

Jabbour ME et al: Percutaneous management of grade II upper urinary tract transitional cell carcinoma: The long-term outcome. J Urol 2000;163:1105.

Kapoor R et al: Endopyelotomy in poorly functioning kidney: Is it worthwhile? J Endourol 2001;15(7):725.

Kumar R et al: Optimum duration of splinting after endopyelotomy. J Endourol 1999;13(2):89.

Meretyk I, Meretyk S, Clayman RV: Endopyelotomy: Comparison of ureteroscopic retrograde and antegrade percutaneous techniques. J Urol 1992;148:775.

Nakada SY et al: Retrospective analysis of the effect of crossing vessels on successful retrograde endopyelotomy outcomes using spiral computerized tomography angiography. J Urol 1998; 159:62.

Okubo K et al: Intrarenal bacillus Calmette-Guérin therapy for carcinoma in situ of the upper urinary tract: Long-term follow-up and natural course in cases of failure. BJU Int 2001;88(4):343.

Potter SR, Chow GK, Jarrett TW: Percutaneous endoscopic management of urothelial tumors of the renal pelvis. Urology 2001;58(3):457.

Rosdy E: Percutaneous transrenal ureteroneocystostomy. J Endourol 1999;13(5):369.

Savage SJ, Streem SB: Simplified approach to percutaneous endopyelotomy. Urology 2000;56:848.

Schenkman EM, Terry WF: Comparison of percutaneous endopyelotomy with open pyeloplasty for pediatric ureteropelvic junction obstruction. J Urol 1998;159:1013.

Schwartz BF et al: Treatment of refractory kidney transplant ureteral strictures using balloon cautery endoureterotomy. Urology 2001;58(4):536.

Segura JW: Antegrade endopyelotomy. Urol Clin North Am 1998; 25:311.

Shalhav AL et al: Adult endopyelotomy: Impact of etiology and antegrade versus retrograde approach on outcome. J Urol 1998; 160:685.

Shalhav AL et al: Endopyelotomy for high-insertion ureteropelvic junction obstruction [review]. J Endourol 1998;12(2):127.

Streem SB: Percutaneous endopyelotomy [review]. Urol Clin North Am 2000;27(4):685, ix.

Van Cangh PJ, Nesa S: Endopyelotomy. Urol Clin North Am 1998;25:281.

Watterson JD et al: Holmium:YAG laser endoureterotomy for ureterointestinal strictures. J Urol 2002;167(4):1692.

Wolf JS: Retrograde Acucise endopyelotomy. Urology 1998, 51:859.

Yohannes P, Smith AD: The endourological management of complications associated with horseshoe kidney. J Urol 2002; 168(1):5.

Percutaneous Aspiration & Biopsy

Bodner L et al: The role of interventional radiology in the management of intra- and extra-peritoneal leakage in patients who have undergone continent urinary diversion. Cardiovasc Intervent Radiol 1997;20:274.

Bush WH Jr, Burnett LL, Gibbons RP: Needle tract seeding of renal cell carcinoma. AJR 1977;129:725.

Coptcoat MJ, Ison KT, Wickham JE: Endoscopic tissue liquidization and surgical aspiration. J Endourol 1988;2:321.

De Dominicis C et al: Percutaneous sclerotization of simple renal cysts with 95% ethanol followed by 24–48 h drainage with nephrostomy tube. Urol Int 2001;66(1):18.

Diaz-Buxo JA, Donadio JV Jr: Complications of percutaneous renal biopsy: An analysis of 1,000 consecutive biopsies. Clin Nephrol 1975;4:223.

Ferrucci JT et al: Malignant seeding of the tract after thin-needle aspiration biopsy. Radiology 1979;130:345.

Gibbons RP, Bush WH Jr, Burnett LL: Needle tract seeding following aspiration of renal cell carcinoma. J Urol 1977;118: 865.

Hara I et al: Role of percutaneous image-guided biopsy in the evaluation of renal masses. Urol Int 2001;67(3):199.

Michael JM et al: Angiomyolipoma of the renal sinus: Diagnosis by percutaneous biopsy. Urology 2000;55(2):286.

Sadi MV, Nardozza A, Gianotti J: Percutaneous drainage of retroperitoneal abscesses. J Endourol 1988;2:293.

Stiles KP et al: The impact of bleeding times on major complication rates after percutaneous real-time ultrasound-guided renal biopsies. J Nephrol 2001;14(4):275.

Wehle MJ, Grabstald H: Contraindications to needle aspiration of a solid renal mass: Tumor dissemination by renal needle aspiration. J Urol 1986;136:446.

Stone Basketing, Ureterorenoscopy

Al-Awadi KA et al: Steinstrasse: A comparison of incidence with and without 'J' stenting and the effect of 'J' stenting on subsequent management. BJU Int 1999;84:618.

Borboroglu PC et al: Ureteral stenting after ureteroscopy for distal ureteral calculi: A multi-institutional prospective randomized controlled study assessing pain, outcomes and complications. J Urol 2001;166(5):1651.

Chen CL, Bagley DH: Ureteroscopic management of upper tract transitional cell carcinoma in patients with normal contralateral kidneys. J Urol 2000;164:1173.

Conlin MJ, Marberger M, Bagley DH: Ureteroscopy, development and instrumentation. Urol Clin North Am 1997;24:25.

Denstedt JD et al: A prospective randomized controlled trial comparing nonstented versus stented ureteroscopic lithotripsy. J Urol 2001;165(5):1419.

Dourmashkin RL: Cystoscopic treatment of stones in the ureter with special reference to large calculi: Based on a study of 1550 cases. J Urol 1945;54:245.

Dretler SP: Clinical experience with electromechanical impactor. J Urol 1993;150:1402.

El-Anany et al: Retrograde ureteropyeloscopic holmium laser lithotripsy for large renal calculi. BJU Int 2001;88(9):850.

Goldfischer ER, Gerber GS: Endoscopic management of ureteral strictures. J Urol 1997;157:770.

Grasso M, Fraiman M, Levine M: Ureteropyeloscopic diagnosis and treatment of upper urinary tract urothelial malignancies. Urology 1999;54:240.

Hafner C et al: Evidence for oligoclonality and tumor spread by intraluminal seeding in multifocal urothelial carcinomas of the upper and lower urinary tract. Oncogene 2001;20(35):4910.

Hara I et al: Usefulness of ureteropyeloscopy for diagnosis of upper urinary tract tumors. J Endourol 2001;15(6):601.

Hollenbeck BK et al: Flexible ureteroscopy in conjunction with in situ lithotripsy for lower pole calculi. Urology 2001; 58(6):859.

Hosking DH, McColm SH, Smith WE: Is stenting following ureteroscopy for removal of distal ureteral calculi necessary? J Urol 1999;161(1):48.

Larizgoitia I, Pons JMV: A systematic review of the clinical efficacy and effectiveness of the holmium:YAG laser in urology. Br J Urol Int 1999;84:1.

Lechevallier E et al: Retrograde Acucise endopyelotomy: Long term results. J Endourol 1999;13:575.

Nakada SY et al: Long-term outcome of flexible ureterorenoscopy in the diagnosis and treatment of lateralizing essential hematuria. J Urol 1997;157:776.

Netto NR et al: Ureteroscopic stone removal in the distal ureter. Why change? J Urol 1997;157:2081.

Richter F et al: Endourologic management of benign ureteral strictures with and without compromised vascular supply. Urology 2000;55:652.

Singal RK, Denstedt JD: Contemporary management of ureteral stones. Urol Clin North Am 1997;24:59.

Sofer M et al: Holmium:YAG laser lithotripsy for upper urinary tract calculi in 598 patients. J Urol 2002;167:31.

Thomas R et al: Safety and efficacy of pediatric ureteroscopy for management of calculous disease. J Urol 1993;149:1082.

Zheng W, Denstedt JD: Intracorporeal lithotripsy: Update on technology. Urol Clin North Am 2000;27:301.

Laparoscopic Surgery

J. Stuart Wolf, Jr, MD, FACS, & Marshall L. Stoller, MD

Since the last edition of this textbook, laparoscopy in urology has gone through an impressive transformation. At that point, major laparoscopic procedures in urology were performed almost solely at academic and other large medical centers. The proponents of laparoscopy gushed with support for the techniques, but for the most part their pleas fell on deaf ears. Since that time, some important developments have brought laparoscopy to a prominent position in urology. Hand-assisted techniques have simplified many procedures and allowed them to be adopted more effectively by physicians already in practice. The number of centers performing laparoscopic donor nephrectomy reached a critical mass, such that in order to compete most remaining centers also adopted the technique. Finally, 5-year data supporting the efficacy of laparoscopic radical nephrectomy for renal cell carcinoma, combined with well-publicized support of the procedure by prominent urologic oncologists, has enhanced interest in this procedure as well.

This chapter is an overview of urologic laparoscopy, including the physiology of laparoscopy, laparoscopic instrumentation and techniques, and a review of urologic laparoscopic procedures. The reader is referred to the laparoscopic textbooks listed in the reference list for additional information.

PHYSIOLOGY OF LAPAROSCOPY

During laparoscopy with pneumoperitoneum, the patient is exposed to unusual physiologic challenges. Although most challenges are met successfully with minor modifications of anesthetic management, the laparoscopic surgeon must be aware of them to prevent and manage complications.

Physiology: Cardiovascular

As intra-abdominal pressure increases with pneumoperitoneum, the systemic vascular resistance increases and venous return decreases, which affects cardiac output. The degree of intra-abdominal pressure and the circulating blood volume determine the cardiovascular effects of pneumoperitoneum. A small increase in intra-abdominal pressure increases venous pressure more than resistance, thereby augmenting venous return and cardiac output. As intra-abdominal pressure rises above a certain point, the increase in resistance exceeds the increase in pressure and venous return (and therefore cardiac output) falls (Figure 9–1). This transition point occurs at a low intra-abdominal pressure in the hypovolemic state and at a greater pressure in the normovolemic and hypervolemic state. Given normovolemia, an intra-abdominal pressure of 15 mm Hg is not usually associated with significant reductions of venous return and cardiac output.

The absorption of carbon dioxide (CO_2), the most commonly used insufflant gas, has several cardiovascular effects. The direct ones are primarily inhibitory, but CO_2 also stimulates the sympathetic nervous system. If acidosis is allowed to develop, parasympathetic effects may be enhanced as well. Moderate hypercapnia produces an increase in cardiac output and blood pressure and a decrease in systemic vascular resistance, which counteract the mechanical effects of pneumoperitoneum.

Overall, an intra-abdominal pressure of 15 mm Hg and moderate hypercapnia in healthy patients produces a hyperdynamic state (increased central venous pressure, systemic vascular resistance, heart rate, and blood pressure) without significant alteration of cardiac output.

Physiological Complications: Cardiovascular

The cardiovascular complications of laparoscopy include tension pneumoperitoneum, cardiac dysrhythmias, fluid overload, and venous thrombosis.

When the intra-abdominal pressure is excessive, usually > 40 mm Hg, the rise in vascular resistance becomes overwhelming and "tension pneumoperitoneum" can occur. Venous return, cardiac output, and blood pressure drop precipitously. Volume status must be optimized before laparoscopy to prevent tension pneumoperitoneum at even lower pressures. Brief periods of elevated intra-abdominal pressure during laparoscopy usually are tolerated well, but the pressure should not be allowed to rise above 20 mm Hg for more than a few minutes. Whenever hemodynamic compromise due to excessive intra-abdominal pressure is suspected, immediate desufflation will quickly improve the situation, and the surgeon may be able to

Figure 9–1. Reduction of venous return and cardiac output during laparoscopy. (Borrowed with permission from Wolf JS Jr, Stoller ML: The physiology of laparoscopy: Basic principles, complications, and other considerations. J Urol 1994;152:294.)

complete the procedure at a lower intra-abdominal pressure.

Tachycardia and ventricular extrasystoles due to CO_2 are usually benign, but fatal dysrhythmias can occur with very high arterial partial pressure of CO_2 ($PaCO_2$). Avoidance of hypercapnia will prevent tachydysrhythmias. Since hypercapnia may also potentiate parasympathetic actions, vagal stimulation by peritoneal manipulation or distention during CO_2 laparoscopy can occasionally produce bradydysrhythmias.

With decreases in both insensible fluid losses and urine output during laparoscopy, owing to lack of evaporation and renal parenchymal compression respectively, there is a predisposition to volume overloading. In an effort to prevent this volume overload, however, patients must not be allowed to become hypovolemic. The volume status of the patient should be optimized before insufflation, and then intraoperative fluid administration should be limited to appropriate replacement for blood loss plus a maintenance rate of 5 mL/kg/hr.

The increased abdominal pressure during laparoscopy restricts lower extremity venous return. Mechanical pressure forces blood out of the splanchnic circulation into the lower extremities, where venous stasis during laparoscopy can be demonstrated with Doppler flow studies. It is not known if laparoscopy poses a greater risk for venous thrombosis than open operation, and the optimal prophylaxis has not been determined.

Physiology: Pulmonary, Acid–Base, & Insufflant-related

Pneumoperitoneum adversely affects pulmonary function. The increased intra-abdominal pressure and volume elevates the diaphragm, which reduces both lung capacity and compliance. When the peritoneal cavity is filled with gas by insufflation, the direction and rate of gas movement is determined by partial pressure gradients, the tissue permeance of the gas, the nature and vascularity of the surrounding tissue, the temperature, and the amount of tissue surface area exposed. Gases with high tissue permeance are absorbed readily, and CO_2 has the highest tissue permeance of the gases used for insufflation during laparoscopy. When instilled into the peritoneal cavity, CO_2 rapidly diffuses into the bloodstream. The amount of CO_2 absorbed from the peritoneal cavity during intraperitoneal CO_2 laparoscopy at typical pressures is equivalent to adding 5–25% to the body's baseline production of CO_2. Clinical studies have suggested that subcutaneous emphysema, elevated intra-abdominal pressure, extraperitoneal insufflation, and increased duration of insufflation all increase the rate of CO_2 absorption.

Physiological Complications: Pulmonary, Acid–Base, & Insufflant-related

The pulmonary, acid-base, and insufflant-related complications of laparoscopy include hypercapnia, intra-abdominal explosion, acidosis, extraperitoneal gas collections, and venous gas embolism.

Hypercapnia, an excess of CO_2 in the bloodstream, occurs when CO_2 production and absorption exceed its elimination. Moderate hypercapnia is stimulatory overall, but if $PaCO_2$ exceeds 60 mm Hg, cardiodepressive effects predominate. Cardiovascular collapse, severe acidosis, and fatal dysrhythmias can occur. In clinical practice, increasing ventilation rates and tidal volumes will elevate CO_2 elimination adequately. $P(et)CO_2$ is monitored intraoperatively with capnography. $P(et)CO_2$ runs 3–5 mm Hg lower than the $PaCO_2$ during general anesthesia in most patients. However, during prolonged operations or in patients with pulmonary disease the $P(et)CO_2$ increases more than $PaCO_2$ in an unpredictable manner, and arterial blood gases should be obtained for accurate monitoring.

Additional measures to prevent hypercapnia include reduction of intra-abdominal pressure (which both decreases the CO_2 absorption and allows more effective CO_2 elimination) and use of alternative gases for insufflation. CO_2 is the most popular gas for insufflation because of its rapid absorption (which offsets some of the hemodynamic burden imposed by the pneumoperitoneum and minimizes the effect of venous gas embolism) and its inability to support combustion. Since excessive levels of hypercapnia are dangerous, however, alternative gases for insufflation have been considered. Nitrous oxide (N_2O) is rapidly absorbed, but it has few physiologic effects at the blood concentration achieved with insufflation and is less irritating than CO_2. Unlike CO_2, however, it can support combustion in the abdominal cavity and is explosive in the presence of hydrogen or methane. N_2O used as an inhaled gas during laparoscopy (which should be avoided to minimize bowel distention) can diffuse into the peritoneal cavity, and theoretically bowel gas could be explosive in this N_2O-enriched pneumoperitoneum even if CO_2 is used for insufflation. Both inhaled and insufflated N_2O should be avoided when electrocautery or laser will be used. Other gases proposed as alternatives to CO_2 include helium and argon, which are absorbed slowly. Hypercapnia is obviated, but the clinical effects of a venous gas embolism may be exacerbated (see below).

Laparoscopy with CO_2 insufflation causes a mild respiratory acidosis due to the absorption of CO_2. With gas insufflation pressures > 20 mm Hg, a metabolic acidosis can also develop, likely related to retained acids from the decreased urine output. At typical pneumoperitoneum pressures this usually is not a clinical problem.

Gases insufflated into the peritoneal cavity may leak into several extraperitoneal tissue planes or spaces. Subcutaneous emphysema is the most common site of extraperitoneal gas. Subcutaneous gas is generally innocuous, but since it is a risk factor for hypercapnia, its presence should prompt an assessment for hypercapnia. Gas that is insufflated inadvertently into the properitoneal space or omentum will interfere with visualization during intraperitoneal laparoscopy and is one of the more common reasons for aborting a laparoscopic procedure. Pneumopericardium, pneumomediastinum, and pneumothorax can inhibit cardiac filling, limit lung excursion, or both. If CO_2 or N_2O has been insufflated, pneumothorax will usually resolve spontaneously, but thoracostomy should be performed for a large or symptomatic pneumothorax.

Venous gas embolism (VGE) is the passage of gas bubbles through the venous system into the heart and pulmonary circulation. When VGE is clinically significant, the outflow tract of the right side of the heart is blocked, producing hypoxemia, hypercapnia, and depressed cardiac output. Clinically detectable VGE may be noted in almost 1% of laparoscopic cases when careful surveillance is used. Many VGEs during laparoscopy have been fatal. VGE is indicated by hypoxemia, evidence of pulmonary edema, increased airway pressure, hypotension, jugular venous distention, facial plethora, dysrhythmias, and a mill-wheel murmur. The capnometer will register a sudden fall in $P(et)CO_2$ if the CO_2 embolus is large and an abrupt but transient increase if it is small. Swift response is required, and this includes immediate desufflation, rapid ventilation with 100% oxygen, steep head-down tilt with the right side up, and general resuscitative maneuvers. The type of the gas comprising the embolus determines in part the outcome. Helium and argon are much less soluble in blood than CO_2. This fact argues against their use for initial insufflation (Figure 9–2), but their insufflation (to avoid hypercapnia) after the pneumoperitoneum has been safely created with CO_2 would appear to be safe, because VGE rarely occurs beyond the first few minutes of insufflation.

LAPAROSCOPIC INSTRUMENTATION & BASIC TECHNIQUES

Along with the increased acceptance of and experience with urologic laparoscopy, many of the dictums that prevailed during the first decade of operative laparoscopy in urology have been revised. No longer is it considered necessary that 2 experienced surgeons scrub on every procedure, and no longer is it mandatory that an open surgical set be open in the room during every case (although having it available within a few minutes is still prudent). For those who are performing laparoscopy frequently, it is a more or less routine endeavor, but for the novice laparoscopic surgery is still quite different from open surgery. The instruments and equipment are unfamiliar, and even the basic tasks are initially very awkward.

Preoperative Preparation

The considerations made in the selection of patients for laparoscopy are a bit more stringent than for open surgery. Although any operation in a patient with obesity, previous abdominal surgery, and abnormal anatomy is more difficult than in a patient lacking these features, laparoscopy is rendered relatively more difficult by these factors than is open surgery. In addition, the physiological considerations discussed above suggest that open surgery may be favored over laparoscopy in patients with severe pulmonary disease or congestive heart failure. The patient being offered laparoscopic intervention should be fully informed of the risks and benefits, most appropriately in the context of a comparison to the spectrum of risks and benefits of open

Figure 9–2. Arterial tracing after rapid intravenous injection of 7.5 cc/kg CO_2 (**top**) and helium (**bottom**) in a dog. There is recovery within 1 minute after the CO_2 injection but complete cardiovascular collapse after helium injection. (Borrowed with permission from Wolf JS Jr, Carrier S, Stoller ML: Gas embolism: Helium is more lethal than carbon dioxide. J Laparoendoscopic Surg 1994;4:173.)

surgery for the particular procedure. It is important to inform the patient of the surgeon's experience with the particular laparoscopic procedure, and that conversion to open surgery may be required.

For transperitoneal laparoscopic surgery without intended bowel resection, patient preparation with a clear liquid diet and oral magnesium citrate on the preoperative day is adequate. This reduces the volume of the bowel contents, which simplifies operative exposure and minimizes problems with postoperative bowel dysfunction. For retroperitoneoscopic surgery, bowel preparation is not necessary.

With all of the equipment required for laparoscopy, a logical operating room setup is required. The primary laparoscopic cart (see below) is positioned opposite the surgeon. For an upper abdominal or retroperitoneal procedure, a secondary monitor for nursing staff or assistants placed on the opposite side of the patient is useful, but for a pelvic procedure only the primary laparoscopic tower at the patient's feet is required. Operating rooms with booms from the ceiling that hold the primary equipment minimize clutter and reduce setup time (Figure 9–3). The laparoscope, camera and video unit, working instruments, insufflator, tubing, and the rest of the extensive equipment required for laparoscopy should be checked for function preoperatively or during setup. Adequate pressure in the CO_2 tank should be verified, and a second tank should be available.

After induction of the general anesthesia and endotracheal intubation, insert a urethral catheter and oro-

gastric tube. The operative procedure determines patient positioning. For a pelvic procedure, the patient is placed supine (or in some cases dorsal lithotomy), with the chest securely taped to allow steep Trendelenburg tilt of the table. For transperitoneal procedures into the retroperitoneum, a partial right flank position (45 degrees) without flexion of the table is safer in terms of patient injury than a full flank position with table flexion and offers similar exposure. Subsequent rotation of the table can provide near supine or near flank position. Upper retroperitoneoscopic procedures do benefit from full flank position with table flexion.

Entry: Obtaining Pneumoperitoneum

Transperitoneal surgery usually begins with insufflation of CO_2 to create pneumoperitoneum, with the 2 most common methods being the closed (Veress needle) and open (Hassan cannula) techniques. Either is acceptable as the first choice, but if the Veress needle is the surgeon's typical first choice then the open technique should be learned as well, since sometimes the former approach is contraindicated or fails.

The Veress needle is the quickest technique but is relatively contraindicated in a previously operated-on abdomen unless the needle can be placed in a quadrant away from prior incisions. The Veress needle has a solid spring-loaded stylet that retracts back only under pressure from firm tissue (ie, fascia) to expose the sharp cannula; once the tip is free in the intraperitoneal space the stylet springs forward and protects against visceral

Figure 9–3. State-of-the-art laparoscopic surgery suite.

injury. The Veress needle is placed through a small incision in the abdominal skin at the chosen location of the first port, which is usually the port for the laparoscope. Held like a dart, it is inserted firmly almost perpendicular to the abdominal wall, tilting slightly away from the large midline vessels. An exception on orientation is when the needle is being placed at the umbilical location in thin individuals, in which case it needs to be angled caudal almost 45°. There are usually 2 "pops" of resistance as the fascial layer and then the peritoneal membrane are penetrated (Figure 9–4).

Once it is thought that the tip of needle is in the intraperitoneal space, there are a series of maneuvers to perform before starting insufflation. First, place a 10-cc syringe half-filled with saline on the hub of the needle and aspirate back. There should be no aspirated gas or liquid. Next, inject almost all of the saline in through the needle and attempt to aspirate it back. It should flow in easily and not return on aspiration. Finally, place a drop of saline at the hub of the Veress needle. If the tip is intraperitoneal, it should drop rapidly into the abdomen. These maneuvers assess for the possibility that the needle tip is in a lumen structure (bowel, blad-

Figure 9–4. Insertion of the Veress needle into the peritoneal cavity.

der, blood vessel), but will all be "normal" if the needle is preperitoneal—which is the most common erroneous placement (Figure 9–5). This possibility is assessed by the final test, the "opening pressure." Gas insufflation is commenced through the needle held carefully in place. The pressure should not rise above 8 mm Hg within the first ½ liter of gas, or if it does it should only be momentary and quickly correctable by a twist, slight withdrawal, and tilting up of the needle (which will free the needle tip from omental or mesenteric fat). If these conditions are met, insufflation is continued until the intra-abdominal pressure stabilizes at the chosen level. If these conditions are not met, then it is presumed that the needle is incorrectly placed. Disconnect the insufflation tubing, allow the gas to escape, and withdraw the needle. Persistence when the pressure is too high initially risks extensive extraperitoneal gas collection that will interfere with surgery. We usually will make 3 attempts with the Veress needle, and if safe insufflation is not achieved, an alternative method is chosen.

The most common non-Veress entry method, the Hassan technique, is placement of a laparoscopic port through a small incision made all the way down into the intraperitoneal space under direct vision. This technique is used if the Veress needle fails or is contraindicated, but some surgeons use it in all cases. A 1.5- to 3-cm incision is made at a chosen site and deepened down to the peritoneal membrane, which is opened under direct vision. One stay suture is placed on each side of the fascial incision, and the Hassan port (10/12 cannula containing a blunt obturator, with a conical adjustable sleeve, Figure 9–6) is inserted. The sutures are tied down tightly on the arms of the device, such that the conical sleeve is cinched down against the fascia. Gas is then insufflated. One modification of this technique is the use of a port with a retaining balloon that inflates intra-abdominally and is held up tight against the fascia by an adjustable retaining ring. Another modification is to make just a small nick in the

fascia and insert a blunt port that dilates rather than cuts the fascia (see below). This technique obviates the need for fascial sutures and reduces gas leak—which is often a problem with the Hassan technique. An additional alternative is to use a visualizing trocar (see below) for initial abdominal entry.

Entry: Port Placement

Selection of port sites is critical, because this determines the access of instruments to the operative. The general scheme is to surround the operative field with the necessary number of instruments placed widely enough apart that they do not "sword fight" in the abdomen and with the laparoscope situated so that a good visual angle can be attained.

There are a variety of ports available, with the standard sizes being 5, 10, and 12 mm. "Needlescopic" ports (3 mm) as well as extra-wide ports (18 and 30 mm) are available for specialized use. Ports can be completely disposable, completely reusable, or "re-posable" ports, which contain both reusable and disposable components. The disposable ports have sharp tips that are shielded to prevent viscus injury (Figure 9–7). They are the most expensive ports over the long term, but do have the advantage of being in good condition at the outset of every case. Reusable ports most commonly have a metal trocar with a metal or plastic cannula (or both). They require maintenance but are less expensive over the long term. Most of the reusable 10/12 mm ports are very heavy, but newer models are improving in this regard. Finally, there are the "re-posable" ports. The cannulae are reusable and the trocars, blades, and diaphragms are mixed: disposable and reusable.

Additionally, trocars can be cutting or noncutting. The most commonly used are the disposable, shielded sharp trocars. Some reusable trocars have nonshielded sharp tips. The Hassan-type ports employ blunt tips. There are ports with clear plastic tips, including the

Figure 9–5. Preperitoneal location of the tip of Veress needle.

Anterior peritoneal membrane

Post peritoneal membrane

Figure 9–6. Hassan cannula.

Endopath nonbladed trocar (Ethicon Endo-Surgery, Cincinnati, OH, Figure 9–8) and the Visi-Port (Auto-Suture Co, Norwalk, CT) that allow visualization with the laparoscope as the port is being inserted. The Step system (AutoSuture Co, Norwalk, CT, Figure 9–9) employs an expandable sheath that is inserted with a Veress needle. The needle is removed and a dilating tro-

Figure 9–8. Endopath nonbladed trocar, with clear plastic tip that allows visualization as the abdominal wall is penetrated (Ethicon Endo-Surgery, Cincinnati, OH).

car is used to insert the port. This and other ports that dilate or screw into the fascia are increasing in popularity because the fascia defect is smaller and there is less risk of visceral injury than with sharp-tipped ports.

If the Veress needle has been used for abdominal entry, the next step is to place the first port. This is usually the port for the laparoscope, inserted at the site of Veress needle placement. Make sure the intraperitoneal

Figure 9–7. Disposable ports with shielded sharp tips (Applied Medical, Rancho Santa Margarita, CA).

Figure 9–9. Step System port (AutoSuture Co, Norwalk, CT).

pressure is stable at 15 mm Hg (some surgeons increase to 20 mm Hg for placement of the first port for safety, and then decrease to 12–15 mm Hg for the rest of the procedure) before removing the Veress needle. Enlarge the skin incision as necessary, and using a firm but controlled motion to drive the port into the abdomen. To avoid inadvertent removal of the port during the procedure, anchor to the skin with suture. Alternatively, special sheaths will hold the port firmly into the fascia. Insert the laparoscope and inspect the intraperitoneal contents. Subsequent ports are placed under visual control through the laparoscope. With cutting ports, take care to inspect for vessels that might be injured, by shining the light of the laparoscope up against the abdominal wall.

Entry: Extraperitoneal Approach

The retroperitoneal route is well suited to many urologic procedures because the organ of interest is in the retroperitoneum. The advantages of the retroperitoneal route are faster access to the renal hilum for nephrectomy and avoidance of intra-abdominal contents with associated reduced risk of ileus and injury. Disadvantages of the route are unfamiliar anatomy and a smaller working space. For flank retroperitoneoscopic surgery, a 2-cm incision is made below the tip of the 12th rib and taken down through the lumbodorsal fascia under direct vision. The retroperitoneal space is dilated with a finger, and then a dilating balloon (commercially available, Figure 9–10, or self-made) is used to dilate the working space. A self-retaining port, such as the Hassan cannula or one with a balloon tip, is inserted at this location. Additional ports are placed at the base of the 12th rib, at the tip of the 11th rib, and in the mid axillary line above the iliac crest. For pelvic extraperitoneal surgery, the dilating balloon is placed directly into an infraumbilical incision and then slid down the inside of

the rectus sheath to the pubic bone, where is it used to enlarge the preperitoneal space.

Hand Assistance

Hand-assisted laparoscopic surgery (HALS) entails the insertion of a hand into the laparoscopic field while maintaining pneumoperitoneum and visualization. Several hand-assistance devices are currently available commercially, all of which employ an adhesive or compressive mechanism to affix the device to the abdomen and a locking or compressive mechanism to prevent leakage of pneumoperitoneum around the intra-abdominal hand (Figure 9–11). Early devices incorporated a sleeve, which was placed around the surgeon's forearm to maintain pneumoperitoneum, whereas the newest devices employ a compressive balloon, gel, or disk that forms a seal. These newer devices have the advantage of accepting instruments directly through the device, thus adding another port without the need of another incision. HALS is predominantly used for transperitoneal laparoscopic procedures, because the limited working space during an extraperitoneal procedure is prohibitive in most patients. The intra-abdominal hand is used for dissection, tissue identification, retraction, and control of injuries. The benefits of HALS include shorter operative times than for similar standard laparoscopic transperitoneal procedures, ease of learning by inexperienced surgeons, and enhanced ability to manage difficult surgical situations such as vascular injuries or reoperative or inflamed operative fields where tissue planes are obliterated. Disadvantages of HALS include problems with the devices, such as gas leakage or interference with port placement, physical strain on the hand, interference of the hand in the operative field, and the need for a larger incision than might otherwise be

Figure 9–10. Trocar-mounted preperitoneal distention balloon (Origin Medsystems, Menlo Park, CA).

Figure 9–11. Surgeon's hand inside Omniport (Weck Closure, Raleigh, NC).

required for a standard laparoscopic procedure. With regard to the latter consideration, if intact specimen removal is recommended (ie, nephroureterectomy for urothelial neoplasm, donor nephrectomy, and some cases of radical nephrectomy), then the incision that needs to be made for specimen removal at the end of an otherwise purely laparoscopic procedure can instead be made at the outset of the procedure to facilitate the entire operation.

Some urologic surgeons use HALS almost exclusively, and some never use it. Given the spectrum of its advantages and disadvantages, HALS is probably best used selectively. The most effective uses for HALS include cases where intact specimen removal is required, when difficult dissection is anticipated, early in a surgeon's experience, or for large specimens. Most simple and radical nephrectomies, as well as pyeloplasties, adrenalectomies, renal cyst resections, and pelvic procedures, can be performed well by experienced surgeons without HALS.

Laparoscopic Video Instrumentation & Cart

The standard adult laparoscope is 10 mm in diameter, although 5-mm laparoscopes are improving in light transmission capability. For pediatric surgery, a 5-mm laparoscope typically is used, but 2-mm laparoscopes are also available. Most laparoscopes employ a 0- or 30-degree lens, with the latter providing more viewing angles. Zero-degree laparoscopes can have the camera chip (CCD, charged-coupled device) on the tip of the instrument, which removes an interface and enhances resolution. Currently these "chips on a stick" are not available in 30-degree configurations, and for these laparoscopes a camera adaptor is used to interface the CCD with the laparoscope. Flexible-tip laparoscopes are also available. One or two large monitors, a strong light source with cables in good condition, and the digital image converter (camera box) complete the video apparatus. Still-image and video-capture devices provide useful ability to document the operative procedure and findings. Other equipment on the laparoscopic cart includes the high-flow insufflator and an electrocautery unit.

Laparoscopic Instrumentation

Laparoscopic operating instruments include ones for grasping and dissection, cutting, hemostasis, retraction, irrigation and aspiration, suturing, clipping or stapling, specimen entrapping, morcellating, and intraoperative imaging. Many are available in both disposable and reusable versions. Most standard instruments are 5 or 10 mm in diameter and 35 cm in length, but there are "needlescopic" 2-mm instruments as well as larger (15–18 mm) devices for particular uses. A thorough understanding of each instrument, especially the clip appliers and staplers, is necessary for their safe and effective use.

Exiting the Abdomen

After a laparoscopic procedure is completed, the operative field is inspected at 5-mm Hg pressure to allow exposure of any disrupted small venules that may have been compressed by the working pneumoperitoneum pressure. The ports are removed under vision so that any bleeding from the abdominal wall can be detected. All port sites 10 mm or larger are closed in the fascial layer with suture. The Carter-Thomason Needle-Suture Passer (Figure 9–12) (Inlet Medical Inc, Eden Prairie, MN) or similar devices simplify the often-difficult task of fascial closure. In children, even 5-mm port sites should be closed. Because the CO_2 is irritating to the abdomen and may be responsible for a considerable portion of pain after laparoscopy, attempts should be made to desufflate all gas before removing the last port. Close the port incisions with a subcuticular stitch or wound glue and apply sterile tape.

Postoperative Care

For urologic laparoscopic procedures that do not involve bowel resection, hospital stay can be limited to one or two days in most patients with aggressive postoperative management. Offer parenteral narcotics the afternoon and evening after the procedure. Unless contraindicated, use intravenous ketorolac around the clock (not as needed) for the first 24 h, including a dose at skin closure in the operating room. Start a clear liquid diet postoperatively, but if nausea develops then hold off on intake for a few hours before trying again. On the morning of postoperative day 1, advance to a regular diet as tolerated and switch from parenteral to oral pain medication. Get the patient up to a chair on the day of the operation, and start ambulation in the hallway the next day.

SPECIFIC PROCEDURES

Pelvic Lymph Node Dissection

Pelvic lymph node dissection (PLND) was the first adult laparoscopic urologic procedure to gain widespread interest and acceptance. The technique was initially described in 1990, and most cases in the early series were performed before the generalized use of prostate-specific antigen testing, when PLND had positive results in up to one-third of patients. Due to stage migration, modern series of prostate cancer patients re-

Cleaning port (luer lock fitting):
- Open to clean and sterilize
- Close after sterilization

Pull ring to open jaw

Push ring to maintain needle point

Set screws

Entry holes (adjust the angle of entry and exit to obtain more or less fascia for closure)

Exit holes (should not protrude below peritoneum)

A   B

Figure 9–12. Carter-Thomason device (Inlet Medical Inc, Eden Prairie, MN). **A:** Needle point suture passer. **B:** Fascial closure guide.

veal that less than 10% of patients with localized disease will have nodes with a positive result. This has greatly decreased the number of stand-alone PLNDs being performed. The interest in learning and perfecting laparoscopic PLND therefore has declined. The interest may once again increase in the future, however, as more laparoscopic radical prostatectomies and laparoscopic cystectomies are performed.

Laparoscopic PLND is indicated for assessment of pelvic nodal metastasis from prostate, bladder, or other pelvic malignancies. In prostate cancer patients, PLND is generally reserved for those with a prostate-specific antigen level greater than 20, those with high-grade disease (Gleason ≥ 8), those with clinical stage T3 or T4 disease, or those with suspicious nodal enlargement as seen on computed tomography scan, before definitive therapy is initiated (ie, radiation, cryotherapy, hormonal ablation, or prostatectomy). There are no contraindications specific to PLND other than those general to laparoscopy. Prior laparoscopic hernia repair can result in severe adhesions, limiting both open and laparoscopic pelvic procedures.

The patient is positioned supine, with Trendelenburg tilt, as would be used for open PLND. Laparoscopic PLND can be performed transperitoneal or extraperitoneal (Figure 9–13). Initial access is typically through an umbilical port followed by 2–4 additional ports in a diamond or fan-shaped pattern (Figure 9–14). Key landmarks are the obliterated umbilical ligament, gonadal vessels, and internal inguinal ring (Figure 9–15), with the limits of the nodal dissection being the iliac bifurcation, the pubis, the obturator nerve, the pelvic side wall and the medial umbilical ligament. The distal and proximal lymphatics are typically clipped to decrease lymphatic leakage. Dissection for bladder, pe-

nile, or urethral cancer usually involves a more extended field, bounded by the common iliac artery, the genitofemoral nerve, and the bladder.

Complications are similar with laparoscopic and open PLND. Specifically, injuries to the obturator nerve, iliac and epigastric vessels, and ureter have been reported but are uncommon. Other potential complications include lymphocele, bowel or bladder injury, subcutaneous emphysema, and scrotal swelling. Comparison studies of open versus laparoscopic PLND reveal a similar number of nodes retrieved. Patients treated with laparoscopic PLND enjoy an earlier time to oral intake, less postoperative pain, a shorter length of stay, and decreased recovery time. The disadvantages include prolonged operative time and higher complication rates in some series, especially early in one's experience.

Figure 9–13. Balloon device inflated in the preperitoneal space for extraperitoneal laparoscopic pelvic lymph node dissection.

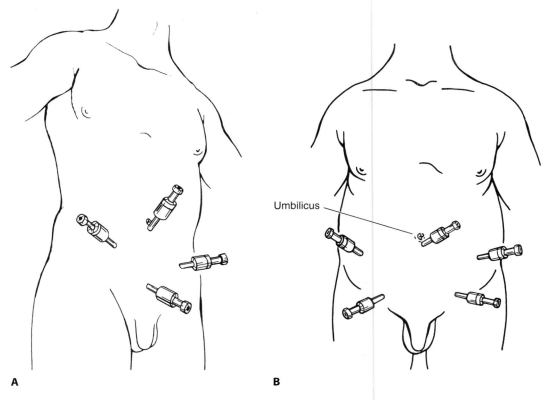

Figure 9–14. Port placements for laparoscopic pelvic lymph node dissection. **A:** Diamond configuration typically used. **B:** Fan configuration for use in obese patients.

Varicocelectomy

As many as 15% of adolescent males will have clinically evident varicoceles. Most of these, however, do not need treatment. Varicocelectomy is reserved for those with asymmetrical testicular growth, infertility, or pain. The laparoscopic technique typically involves 3 ports. The initial camera port is placed at the umbilicus and additional ports are placed lateral to the rectus muscle. The gonadal veins are flattened by the pneumoperitoneum and therefore the artery appears more tubular than surrounding structures. After incising through the posterior peritoneum (Figure 9–16), gonadal veins are clipped and transected. Some series report meticulous dissection and salvage of lymphatic and arterial vessels; others have promoted transection of all vessels, including the artery. One study documents that testicular catch-up growth after artery-sparing varicocelectomy is the same as with non-artery-sparing procedures, therefore questioning the need to salvage the gonadal artery. Outcomes after laparoscopic varicocelectomy are comparable to those with open techniques. Recurrence rates

are 2–15% depending on technique and follow-up. Complications include hydrocele formation and injury to the vas deferens as well as those generally associated with laparoscopic surgery. Unilateral laparoscopic varicocelectomy is rarely performed today due to the refinements in the subinguinal open technique.

Orchidopexy

Laparoscopy has been judged by many pediatric urologists to be the gold-standard diagnostic tool for nonpalpable testes. Although somewhat controversial, laparoscopic orchidopexy has been shown to be comparable to if not better than open orchidopexy in a recent multi-institutional analysis. A laparoscopic approach may be used for intersex evaluations. There are no specific contraindications for laparoscopic orchidopexy other than those for general laparoscopic procedures.

Positioning is usually supine with the legs froglegged. A small laparoscope is inserted through a peri-umbilical site. The first step involves identifying the inguinal ring with the corresponding gonadal vessels and

Figure 9–15. Key landmarks for laparoscopic pelvic lymph node dissection are the obliterated umbilical ligament, gonadal vessels, and internal inguinal ring.

vas deferens. If the vas and vessels are seen entering the inguinal ring, the laparoscope is removed and an open inguinal exploration is performed as would be for a palpable cryptorchid testis. If the gonadal vessels are blind ending, the procedure is terminated. If an unsalvageable testis is identified, laparoscopic orchiectomy can be performed. If a salvageable testis is identified intra-abdominally, working ports are placed and the testis is freed from its nonvital attachments (Figure 9–17). If sufficient cord length can be gained, a scrotal incision is made and the testis is pexed. If there is insufficient cord length, a 1 or 2-stage Fowler-Stephens procedure may be performed. A multi-institutional review found decreased testicular atrophy and a higher rate of postoperative scrotal testicular positioning after the 2-stage procedure. Fifteen complications were noted in 310 procedures, with an overall success rate of 93%.

Renal Cyst Decortication

Although simple renal cysts are common, they rarely require surgical intervention. Occasionally, pain, infection, or secondary obstruction can develop, necessitating laparoscopic renal cyst decortication. Infrequently, a cystic mass may need to be explored for diagnostic purposes. Decortication can also be performed for pain relief in patients with polycystic kidney disease who still have good renal function. There are no specific contraindications other than that for general laparoscopic techniques.

If there is suspicion of a connection to the collecting system, a retrograde ureteral catheter may be placed. A 3-port approach is often sufficient. The colon is reflected medially to expose the kidney, and Gerota's fascia is

Figure 9–16. T-shaped incision is made through the posterior peritoneum to gain access to the gonadal vessels.

Figure 9–17. Dashed lines indicate incisions into posterior peritoneum for orchidopexy of a left intra-abdominal testis.

incised to expose the cyst(s). Laparoscopic ultrasound may be used if necessary to help localize the lesions. The roof of the cyst typically appears blue before excision (Figure 9–18). The roof is excised, minimizing the removal of the surrounding renal parenchyma that can result in troublesome hemorrhage. A biopsy specimen of the base of the cyst may be taken and then coagulated with the argon beam coagulator or electrocautery. Retained perirenal fat may be fixed to the cyst base. Complications specific to renal cyst decortication include worsening of patient's symptoms, infection, or urine leak.

Nephrectomy

A. HISTORY AND INDICATIONS

Widespread interest in urologic laparoscopy was rekindled when the first total laparoscopic nephrectomy was performed in 1990. Laparoscopic nephrectomy has become the most common laparoscopic urologic procedure. First popularized for the removal of benign, nonfunctioning renal units, laparoscopy has now become a well-accepted technique for renal malignancies. Indications for laparoscopic nephrectomy include nonfunctioning kidneys, chronic infections, symptomatic polycystic kidney disease, and tumors. Initially, large tumor size was considered a contraindication for laparoscopic nephrectomy, but with experience tumor size has become less of an issue. The only limitation is the expertise of the laparoscopic urologist. Laparoscopic excision of a level 1 venous thrombus has been reported. Relative contraindications include large venous thrombus, adjacent organ involvement, and widespread metastatic disease.

B. APPROACHES

Transperitoneal or retroperitoneal approaches are used, depending on surgeon preference. Each technique has advantages and disadvantages. The transperitoneal route provides a capacious working space and allows direct visualization of familiar intraperitoneal anatomy compared to the retroperitoneal technique. Transperitoneal access may be difficult, however, in patients who have had extensive abdominal surgery. The retroperitoneal approach allows easier and more rapid access to the renal artery from the posterior aspect and avoidance of intra-abdominal organs and adhesions. The disadvantage of the retroperitoneal technique is the limited working space. Comparisons of the 2 techniques have shown no difference in operative times, cost, length of stay, or postoperative convalescence. The approach therefore is dictated by the familiarity of the surgeon and the patient's condition.

Hand-assisted laparoscopic nephrectomy has been accepted as the technique of choice by many urologists. This technique has the advantage of using the surgeon's hand to retract, dissect, and guide the laparoscopic tools during laparoscopic nephrectomy. A small (approximately 7–8 cm) incision is required for the hand-assistance device, which maintains pneumoperitoneum. Numerous retrospective comparison studies between pure laparoscopic and hand-assisted laparoscopic nephrectomy show similar postoperative pain, time to oral intake, and convalescence. Operative times for hand-assisted laparoscopic nephrectomy are shorter than laparoscopic nephrectomy in some series.

C. TECHNIQUES

Positioning for laparoscopic nephrectomy is similar to that of flank approaches for open renal surgery. If a Pfannenstiel incision is to be used for specimen extraction, it is best marked in the supine position because its location often changes when the patient is positioned and the abdomen insufflated. Sequential compression stockings are placed. After initiation of general anesthesia, a Foley catheter and oral/nasogastric tube are placed and the patient is turned into a (modified) lateral decubitus position (45 to 90 degrees with lesion side up, depending on the specific approach and surgeon preference). The lower knee is flexed and the upper leg is straight (figure of 4 position). All pressure points are adequately padded. The table may or may not require flexion depending on the specific approach and surgeon preference, and the patient is secured. The ipsilateral arm is flexed and secured with a pillow or arm supporter. The surgeon and assistant both stand toward the patient's anterior body wall for the transperitoneal approach.

The techniques for a laparoscopic nephrectomy will be discussed in detail as a template for other common laparoscopic urologic procedures. Many variations on port placement have been used. For transperitoneal laparoscopic nephrectomy, a 4-port "L"-shaped configu-

Figure 9–18. Bluish hue of renal cyst.

ration for left nephrectomy and a reversed "L"-shaped pattern for right nephrectomy is commonly used. The initial trocar is placed 2 fingerbreadths below the costal margin at the lateral edge of the rectus muscle and the abdomen is insufflated initially to 15–18 mm Hg. Intra-abdominal organs are inspected for inadvertent injury. Another port is placed in the mid-axillary line 2 fingerbreadths above the iliac crest. One to two additional ports are placed along the lateral edge of the rectus muscle including one able to accept the endoscopic stapler if one anticipates its use. Depending on the patient's body habitus and relative position of the kidney and spleen/liver, other configurations may be chosen (Figure 9–19).

If hand assistance is chosen, port placement is altered to allow room for the hand-assistance device template. For left-sided lesions, the hand-assistance device is typically placed in the midline and may incorporate the umbilicus. For obese patients, the device may be placed paramedian, closer to the pathology. For right-sided lesions, the device may be placed in the midline or alternatively in the right lower quadrant using a muscle-splitting diagonal incision (Gibson). Placement of the hand-assistance device is dependent on the surgeon's arm length, optimal position of the surgeon's nondominant hand, and the patient's body habitus. Some devices are designed for placement before insufflation, whereas others may be added later in the procedure.

For left-sided lesions, the left colon is mobilized from the splenic flexure toward the iliac vessels, leaving the anterior fascicle of Gerota's fascia intact. The lienophrenic ligament is incised, allowing medial rotation of the spleen. Further medial rotation is achieved

by mobilizing the pancreas, thus revealing the renal hilum. The ureter is identified lateral to the gonadal vein on top of the psoas muscle. The ureter can be transected with a variety of instruments. Following the gonadal vein superiorly will help identify the renal vein. The renal vein is dissected over the aorta to help avoid damage to the adrenal or lumbar veins. One should be careful using clips on vascular branches near the renal hilum because these can interfere with subsequent utilization of the endoscopic stapler. The renal artery is typically found posterior to the renal vein and is transected after securing it with locking plastic, titanium clips, or the endoscopic stapler. Once the artery is transected, the renal vein is secured and transected in a similar fashion. Rarely, if the hilar dissection is difficult and the vein and artery cannot be separated, the endoscopic stapler can be used to transect the artery and vein en bloc. The superior border of the kidney is dissected, either incorporating the adrenal or below the adrenal if salvage is planned. A definite adrenal artery is rarely identified. The lateral renal attachments are the last to be transected, because they help suspend the kidney and ease hilar dissection.

The kidney can be removed intact or morcellated after being placed into a specimen retrieval bag. If intact extraction is desired, a premarked incision is utilized, or a port site may be extended for extraction. For morcellation, the neck of the bag is brought through the port site. Appropriate drapings should be used to prevent potential tumor seeding. Blunt forceps are used to remove the specimen piecemeal, and laparoscopic monitoring is used to help prevent injuries. These instruments are then considered contaminated and are removed from the field. As with all laparoscopic procedures, insufflation pressures should be reduced to 5 mm Hg for final evaluation of hemostasis. Port sites greater than 5 mm that utilized cutting trocars require fascial closure. The skin is approximated with subcuticular suture or liquid incisional sealant.

The technique for right-sided transperitoneal nephrectomy is similar. The ascending colon is mobilized from the hepatic flexure toward the iliac bifurcation. The triangular ligament is incised, with care not to injure the diaphragm. The liver is retracted with a blunt-tipped instrument. If necessary, the duodenum is mobilized medially to help expose the inferior vena cava (IVC). Entering the plane of Leriche directly anterior to the IVC will direct one to the right renal vein. Dissection lateral to the lower edge of the IVC will reveal the psoas muscle and ureter. Although the right renal vein is shorter, it rarely has branches, as typically seen on the left side. The remainder of the technique is analogous to that for the left side, as previously described.

Retroperitoneal nephrectomy begins with the patient in a full lateral decubitus position with similar

Figure 9–19. One of the possible port configurations for right transperitoneal laparoscopic nephrectomy.

padding and bed adjustments. In contrast to the transperitoneal approach, the surgeon and the assistant stand on the dorsal side of the patient. After an incision is made over Petit's triangle, blunt dissection through the lumbodorsal fascia is performed and a plane is developed over the psoas muscle. A dissecting balloon trocar is placed into this space. There are commercially available dissecting balloon trocars for this purpose, or a "homemade" version can be constructed by attaching a glove to a catheter. The commercially available dissecting trocar has the added advantage of allowing the laparoscopist to visually inspect the dissecting process and ensure proper location. This expansion typically requires 500–1000 cc of balloon inflation. The renal artery, ureter, or both may be seen through the balloon's wall. Pneumoretroperitoneum is then created and 2–3 additional port sites are placed according to surgeon preference (Figure 9–20). The kidney is retracted anteriorly to allow direct access to the hilum. Blunt dissection easily exposes the artery, which is clipped and transected. Anterior to the arterial stump, the vein is identified, dissected, and controlled in a similar fashion as previously described. After hilar control, the ureter is identified and transected. Further dissection is similar to that of transperitoneal techniques. Many laparoscopists remove the specimen intact when performing retroperitoneoscopic nephrectomy due to the limited working space. If morcellation is preferred, specimen-bag entrapment may require incising the peritoneum if the specimen is large. The final steps of ensuring hemostasis under low-pressure insufflation and inspecting the port sites remain the same.

The technique for hand-assisted laparoscopic nephrectomy is similar to that for transperitoneal laparoscopic nephrectomy. The hand-assistance device incision is made according to the manufacturer's directions, and 2–3 subsequent ports are placed according to surgeon preference. Dissection is similar to the transperitoneal description above. Lateral renal attachments can be transected earlier because the hand can provide countertraction, facilitating hilar dissection. Specimen extraction is rapidly performed through the hand-assist incision.

D. Complications

The complication rate from laparoscopic nephrectomy ranges from 8% to 17%. Open conversion is required in 1.7–4% of cases. Minor complications include ileus, mild hemorrhage, urinary tract infection, hernia, and wound infection. Major complications include pulmonary embolus; pneumothorax; injury to the duodenum, spleen, liver, or pancreas; and major hemorrhage from the aorta, IVC, or iliac, gonadal, lumbar, or renal vessels. Technical complications are more common during the first 30–50 cases of a surgeon's experience.

E. Outcomes

Numerous studies have attempted to compare laparoscopic nephrectomy with open nephrectomy. Overall, laparoscopic nephrectomy offers shorter length of hospital stay, earlier time to oral intake, and less pain medication requirement with similar complication and cancer-control rates. Numerous studies have documented longer operative times for laparoscopic approaches; however, with surgeon experience, operative times may even be shorter than with open techniques. Studies comparing different laparoscopic techniques show similar outcomes, suggesting that no one approach is uni-

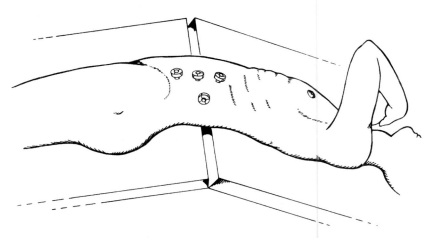

Figure 9–20. One of the possible port configurations for left retroperitoneal laparoscopic nephrectomy.

formly superior. The surgeon should be familiar with the various techniques so that the optimal procedure can be performed.

Nephroureterectomy

Open nephroureterectomy has been the gold-standard treatment for upper tract urothelial carcinoma. This procedure is performed through a long curved flank incision or 2 separate incisions, leading to significant postoperative morbidity. Laparoscopic nephroureterectomy (LNUx) incorporates the benefits of cancer control with less postoperative pain and earlier return to normal activity. Indications include urothelial carcinoma of the renal pelvis (T1–3) and ureter (T1–2). LNUx can be employed for nonfunctioning kidneys due to reflux nephropathy, although control of the intramural ureter is not as critical as in cases of carcinoma. Transperitoneal, retroperitoneal, and hand-assisted techniques have been described.

Management of the distal ureter remains controversial. Initially, the distal ureter was transurethrally excised from the bladder using a resectoscope and delivered into the retroperitoneum. This procedure resulted in numerous reports of local recurrence. Other techniques to manage the distal ureter have since been described. Some perform a laparoscopic nephrectomy and proceed with a Pfannenstiel incision for open bladder cuff excision and specimen extraction. Alternatively, some authors have described transurethral mobilization and cauterization of the distal ureter in hopes of sealing the ureter. Other techniques involve 1- or 2-port transvesical dissection of the distal ureter (Figure 9–21) with (2-port) or without (1-port) transvesical closure of the ureteral orifice. Others have described using an endoscopic stapler or clips to secure the bladder cuff with subsequent transurethral cauterization of the ureteral orifice. Cancer-control rates appear adequate and complication rates are similar to those for laparoscopic radical nephrectomy. However, only short-term follow-up data are available.

Partial Nephrectomy

Open partial nephrectomy is performed in patients with renal lesions and risk for postoperative renal insufficiency (anatomically solitary kidney, bilateral lesions, significant preoperative renal insufficiency) or risk factors for future renal disease. Patients who are candidates for open partial nephrectomy have been treated with laparoscopic radical nephrectomy because of the decreased morbidity. Recently, reports of laparoscopic partial nephrectomy have become more common.

Transperitoneal, retroperitoneal, and hand-assisted techniques have been described. Although the overall technique is similar to that for laparoscopic radical

Figure 9–21. Transvesical dissection of the distal ureter performed with a Colling's knife on a resectoscope placed through a 10-mm port inserted suprapubically into the bladder. After the nephrectomy portion of the procedure and clipping of the ureter, incision (dotted black line) is gradually made around the ureteral orifice (white arrowhead) until the distal ureter can be pulled free of the bladder.

nephrectomy, a few modifications are required. Some physicians perform preoperative ureteral catheterization to help ensure adequate collecting system closure. Laparoscopic ultrasound may be useful to delineate tumor margins and multifocality. The kidney is dissected from Gerota's fascia and perirenal fat, except for the fatty tissue directly over the lesion. The renal artery may be occluded with a laparoscopic bulldog or, alternatively, a loop or hand can be used for localized compression. Intracorporeal cooling with ice slush has been described. Maneuvers to minimize reperfusion injury (intravenous fluids, mannitol) can be used as with open partial nephrectomy. Enucleation or wedge resection can be performed with endoscopic scissors, electrocautery (Figure 9–22), or coagulating shears. Frozen section may be used to assess tumor margins. Biopsies of the base of the resection bed are recommended by some authors. Vessels and collecting system entry sites are closed using manual intracorporeal suturing techniques or with a variety of tissue glues. The overlying parenchyma is frequently coagulated using the laparoscopic argon beam coagulator. Tissue glues and bulking agents (collagen, gelatin, etc) may be placed on the resection bed to help ensure hemostasis. Bolstering sutures can be placed to compress and reconstruct the remaining renal tissue. Once reperfused, the surgical area is inspected for hemostasis. This is a procedure in evolution, and the optimal technique is yet to be determined.

Complications of laparoscopic partial nephrectomy, including delayed hemorrhage and urinary leak, are similar to those of open partial nephrectomy. Port site

Figure 9–22. Partial nephrectomy for small lower pole tumor (white arrow), using bipolar electrocautery to maintain hemostasis in the resection bed (black arrow) without clamping of the renal artery. The intra-abdominal hand for hand assistance is visible on the left side.

recurrences have not been documented. Long-term follow-up is needed to ascertain if cancer-control rates are equivalent to those of open partial nephrectomy.

Modifications to laparoscopic partial nephrectomy include cryoablation and radiofrequency coagulation of small peripheral renal lesions. The dissection techniques are similar to that for laparoscopic partial nephrectomy. A biopsy specimen is frequently taken to document localized renal cell carcinoma. For cryoablation, the probe is passed into the tumor and the lesion is frozen to −20 °C, thawed, and then refrozen to ensure adequate tissue destruction. This process can be monitored by laparoscopic ultrasound to ensure that the "ice ball" extends 1 cm beyond the tumor margin. The probe is gently released after the lesion has thawed. Pressure, fibrin sealant, and gelatinized foam help to ensure hemostasis. The radiofrequency ablative technique is similar. A percutaneous radiofrequency probe is introduced into the lesion after adequate mobilization and biopsy. The probe delivers 50–100 W of energy and is preset to the estimated tumor volume plus a margin of normal surrounding tissue. Temperature at the tip of the probe is 100 °C. After treatment, the lesion may be resected and a biopsy specimen taken from the base, or the coagulated mass can be left in situ. Postresection techniques for hemostasis are similar to those for laparoscopic partial nephrectomy. Cryoablation and radiofrequency coagulation techniques may decrease blood loss and operative times compared to partial nephrectomy. Renal arterial clamping is unnecessary, thus avoiding possible ischemia and reperfusion injuries associated with traditional partial nephrectomy.

Complications are similar to those of laparoscopic partial nephrectomy. Long-term data are unavailable, and close follow-up is required.

Donor Nephrectomy

Approximately 53,000 people await kidney transplantation, but only 15,000 transplants were performed in 2001, according to the United Network for Organ Sharing data registry. Of these, less than 6000 kidneys came from living donors. Open donor nephrectomy has many disincentives, including pain, cosmetic concerns, and a long recuperation time. Laparoscopic techniques reduce these disincentives, and data suggest that their availability may have increased the number of living renal donors at centers that have incorporated this technique. The first laparoscopic donor nephrectomy was performed in 1995. Donors are able to return to their normal responsibilities of family and work after only 1–2 days of postoperative hospital stay. Most centers begin their series with left-sided, single-artery kidneys, but multiple arteries and right-sided donation have been documented with excellent graft survival rates. The positioning and dissection technique is similar to that of laparoscopic nephrectomy, except that the ligation of the vasculature is one of the last steps. The ureter, vein, and artery are circumferentially dissected and tagged. For the pure laparoscopic technique, a pre-marked low transverse incision is carried down to the peritoneum. The ureter, artery, and vein are clipped and transected in sequential order. To optimize renal vein length, especially on the right side, an endoscopic stapler that lays down 3 rows of staples without cutting can be used, in place of the more commonly used stapler that lays down 6 rows of staples and cuts in between rows 3 and 4. A peritoneotomy is made and the kidney is passed to the recipient team.

Many centers use hand-assisted laparoscopic techniques for live renal donation. Proponents of hand-assisted approaches argue that the incision should be made at the beginning of the procedure and utilized for assistance in dissection. Others use the retroperitoneal approach for laparoscopic donor nephrectomy, claiming decreased operative times. Surgeon experience and comfort level will dictate the laparoscopic technique. Laparoscopic donor nephrectomy produces renal units that function as well as those from open donation procedures, with similar complication rates. With widespread use of laparoscopic renal donation, it is hoped that kidney supply will match the demand for these lifesaving organs.

Pyeloplasty

Laparoscopic pyeloplasty was first introduced in 1993. Since that time, it has become a favored approach to treating ureteropelvic junction obstruction by many physicians. Transperitoneal, retroperitoneal, and hand-assisted techniques have been described. Common to all approaches is the need to be well skilled in laparoscopic suturing, a difficult intracorporeal task. Port placement is similar to that for laparoscopic transperitoneal or retroperitoneal nephrectomy. Dissection and reconfiguration of the ureteropelvic junction is similar to that of open techniques and is dependent on intraoperative findings. The Anderson-Hynes dismembered pyeloplasty, Y-V plasty, Heineke-Mikulicz reconstruction, Davis intubated ureterotomy, Hellstrom vascular relocation, and tubularized flap pyeloplasty have all been described laparoscopically. The procedure has been performed in infants, children, adults, and the elderly. Some physicians use fibrin sealant to cover the repair with only minimal suturing.

The largest laparoscopic pyeloplasty series to date with 100 cases reveals a 96% obstruction-free rate with 2 years' follow-up. A comparison of open versus laparoscopic pyeloplasty revealed equivalent pain relief, activity level improvement, and relief of obstruction. These outcomes are better than other minimally invasive approaches to ureteropelvic junction obstruction, including retrograde and antegrade endopyelotomy or balloon dilation. The higher success of laparoscopic techniques compared to these other procedures is based on direct laparoscopic visualization of the pathologic areas, thus directing an appropriate repair. Although endopyelotomy may be successful in patients with an intrinsic obstruction, delayed failure is not uncommon in those with crossing vessels (Figure 9–23). Laparoscopic pyeloplasty is associated with decreased blood loss compared to open techniques. Postoperative pain and con-

valescence are similar to those in endopyelotomy; however, operative times are longer. Newer techniques with fibrin sealant and fewer sutures may decrease operative times. Robotic-assisted laparoscopic approaches may facilitate complex fine suturing. Complications are similar to that for laparoscopic nephrectomy. In addition, fistula, urine leak, and infection have been reported.

Adrenalectomy

Laparoscopic adrenalectomy is the standard approach for most adrenal lesions. Indications include aldosteronomas, pheochromocytomas, Cushing's adenomas, incidentalomas, metastatic lesions, symptomatic myelolipomas, and feminizing/virilizing tumors. Large (> 6 cm), invasive carcinomas are considered by most to be the only contraindication to laparoscopic adrenalectomy. Reports of laparoscopic adrenalectomy for up to 15-cm lesions have been reported by experienced laparoscopists. A complete endocrine workup is required preoperatively to help prevent the intraoperative hemodynamic lability associated with functional adrenal lesions. Hydration and medications may be needed 2–4 weeks preoperatively in some cases (calcium channel, alpha or beta blockers for pheochromocytomas, spironolactone and potassium for aldosteronomas).

Transperitoneal (anterior or lateral), retroperitoneal (posterior or lateral), hand-assisted, and transthoracic laparoscopic approaches have been reported. Bilateral synchronous adrenalectomy and partial adrenalectomy have been performed. The laparoscopic approach to the adrenal gland is similar to that previously described for transperitoneal laparoscopic nephrectomy. Instead of the "L"-shaped port configuration, however, 2–3 additional ports are placed in a subcostal location (Figure 9–24). The dissection can be compared to opening a book. For left-sided lesions, the spleen is mobilized medially while the characteristic yellow adrenal tissue is mobilized to the right. Dissection continues in a

Figure 9–23. Ureteropelvic junction obstruction associated with crossing vessel before laparoscopic pyeloplasty.

Figure 9–24. One of the possible port configurations for right transperitoneal laparoscopic adrenalectomy.

counterclockwise direction. Small lesions may be difficult to identify within the overlying adipose tissue. As one mobilizes the spleen and pancreas medially, the adrenal vein will be seen entering the renal vein. One should be cautious superomedially because the inferior phrenic vein will join the adrenal vein before entering the left renal vein and must be controlled. After one ligates and transects the adrenal vein, blunt and sharp dissection will allow mobilization of the adrenal gland from the psoas muscle and superior aspect of the kidney.

On the right side, the surgical approach is again analogous to opening a book, and dissection proceeds in a clockwise direction. The triangular ligament is incised with the posterior peritoneum, allowing medial retraction of the liver and colon. This exposes the IVC, and the adrenal is mobilized to the left. The adrenal vein is identified, ligated, and transected. Caution is necessary because an anomalous adrenal vein (10% incidence) may be identified connecting to the hepatic vein.

Complication rates from laparoscopic adrenalectomy are 8–29%. Open conversion rates range from 0% to 5%. Vascular injuries (transfusion rate 3%), visceral injury (3%), heart failure (pheochromocytoma), infections (Cushing's syndrome), pneumothorax (< 1%), and deep venous thrombosis have been reported. Subclinical Cushing's syndrome may result in an Addisonian crisis, typically within the first 10 postoperative days. Laparoscopic adrenalectomy offers significantly less postoperative pain, earlier time to oral intake, shorter length of hospital stay, and more rapid recovery when compared to open adrenalectomy.

Retroperitoneal Lymph Node Dissection

Retroperitoneal lymph node dissection (RPLND) is indicated for patients with stage I, marker-negative high-risk nonseminomatous germ cell tumors and for residual disease in patients with stage I–IIB nonseminomatous germ cell tumors after chemotherapy. The open version of this procedure involves a xiphoid-to-pubis midline incision and significant morbidity related to ileus, blood loss, and postoperative pain. The laparoscopic RPLND was initiated in 1992 in an effort to reduce morbidity. The dissection template is the same as in the open approach. For left-sided lesions, the para-aortic, preaortic, and retroaortic nodes are removed. The boundaries are the renal vessels, the medial edge of the aorta, and the ureter inferiorly down to the iliac vessels. For right-sided lesions, the interaortocaval, precaval, retrocaval, and preaortic nodes are removed (Figure 9–25). The boundaries are the renal vessels, the aorta, and the ureter inferiorly down to the iliac vessels. Additionally, the para-aortic nodes between the renal hilum and the inferior mesenteric artery are removed.

Figure 9–25. Exposure of paraspinous tissue during right-sided laparoscopic retroperitoneal lymph node dissection.

Laparoscopic RPLND should be approached with caution in patients with bulky nodal disease.

The patient is positioned in a modified lateral decubitus fashion. The initial port is placed near the umbilicus. Three to five additional ports are placed to optimize dissection and retraction. As with open RPLND, strict hemostasis is vital to identify the planes of dissection.

The dissection is similar to the previously described transperitoneal laparoscopic nephrectomy except that on the left side, the spleen and pancreas are rotated further medially and the descending colon is mobilized lower into the pelvis. This gives excellent exposure to the retroperitoneum. On the right side, the posterior peritoneum is incised under the liver to reveal the superior margin of the IVC, and the colon and duodenum are mobilized further medially to expose the retroperitoneal area of interest. A methodical approach, using the same split-and-roll technique as in open RPLND, is performed. Nerve-sparing techniques are similar to the open approach in hopes of preserving ejaculatory function.

The largest series of laparoscopic RPLND includes 125 patients. There were 2 conversions to open surgery. Other complications encountered were hemorrhage, lymphocele (7), chylous ascites (6), injury to renal and lumbar veins, and bowel injury. Post-chemotherapy dissections are more difficult, with higher morbidity and open conversion rates. Follow-up studies at an average of 3–4 y show excellent relapse-free survival, comparable to that of open techniques.

Radical Prostatectomy

Interest in laparoscopic urologic surgery has intensified with successful laparoscopic techniques for radical prostatectomy. The first laparoscopic prostatectomies, described in 1992, required a mean operative time of

9.4 h and offered no obvious advantages. The technique was modified in Europe and has become routine in some centers, with operative times similar to those for open prostatectomy. The indications for laparoscopic radical prostatectomy are similar to the open approach in patients with localized prostate cancer. Contraindications to this procedure are the same as those for general laparoscopy.

The patient is positioned in a modified lithotomy fashion with the thighs abducted for access to the perineum and the table in steep Trendelenburg position. A periumbilical insufflation port is placed with 4–5 additional ports in a fan-shaped pattern. Typically, laparoscopic dissection begins by incising the peritoneum posterior to the bladder to expose the seminal vesicles and transect the vas deferentia. Denonvillier's fascia is incised, allowing dissection anterior to the rectum in a caudal direction toward the prostatic apex. Retropubic dissection is then performed to expose the endopelvic fascia and control the dorsal vein complex. Dissection can be approached from the bladder neck distally to the apex or from the apex proximally to the bladder neck. The lateral pedicles can be controlled with electrocautery, clips, coagulating shears, or endoscopic staplers. If nerve sparing is desired, electrocautery is limited in this area. The bladder neck is inspected and any necessary reconstruction is performed. The laparoscopic approach has the advantage of performing the anastomosis under direct magnified vision. Robotic assistance may facilitate the vesicourethral anastomosis.

Although the reported data for laparoscopic radical prostatectomy are still preliminary, oncologic results seem comparable to those in open radical prostatectomy. Three-year biochemical recurrence-free survival was 91% for T2 patients and 81% for T3 patients. A retrospective comparison of open retropubic, open perineal, and laparoscopic prostatectomy showed comparable prostate-specific antigen-free survival. Positive margin, incontinence, and sexual dysfunction rates are comparable with those of open techniques. Blood loss is less than with open techniques because the pneumoperitoneum helps reduce venous hemorrhage. Conversion to open surgery is rare after the initial learning curve. Many centers remove the urethral catheter earlier than with open techniques. The benefits of laparoscopic radical prostatectomy as compared with open surgery remain unclear, however, because open surgical prostatectomy provides excellent results. The relative benefit of laparoscopy over open surgery in the duration and intensity of convalescence is likely much less in the case of prostatectomy than it is for upper retroperitoneal procedures such as nephrectomy and adrenalectomy. Future refinement of the technique may allow for better neurovascular bundle and urethral dissection and thus improved postoperative outcomes. Survival rates after 10–15 years will determine if laparoscopic radical prostatectomy is comparable to open techniques.

Cystectomy/Cystoprostatectomy with Urinary Diversion

Laparoscopic cystectomy/cystoprostatectomy is feasible, yet experience is limited. The first laparoscopic cystectomy was performed for pyocystis in a patient with an existing urinary diversion. In 1995, the first series of laparoscopic cystectomies for bladder cancer was reported. Initial reports included diversions performed entirely extracorporeally, but intracorporeal ileal conduit (1995), rectal sigmoid pouch (2001), and Studer ileal neobladder (2002) are now being performed.

The technique for laparoscopic cystectomy/cystoprostatectomy is similar to that of laparoscopic radical prostatectomy, with minor modifications including controlling the pedicles of the bladder with the endoscopic stapler and transecting the ureters. Bowel diversion requires division and reanastomosis as in open surgery. Endoscopic staplers and free-hand laparoscopic suturing facilitate the creation of the urinary diversion. Totally intracorporeal cystectomy with neobladder reconstruction highlights the rapid advances made in the field of laparoscopic urology; these techniques will continue to evolve.

Miscellaneous Laparoscopic Procedures

Numerous other laparoscopic procedures have been described. Interesting examples include laparoscopic ureteroneocystostomy for vesicoureteral reflux, augmentation enterocystoplasty with or without biodegradable grafts, ileal ureter, Boari flap, flank herniorrhaphy, and catheterizable cecal tubes (ACE Malone). Continued improvement in technology, surgical skills, and patient demand will likely deliver laparoscopic approaches into mainstream urology.

COMPLICATIONS

During the first decade of urologic laparoscopy, much attention was paid to its "steep learning curve." Many large reports indicate a considerable complication rate at the outset of a center's series, which falls markedly as experience is accrued. The surgeons in these series were usually some of the first to perform advanced laparoscopy. More recent data suggest that when the surgeons have received laparoscopic training during their residency or fellowship, this "learning curve" is less dramatic. In general, the rates of minor and major complications of laparoscopy are similar to those in open surgery. The intraoperative complications that are most feared during laparoscopy, just as in open surgery, are vascular and viscus injury. The problem in laparoscopy

Figure 9–26. Da Vinci surgical robot (Intuitive Surgical, Mountain View, CA).

is that such injuries may require an emergent change in the approach (ie, conversion to hand-assistance or open surgery), whereas in open surgery the problem can be managed right there. As such, maneuvers during laparoscopic surgery must be more deliberate and careful, not because complications are easier to create but because they may be harder to manage.

FUTURE OF LAPAROSCOPY

Laparoscopy is now well established in urology. Certainly there are many applications for which laparoscopy has not yet reached its fullest potential, most notably radical prostatectomy and radical cystectomy with urinary diversion. In addition, new and evolving technologies such as surgical robots (Figure 9–26), virtual reality, and telemedicine will likely enhance not only laparoscopy but also all surgical endeavors. The challenge for the next decade is not only to continue developing procedures and techniques but also to integrate laparoscopy into urologic practice such that it is no longer viewed as a technique for technical specialists but rather a technique for disease specialists. In other words, rather than having endourologists or other minimally invasive specialists perform all of the laparoscopic procedures, those with subspecialization in oncology should perform laparoscopic oncologic procedures, those with subspecialization in reconstructive urology should perform reconstructive laparoscopic procedures, and so on. In this way the urologic patient will benefit most from minimally invasive surgery.

REFERENCES

General and Instrumentation

Breda G, Nakada S, Rassweiler J: Future developments and perspectives in laparoscopy. Eur Urol 2001;40:84.

Fadden PT, Nakada SY: Hand-assisted laparoscopic renal surgery. Urol Clin North Am 2001;8:167.

Gaur D et al: A single-centre experience of retroperitoneoscopy using the balloon technique. BJU International 2001;87:602.

Gill I, Rassweiler J: Retroperitoneoscopic renal surgery: Our approach. Urology 1999;54:734.

Hedican S: Laparoscopy in urology. Surg Clin North Am 2000; 80:1465.

Jackson C: Urologic laparoscopy. Surg Oncol Clin North Am 2001;10:571.

Link R, Schulam P, Kavoussi L: Telesurgery: Remote monitoring and assistance during laparoscopy. Urol Clin North Am 2001;28:177.

McGinnis D, Strup S, Gomella L: Management of hemorrhage during laparoscopy. J Endourol 2000;14:915.

McNeill S, Tolley D: Laparoscopy in urology: Indications and training. BJU International 2002;89:169.

Nelson CP, Wolf JS Jr: Comparison of hand-assisted versus standard laparoscopic radical nephrectomy for suspected renal cell carcinoma. J Urol 2002;167:1989.

Philips P, Amaral J: Abdominal access complications in laparoscopic surgery. J Am Coll Surg 2001;192:525.

Pietrow P, Albala D: Hand-assisted urological laparoscopy. Curr Opin Urol 2002;12:233.

Shah J, Vale J, Darzi A: Laparoscopy for urological cancers. BJU International 2001;88:493.

Shah J et al: Urorobotics: Robots in urology. BJU International 2001;88:313.

Smith AD et al (editors): *Smith's Textbook of Endourology.* Quality Medical Publishing, 1996.

Wolf JS Jr et al: Survey of neuromuscular injuries to the patient and surgeon during urologic laparoscopic surgery. Urology 2000;55:831.

Wolf JS Jr, Marcovich R: Laparoscopic tissue approximation. World J Urol 2000;18:257.

Physiology

Dunn MD, McDougall EM: Renal physiology: Laparoscopic considerations. Urol Clin North Am 2000;27:609.

Odeberg-Wernerman S: Laparoscopic surgery—effects on circulatory and respiratory physiology: An overview. Eur J Surg 2000;Suppl 585:4.

O'Malley C, Cunningham A: Physiologic changes during laparoscopy. Anesthesiology Clin North Am 2001;19:1.

Schafer M, Krahenbuhl L: Effect of laparoscopy on intra-abdominal blood flow. Surgery 2001;129:385.

Seiba M, Schulsinger D, Sosa E: The renal physiology of laparoscopic surgery. AUA Update Series 2000;19:178.

Specific Procedures

Anderson KR, Clayman RV: Laparoscopic lower urinary tract reconstruction. World J Urol 2000;18:349.

Baker LA et al: A multi-institutional analysis of laparoscopic orchidopexy. BJU 2001;87:484.

Bauer JJ et al: Laparoscopic versus open pyeloplasty: Assessment of objective and subjective outcome. J Urol 1999;162:692.

Cadeddu JA et al: Laparoscopic nephrectomy for renal cell cancer: Evaluation of efficacy and safety: A multicenter experience. Urology 1998;52:773.

Chan DY et al: Laparoscopic radical nephrectomy: Cancer control for renal cell carcinoma. J Urol 2001;166:2095.

Cheah WK et al: Laparoscopic adrenalectomy for pheochromocytoma. World J Surg 2002;26 [epub].

Chen RN et al: Laparoscopic cryoablation of renal masses. Urol Clin North Am 2000;27:813.

Chen RN et al: Laparoscopic pyeloplasty: Indications, techniques, and long-term outcome. Urol Clin North Am 1998;25:323.

Clayman RV et al: Laparoscopic nephrectomy. N Engl J Med 1991;324:1370.

Dunn MD et al: Laparoscopic versus open radical nephrectomy: A 9-year experience. J Urol 2000;164:1153.

Elliot SP et al: Complete laparoscopic ileal cystoplasty. Urology 2002;59:939.

Fugita OE et al: The laparoscopic Boari flap. J Urol 2001;166:51.

Gettman MT et al: Hemostatic laparoscopic partial nephrectomy: Initial experience with the radiofrequency coagulation-assisted technique. Urology 2001;58:8.

Gill IS: Needlescopic urology: Current status. Urol Clin North Am 2001;28:71.

Gill IS et al: Laparoscopic cross-trigonal Cohen ureteroneocystostomy: Novel technique. J Urol 2001;166:1811.

Gill IS et al: Laparoscopic ileal ureter. J Urol 2000;163:1199.

Gill IS et al: Laparoscopic nephroureterectomy for upper tract transitional cell carcinoma: The Cleveland Clinic experience. J Urol 2000;164:1513.

Gill IS et al: Laparoscopic partial nephrectomy for renal tumor: Duplicating open surgical techniques. J Urol 2002;167:469.

Gill IS et al: Laparoscopic radical cystectomy and continent orthotopic ileal neobladder performed completely intracorporeally: The initial experience. J Urol 2002;168:13.

Gill IS et al: Laparoscopic renal cryoablation in 32 patients. Urology 2000;56:748.

Gill IS et al: Thoracoscopic transdiaphragmatic adrenalectomy: The initial experience. J Urol 2001;165:1875.

Guillonneau B, Vallencian G: Laparoscopic radical prostatectomy: The Montsouris technique. J Urol 2000;162:1643.

Guillonneau B et al: Laparoscopic radical prostatectomy: Assessment after 240 procedures. Urol Clin North Am 2001; 28:189.

Guillonneau B et al: Robot assisted laparoscopic nephrectomy. J Urol 2001;166:200.

Henry JF: Complications of laparoscopic adrenalectomy: Results of 169 consecutive procedures. World J Surg 2000;24:1342.

Hirsch IH et al: Postsurgical outcomes assessment following varicocele ligation: Laparoscopic versus subinguinal approach. Urology 1998;51:810.

Hollenbeck BK, Wolf JS: Laparoscopic partial nephrectomy. Semin Urol Oncol 2001;19:123.

Hoznek A et al: Laparoscopic radical prostatectomy: The Creteil experience. Eur Urol 2001;40:38.

Hsu TH, Gill IS: Bilateral laparoscopic adrenalectomy: Retroperitoneal and transperitoneal approaches. Urology 2002;59:184.

Hsu TH et al: Radiofrequency ablation of the kidney: Acute and chronic histology in porcine model. Urology 2000;56:872.

Janetschek G: Laparoscopic retroperitoneal lymph node dissection: Evolution of a new technique. World J Urol 2000;18:267.

Janetschek G et al: Laparoscopic retroperitoneal lymph node dissection for clinical stage I nonseminomatous testicular carcinoma: Long-term outcome. J Urol 2000;163:1793.

Jarrett TW et al: Laparoscopic nephroureterectomy for the treatment of transitional cell carcinoma of the upper urinary tract. Urology 2001;57:448.

Jarrett TW et al: Laparoscopic pyeloplasty: The first 100 cases. J Urol 2002;167:1253.

Johnson DB, Nakada SY: Cryosurgery and needle ablation of renal lesions. J Endourol 2001;15:361.

Kaouk JH et al: Laparoscopic dismembered tubularized flap pyeloplasty: A novel technique. J Urol 2002;l67:229.

Kaouk JH et al: Retroperitoneal laparoscopic nephroureterectomy and management options for the distal ureter. J Endourol 2001;15:385.

Katz EE et al: Bilateral laparoscopic inguinal hernia repair can complicate subsequent radical retropubic prostatectomy. J Urol 2002;167:637.

Kava BR et al: Results of laparoscopic pelvic lymphadenectomy in patients at high risk for nodal disease from prostate cancer. Ann Surg Oncol 1998;5:173.

Kebebew E et al: Laparoscopic adrenalectomy: The optimal surgical approach. J Laparoendosc Adv Surg Tech A 2001;11:409.

Kozlowski PM, Winfield HN: Laparoscopic partial nephrectomy and wedge resection for the treatment of renal malignancy. J Endourol 2001;15:369.

Kumar U, Albala DM: Laparoscopic approach to adrenal carcinoma. J Endourol 2001;15:229.

Kurian MS et al: Hand-assisted laparoscopic surgery: An emerging technique. Surg Endosc 2001;15:1277.

Lund L et al: Testicular catch-up growth after varicocele correction in adolescents. Pediatr Surg Int 1999;15:234.

Meng MV et al: Pure laparoscopic enterocystoplasty. J Urol 2002;167:1386.

Montgomery RA et al: Improved recipient results after 5 years of performing laparoscopic donor nephrectomy. Transplant Proc 2001;33:1108.

Nelson CP, Wolf JS: Comparison of hand assisted versus standard laparoscopic radical nephrectomy for suspected renal carcinoma. J Urol 2002;167:1989.

Nelson JB et al: Laparoscopic retroperitoneal lymph node dissection for clinical stage I nonseminomatous germ cell testicular tumors. Urology 1999;54:1064.

Ono Y: The long-term outcome of laparoscopic radical nephrectomy for small renal cell carcinoma. J Urol 2001;165:1867.

Palese MA et al: Laparoscopic retroperitoneal lymph node dissection after chemotherapy. Urology 2002;60:130.

Parra RO et al: Laparoscopic cystectomy: Initial report on a new technique for the retained bladder. J Urol 1992;148:1140.

Patteras JG, Moore RG: Laparoscopic pyeloplasty. J Endourol 2000;14:895.

Podkamenev VV et al: Laparoscopic surgery for pediatric varicoceles: Randomized controlled trial. J Pediatr Surg 2002;37: 727).

Portis AJ et al: Laparoscopic radical/total nephrectomy: A decade of progress. J Endourol 2001;15:345.

Potter SR et al: Laparoscopic ileal conduit: Five-year follow-up. Urology 2000;56:22.

Rabban JT et al: Kidney morcellation in laparoscopic nephrectomy for tumor: Recommendations for specimen sampling and pathologic tumor staging. Am J Surg Pathol 2001;25:1158.

Rassweiler JJ et al: Laparoscopic partial nephrectomy: The European experience. Urol Clin North Am 2000;27:721.

Rassweiler JJ et al: Long-term experience with laparoscopic retroperitoneal lymph node dissection in the management of low-stage testis cancer. Eur Urol 2000;37:251.

Ratner LE: Laparoscopic live donor nephrectomy: A review of the first 5 years. Urol Clin North Am 2001;28:709.

Salomon L et al: Experience with retroperitoneal laparoscopic adrenalectomy in 115 procedures. J Urol 2001;166:38.

Savage SJ, Gill IS: Laparoscopic radical nephrectomy for renal cell carcinoma in a patient with level I renal vein tumor thrombus. J Urol 2000 163;1243.

Schuessler WW et al: Transperitoneal endosurgical lymphadenectomy in patients with localized prostate cancer. J Urol 1991; 145:988.

Shalhav AL et al: Laparoscopic nephroureterectomy for upper tract transitional cell carcinoma: The Washington University experience. J Urol 2000;163:1100.

Shekarriz B et al: Laparoscopic nephrectomy for inflammatory renal conditions. J Urol 2001;166:2091.

Shekarriz B et al: Transperitoneal prepubertal laparoscopic lumbar incisional herniorrhaphy. J Urol 2001;166:1267.

Stifelman MD et al: Hand-assisted laparoscopic nephroureterectomy versus open nephroureterectomy for the treatment of transitional-cell carcinoma of the upper urinary tract. J Endourol 2001;15:391.

Suzuki K: Comparison of 3 surgical approaches to laparoscopic adrenalectomy: A nonrandomized, background matched analysis. J Urol 2001;166:437.

Turk I et al: Laparoscopic radical cystectomy with continent urinary diversion (rectal sigmoid pouch) performed completely intracorporeally: The initial 5 cases. J Urol 2001;165:1863.

Yeung CK: Retroperitoneoscopic dismembered pyeloplasty for periureteric junction obstruction in infants and children. BJU International 2001;87:509.

Yoshimura K et al: Laparoscopic partial nephrectomy with a microwave tissue coagulator for small renal tumor. J Urol 2001; 165:1893.

Retrograde Instrumentation of the Urinary Tract

10

Marshall L. Stoller, MD

The ability to manipulate the urinary tract without the need for an open surgical incision differentiates urology from other disciplines. Such intervention may be required for diagnostic or therapeutic purposes (or both). Understanding the various catheters, guidewires, stents, endoscopes, and associated instrumentation is key in helping physicians accomplish their desired tasks. Manipulation of the urinary tract should be performed in a gentle fashion; instruments need not be forced. An understanding of anatomy and alternative instrumentation should allow physicians to accomplish their tasks with finesse. The patient should understand the proposed procedure and potential complications. For example, the attempt to place a retrograde ureteral catheter to drain an infected kidney may ultimately lead to a percutaneous nephrostomy if the surgeon is unable to achieve retrograde drainage. Knowing when to stop is as important as knowing when to start.

Many procedures are performed at the bedside or in a cystoscopy suite under local anesthesia. A patient who is comfortable, informed, and assured will more likely cooperate and tolerate the procedure. A physician who is familiar with the proposed instrumentation and understands its limitations and alternatives will win the patient's confidence.

Manipulation of the urinary tract can result in significant injury. Anticipated prolonged procedures should be covered with appropriate antibiotics directed by preoperative urine cultures and sensitivities. Generous use of a water-soluble lubricant and low-pressure irrigation decreases the likelihood of significant iatrogenic infections. Patient positioning is as important as proper choice of instrumentation. Pressure points must be identified and adequately padded, especially when the patient is placed in the dorsal lithotomy position. Additionally, the legs should be secured in their stirrups to prevent accidental injury, such as might result from a leg hitting the surgeon after an unexpected obturator reflex during endoelectric surgery.

URETHRAL CATHETERIZATION

Urethral catheterization is the most frequent retrograde manipulation performed on the urinary tract. Catheters are placed to drain the bladder during and after surgical procedures requiring anesthetics, to assess urinary output in critically ill patients, to collect reliable urine specimens, for urodynamic evaluation, for radiographic studies (eg, cystograms), and to assess residual urine. Such catheters can be left indwelling with a self-retaining balloon, as is done with a Foley catheter. An in-and-out procedure to drain a bladder does not require a self-retaining device. Adequate lubrication and sufficient frequency to keep the bladder at reasonable volumes are critical and must be emphasized to the patient performing self-intermittent catheterization; sterility is secondary. In contrast, when a catheter is left indwelling it is important to use sterile technique.

Technique of Catheterization

A. IN MEN

The penis should be positioned pointing toward the umbilicus to decrease the acute angulation as the catheter traverses the bulbar urethra. On most occasions, the catheter passes without difficulty. When difficulties arise, a careful history relating to previous urologic manipulations is critical. Strictures are not infrequent. Soon after endourologic surgery, urethral strictures can be found, initially at the meatus and 1–2 months postoperatively at the bladder neck. History of a straddle injury may suggest a bulbar urethral stricture. Adequate lubrication injected into the urethra and instruction of the patient to relax his pelvic floor eases the passage beyond the striated rhabdosphincter. A large-caliber catheter of approximately 18F should be used. Narrow, stiff, small catheters have greater potential of creating false passages and possible perforation. Coudé (elbowed) tipped catheters frequently help negotiate a high bladder neck, as seen with benign prostatic hyperplasia. With self-retaining Foley catheters, complete advancement until the elbowed valve is at the meatus or until the urine returns is important. Inflating the balloon prematurely (while it is in the urethra) may result in severe pain and possible urethral rupture. This must be emphasized to ancillary nursing personnel dealing with demented patients unable to communicate effectively, because under such circumstances, urethral rupture may present only after severe infection is evident.

B. In Women

It may be difficult to identify the meatus, especially in patients with hypospadias. Lateral traction on the labia and a vaginal speculum may be needed. With adequate instruction and a mirror to visualize the meatus, women can learn to catheterize themselves. For repeat catheterizations, a finger inserted into the vagina can help to guide the catheter.

C. Difficult Placement and Removal

When a urethral catheter cannot be placed, filiforms and followers may be used with caution; the narrow filiform leaders are stiff and can easily puncture the urethra. Gentle advancement should stop when resistance is encountered, and the initial filiform should be left in place. A second and third filiform, and possibly additional ones, should be placed next to the previously placed catheters in hopes that the existing catheter occupies false passages or tortuous kinks. Eventually, one of the filiforms should pass and coil into the bladder. A female screw mount can be secured to the end of the filiform and used to progressively dilate the narrowed urethra. After adequate dilatation, an open-tipped Councill catheter can be placed over the filiform and into the bladder. If at any stage a problem or resistance is encountered, the procedure should be aborted and a suprapubic cystostomy should be performed to achieve adequate drainage.

Indwelling catheters should be secured to a closed gravity drainage system. For long-term requirements in males, the catheter should be secured to the abdominal wall to decrease the likelihood of stricture formation. Meatal care is needed to ensure adequate egress of urethral secretions.

Difficulty is much less common when removing indwelling urethral catheters, which are usually balloon retaining types. Inspection of the valve frequently reveals any problem. One may attempt to cut proximal to the valve in hopes of evacuating the balloon contents, but this is not always successful. Other options include transperineal or transabdominal puncture, or injection of an organic agent such as ether through the balloon port (with a full bladder to prevent chemical cystitis) to dissolve the balloon wall. Occasionally, a narrow endoscope must be placed next to the catheter in the urethra and an unintended retaining suture cut after an open surgical procedure. Another complication of urethral catheters is incrustation, especially when a catheter is left indwelling for a long time.

Catheter Design

Catheters differ in size, shape, type of material, number of lumens, and type of retaining mechanism (Figure 10–1). Standard sizes of external catheter diameters and most endoscopic instruments are given according to Charriére's French scale (units of 0.33 mm = 1 French [F] or 1 Charriére [Charr]). Thus, 3F equals 1 mm in diameter and 30F equals 10 mm in diameter.

The choice of catheter size is dependent on the patient and the purpose. Large-caliber catheters are used to evacuate potential blood clots. Other catheters are used to stabilize grafts after open urethroplasties, for stenting after endoscopic incisions of strictures, for support of external ureteral catheters, or to assess urinary output. Triple-lumen catheters (one port for balloon inflation and deflation, and one each for inflow and outflow) have smaller lumens than 2-way catheters. Other catheter variables include balloon size and construction materials; smaller catheters have smaller balloons. Large balloons (eg, 30 mL) can be inflated well over 50 mL to decrease the likelihood of the balloon migrating into the prostatic fossa, especially after transurethral resection of the prostate, and can be used as traction devices against the bladder neck in hopes of controlling hemorrhage from the prostatic fossa.

The rigidity of the catheter, the ratio between internal and external diameters, and the biocompatibility depend on the material with which the catheter is made. The standard latex catheter can result in severe reactions in patients with latex allergies, most commonly those with myelomeningoceles. Silicone varieties are good alternatives in such situations. Mucosal irritation is decreased when catheters with a low coefficient of friction are used. Hydromers are placed onto catheters to allow for transient coating, creating an interface between biologic tissues and the foreign catheter; this interface lasts for only approximately 5 days. Permanent hydrogel coatings last the life of the catheter. Decreasing the coefficient of friction of these catheters brings about a decrease in mucosal irritation and better biocompatibility. Catheters with a longer lasting interface result in decreased incrustation.

URETHROSCOPY

To identify and aid in treating urethral pathology, endoscopic inspection via a urethroscope with a 0-degree lens is helpful. Stricture disease can be identified or confirmed after radiographic studies. Strictures are characterized by circumferential narrowing. Sequential dilation of urethral strictures by inserting catheters of increasing size exerts shear and tear forces to the mucosa and is likely to produce extended scarring. Thus, stricture recurrence is common if periodic urethral dilation is terminated. Balloon dilation of a stricture with 7–9F balloon dilators (which can be passed over guidewires and inflated up to 30F with pressures of up to 15 atm) does not exert shear force, but the long-term results are poor. Limited circumferential strictures can

Figure 10–1. Urethral catheters, metal stylet, catheter and guidewire techniques for catheter insertion.

be incised under direct vision with a cold knife. The incision is usually made at the 12 o'clock position, adequate to allow passage of the urethroscope. The bladder then can be evacuated and adequate irrigation used if further incision results in hemorrhage. It is difficult to identify the true limits of a stricture solely by vision.

A urethral diverticulum can be confirmed with urethroscopy. If it has been identified, a catheter can be placed through the neck of the diverticulum to help identify it during definitive open surgical repair. Urethroscopy can be used to inject dye into rare retained müllerian duct cysts, to identify and extract foreign bodies or rare calculi, and to access biopsy-suspicious lesions. Urethroscopy allows endoscopic access to treat urethral condylomata.

CYSTOSCOPY

Endoscopic inspection of the lower urinary tract requires irrigation, illumination (fiberoptics), and optics.

The optics and illumination are offset by the irrigating and working port. To optimize a complete examination, the rigid endoscope should be rotated, and 0-, 30-, 70-, and 120-degree lenses may be required. Suprapubic pressure facilitates inspection of the bladder dome, which frequently has an air bubble. A systematic approach is required when evaluating the urethra, prostate, bladder walls, dome and neck, and ureteral orifices (including location, number, shape, and character of efflux). The bladder should be evaluated at different levels of filling. It is only after full distention of the bladder that characteristic glomerulations and ecchymoses are seen in interstitial cystitis. Rectal examination with the endoscope in place is informative, especially in assessing prostate size and length of prostatic urethra.

Choice of irrigant during endoscopic manipulation is important. There are conductive and nonconductive irrigants. Conductive irrigants, which include saline and lactated Ringer's solution, would be inappropriate during endoelectric surgery. Nonconductive irrigants include water and glycine. Water has a theoretic advantage of increasing visibility, and because it is hypotonic, it can lyse tumor cells. If the potential exists for increased intravascular absorption, isoosmotic or other nonhemolyzing agents are preferred to hypotonic solutions.

Rigid endoscopy results in discomfort, which can be minimized with 1% lidocaine per urethra as a local anesthetic. Flexible endoscopes that decrease patient discomfort and allow for instrumentation in the supine rather than the routine dorsal lithotomy position are popular. They are now used routinely in an office setting, especially for hematuria/tumor surveillance and double-J stent retrieval. Videoendoscopy with flexible scopes allows patients to visualize normal and abnormal anatomy and thus helps them understand their pathology. Videoendoscopy reduces fluid contact to the urologist and can help reduce cervical neck disease. Such scopes have smaller irrigating ports that decrease maximal irrigation and they do not have a working sheath. As a result, changing lenses, assessing residual urine, and repeat evacuation of irrigant cannot be completed without entirely removing the endoscope. Rigid endoscopy allows for a greater variety of instrumentation, better optics, and increased durability.

Instrumentation similar to that used to evaluate the urethra and bladder can be used to inspect continent urinary reservoirs or conventional ileal loops. A Robinson or a Foley catheter placed prior to the endoscope gives the operator a visual landmark and an exit port for irrigation to keep the procedure at a low pressure. Alternatively, the Foley balloon can be inflated and the catheter plugged to transiently expand the intestinal segment in hopes of helping to identify landmarks or pathologic lesions. Endoscopic inspection allows for identification of calculi, foreign bodies, mucous plugs, and eroded Marlex collars and also has the potential for intubation of ureterointestinal anastomoses.

URETERAL CATHETERIZATION

Ureteral catheterization is required in performing retrograde pyelography, collecting urine for cytologic examination or appropriate cultures, performing brush biopsies (Figure 10–2), and placing a ureteral catheter. Other procedures (Figure 10–3) that require ureteral catheterization include draining an obstructed kidney due to either intrinsic or extrinsic compressions and placement of an internal double-J catheter. Finding the ureteral orifice can be difficult. Long-term indwelling Foley catheters, infection, history of a psoas hitch and ureteral reimplantation, or renal transplantation can hinder identification of the ureteral orifice. One must first try to identify the interureteric ridge and then look for a jet of efflux. Varying bladder volumes can facili-

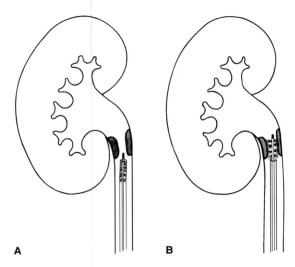

Figure 10–2. Brushing of a proximal ureteral lesion. **A:** Insertion of the brush covered by a catheter. **B:** Advancement of the brush through the lesion.

tate localizing ureteral orifices. Intravenous methylene blue may be helpful once it is excreted out of the ureteral orifice (it usually takes longer than anticipated). Once the orifice is identified, catheters usually are placed uneventfully. However, in the setting of benign prostatic hyperplasia with J-hooking of the distal ureter, previous retroperitoneal surgery, reimplantation of the ureter, decreased lower extremity mobility or other skeletal abnormalities, or edema or kinking secondary to long-standing impacted ureteral calculi, catheterization procedures can be difficult or impossible. An Albiron bridge may help direct catheters and guidewires.

There are many configurations of catheter tips (Figure 10–4). Acorn or cone-tipped catheters are excellent for routine retrograde pyelography. Care should be taken to eliminate air in the catheter before injection to avoid confusing air with a filling defect. Fluoroscopy helps determine the appropriate volume of radiocontrast material to decrease the likelihood of pyelolymphatic or pyelovenous reflux or forniceal rupture. The average collecting system holds 7–9 mL of contrast material. If performed under local anesthesia, overdistention is recognized by severe ipsilateral flank pain. With low-pressure injections, there is no systemic absorption of contrast material. A coudé-tipped catheter allows for dramatic mobility of the tip of the catheter by merely twisting it; there is no need for exaggerated motion of the endoscope. This is helpful in orifices that are difficult to identify because of edema or tumor infiltration.

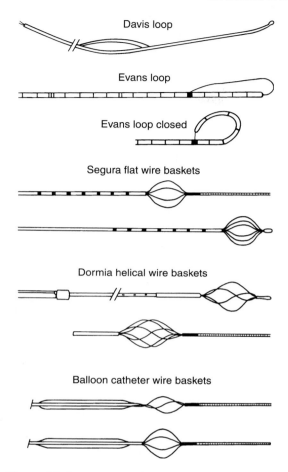

Davis loop

Evans loop

Evans loop closed

Segura flat wire baskets

Dormia helical wire baskets

Balloon catheter wire baskets

Figure 10–3. Loops, wire baskets, and wire baskets with balloon catheters for extraction of ureteral stones.

To bypass severe angulations, passage of a guidewire must first be attempted. Straight guidewires can be made floppy if they have removable cores, and frequently this allows easy passage. At times, hydrophilic coudé-tipped torque guidewires are helpful. If the orifice can be engaged with the tip of the guidewire but the guidewire cannot be advanced, the tip of the endoscope should be pivoted toward the contralateral orifice while the guidewire is advanced through the endoscope just enough to keep the guidewire engaged in the orifice. The guidewire should then be advanced against the back wall of the bladder, effectively changing the vector force so that the wire can be advanced through a severe J deformity (Figure 10–5). With the guidewire advanced, an exchange catheter can be advanced over the guidewire for injection of contrast material, to be

exchanged later for another guidewire or an open-ended catheter. A coudé-tipped guidewire or floppy-tipped guidewire (with a removable core guide) can be advanced through such exchange catheters to facilitate bypassing stones or severe kinks. A push-pull maneuver (pulling the exchange catheter while pushing the guidewire) frequently straightens the ureter as a result of resistance from the exchange catheter, allowing advancement of the guidewire. To increase resistance, an occlusion balloon ureteral catheter can be inflated and with gentle traction can help straighten a kinked or tortuous ureter. Additional helpful maneuvers include deep exhalation, thus elevating the diaphragm, external cephalad pressure by an assistant, or Trendelenburg patient positioning.

Double-J catheters are used to facilitate internal drainage due to obstruction from ureteral angulation and internal or external ureteral compression; they are also used to help decrease the likelihood of sepsis or obstruction in the presence of steinstrasse after extracorporeal shock wave lithotripsy. Double-J stents increase the internal lumen of the ureter. This increase may be used to one's advantage after attempts at ureteroscopy have been unsuccessful because of a narrow ureter. Placing a double-J catheter and postponing the ureteroscopy for a few days significantly decreases the difficulty of the procedure. Double-J stents disrupt normal ureteral peristalsis.

Double-J catheters can be placed over a guidewire or with a closed leading end. With proper placement of the proximal end into the renal pelvis, the J should project in the lateral position when seen on fluoroscopy or x-ray. Projecting in an anterior-posterior position suggests a proximal ureteral location. Proximal J stent placement can be confirmed by renal ultrasonography during placement in pregnant patients. If it is too long, the distal end in the bladder can result in severe irritative voiding symptoms; if too short, it is more likely to advance inadvertently beyond the ureteral orifice into the ureter. In such situations, drainage cannot be ensured, and thus the catheter must be extracted with a ureteroscope or snared with a ureteral stone basket. Patients must be informed that such stents have been placed. Frequently, they will not feel the stent. However, if the stent is left in place for long periods, the likelihood of incrustations, with potentially poor drainage and difficult extraction, is increased. It is unclear whether double-J stents facilitate drainage because of drainage around the catheter or via the numerous side holes communicating with the internal lumen. New helically ridged double-J ureteral stents likely enhance ureteral stone passage through unidirectional ratchetlike motion over the external ridges during respiratory and body wall motion. Additional potential

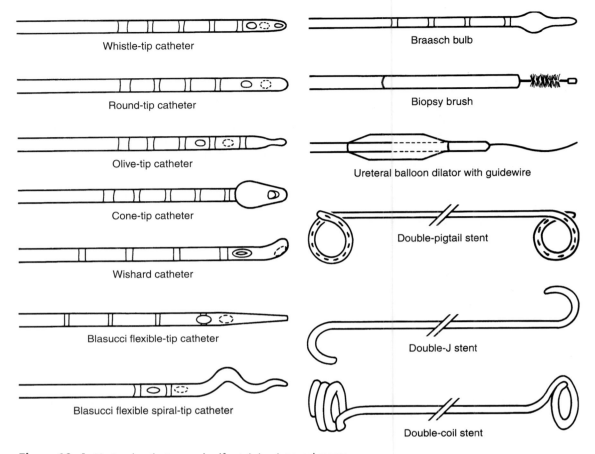

Figure 10–4. Ureteral catheters and self-retaining internal stents.

complications include distal migration into the bladder, distal migration beyond the bladder neck (resulting in total urinary incontinence), and flank pain during micturition secondary to reflux. The catheter can be removed with cold cup forceps via a flexible or rigid cystoscope or by pulling a string that has been attached to the distal end of the catheter and left exiting through the meatus. Although double-J catheters have potential complications, they can help ensure internal urinary drainage.

Balloon dilators can be used to ease passage of ureteroscopes (rigid or flexible; see Chapter 8) and extract intact large calculi. Balloons are routinely passed over a guidewire. Woven balloons have a tight, unfolded outer surface that shortens in longitudinal length when inflated. In contrast, nonwoven varieties are folded and may be difficult to pass after initial inflation and deflation; however, they do not shorten in length with inflation. Balloons inflated alongside distal uret-

eral calculi can result in balloon perforation or extrusion of the calculus outside the ureteral lumen. Balloon inflation is best achieved with ratcheted or torqued syringe aids directed with pressure gauges.

Retrograde endopyelotomy is an alternative to open surgical repair and percutaneous antegrade approaches. After documentation of the exact location of the ureteropelvic junction obstruction under fluoroscopic control, a 150-cm superstiff Linderquist guidewire is advanced into the renal pelvis. The endoscope is removed and the retrograde endopyelotomy device is advanced over the guidewire under fluoroscopic control. After the incising wire is directed laterally, the balloon is inflated during cautery. Successful results are seen in approximately 80% of patients. An internal endopyelotomy double-J stent, 14F at the proximal end, straddling the ureteropelvic junction, and tapered to 6–8F as it enters and coils in the bladder, or a routine 7F double-J ureteral stent is then placed over the stiff guide-

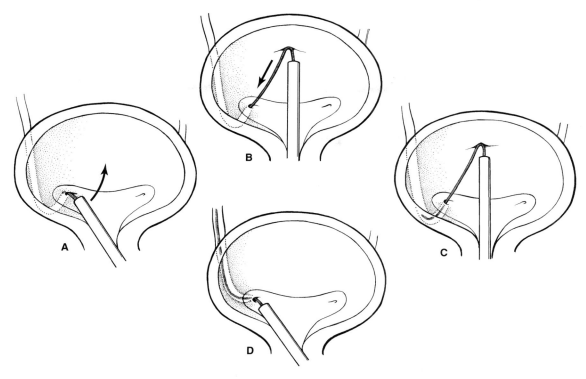

Figure 10–5. Negotiating a difficult ureteral orifice. **A:** Guidewire engaged in orifice, cannot be advanced. **B:** Endoscope is rotated toward contralateral orifice. Guidewire remains engaged in orifice. **C:** Guidewire is advanced against bladder wall. **D:** Guidewire negotiated beyond angulation.

wire and left in place for 6 weeks. Placing a standard double-J catheter before this procedure dilates the ureter and eases passage of the balloon cutting device (Acucise) and the endopyelotomy double-J catheter.

A large selection of endoscopic baskets are available to entrap and remove material including calculi, sloughed papillae, bulky tumors, fungal bezoars, and other foreign bodies. Baskets are designed with and without filiform leaders and can be advanced on their own or, more commonly, through the working ports of flexible and rigid ureteroscopes. Round wire baskets can be torqued to help entrap the target material. A few (2–3) wired baskets are used for large material, while numerous (4–6) wired baskets are used for small or numerous objects. Flat wired baskets can engage stones effectively. If twisted, however, the wire can fold and transform into a knifelike edge. Once the basket is engaged, one should ensure that the endothelium is not entrapped. Gentle traction helps extract these foreign materials. Engaged baskets may be difficult to disengage. Occasionally, one must cut the handle and place a ureteroscope alongside the basket to facilitate stone and basket extraction. Nitinol baskets have rounded tops and decrease potential endothelial trauma.

TRANSURETHRAL SURGERY

Resectoscopes are endoscopes with sheaths of 10–30F (Figure 10–6) designed for transurethral surgery; they allow urologists to excise, fulgurate, or vaporize tissue from the lower genitourinary tract. Applying an alternating current at high frequencies decreases muscular contractions and allows for cutting and coagulation properties. A pure sine wave is optimal for cutting, whereas dampened oscillating waveforms are best for coagulation. It is possible to combine the 2 waves to allow for simultaneous cutting and coagulation. A ground plate, as an indifferent electrode, usually applied over the hip, is required. The cutting current results in rapid vaporization of tissue, allowing the cutting loop to move easily through tissue with minimal resistance, and separates the chip, enabling easy flow into the bladder. Rapid succession of cutting sweeps allows rapid surgical excision. In contrast, a coagulation

Figure 10–6. Transurethral resectoscope. **Left:** Continuous-flow sheath, standard sheath, working element with cutting loop, telescope. **Right:** Instrument assembled.

current results in less rapid vaporization and thus decreased separation of tissue from the cutting current. If a resectoscope does not cut tissue, the operator should check for a broken resecting loop, a broken or disconnected cable or generator, or a conductive irrigant (as with saline) that diffuses the current.

Before endoelectric surgery, the urethra should be calibrated with sounds to ensure ease in placing the resectoscope. Urethral sounds and probes come in numerous varieties (Figure 10–7). An Otis urethrotome can be used to incise the urethra at the 12 o'clock position, thereby decreasing the potential for stricture disease in narrow urethras. Generous use of a water-soluble lubricant is indicated. Before placement of the resectoscope, the loop should be inspected for defects and for appropriate engagement to ensure complete retraction into the sheath, thereby allowing resected tissue to flow easily into the bladder. The endoscope can be placed under direct vision, especially if the patient has not recently been cystoscoped. Alternatively, a Timberlake obturator allows for blind placement of the resectoscope sheath. Most endoscopes require the operator to intermittently remove the working element to allow evacuation of bladder contents. Other endoscopes have an additional channel for continuous operation. An alternative is a percutaneous suprapubic drainage catheter, which allows for continuous flow. Orientation with identification of landmarks, such as the verumontanum and the ureteral orifices, before resection dramatically decreases the potential for complications. Bladder lesions are best resected with minimal bladder distention to decrease the likelihood of perforation. A Bugbee electrode can be used for point coagulation of bleeding points or pathologic lesions. A rollerball can be used to coagulate large areas. Transurethral resection can be used to resect an obstructing prostate gland, to drain prostatic abscesses, or to unroof the ejaculatory duct in select infertility patients.

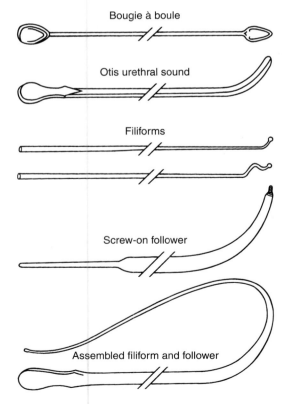

Figure 10–7. Urethral probes and sounds.

Transurethral resection of the prostate (TURP) is a time-tested procedure for resecting prostatic tissue and decreasing symptoms of urinary obstruction. In experienced hands, this can be done with minimal complications. New, alternative procedures are being investigated, especially with patients who are poor anesthetic risks, whose life expectancy is limited, or who are averse to TURP. Those with small glands or with bladder neck contractures have been treated by transurethral incision of the prostate from a point just distal to the ureteral orifices to the verumontanum. Transcystoscopic urethroplasty, also known as prostatic balloon dilatation, dilates the prostatic urethra under visual and fluoroscopic control. Intraurethral coils can be placed in high-risk patients to avoid permanent catheter drainage. Thermotherapy treatment delivers temperatures of 41–44 °C for 60 min. Obstructing median lobes are unsuited for such newer techniques. Transurethral laser ablation of the prostate gland is another method for the management of prostatic enlargement. Long-term studies are required to compare this technique with TURP.

There are various cutting techniques for resecting an obstructing prostate gland during TURP. All require good vision, a comfortable operator, identification of the surgical capsule, and established goals that are met before starting additional stages of the procedure. Pulsatile arterial bleeders should be coagulated first and venous hemorrhage next. Occasionally, arterial bleeders cannot be coagulated without additional resection of tissue. An Ellik bulb or piston syringe should be available to evacuate resected tissue. At the conclusion of the procedure, one should ensure adequate resection and hemostasis, and perform an inspection for forgotten chips of tissue and possible injuries. A Foley catheter should be placed into the bladder and irrigated to confirm unobstructed flow and adequate hemostasis. If an undermined trigone is suspected, a coudé-tipped catheter, a finger in the rectum, or a stylet inserted into the catheter can help in proper placement. The Foley balloon should be inflated 20 mL plus 1 mL for each gram of resected tissue. Gentle traction on the catheter can aid hemostasis.

Video cameras can be attached to the optical eyepiece while transurethral surgery is performed. Use of the camera can reduce the risk of cervical disc disease and distance the surgeon from blood products. It is an excellent resource to improve the teaching of endoscopic surgery.

Acute complications include intra- or extraperitoneal rupture of the bladder, rectal perforation, incontinence, incision of a ureteral orifice with possible reflux or stricture, hemorrhage, gas explosion (especially during resection of a bladder lesion at the dome in the presence of accumulated gas), epididymitis, sepsis, and transurethral resection syndrome. The transurethral resection syndrome is characterized by delusional hyponatremia resulting in possible confusion, congestive heart failure, or pulmonary edema. It is secondary to a large amount of fluid being absorbed, usually through a perforation of a low-pressure system such as the venous sinusoids. If perforations are noted, especially into a sinus, the height of the irrigating solution should be lowered, hemostasis achieved, and the procedure brought to a rapid conclusion. Other complications include impotence (with excessive coagulation) and urethral stricture disease. After an adequate transurethral resection of the prostate, retrograde ejaculation almost always occurs.

LOWER TRACT CALCULI

Most bladder calculi originating from the upper tract pass spontaneously through the urethra. In contrast, bladder calculi resulting from outlet obstruction may require endoscopic extraction. Many of these calculi can be washed out or extracted with the aid of various forceps or a resectoscope loop. Calculi too large to pass through an endoscopic sheath first require fragmentation. Visual lithotrites with crushing jaws or a punch-type mechanism are effective. Introduction of these bulky devices is potentially dangerous. A distended bladder facilitates effective engagements of the stone without injuring the bladder wall. Twisting the lithotrite before crushing ensures that the bladder wall is free from the instrument.

Other methods available to fragment bladder calculi include ultrasonic, electrohydraulic, laser, and pneumatic lithotrites. Ultrasonic lithotrites use vibratory energy delivered via a rigid metal transducer. An offset endoscopic lens is required. Gentle pressure of the transducer against the stone facilitates fragmentation; excessive pressure can erode or perforate the bladder wall. A hollow core with suction extracts the fragments. Electrohydraulic lithotripsy generates a spark-gap, resulting in a shock wave. It is delivered at the end of a flexible catheter and can be applied as single or repetitive shocks. Fragmentation can be performed with normal saline. A rheostat can adjust the power output. A high setting can result in the stone caroming to various locations in the bladder; lower settings result in suboptimal fragmentation. To optimize fragmentation, the tip of the lithotrite should be a few millimeters away from the stone. To protect the endoscopic optics, the endoscope should be kept at a distance. Shock waves fragment brittle material, such as the stone or a lens. Biologic tissues are elastic and are unharmed as long as the spark-gap does not touch them. Air-driven, jackhammer-like devices (rigid and flexible) can be used for stone fragmentation. The photothermal mechanism of holmium lasers is effective in fragmenting very large bladder stones. Uric acid calculi produce small amounts of cyanide gas when fragmented with holmium lasers; no clinical sequelae have been documented. Pneumatic lithotrites are effective with minimal tissue trauma, use reusable probes, and are powered by compressed gas.

ADVANCED INSTRUMENTATION

Lasers

Lasers (light amplification by stimulated emission of radiation) have recently been used through flexible and rigid endoscopes. Carbon dioxide and argon lasers result in tissue penetration that is inadequate for the needs of urology. Neodymium:YAG lasers give adequate tissue coagulation and are useful for various lesions. The holmium:YAG system is excellent for stone fragmentation and tissue ablation and is now the most popular system in use. Disadvantages are the lack of adequate tissue for histopathologic evaluation and the initial cost of machinery.

Ultrasonography

Ultrasound has found increased application to the lower genitourinary tract. It results in minimal discomfort; gives a 3-dimensional appreciation of the shape, size, and volume of organs and disease; and can provide direct intervention. Various transducers are available; high-megahertz transducers are required for superficial structures (for example, scrotal structures) to assess testicular disease (including tumors and torsion), while low-megahertz transducers are reserved for deep structures (for example, guiding percutaneous access for kidneys and bladders). Intervening tissue can significantly reduce image quality.

Transrectal ultrasound is valuable in evaluating the prostate to determine size and confirm digital information on the presence and stage of a suspected malignant tumor. Because of the low incidence of detecting malignancies (1.6–7%), mass screening programs are not cost-effective. Direct needle biopsies, with automatic biopsy mechanisms, are quick, well-tolerated, and result in reliable tissue cores and less pain than traditional needles (such as Tru-Cut) directed under digital palpation. Percutaneous drainage tubes, radioactive seed implants, and temperature coils used for cryosurgery of the prostate can be placed safely under transrectal ultrasonic guidance. Transrectal ultrasonography can yield unreliable images that often are misinterpreted by the novice. Pitfalls include faulty instrument settings, poor coupling caused by feces or gas, and unrecognized artifacts resulting from reverberation, deflection, shadowing, or enhancement.

Suprapubic ultrasonography can help to assess prostate anatomy, especially size and intravesical extension. It can help to evaluate the bladder for residual urine and for calculi that are questionable on plain abdominal radiographs. (Changing the patient's position can shift the position of a calculus.) Distal ureteral stones can be identified, especially when visualized through a full bladder used as an acoustic window. Double-J stents, incrustations, diverticula, and large malignant lesions can be identified. The procedure also can direct placement of suprapubic cystostomy drainage catheters.

Additional applications include endocavitary, color, Doppler, and dynamic ultrasonography. Endocavitary

Figure 10–8. Multifocal bladder cancer. **Left:** Transurethral ultrasound. **Right:** Cystectomy specimen.

ultrasound, which includes transvaginal, transurethral (Figure 10–8), and transcystoscopic techniques, can delineate vaginal, urethral, and bladder disease. Endoureteral ultrasound can help in the identification of crossing vessels, preferably before an endopyelotomy. Color and Doppler ultrasound can assess blood flow as related to erectile dysfunction. Dynamic ultrasound can supplement urodynamic findings. Ultrasound applied to the lower genitourinary tract causes minimal discomfort and provides valuable information.

REFERENCES

Urethral Catheterization Cystoscopy

Berci G: Instrumentation 1: Rigid endoscopes. In: Berci G (editor): *Endoscopy.* Appleton-Century-Crofts, 1976.

Berci G: Instrumentation 2: Flexible fiber endoscopes. In: Berci G (editor): *Endoscopy.* Appleton-Century-Crofts, 1976.

Bloom DA, McGuire EJ, Lapides J: A brief history of urethral catheterization. J Urol 1994;151:317.

Brocklehurst JC: The management of indwelling catheters. Br J Urol 1978;50:102.

Choong S et al: A prospective, randomized, double-blind study comparing lignocaine gel and plain lubricating gel in relieving pain during flexible cystoscopy. Br J Urol 1997;80:69.

Clayman RV, Reddy P, Lange PH: Flexible fiberoptic and rigid-rod lens endoscopy of the lower urinary tract: A prospective controlled comparison. J Urol 1984;131:715.

Cox CE, Hinman F Jr: Experiments with induced bacteriuria, vesical emptying and bacterial growth on the mechanism of bladder defense to infection. J Urol 1961;86:739.

Fuselier HA Jr, Mason C: Liquid sterilization versus high level disinfection in the urologic office. Urology 1997;50:337.

Koss EH, Schneiderman JJ: Entry of bacteria in urinary tracts of patients with in-lying catheter. N Engl J Med 1957;256:556.

Lapides J et al: Clean, intermittent self-catheterization in the treatment of urinary tract disease. J Urol 1972;107:458.

Madsen FA, Bruskewitz RC: Cystoscopy in the evaluation of benign prostatic hyperplasia. World J Urol 1995;13:14.

Simonato A, Galli S, Carmignani G: Simple, safe and inexpensive retrieval of JJ stents with a flexible cystoscope. Br J Urol 1998;81:490.

Williams JC et al: Deflation techniques for faulty Foley catheter balloons: Presentation of a cystoscopic technique. Tech Urol 1996;2:174.

Transrectal & Transurethral Ultrasound

Hernandez AD, Smith JA Jr: Transrectal ultrasonography for the early detection and staging of prostate cancer. Urol Clin North Am 1990;17:45.

Nash PA et al: Sono-urethrography in the evaluation of anterior urethral strictures. J Urol 1995;154:72.

Rickards D: Transrectal ultrasound 1992. Br J Urol 1992;69:449.

Ureteral Catheterization

Bigongiari LR: Transluminal dilatation of ureteral strictures. In: Lang EK (editor): *Percutaneous and Interventional Urology and Radiology.* Springer-Verlag, 1986.

Finney RP: Double-J and diversion stents. Urol Clin North Am 1982;9:89.

Fritzche PJ: Antegrade and retrograde ureteral stenting. In: Lang EK (editor): *Percutaneous and Interventional Urology and Radiology.* Springer-Verlag, 1986.

Gibbons RP et al: Experience with indwelling ureteral stent catheters. J Urol 1976;115:22.

Huffman JL, Bagley DH, Lyon ES: Ureteral catheterization, retrograde ureteropyelography and self retaining ureteral stents. In: Bagley DH, Huffman JL, Lyon ES (editors): *Urologic Endoscopy: A Manual and Atlas.* Little, Brown, 1985.

Irby PI et al: Long term followup of ventriculoureteral shunts for the treatment of hydrocephalus. Urology 1993;42:193.

Mardis HK, Hepperlen TW, Kammandel H: Double pigtail ureteral stent. Urology 1979;14:23.

Oswalt GC Jr, Bueschen AJ, Lloyd IK: Upward migration of indwelling ureteral stents. J Urol 1979;122:249.

Phan CN, Stoller ML: Helically ridged ureteral stent facilitates the passage of stone fragments in an experimental porcine model. Br J Urol 1993;72:17.

Ramsay JWA et al: The effects of double J stenting on unobstructed ureters: An experimental and clinical study. Br J Urol 1985;57:630.

Stone Basketing, Ureterorenoscopy

Abdelsayed M, Onal E, Wax SH: Avulsion of the ureter caused by stone basket manipulation. J Urol 1977;118:868.

Aslan P, Malloy B, Preminger GM: Access to the distal ureter after failure of direct visual ureteroscopy. Br J Urol 1998;82:290.

Dourmashkin RL: Cystoscopic treatment of stones in the ureter with special reference to large calculi: Based on a study of 1550 cases. J Urol 1945;54:245.

Fabrizio MD, Behari A, Bagley DH: Ureteroscopic management of intrarenal calculi. J Urol 1998;159:1139.

Hofmann R, Hartung R: Laser-induced shock-wave lithotripsy of ureteric calculi. World J Urol 1989;7:142.

Low RK, Stoller ML: Endoscopic mapping of renal papillae for Randall's plaques in patients with urinary stone disease. J Urol 1997;158:2062.

Perez-Castro Ellendt E, Martinez-Pineiro JA: Ureteral and renal endoscopy: A new approach. Eur Urol 1982;8:117.

Rutner AB: Ureteral balloon dilatation and stone basketing. Urology 1985;23(5 Spec No.):44.

Rutner AB, Fucilla IS: An improved helical stone basket. J Urol 1976;116:784.

Schwartz BA, Wise HA II: Endourologic techniques for the bladder and urethra. Urol Clin North Am 1982;9:165.

Shihata AA, Greene JE: Ureteric stone extraction by a new double-balloon catheter: An experimental study. J Urol 1983;129:616.

Stoller ML et al: Endoscopic management of upper tract urothelial tumors. Tech Urol 1997;3:1.

Wolf JS Jr, Carroll PR, Stoller ML: Cost-effectiveness v patient preference in the choice of treatment for distal ureteral calculi: A literature-based decision analysis. J Endourol 1995; 9:243.

Cytology, Biopsy Histology

Barry JM et al: The influence of retrograde contrast medium on urinary cytodiagnosis: A preliminary report. J Urol 1978; 119:633.

Crawford ED et al: Prevention of urinary tract infection and sepsis following transrectal prostatic biopsy. J Urol 1982;127:449.

Dodd LG et al: Endoscopic brush cytology of the upper urinary tract: Evaluation of its efficacy and potential limitations in diagnosis. Acta Cytol 1997;41:377.

Epsoti PL: Cytologic malignancy grading for prostatic carcinoma for transurethral aspiration biopsy. Scand J Urol Nephrol 1971;5:199.

Epstein NA: Prostatic biopsy: A morphologic correlation of aspiration cytology with needle biopsy histology. Cancer 1976; 38:2078.

Gill WB, Lu C, Bibbo M: Retrograde brush biopsy of the ureter and renal pelvis. Urol Clin North Am 1979;6:573.

Lieberman RP, Cummins KB, Leslie SW: Sheathed catheter system for fluoroscopically guided retrograde catheterization, and brush and forceps biopsy of the upper urinary tract. J Urol 1984;131:450.

Endoscopy

Hopkins HH: The modern urological endoscope. In: *A Handbook of Urological Endoscopy.* Churchill Livingstone, 1978.

Merkle EM et al: Virtual cystoscopy based on helical CT scan datasets: Perspectives and limitations. Br J Radiol 1998; 71:262.

Nicholson P: Problems encountered by early endoscopists. Urology 1982;19:114.

Reuter MA, Reuter HJ: The development of the cystoscope. J Urol 1998;159:638.

Lithotripsy

Bapat SS: Endoscopic removal of bladder stones in adults. Br J Urol 1977;49:527.

Bigelow HJ: Lithotripsy by a single operation. Am J Med Sci 1978; 75:117.

Reuter HJ: Electronic lithotripsy: Transurethral treatment of bladder stones in 50 cases. J Urol 1970;104:834.

Vassar GJ, Teichman JM, Glickman RD: Holmium:YAG lithotripsy efficiency varies with energy density. J Urol 1998; 160:471.

Urinary Obstruction & Stasis

Emil A. Tanagho, MD

Because of their damaging effect on renal function, obstruction and stasis of urinary flow are among the most important of urologic disorders. Either leads eventually to hydronephrosis, a peculiar type of atrophy of the kidney that may terminate in renal insufficiency or, if unilateral, complete destruction of the organ. Furthermore, obstruction leads to infection, which causes additional damage to the organs involved.

Classification

Obstruction may be classified according to cause (congenital or acquired), duration (acute or chronic), degree (partial or complete), and level (upper or lower urinary tract).

Etiology

Congenital anomalies, more common in the urinary tract than in any other organ system, are generally obstructive. In adult life, many types of acquired obstruction can occur.

A. CONGENITAL

The common sites of congenital narrowing are the external meatus in boys (meatal stenosis) or just inside the external urinary meatus in girls, the distal urethra (stenosis), posterior urethral valves, ectopic ureters, ureteroceles, and the ureterovesical and ureteropelvic junctions. Another congenital cause of urinary stasis is damage to sacral roots 2–4 as seen in spina bifida and myelomeningocele. Vesicoureteral reflux causes both vesical and renal stasis (see Chapter 12).

B. ACQUIRED

Acquired obstructions are numerous and may be primary in the urinary tract or secondary to retroperitoneal lesions that invade or compress the urinary passages. Among the common causes are (1) urethral stricture secondary to infection or injury; (2) benign prostatic hyperplasia or cancer of the prostate; (3) vesical tumor involving the bladder neck or one or both ureteral orifices; (4) local extension of cancer of the prostate or cervix into the base of the bladder, occluding the ureters; (5) compression of the ureters at the pelvic brim by metastatic nodes from cancer of the

prostate or cervix; (6) ureteral stone; (7) retroperitoneal fibrosis or malignant tumor; and (8) pregnancy.

Neurogenic dysfunction affects principally the bladder. The upper tracts are damaged secondarily by ureterovesical obstruction or reflux and, often, complicating infection. Severe constipation, especially in children, can cause bilateral hydroureteronephrosis from compression of the lower ureters.

Elongation and kinking of the ureter secondary to vesicoureteral reflux commonly lead to ureteropelvic obstruction and hydronephrosis. Unless a voiding cystourethrogram is obtained in children with this lesion, the primary cause may be missed and improper treatment given.

Pathogenesis & Pathology

Obstruction and neuropathic vesical dysfunction have the same effects on the urinary tract. These changes can best be understood by considering (1) the effects on the lower tract (distal to the bladder neck) of severe external urinary meatal stricture and (2) the effects on the mid tract (bladder) and upper tract (ureter and kidney) of benign prostatic hyperplasia.

A. LOWER TRACT (EG, URETHRAL STRICTURE)

Hydrostatic pressure proximal to the obstruction causes dilation of the urethra. The wall of the urethra may become thin, and a diverticulum may form. If the urine becomes infected, urinary extravasation may occur, and periurethral abscess can result. The prostatic ducts may become widely dilated.

B. MID TRACT (EG, PROSTATIC HYPERPLASIA)

In the earlier stages (compensatory phase), the muscle wall of the bladder becomes hypertrophied and thickened. With decompensation, it becomes less contractile and, therefore, weakened.

1. Stage of compensation—To balance the increasing outlet resistance, the bladder musculature hypertrophies. Its thickness may double or triple. Complete emptying of the bladder is thus made possible.

Hypertrophied muscle may be seen microscopically. With secondary infection, the effects of infection are often superimposed. There may be edema of the submucosa, which may be infiltrated with plasma cells, lymphocytes, and polymorphonuclear cells.

At cystoscopy, surgery, or autopsy, the following evidence of this compensation may be visible (Figure 11–1):

a. Trabeculation of the bladder wall—The wall of the distended bladder is normally quite smooth. With hypertrophy, individual muscle bundles become taut and give a coarsely interwoven appearance to the mucosal surface. The trigonal muscle and the interureteric ridge, which normally are only slightly raised above the surrounding tissues, respond to obstruction by hypertrophy of their smooth musculature. The ridge then becomes prominent. This trigonal hypertrophy causes increased resistance to urine flow in the intravesical ureteral segments owing to accentuated downward pull on them. It is this mechanism that causes relative functional obstruction of the ureterovesical junctions, leading to back pressure on the kidney and hydroureteronephrosis. The obstruction increases in the presence of significant residual urine, which further stretches the ureterotrigonal complex. (A urethral catheter relieves the obstruction somewhat by eliminating the trigonal stretch. Definitive prostatectomy leads to permanent release of stretch and gradual softening of trigonal hypertrophy with relief of the obstruction.)

b. Cellules—Normal intravesical pressure is about 30 cm of water at the beginning of micturition. Pressures 2–4 times as great may be reached by the trabeculated (hypertrophied) bladder in its attempt to force urine past the obstruction. This pressure tends to push mucosa between the superficial muscle bundles, causing the formation of small pockets, or cellules (Figure 11–1).

c. Diverticula—If cellules force their way entirely through the musculature of the bladder wall, they become saccules, then actual diverticula, which may be embedded in perivesical fat or covered by peritoneum, depending on their location. Diverticula have no muscle wall and are therefore unable to expel their contents into the bladder efficiently even after the primary obstruction has been removed. When secondary infection occurs, it is difficult to eradicate; surgical removal of the diverticula may be required. If a diverticulum pushes through the bladder wall on the anterior surface of the ureter, the ureterovesical junction will become incompetent (see Chapter 12).

d. Mucosa—In the presence of acute infection, the mucosa may be reddened and edematous. This may lead to temporary vesicoureteral reflux in the presence of a "borderline" junction. The chronically inflamed membrane may be thinned and pale. In the absence of infection, the mucosa appears normal.

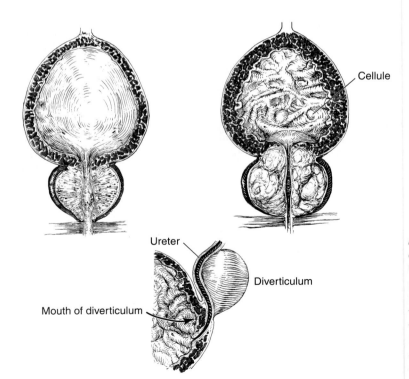

Ureter

Diverticulum

Mouth of diverticulum

Figure 11–1. Changes in the bladder developing from obstruction. **Upper left:** Normal bladder and prostate. **Upper right:** Obstructing prostate causing trabeculation, cellule formation, and hypertrophy of the interureteric ridge. **Bottom:** Marked trabeculation (hypertrophy) of the vesical musculature; diverticulum displacing left ureter.

Cellule

2. Stage of decompensation—The compensatory power of the bladder musculature varies greatly. One patient with prostatic enlargement may have only mild symptoms of prostatism but a large obstructing gland that can be palpated rectally and observed cystoscopically; another may suffer acute retention and yet have a gland of normal size on rectal palpation and what appears to be only a mild obstruction cystoscopically.

In the face of progressive outlet obstruction, possibly aggravated by prostatic infection with edema or by congestion from lack of intercourse, decompensation of the detrusor may occur, resulting in the presence of residual urine after voiding. The amount may range up to 500 mL or more.

C. UPPER TRACT

1. Ureter—In the early stages of obstruction, intravesical pressure is normal while the bladder fills and is increased only during voiding. The pressure is not transmitted to the ureters and renal pelves because of the competence of the ureterovesical "valves." (A true valve is not present; the ureterotrigonal unit, by virtue of its intrinsic structure, resists the retrograde flow of urine.) However, owing to trigonal hypertrophy (see the section Trabeculation of the Bladder Wall) and to the resultant increase in resistance to urine flow across the terminal ureter, there is progressive back pressure on the ureter and kidney, resulting in ureteral dilatation and hydronephrosis. Later, with the phase of decompensation accompanied by residual urine, there is an added stretch effect on the already hypertrophied trigone that increases appreciably the resistance to flow at the lower end of the ureter and induces further hydroureteronephrosis. With decompensation of the ureterotrigonal complex, the valvelike action may be lost, vesicoureteral reflux occurs, and the increased intravesical pressure is transmitted directly to the renal pelvis, aggravating the degree of hydroureteronephrosis.

Secondary to the back pressure resulting from reflux or from obstruction by the hypertrophied and stretched trigone or by a ureteral stone, the ureteral musculature thickens in its attempt to push the urine downward by increased peristaltic activity (stage of compensation). This causes elongation and some tortuosity of the ureter (Figure 11–2). At times, this change becomes marked, and bands of fibrous tissue develop. On contraction, the bands further angulate the ureter, causing secondary ureteral obstruction. Under these circumstances, removal of the obstruction below may not prevent the kidney from undergoing progressive obstruction due to the secondary ureteral obstruction.

Finally, because of increasing pressure, the ureteral wall becomes attenuated and therefore loses its contractile power (stage of decompensation). Dilatation may be so extreme that the ureter resembles a loop of bowel (Figures 11–3 and 12–8, upper right).

2. Kidney—The pressure within the renal pelvis is normally close to zero. When this pressure increases because of obstruction or reflux, the pelvis and calyces dilate. The degree of hydronephrosis that develops depends on the duration, degree, and site of the obstruction (Figure 11–4). The higher the obstruction, the greater the effect on the kidney. If the renal pelvis is entirely intrarenal and the obstruction is at the ureteropelvic junction, all the pressure will be exerted on the parenchyma. If the renal pelvis is extrarenal, only part of the pressure produced by a ureteropelvic stenosis is exerted on the parenchyma; this is because the extrarenal renal pelvis is embedded in fat and dilates more readily, thus "decompressing" the calyces (Figure 11–2).

In the earlier stages, the pelvic musculature undergoes compensatory hypertrophy in its effort to force urine past the obstruction. Later, however, the muscle becomes stretched and atonic (and decompensated).

The progression of hydronephrotic atrophy is as follows:

(1) The earliest changes in the development of hydronephrosis are seen in the calyces. The end of a normal calyx is concave because of the papilla that projects into it; with increase in intrapelvic pressure, the fornices become blunt and rounded. With persistence of increased intrapelvic pressure, the papilla becomes flattened, then convex (clubbed) as a result of compression enhanced by ischemic atrophy (Figure 11–5). The parenchyma between the calyces is affected to a lesser extent. The changes in the renal parenchyma are due to (1) compression atrophy from increase in intrapelvic pressure (more accentuated with intrarenal pelves) and (2) ischemic atrophy from hemodynamic changes, mainly manifested in arcuate vessels that run at the base of the pyramids parallel to the kidney outline and are more vulnerable to compression between the renal capsule and the centrally increasing intrapelvic pressure.

This spotty atrophy is caused by the nature of the blood supply of the kidney. The arterioles are "end arteries"; therefore, ischemia is most marked in the areas farthest from the interlobular arteries. As the back pressure increases, hydronephrosis progresses, with the cells nearest the main arteries exhibiting the greatest resistance.

This increased pressure is transmitted up the tubules. The tubules become dilated, and their cells atrophy from ischemia.

It should be pointed out that a few instances of dilated renal pelves and calyces are not due to the presence of obstruction. Rarely, the renal cavities are congenitally capacious and thus simulate hydronephrosis.

Figure 11–2. Mechanisms and results of obstruction. **Upper left:** Early stage. Elongation and dilatation of ureter due to mild obstruction. **Upper center:** Later stage. Further dilatation and elongation with kinking of the ureter; fibrous bands cause further kinking. **Upper right:** Intrarenal pelvis. Obstruction transmits all back pressure to parenchyma. **Lower:** Extrarenal pelvis, when obstructed, allows some of the increased pressure to be dissipated by the pelvis.

Figure 11–3. Pathogenesis of bilateral hydronephrosis. Progressive changes in bladder, ureters, and kidneys from obstruction of an enlarged prostate: thickening of bladder wall, dilatation and elongation of ureters, and hydronephrosis.

Figure 11–4. Hydronephrotic left renal pelvis. Low-density mass (P) in left renal sinus had attenuation value similar to that of water, suggesting the correct diagnosis. Unless intravenous contrast material is used, differentiation from peripelvic cyst may be difficult.

Figure 11–5. Lower right ureteral obstruction. Mild-to-moderate dilatation of the collecting system with rounded blunting of the calyces.

More commonly, hydronephrosis may occur in childhood owing to the back pressure associated with vesicoureteral reflux. If the valvular incompetence resolves (and this is common), some degree of the hydronephrotic changes may persist. These persisting changes may cause the physician to suspect the presence of obstruction, which may lead to unnecessary surgery. An isotope renogram or the Whitaker test can be performed to determine whether organic obstruction is present.

(2) Only in unilateral hydronephrosis are the advanced stages of hydronephrotic atrophy seen. Eventually the kidney is completely destroyed and appears as a thin-walled sac filled with clear fluid (water and electrolytes) or pus (Figure 11–6).

If obstruction is unilateral, the increased intrarenal pressure causes some suppression of renal function on that side. The closer the intrapelvic pressure approaches the glomerular filtration pressure (6–12 mm Hg), the less urine can be secreted. Glomerular filtration rate and renal plasma flow are reduced, concentrating power is gradually lost, and the urea-creatinine concentration ratio of urine from the hydronephrotic kidney is lower than that of urine from the normal kidney.

Hydronephrotic atrophy is an unusual type of pathologic change. Other secretory organs (eg, the submaxillary gland) cease secreting when their ducts are obstructed. This causes primary (disuse) atrophy. The completely obstructed kidney, however, continues to secrete urine. (If this were not so, hydronephrosis could not occur, since it depends on increased intrarenal pressure.) As urine is excreted into the renal pelvis, fluid and, particularly, soluble substances are reabsorbed, through either the tubules or the lymphatics. This has been demonstrated by injecting phenolsulfonphthalein (PSP) into the obstructed renal pelvis. It disappears (is reabsorbed) in a few hours and is excreted by the other kidney. If the intrapelvic pressure in the hydronephrotic kidney rapidly increases to a level approaching filtration pressure (resulting in cessation of filtration), a safety mechanism is activated that produces a break in the surface lining of the collecting structure at the weakest point—the fornices. This leads to escape and extravasation of urine from the renal pelvis into the parenchymal interstitium (pyelointerstitial backflow). The extravasated fluid is absorbed by the renal lymphatics, and the pressure in the renal pelvis drops, allowing further filtration of urine. This explains the process by which the markedly hydronephrotic kidney continues to function. Further evidence of the occurrence of extravasation and reabsorption is that the markedly hydronephrotic kidney does not contain urine in the true sense; only water and a few salts are present.

Figure 11–6. Pathogenesis of unilateral hydronephrosis. Progressive changes in ureter and kidney secondary to obstructing calculus (arrowheads). As the right kidney undergoes gradual destruction, the left kidney gradually enlarges (compensatory hypertrophy).

Functional impairment in unilateral hydronephrosis, as measured by excretory urograms or renal scans, is greater and increases faster than that seen in bilateral hydronephrotic kidneys showing comparable damage on urography. As unilateral hydronephrosis progresses, the normal kidney undergoes compensatory hypertrophy (particularly in children) of its nephrons (renal counterbalance), thereby assuming the function of the diseased kidney in order to maintain normal total renal function. For this reason, successful anatomic repair of the ureteral obstruction of such a kidney may fail to improve its powers of waste elimination.

If both kidneys are equally hydronephrotic, a strong stimulus is continually being exerted on both to maintain maximum function. This is also true of a hydronephrotic solitary kidney. Consequently, the return of function in these kidneys after repair of their obstructions is at times remarkable.

Experimental studies have shown recovery of function after release of complete obstruction of up to 4 weeks' duration. In 2 well-documented human cases, function was recovered after obstruction of 56 and 69 days. However, irreversible loss of function can begin as early as 7 days, as evidenced by dilatation and necrosis of the proximal tubules, which progressively increase with time.

The extent of recovery after partial obstruction is difficult to determine preoperatively. Renal scanning with DMSA (dimercaptosuccinic acid) is most helpful. Temporary drainage, especially by nephrostomy, followed by tests to assess renal function is the best measure.

Physiologic Explanation of Symptoms of Bladder Neck Obstruction

The following hypothesis has been proposed to explain the syndrome known as "prostatism," which occurs with progressive vesical obstruction:

The bladder, like the heart, is a hollow muscular organ that receives fluid and forcefully expels it. And, like the heart, it reacts to an increasing work load by going through the successive phases of compensation and finally decompensation.

Normally, contraction of the detrusor muscle and the trigone pulls the bladder neck open and forms a funnel through which the urine is expelled. The intravesical pressure generated in this instance varies between 20 and 40 cm of water; this force further widens the bladder neck.

With bladder neck obstruction, hypertrophy of the vesical musculature develops, allowing the intravesical voiding pressure to rise to 50–100 cm or more of water in order to overcome the increased outlet resistance. Despite this, the encroaching prostate appears to interfere with the mechanisms that ordinarily open the internal orifice. Also, the contraction phase may not last long enough for all of the urine to be expelled; "exhaustion" of the muscle occurs prematurely. The refractory phase then sets in, and the detrusor is temporarily unable to respond to further stimuli. A few minutes later, voiding may be initiated again and completed.

A. COMPENSATION PHASE

1. Stage of irritability—In the earliest stages of obstruction of the bladder neck, the vesical musculature begins to hypertrophy. The force and size of the urinary stream remain normal because the balance is maintained between the expelling power of the bladder and urethral resistance. During this phase, however, the bladder appears to be hypersensitive. As the bladder is distended, the need to void is felt. In patients with a normal bladder, these early urges can be inhibited, and the bladder relaxes and distends to receive more urine. However, in patients with a hypertrophied detrusor, the contraction of the detrusor is so strong that it virtually goes into spasm, producing the symptoms of an irritable bladder. The earliest symptoms of bladder neck obstruction, therefore, are urgency (even to the point of incontinence) and frequency, both day and night.

2. Stage of compensation—As the obstruction increases, further hypertrophy of the muscle fibers of the bladder occurs, and the power to empty the bladder completely is thereby maintained. During this period, in addition to urgency and frequency, the patient notices hesitancy in initiating urination while the bladder develops contractions strong enough to overcome resistance at the bladder neck. The obstruction causes some loss in the force and size of the urinary stream, and the stream becomes slower as vesical emptying nears completion (exhaustion of the detrusor as it nears the end of the contraction phase).

B. DECOMPENSATION PHASE

If vesical tone becomes impaired or if urethral resistance exceeds detrusor power, some degree of decompensation (imbalance) occurs. The contraction phase of the vesical muscle becomes too short to completely expel the contents of the bladder, and some urine remains in the bladder (residual urine).

1. Acute decompensation—The tone of the compensated vesical muscle can be temporarily embarrassed by rapid filling of the bladder (high fluid intake) or by overstretching of the detrusor (postponement of urination though the urge is felt). This may cause increased difficulty of urination, with marked hesitancy and the need for straining to initiate urination; a very weak and small stream; and termination of the stream before the bladder completely empties (residual urine). Acute and sudden complete urinary retention may also occur.

2. Chronic decompensation—As the degree of obstruction increases, a progressive imbalance between the power of the bladder musculature and urethral resistance develops. Therefore, it becomes increasingly difficult to expel all the urine during the contraction phase of the detrusor. The symptoms of obstruction become more marked. The amount of residual urine gradually increases, and this diminishes the functional capacity of the bladder. Progressive frequency of urination is noted. On occasion, as the bladder decompensates, it becomes overstretched and attenuated. It may contain 1000–3000 mL of urine. It loses its power of contraction, and overflow (paradoxic) incontinence results.

Clinical Findings

A. SYMPTOMS

1. Lower and mid tract (urethra and bladder)— Symptoms of obstruction of the lower and mid tract are typified by the symptoms of urethral stricture, benign prostatic hyperplasia, neurogenic bladder, and tumor of the bladder involving the vesical neck. The principal symptoms are hesitancy in starting urination, lessened force and size of the stream, and terminal dribbling; hematuria, which may be partial, initially, with stricture or total with prostatic obstruction or vesical tumor; and burning on urination, cloudy urine (due to complicating infection), and occasionally acute urinary retention.

2. Upper tract (ureter and kidney)—Symptoms of obstruction of the upper tract are typified by the symptoms of ureteral stricture or ureteral or renal stone. The principal complaints are pain in the flank radiating along the course of the ureter, gross total hematuria (from stone), gastrointestinal symptoms, chills, fever, burning on urination, and cloudy urine with onset of infection, which is the common sequel to obstruction or vesicoureteral reflux. Nausea, vomiting, loss of weight and strength, and pallor are due to uremia secondary to bilateral hydronephrosis. A history of vesicoureteral reflux in childhood may be significant. Obstruction of the upper tract may be silent even when uremia supervenes.

B. SIGNS

1. Lower and mid tract—Palpation of the urethra may reveal induration about a stricture. Rectal examination may show atony of the anal sphincter (damage to the sacral nerve roots) or benign or malignant enlargement of the prostate. Vesical distention may be found.

Although observation of the force and caliber of the urinary stream affords a rough estimate of maximum flow rate, the rate can be measured accurately with a urine flowmeter or, even more simply, by the following technique: Have the patient begin to void. When ob-

served maximum flow has been reached, interpose a container to collect the urine and simultaneously start a stopwatch. After exactly 5 s, remove the container. The flow rate in milliliters per second can easily be calculated. The normal urine flow rate is 20–25 mL/s in males and 25–30 mL/s in females. Any flow rate under 15 mL/s should be regarded with suspicion. A flow rate under 10 mL/s is indicative of obstruction or weak detrusor function. Flow rates associated with an atonic neurogenic (neuropathic) bladder (diminished detrusor power), or with urethral stricture or prostatic obstruction (increased urethral resistance) may be as low as 3–5 mL/s. A cystometrogram can differentiate between these 2 causes of impaired flow rate. After definitive treatment of the cause, the flow rate should return to normal.

In the presence of a vesical diverticulum or vesicoureteral reflux, although detrusor power is normal, the urinary stream may be impaired because of the diffusion of intravesical pressure into the diverticulum and vesicoureteral junction as well as the urethra. Excision of the diverticulum or repair of the vesicoureteral junctions leads to efficient expulsion of urine via the urethra.

2. Upper tract—An enlarged kidney may be discovered by palpation or percussion. Renal tenderness may be elicited if infection is present. Cancer of the cervix may be noted; it may invade the base of the bladder and occlude one or both ureteral orifices, or its metastases to the iliac lymph nodes may compress the ureters. A large pelvic mass (tumor, pregnancy) can displace and compress the ureters. Children with advanced urinary tract obstruction (usually due to posterior urethral valves) may develop ascites. Rupture of the renal fornices allows leakage of urine retroperitoneally; with rupture of the bladder, urine may pass into the peritoneal cavity through a tear in the peritoneum.

C. LABORATORY FINDINGS

Anemia may be found secondary to chronic infection or in advanced bilateral hydronephrosis (stage of uremia). Leukocytosis is to be expected in the acute stage of infection. Little if any elevation of the white blood count accompanies the chronic stage.

Large amounts of protein are usually not found in the obstructive uropathies. Casts are not common from hydronephrotic kidneys. Microscopic hematuria may indicate renal or vesical infection, tumor, or stone. Pus cells and bacteria may or may not be present.

In the presence of significant bilateral hydronephrosis, urine flow through the renal tubules is slowed. Thus, urea is significantly reabsorbed but creatinine is not. Blood chemistry therefore reveals a urea-creatinine ratio well above the normal 10:1.

D. X-Ray Findings (Figure 11–7)

A plain film of the abdomen may show enlargement of renal shadows, calcific bodies suggesting ureteral or renal stone, or tumor metastases to the bones of the spine or pelvis. Metastases in the spine may be the cause of spinal cord damage (neuropathic bladder); if they are osteoblastic, they are almost certainly from cancer of the prostate.

Excretory urograms reveal almost the entire story unless renal function is severely impaired. They are more informative when obstruction is present because the radiopaque material is retained. These urograms demonstrate the degree of dilatation of the pelves, calyces, and ureters. The point of ureteral stenosis is revealed. Segmental dilatation of the lower end of a ureter implies the possibility of vesicoureteral reflux (Figure 11–7), which can be revealed by cystography. The cystogram may show trabeculation as an irregularity of the vesical outline and may show diverticula. Vesical tumors, nonopaque stones, and large intravesical prostatic lobes may cause radiolucent shadows. A film taken immediately after voiding will show residual urine. Few tests that are as simple and inexpensive give the physician so much information.

Retrograde cystography shows changes of the bladder wall caused by distal obstruction (trabeculation, diverticula) or demonstrates the obstructive lesion itself (enlarged prostate, posterior urethral valves, cancer of the bladder). If the ureterovesical valves are incompetent, ureteropyelograms are obtained by reflux.

Retrograde urograms may show better detail than the excretory type, but care must be taken not to overdistend the passages with too much opaque fluid; small hydronephroses can be made to look quite large. The degree of ureteral or ureterovesical obstruction can be judged by the degree of delay of drainage of the radiopaque fluid instilled.

Computed tomography scanning and sonography can also help determine the extent of dilatation and parenchymal atrophy.

E. Isotope Scanning

In the presence of obstruction, the radioisotope renogram may show depression of both the vascular and secretory phases and a rising rather than a falling excretory phase due to retention of the radiopaque urine in the renal pelvis.

The ^{131}I activity recorded on the gamma camera will show that the isotope is poorly taken up, slowly transported through the parenchyma, and accumulated in the renal pelvis.

F. Instrumental Examination

Exploration of the urethra with a catheter or other instrument is a valuable diagnostic measure. Passage may be blocked by a stricture or tumor. Spasm of the external sphincter may make passage difficult. Passage of the catheter immediately after voiding allows estimation of the amount of residual urine in the bladder. Residual urine is common in bladder neck obstruction (enlarged prostate), cystocele, and neurogenic (neuropathic) bladder. Residual urine is usually absent with urethral stricture, even though the urinary stream may be markedly impaired.

Measurement of vesical tone by means of cystometry is helpful in diagnosing neurogenic bladder and in differentiating between bladder neck obstruction and vesical atony.

Inspection of the urethra and bladder by means of cystoscopy and panendoscopy may reveal the primary obstructive agent. Catheters may be passed to the renal pelves and urine specimens obtained. The function of each kidney may be measured and retrograde ureteropyelograms can be obtained.

G. Interventional Uroradiology

If there is doubt about the presence of true obstruction, either the Whitaker test or an isotope renogram can be done. However, Whitaker and Buxton-Thomas (1984) have shown that neither test is without error.

Differential Diagnosis

A thorough examination usually leaves no doubt about the diagnosis. The differential diagnosis under these circumstances is rarely difficult. If seemingly simple infection does not respond to medical therapy or if infection recurs, obstruction, a foreign body, or vesicoureteral reflux is the probable cause, and complete study of the urinary tract is indicated.

Complications

Stagnation of urine leads to infection, which then may spread throughout the entire urinary system. Once established, infection is difficult and at times impossible to eradicate even after the obstruction has been relieved.

Often the invading organisms are urea-splitting (*Proteus,* staphylococci), which causes the urine to become alkaline. Calcium salts precipitate and form bladder or kidney stones more easily in alkaline urine.

If both kidneys are affected, the result may be renal insufficiency. Secondary infection increases renal damage.

Pyonephrosis is the end stage of a severely infected and obstructed kidney. The kidney is functionless and filled with thick pus. At times, a plain film of the abdomen may show an air urogram caused by gas liberated by infecting organisms.

Figure 11–7. Changes in bladder, ureters, and kidneys caused by obstruction. **Upper left:** Cystogram showing benign prostatic enlargement and multiple diverticula. Arrows point to femoral hernia that probably developed as a result of straining to urinate. **Upper right:** Pregnancy. Significant dilatation and elongation of upper right ureter due to compression at the pelvic line. Left side normal. **Lower left:** Excretory urogram, 70 min after injection. Advanced right hydronephrosis secondary to ureteropelvic obstruction. Mild ureteropelvic obstruction on left. **Lower right:** Stone in left ureter (at arrow) with mild hydronephrosis.

Treatment

A. RELIEF OF OBSTRUCTION

Treatment of the main causes of obstruction and stasis (benign prostatic hyperplasia, cancer of the prostate, neurogenic bladder, ureteral stone, posterior urethral valves, and ureteral stenosis) is described in detail elsewhere in this book.

1. Lower tract obstruction (distal to the bladder)— With patients in whom secondary renal or ureterovesical damage (reflux in the latter) is minimal or nonexistent, correction of the obstruction is sufficient. If significant reflux is demonstrated and does not subside spontaneously after relief of obstruction, surgical repair may be needed. Repair becomes imperative if there is considerable hydronephrosis in addition to reflux. Preliminary drainage of the bladder by an indwelling catheter or other means of diversion (eg, loop ureterostomy) is indicated in order to preserve and improve renal function. If, after a few months of drainage, reflux persists, the incompetent ureterovesical junction should be surgically repaired.

2. Upper tract obstruction (above the bladder)—If tortuous, kinked, dilated, or atonic ureters have developed secondary to lower tract obstruction (so that they are themselves obstructive), vesical drainage will not protect the kidneys from further damage; the urine proximal to the obstruction must be diverted by nephrostomy or ureterostomy. The kidneys then may regain some function. Over a period of many months, the ureter may become less tortuous and less dilated; its obstructive areas may open up. If radiopaque material instilled into the nephrostomy tube passes readily to the bladder, it may be possible to remove the nephrostomy tube. If obstruction or reflux persists, surgical repair is indicated. Permanent urinary diversion (eg, ureteroileal conduit) may be necessary.

If one kidney has been irreversibly damaged, as measured by kidney function tests, urography, sonography, computed tomography scan, or scintigraphy, nephrectomy may be necessary.

B. ERADICATION OF INFECTION

Once the obstruction is removed, every effort should be made to eradicate infection. If the infection has been severe and prolonged, antibiotics may fail to sterilize the urinary tract.

Prognosis

No simple statement can be made about the prognosis in this group of patients. The outcome depends on the cause, site, degree, and duration of the obstruction. The prognosis is also definitely influenced by complicating infection, particularly if the infection has been present for a long time.

If renal function is fair to good, if the obstruction or other causes of stasis can be corrected, and if complicating infection can therefore be eradicated, the prognosis is generally excellent.

REFERENCES

Abrams P: Objective evaluation of bladder outlet obstruction. Br J Urol 1995;76(Suppl 1):11.

Andrich DE, Mundy AR: Urethral strictures and their surgical treatment. BJU Int 2000;86:571.

Barry MJ: Evaluation of symptoms and quality of life in men with benign prostatic hyperplasia. Urology 2001;58(6 Suppl 1):25.

Bauer SB, Joseph DB: Management of the obstructed urinary tract associated with neurogenic bladder dysfunction. Urol Clin North Am 1990;17:395.

Belman AB, King LR: Vesicostomy: Useful means of reversible urinary diversion in selected infants. Urology 1973;1:208.

Bloom DA, Lebowitz RL, Bauer SB: Correlation of cystographic bladder morphology and neuroanatomy in boys with posterior urethral valves. Pediatr Radiol 1997;27:553.

Blyth B, Snyder HM, Duckett JW: Antenatal diagnosis and subsequent management of hydronephrosis. J Urol 1993;149:693.

Bomalaski MD, Hirschl RB, Bloom DA: Vesicoureteral reflux and ureteropelvic junction obstruction: Association, treatment options and outcome. J Urol 1997;157:969.

Bratt CG et al: Long-term followup of maximum concentrating ability and glomerular filtration rate in adult obstructed kidneys after pyeloplasty. J Urol 1988;140:273.

Cardenas DD, Mayo ME, Turner LR: Lower urinary changes over time in suprasacral spinal cord injury. Paraplegia 1995;33:326.

Carr LK, Webster GD: Bladder outlet obstruction in women. Urol Clin North Am 1996;23:385.

Cartwright PC et al: Managing apparent ureteropelvic junction obstruction in the newborn. J Urol 1992;148:1224.

Chapple CR, Png D: Contemporary management of urethral trauma and the post-traumatic stricture. Curr Opin Urol 1999;9:253.

Clark WR, Malek RS: Ureteropelvic junction obstruction. I. Observations on the classic type in adults. J Urol 1987;138:276.

Colodny AH: Antenatal diagnosis and management of urinary abnormalities. Pediatr Clin North Am 1987;34:1365.

Coplen DE, Barthold JS: Controversies in the management of ectopic ureteroceles. Urology 2000;56:665.

DeMaeyer P et al: Clinical study of technetium dimercaptosuccinic acid uptake in obstructed kidneys: Comparison with creatinine clearance. J Urol 1982;128:8.

Dinneen MD, Duffy PG: Posterior urethral valves. Br J Urol 1996;78:275.

Dowling KJ et al: Ureteropelvic junction obstruction: The effect of pyeloplasty on renal function. J Urol 1988;140:1227.

Elbadawi A: Voiding dysfunction in benign prostatic hyperplasia: Trends, controversies and recent revelations. I. Symptoms and urodynamics. Urology 1998;51(Suppl 5A):62.

Elbadawi A: Voiding dysfunction in benign prostatic hyperplasia: Trends, controversies and recent revelations. II. Pathology and pathophysiology. Urology 1998;51(Suppl 5A):73.

Emmott RC, Tanagho EA: Ureteral obstruction due to fecal impaction in patient with colonic loop urinary diversion. Urology 1980;15:496.

Ewalt DH, Bauer SB: Pediatric neurourology. Urol Clin North Am 1996;23:501.

Gatti JM, Kirsch AJ: Posterior urethral valves: Pre- and postnatal management. Curr Urol Rep 2001;2:138.

Gerber GS, Cromie WJ: Endoscopic management of ureteropelvic junction obstruction in children. Tech Urol 1999;5:210.

Glassberg KI: The valve bladder syndrome: 20 years later. J Urol 2001;166:1406.

Gonzalez R, Schimke CM: Ureteropelvic junction obstruction. Pediatr Clin N Amer 2001;48:1505.

Hanna MK: Antenatal hydronephrosis and ureteropelvic junction obstruction: The case for early intervention. Urology 2000;55:612.

Hines JE: Symptom indices in bladder outlet obstruction. Br J Urol 1996;77:494.

Hollowell JG et al: Coexisting ureteropelvic junction obstruction and vesicoureteral reflux: Diagnostic and therapeutic implications. J Urol 1989;142:490.

Hutch JA, Tanagho EA: Etiology of non-occlusive ureteral dilatation. J Urol 1965;93:177.

Jacobsen SJ, Girman CJ, Lieber MM: Natural history of benign prostatic hyperplasia. Urology 2001;58(6 Suppl 1):5.

Jepsen JV, Bruskewitz RC: Comprehensive patient evaluation for benign prostatic hyperplasia. Urology 1998;51(4A Suppl):13.

Karmarkar SJ: Long-term results of surgery for posterior urethral valves: A review. Pediatr Surg Int 2001;17:8.

Keating MA et al: Changing concepts in management of primary obstructive megaureter. J Urol 1989;142:636.

Kirby RS: The natural history of benign prostatic hyperplasia: What have we learned in the last decade? Urology 2000;56(5 Suppl 1):3.

Klahr S: Obstructive nephropathy. Intern Med 2000;39:355.

Koff SA: Pathophysiology of ureteropelvic junction obstruction: Clinical and experimental observations. Urol Clin North Am 1990;17:263.

Levin RM et al: Genetic and cellular characteristics of bladder outlet obstruction. Urol Clin North Am 1995;22:263.

Maizels M et al: Grading nephroureteral dilatation detected in the first year of life: Correlation with obstruction. J Urol 1992;148:609; discussion 615.

Mandell J et al: Prenatal diagnosis of the megacystis-megaureter association. J Urol 1992;148:1487.

McGrath MA, Estroff J, Lebowitz RL: The coexistence of obstruction at the ureteropelvic and ureterovesical junctions. AJR 1987;149:403.

McNicholas TA: Lower urinary tract symptoms suggestive of benign prostatic obstruction: What are the current practice patterns? Eur Urol 2001;39(Suppl 3):26.

Michel MC, Goepel M: Lower urinary tract symptoms suggestive of benign prostatic obstruction: What's the long-term effectiveness of medical therapies? Eur Urol 2001;39(Suppl 3):20.

Nguyen HT, Kogan BA: Upper urinary tract obstruction: Experimental and clinical aspects. Br J Urol 1998;81(Suppl 2):13.

O'Reilly PH: Functional outcome of pyeloplasty for ureteropelvic junction obstruction: Prospective study in 30 consecutive cases. J Urol 1989;142:273.

Patel R, Nitti V: Bladder outlet obstruction in women: Prevalence, recognition, and management. Curr Urol Rep 2001;2:379.

Peters CA et al: The response of the fetal kidney to obstruction. J Urol 1992;148:503.

Platt JF et al: Duplex Doppler US of the kidney: Differentiation of obstructive from nonobstructive dilatation. Radiology 1989;171:515.

Rawashdeh YF et al: The intrarenal resistive index as a pathophysiological marker of obstructive uropathy. J Urol 2001;165:1397.

Reinberg Y, Gonzalez R: Upper urinary tract obstruction in children: Current controversies in diagnosis. Pediatr Clin North Am 1987;34:1291.

Ross JH, Kay R: Ureteropelvic junction obstruction in anomalous kidneys. Urol Clin North Am 1998;25:219.

Sacks SH et al: Late renal failure due to prostatic outflow obstruction: A preventable disease. Br Med J 1989;298:156.

Sherer DM: Is fetal hydronephrosis overdiagnosed? Ultrasound Obstet Gynecol 2000;16:601.

Shokeir AA, Nijman RJ: Primary megaureter: Current trends in diagnosis and treatment. BJU Int 2000;86:861.

Skinner DG, Lieskovsky G, Boyd S: Continent urinary diversion. J Urol 1989;141:1323.

Staskin DR: Hydroureteronephrosis after spinal cord injury: Effects of lower urinary tract dysfunction on upper tract anatomy. Urol Clin North Am 1991;18:309.

Sutaria PM, Staskin DR: Hydronephrosis and renal deterioration in the elderly due to abnormalities of the lower urinary tract and ureterovesical junction. Int Urol Nephrol 2000;32:119.

Tanagho EA: Congenitally obstructed bladders: Fate after defunctionalization. J Urol 1974;111:102.

Tanagho EA: The pathogenesis and management of megaureter. In: Johnson JH, Goodwin WF (editors): *Excerpta Medica in Paediatric Urology*. North Holland, 1974.

Tanagho EA, Meyers FH: Trigonal hypertrophy: A cause of ureteral obstruction. J Urol 1965;93:678.

Tanagho EA, Smith DR, Guthrie TH: Pathophysiology of functional ureteral obstruction. J Urol 1970;104:73.

Thomas AW, Abrams P: Lower urinary tract symptoms, benign prostatic obstruction and the overactive bladder. BJU Int 2000;85(Suppl 3):57.

Van Cangh PJ, Nesa S, Tombal B: The role of endourology in ureteropelvic junction obstruction. Curr Urol Rep 2001;2:149.

Wein AJ: Bladder outlet obstruction—an overview. Adv Exp Med Biol 1995;385:3, 75.

Whitaker RH, Buxton-Thomas M: A comparison of pressure flow studies and renography in equivocal upper urinary tract obstruction. J Urol 1984;131:446.

Witherow RO, Whitaker RH: The predictive accuracy of antegrade pressure flow studies in equivocal upper tract obstruction. Br J Urol 1982;53:496.

Vesicoureteral Reflux

Emil A. Tanagho, MD

Under normal circumstances, the ureterovesical junction allows urine to enter the bladder but prevents urine from regurgitating into the ureter, particularly at the time of voiding. In this way, the kidney is protected from high pressure in the bladder and from contamination by infected vesical urine. When this valve is incompetent, the chance for development of urinary infection is significantly enhanced, and pyelonephritis is inevitable. With few exceptions, pyelonephritis—acute, chronic, or healed—is secondary to vesicoureteral reflux.

ANATOMY OF THE URETEROVESICAL JUNCTION

An understanding of the causes of vesicoureteral reflux requires a knowledge of the anatomy of the ureterovesical valve. Anatomic studies performed by Hutch (1972) and by Tanagho and Pugh (1963) (Figure 12–1) are incorporated into the following discussion.

Mesodermal Components

The mesodermal component, which arises from the wolffian duct, is made up of 2 parts that are innervated by the sympathetic nervous system:

A. The Ureter and the Superficial Trigone

The smooth musculature of the renal calyces, pelvis, and extravesical ureter is composed of helically oriented fibers that allow for peristaltic activity. As these fibers approach the vesical wall, they are reoriented into the longitudinal plane. The ureter passes obliquely through the vesical wall; the intravesical ureteral segment is thus composed of longitudinal muscle fibers only and therefore cannot undergo peristalsis. As these smooth-muscle fibers approach the ureteral orifice, those that form the roof of the ureter swing to either side to join those that form its floor. They then spread out and join equivalent muscle bundles from the other ureter and also continue caudally, thus forming the superficial trigone. The trigone passes over the neck of the bladder, ending at the verumontanum in the male and just inside the external urethral meatus in the female. Thus, the ureterotrigonal complex is one structure. Above the ureteral orifice, it is tubular; below that point, it is flat.

B. Waldeyer's Sheath and the Deep Trigone

Beginning at a point about 2–3 cm above the bladder, an external layer of longitudinal smooth muscle surrounds the ureter. This muscular sheath passes through the vesical wall, to which it is connected by a few detrusor fibers. As it enters the vesical lumen, its roof fibers diverge to join its floor fibers, which then spread out, joining muscle bundles from the contralateral ureter and forming the deep trigone, which ends at the bladder neck.

Endodermal Component

The vesical detrusor muscle bundles are intertwined and run in various directions. As they converge on the internal orifice of the bladder, however, they tend to become oriented into 3 layers:

A. Internal Longitudinal Layer

The internal longitudinal layer continues into the urethra submucosally and ends just inside the external meatus in the female and at the caudal end of the prostate in the male.

B. Middle Circular Layer

The middle circular layer is thickest anteriorly and stops at the vesical neck.

C. Outer Longitudinal Layer

The muscle bundles of the outer longitudinal layer take a circular and spiral course about the external surface of the female urethra and are incorporated within the peripheral prostatic tissue in the male. They constitute the true vesicourethral sphincter.

The vesical detrusor muscle is innervated by the parasympathetic nerves (S_2–S_4).

PHYSIOLOGY OF THE URETEROVESICAL JUNCTION

Although many investigators had suspected that normal trigonal tone tended to occlude the intravesical ureter,

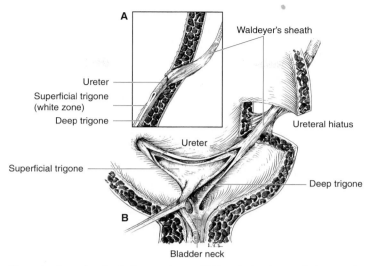

A

Waldeyer's sheath

Ureter

Superficial trigone
(white zone)

Deep trigone

Ureteral hiatus

Ureter

Superficial trigone

Deep trigone

B

Bladder neck

The ureteral muscle extends downward
and becomes the superficial trigone.

Waldeyer's sheath extends downward
and becomes the deep trigone.

Figure 12–1. Normal ureterotrigonal complex. **A:** Side view of ureterovesical junction. Waldeyer's muscular sheath invests the juxtavesical ureter and continues downward as the deep trigone, which extends to the bladder neck. The ureteral musculature becomes the superficial trigone, which extends to the verumontanum in the male and stops just short of the external meatus in the female. **B:** Waldeyer's sheath is connected by a few fibers to the detrusor muscle in the ureteral hiatus. This muscular sheath, inferior to the ureteral orifices, becomes the deep trigone. The musculature of the ureters continues downward as the superficial trigone. (Redrawn and modified, with permission, from Tanagho EA, Pugh RCB: The anatomy and function of the ureterovesical junction. Br J Urol 1963;35:151.)

it remained for Tanagho et al (1965) to prove it. Using nonrefluxing dogs, they demonstrated the following:

(1) Interruption of the continuity of the trigone resulted in reflux. An incision was made in the trigone 3 mm below the ureteral orifice, resulting in an upward and lateral migration of the ureteral orifice with shortening of the intravesical ureter. Reflux was demonstrable. After the incision healed, reflux ceased.

(2) Unilateral lumbar sympathectomy resulted in paralysis of the ipsilateral trigone. This led to lateral and superior migration of the ureteral orifice and reflux.

(3) Electrical stimulation of the trigone caused the ureteral orifice to move caudally, thus lengthening the intravesical ureter. This maneuver caused a marked rise in resistance to flow through the ureterovesical junction. Ureteral efflux of urine ceased. Intravenous injection of epinephrine caused the same reaction. On the

other hand, isoproterenol caused the degree of occlusion to drop below normal. If the trigone was incised, however, electrical stimulation of the trigone or the administration of epinephrine failed to increase ureteral occlusive pressure.

(4) During gradual filling of the bladder, intravesical pressure increased only slightly, whereas pressure within the intravesical ureter rose progressively—owing, apparently, to increasing trigonal stretch. A few seconds before the expected sharp rise in intravesical pressure generated for voiding, the closure pressure in the intravesical ureter rose sharply and was maintained for 20 s after detrusor contraction had ceased. This experiment demonstrated that ureterovesical competence is independent of detrusor action and is governed by the tone of the trigone, which contracts vigorously just before voiding, thus helping to open and funnel the vesical neck. At the same time, significant pull is placed on the intravesical ureter, so that it is occluded during the period when intravesical pressure is high. During the voiding phase, there is naturally no efflux of ureteral urine.

One may liken this function to the phenomenon of the Chinese thimble: The harder the finger (trigone) pulls, the tighter the thimble (intravesical ureter) becomes. Conversely, a deficient pull may lead to incomplete closure of the ureterovesical junction.

It was concluded from these experiments that normal ureterotrigonal tone prevents vesicoureteral reflux. Electrical or pharmacologic stimulation of the trigone caused increased occlusive pressure in the intravesical ureter and increased resistance to flow down the ureter, whereas incision or paralysis of the trigone led to reflux. The theory that ureterovesical competence was maintained by intravesical pressure compressing the intravesical ureter against its backing of detrusor muscle was thereby disproved.

Biopsy of the trigone (and the intravesical ureter) in patients with primary reflux revealed marked deficiency in the development of its smooth muscle (Figure 12–2). Electrical stimulation of such a trigone caused only a minor contraction of the ureterotrigonal complex. This

work led to the conclusion that the common cause of reflux, particularly in children, is congenital attenuation of the ureterotrigonal musculature.

■ VESICOURETERAL REFLUX

CAUSES

The major cause of vesicoureteral reflux is attenuation of the trigone and its contiguous intravesical ureteral musculature. Any condition that shortens the intravesical ureter may also lead to reflux, but this is less common. Familial vesicoureteral reflux has been observed by a number of authors. It appears to be a genetic trait.

Congenital Causes

A. TRIGONAL WEAKNESS (PRIMARY REFLUX)

Trigonal weakness is by far the most common cause of ureteral reflux. It is most often seen in young girls, though it occurs occasionally also in boys. Reflux in adults—usually women—probably represents the same congenital defect. Weakness of one side of the trigone leads to a decrease in the occlusive pressure in the ipsilateral intravesical ureter. Diffuse ureterotrigonal weakness causes bilateral reflux.

It is postulated that ureteral trigonal weakness is related to the development of the ureteral bud on the mesonephric duct. It is known that the ureter acquires its musculature from its cranial end caudally, so that if a segment is muscularly deficient, it is deficient in its most caudal part. It is also postulated that if the ureter is too close to the urogenital sinus on the mesonephric duct, it will join the latter relatively early in embryonic life, before acquiring adequate mesenchymal tissue around itself to be differentiated later into proper trigonal musculature as well as lower ureter. This embryologic hypothesis explains all the known features of refluxing ureters: their muscular weakness, their lateral placement on the bladder base with a very short submucosal segment, and their usual association with weak ureteral musculature and gaping ureteral orifices (which, in severe cases, ensures a golf-hole endoscopic appearance at their junction with the bladder wall). It also explains why, in duplicated systems, if there is only one refluxing unit, it is the upper orifice (which originated closer to the urogenital sinus on the mesonephric duct and thus has the least muscular development).

In the normal state, the intravesical ureterotrigonal muscle tone exerts a downward pull, whereas the extravesical ureter tends to pull cephalad (Figure 12–3). If

Figure 12–2. Histology of the trigone in primary reflux. **Top:** Normal trigone demonstrating wealth of closely packed smooth-muscle fibers. **Bottom:** The congenitally attenuated trigonal muscle that accompanies vesicoureteral reflux. Note absence of inflammatory cells. (Reproduced, with permission, from Tanagho EA et al: Primary vesicoureteral reflux: Experimental studies of its etiology. J Urol 1965;93:165.)

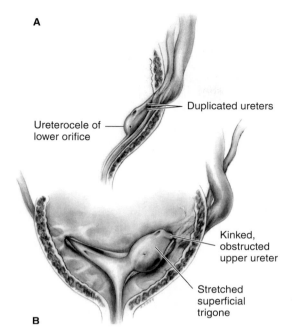

A

B

Figure 12–3. **A:** Small ureterocele developing in a duplicated system (where it always involves a lower ureteral orifice). **B:** Expansion of submucosal segment leads to lifting and angulation of ipsilateral lower pole ureteral orifice. Duplicated system ureteroceles are rarely so small. (Diagrammatic representation.) (Reproduced, with permission, from Tanagho EA: Ureteroceles: Embryogenesis, pathogenesis and management. J Cont Educ Urol [Feb] 1979;18:13.)

trigonal development is deficient, not only is its occlusive power diminished but the ureteral orifice tends to migrate upward toward the ureteral hiatus. The degree of this retraction relates to the degree of incompetence of the junction (Figure 12–4). If the ureteral orifice lies over the ureteral hiatus in the bladder wall (so-called golf-hole orifice), it is completely incompetent. The degree of incompetence is judged by the findings on excretory urography and cystography and the cystoscopic appearance of the ureteral orifices.

B. URETERAL ABNORMALITIES

1. Complete ureteral duplication (Figure 12–5)— The intravesical portion of the ureter to the upper renal segment is usually of normal length, whereas that of the ureter to the lower pole is abnormally short; this orifice is commonly incompetent. However, Stephens (1957) demonstrated that the musculature of the superiorly

placed orifice is attenuated, which further contributes to its weakness.

2. Ectopic ureteral orifice— single ureter or one of a pair may open well down on the trigone, at the vesical neck, or in the urethra. In this instance, vesicoureteral reflux is the rule. This observation makes it clear that the length of the intravesical ureter is not the sole factor in reflux. Such intravesical ureteral segments are usually devoid of smooth muscle. Thus, they have no occlusive force.

3. Ureterocele— A ureterocele involving a single ureter rarely allows reflux, but this lesion usually involves the ureter that drains the upper pole of a duplicated kidney. Because the ureteral orifice is obstructed, the intramural ureter becomes dilated. This increases the diameter of the ureteral hiatus, further shortening the intravesical segment of the other ureter, which therefore may become incompetent. Resection of the ureterocele usually causes its ureter to reflux freely as well.

Vesical Trabeculation

Occasionally, a heavily trabeculated bladder may be associated with reflux. The causes include spastic neurogenic bladder and severe obstruction distal to the bladder. These lesions, however, are associated with trigonal hypertrophy as well; the resultant extra pull on the ureterotrigonal muscle tends to protect the junction from incompetence. In a few such cases, however, the vesical mucosa may protrude through the ureteral hiatus just above the ureter to form a diverticulum, or saccule (Figure 12–6). The resulting dilatation of the hiatus shortens the intravesical segment; reflux may then occur.

Edema of the Vesical Wall Secondary to Cystitis

As noted previously, valves vary in their degrees of incompetence. A "borderline" junction may not allow reflux when the urine is sterile, but valvular function may be impaired when cystitis causes associated edema involving the trigone and intravesical ureter. In addition, the abnormally high voiding pressure may lead to reflux, in which case secondary pyelonephritis may ensue. After cure of the infection, cystography again reveals no reflux. It is believed that a completely normal junction will not decompensate even under these circumstances.

It has been shown that pyelonephritis of pregnancy is associated with vesicoureteral reflux. Many patients give a history of urinary tract infections during childhood. The implication is that they "outgrew" reflux at puberty, but if bacteriuria becomes established during pregnancy, their "borderline" valves may become in-

Figure 12–4. Histology of the various grades of submucosal muscular weakness of the ureteral orifice. (See also Figure 12–9.) **A:** Normal. Minimal deficiency. (Cone orifice.) **B:** More marked muscular weakness. (Stadium orifice.) **C:** Marked muscular deficiency. (Horseshoe orifice.) **D:** Extreme muscular deficiency. Only a few muscle fibers can be seen; the rest is collagen tissue.

competent. This condition may be aggravated by the hormones of pregnancy, which may contribute to a further loss of tone of the ureterotrigonal complex. After delivery, reflux is usually no longer demonstrable (Hutch and Amar, 1972).

Eagle-Barrett (Prune Belly) Syndrome

The Eagle-Barrett syndrome is a relatively rare condition in which there is failure of normal development of the abdominal muscles and the smooth muscle of the ureters and bladder. Bilateral cryptorchidism is the rule. At times, talipes equinovarus and hip dislocation are also noted. Because the smooth muscle of the ureterotrigonal complex is deficient, reflux is to be ex-

pected; advanced hydroureteronephrosis is therefore found.

Iatrogenic Causes

Certain operative procedures may lead to either temporary or permanent ureteral regurgitation.

A. PROSTATECTOMY

With any type of prostatectomy, the continuity of the superficial trigone is interrupted at the vesical neck. If the proximal trigone moves upward, temporary reflux may occur. This mechanism may account for the high fever (and even bacteremia) that is sometimes observed when the catheter is finally removed. Fortunately, in

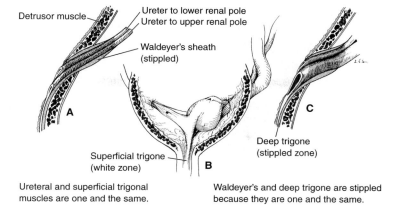

Detrusor muscle

Ureter to lower renal pole
Ureter to upper renal pole

Waldeyer's sheath
(stippled)

A

Deep trigone
(stippled zone)

C

Superficial trigone
(white zone)

B

Ureteral and superficial trigonal
muscles are one and the same.

Waldeyer's and deep trigone are stippled
because they are one and the same.

Figure 12–5. Ureteral duplication and ureterocele as causes of vesicoureteral reflux. **A:** Ureteral duplication showing juxtavesical and intravesical ureters encased in common sheath (Waldeyer's). The superior ureter, which always drains the lower renal pole, has a shorter intravesical segment; in addition, it is somewhat devoid of muscle. It therefore tends to allow reflux. **B:** Duplication with ureterocele that always involves caudal ureter, which drains upper renal pole. Pinpoint orifice is obstructive, causing hydroureteronephrosis. Resulting wide dilatation of ureter and ureteral hiatus shortens the intravesical segment of the other ureter, often causing it to reflux. **C:** Resection of ureterocele allows reflux into that ureter.

Figure 12–6. Development of ureteral saccule, seen occasionally in cases of primary reflux but more commonly in obstructed or neurogenic bladders with marked trabeculation. Note that the vesical mucosa herniates through the ureteral hiatus, pulling the ureteral orifice upward with it. The orifice may ultimately open in the saccule rather than in the bladder.

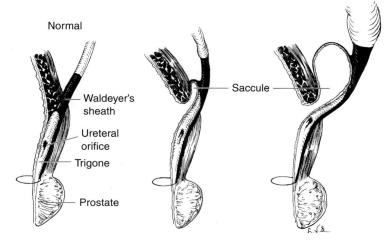

Normal

Waldeyer's
sheath

Ureteral
orifice

Trigone

Prostate

Saccule

2–3 weeks the trigone again becomes anchored and reflux ceases.

Preexisting trigonal hypertrophy (due to prostatic obstruction) helps to compensate for the effect of trigonal interruption; thus, reflux may never occur.

B. Wedge Resection of the Posterior Vesical Neck

Wedge resection of the posterior vesical neck, often ill-advised when performed in conjunction with plastic revision of the vesical neck for supposed vesical neck stenosis or dysfunction, may also upset trigonal continuity and allow reflux.

C. Ureteral Meatotomy

Extensive ureteral meatotomy may be followed by reflux. Fortunately, however, limited incision of the roof of the intravesical ureter divides few muscle fibers, since the fibers have left the roof to join muscle fibers on the floor. Wide resection for treatment of vesical cancer is often followed by ureteral reflux.

D. Resection of Ureterocele

If the ureteral hiatus is widely dilated, this procedure is often followed by reflux.

Contracted Bladder

A bladder that is contracted secondary to interstitial cystitis, tuberculosis, radiotherapy, carcinoma, or schistosomiasis may be associated with ureteral reflux.

COMPLICATIONS

Vesicoureteral reflux damages the kidney through one or both of 2 mechanisms: (1) pyelonephritis and (2) hydroureteronephrosis.

Pyelonephritis

Vesicoureteral reflux is one of the common contributing factors leading to the development of cystitis, particularly in females. When reflux is present, bacteria reach the kidney and the urinary tract cannot empty itself completely, so infection is perpetuated. Pyelonephritis is discussed in more detail in Chapter 13.

Hydroureteronephrosis (See also Chapter 11)

Dilation of the ureter, renal pelvis, and calyces is usually observed in association with reflux (Figure 12–7), sometimes to an extreme degree (Figure 12–8). In males, because they have a relatively long segment of sterile urethra, such changes are often seen in the absence of infection. Sterile reflux is less damaging than infected reflux.

There are 3 reasons for the dilatation:

(1) Increased work load: The ureter is meant to transport the urine secreted by the kidney to the bladder only once. In the presence of reflux, variable amounts of urine go back and forth, and the work load may be doubled, quadrupled, or increased 10-fold or even more. Eventually, the ureter is not able to transport the increased volume of urine, and stasis and dilatation result.

(2) High hydrostatic pressure: The ureter is protected from the high pressures of the urinary bladder by a competent ureterovesical junction. If there is free reflux, the high intravesical pressure is directly transmitted to the ureteral and pelvic walls, which results in marked stretching and dilation.

(3) Weak ureteral musculature: In reflux, the ureteral wall is invariably deficient in musculature to some degree. The more severe the reflux, the more apparent the muscular deficiency. Some cases show more massive dilatation than others. The properly muscularized ureter is better able to resist and compensate for overwork and hydrostatic pressure than the muscularly deficient ureter. The latter tends to undergo further dilatation once it is subjected to any increased intraluminal pressure.

Whether sterile reflux is harmful is the subject of controversy. My colleagues and I believe there is conclusive evidence that severe sterile reflux can lead to parenchymal damage. Pyelointerstitial backflow or pyelotubular backflow under the high pressures of reflux (not infrequently seen during cystographic studies) leads to extravasation of urine in the interstitium of the kidney. The presence of urine in any interstitium will result in a marked inflammatory response with cellular infiltration, resulting finally in fibrosis and scarring. On a long-term basis, this can lead to parenchymal changes indistinguishable from pyelonephritic scarring caused by inflammation due to bacterial infection. This damage may be termed **reflux nephropathy.** If severe, it will produce parenchymal damage serious enough to lead to end-stage kidney disease.

Ransley's studies (1976) indicate that intrarenal reflux is more likely to occur in the presence of flat, concave, or compound papillae, because their collecting ducts tend to open with an increase in intrapelvic pressure and reflux. Papillae prone to reflux are more commonly seen in the polar segments of the kidney. Normal papillae might also permit intrarenal reflux if flattened as a result of the changes due to reflux.

Intravesical pressure is transmitted through the incompetent ureteral orifice. This back pressure is quite

Figure 12–7. Excretory urogram with changes that imply right vesicoureteral reflux. **Upper left:** Excretory urogram showing normal right urogram and a ureter that is mildly dilated and remains full through its entire length. The ureteral change implies reflux. **Upper right:** Cystogram demonstrates the reflux. Note, now, the degree of dilatation of the ureter, pelvis, and calyces. **Lower left:** Excretory urogram shows bilateral hydroureteronephrosis with pyelonephritic scarring. These findings imply the presence of reflux. **Lower right:** Voiding cystourethrogram. Free reflux bilaterally.

high at the time of voiding. Furthermore, the ureteropelvic and ureterovesical junctions are less distensible than the rest of the ureter. Either junction may have trouble passing the normal amount of secreted urine plus the refluxed urine; functional obstruction may result. A common cause of ureteropelvic and ureterovesical "obstruction" is vesicoureteral reflux. Such changes indicate the need for cystography.

INCIDENCE

Vesicoureteral reflux occurs in 50% of children with urinary tract infection but in only 8% of adults with bacteriuria. This discrepancy is explained by the fact that girls usually have pyelonephritis, whereas women usually have cystitis only. Bacteriuria does not always imply pyelonephritis.

Figure 12–8. Cystograms revealing vesicoureteral reflux. **Upper left:** Saccule at right ureterovesical junction. **Upper right:** Meningomyelocele. Reflux with severe bilateral hydroureteronephrosis; serum creatinine, 0.6 mg/dL; phenolsulfonphthalein excretion, 5% in 1 h. **Lower left:** Post-prostatectomy patient with reflux on left and bilateral saccules. **Lower right:** Ten-year-old boy with meningomyelocele. Bladder has been emptied. Impairment of drainage at ureterovesical junctions is demonstrated. (Courtesy of JA Hutch.)

The fairly competent (borderline) valve refluxes only during an acute attack of cystitis. Since cystography is performed in such cases only after the infection has been eradicated, the incidence of reflux found on cystography is abnormally low. On the other hand, reflux is demonstrable in 85% of patients whose excretory urograms reveal significant changes typical of healed pyelonephritis.

When infection associated with reflux occurs during the first few weeks of life, many patients are septic and uremic. Most are boys with posterior urethral valves. After age 6 months, the female-male ratio of infection with reflux is 10:1.

CLINICAL FINDINGS

A history compatible with acute pyelonephritis implies the presence of vesicoureteral reflux. This is most commonly seen in females, particularly young girls. Persistence of recurrent "cystitis" should suggest the possibility of reflux. Such patients often have asymptomatic low-grade pyelonephritis.

Symptoms Related to Reflux

A. SYMPTOMATIC PYELONEPHRITIS

The usual symptoms in adults are chills and high fever, renal pain, nausea and vomiting, and symptoms of cystitis. In children, only fever, vague abdominal pains, and sometimes diarrhea are apt to occur.

B. ASYMPTOMATIC PYELONEPHRITIS

The patient may have no symptoms whatsoever. The incidental findings of pyuria and bacteriuria may be the only clues. This fact points up the need for a screening urinalysis in all children.

C. SYMPTOMS OF CYSTITIS ONLY

In cases of symptoms of cystitis only, bacteriuria is resistant to antimicrobial drugs, or infection quickly recurs following treatment. These patients may have reflux with asymptomatic chronic pyelonephritis.

D. RENAL PAIN ON VOIDING

Surprisingly, renal pain on voiding is a rare complaint in patients with vesicoureteral reflux.

E. UREMIA

The last stage of bilateral reflux is uremia due to destruction of the renal parenchyma by hydronephrosis or pyelonephritis (or both). The patient often adjusts to renal insufficiency and may appear quite healthy. Many renal transplants are performed in patients whose kidneys have deteriorated secondarily to reflux and accompanying infection. Early diagnosis, based on careful urinalysis, would have led to the proper diagnosis in childhood. Progressive pyelonephritis is, with few exceptions, preventable.

F. HYPERTENSION

In the later stages of atrophic pyelonephritis, a significant incidence of hypertension is observed.

Symptoms Related to the Underlying Disease

The clinical picture is often dominated by the signs and symptoms of the primary disease.

A. URINARY TRACT OBSTRUCTION

Young girls may have hesitancy in initiating the urinary stream and an impaired or intermittent stream secondary to spasm of the periurethral striated muscle (see Distal Urethral Stenosis in Chapter 39). In males, the urinary stream may be slow as a result of posterior urethral valves (infants) or prostatic enlargement (men over age 50).

B. SPINAL CORD DISEASE

The patient may have a serious neurogenic disease such as paraplegia, quadriplegia, multiple sclerosis, or meningomyelocele. Symptoms may be limited to those of neurogenic bladder: incontinence of urine, urinary retention or large residual volume, and vesical urgency.

Physical Findings

During an attack of acute pyelonephritis, renal tenderness may be noted. Its absence, however, does not rule out chronic renal infection. Palpation and percussion of the suprapubic area may reveal a distended bladder secondary to obstruction or neurogenic disease. The finding of a hard midline mass deep in the pelvis in a male infant is apt to represent a markedly thickened bladder caused by posterior urethral valves. Examination may reveal a neurologic deficit compatible with a paretic bladder.

Laboratory Findings

The most common complication of reflux, particularly in females, is infection. Bacteriuria without pyuria is not uncommon. In males, the urine may be sterile because of the long, sterile urethra.

The serum creatinine may be elevated in the advanced stage of renal damage, but it may be normal even when the degree of reflux and hydronephrosis is marked (Figure 12–8, upper right).

X-Ray Findings

The plain film may reveal evidence of spina bifida, meningomyelocele, or absence of the sacrum and thus point to a neurologic deficit. Even in vesicoureteral reflux, excretory urograms may be normal, but usually one or more of the following clues to the presence of reflux is noted (Figure 12–7): (1) a persistently dilated lower ureter, (2) areas of dilatation in the ureter, (3) ureter visualized throughout its entire length, (4) presence of hydroureteronephrosis with a narrow juxtavesical ureteral segment, or (5) changes of healed pyelonephritis (caliceal clubbing with narrowed infundibula or cortical thinning). A normal intravenous urogram does not rule out reflux.

The presence of ureteral duplication suggests the possibility of reflux into the lower pole of the kidney. In this case, hydronephrosis or changes compatible with pyelonephritic scarring may be seen. Abnormality of the upper segment of a duplicated system can be caused by the presence of an ectopic ureteral orifice with reflux or by obstruction secondary to a ureterocele.

Reflux is diagnosed by demonstration of its existence with one of the following techniques: simple or delayed cystography, voiding cystourethrography, or voiding cinefluoroscopy. Radionuclide scanning can be used: 1 mCi of ^{99m}Tc is instilled into the bladder along with sterile saline solution, and the gamma camera will reveal ureteral reflux.

Reflux can be demonstrated by a technique using indigotindisulfonate sodium (indigo carmine), a blue dye. The bladder is filled with sterile water containing 5 mL of indigo carmine per 100 mL, after which the patient voids and the bladder is thoroughly flushed out with sterile water. The ureteral orifices are then viewed cystoscopically for blue-tinged efflux. This technique has the advantage that no ionizing radiation is used, and its efficiency is equal to that of voiding cystourethrography. In general, reflux demonstrable only with voiding implies a more competent valve than does reflux that occurs at low pressures. As has been pointed out, failure to demonstrate reflux on one study does not rule out intermittent reflux.

The voiding phase of the cystogram may reveal changes compatible with distal urethral stenosis with secondary spasm of the voluntary periurethral muscles in girls (Figure 39–1) or changes diagnostic of posterior urethral valves in young boys.

Instrumental Examination

A. Urethral Calibration

In females, urethral calibration using bougies à boule should be done. Distal urethral stenosis is almost routinely found in young girls who have urinary infection. Dilation of the ring of stenosis is an important step in improving the hydrodynamics of voiding: lowering intravesical voiding pressure and eliminating the presence

of residual vesical urine (see Chapter 39). Less commonly, urethral stenosis is discovered in women and should be treated.

B. Cystoscopy

Most young girls with reflux have smooth-walled or only slightly trabeculated bladders. Chronic cystitis, ureteral duplication, or ureterocele may be evident. An orifice may be ectopic and be found at the bladder neck or even in the urethra. As the bladder is filled, a small diverticulum may form on the roof of the ureteral orifice (Figure 12–6). These findings imply the possibility of reflux. The major contribution of cystoscopy is to allow study of the morphologic characteristics of the ureteral orifice and its position in relation to the vesical neck (Figure 12–9).

1. Morphology—The orifice of a normal ureter has the appearance of a volcanic cone. That of a slightly weaker valve looks like a football stadium; an even weaker one has the appearance of a horseshoe with its open end pointing toward the vesical neck. The completely incompetent junction has a golf-hole orifice that lies over the ureteral hiatus.

2. Position—By and large, the more defective the appearance of the ureteral orifice, the farther from the vesical neck it lies. The degree of lateralization of the orifice reflects the degree of ureterotrigonal deficiency.

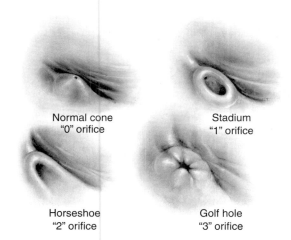

Normal cone
"0" orifice

Stadium
"1" orifice

Horseshoe
"2" orifice

Golf hole
"3" orifice

Figure 12–9. Cystoscopic appearance of the normal ureteral orifice and 3 degrees of incompetence of the ureterovesical junction. (See also Figure 12–4.) (Reproduced, with permission, from Lyon RP, Marshall SK, Tanagho EA: The ureteral orifice: Its configuration and competency. J Urol 1969;102:504.)

DIFFERENTIAL DIAGNOSIS

Functional (nonocclusive) vesicoureteral obstruction may cause changes similar to those suggesting the presence of reflux on excretory urography. Multiple cystograms fail to show reflux. Tanagho, Smith, and Guthrie (1970) showed that this congenital obstruction is due to an abundance of circularly oriented smooth-muscle fibers in the ureteral musculature at this point. Its action is sphincteric.

Significant obstruction distal to the vesical neck leads to hypertrophy of both the detrusor and trigonal muscles. The latter exert an exaggerated pull on the intravesical ureter and thus cause functional obstruction (Tanagho and Meyers, 1965). Hydroureteronephrosis is therefore to be expected; vesicoureteral reflux is uncommon.

Other lesions that may cause hydroureteronephrosis without reflux include low ureteral stone, occlusion of the ureter by cervical or prostatic cancer, urinary tract tuberculosis, and schistosomiasis.

TREATMENT

It is impossible to give a concise and definitive discourse on the treatment of vesicoureteral reflux because of the many factors involved and because there is no unanimity of opinion among urologists on this subject. In general, probably more than half of the cases of primary reflux that occur in children can be controlled by nonsurgical means; the rest require some form of operative procedure. Adults with reflux usually require vesicoureteroplasty.

Medical Treatment

A. INDICATIONS

A child with primary reflux (attenuated trigone) who has fairly normal upper tracts on urographic study and whose ureterovesical valves appear fair to good on cystoscopy has an excellent chance of "outgrowing" the defect, particularly if cystograms show only transient or "high-pressure" reflux. A boy with posterior urethral valves may cease to have reflux once these valves are destroyed.

In a woman who occasionally develops acute pyelonephritis following intercourse but whose urine quickly clears on antimicrobial therapy, reflux will probably be controlled if she takes steps to prevent vesical infections. This is particularly true if reflux cannot be demonstrated cystographically when her urine is sterile. The maintenance of sterile urine allows her "borderline" valve to remain competent.

B. METHODS OF TREATMENT

Dilation of the ring of distal urethral stenosis in young girls or of posterior urethral valves in boys usually gives excellent results, reducing intravesical voiding pressure and abolishing vesical residual urine and reflux.

Urinary infection should be definitively treated with antimicrobial drugs, after which chronic suppressive therapy should be continued for 6 months or more.

Triple voiding is the least effective method of treating reflux. Since vesicoureteral reflux prevents the urinary tract from emptying itself completely, thus destroying the vesical defense mechanism, triple voiding once a day is helpful if the child is old enough to be trained. When reflux is present, the bladder empties itself on voiding, but some urine ascends to the kidneys and then returns to the bladder. Voiding again a few minutes later pushes less urine into the ureters. A third voiding usually completely empties the urinary tract. This allows the patient's own natural resistance to operate to a maximum degree.

Children with reflux often have thin-walled bladders and do not perceive the normal urge to void when the bladder is full. Further detrusor tone is lost with overfilling, increasing the likelihood of residual urine. Such children should "void by the clock" every 3–4 h whether they have the urge or not. Vesical residual urine may then be minimized.

Infant girls with markedly dilated upper urinary tracts may be tided over by means of an indwelling urethral catheter. Over a period of months, ureteral dilation and elongation may regress; renal function is protected. At a convenient and strategic time, more definitive therapy can be accomplished.

C. EVALUATION OF SUCCESS OF MEDICAL TREATMENT

Urinalysis should be done at least once a month for a year or more. Maintenance of sterile urine is an encouraging sign. Cystograms should be repeated every 4–6 months. Excretory urography or nuclear renal scan should be performed at 6 and 12 months to be sure that renal deterioration does not occur. About half of children with reflux are cured by medical treatment.

Surgical Treatment

A. INDICATIONS

Reflux caused by the following abnormalities will not disappear spontaneously: (1) ectopic ureteral orifice, (2) ureteral duplication, (3) ureterocele associated with ureteral duplication and reflux into the uninvolved ureter, (4) golf-hole ureteral orifice, and (5) low-pressure reflux with significant hydroureteronephrosis.

Surgery is indicated (1) if it is not possible to keep the urine sterile and reflux persists; (2) if acute pyelonephritis recurs despite a strict medical regimen and chronic suppressive antimicrobial therapy; or (3) if increased renal damage is demonstrated by serial excretory urograms or nuclear scan.

B. TYPES OF SURGICAL TREATMENT

In cases of markedly impaired kidney function and massively dilated ureters, preliminary urinary diversion may be required to improve renal function and to allow dilated ureters to regain tone, after which definitive relief of obstruction (eg, posterior urethral valves) and ureterovesicoplasty can be performed at the optimum time. Some patients with irreversible lesions causing reflux (eg, meningomyelocele) or badly damaged and atonic ureters may require permanent diversion of the urine (ie, ureteroileocutaneous anastomosis).

1. Temporary urinary diversion—If refluxed urine drains freely into the bladder, cystostomy (or an indwelling urethral catheter in girls) may prove helpful. If the ureters are dilated and kinked, a low redundant loop can be brought to the skin. The ureter is opened at this point and urine collected into an ileostomy bag. Later, the loop and the section of ureter distal to it can be resected and the ureter proximal to the loop reimplanted into the bladder. Nephrostomy may be necessary if there is no ureteral redundancy.

2. Permanent urinary diversion—If it is felt that successful ureterovesicoplasty cannot be accomplished, a Bricker type of diversion is indicated. If renal function is poor and the ureters are widely dilated and atonic, ureterocutaneous diversion may be the procedure of choice.

3. Other surgical procedures—
a. If reflux is unilateral, with the affected kidney badly damaged and the other kidney normal, nephrectomy is indicated.

b. If one renal pole of a duplicated system is essentially functionless, heminephrectomy with removal of its entire ureter should be done. If there is moderate hydronephrosis of one renal pole with duplication, an alternative is anastomosis of the dilated ureter or pelvis to the normal ureter or pelvis. The remainder of the dilated refluxing ureter should be removed.

c. In unilateral reflux, anastomosis of the lower end of the refluxing ureter into the side of its normal mate (transureteroureterostomy) has a few proponents.

4. Definitive repair of ureterovesical junction (ureterovesicoplasty)—

a. Principles of repair (Tanagho, 1970)—

1. Resect the lower 2–3 cm of the ureter in which the muscle is underdeveloped.

2. Free up enough extravesical ureter so that an intravesical segment 2.5 cm long can be formed.

3. Place the intravesical ureter in a submucosal position.

4. Suture the wall of the new ureteral orifice to the cut edge of the trigonal muscle.

b. Types of operation—The following procedures satisfy the preceding principles and have been successful in a high percentage of cases: suprahiatal repair, increasing the length of intravesical ureter above the level of the ureteral hiatus (Paquin, 1959; Politano and Leadbetter, 1958); infrahiatal repair, the advancement procedures of Hutch (1963) and Glenn and Anderson (1967); combined supra- and infrahiatal repair, which is the most attractive; and transtrigonal repair (Cohen, 1975).

If the ureters are unduly tortuous, the redundant portions must be resected. If they are widely dilated, the lower ends must be tailored to a more normal size.

c. Results of ureterovesicoplasty—About 93% of patients no longer show reflux after ureterovesicoplasty. About 3% develop ureterovesical stenosis that requires reoperation. At least 75% have and maintain sterile urine without antimicrobial drugs 3–6 months after surgery. Many patients in whom bacteriuria persists have cystitis only. This has been demonstrated by the finding that renal urine specimens collected by ureteral catheters are sterile. Febrile attacks cease. Considering that only the most severe and advanced cases are submitted to surgical repair, these are impressive results, and they exceed by far the cure rates reported when only antimicrobial drugs are used (10–15%). This operation is rightly considered one of the most significant accomplishments of modern urology.

PROGNOSIS

In patients with reflux who are judged to have fairly competent valves, conservative therapy as outlined previously is highly successful in the cure of the reflux and therefore of infection.

Patients with very incompetent ureterovesical valves subjected to surgical repair also have an excellent prognosis. A few children, however, have such badly damaged urinary tracts when finally submitted to diagnostic procedures that little help other than permanent urinary diversion can be offered.

REFERENCES

Ahmed S, Boucaut HA: Vesicoureteral reflux in complete ureteral duplication: Surgical options. J Urol 1988;140:1092.

Agarwal S: Vesicoureteral reflux and urinary tract infections. Curr Opin Urol 2000;10:587.

Arap S, Abrao EG, Menezes de Goes G: Treatment and prevention of complications after extravesical antireflux technique. Eur Urol 1981;7:263.

Atwell JD, Allen NH: The interrelationship between paraureteric diverticula, vesicoureteric reflux and duplication of the pelvicaliceal collecting system: A family study. Br J Urol 1980; 52:269.

Atwell JD, Cox PA: Growth of the kidney following unilateral antireflux surgery. Eur Urol 1981;7:257.

Bailey RR, Rolleston GL: Vesicoureteric reflux and reflux nephropathy: The Christchurch contribution. N Z Med J 1997;110:266.

Bakshandeh K, Lynne C, Carrion H: Vesicoureteral reflux and end stage renal disease. J Urol 1976;116:557.

Belman AB: Vesicoureteral reflux. Pediatr Clin North Am 1997; 44:1171.

Birmingham Reflux Study Group. Operative versus non-operative treatment of severe vesicoureteric reflux in children: Five years' observation. Br Med J Clin Res 1987;295:237.

Bjorgvinsson E, Jajd M, Eggli KD: Diagnosis of acute pyelonephritis in children: Comparison of sonography and ^{99m}Tc-DMSA scintigraphy. AJR 1991;157:539.

Blake NS, O'Connell E: Endoscopic correction of vesicoureteric reflux by subureteric Teflon injection: Follow-up ultrasound and voiding cystography. Br J Radiol 1989;62:443.

Bomalaski MD, Hirschl RB, Bloom DA: Vesicoureteral reflux and ureteropelvic junction obstruction: Association, treatment options and outcome. J Urol 1997;157:969.

Bourne HH et al: Intrarenal reflux and renal damage. J Urol 1976;115:304.

Cohen SJ: Ureterocystoneostomie: Eine neue antireflux Technik. [Ureterocystoneostomy: A new technique for reflux prevention.] Aktuelle Urologie 1975;6:1.

Darge K: Diagnosis of vesicoureteral reflux with ultrasonography. Pediatr Nephrol 2002;17:52.

DeKlerk DP, Reiner WG, Jeffs RD: Vesicoureteral reflux and ureteropelvic junction obstruction: Late occurrence of ureteropelvic obstruction after successful ureteroneocystostomy. J Urol 1979;121:816.

Devriendt K et al: Vesico-ureteral reflux: A genetic condition? Eur J Pediatr 1998;157:265.

Dewan PA: Ureteric reimplantation: A history of the development of surgical techniques. BJU Int 2000;85:1000.

Dewan PA, Anderson P: Ureterocystoplasty: The latest developments. BJU Int 2001;88:744.

Duckett JW, Bellinger MF: A plea for standardized grading of vesicoureteral reflux. Eur Urol 1982;8:74.

Duckett JW Jr: Ureterovesical junction and acquired vesicoureteral reflux. J Urol 1982;127:249.

Garin EH, Campos A, Homsy Y: Primary vesicoureteral reflux: Review of current concepts. Pediatr Nephrol 1998;12:249.

Glenn JF, Anderson EE: Distal tunnel ureteral reimplantation. J Urol 1967;97:623.

Greenfield SP, Wan J: The relationship between dysfunctional voiding and congenital vesicoureteral reflux. Curr Opin Urol 2000;10:607.

Hendren WH: Complications of megaureter repair in children. J Urol 1975;113:228.

Holland NH et al: Relation of urinary tract infection and vesicoureteral reflux to scars: Follow-up of thirty-eight patients. J Pediatr 1990;116:S65.

Huland H et al: Vesicoureteral reflux in end stage renal disease. J Urol 1979;121:10.

Hutch JA: The mesodermal component: Its embryology, anatomy, physiology and role in prevention of vesicoureteral reflux. J Urol 1972;108:406.

Hutch JA: Ureteric advancement operation: Anatomy, technique, and early results. J Urol 1963;89:180.

Hutch JA, Amar AD: *Vesicoureteral Reflux and Pyelonephritis.* Appleton-Century-Crofts, 1972.

Jodal U, Hansson S, Hjalmas K: Medical or surgical management for children with vesico-ureteric reflux? Acta Paediatr Suppl 1999;88:53.

Johnston JH: Vesicoureteric reflux with urethral valves. Br J Urol 1979;51:100.

Kallen RJ: Paleonephrology and reflux nephropathy: From the "big bang" to end-stage renal disease. Am J Dis Child 1991; 145:860.

Kershen RT, Atala A: New advances in injectable therapies for the treatment of incontinence and vesicoureteral reflux. Urol Clin North Am 1999;26:81.

Koff SA: Relationship between dysfunctional voiding and reflux. J Urol 1992;148:1703.

Koff SA, Murtagh DS: The uninhibited bladder in children: Effect of treatment of recurrence of urinary infection and on vesicoureteral reflux resolution. J Urol 1983;130:1138.

Koo HP, Bloom DA: Lower ureteral reconstruction. Urol Clin North Am 1999;26:167.

Lerner GR, Fleischmann LE, Perlmutter AD: Reflux nephropathy. Pediatr Clin North Am 1987;34:747.

Lyon RP, Marshall SK, Scott MP: Treatment of vesicoureteral reflux: Point system based on 20 years of experience. Trans Am Assoc Genitourin Surg 1979; 71:146.

Lyon RP, Marshall SK, Tanagho EA: The ureteral orifice: Its configuration and competency. J Urol 1969; 102:504.

Mundy AR et al: Improvement in renal function following ureteric reimplantation for vesicoureteric reflux. Br J Urol 1982; 53:542.

O'Donnell B: Management of urinary tract infection and vesicoureteric reflux in children. 2. The case for surgery. Br Med J 1990;300:1393.

Paltiel HJ, Lebowitz RL: Neonatal hydronephrosis due to primary vesicoureteral reflux: Trends in diagnosis and treatment. Radiology 1989;170:787.

Paquin AJ Jr: Ureterovesical anastomosis: The description and evaluation of a technique. J Urol 1959;82:573.

Politano VA, Leadbetter WF: An operative technique for correction of vesicoureteral reflux. J Urol 1958;79:932.

Pope JC IV et al: How they begin and how they end: Classic and new theories for the development and deterioration of congenital anomalies of the kidney and urinary tract, CAKUT. J Am Soc Nephrol 1999;10:2018.

Ransley PG: The renal papilla and intrarenal reflux. In: Williams PI, Chisholm GD (editors): *Scientific Foundations of Urology.* Year Book, 1976.

Ransley PG: Vesicoureteral reflux: Continuous surgical dilemma. Urology 1978;12:246.

Roberts JA: Experimental pyelonephritis in the monkey. 4. Vesicoureteral reflux and bacteria. Invest Urol 1976;14:198.

Rolleston GL, Maling TMJ, Hodson CJ: Intrarenal reflux and the scarred kidney. Arch Dis Child 1974;49:531.

Rose JS, Glassberg KI, Waterhouse K: Intrarenal reflux and its relationship to renal scarring. J Urol 1975; 113;400.

Salvatierra O Jr, Kountz SL, Belzer FO: Primary vesicoureteral reflux and end-stage renal disease. JAMA 1973;226:1454.

Salvatierra O Jr, Tanagho EA: Reflux as a cause of end stage kidney disease: Report of 32 cases. J Urol 1977;117:441.

Seruca H: Vesicoureteral reflux and voiding dysfunction: A prospective study. J Urol 1989;142:494.

Shimada K et al: Renal growth and progression of reflux nephropathy in children with vesicoureteral reflux. J Urol 1988;140:1097.

Sillen U: Bladder dysfunction in children with vesico-ureteric reflux. Acta Paediatr Suppl 1999;88:40.

Skoog SJ, Belman AB, Majd M: A nonsurgical approach to the management of primary vesicoureteral reflux. J Urol 1987;138:941.

Smellie JM: Vesico-ureteric reflux. Acta Paediatr 1999;88:1182.

Smith JW: Prognosis in pyelonephritis: Promise or progress? Am J Med Sci 1989;297:53.

Soulen MC, Fishman EK, Goldman SM: Sequelae of acute renal infections: CT evaluation. Radiology 1989;173:423.

Stephens FD: Treatment of megaloureters by multiple micturition. Aust N Z J Surg 1957;27:130.

Tanagho EA: The pathogenesis and management of megaureter. In: Johnston JH, Goodwin WE (editors): *Reviews in Paediatric Urology.* North Holland, 1974.

Tanagho EA: Surgical revision of the incompetent ureterovesical junction: A critical analysis of techniques and requirements. Br J Urol 1970;42:410.

Tanagho EA: Ureteral tailoring. J Urol 1971;106:194.

Tanagho EA, Guthrie TH, Lyon RP: The intravesical ureter in primary reflux. J Urol 1969;101:824.

Tanagho EA, Jonas U: Reduced bladder capacity: Cause of ureterovesical reflux. Urology 1974;4:421.

Tanagho EA, Meyers FH: Trigonal hypertrophy: A cause of ureteral obstruction. J Urol 1965;93:678.

Tanagho EA, Pugh RCB: The anatomy and function of the ureterovesical junction. Br J Urol 1963;35:151.

Tanagho EA, Smith DR, Guthrie TH: Pathophysiology of functional ureteral obstruction. J Urol 1970;104:73.

Tanagho EA et al: Primary vesicoureteral reflux: Experimental studies of its etiology. J Urol 1965;93:165.

Van den Abbeele AD et al: Vesicoureteral reflux in asymptomatic siblings of patients with known reflux: Radionuclide cystography. Pediatrics 1987;79:147.

Verber IG, Strudley MR, Meller ST: ^{99m}Tc dimercaptosuccinic acid (DMSA) scan as first investigation of urinary tract infection. Arch Dis Child 1988;63:1320.

Weiss RA: Update on childhood urinary tract infections and reflux. Semin Nephrol 1998;18:264.

Weiss RM, Biancani P: Characteristics of normal and refluxing ureterovesical junctions. J Urol 1983;129:858.

Whitaker RH: Reflux induced pelvi-ureteric obstruction. Br J Urol 1976;48:555.

Whitaker RH, Flower CDR: Ureters that show both reflux and obstruction. Br J Urol 1979;51:471.

White RH: Management of urinary tract infection and vesicoureteric reflux in children. 1. Operative treatment has no advantage over medical management. Br Med J 1990;300:1391.

White RH: Vesicoureteric reflux and renal scarring. Arch Dis Child 1989;64:407.

Williams DI: The natural history of reflux. Urol Int 1971;26:350.

Woodard JR, Rushton HG: Reflux uropathy. Pediatr Clin North Am 1987;34:1349.

Woodard JR, Zucker I: Current management of the dilated urinary tract in prune belly syndrome. Urol Clin North Am 1990;17:407.

Bacterial Infections of the Genitourinary Tract

13

Hiep T. Nguyen, MD

Urinary tract infection (UTI) is a term that is applied to a variety of clinical conditions ranging from the asymptomatic presence of bacteria in the urine to severe infection of the kidney with resultant sepsis. UTI is one of the more common medical problems. It is estimated that 150 million patients are diagnosed with a UTI yearly, resulting in at least $6 billion in health care expenditures (Stamm and Norrby, 2001). UTIs are at times difficult to diagnose; some cases respond to a short course of a specific antibiotic, while others require a longer course of a broad-spectrum antibiotic. Accurate diagnosis and treatment of a UTI is essential to limit its associated morbidity and mortality and avoid prolonged or unnecessary use of antibiotics. Advances in our understanding of the pathogenesis of UTI, the development of new diagnostic tests, and the introduction of new antimicrobial agents have allowed physicians to appropriately tailor specific treatment for each patient.

EPIDEMIOLOGY

The epidemiology of UTI grouped by age and sex is shown in Table 13–1. In newborns up to 1 year of age, bacteriuria is present in 2.7% of boys and 0.7% in girls (Wettergren, Jodal, and Jonasson, 1985). The incidence of UTI in uncircumcised males is higher than in circumcised males (1.12% compared to 0.11%) during the first 6 months of life(Wiswell and Roscelli, 1986). In children between 1 and 5 years of age, the incidence of bacteriuria in girls increases to 4.5%, while it decreases in boys to 0.5% (Randolph and Greenfield, 1964). Most UTIs in children younger than 5 years are associated with congenital abnormalities of the urinary tract, such as vesicoureteral reflux or obstruction. The incidence of bacteriuria remains relatively constant in children 6–15 years of age. However, the UTIs in these children are more likely to be associated with functional abnormalities of the urinary tract, such as dysfunctional voiding. During adolescence, the incidence of UTI significantly increases (to 20%) in young women, while remaining constant in young men (Sanford, 1975).

Approximately 7 million cases of acute cystitis are diagnosed yearly in young women (Schappert, 1999); this likely is an underestimate of the true incidence of UTI because at least 50% of all UTIs do not come to medical attention. The major risk factors for women 16–35 years of age are related to sexual intercourse and diaphragm use. Later in life, the incidence of UTI increases significantly for both males and females. For women between 36 and 65 years of age, gynecologic surgery and bladder prolapse appear to be important risk factors. In men of the same age group, prostatic hypertrophy/obstruction, catheterization, and surgery are relevant risk factors. For patients older than 65 years, the incidence of UTI continues to increase in both sexes. Incontinence and chronic use of urinary catheters are important risk factors in these patients. In those younger than 1 year and those older than 65 years, the morbidity and mortality of UTI are the greatest (Shortliffe and McCue, 2002).

PATHOGENESIS

Bacterial Entry

Understanding of the mode of bacterial entry, host susceptibility factors, and bacterial pathogenic factors is essential to tailoring appropriate treatment for the diverse clinical manifestations of UTI. There are 4 possible modes of bacterial entry into the genitourinary tract. It is generally accepted that periurethral bacteria ascending into the urinary tract causes most UTI. Most cases of pyelonephritis are caused by the ascent of bacteria from the bladder, through the ureter and into the renal parenchyma. Consequently, the short nature of the female urethra combined with its close proximity to the vaginal vestibule and rectum likely predisposes women to more frequent UTIs than men (Nicolle et al, 1982).

Other modes of bacterial entry are uncommon causes of UTI. Hematogenous spread can occur in immunocompromised patients and in neonates. *Staphylococcus aureus, Candida* species, and *Mycobacterium tuberculosis* are common pathogens that travel through the blood to infect the urinary tract. Lymphatogenous spread through the rectal, colonic, and periuterine lymphatics has been postulated as a cause for UTI; however, currently there is little scientific support to suggest that dissemination of bacteria through lymphatic

Table 13–1. Epidemiology of UTI by age group and sex.

Age (y)	Incidence (%) Female	Male	Risk Factors
< 1	0.7	2.7	Foreskin, anatomic GU abnormalities
1–5	4.5	0.5	Anatomic GU abnormalities
6–15	4.5	0.5	Functional GU abnormalities
16–35	20	0.5	Sexual intercourse, diaphragm use
36–65	35	20	Surgery, prostate obstruciton, catheterization
> 65	40	35	Incontinence, catheterization, prostate obstruction

GU, genitourinary.

channels plays a role in the pathogenesis of UTI. Direct extension of bacteria from adjacent organs into the urinary tract can occur in patients with intraperitoneal abscesses or vesicointestinal or vesicovaginal fistulas. Relapsing infection from an inadequately treated focus in the prostate or kidney may seed other parts of the urinary tracts.

Host Defenses

Host factors have an essential role in the pathogenesis of UTI. Unobstructed urinary flow with the subsequent washout of ascending bacteria is essential in preventing UTI. In addition, the urine itself has specific characteristics (its osmolality, urea concentration, organic acid concentration, and pH) that inhibit bacterial growth and colonization (Sobel, 1997). It also contains factors that inhibit bacterial adherence, such as Tamm-Horsfall glycoprotein (Duncan, 1988; Pak et al, 2001). Urinary retention, stasis, or reflux of urine into the upper urinary tract can promote bacterial growth and subsequent infection. Consequently, any anatomic or functional abnormalities of the urinary tract that impede urinary flow can increase the host's susceptibility to UTI. These abnormalities include obstructive conditions at any level of the urinary tract, neurologic diseases affecting the function of the lower urinary tract, diabetes, and pregnancy. Similarly, the presence of foreign bodies (such as stones, catheters, and stents) allows the bacteria to hide from these host defenses.

In response to the presence of bacteria, cells lining the urinary tract secrete chemoattractants such as interleukin-8 to recruit neutrophils to the area and limit tissue invasion (Frendeus et al, 2001). Specific serum and urinary antibodies are produced by the kidney to enhance bacterial opsonization and phagocytosis and to inhibit bacterial adherence. The protective role of both cellular and humoral-mediated immunity in preventing UTIs remains unclear; deficiency in B-cell or T-cell function has not been associated with the increased frequency of UTI or altered the course of the infection (Schaeffer, 2001; Svanborg Eden et al, 1988).

Many studies have demonstrated that there is selectivity in bacterial adherence to cells lining the urinary tract, and the degree of adherence correlates with colonization and infection. Women with recurrent UTIs have higher adherence of bacteria to their mucosal cells in vitro compared to women who never had an infection (Navas et al, 1994). The increased adherence may be due to having more binding sites for bacterial adhesins on their mucosal cells. Alternatively, these patients may not secrete soluble compounds, which normally compete for the same receptors that bind bacterial adhesins. Blood group antigens may constitute one group of these soluble compounds that inhibit bacterial adherence (Lomberg et al, 1986). These findings would suggest a genetic predisposition for UTI.

Other important host factors include the normal flora of the periurethral area or the prostate and the presence of vesicoureteral reflux. In women, the normal flora of the periurethral area composed of organisms such as lactobacillus provide a defense against the colonization of uropathogenic bacteria (Osset et al, 2001). Alterations in the periurethral environment (such as changes in the pH or estrogen levels or the use of antibiotics) can damage the periurethral flora, allowing uropathogens to colonize and subsequently to infect the urinary tract (Schaeffer et al, 1999). In men, the prostate secretes fluid containing zinc, which has potent antimicrobial activity (Fair, Couch, and Wehner, 1976). Finally, in children, the presence of vesicoureteral reflux does not increase their susceptibility to UTI but does allow bacteria to be inoculated into the upper tract and the infection to progress.

Aging is associated with an increased susceptibility to UTI, in part because of the increased incidence of obstructive uropathy in men (Matsumoto, 2001; Nicolle, 2002) and alteration in the vaginal and periurethral flora from menopause in women (Foxman et al, 2001). Other causes include soiling of the perineum from fecal incontinence, neuromuscular diseases, increased instrumentation, and bladder catheterization (Ronald, 2002).

Bacterial Pathogenic Factors

Not all bacteria are capable of adhering to and infecting the urinary tract. Of the many strains of *Escherichia coli,* the uropathogens belong to a limited number of O, K, and H serogroups. They have increased adherence properties to uroepithelial cells (Blanco et al, 1996; Hovanec and Gorzynski, 1980; Orskov et al,

1982), resistance to the bactericidal activity of human serum (Bjorksten and Kaijser, 1978), production of hemolysin (Hughes et al, 1983; Koronakis and Hughes, 1996), and the increased expression of K capsular antigen (Whitfield and Roberts, 1999). The ability of *E coli* to adhere to epithelial cells is mediated by ligands located on the tips of the bacterial fimbriae (pili). The ligands bind to glycolipids or glycoprotein receptors on the surface membrane of uroepithelial cells. The pili are classified by their ability to cause hemagglutination and the type of sugar that can block this process. P pili, which can agglutinate human blood, bind to glycolipid receptors on uroepithelial cells, erythrocytes (P-blood group antigens), and renal tubular cells (Svenson et al, 1983). Type 1 pili, which can agglutinate guinea pig blood, bind to mannoside residues on uroepithelial cells (Ofek et al, 2000). P pili are observed in over 90% of the *E coli* strains causing pyelonephritis but less than 20% of the strains causing lower urinary tract infections (Kallenius et al, 1981; JA Roberts et al, 1997). In contrast, type 1 pili may help bacteria to adhere to bladder mucosa (Connell et al, 1996; Martinez et al, 2000). Most uropathogenic *E coli* have both types of pili. Once attachment to the uroepithelial cells occurs, other bacterial pathogenic factors become important. Most uropathogenic *E coli* strains produce hemolysin, which initiates tissue invasion and makes iron available for the infecting pathogens (Hughes et al, 1983; Koronakis and Hughes, 1996). The presence of K antigen on the invading bacteria protects them from phagocytosis by neutrophils (Bortolussi et al, 1979; Evans et al, 1981). These factors allow the infecting pathogens to escape the various host defenses (Svanborg et al, 1996).

CAUSATIVE PATHOGENS

Most UTIs are caused by a single bacterial species. At least 80% of the uncomplicated cystitis and pyelonephritis are due to *E coli,* with most of pathogenic strains belong to the O serogroups (Orskov et al, 1982). Other less common uropathogens include *Klebsiella, Proteus,* and *Enterobacter* spp. and enterococci. In hospital-acquired UTIs, a wider variety of causative organisms is found, including *Pseudomonas* and *Staphylococcus* spp. (Wagenlehner and Naber, 2000). UTIs caused by *S aureus* often result from hematogenous dissemination. Group B β-hemolytic streptococci can cause UTIs in pregnant women (Wood and Dillon, 1981). *Staphylococcus saprophyticus,* once often thought of as urinary contaminants, can cause uncomplicated UTIs in young women (Hovelius and Mardh, 1984). In children, the causative bacterial spectrum is slightly different from that of adults, with *Klebsiella* and *Enterobacter* spp. being more common causes of UTI (Jeena et al, 1996; Ronald, 2002; Schlager, 2001). Anaerobic bacteria, lactobacilli, corynebacteria, streptococci (not including enterococci) and *Staphylococcus epidermidis* are found in normal periurethral flora. They do not commonly cause UTIs in healthy individuals and are considered common urinary contaminants.

DIAGNOSIS

The diagnosis of UTI is sometimes difficult to establish and relies on urinalysis and urine culture. Occasionally, localization studies may be required to identify the source of the infection. Most often, the urine is often obtained from a voided specimen. In children who are not toilet-trained, a urine collection device, such as a bag, is placed over the genitalia, and the urine is cultured from the bagged specimen. These 2 methods of urine collection are easy to obtain, but potential contamination from the vagina and perirectal area may occur. There is a high false-positive rate, especially from bagged specimens (Al-Orifi et al, 2000). Suprapubic aspiration avoids potential contamination; however, due to its invasiveness, it is rarely used except in children and selected patients. Urine obtained from a urinary catheter is less invasive than a suprapubic aspiration and is less likely to be contaminated than that from a voided specimen. If a patient has an indwelling catheter, a urine specimen should be obtained from the collection port on the catheter.

Urinalysis

Urinalysis provides a rapid screen for UTIs. The urine can be immediately evaluated for leukocyte esterase, a compound produced by the breakdown of white blood cells (WBCs) in the urine. Urinary nitrite is produced by reduction of dietary nitrates by many gram-negative bacteria. Esterase and nitrite can be detected by a urine dipstick and are more reliable when the bacterial count is greater than 100,000 colony-forming units (CFU) per milliliter. Microscopic examination of the urine for WBCs and bacteria is performed after centrifugation. When bacteria counts are greater than 100,000 CFU/mL, bacteria can be detected microscopically (Jenkins, Fenn, and Matsen, 1986). More than 3 WBCs per high-power field suggests a possible infection. The sensitivity and specificity of these tests are shown in Table 13–2. The urinary nitrite test is highly specific but not sensitive, whereas the other 3 tests have a sensitivity and specificity approximately 80%. A combination of these tests may help to identify those patients in whom urine culture will be positive.

Urine Culture

The gold standard for identification of UTI is the quantitative culture of urine for specific bacteria. The

Table 13–2. Sensitivity and specificity of urinalysis.

Tests	Sensitivity (%)	Specificity (%)
Esterase	83 (67–94)	78 (64–92)
Nitrite	53 (15–82)	98 (90–100)
E or N	93 (90–100)	72 (58–91)
White blood cells	73 (32–100)	81 (45–98)
Bacteria	81 (16–99)	83 (11–100)
Any above	99.8 (99–100)	70 (60–92)

urine should be collected in a sterile container and cultured immediately after collection. When this is not possible, the urine can be stored in the refrigerator for up to 24 hours. The sample is then diluted and spread on culture plates. Each bacterium will form a single colony on the plates. The number of colonies is counted and adjusted per milliliter of urine (CFU/mL). Defining the CFU/mL that represents clinically significant infection can be difficult. It is dependent on the method of collection, the sex of the patient, and the type of bacteria isolated (Table 13–3). Traditionally, greater than 100,000 CFU/mL is used to exclude contamination. However, studies have clearly demonstrated that clinically significant UTI can occur with less than 100,000 CFU/mL bacteria in the urine (Stamm et al, 1982).

Table 13–3. Probability of UTIs based on urine culture.

Collection	CFU	Probability of Infection (%)
Suprapubic	Gram neg. any	> 99
	Gram pos. > 1000	
Catheterization	> 10^5	95
	10^{4-5}	Likely
	10^{3-4}	Repeat
	< 10^3	Unlikely
Clean catch		
Male	> 10^4	Likely
Female	3 specimens: > 10^5	95
	2 specimens: > 10^5	90
	1 specimen: > 10^5	80
	5×10^4–10^5	Repeat
	1–5×10^4 sympt.	Repeat
	1–5×10^4 nonsympt.	Unlikely
	< 10^4	Unlikely

CFU, colony-forming unit; gram neg, gram-negative; gram pos., gram-positive; nonsympt, nonsymptomatic; sympt, symptomatic.

Localization Studies

Occasionally, it is necessary to localize the site of infection. For upper urinary tract localization (Lorentz, 1979), the bladder is irrigated with sterile water and a ureteral catheter is placed into each ureter. A specimen is collected from the renal pelvis. Culture of this specimen will indicate whether infection in the upper urinary tract is present. In men, infection in the lower urinary tract can be differentiated (Figure 13–1) (Meares and Stamey, 1968). A specimen is collected at the beginning of the void and represents possible infection in the urethra. A midstream specimen is next collected and represents possible infection in the bladder. The prostate is then massaged and the patient is asked to void again. This specimen represents possible infection of the prostate.

ANTIBIOTICS

Treatment with antimicrobial agents has minimized the morbidity and mortality associated with UTIs. The goal in treatment is to eradicate the infection by selecting the appropriate antibiotics that would target specific bacterial susceptibility. However, choosing the appropriate antimicrobial agents is often difficult. Many antibiotics are available, and the lowest effective dose and length of therapy are not well defined. Many con-

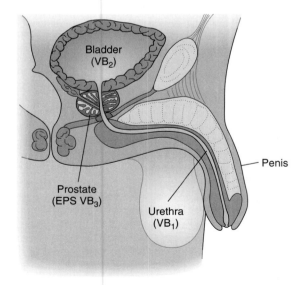

Figure 13–1. Localization of lower urinary tract infection. A positive culture in the VB1 specimen suggests infection of the urethra, while in VB2 an infection of the bladder, and in EPS or VB3 an infection of the prostate.

ventions for the treatment of UTI are arbitrary. The general principles for selecting the appropriate antibiotics include consideration of the infecting pathogen (antibiotic susceptibility, single-organism vs. poly-organism infection, pathogen vs. normal flora, community vs. hospital-acquired infection); the patient (allergies, underlying diseases, age, previous antibiotic therapy, other medications currently taken, outpatient vs. inpatient status, pregnancy); and the site of infection (kidney vs. bladder vs. prostate). Because most antibiotics are cleared from the body by the liver or the kidney, certain antimicrobial agents need to be adjusted in the presence of liver or renal diseases (Table 13–4). Table 13–5 lists the common uropathogens and the recommended oral and intravenous antimicrobial agents for treatment. Table 13–6 lists the common sites of UTI, the recommended treatment, and the duration of therapy. In patients with recurrent UTIs or those who are at risk for UTI (such as children with vesicoureteral reflux), prophylactic antibiotics may be used. Table 13–7 lists common prophylactic regimens.

Trimethoprim-Sulfamethoxazole

Trimethoprim-sulfamethoxazole (TMP-SMX) is commonly used to treat many UTIs, except those caused by

Table 13–4. Antibiotics that require dosage adjustments for liver and renal diseases.

Renal diseases (Creatinine clearance < 30 mL/min)
Aminoglycosides
β-Lactams

Cefoxitin	Ceftizoxime
Cefonacid	Ceftazidime
Cefuroxime	Cefepime
Cepirome	Moxalactam

Carbenicillin, ticarcillin, ticarcillin-clavulanate
Vancomycin
Tetracycline (except doxycycline)
Sulfonamides

Hepatic diseases (with elevated bilirubin)
Chloramphenicol
Tetracyclines
Clindamycin, rifampin, pefloxacin

Renal-hepatic diseases
Ceftriaxone
Cefoperazone
Carbenicillin
Ticarcillin
Azlocillin
Mezlocillin
Piperacillin

Enterococcus and *Pseudomonas* spp. It interferes with the bacterial metabolism of folate. Trimethoprim-sulfamethoxazole is highly effective and relatively inexpensive. Adverse reactions occur in 6–8% of patients using this medication; they include hypersensitivity reactions, rashes, gastrointestinal upset, leukopenia, thrombocytopenia, and photosensitivity. Trimethoprim-sulfamethoxazole should not be used in patients who have a folic acid deficiency state, glucose-6-phosphate dehydrogenase deficiency, or AIDS, or in pregnant patients. It is the most frequently prescribed antibiotic for uncomplicated UTI (Huang and Stafford, 2002). Recently, the use of TMP-SMX has declined due to the increased incidence of bacterial resistance (Brown et al, 2002) and physicians' preference for other newer antibiotics (Huang and Stafford, 2002).

Fluoroquinolones

Fluoroquinolones have a broad spectrum of activity, especially against gram-negative bacteria. Although they have adequate activity against *Staphylococci* species, fluoroquinolones do not have good activity against *Streptococci* species and anaerobic bacteria. They interfere with the bacterial DNA gyrase, preventing bacterial replication. Although they are highly effective in the treatment of UTI, fluoroquinolones are relative expensive. Adverse reactions are infrequent and include mild gastrointestinal effects, dizziness, and lightheadedness. Fluoroquinolones should not be used in patients who are pregnant and should be used judiciously in children because of potential damage to developing cartilage. Due to their broad spectrum of activity, fluoroquinolones have gained popularity in the empiric treatment of both uncomplicated and complicated UTIs (Schaeffer, 2002).

Nitrofurantoin

Nitrofurantoin has good activity against most gram-negative bacteria (except for *Pseudomonas* and *Proteus* spp.), *Staphylococci,* and *Enterococci* species. It inhibits bacterial enzymes and DNA activity. Nitrofurantoin is highly effective in the treatment of UTI and is relative inexpensive. Adverse reactions are relatively common and include gastrointestinal upset, peripheral polyneuropathy, and hepatotoxicity. Long-term use may result in pulmonary hypersensitivity reaction and interstitial changes. With increasing awareness of this antibiotic and its activity against common uropathogens, nitrofurantoin usage in the treatment of uncomplicated UTIs has increased from 14% to 30% in the past 5 years (Huang and Stafford, 2002).

Table 13–5. Recommended antimicrobial agents for common genitourinary pathogens.

Bacteria	Oral Therapy	Parenteral Therapy
Gram-positive cocci		
Staphylococcus aureus	Nafcillin, nitrofurantoin, ciprofloxacin	Nafcillin, vancomycin
Staphylococcus epidermidis	Ampicillin, nitrofurantoin, ciprofloxacin	Ampicillin, penicillin G
Staphylococcus saprophyticus	Ampicillin, nitrofurantoin, ciprofloxacin	Ampicillin, penicillin G
Streptococcus, group D		
S faecalis (enterococci)	Ampicillin, nitrofurantoin	Ampicillin plus gentamicin
S bovis	Penicillin G, ampicillin	Ampicillin, vancomycin
Streptococcus, group B	Ampicillin, cephalosporin	Ampicillin, cephalosporin
Gram-negative cocci		
Neisseria gonorrhoeae	Ciprofloxacin plus doxycycline	Ceftriaxone
Gram-negative rods		
Escherichia coli	TMP-SMX, ciprofloxacin, nitrofurantoin	Gentamicin
Enterobacter sp.	TMP-SMX, ciprofloxacin, nitrofurantoin	Gentamicin plus piperacillin
Gardnerella vaginalis	Metronidazole, ampicillin	Metronidazole
Klebsiella sp.	TMP-SMX, ciprofloxacin	Gentamicin plus cephalosporin
Proteus sp.	Ampicillin, TMP-SMX, ciprofloxacin	Ampicillin, gentamicin
Pseudomonas aeruginosa	Carbenicillin, tetracycline, ciprofloxacin	Gentamicin plus piperacillin
Serratia sp.	TMP-SMX, carbenicillin	TMP-SMX, amikacin
Other pathogens		
Chlamydiae	Tetracycline, erythromycin	Tetracycline, erythromycin
Mycoplasmas, ureaplasmas	Tetracycline, erythromycin	Tetracycline, erythromycin
Obligate anaerobes	Metronidazole, clindamycin	Metronidazole, clindamycin

TMP-SMX, trimethoprim plus sulfamethoxazole.

Table 13–6. Recommended antimicrobial agents and duration of therapy based on the type of UTI.

Diagnosis	Pathogen	Choice of Antibiotics	Duration of Therapy
Cystitis	*E coli* *Klebsiella* *Proteus*	1st: TMP/SMX 2nd: Fluoroquinolone	1–3 days
Pyelonephritis	*E coli* *Proteus* *Klebsiella* *Enterobacteria*	1st: Gluoroquinolone 2nd: 2nd generation cephalosporin 3rd: Aminopenicillin/BLI	7–10 days
Complicated UTI	*E coli* *Enterococci* *Pseudomonas* *Staphylococci*	1st Fluoroquinolone 2nd: Aminopenicillin/BLI 3rd: 3rd generation cephalosporin Aminoglycosides	3–5 days after afebrile
Prostatitis	*E coli* *Enterobacteria* *Pseudomonas* *Enterococci*	1st: Fluoroquinolone 2nd: 2nd generation cephalosporin 3rd: 3rd generation cephalosporin	Acute: 2 weeks Chronic: 4–6 weeks
Epididymitis	*E coli* *Enterobacteria* *Enterococci* *Chlmaydia* *Ureaplasma*	1st: Fluoroquinolone 2nd: 2nd generation cephalosporin 1st: Doxycycline 2nd: Macrolide	2 weeks

BLI, beta-lactamase inhibitor; TMP/SMX, trimethoprim-sulfamethoxazole.
(Adapted from table 2 from Wagenlehner and Naber, 2000.)

Table 13–7. Prophylactic antibiotics regimen.

Nitrofurantoin, 50 or 100 mg daily
Nitrofurantoin macrocrystals, 100 mg daily
TMP-SMX, 40/200 mg daily
Cephalexin, 250 mg daily
Ciprofloxacin, 250 mg daily
Trimethoprim, 100 mg daily

TMP-SMX, trimethoprim-sulfamethoxazole.

Aminoglycosides

Aminoglycosides are commonly used in the treatment of complicated UTI. They are highly effective against most gram-negative bacteria. When combined with ampicillin, they are effective against enterococci. They inhibit bacterial DNA and RNA synthesis. The principal adverse effects of aminoglycosides are nephrotoxicity and ototoxicity. Aminoglycosides are primarily used in patients with complicated UTIs who require intravenous antibiotics (Santucci and Krieger, 2000). Aminoglycosides can be given as a single daily dosing; this regimen is directed toward obtaining higher peak and lower trough levels in order to achieve more effective microbial killing while reducing toxicity (Carapetis et al, 2001).

Cephalosporins

Cephalosporins have good activity against most uropathogens (Garcia-Rodriguez and Munoz Bellido, 2000). First-generation cephalosporins have good activity against gram-positive bacteria, *E coli,* and *Proteus* and *Klebsiella* spp. Second-generation cephalosporins have increased activity against anaerobes and *Haemophilus influenzae.* Third-generation cephalosporins have broader coverage against gram-negative bacteria but less against gram-positive bacteria. The cephalosporins inhibit bacterial cell wall synthesis. Adverse reactions include hypersensitivity and gastrointestinal upset. Oral cephalosporins have been used effectively in the empiric treatment of uncomplicated UTIs (Lawrenson and Logie, 2001); in children with febrile UTI/pyelonephritis, oral third-generation cephalosporins such as cefixime have been shown to be safe and effective (Hoberman et al, 1999).

Penicillins

First-generation penicillins are ineffective against most uropathogens and are not commonly used in the treatment of UTI. However, the aminopenicillins (amoxicillin and ampicillin) have good activity against *Enterococci, Staphylococci, E coli,* and *Proteus mirabilis.* However, gram-negative bacteria can quickly develop resistance to many aminopenicillins. The addition of β-lactamase inhibitors such as clavulanic acid makes the aminopenicillins more active against the gram-negative bacteria. Although penicillins and aminopenicillins are inexpensive, the addition of the β-lactamase inhibitors makes them more expensive. Adverse reactions include hypersensitivity (which can be immediate or delayed), gastrointestinal upset, and diarrhea. In general, penicillins are not commonly used in the treatment of UTI unless they are combined with β-lactamase inhibitors (Sotto et al, 2001).

■ CLINICAL PRESENTATION

KIDNEY INFECTION

Acute Pyelonephritis

Acute pyelonephritis is defined as inflammation of the kidney and renal pelvis, and its diagnosis is usually made clinically.

A. PRESENTATION AND FINDINGS

Patients with acute pyelonephritis present with chills, fever, and costovertebral angle tenderness. They often have accompanying lower-tract symptoms such as dysuria, frequency, and urgency. Sepsis may occur, with 20–30% of all systemic sepsis resulting from a urine infection. Urinalysis commonly demonstrates the presence of WBCs and red blood cells in the urine. Leukocytosis, increased erythrocyte sedimentation, and elevated levels of C-reactive protein are commonly seen on blood analysis. Bacteria are cultured from the urine when the culture is obtained before antibiotic treatment is instituted. *E coli* is the most common causative organism, accounting for 80% of the cases. *Klebsiella, Proteus, Enterobacter, Pseudomonas, Serratia,* and *Citrobacter* spp. account for the remaining cases. Of the gram-positive bacteria, *Streptococcus faecalis* and *S aureus* can be important causes of pyelonephritis.

B. RADIOGRAPHIC IMAGING

Contrast-enhanced computed tomography (CT) scans can accurately demonstrate findings, confirming the diagnosis of pyelonephritis (Dacher et al, 1993). Acute bacterial infection causes constriction of peripheral arterioles and reduces perfusion of the affected renal segments. Perfusion defects, which can be segmental, multifocal, or diffuse, are seen as areas of reduced signal density (Figure 13–2). Renal enlargement, attenuated parenchyma, and a compressed collecting system are other characteristic findings on CT scan. However, CT scan is not necessary unless the diagnosis is unclear or

Figure 13–2. Acute pyelonephritis. Computed tomography scan with intravenous contrast demonstrates a perfusion defect (white arrow) and enlargement of the affected kidney.

the patient is not responding to therapy. Radionuclide study with ^{99m}Tc-dimercaptosuccinic acid is equally sensitive in detecting the perfusion defects of pyelonephritis (Levtchenko et al, 2001). In patients with acute pyelonephritis, renal ultrasonography is important to rule out concurrent urinary tract obstruction but cannot reliably detect inflammation or infection of the kidney.

C. MANAGEMENT

The management of acute pyelonephritis depends on the severity of the infection (Ghiro et al, 2002; Nickel, 2001). In patients who have toxicity because of associated septicemia, hospitalization is warranted. Empiric therapy with intravenous ampicillin and aminoglycosides is effective against a broad range of uropathogens, including enterococci and *Pseudomonas* species. Alternatively, amoxicillin with clavulanic acid or a third-generation cephalosporin can be used. Fever from acute

pyelonephritis may persist for several days despite appropriate therapy. Parenteral therapy should be maintained until the patient defervesces. If bacteremia is present, parenteral therapy should be continued for an additional 7–10 days and then the patient should be switched to oral treatment for 10–14 days. In patients who are not severely ill, outpatient treatment with oral antibiotics is appropriate. For adults, treatment with fluoroquinolones or TMP-SMX is well tolerated and effective. Therapy should continue for 10–14 days. Some patients in whom acute pyelonephritis develops will require follow-up radiologic examination such as voiding cystourethrogram or cystoscopy.

Emphysematous Pyelonephritis

Emphysematous pyelonephritis is a necrotizing infection characterized by the presence of gas within the renal parenchyma or perinephric tissue. Eighty to ninety percent of patients with emphysematous pyelonephritis have diabetes; the rest of the cases are associated with urinary tract obstruction from calculi or papillary necrosis (Shokeir et al, 1997).

A. Presentation and Findings

Patients with emphysematous pyelonephritis present with fever, flank pain, and vomiting that fails initial management with parenteral antibiotics (Tang et al, 2001). Pneumaturia may be present. Bacteria most frequently cultured from the urine include *E coli, Klebsiella pneumoniae,* and *Enterobacter cloacae.*

B. Radiographic Imaging

The diagnosis of emphysematous pyelonephritis is made after radiographic examination. Gas overlying the affected kidney may be seen on a plain abdominal radiograph (KUB). CT scan is much more sensitive in detecting the presence of gas in the renal parenchyma than renal ultrasonography.

C. Management

In the management of emphysematous pyelonephritis, prompt control of blood glucose and relief of urinary obstruction is essential, in addition to fluid resuscitation and parenteral antibiotics. The mortality rate is 11–54% (Michaeli et al, 1984). Poor prognostic factors include high serum creatinine level, low platelet count, and the presence of renal/perirenal fluid in association with a bubbly/loculated gas pattern or gas in the collecting system (Wan et al, 1998). In combination with medical treatment, percutaneous drainage appears to be helpful in accelerating resolution of the infection and minimizing the morbidity and mortality of the infection (Chen et al, 1997). Nephrectomy may be required if there is no function in the affected kidney. Three to four weeks of parenteral antibiotic therapy is usually required.

Chronic Pyelonephritis

Chronic pyelonephritis results from repeated renal infection, which leads to scarring, atrophy of the kidney, and subsequent renal insufficiency. The diagnosis is made by radiologic or pathologic examination rather than from clinical presentation.

A. Presentation and Findings

Many individuals with chronic pyelonephritis have no symptoms, but they may have a history of frequent UTIs. In children, there is a strong correlation between renal scarring and recurrent UTIs (Wennerstrom et al, 2000). The developing kidney appears to be very susceptible to damage, and this susceptibility appears to be age-dependent. Renal scarring induced by UTIs is

rarely seen in adult kidneys. Because patients with chronic pyelonephritis often are asymptomatic, the diagnosis is made incidentally when radiologic investigation is initiated to evaluate for the complications associated with renal insufficiency, such as hypertension, visual impairments, headaches, fatigue, and polyuria. In these patients, urinalysis may show leukocytes or proteinuria but is likely to be normal. Serum creatinine levels reflect the severity of the renal impairment. Urine cultures are only positive when there is an active infection.

B. Radiographic Imaging

Intravenous pyelogram or CT scan can readily demonstrate a small and atrophic kidney on the affected side. Focal coarse renal scarring with clubbing of the underlying calyx is characteristic. Ultrasonography similarly can demonstrate these findings. DMSA is the best imaging modality to look for renal scarring (Figure 13–3A–B) (Stoller and Kogan, 1986). Areas of scarring can be seen as photopenic areas.

C. Management

The management of chronic pyelonephritis is somewhat limited because renal damage incurred by chronic pyelonephritis is not reversible. Eliminating recurrent UTIs and identifying and correcting any underlying anatomic or functional urinary problems such as obstruction or urolithiasis can prevent further renal damage. In children, evaluation for vesicoureteral reflux with a voiding cystourethrogram is important to eliminate a risk factor for recurrent pyelonephritis and renal scarring. Long-term use of continuous prophylactic antibiotic therapy may be required to limit recurrent UTIs and renal scarring. Rarely, removal of the affected kidney may be necessary due to hypertension or having a large stone burden in a nonfunctioning kidney.

Renal Abscesses

Renal abscesses result from a severe infection that leads to liquefaction of renal tissue; this area is subsequently sequestered, forming an abscess. They can rupture out into the perinephric space, forming **perinephric abscesses.** When the abscesses extend beyond the Gerota's fascia, **paranephric abscesses** develop. Historically, most renal/perinephric abscesses result from hematogenous spread of staphylococci, in particular from infected skin lesions. Patients with diabetes, those undergoing hemodialysis, or intravenous drug abusers were at high risk for developing renal abscesses. With the development of effective antibiotics and better management of diseases such as diabetes and renal failure, renal/perinephric abscesses due to gram-positive bacteria are less prevalent; those caused by *E coli* or *Proteus* species are

A

B

Figure 13–3. Chronic pyelonephritis. Multiple parenchymal defects (white and black arrows) are seen on DMSA scan (**A**), suggestive of scarring from recurrent infection. Voiding cystourethrogram (**B**) revealed high-grade reflux in this patient.

becoming more common (Merimsky and Feldman, 1981; Thorley, Jones, and Sanford, 1974). Abscesses that form in the renal cortex are likely to arise from hematogenous spread, whereas those in the corticomedullary junction are caused from gram-negative bacteria in conjunction with some other underlying urinary tract abnormalities, such as stones or obstruction.

A. Presentation and Findings

The most common presenting symptoms in patients with renal/perinephric abscesses include fever, flank or abdominal pain, chills, and dysuria. Many of the symptoms have lasted for more than 2 weeks. A flank mass may be palpated in some patients. Urinalysis usually demonstrates WBCs; however, it may be normal in approximately 25% of the cases (Thorley, Jones, and Sanford, 1974). Urine cultures only identify the causative organisms in about one-third of cases and blood cultures in only about half of cases (Edelstein and Mc-Cabe, 1988).

B. Radiographic Imaging

Renal abscesses can be accurately detected using ultrasonography or CT scans. There is a wide range of ultrasonographic findings ranging from an anechoic mass within or displacing the kidney to an echogenic fluid collection that tends to blend with the normally echogenic fat within Gerota's fascia (Corriere and Sandler, 1982). With high sensitivity, CT scans can demon-strate an enlarged kidney with focal areas of hypoattenuation early on during the course of the infection. Once the inflammatory wall forms around the fluid collection, the abscess appears as a mass with a rim of contrast enhancement, the "ring" sign (Figure 13–4). CT scans may also demonstrate thickening of Gerota's fascia, stranding of the perinephric fat, or obliteration of the surrounding soft-tissue planes (Dalla Palma, Pozzi-Mucelli, and Ene, 1999). Intravenous pyelogram and kidneys, ureter, and bladder tests are less sensitive tests in detecting renal/perinephric abscesses, with results being normal in about 20% of the cases (Thorley et al, 1974).

C. Management

The appropriate management of renal abscess first must include appropriate antibiotic therapy. Because it is often very difficult to identify the correct causative organisms from the urine or blood, empiric therapy with broad-spectrum antibiotics (ampicillin or vancomycin in combination with an aminoglycoside or third-generation cephalosporin) is usually recommended. If the patient does not respond within 48 h of treatment, percutaneous drainage under CT or ultrasound guidance is indicated (Siegel, Smith, and Moldwin, 1996). The drained fluid should be cultured for the causative organisms. If the abscess still does not resolve, then open surgical drainage or nephrectomy may be necessary. Follow-up imaging is needed to confirm resolution of the abscesses. These patients will also require evaluation

Figure 13–4. Renal abscess. CT scan with intravenous contrast demonstrates a large perinephric fluid collection with rim enhancement (white arrow). The parenchyma defect in the right kidney is suggestive of pyelonephritis.

for underlying urinary tract abnormalities such as stone or obstruction after the infection has resolved.

Xanthogranulomatous Pyelonephritis

Xanthogranulomatous pyelonephritis (XGP) is a form of chronic bacterial infection of the kidney. The affected kidney is almost always hydronephrotic and obstructed. In most cases, XGP occurs unilaterally. Severe inflammation and necrosis obliterate the kidney parenchyma. Characteristically, foamy lipid-laden histiocytes (xanthoma cells) are present and may be mistaken for renal clear cell carcinoma (Iskandar, Prahlow, and White, 1993; Lorentzen and Nielsen, 1980).

A. PRESENTATION AND FINDINGS

Patients with XGP commonly present with flank pain, fever, chills, and persistent bacteriuria. A history of urolithiasis is present in about 35% of the patients (Malek and Elder, 1978). On physical examination, a flank mass can often be palpated. Urinalysis commonly demonstrates WBCs and protein. Serum blood analysis reveals anemia and may show hepatic dysfunction in approximately 50% of the patients (Malek and Elder, 1978). Because XGP primarily occurs unilaterally, azotemia or renal failure is not often seen (Goodman et al, 1979). *E coli* or *Proteus* species are commonly cultured from the urine. However, one-third of patients with XGP have no growth in their urine, most likely because they have recently received antibiotic therapy. Approximately 10% of the patients with XGP have mixed organisms or anaerobic bacteria identified in their urine. Culture of the affected renal tissue can reliably identify the causative organism.

B. RADIOGRAPHIC IMAGING

CT scan is the most reliable method in imaging patients suspected of having XGP. It usually demonstrates a large heterogeneous, reniform mass. The renal parenchyma is often marked with multiple water-density lesions, representing dilated calyces or abscesses (Figure 13–5A–B) (Goldman et al, 1984). On contrast-enhanced images, these lesions will have a prominent blush peripherally, while the central areas, which are filled with pus and debris, do not enhance. An area of central calcification surrounded by a contracted pelvis may also be seen (Eastham, Ahlering, and Skinner, 1994). The inflammatory process may be seen extending to the perinephric fat, the retroperitoneum, and adjacent organs such as the psoas muscle, spleen, colon, or the great vessels. Because of the association of urolithiasis and XGP, renal calculi may be seen (Parsons, 1993). Renal ultrasonography can also be used in performing imaging on patients with XGP (Tiu et al, 2001). It usually reveals an enlarged kidney with a large central echogenic area and anechoic parenchyma. However, ultrasonography does not provide comparable anatomic details to those obtained from CT scan. It is not uncommon for XGP to be misdiagnosed as a renal tumor because of their similar appearances on radiologic imaging (Zorzos et al, 2002).

C. MANAGEMENT

The management of XGP is dependent on accurate diagnosis. In some cases, XGP is misdiagnosed as a renal tumor. A nephrectomy is performed and a diagnosis is made pathologically. In those in whom a diagnosis of XGP is suspected, kidney-sparing surgery such as a partial nephrectomy is indicated. However, when the infection is extensive, a nephrectomy with excision of all involved tissue is warranted. There are reported cases of treating XGP with antibiotic therapy alone (Brown, Dodson, and Weintrub, 1996) or in combination with percutaneous drainage; however, these treatments are not likely to be curative in most patients and may lead to complications such as renal cutaneous fistula.

Pyonephrosis

Pyonephrosis refers to bacterial infection of a hydronephrotic, obstructed kidney, which leads to suppurative destruction of the renal parenchyma and potential loss of renal function. Because of the extent of the infection and the presence of urinary obstruction, sepsis may rapidly ensue, requiring rapid diagnosis and management.

A. PRESENTATION AND FINDINGS

Patients with pyonephrosis are usually very ill, with high fever, chills, and flank pain. Lower-tract symptoms are not usually present. Bacteriuria and pyuria may not be present when there is complete obstruction of the affected kidney.

B. RADIOGRAPHIC IMAGING

Imaging with renal ultrasonography can be performed to rapidly diagnose pyonephrosis. Ultrasonographic findings include persistent echoes in the inferior portion of the collecting system, fluid-debris level with dependent echoes that shift with positional changes (Figure 13–6), strong echoes with acoustic shadowing from air in the collecting system, and weak echoes throughout a dilated collecting system. Renal or ureteral calculi may also be identified on ultrasonography.

C. MANAGEMENT

Management of pyonephrosis includes immediate institution of antibiotic therapy and drainage of the infected collecting system. Broad-spectrum antimicrobials are indicated to prevent sepsis while the causative organism is being identified; antibiotics should be started before manipulation of the urinary tract. Performing drainage of the obstruction through the lower urinary tract (such as using a ureteral stent) should be reserved for patients who are not septic. Extensive manipulation may rapidly induce sepsis and toxemia. In the ill patient, drainage of the collecting system with a percutaneous nephrostomy tube is preferable. Once the infection is treated, additional imaging evaluation is required to identify the cause of the urinary obstruction, such as urolithiasis or ureteropelvic junction obstruction.

BLADDER INFECTION

Acute Cystitis

Acute cystitis refers to urinary infection of the lower urinary tract, principally the bladder. Acute cystitis

---

Figure 13–5. Xanthogranulomatous pyelonephritis. CT scan (**A**) demonstrates a large heterogeneous left kidney, with dilated calyces and areas filled with lipid-laden macrophages. Xanthogranulomatous pyelonephritis is often associated with the presence of renal stones. Pathology specimen (**B**) better demonstrated the pockets of intraparenchymal abscesses and deposition of macrophages (arrows). PNS, percutaneous nephrostomy.

A

B

Figure 13–6. Pyonephrosis. US demonstrates fluid-debris level (white arrow) within the dilated renal pelvis.

more commonly affects women than men. The primary mode of infection is ascending from the periurethral/vaginal and fecal flora. The diagnosis is made clinically. In children, the distinction between upper and lower UTI is important. In general, those in whom acute cystitis developed do not usually require any extensive radiologic investigation (such as a voiding cystourethrogram), but those in whom pyelonephritis developed do (American Academy of Pediatrics, 1999).

A. PRESENTATION AND FINDINGS

Patients with acute cystitis present with irritative voiding symptoms such as dysuria, frequency, and urgency. Low back and suprapubic pain, hematuria, and cloudy/foul-smelling urine are also common symptoms. Fever and systemic symptoms are rare. Typically, urinalysis demonstrates WBCs in the urine, and hematuria may be present. Urine culture is required to confirm the diagnosis and identify the causative organism. How-

ever, when the clinical picture and urinalysis are highly suggestive of the diagnosis of acute cystitis, urine culture may not be needed. *E coli* causes most of the acute cystitis. Other gram-negative (*Klebsiella* and *Proteus* spp.) and gram-positive (*Staphylococcus saprophyticus* and enterococci) bacteria are uncommon pathogens (Gupta et al, 1999).

B. RADIOGRAPHIC IMAGING

In uncomplicated infection of the bladder, radiologic evaluation is often not necessary.

C. MANAGEMENT

Management for acute cystitis consists of a short course of oral antibiotics. Trimethoprim-sulfamethoxazole, nitrofurantoin, and fluoroquinolones have excellent activity against most pathogens that cause cystitis. Trimethoprim-sulfamethoxazole and nitrofurantoin are less expensive and thus are recommended for the treatment of uncomplicated cystitis (Huang and Stafford, 2002). However, it is estimated that resistance to TMP-SMX by *E coli* isolates causing uncomplicated acute cystitis is approximately 20%, compared to less than 2% to nitrofurantoin (Gupta, Scholes, and Stamm, 1999). In adults and children, the duration of treatment is usually limited to 3–5 days (Abrahamsson et al, 2002; Naber, 1999). Longer therapy is not indicated. Single-dose therapy for the treatment of recurrent cystitis/UTI appears to be less effective (Philbrick, 1986); however, fluoroquinolones with long half-lives (fleroxacin, pefloxacin, and rufloxacin) may be suitable for single-dose therapy (Naber, 1999). Resistance to penicillins and aminopenicillins is high and thus they are not recommended for treatment.

Recurrent Cystitis/UTI

A. Presentation and Findings

Recurrent cystitis/UTI is caused either by bacterial persistence or reinfection with another organism. Identification of the cause of the recurrent infection is important, because the management of bacterial persistence and reinfection are distinct. If bacterial persistence is the cause of recurrent UTI, the removal of the infected source is often curative, whereas preventative therapy is effective in treating reinfection.

B. Radiographic Imaging

When bacterial persistence is the suspected cause, radiologic imaging is indicated. Ultrasonography can be obtained to provide a screening evaluation of the genitourinary tract. More detailed assessment with intravenous pyelogram, cystoscopy, and CT scans may occasionally be necessary. In patients who have frequent, recurrent UTI, bacterial localization studies and more extensive radiologic evaluation (such as retrograde pyelograms) is warranted. When bacterial reinfection is the suspected cause of recurrent cystitis, the patient should be carefully evaluated for evidence of vesicovaginal or vesicoenteric fistula. Otherwise, radiologic examination is often not necessary in these patients.

C. Management

Management of recurrent cystitis, again, depends on its cause. Surgical removal of the infected source (such as urinary calculi) is needed to treat bacterial persistence. Similarly, fistulas need to be repaired surgically to prevent bacterial reinfection. In most cases of bacterial reinfection, medical management with prophylactic antibiotics is indicated. Low-dose continuous prophylactic antibiotic has been shown to reduce the recurrences of UTI by 95% compared to placebo or historical controls (Mangiarotti, Pizzini, and Fanos, 2000; Nicolle and Ronald, 1987). Alternatively, intermittent self-start an-

tibiotic therapy can be used in treating recurrent cystitis in some women. Motivated patients self-identify episodes of infection on the basis of their symptoms and treat themselves with a single dose of antibiotics such as TMP-SMX. This regimen has been shown to be effective and economical in selected patients (Pfau and Sacks, 1993; Raz et al, 1991). When the recurrent cystitis/UTI is related to sexual activity, frequent emptying of the bladder and a single dose of antibiotic taken after sexual intercourse can significantly reduce the incidence of recurrent infection (Pfau and Sacks, 1994). Alternatives to antibiotic therapy in the treatment of recurrent cystitis/UTI include intravaginal estriol (Raz and Stamm, 1993), lactobacillus vaginal suppositories (Reid and Burton, 2002), and cranberry juice taken orally (Lowe and Fagelman, 2001).

Malacoplakia

Malacoplakia is an uncommon inflammatory disease of the bladder that can also affect other parts of the urinary tract, including the ureters and kidneys (Stanton and Maxted, 1981). In the bladder, it manifests as plaques or nodules made of large histiocytes (von Hansemann cells) with laminar inclusion bodies (Michaelis-Gutmann bodies) (McClure, Cameron, and Garrett, 1981).

A. Presentation and Findings

Malacoplakia more commonly affects women than men (Stanton and Maxted, 1981) and is associated with a history of UTI. Patients with malacoplakia often have chronic illness or are immunosuppressed. In patients with malacoplakia of the bladder, irritative voiding symptoms (urgency and frequency) and hematuria are common (Curran, 1987). When the disease affects the ureter or kidney, the patient may present with fever, flank pain, or flank mass. When it affects both kidneys, signs or symptoms of azotemia or renal failure may be present (Dobyan, Truong, and Eknoyan, 1993).

B. Radiologic Imaging

Radiologic imaging with ultrasonography or CT may demonstrate a mass in the bladder and evidence of obstruction if the disease extends to the ureter (Vas et al, 1985). When the disease involves the kidney, focal or diffuse, hypodense, parenchymal masses may be seen on CT imaging (Frederic, D'Hondt, and Potvliege, 1981). It is often difficult to distinguish malacoplakia from malignancy (transitional cell or renal cell carcinoma) with radiologic imaging. The diagnosis is often established after biopsy.

C. Management

Management of malacoplakia primarily consists of antibiotic therapy, in particular those that produce high intracellular levels. Consequently, TMP-SMX and fluoroquinolones are recommended in the treatment of malacoplakia. Bethanecol and ascorbic acid, which enhance phagolysosomal activity, may have some benefits (Stanton and Maxted, 1981; Trujillo-Santos et al, 1999). In patients with malacoplakia limited to the lower urinary tract, antibiotic therapy alone is usually sufficient. However, when malacoplakia involves the ureter or kidney, surgical excision may be needed in addition to the antibiotic therapy (Dasgupta et al, 1999; Long and Althausen, 1989). The prognosis is poor and the mortality rate is high in patients who have bilateral renal involvement, regardless of treatment.

PROSTATE INFECTION

Acute Bacterial Prostatitis

Acute bacterial prostatitis refers to inflammation of the prostate associated with a UTI. It is thought that infection results from ascending urethral infection or reflux of infected urine from the bladder into the prostatic ducts. In response to bacterial invasion, leukocytes (polymorphonuclear leukocytes, lymphocytes, plasma cells, and macrophages) are seen within and surrounding the acini of the prostate. Edema and hyperemia of the prostatic stroma frequently develop. With prolonged infection, variable degree of necrosis and abscess formation can occur.

A. PRESENTATION AND FINDINGS

 Acute bacterial prostatitis is uncommon in prepubertal boys but frequent affects adult men. It is the most common urologic diagnosis in men younger than 50 years (Collins et al, 1998). Patients with acute bacterial prostatitis usually present with an abrupt onset of constitutional (fever, chills, malaise, arthralgia, myalgia, lower back/rectal/perineal pain) and urinary symptoms (frequency, urgency, dysuria). They may also present with urinary retention due to swelling of the prostate. Digital rectal examination reveals tender, enlarged glands that are irregular and warm. Urinalysis usually demonstrates WBCs and occasionally hematuria. Serum blood analysis typically demonstrates leukocytosis. Prostate-specific antigen levels are often elevated. The diagnosis of prostatitis is made with microscopic examination and culture of the prostatic expressate and culture of urine obtained before and after prostate massage. In patients with acute prostatitis, fluid from the prostate massage often contains leukocytes with fat-laden macrophages. However, at the onset of acute prostatitis, prostatic massage is usually not suggested because the prostate is quite tender and the massage may lead to bacteremia. Similarly, urethral catheterization should be avoided. Culture of urine and prostate expressate usually identifies a single organisms, but occasionally,

polymicrobial infection may occur. *E coli* is the most common causative organism in patients with acute prostatitis. Other gram-negative bacteria (*Proteus, Klebsiella, Enterobacter, Pseudomonas,* and *Serratia* spp.) and enterococci are less frequent pathogens. Anaerobic and other gram-positive bacteria are rarely a cause of acute prostatitis (RO Roberts et al, 1997).

B. RADIOLOGIC IMAGING

Radiologic imaging is rarely indicated in patients with acute prostatitis. Bladder ultrasonography may be useful in determining the amount of residual urine. Transrectal ultrasonography is only indicated in patients who do not respond to conventional therapy.

C. MANAGEMENT

Treatment with antibiotics is essential in the management of acute prostatitis. Empiric therapy directed against gram-negative bacteria and enterococci should be instituted immediately, while awaiting the culture results. Trimethoprim and fluoroquinolones have high drug penetration into prostatic tissue and are recommended for 4–6 weeks. The long duration of antibiotic treatment is to allow complete sterilization of the prostatic tissue to prevent complications such as chronic prostatitis and abscess formation (Childs, 1992; Nickel, 2000). Patients who have sepsis, are immunocompromised or in acute urinary retention, or have significant medical comorbidities would benefit from hospitalization and treatment with parenteral antibiotics. Ampicillin and an aminoglycoside provide effective therapy against both gram-negative bacteria and enterococci. Patients with urinary retention secondary to acute prostatitis should be managed with a suprapubic catheter because transurethral catheterization or instrumentation is contraindicated.

Chronic Bacterial Prostatitis

In contrast to the acute form, chronic bacterial prostatitis has a more insidious onset, characterized by relapsing, recurrent UTI caused by the persistence of pathogen in the prostatic fluid despite antibiotic therapy.

A. PRESENTATION AND FINDINGS

Most patients with chronic bacterial prostatitis typically present with dysuria, urgency, frequency, nocturia, and low back/perineal pain. Others are asymptomatic, but the diagnosis is made after investigation for bacteriuria. In patients with chronic bacterial prostatitis, digital rectal examination of the prostate is often normal; occasionally, tenderness, firmness, or prostatic calculi may be found on examination. Urinalysis demonstrates a variable degree of WBCs and bacteria in the urine, depending on the extent of the disease. Serum blood analysis normally does not show any evidence of leukocytosis. Prostate-specific antigen levels may be elevated. Diagnosis is made after identification of bacteria from prostate expressate or urine specimen after a prostatic massage, using the 4-cup test (Table 13–8). The causative organisms are similar to those of acute bacterial prostatitis. It is currently believed that other gram-positive bacteria, *Mycoplasma, Ureaplasma,* and *Chlamydia* spp. are not causative pathogens in chronic bacterial prostatitis.

B. RADIOLOGIC IMAGING

Radiologic imaging is rarely indicated in patients with chronic prostatitis. Transrectal ultrasonography is only indicated if a prostatic abscess is suspected.

C. MANAGEMENT

Antibiotic therapy is similar to that for acute bacterial prostatitis (Bjerklund Johansen et al, 1998). Interestingly, the presence of leukocytes or bacteria in the urine and prostatic massage does not predict antibiotic response in patients with chronic prostatitis (Nickel et al, 2001). In patients with chronic bacterial prostatitis, the

Table 13–8. Technique of localization cultures (4-cup test) for the diagnosis of prostatitis.

- **Preparation:**
  - Require that the patient have a full bladder
  - Retract foreskin of uncircumcised men
  - Clean glans with soap/water or providone-iodine
- **Collection:**
  - Collect first 10 mL of voided urine (VB1)
  - Discard the next 100 mL
  - Collect the next 10 mL of voided urine (VB2)
  - Massage prostate and collect prostate expressate (EPS)
  - Collect first 10 mL of voided urine after massage (VB3)
  - Immediately culture and microscopically examine all specimens
- **Interpretation:**
  - All specimens $< 10^3$ CFU/mL $\rightarrow$ not bacterial prostatitis
  - VB3 or EPS $> 10 \times$ CFU of VB1 $\rightarrow$ chronic bacterial prostatitis
  - VB1 $>$ other specimens $\rightarrow$ urethritis or specimen contamination
  - All specimens $> 10^3$ CFU/mL $\rightarrow$ treat for UTI and repeat test
- **Caution:**
  - Sensitivity of the test may not be high (Lipsky, 1999)
  - Time-consuming and expensive
- **Alternative:**
  - Voided specimen before and after prostate massage (Nickel, 1997)

CFU, colony-forming unit.

duration of antibiotic therapy may be 3–4 months. Using fluoroquinolones, some patients may respond after 4–6 weeks of treatment. The addition of an alpha blocker to antibiotic therapy has been shown to reduce symptom recurrences (Barbalias, Nikiforidis, and Liatsikos, 1998). Despite maximal therapy, cure is not often achieved due to poor penetration of antibiotic into prostatic tissue and relative isolation of the bacterial foci within the prostate. When recurrent episodes of infection occur despite antibiotic therapy, suppressive antibiotic (TMP-SMX 1 single-strength tablet daily, nitrofurantoin 100 mg daily, or ciprofloxacin 250 mg daily) may be used (Meares, 1987). Transurethral resection of the prostate has been used to treat patients with refractory disease; however, the success rate has been variable and this approach is not generally recommended (Barnes, Hadley, and O'Donoghue, 1982).

Granulomatous Prostatitis

Granulomatous prostatitis is an uncommon form of prostatitis. It can result from bacterial, viral, or fungal infection, the use of bacillus Calmette-Guérin therapy (Rischmann et al, 2000), malacoplakia, or systemic granulomatous diseases affecting the prostate. Two-thirds of the cases have no specific cause. There are two distinct forms of nonspecific granulomatous prostatitis: noneosinophilic and eosinophilic. The former represents an abnormal tissue response to extravasated prostatic fluid (O'Dea, Hunting, and Greene, 1977). The latter is a more severe, allergic response of the prostate to some unknown antigen.

A. PRESENTATION AND FINDINGS

Patients with granulomatous prostatitis often present acutely, with fever, chills, and obstructive/irritative voiding symptoms. Some may present with urinary retention. Patients with eosinophilic granulomatous prostatitis are severely ill and have high fevers. Digital rectal examination in patients with granulomatous prostatitis demonstrates a hard, indurated, and fixed prostate, which is difficult to distinguish from prostate carcinoma. Urinalysis and culture do not show any evidence of bacterial infection. Serum blood analysis typically demonstrates leukocytosis; marked eosinophilia is often seen in patients with eosinophilic granulomatous prostatitis. The diagnosis is made after biopsy of the prostate.

B. MANAGEMENT

Some patients respond to antibiotic therapy, corticosteroids, and temporary bladder drainage. Those with eosinophilic granulomatous prostatitis dramatically response to corticosteroids (Ohkawa, Yamaguchi, and Kobayashi, 2001). Transurethral resection of the prostate may be required in patients who do not respond to treatment and have significant outlet obstruction.

Prostate Abscess

Most cases of prostatic abscess result from complications of acute bacterial prostatitis that were inadequately or inappropriately treated. Prostatic abscesses are often seen in patients with diabetes; those receiving chronic dialysis; or patients who are immunocompromised, undergoing urethral instrumentation, or who have chronic indwelling catheters.

A. PRESENTATION AND FINDINGS

Patients with prostatic abscess present with similar symptoms to those with acute bacterial prostatitis. Typically, these patients were treated for acute bacterial prostatitis previously and had a good initial response to treatment with antibiotics. However, their symptoms recurred during treatment, suggesting development of prostatic abscesses. On digital rectal examination, the prostate is usually tender and swollen. Fluctuance is only seen in 16% of patients with prostatic abscess (Weinberger et al, 1988).

B. RADIOLOGIC IMAGING

Imaging with transrectal ultrasonography (Figure 13–7) or pelvic CT scan is crucial for diagnosis and treatment.

C. MANAGEMENT

Antibiotic therapy in conjunction with drainage of the abscess is required. Transrectal ultrasonography or CT scan can be used to direct transrectal drainage of the abscess (Barozzi et al, 1998). Transurethral resection and drainage may be required if transrectal drainage is inadequate. When properly diagnosed and treated, most

Figure 13–7. Prostatic abscess. Transrectal ultrasonography demonstrates hypoechoic lesions (black and white arrows) in the prostate consistent with abscesses.

cases of prostatic abscess resolve without significant sequelae (Weinberger et al, 1988).

URETHRITIS

Types of Urethritis

Infection/inflammation of the urethra can be categorized into those types caused by *Neisseria gonorrhoeae* and by other organisms (*Chlamydia trachomatis, Ureaplasma urealyticum, Trichomonas vaginalis,* and herpes simplex virus) (Dixon, Pearson, and Clutterbuck, 2002). Most cases are acquired during sexual intercourse.

A. PRESENTATION AND FINDINGS

Patients with urethritis may present with urethral discharge and dysuria. The amount of discharge may vary significantly, from profuse to scant amounts. Obstructive voiding symptoms are primarily present in patients with recurrent infection, in whom urethral strictures subsequently develop. It is important to note that approximately 40% of patients with gonococcal urethritis are asymptomatic (John and Donald, 1978). The diagnosis is made from examination and culture of the urethra. It is important to obtain the specimen from within the urethra, rather than from just the discharge. Approximately 30% of men infected with *N gonorrhoeae* will have concomitant infection with *C trachomatis.*

B. RADIOLOGIC IMAGING

Retrograde urethrogram is only indicated in patients with recurrent infection and obstructive voiding symptoms. Most patients with uncomplicated urethritis do not require any radiologic imaging.

C. MANAGEMENT

Pathogen-direct antibiotic therapy is required. In patients with gonococcal urethritis, ceftriaxone (250 mg intramuscularly) or fluoroquinolones (ciprofloxacin 250 mg) (David, Wildman, and Rajamanoharan, 2000) or norfloxacin 800 mg) may be used. For patients with nongonococcal urethritis, treatment is with tetracycline or erythromycin (500 mg 4 times daily) or doxycycline (100 mg twice daily) for 7–14 days (O'Mahony, 1999). However, the most essential component of treatment is prevention. Sexual partners of the affected patients should be treated, and protective sexual practices (such as using condoms) are recommended.

EPIDIDYMITIS

Causes of Epididymitis

Infection and inflammation of the epididymis most often result from an ascending infection from the lower urinary tract. Most cases of epididymitis in men younger than 35 years are due to sexually transmitted organisms (*N gonorrhoeae* and *C trachomatis*); those in children and older men are due to urinary pathogens such as *E coli*. In homosexual men who practice anal intercourse, *E coli* and other coliform bacteria are common causative organisms. The infection in the epididymis may spread to involve the testis.

A. PRESENTATION AND FINDINGS

Patients with epididymitis present with severe scrotal pain that may radiate to the groin or flank. Scrotal enlargement due to the inflammation of the epididymis/testis or a reactive hydrocele may develop rapidly. Other symptoms of urethritis, cystitis, or prostatitis may be present before or concurrent with the onset of scrotal pain. On physical examination, an enlarged and red scrotum is present, and it is often difficult to distinguish the epididymis from the testis during the acute infection. A thickened spermatic cord can occasionally be palpated. Urinalysis typically demonstrates WBCs and bacteria in the urine or urethral discharge. Serum blood analysis often reveals leukocytosis.

B. RADIOLOGIC IMAGING

Frequently, it is difficult to distinguish epididymitis from acute testicular torsion based on the history and physical examination alone (Petrack and Hafeez, 1992). Scrotal Doppler ultrasonography or radionuclide scanning can be used to confirm the diagnosis (Paltiel et al, 1998). The presence of blood flow in the testis on Doppler ultrasonography or uptake of the tracers into the center of the testis on radionuclide scanning rules out torsion. On scrotal ultrasonography, patients with epididymitis commonly have an enlarged epididymis with increased blood flow. A reactive hydrocele or testicular involvement may also be seen. Prepubertal children who are diagnosed with epididymitis will require radiologic investigation for urinary tract anomalies such as reflux or ureteral ectopia (Likitnukul et al, 1987). Postpubertal children who are diagnosed with epididymitis should be educated about sexually transmitted diseases and safe sexual practices.

C. MANAGEMENT

Oral antibiotic treatment is directed against specific causative organisms, as mentioned in the previous sections on urethritis and UTI. In addition, bed rest, scrotal elevation, and the use of nonsteroidal anti-inflammatory agents are helpful in reducing the duration of the symptoms. In patients with epididymitis caused by sexually transmitted organisms, treatment of their sexual partners is recommended to prevent reinfection. For patients with sepsis or severe infection, hospitalization and parenteral antibiotic therapy may be needed. Open drainage is indicated in cases in which an abscess develops. Occasionally, patients with chronic, relapsing epididymitis and scrotal pain may require epididymectomy for relief of their symptoms.

SPECIAL CIRCUMSTANCES

Urinary Tract Infection related to Pregnancy

With pregnancy, there are anatomic and physiologic changes to the urinary tract due to compression by the gravid uterus and alterations in the hormonal milieu. Renal length increases approximately by 1 cm during normal pregnancy as a result of increased vascular and interstitial volume (Waltzer, 1981). The glomerular filtration rate increases by 30–50%, most likely secondary to the increase in cardiac output (Waltzer, 1981). Typically, there is significant ureteral dilation with resultant urinary stasis during the second and third trimesters of gestation. This hydroureter is attributed to the smooth muscle–relaxing effects of progesterone and the mechanical compression of the ureters by the uterus at the level of the pelvic brim (Waltzer, 1981). The bladder is also affected, both physically and physiologically. The enlarged uterus displaces the bladder superiorly and anteriorly. The bladder becomes hyperemic, and its capacity is increased, most likely due to the effects of progesterone (Waltzer, 1981).

Because of these changes in the urinary tract during normal pregnancy, bacteriuria is a clinically relevant finding in pregnant women. It is estimated that the prevalence of bacteriuria is 4–6% (Sweet, 1977), which is not significantly different from that in nonpregnant women of comparable age. Interestingly, approximately 30% of those who have bacteriuria on screening evaluation later have pyelonephritis, compared to only 1–2% in those who do not have bacteriuria (Sweet, 1977). Treatment of bacteriuria decreases the incidence of pyelonephritis during pregnancy to approximately 3% (Christensen, 2000; Sweet, 1977).

Overall, the incidence of acute bacterial pyelonephritis is 1–4% in pregnant women (Gilstrap, Cunningham, and Whalley, 1981; Wing, 1998). Sixty to seventy percent of the episodes of pyelonephritis occur during the second and third trimesters of pregnancy, when urinary stasis is the greatest. In 10–20%, recurrent episodes of pyelonephritis develop before delivery (Gilstrap, Cunningham, and Whalley, 1981). Significant maternal risk factors include diabetes and history of UTI. When left untreated, pyelonephritis during pregnancy is associated with a high rate of infant prematurity and its associated perinatal mortality (Lock-smith and Duff, 2001; McGregor and French, 1998; Schieve et al, 1994). It remains unclear whether treated pyelonephritis during pregnancy has any effects on the developing fetus (Gilstrap and Ramin, 2001).

Consequently, it is recommended that women be screened for bacteriuria during pregnancy to prevent the development of pyelonephritis. A voided urine specimen should be obtained at the first prenatal visit and at 16 weeks of gestation (Stenqvist et al, 1989). For asymptomatic individuals, significant bacteriuria is defined as 2 voided urine cultures with greater than 10^5 CFU/mL of a single organism. For symptomatic pregnant women, greater than 10^3 CFU/mL is considered to be significant (Rubin, Beam, and Stamm, 1992). Pregnant women who are found to have bacteriuria should be treated with penicillins, oral cephalosporins (Christensen, 2000; Wing et al, 1999), or fosfomycin trometamol (Minassian et al, 1998). Table 13–9 lists the antibiotics and their effects on pregnancy. However, amoxicillin is not recommended because of the rate of bacterial resistance (Hart et al, 2001). A 3-day course is suggested, although single-dose therapy may be effective in some patients (Tincello and Richmond, 1998). Repeat urine culture to document eradication of bacteriuria is necessary in all patients. Patients with acute bacterial pyelonephritis should be treated with parenteral cephalosporins, penicillins with β-lactamase inhibitors, or monolactams (Rubin, Beam, and Stamm, 1992). Periodic surveillance urine culture is recommended because many of these women will have recurrent episodes of pyelonephritis.

Table 13–9. Antibiotics and their effects on pregnancy.

Drugs	Side Effects on the Developing Fetus
Sulfonamides	Kernicterus
Trimethoprim	Interferes with neural tube development
Tetracyclines	Dysplasia and discoloration of teeth and bones
Nitrofurantoin	Hemolysis and G6PD deficiency
Aminoglycosides	Nerve damage
Fluoroquinolones	Interferes with cartilage formation
Penicillins	Safe
Cephalosporins	Safe
β-Lactamase inhibitors	Safe
Monobactams	Safe
Fosfomycin trometamol	Safe

UTI in Patients With Human Immunodeficiency Virus or Acquired Immunodeficiency Syndrome

Human immunodeficiency virus alters the normal host defense against bacterial infection. When the CD4 lymphocyte count falls to less than $200/mm^3$, the risk of bacterial and opportunistic UTI increases dramatically (Evans et al, 1995; Hoepelman et al, 1992). In addition, antiretroviral medications used to treat HIV (eg, zidovudine) can further suppress normal immune response and increase the risk of UTI in these patients.

A. UTI/CYSTITIS

Hoepelman et al (1992) obtained urine cultures from HIV-positive men prospectively and when they had symptoms suggestive of a UTI. They observed that positive urine cultures were identified in 30% of HIV-infected men with CD4 < $200/mm^3$ and in 11% with CD4 = $200-500/mm^3$, while none with CD4 > $500/mm^3$ had evidence of a urine infection. Gugino et al (1998) similarly observed that the incidence of bacteriuria in asymptomatic HIV-infected women was the same as that in uninfected women. Causative organisms include common uropathogens such as *E coli* and *Klebsiella and Enterococcus* spp. Urinary infection with *S aureus* and *Pseudomonas aeruginosa* is more common in HIV-infected patients (Schonwald, Begovac, and Skerk, 1999). Because of the common prophylactic use of TMP-SMX to prevent *Pneumocystis carinii* pneumonia in AIDS patients, the incidence of UTI in this group is decreased. However, when a UTI develops in these patients, the infecting organism is typically resistant to TMP-SMX (van Dooyeweert et al, 1996).

B. PROSTATITIS

In HIV patients, the incidence of bacterial prostatitis is approximately 3% and is 14% in patients with AIDS, compared to 1–2% in noninfected men of similar age (Leport et al, 1989). Causative organisms include common prostatitis pathogens such as *E coli* and *Proteus* spp. and other less common organisms such as *Salmonella typhi, S aureus, P aeruginosa, and N gonorrhoeae* (Staiman and Lowe, 1995). Prolonged treatment (4–6 weeks) with fluoroquinolones may be necessary because of a high risk of reinfection and lower immunity status in these patients. Prostatic abscess is more common in patients with AIDS compared to that in the general population (Staiman and Lowe, 1995; Trauzzi et al, 1994). Causative organisms include *E coli* and other gram-negative bacteria or opportunistic fungus or mycobacterial infection (Lee, Dinneen, and Ahmad, 2001). Effective drainage and prolonged antimicrobial or antifungal therapy are needed.

C. EPIDIDYMITIS AND URETHRITIS

In HIV-infected men, epididymitis may be caused by *N gonorrhoeae* and *C trachomatis*. However, infection by coliform bacteria such as *E coli* is more common, especially in patients having unprotected anal intercourse (Berger et al, 1987). In HIV-infected patients with suppurative or antibiotic-resistant epididymitis, infection with fungi or mycobacteria should be considered (Desmond et al, 1993). In HIV-infected men who present with urethritis, treatment for both *Chlamydia* and *N gonorrhoeae* is indicated even when gonococcus is only isolated from culture. Due to increased viral shedding with genital infections, it is recommended that HIV-infected patients abstain from sexual intercourse until 7 days after treatment is completed.

D. INFECTION BY UNCOMMON ORGANISMS

Urinary infection with *Mycobacterium* species can develop in HIV-infected patients. The kidneys are first infected and the infection spreads to the lower urinary tract. In patients with AIDS, it is estimated that 6–23% have renal tuberculosis (Marques et al, 1996). *M tuberculosis* is the most common pathogen, with *M avium and M intracellulare* being less common (Sepkowitz et al, 1995). In HIV-infected patients who present with irritative/obstructive voiding symptoms but have no evidence of bacterial infection on culture, infection of the lower urinary tract by *Mycobacterium* species should be considered. Treatment with at least 2 antituberculosis agents is needed for 6–9 months.

REFERENCES

Abrahamsson K et al: Antibiotic treatment for five days is effective in children with acute cystitis. Acta Paediatr 2002;91:55.

Al-Orifi F et al: Urine culture from bag specimens in young children: Are the risks too high? J Pediatr 2000;137:221.

American Academy of Pediatrics. Committee on Quality Improvement. Subcommittee on Urinary Tract Infection: Practice parameter: The diagnosis, treatment, and evaluation of the initial urinary tract infection in febrile infants and young children. Pediatrics 1999;103:843.

Barbalias GA, Nikiforidis G, Liatsikos EN: Alpha-blockers for the treatment of chronic prostatitis in combination with antibiotics. J Urol 1998;159:883.

Barnes RW, Hadley HL, O'Donoghue EP: Transurethral resection of the prostate for chronic bacterial prostatitis. Prostate 1982; 3:215.

Barozzi L et al: Prostatic abscess: Diagnosis and treatment. AJR 1998;170:753.

Berger RE, Kessler D, Holmes KK: Etiology and manifestations of epididymitis in young men: Correlations with sexual orientation. J Infect Dis 1987;155:1341.

Bjerklund Johansen TE et al: The role of antibiotics in the treatment of chronic prostatitis: A consensus statement. Eur Urol 1998;34:457.

Bjorksten B, Kaijser B: Interaction of human serum and neutrophils with *Escherichia coli* strains: Differences between strains isolated from urine of patients with pyelonephritis or asymptomatic bacteriuria. Infect Immun 1978;22:308.

Blanco M et al: Virulence factors and O groups of *Escherichia coli* isolates from patients with acute pyelonephritis, cystitis and asymptomatic bacteriuria. Eur J Epidemiol 1996;12:191.

Bortolussi R et al: Capsular K1 polysaccharide of *Escherichia coli*: Relationship to virulence in newborn rats and resistance to phagocytosis. Infect Immun 1979;25:293.

Brown PD, Freeman A, Foxman B: Prevalence and predictors of trimethoprim-sulfamethoxazole resistance among uropathogenic *Escherichia coli* isolates in Michigan. Clin Infect Dis 2002;34:1061.

Brown PS Jr, Dodson M, Weintrub PS: Xanthogranulomatous pyelonephritis: Report of nonsurgical management of a case and review of the literature. Clin Infect Dis 1996;22:308.

Carapetis JR et al: Randomized, controlled trial comparing once daily and three times daily gentamicin in children with urinary tract infections. Pediatr Infect Dis J 2001;20:240.

Chen MT et al: Percutaneous drainage in the treatment of emphysematous pyelonephritis: 10-year experience. J Urol 1997; 157:1569.

Childs S: Current diagnosis and treatment of urinary tract infections. Urology 1992;40:295.

Christensen B: Which antibiotics are appropriate for treating bacteriuria in pregnancy? J Antimicrob Chemother 2000;46:29; discussion 63.

Collins MM et al: How common is prostatitis? A national survey of physician visits. J Urol 1998;159:1224.

Connell I et al: Type 1 fimbrial expression enhances *Escherichia coli* virulence for the urinary tract. Proc Natl Acad Sci U S A 1996;93:9827.

Corriere JN Jr, Sandler CM: The diagnosis and immediate therapy of acute renal and perirenal infections. Urol Clin North Am 1982;9:219.

Curran FT: Malakoplakia of the bladder. Br J Urol 1987;59:559.

Dacher JN et al: Rational use of CT in acute pyelonephritis: Findings and relationships with reflux. Pediatr Radiol 1993; 23:281.

Dalla Palma L, Pozzi-Mucelli F, Ene V: Medical treatment of renal and perirenal abscesses: CT evaluation. Clin Radiol 1999; 54:792.

Dasgupta P et al: Malacoplakia: von Hansemann's disease. BJU Int 1999;84:464.

David N, Wildman G, Rajamanoharan S: Ciprofloxacin 250 mg for treating gonococcal urethritis and cervicitis. Sex Transm Infect 2000;76:495.

Desmond N et al: Tuberculous epididymitis: A case report in an HIV seropositive male. Int J STD AIDS 1993;4:178.

Dixon L, Pearson S, Clutterbuck DJ: *Chlamydia trachomatis* infection and non-gonococcal urethritis in homosexual and heterosexual men in Edinburgh. Int J STD AIDS 2002;13:425.

Dobyan DC, Truong LD, Eknoyan G: Renal malacoplakia reappraised. Am J Kidney Dis 1993;22:243.

Duncan JL: Differential effect of Tamm-Horsfall protein on adherence of *Escherichia coli* to transitional epithelial cells. J Infect Dis 1988;158:1379.

Eastham J, Ahlering T, Skinner E: Xanthogranulomatous pyelonephritis: Clinical findings and surgical considerations. Urology 1994;43:295.

Edelstein H, McCabe RE: Perinephric abscess: Modern diagnosis and treatment in 47 cases. Medicine (Baltimore) 1988;67: 118.

Evans DJ Jr et al: Hemolysin and K antigens in relation to serotype and hemagglutination type of *Escherichia coli* isolated from extraintestinal infections. J Clin Microbiol 1981;13:171.

Evans JK et al: Incidence of symptomatic urinary tract infections in HIV seropositive patients and the use of cotrimoxazole as prophylaxis against *Pneumocystis carinii* pneumonia. Genitourin Med 1995;71:120.

Fair WR, Couch J, Wehner N: Prostatic antibacterial factor: Identity and significance. Urology 1976;7:169.

Foxman B et al: Urinary tract infection among women aged 40 to 65: Behavioral and sexual risk factors. J Clin Epidemiol 2001; 54:710.

Frederic N, D'Hondt M, Potvliege P: Renal malakoplakia: Ultrasonic and computed appearances. J Belge Radiol 1981;64: 361.

Frendeus B et al: Interleukin-8 receptor deficiency confers susceptibility to acute pyelonephritis. J Infect Dis 2001;183:S56.

Garcia-Rodriguez JA, Munoz Bellido JL: Oral cephalosporins in uncomplicated urinary tract infections. Clin Microbiol Infect 2000;6:73.

Ghiro L et al: Retrospective study of children with acute pyelonephritis: Evaluation of bacterial etiology, antimicrobial susceptibility, drug management and imaging studies. Nephron 2002;90:8.

Gilstrap LC III, Cunningham FG, Whalley PJ: Acute pyelonephritis in pregnancy: An anterospective study. Obstet Gynecol 1981;57:409.

Gilstrap LC III, Ramin SM: Urinary tract infections during pregnancy. Obstet Gynecol Clin North Am 2001;28:581.

Goldman SM et al: CT of xanthogranulomatous pyelonephritis: Radiologic-pathologic correlation. AJR 1984;142:963.

Goodman M, Curry T, Russell T: Xanthogranulomatous pyelonephritis (XGP): A local disease with systemic manifestations. Report of 23 patients and review of the literature. Medicine (Baltimore) 1979;58:171.

Gugino L et al: Asymptomatic bacteriuria in human immunodeficiency (HIV)-infected women. Prim Care Update Ob Gyns 1998;5:146.

Gupta K, Scholes D, Stamm WE: Increasing prevalence of antimicrobial resistance among uropathogens causing acute uncomplicated cystitis in women. JAMA 1999;281:736.

Gupta K et al: The prevalence of antimicrobial resistance among uropathogens causing acute uncomplicated cystitis in young women. Int J Antimicrob Agents 1999;11:305.

Hart A et al: Ampicillin-resistant *Escherichia coli* in gestational pyelonephritis: Increased occurrence and association with the colonization factor Dr adhesin. J Infect Dis 2001;183:1526.

Hoberman A et al: Oral versus initial intravenous therapy for urinary tract infections in young febrile children. Pediatrics 1999;104:79.

Hoepelman AI et al: Bacteriuria in men infected with HIV-1 is related to their immune status (CD4+ cell count). AIDS 1992;6:179.

Hovanec DL, Gorzynski EA: Coagglutination as an expedient for grouping *Escherichia coli* associated with urinary tract infections. J Clin Microbiol 1980;11:41.

Hovelius B, Mardh PA: *Staphylococcus saprophyticus* as a common cause of urinary tract infections. Rev Infect Dis 1984;6:328.

Huang ES, Stafford RS: National patterns in the treatment of urinary tract infections in women by ambulatory care physicians. Arch Intern Med 2002;162:41.

Hughes C et al: Hemolysin production as a virulence marker in symptomatic and asymptomatic urinary tract infections caused by *Escherichia coli*. Infect Immun 1983;39:546.

Iskandar SS, Prahlow JA, White WL: Lipid-laden foamy macrophages in renal cell carcinoma: Potential frozen section diagnostic pitfall. Pathol Res Pract 1993;189:549.

Jeena PM, Coovadia HM, Adhikari MA: Bacteriuria in children attending a primary health care clinic: A prospective study of catheter stream urine samples. Ann Trop Paediatr 1996; 16:293.

Jenkins RD, Fenn JP, Matsen JM: Review of urine microscopy for bacteriuria. JAMA 1986;255:3397.

John J, Donald WH: Asymptomatic urethral gonorrhoea in men. Br J Vener Dis 1978;54:322.

Kallenius G et al: Occurrence of P-fimbriated *Escherichia coli* in urinary tract infections. Lancet 1981;2:1369.

Koronakis V, Hughes C: Synthesis, maturation and export of the *E. coli* hemolysin. Med Microbiol Immunol (Berl) 1996; 185:65.

Lawrenson RA, Logie JW: Antibiotic failure in the treatment of urinary tract infections in young women. J Antimicrob Chemother 2001;48:895.

Lee LK, Dinneen MD, Ahmad S: The urologist and the patient infected with human immunodeficiency virus or with acquired immunodeficiency syndrome. BJU Int 2001;88:500.

Leport C et al: Bacterial prostatitis in patients infected with the human immunodeficiency virus. J Urol 1989;141:334.

Levtchenko EN et al: Role of Tc-99m DMSA scintigraphy in the diagnosis of culture negative pyelonephritis. Pediatr Nephrol 2001;16:503.

Likitnukul S et al: Epididymitis in children and adolescents: A 20-year retrospective study. Am J Dis Child 1987;141:41.

Lipsky BA: Prostatitis and urinary tract infection in men: What's new; what's true? Am J Med 1999;106:327.

Locksmith G, Duff P: Infection, antibiotics, and preterm delivery. Semin Perinatol 2001;25:295.

Lomberg H et al: Influence of blood group on the availability of receptors for attachment of uropathogenic *Escherichia coli*. Infect Immun 1986;51:919.

Long JP Jr, Althausen AF: Malacoplakia: A 25-year experience with a review of the literature. J Urol 1989;141:1328.

Lorentz WB: Localization of urinary tract infection. Urol Clin North Am 1979;6:519.

Lorentzen M, Nielsen HO: Xanthogranulomatous pyelonephritis. Scand J Urol Nephrol 1980;14:193.

Lowe FC, Fagelman E: Cranberry juice and urinary tract infections: What is the evidence? Urology 2001;57:407.

Malek RS, Elder JS: Xanthogranulomatous pyelonephritis: A critical analysis of 26 cases and of the literature. J Urol 1978; 119:589.

Mangiarotti P, Pizzini C, Fanos V: Antibiotic prophylaxis in children with relapsing urinary tract infections: Review. J Chemother 2000;12:115.

Marques LP et al: AIDS-associated renal tuberculosis. Nephron 1996;74:701.

Martinez JJ et al: Type 1 pilus-mediated bacterial invasion of bladder epithelial cells. Embo J 2000;19:2803.

Matsumoto T: Urinary tract infections in the elderly. Curr Urol Rep 2001;2:330.

McClure J, Cameron CH, Garrett R: The ultrastructural features of malakoplakia. J Pathol 1981;134:13.

McGregor JA, French JI: Prevention of preterm birth. N Engl J Med 1998;339:1858; discussion 1860.

Meares EM Jr: Acute and chronic prostatitis: Diagnosis and treatment. Infect Dis Clin North Am 1987;1:855.

Meares EM, Stamey TA: Bacteriologic localization patterns in bacterial prostatitis and urethritis. Invest Urol 1968;5:492.

Merimsky E, Feldman C: Perinephric abscess: Report of 19 cases. Int Surg 1981;66:79.

Michaeli J et al: Emphysematous pyelonephritis. J Urol 1984; 131:203.

Minassian MA et al: A comparison between single-dose fosfomycin trometamol (Monuril) and a 5-day course of trimethoprim in the treatment of uncomplicated lower urinary tract infection in women. Int J Antimicrob Agents 1998;10:39.

Naber KG: Short-term therapy of acute uncomplicated cystitis. Curr Opin Urol 1999;9:57.

Navas EL et al: Blood group antigen expression on vaginal cells and mucus in women with and without a history of urinary tract infections. J Urol 1994;152:345.

Nickel JC: Antibiotics for bacterial prostatitis. J Urol 2000;163: 1407.

Nickel JC: The management of acute pyelonephritis in adults. Can J Urol 2001;8:29.

Nickel JC: The Pre and Post Massage Test (PPMT): A simple screen for prostatitis. Tech Urol 1997;3:38.

Nickel JC et al: Predictors of patient response to antibiotic therapy for the chronic prostatitis/chronic pelvic pain syndrome: A prospective multicenter clinical trial. J Urol 2001;165:1539.

Nicolle LE: Urinary tract infection in geriatric and institutionalized patients. Curr Opin Urol 2002;12:51.

Nicolle LE, Ronald AR: Recurrent urinary tract infection in adult women: Diagnosis and treatment. Infect Dis Clin North Am 1987;1:793.

Nicolle LE et al: The association of urinary tract infection with sexual intercourse. J Infect Dis 1982;146:579.

O'Dea MJ, Hunting DB, Greene LF: Non-specific granulomatous prostatitis. J Urol 1977;118:58.

Ofek I et al: Role of bacterial lectins in urinary tract infections: Molecular mechanisms for diversification of bacterial surface lectins. Adv Exp Med Biol 2000;485:183.

Ohkawa M, Yamaguchi K, Kobayashi M: Non-specific eosinophilic granulomatous prostatitis responded favorably to an antimicrobial agent and a hydrocortisone. Int J Urol 2001; 8:578.

O'Mahony C: Treatment of non-specific urethritis should be two weeks, not 1. Sex Transm Infect 1999;75:449.

Orskov I et al: O, K, H and fimbrial antigens in *Escherichia coli* serotypes associated with pyelonephritis and cystitis. Scand J Infect Dis Suppl 1982;33:18.

Osset J et al: Assessment of the capacity of *Lactobacillus* to inhibit the growth of uropathogens and block their adhesion to vaginal epithelial cells. J Infect Dis 2001;183:485.

Pak J et al: Tamm-Horsfall protein binds to type 1 fimbriated *Escherichia coli* and prevents *E. coli* from binding to uroplakin Ia and Ib receptors. J Biol Chem 2001;276:9924.

Paltiel HJ et al: Acute scrotal symptoms in boys with an indeterminate clinical presentation: Comparison of color Doppler sonography and scintigraphy. Radiology 1998;207:223.

Parsons MA: Xanthogranulomatous gastritis: An entity or a secondary phenomenon? J Clin Pathol 1993;46:580.

Petrack EM, Hafeez W: Testicular torsion versus epididymitis: A diagnostic challenge. Pediatr Emerg Care 1992;8:347.

Pfau A, Sacks TG: Effective postcoital quinolone prophylaxis of recurrent urinary tract infections in women. J Urol 1994; 152:136.

Pfau A, Sacks TG: Single dose quinolone treatment in acute uncomplicated urinary tract infection in women. J Urol 1993; 149:532.

Philbrick JT: Single dose for urinary tract infections. J Gen Intern Med 1986;1:207.

Randolph MF, Greenfield M: The incidence of asymptomatic bacteriuria and pyuria in infancy: A study of 400 infants in private practice. J Pediatr 1964;65:57.

Raz R, Stamm WE: A controlled trial of intravaginal estriol in postmenopausal women with recurrent urinary tract infections. N Engl J Med 1993;329:753.

Raz R et al: Comparison of single-dose administration and three-day course of amoxicillin with those of clavulanic acid for treatment of uncomplicated urinary tract infection in women. Antimicrob Agents Chemother 1991;35:1688.

Reid G, Burton J: Use of Lactobacillus to prevent infection by pathogenic bacteria. Microbes Infect 2002;4:319.

Rischmann P et al: BCG intravesical instillations: Recommendations for side-effects management. Eur Urol 2000;37:33.

Roberts JA et al: Epitopes of the P-fimbrial adhesin of E. coli cause different urinary tract infections. J Urol 1997;158:1610.

Roberts RO et al: A review of clinical and pathological prostatitis syndromes. Urology 1997;49:809.

Ronald A: The etiology of urinary tract infection: Traditional and emerging pathogens. Am J Med 2002;113:14.

Rubin RH, Beam TR Jr, Stamm WE: An approach to evaluating antibacterial agents in the treatment of urinary tract infection. Clin Infect Dis 1992;14:S246; discussion S253.

Sanford JP: Urinary tract symptoms and infections. Annu Rev Med 1975;26:485.

Santucci RA, Krieger JN: Gentamicin for the practicing urologist: Review of efficacy, single daily dosing and "switch" therapy. J Urol 2000;163:1076.

Schaeffer AJ: The expanding role of fluoroquinolones. Am J Med 2002;113:45.

Schaeffer AJ: What do we know about the urinary tract infection-prone individual? J Infect Dis 2001;183:S66.

Schaeffer AJ et al: Role of vaginal colonization in urinary tract infections (UTIs). Adv Exp Med Biol 1999;462:339.

Schappert SM: Ambulatory care visits to physician offices, hospital outpatient departments, and emergency departments: United States, 1997. Vital Health Stat 13 1999;i–iv, 1–39.

Schieve LA et al: Urinary tract infection during pregnancy: Its association with maternal morbidity and perinatal outcome. Am J Public Health 1994;84:405.

Schlager TA: Urinary tract infections in children younger than 5 years of age: Epidemiology, diagnosis, treatment, outcomes and prevention. Paediatr Drugs 2001;3:219.

Schonwald S, Begovac J, Skerk V: Urinary tract infections in HIV disease. Int J Antimicrob Agents 1999;11:309.

Sepkowitz KA et al: Tuberculosis in the AIDS era. Clin Microbiol Rev 1995;8:180.

Shokeir AA et al: Emphysematous pyelonephritis: A 15-year experience with 20 cases. Urology 1997;49:343.

Shortliffe LM, McCue JD: Urinary tract infection at the age extremes: Pediatrics and geriatrics. Am J Med 2002;113:55.

Siegel JF, Smith A, Moldwin R: Minimally invasive treatment of renal abscess. J Urol 1996;155:52.

Sobel JD: Pathogenesis of urinary tract infection: Role of host defenses. Infect Dis Clin North Am 1997;11:531.

Sotto A et al: Risk factors for antibiotic-resistant Escherichia coli isolated from hospitalized patients with urinary tract infections: A prospective study. J Clin Microbiol 2001;39:438.

Staiman VS, Lowe FC: Prostatic disease in HIV infected patients. AIDS Reader 1995;5:165.

Stamm WE, Norrby SR: Urinary tract infections: Disease panorama and challenges. J Infect Dis 2001;183:S1.

Stamm WE et al: Diagnosis of coliform infection in acutely dysuric women. N Engl J Med 1982;307:463.

Stanton MJ, Maxted W: Malacoplakia: A study of the literature and current concepts of pathogenesis, diagnosis and treatment. J Urol 1981;125:139.

Stenqvist K et al: Bacteriuria in pregnancy: Frequency and risk of acquisition. Am J Epidemiol 1989;129:372.

Stoller ML, Kogan BA: Sensitivity of ^{99m}technetium-dimercaptosuccinic acid for the diagnosis of chronic pyelonephritis: Clinical and theoretical considerations. J Urol 1986;135:977.

Svanborg C et al: Bacterial adherence and mucosal cytokine responses: Receptors and transmembrane signaling. Ann N Y Acad Sci 1996;797:177.

Svanborg Eden C et al: Host-parasite interaction in the urinary tract. J Infect Dis 1988;157:421.

Svenson SB et al: P-fimbriae of pyelonephritogenic Escherichia coli: Identification and chemical characterization of receptors. Infection 1983;11:61.

Sweet RL: Bacteriuria and pyelonephritis during pregnancy. Semin Perinatol 1977;1:25.

Tang HJ et al: Clinical characteristics of emphysematous pyelonephritis. J Microbiol Immunol Infect 2001;34:125.

Thorley JD, Jones SR, Sanford JP: Perinephric abscess. Medicine (Baltimore) 1974;53:441.

Tincello DG, Richmond DH: Evaluation of reagent strips in detecting asymptomatic bacteriuria in early pregnancy: Prospective case series. BMJ 1998;316:435.

Tiu CM et al: Sonographic features of xanthogranulomatous pyelonephritis. J Clin Ultrasound 2001;29:279.

Trauzzi SJ et al: Management of prostatic abscess in patients with human immunodeficiency syndrome. Urology 1994;43: 629.

Trujillo-Santos AJ et al: Therapeutic options for malacoplakia secondary to Escherichia coli infection. Clin Infect Dis 1999; 29:444.

van Dooyeweert DA et al: The influence of PCP prophylaxis on bacteriuria incidence and resistance development to trimethoprim/sulfamethoxazole in HIV-infected patients. Neth J Med 1996;49:225.

Vas W et al: Computed tomography and ultrasound appearance of bladder malacoplakia. J Comput Tomogr 1985;9:119.

Wagenlehner FM, Naber KG: Hospital-acquired urinary tract infections. J Hosp Infect 2000;46:171.

Waltzer WC: The urinary tract in pregnancy. J Urol 1981;125:271.

Wan YL et al: Predictors of outcome in emphysematous pyelonephritis. J Urol 1998;159:369.

Weinberger M et al: Prostatic abscess in the antibiotic era. Rev Infect Dis 1988;10:239.

Wennerstrom M et al: Primary and acquired renal scarring in boys and girls with urinary tract infection. J Pediatr 2000;136:30.

Wettergren B, Jodal U, Jonasson G: Epidemiology of bacteriuria during the first year of life. Acta Paediatr Scand 1985;74:925.

Whitfield C, Roberts IS: Structure, assembly and regulation of expression of capsules in *Escherichia coli*. Mol Microbiol 1999;31:1307.

Wing DA et al: Outpatient treatment of acute pyelonephritis in pregnancy after 24 weeks. Obstet Gynecol 1999;94:683.

Wing DA: Pyelonephritis. Clin Obstet Gynecol 1998;41:515.

Wiswell TE, Roscelli JD: Corroborative evidence for the decreased incidence of urinary tract infections in circumcised male infants. Pediatrics 1986;78:96.

Wood EG, Dillon HC Jr: A prospective study of group B streptococcal bacteriuria in pregnancy. Am J Obstet Gynecol 1981;140:515.

Zorzos I et al: Xanthogranulomatous pyelonephritis—the "great imitator" justifies its name. Scand J Urol Nephrol 2002;36:74.

Specific Infections of the Genitourinary Tract

Emil A. Tanagho, MD

Specific infections are those caused by specific organisms, each of which causes a clinically unique disease that leads to specific pathologic tissue reactions. See also Chapter 15.

TUBERCULOSIS

Tubercle bacilli may invade one or more (or even all) of the organs of the genitourinary tract and cause a chronic granulomatous infection that shows the same characteristics as tuberculosis in other organs. Urinary tuberculosis is a disease of young adults (60% of patients are between the ages of 20 and 40) and is a little more common in males than in females.

Etiology

The infecting organism is *Mycobacterium tuberculosis,* which reaches the genitourinary organs by the hematogenous route from the lungs. The primary site is often not symptomatic or apparent.

The kidney and possibly the prostate are the primary sites of tuberculous infection in the genitourinary tract. All other genitourinary organs become involved by either ascent (prostate to bladder) or descent (kidney to bladder, prostate to epididymis). The testis may become involved by direct extension from epididymal infection.

Pathogenesis (Figure 14–1)

A. KIDNEY AND URETER

When a shower of tubercle bacilli hits the renal cortex, the organisms may be destroyed by normal tissue resistance. Evidence of this is commonly seen in autopsies of persons who have died of tuberculosis; only scars are found in the kidneys. However, if enough bacteria of sufficient virulence become lodged in the kidney and are not overcome, a clinical infection is established.

Tuberculosis of the kidney progresses slowly; it may take 15–20 years to destroy a kidney in a patient who has good resistance to the infection. As a rule, therefore, there is no renal pain and little or no clinical disturbance of any type until the lesion has involved the ca-

lyces or the pelvis, at which time pus and organisms may be discharged into the urine. It is only at this stage that symptoms (of cystitis) are manifested. The infection then proceeds to the pelvic mucosa and the ureter, particularly its upper and vesical ends. This may lead to stricture and back pressure (hydronephrosis).

As the disease progresses, a caseous breakdown of tissue occurs until the entire kidney is replaced by cheesy material. Calcium may be laid down in the reparative process. The ureter undergoes fibrosis and tends to be shortened and therefore straightened. This change leads to a "golf-hole" (gaping) ureteral orifice, typical of an incompetent valve.

B. BLADDER

Vesical irritability develops as an early clinical manifestation of the disease as the bladder is bathed by infected material. Tubercles form later, usually in the region of the involved ureteral orifice, and finally coalesce and ulcerate. These ulcers may bleed. With severe involvement, the bladder becomes fibrosed and contracted; this leads to marked frequency. Ureteral reflux or stenosis and, therefore, hydronephrosis may develop. If contralateral renal involvement occurs later, it is probably a separate hematogenous infection.

C. PROSTATE AND SEMINAL VESICLES

The passage of infected urine through the prostatic urethra ultimately leads to invasion of the prostate and one or both seminal vesicles. There is no local pain.

On occasion, the primary hematogenous lesion in the genitourinary tract is in the prostate. Prostatic infection can ascend to the bladder and descend to the epididymis.

D. EPIDIDYMIS AND TESTIS

Tuberculosis of the prostate can extend along the vas or through the perivasal lymphatics and affect the epididymis. Because this is a slow process, there is usually no pain. If the epididymal infection is extensive and an abscess forms, it may rupture through the scrotal skin, thus establishing a permanent sinus, or it may extend into the testicle.

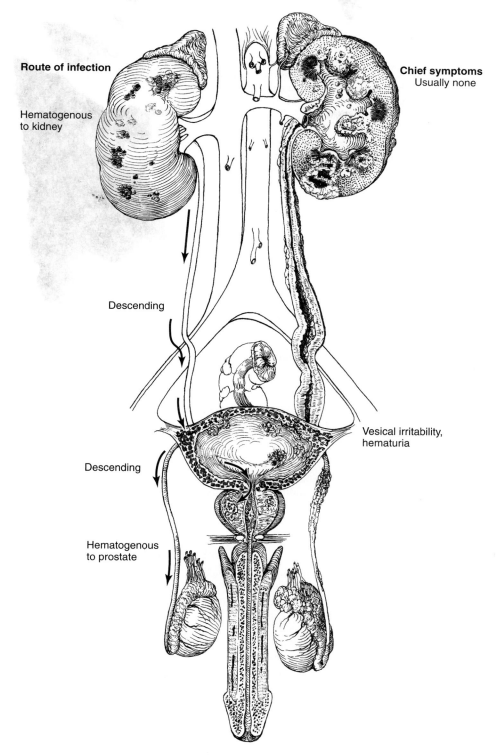

Route of infection

Hematogenous
to kidney

Descending

Descending

Hematogenous
to prostate

Chief symptoms
Usually none

Vesical irritability,
hematuria

Figure 14–1. Pathogenesis of tuberculosis of the urinary tract.

Pathology

A. KIDNEY AND URETER

The gross appearance of the kidney with moderately advanced tuberculosis is often normal on its outer surface, although the kidney is usually surrounded by marked perinephritis. Usually, however, there is a soft, yellowish localized bulge. On section, the involved area is seen to be filled with cheesy material (caseation). Widespread destruction of parenchyma is evident. In otherwise normal tissue, small abscesses may be seen. The walls of the pelvis, calyces, and ureter may be thickened, and ulceration appears frequently in the region of the calyces at the point at which the abscess drains. Ureteral stenosis may be complete, causing "autonephrectomy." Such a kidney is fibrosed and functionless. Under these circumstances, the bladder urine may be normal and symptoms absent.

Tubercle foci appear close to the glomeruli. These are an aggregation of histiocytic cells possessing a vesicular nucleus and a clear cell body that can fuse with neighboring cells to form a small mass called an epithelioid reticulum. At the periphery of this reticulum are large cells with multiple nuclei (giant cells). This pathologic reaction, which can be seen macroscopically, is the basic lesion in tuberculosis. It can heal by fibrosis or coalesce and reach the surface and ulcerate, forming an ulcerocavernous lesion. Tubercles might undergo a central degeneration and caseate, creating a tuberculous abscess cavity that can reach the collecting system and break through. In the process, progressive parenchymal destruction occurs. Depending on the virulence of the organism and the resistance of the patient, tuberculosis is a combination of caseation and cavitation and healing by fibrosis and scarring.

Microscopically, the caseous material is seen as an amorphous mass. The surrounding parenchyma shows fibrosis with tissue destruction, small round cell and plasma cell infiltration, and epithelial and giant cells typical of tuberculosis. Acid-fast stains will usually demonstrate the organisms in the tissue. Similar changes can be demonstrated in the wall of the pelvis and ureter.

In both the kidney and ureter, calcification is common. It may be macroscopic or microscopic. Such a finding is strongly suggestive of tuberculosis but, of course, is also observed in bilharzial infection. Secondary renal stones occur in 10% of patients.

In the most advanced stage of renal tuberculosis, the parenchyma may be completely replaced by caseous substance or fibrous tissue. Perinephric abscess may develop, but this is rare.

B. BLADDER

In the early stages, the mucosa may be inflamed, but this is not a specific change. The bladder is quite resistant to actual invasion. [...] form and can be easily seen endoscopically a[...] yello[...] raised nodules surrounded by a halo of h[...] mural fibrosis and severe vesical contrac[...] ay occur.

Microscopically, the nod[...] tubercles. These break dow[...] cers. At this stage the bladder [...] aling, fibrosis develops that i[...]

C. PROSTATE AND S[...]

Grossly, the exter[...] ns may show nodules and ar[...] osis. Areas of necrosis are co[...] g may end in calcification. [...] ostate should suggest tuberc[...]

D. SPERMATIC CORD, [...] ESTIS

The vas deferens is often gr[...] olved; fusiform swellings represent tubercles that [...] ronic cases are characteristically described as bead[...] he epididymis is enlarged and quite firm. It is usual[ly] separate from the testis, although occasionally it may adhere to it. Microscopically, the changes typical of tuberculosis are seen. Tubular degeneration may be marked. The testis is usually not involved except by direct extension of an abscess in the epididymis.

E. FEMALE GENITAL TRACT

Infections are usually carried by the bloodstream; rarely, they are the result of sexual contact with an infected male. The incidence of associated urinary and genital infection in females ranges from 1% to 10%. The uterine tubes may be affected. Other presentations include endarteritis, localized adnexal masses (usually bilateral), and tuberculous cervicitis, but granulomatous lesions of the vaginal canal and vulva are rare.

Clinical Findings

Tuberculosis of the genitourinary tract should be considered in the presence of any of the following situations: (1) chronic cystitis that refuses to respond to adequate therapy, (2) the finding of pus without bacteria in a methylene blue stain or culture of the urinary sediment, (3) gross or microscopic hematuria, (4) a nontender, enlarged epididymis with a beaded or thickened vas, (5) a chronic draining scrotal sinus, or (6) induration or nodulation of the prostate and thickening of one or both seminal vesicles (especially in a young man). A history of present or past tuberculosis elsewhere in the body should cause the physician to suspect tuberculosis in the genitourinary tract when signs or symptoms are present.

The diagnosis rests on the demonstration of tubercle bacilli in the urine by culture. The extent of the infection is determined by (1) the palpable findings in the epididymides, vasa deferentia, prostate, and seminal vesicles; (2) the renal and ureteral lesions as revealed by excretory urograms; (3) involvement of the bladder as seen through the cystoscope; (4) the degree of renal damage as measured by loss of function; and (5) the presence of tubercle bacilli in one or both kidneys.

A. Symptoms

There is no classic clinical picture of renal tuberculosis. Most symptoms of this disease, even in the most advanced stage, are vesical in origin (cystitis). Vague generalized malaise, fatigability, low-grade but persistent fever, and night sweats are some of the nonspecific complaints. Even vesical irritability may be absent, in which case only proper collection and examination of the urine will afford the clue. Active tuberculosis elsewhere in the body is found in less than half of patients with genitourinary tuberculosis.

1. Kidney and ureter—Because of the slow progression of the disease, the affected kidney is usually completely asymptomatic. On occasion, however, there may be a dull ache in the flank. The passage of a blood clot, secondary calculi, or a mass of debris may cause renal and ureteral colic. Rarely, the presenting symptom may be a painless mass in the abdomen.

2. Bladder—The earl symptoms of renal tuberculosis may arise from seco olvement. These include burning, freq Hematuria is occasionally found a esical origin. At times, par disease, the vesical irrita lcera-tion occurs, suprapu adder becomes full.

3. Genital tract—seminal vesicles usual clue to the presence organs is the onset of a

Tuberculosis of the painless or only mildly pair drain spontaneously th draining sinus should proved otherwise. In ra c and may simulate an acu e

B. Signs

Evidence of extragenital tub (lungs, bone, lymph nodes, tons

1. Kidney—There is usually n derness of the involved kidney.

2. External genitalia—A thic only slightly tender epididymis m

vas deferens often is thickened and beaded. A chronic draining sinus through the scrotal skin is almost pathognomonic of tuberculous epididymitis. In the more advanced stages, the epididymis cannot be differentiated from the testis on palpation. This may mean that the testis has been directly invaded by the epididymal abscess.

Hydrocele occasionally accompanies tuberculous epididymitis. The idiopathic hydrocele should be tapped so that underlying pathologic changes, if present, can be evaluated (epididymitis, testicular tumor). Involvement of the penis and urethra is rare.

3. Prostate and seminal vesicles—These organs may be normal to palpation. Ordinarily, however, the tuberculous prostate shows areas of induration, even nodulation. The involved seminal vesicle is usually indurated, enlarged, and fixed. If epididymitis is present, the ipsilateral seminal vesicle usually shows changes as well.

C. Laboratory Findings

Proper urinalysis affords the most important clue to the diagnosis of genitourinary tuberculosis.

1. Persistent pyuria without organisms on culture or on the smear stained with methylene blue means tuberculosis until proved otherwise. Acid-fast stains done on the concentrated sediment from a 24-h specimen are positive in at least 60% of cases. However, this must be corroborated by a positive culture.

About 15–20% of patients with tuberculosis have secondary pyogenic infection; the clue ("sterile" pyuria) is thereby obscured. If clinical response to adequate treatment fails and pyuria persists, tuberculosis must be ruled out by bacteriologic and roentgenologic eans.

Cultures for tubercle bacilli from the first morn- re positive in a very high percentage of cases fection. If positive, sensitivity tests ce of strong presumptive lures should be re-

how aneotherwise healthy patient speaks against a diagnosis of tuberculosis.

D. X-Ray Findings (Figure 14–2)

A chest film that shows evidence of tuberculosis should cause the physician to suspect tuberculosis of the urogenital tract in the presence of urinary signs and symptoms. A plain film of the abdomen may show enlargement of one kidney or obliteration of the renal and psoas shadows due to perinephric abscess. Punctate calcification in the renal parenchyma may be due to tuberculosis. Renal stones are found in 10% of cases. Calcification of the ureter may be noted, but this is rare (Figure 6–1).

Excretory urograms can be diagnostic if the lesion is moderately advanced. The typical changes include (1) a "moth-eaten" appearance of the involved ulcerated calyces, (2) obliteration of one or more calyces, (3) dilatation of the calyces due to ureteral stenosis from fibrosis, (4) abscess cavities that connect with calyces, (5) single or multiple ureteral strictures, with secondary dilatation, with shortening and therefore straightening of the ureter, and (6) absence of function of the kidney due to complete ureteral occlusion and renal destruction (autonephrectomy).

If the excretory urograms demonstrate gross tuberculosis in one kidney, there is no need to do a retrograde urogram on that side. In fact, there is at least a theoretic danger of hematogenous or lymphogenous dissemination resulting from the increased intrapelvic pressure. Retrograde urography may be carried out on the unsuspected side, however, as a verification of its normality. This is further substantiated if the urine from that side is free of both pus cells and tubercle bacilli.

E. Instrumental Examination

Thorough cystoscopic study is indicated even wh__ the offending organism has been found in th_____ cretory urograms show the_____ study clearly demonstra_____ Cystoscopy may _____ tuberculosis_____

ceration of the bladder wall means tuberculosis. Urograms are usually definitive.

Acute or chronic nonspecific epididymitis may be confused with tuberculosis, since the onset of tuberculosis is occasionally quite painful. It is rare to have palpatory changes in the seminal vesicles with nonspecific epididymitis, but these are almost routine findings in tuberculosis of the epididymis. The presence of tubercle bacilli on a culture of the urine is diagnostic. On occasion, only the pathologist can make the diagnosis by microscopic study of the surgically removed epididymis.

Amicrobic cystitis usually has an acute onset and is often preceded by a urethral discharge. "Sterile" pyuria is found, but tubercle bacilli are absent. Cystoscopy may reveal ulcerations, but these are acute and superficial. Although urograms show mild hydroureter and even hydronephrosis, there is no ulceration of the calyces as seen in renal tuberculosis. Interstitial cystitis is typically characterized by frequency, nocturia, and suprapubic pain with vesical filling. The urine is usually free of pus. Tubercle bacilli are absent.

Multiple small renal stones or nephrocalcinosis seen by x-ray may suggest the type of calcification seen in the tuberculous kidney. In renal tuberculosis, the calcium is in the parenchyma, although secondary stones are occasionally seen.

Necrotizing papillitis, which may involve all of the calyces of one or both kidneys or, rarely, a solitary calyx, shows caliceal lesions (including calcifications) that simulate those of tuberculosis. Careful bacteriologic studies fail to demonstrate tubercle bacilli.

Medullary sponge kidneys may show small calcifications just distal to the calyces. The calyces are sharp, however, and no other stigmas of tuberculosis can be demonstrated.

In disseminated coccidioidomycosis, renal involvement may occur. The renal lesion resembles that of tuberculosis. Coccidioidal epididymitis may be confused with tuberculous involvement.

Urinary bilharziasis is a great mimic of tuberculosis. Both present with symptoms of cystitis and often _____ contraction, seen in both diseases, _____ frequency. Schistosomiasis must be _____ reas; the typical ova are found in _____ and urographic findings are de-_____ fferential diagnosis.

_____CULOS __cause an enlarging mass in the _bscess r_ e abdomen shows obliteration _in film_ hadows. Sonograms and CT _nal and_ l. Renal stones may develop if _y be mor_

Figure 14–2. Radiologic evidence of tuberculosis. **Upper left:** Excretory urogram showing "moth-eaten" calyces in upper renal poles. Calcifications in upper calyces; right upper ureter is straight and dilated. **Upper right:** Excretory urogram showing ulcerated and dilated calyces on the left. **Lower left:** Plain film showing calcifications in right kidney, adrenals, and spleen (tuberculosis of right kidney and Addison disease). **Lower right:** Excretory urogram. Dilatation of calyces; upper right ureter dilated and straight. Arrows point to poorly defined parenchymal abscesses.

secondary nonspecific infection is present. Uremia is the end stage if both kidneys are involved.

B. Ureteral Tuberculosis

Scarring with stricture formation is one of the typical lesions of tuberculosis and most commonly affects the juxtavesical portion of the ureter. This may cause progressive hydronephrosis. Complete ureteral obstruction may cause complete nonfunction of the kidney (autonephrectomy).

C. Vesical Tuberculosis

When severely damaged, the bladder wall becomes fibrosed and contracted. Stenosis of the ureters or reflux occurs, causing hydronephrotic atrophy.

D. Genital Tuberculosis

The ducts of the involved epididymis become occluded. If this is bilateral, sterility results. Abscess of the epididymis may rupture into the testis, through the scrotal wall, or both, in which case the spermatogenic tubules may slough out.

Treatment

Tuberculosis must be treated as a generalized disease. Even when it can be demonstrated only in the urogenital tract, one must assume activity elsewhere. (It is theoretically possible, however, for the primary focus to have healed spontaneously.) This means that the basic treatment is medical. Surgical excision of an infected organ, when indicated, is merely an adjunct to overall therapy.

A. Renal Tuberculosis

A strict medical regimen should be instituted. A combination of drugs is usually desirable. The following drugs are effective in combination: (1) isoniazid, 200–300 mg orally once daily; (2) rifampin, 600 mg orally once daily; (3) ethambutol, 25 mg/kg daily for 2 months, then 15 mg/kg orally once daily; (4) streptomycin, 1 g intramuscularly once daily; and (5) pyrazinamide, l.5–2 g orally once daily. It is preferable to begin treatment with a combination of isoniazid, rifampin, and ethambutol. If resistance to one of these drugs develops, one of the others listed should be chosen as a replacement. The following drugs are usually considered only in cases of resistance to first-line drugs and when expert medical personnel are available to treat toxic side effects, should they occur: aminosalicylic acid (PAS), capreomycin, cycloserine, ethionamide, pyrazinamide, viomycin. *Pyrazinamide may cause serious liver damage.*

B. Vesical Tuberculosis

Tuberculosis of the bladder is always secondary to renal or prostatic tuberculosis; it tends to heal promptly when definitive treatment for the "primary" genitourinary infection is given. Vesical ulcers that fail to respond to this regimen may require transurethral electrocoagulation. Vesical instillations of 0.2% monoxychlorosene (Clorpactin) may also stimulate healing.

Should extreme contracture of the bladder develop, it may be necessary to divert the urine from the bladder or perform augmentation cystoplasty after subtotal cystectomy (ileocystoplasty, ileocecocystoplasty, sigmoidocystoplasty) to increase bladder capacity (Abel and Gow, 1978).

C. Tuberculosis of the Epididymis

This condition never produces an isolated lesion; the prostate is always involved and usually the kidney as well. Only rarely does the epididymal infection break through into the testis. Treatment is medical. If after months of treatment an abscess or a draining sinus exists, epididymectomy is indicated.

D. Tuberculosis of the Prostate and Seminal Vesicles

Although a few urologists advocate removal of the entire prostate and the vesicles when they become involved by tuberculosis, the majority opinion is that only medical therapy is indicated. Control can be checked by culture of the semen for tubercle bacilli.

E. General Measures for All Types

Optimal nutrition is no less important in treating tuberculosis of the genitourinary tract than in the treatment of tuberculosis elsewhere. Bladder sedatives may be given for the irritable bladder.

F. Treatment of Other Complications

Perinephric abscess usually occurs when the kidney is destroyed, but this is rare. The abscess must be drained, and nephrectomy should be done either then or later to prevent development of a chronic draining sinus. Prolonged antimicrobial therapy is indicated. If ureteral stricture develops on the involved side, ureteral dilatations offer a better than 50% chance of cure (Cos and Cockett, 1982). The severely involved bladder may cause incompetence of the ureterovesical junction on the uninvolved side. Ureteroneocystostomy cannot be done in such a bladder; some form of urinary diversion may be required. For this reason, serial excretory urograms are necessary even when the treatment is medical.

AMICROBIC (ABACTERIAL) CYSTITIS

Amicrobic cystitis is a rare disease of abrupt onset with a marked local vesical reaction. Although it acts like an infectious disease, search for the usual urinary bacterial pathogens is negative. It affects adult men and occasionally children, usually boys.

Etiology

The patient usually gives a history of recent sexual exposure. Mycoplasmas and chlamydiae have been isolated or suspected as etiologic agents. An adenovirus has been isolated from the urine in children suffering from acute hemorrhagic cystitis.

Pathogenesis & Pathology

Whatever the source and identity of the invader, the disease is primarily manifested as an acute inflammation of the bladder. Vesical irritability is severe and often associated with terminal hematuria. The mucosa is red and edematous, and superficial ulceration is occasionally seen. A thin membrane of fibrin often lies on the wall. Similar changes may be noted in the posterior urethra. The renal parenchyma is not involved, although the pelvic and ureteral mucosa may show mild inflammatory changes. Some dilatation of the lower ureters is apt to develop. This may be due to an inflammatory reaction about the ureteral orifices, for these changes regress after successful treatment.

Microscopically, there is nothing specific about the reaction. The mucosa and submucosa are infiltrated with neutrophils, plasma cells, and eosinophils. Submucosal hemorrhages are common; superficial ulceration of the mucosa may be noted.

Clinical Findings

A. Symptoms

All symptoms are local. Urethral discharge, which is usually clear and mucoid but may be purulent, may be the initial symptom in men. Symptoms of acute cystitis come on abruptly. Urgency, frequency, and burning may be severe. Terminal hematuria is not uncommon. Suprapubic discomfort or even pain may be noted; it is most apt to be present as the bladder fills and is relieved somewhat by voiding. There is no fever or malaise.

B. Signs

Some suprapubic tenderness may be found. Urethral discharge may be profuse or scanty and may be purulent or thin and mucoid. The prostate is usually normal to palpation. Massage is contraindicated during the acute stage of urinary tract infection. When massage is done later, infection is usually not present.

C. Laboratory Findings

Some leukocytosis may develop. The urine is grossly purulent and may contain blood as well. Stained smears reveal an absence of bacteria. Routine cultures are uniformly negative. In a few cases, mycoplasmas and TRIC agent (*Chlamydia trachomatis*) have been identified, but the significance of this is not yet clear. Search for tubercle bacilli is not successful.

Urethral discharge reveals no bacteria. Renal function is not impaired.

D. X-Ray Findings

Excretory urograms may demonstrate some dilatation of the lower ureters, but these changes regress completely when the disease is cured. The bladder shadow is small because of its markedly diminished capacity. Cystograms may reveal reflux.

E. Instrumental Examination

Cystoscopy is not indicated in acute inflammation of the bladder. It has been done, however, when the diagnosis was obscure and tuberculosis suspected. In such cases it reveals redness and edema of the mucosa. Superficial ulceration may be noted. Bladder capacity is markedly diminished. Biopsy of the wall shows nonspecific changes.

Differential Diagnosis

Tuberculosis causes symptoms of cystitis, which usually come on gradually and become severe only in the stage of ulceration. A painless, nontender enlargement of an epididymis suggests tuberculosis. Although both tuberculosis and amicrobic cystitis produce pus without bacteria, thorough laboratory study demonstrates tubercle bacilli only in the former. On cystoscopy, the tuberculous bladder may be studded with tubercles. The ulcers in this disease are deep and of a chronic type. The changes in amicrobic cystitis are more acute; ulceration, if present, is superficial. Excretory urograms in tuberculosis may show "moth-eaten" calyces typical of infection with acid-fast organisms.

Nonspecific (pyogenic) cystitis may mimic amicrobic cystitis perfectly, but pathogenic organisms are easily found on a smear stained with methylene blue or on culture.

Cystitis secondary to chronic nonspecific prostatitis occasionally produces pus without bacteria. The findings on rectal examination, the pus in the prostatic secretion, and the response to antibiotics point to the proper diagnosis.

Vesical neoplasm may ulcerate, become infected, and bleed; hence it may mimic amicrobic cystitis. Bacteriuria, however, is found. In case of doubt, cystoscopy is indicated.

Interstitial cystitis may be accompanied by severe symptoms of vesical irritability. However, it usually affects women and urinalysis is entirely negative except for a few red cells. Cystoscopy should be diagnostic.

Complications

Amicrobic cystitis is usually self-limited. Rarely, secondary contracture of the bladder develops. Under these circumstances, vesicoureteral reflux may be noted.

Treatment

A. SPECIFIC MEASURES

One of the tetracyclines or chloramphenicol, 1 g/d orally in divided doses for 3–4 days, is said to be curative in 75% of cases. Streptomycin, 1–2 g/d intramuscularly for 3–4 days, may be tried. Neoarsphenamine is also effective and appears to be the drug of choice, but arsenicals are hard to find. The first dose is 0.3 g intravenously; subsequent dosage is 0.45 g intravenously every 3–5 days for a total of 3–4 injections.

Penicillin and the sulfonamides are without effect. In the cases reported in children, cure occurred spontaneously.

B. GENERAL MEASURES

Bladder sedatives are usually of little help if symptoms are severe. Analgesics or narcotics may prove necessary to combat pain. Hot sitz baths may relieve spasm.

The instillation of a 0.1% solution of sodium oxychlorosene (Clorpactin WCS-90) has been recommended.

Prognosis

The prognosis is excellent.

CANDIDIASIS

Candida albicans is a yeastlike fungus that is a normal inhabitant of the respiratory and gastrointestinal tracts and the vagina. The intensive use of potent modern antibiotics is apt to disturb the normal balance between normal and abnormal organisms, thus allowing fungi such as *Candida* to overwhelm an otherwise healthy organ. The bladder and, to a lesser extent, the kidneys have proved vulnerable; candidemia has been observed. Anogenital candidiasis is discussed in Chapter 40.

The patient may present with vesical irritability or symptoms and signs of pyelonephritis. Fungus balls may be passed spontaneously. The diagnosis is made by observing mycelial or yeast forms of the fungus microscopically in a properly collected urine specimen. The diagnosis may be confirmed by culture. Excretory urograms may show caliceal defects and ureteral obstruction (fungus masses).

Vesical candidiasis usually responds to alkalinization of the urine with sodium bicarbonate. A urinary pH of 7.5 is desired; the dose is regulated by the patient, who checks the urine with indicator paper. Should this fail, amphotericin B should be instilled via catheter 3 times a day. One dissolves 50 mg of the drug in 1 L of sterile water.

If there is renal involvement, irrigations of the renal pelvis with a similar concentration of amphotericin B are efficacious. In the presence of systemic manifestations or candidemia, flucytosine (Ancobon) is the drug of choice. The dose is 100 mg/kg/d orally in divided doses given for 1 week. In the face of serious involvement, 600 mg is given intravenously on the first day followed by a shift to the oral form of the drug. Nifuratel, a nitrofuran antibiotic, is superior to flucytosine. The recommended dose is 400 mg 3 times daily for 1 week. The dose must be modified in the face of renal impairment. The drug is more active in acid urine. Graybill et al (1983) reported good results with ketoconazole. The dose is 200–400 mg/d for 2–3 weeks or more depending on the effect as reflected by serial cultures. Its toxicity is relatively low. Amphotericin B (Fungizone) has the disadvantages of requiring parenteral administration and being highly nephrotoxic. It is given intravenously in a dosage of 1–5 mg/d in divided doses dissolved in 5% dextrose. The concentration of the solution should be 0.1 mg/mL.

ACTINOMYCOSIS

Actinomycosis is a chronic granulomatous disease in which fibrosis tends to become marked and spontaneous fistulas are the rule. On rare occasions, the disease involves the kidney, bladder, or testis by hematogenous invasion from a primary site of infection. The skin of the penis or scrotum may become involved through a local abrasion. The bladder may also become diseased by direct extension from the appendix, bowel, or oviduct.

Etiology

Actinomyces israelii (*A bovis*) is the causative organism.

Clinical Findings

There is nothing specifically pathognomonic about the symptoms or signs in actinomycosis. The microscopic demonstration of the organisms, which are visible as yellow bodies called "sulfur granules," makes the diagnosis. If persistently sought, these may be found in the discharge from sinuses or in the urine. Pollock et al (1978) recommend aspiration biopsy performed by a thin needle. They found that in addition to the discovery of sulfur granules, both Gram stain and a modified

Ziehl-Neelsen stain were useful in diagnosis. Definitive diagnosis is established by culture.

Urographically, the lesion in the kidney may resemble tuberculosis (eroded calyces) or tumor (space-occupying lesion).

Treatment

Penicillin G is the drug of choice. The dosage is 10–20 million units/d parenterally for 4–6 weeks, followed by penicillin V orally for a prolonged period. If secondary infection is suspected, a sulfonamide is added; streptomycin is also efficacious. Broad-spectrum antibiotics are indicated only if the organism is resistant to penicillin. Surgical drainage of the abscess or, better, removal of the involved organ is usually indicated.

Prognosis

Removal of the involved organ (eg, kidney or testis) may be promptly curative. Drainage of a granulomatous abscess may cause the development of a chronic draining sinus. Chemotherapy is helpful.

SCHISTOSOMIASIS (BILHARZIASIS)

Schistosomiasis, caused by a blood fluke, is a disease of warm climates. In its 3 forms, it affects about 350 million people. *Schistosoma mansoni* is widely distributed in Africa, South and Central America, Pakistan, and India; *Schistosoma japonicum* is found in the Far East; and *Schistosoma haematobium* (*Bilharzia haematobia*) is limited to Africa (especially along its northern coast), Saudi Arabia, Israel, Jordan, Lebanon, and Syria.

Schistosomiasis is on the increase in endemic areas because of the construction of modern irrigation systems that provide favorable conditions for the intermediate host, a freshwater snail. This disease principally affects the urogenital system, especially the bladder, ureters, seminal vesicles, and, to a lesser extent, the male urethra and prostate gland. Because of emigration of people from endemic areas, the disease is being seen with increasing frequency in both Europe and the United States. Infection with *S mansoni* and *S japonicum* mainly involves the colon.

Etiology

Humans are infected when they come in contact with larva-infested water in canals, ditches, or irrigation fields during swimming, bathing, or farming procedures. Fork-tailed larvae, the cercariae, lose their tails as they penetrate deep under the skin. They are then termed **schistosomules.** They cause allergic skin reactions that are more intense in people infected for the first time. These schistosomules enter the general circulation through the lymphatics and the peripheral veins and reach the lungs. If the infection is massive, they may cause pneumonitis. They pass through the pulmonary circulation, to the left side of the heart, and to the general circulation. The worms that reach the vesicoprostatic plexus of veins survive and mature, whereas those that go to other areas die.

Pathogenesis

The adult *S haematobium* worm, a digenetic trematode, lives in the prostatovesical plexus of veins. The male is about 10×1 mm in size, is folded upon itself, and carries the long, slim 20×0.25 mm female in its "schist," or gynecophoric canal. In the smallest peripheral venules, the female leaves the male and partially penetrates the venule to lay her eggs in the subepithelial layer of the affected viscus, usually in the form of clusters that form tubercles. The ova are seen only rarely within the venules; they are almost always in the subepithelial or interstitial tissues. The female returns to the male, which carries her to other areas to repeat the process.

The living ova, by a process of histolysis and helped by contraction of the detrusor muscle, penetrate the overlying urothelium, pass into the cavity of the bladder, and are extruded with the urine. If these ova reach fresh water, they hatch, and the contained larvae—ciliated miracidia—find a specific freshwater snail that they penetrate. There they form sporocysts that ultimately form the cercariae, which leave the snail hosts and pass into fresh water to repeat their life cycle in the human host.

Pathology

The fresh ova excite little tissue reaction when they leave the human host promptly through the urothelium. The contents of the ova trapped in the tissues and the death of the organisms cause a severe local reaction, with infiltration of round cells, monocytes, eosinophils, and giant cells that form tubercles, nodules, and polyps. These are later replaced by fibrous tissue that causes contraction of different parts of the bladder and strictures of the ureter. Fibrosis and massive deposits of eggs in subepithelial tissues interfere with the blood supply of the area and cause chronic bilharzial ulcerations. Epithelial metaplasia is common, and squamous cell carcinoma is a frequent sequela. Secondary infection of the urinary tract is a common complication and is difficult to overcome. The trapped dead ova become impregnated with calcium salts and form sheets of subepithelial calcified layers in the ureter, bladder, and seminal vesicles.

Clinical Findings

A. SYMPTOMS

Penetration of the skin by the cercariae causes allergic reactions, with cutaneous hyperemia and itching that are more intense in people infected for the first time. During the stage of generalization or invasion, the patient complains of symptoms such as malaise, fatigue and lassitude, low-grade fever, excessive sweating, headache, and backache. When the ova are laid in the bladder wall and begin to be extruded, the patient complains of terminal, slightly painful hematuria that is occasionally profuse. This may remain the only complaint for a long time until complications set in, when vesical symptoms become exaggerated and progressive. Increasing frequency, suprapubic and back pain, urethralgia, profuse hematuria, pyuria, and necroturia are likely to occur, with secondary infection, ulceration, or malignancy. Renal pain may be due to ureteral stricture, vesicoureteral reflux, or secondary stones obstructing the ureter. Fever, rigor, toxemia, and uremia are manifestations of renal involvement.

B. SIGNS

In early uncomplicated cases, there are essentially no clinical findings. Later, a fibrosed, pitted, bilharzial glans penis, a urethral stricture or fistula, or a perineal fibrous mass may be found. A suprapubic bladder mass or a renal swelling may be felt abdominally. Rectal examination may reveal a fibrosed prostate, an enlarged seminal vesicle, or a thickened bladder base.

C. LABORATORY FINDINGS

Urinalysis usually reveals the terminal-spined dead or living ova, blood and pus cells, and bacteria. Malignant squamous cells may be seen. The hemogram usually shows leukocytosis with eosinophilia and hypochromic normocytic anemia. Serum creatinine and blood urea nitrogen measurements may demonstrate some degree of renal impairment.

A variety of immunologic methods have been used to confirm the diagnosis of schistosomiasis. Positive immunologic tests indicate previous exposure but not whether schistosomiasis is currently present. The cercariae, schistosomules, adult worms, and eggs are all potentially antigenic. Adult worms, however, acquire host antigen on their integument that circumvents the immunologic forces of the host. Antibody production may be manifested as hypergammaglobulinemia.

D. X-RAY FINDINGS

A plain film of the abdomen may show areas of grayness in the flank (enlarged hydronephrotic kidney) or in the bladder area (large tumor). Opacifications (stones) may be noted in the kidney, ureter, or bladder. Linear calcification may be seen in the ureteral and bladder walls (Figure 14–3). Punctate calcification of the ureter (ureteritis calcinosa) and a honeycombed calcification of the seminal vesicle may be obvious (Figure 14–3).

Excretory urograms may show either normal or diminished renal function and varying degrees of dilatation of the upper urinary tracts (Figure 14–4). These changes include hydronephrosis, dilated and tortuous ureters, ureteral strictures, or a small contracted bladder having a capacity of only a few milliliters. Gross irregular defects of the bladder wall represent cancer (Figure 14–4).

Retrograde urethrography may reveal a bilharzial urethral stricture. Cystograms often reveal vesicoureteral reflux, particularly if the bladder is contracted.

E. INSTRUMENTAL EXAMINATION

Urethral calibration with a sound may reveal stricture formation.

Cystoscopy may show fresh conglomerate, grayish tubercles surrounded by a halo of hyperemia, old calcified yellowish tubercles, sandy patches of mucous membrane, and a lusterless ground-glass mucosa that lacks the normal vascular pattern. Other obvious lesions include bilharzial polyps, chronic ulcers on the dome that bleed when the bladder is deflated (weeping ulcers), vesical stones, malignant lesions, stenosed or patulous ureteric orifices, and a distorted, asymmetric trigone. All are signs of schistosomal infestation.

Differential Diagnosis

Bilharzial cystitis is unmistakable in endemic areas. The presence of schistosomal ova in the urine, together with radiographic and cystoscopic findings, usually confirms the diagnosis. Nonspecific cystitis usually responds to medical treatment unless there is a complicating factor. Tuberculous cystitis may mimic bilharzial cystitis; the detection of tubercle bacilli, together with the radiographic picture, is confirmatory, but tuberculosis may occur in a bilharzial bladder. Vesical calculi and malignancy should be diagnosed by thorough urologic examination, although both conditions are common in association with bilharzial bladder. Complications of schistosomiasis are the result of fibrosis, which may be extreme and causes contraction of the bladder neck as well as of the bladder itself. It also causes strictures of the urethra and ureter that are usually bilateral. Vesicoureteral reflux is a frequent sequela. Secondary persistent infection and stone formation usually complicate the picture still further. Squamous cell tumors of the

Figure 14–3. Schistosomiasis. Plain films. **Upper left:** Extensive calcification in the wall of a contracted bladder. **Right:** Extensive calcification of the bladder and both ureters up to the renal pelves. The ureters are dilated and tortuous. **Lower left:** Extensive calcification of seminal vesicles and ampullae of vasa.

bladder are common. They are seen as early as the second or third decade of life and are much more common in men than in women.

Treatment

A. MEDICAL MEASURES

Praziquantel, metrifonate, and oxamniquine are the drugs of choice in treating schistosomiasis. These drugs do not have the serious side effects associated with the older drugs (eg, antimonials).

1. Praziquantel is unique in that it is effective against all human schistosome species. It is given orally and is effective in adults and children. Patients in the hepatosplenic stage of advanced schistosomiasis tolerate the drug well. The recommended dosage for all forms of schistosomiasis is 20 mg/kg 3 times in 1 day only.

Figure 14–4. Schistosomiasis. **Upper left:** Excretory urogram showing markedly contracted bladder. Lower right ureter dilated probably secondary to vesicoureteral reflux. **Right:** Excretory urogram at 2 h showing a fairly normal right kidney. The upper ureter is distorted. Arrows point to calcified wall. The lower ureter is quite abnormal. The calyces and pelvis of the left kidney are dilated, but the kidney shows atrophy secondary to nonspecific infection. The upper ureter is dilated and displaced by elongation due to obstruction. Arrows show calcification. Linear calcification can be seen in the periphery of the lower half of the bladder wall (arrows). **Lower left:** Nodular squamous cell carcinoma of the bladder. Dilated left lower ureter probably secondary to obstruction by tumor. Nonvisualization of the right ureter caused by complete occlusion.

2. Metrifonate is also a highly effective oral drug. It is the drug of choice for treatment of *S haematobium* infections but is not effective against *S mansoni* or *S japonicum*. For treatment of *S haematobium* infections, the dosage is 7.5–10 mg/kg (maximum 600 mg) once and then repeated twice at 2-week intervals.

3. Oxamniquine is a highly effective oral drug and is the drug of choice for treatment of *S mansoni* infec-

tions. It is safe and effective in advanced disease. It is not effective in *S haematobium* or *S japonicum* infections. The dosage is 12–15 mg/kg given once; for children under 30 kg, 20 mg/kg is given in 2 divided doses in 1 day, with an interval of 2–8 h between doses. Cure rates are 70–95%.

4. Niridazole, a nitrothiazole derivative, is effective in treating *S mansoni* and *S haematobium* infections. It may be tried against *S japonicum* infections. It is given orally and should be administered only under close medical supervision. The dosage is 25 mg/kg (maximum, 1.5 g) daily in 2 divided doses for 7 days. Side effects may include nausea, vomiting, anorexia, headache, T-wave depression, and temporary suppression of spermatogenesis.

5. Antimonial drugs are no longer used in the treatment of schistosomiasis if praziquantel, oxamniquine, or metrifonate is available. The antimonials (eg, sodium antimony dimercaptosuccinate [stibocaptate], stibophen, tartar emetic) are much more toxic, and a longer course of therapy is needed. Tartar emetic is nonetheless occasionally needed as a third alternative drug in the treatment of *S japonicum* infection.

B. General Measures

Antibiotics or urinary antiseptics are needed to overcome or control secondary infection. Supportive treatment in the form of iron, vitamins, and a high-calorie diet is indicated in selected cases.

C. Complications

Treatment of the complications of schistosomiasis of the genitourinary tract makes demands on the skill of the physician. Juxtavesical ureteral strictures require resection of the stenotic segment with ureteroneocystostomy. If the ureter is not long enough to reimplant, a tube of bladder may be fashioned, turned cephalad, and anastomosed to the ureter. Should the ureter be widely dilated, it must be tailored to approach normal size. Vesicoureteral reflux requires a suitable surgical repair. A contracted bladder neck may need transurethral anterior commissurotomy or a suprapubic Y-V plasty.

A chronic "weeping" bilharzial bladder ulcer necessitates partial cystectomy. The contracted bladder is treated by enterocystoplasty (placing a segment of bowel as a patch on the bladder). This procedure, which significantly increases vesical capacity, is remarkably effective in lessening the severity of symptoms associated with contracted bladder. Preoperative vesicoureteral reflux may disappear.

The most dreaded complication, squamous cell carcinoma, requires total cystectomy with urinary diversion if the lesion is deemed operable. Unfortunately, late diagnosis is the rule.

Prognosis

With energetic treatment, mild and early cases of schistosomiasis are not likely to result in severe damage to the urinary tract. On the other hand, massive repeated infections undermine the function of the urinary tract to such an extent that patients are disabled and become chronic invalids whose life spans are shortened by 1 or 2 decades.

In many endemic areas, attempts have been made to control the disease by mass treatment of patients, proper education, mechanization of agriculture, and various methods of eradication or control of the snail population. All these efforts have failed to be fully effective.

FILARIASIS

Filariasis is endemic in the countries bordering the Mediterranean, in south China and Japan, the West Indies, and the South Pacific islands, particularly Samoa. Limited infection, as seen in American soldiers during World War II, gives an entirely different clinical picture from that seen in the frequent reinfections usually encountered among the native population.

Etiology

Wuchereria bancrofti is a threadlike nematode about 0.5 cm or more in length that lives in the human lymphatics. In the lymphatics, the female gives off microfilariae, which are found in the peripheral blood, particularly at night. The intermediate host (usually a mosquito) bites an infected person and becomes infested with microfilariae, which develop into larvae. These are in turn transferred to another human, in whom they reach maturity. Mating occurs, and microfilariae are again produced. *Brugia malayi,* a nematode that causes filariasis in Southeast Asia and adjacent Pacific islands, acts in a similar fashion.

Pathogenesis & Pathology

The adult nematode in the human host invades and obstructs the lymphatics; this leads to lymphangitis and lymphadenitis. In long-standing cases, the lymphatic vessels become thickened and fibrous; there is a marked reticuloendothelial reaction.

Clinical Findings

A. Symptoms

In mild cases (few exposures), the patient suffers recurrent lymphadenitis and lymphangitis with fever and malaise. Not infrequently, inflammation of the epididymis, testis, scrotum, and spermatic cord occurs. These structures then become edematous, boggy, and at times tender. Hydrocele is common. In advanced cases (many exposures), obstruction of major lymph channels may cause chyluria and elephantiasis.

B. Signs

Varying degrees of painless elephantiasis of the scrotum and extremities develop as obstruction to lymphatics progresses. Lymphadenopathy is common.

C. Laboratory Findings

Chylous urine may look normal if minimal amounts of fat are present, but in an advanced case or following a fatty meal, it is milky. On standing, the urine forms layers: the top layer is fatty, the middle layer is pinkish, and the lower layer is clear. In the presence of chyluria, large amounts of protein are to be expected. Hypoproteinemia is found, and the albumin-globulin ratio is reversed. Both white blood cells (leukocytes) and red blood cells (erythrocytes) are found.

Marked eosinophilia is the rule in the early stages. Microfilariae may be demonstrated in the blood, which should be drawn at night. The adult worm may be found by biopsy. When filariae cannot be found, an indirect hemagglutination titer of 1/128 and a bentonite flocculation titer of 1/5 in combination are considered diagnostic.

D. Cystoscopy

Following a fatty meal, endoscopy to observe the efflux of milky urine from the ureteral orifices may differentiate between unilateral and bilateral cases.

E. X-Ray Findings

Retrograde urography and lymphangiography may reveal the renolymphatic connections in patients with chyluria.

Prevention

In endemic areas, mosquito abatement programs must be intensively pursued.

Treatment

A. Specific Measures

Diethylcarbamazine (Hetrazan) is the drug of choice, but it is toxic. The dose is 2 mg/kg orally 3 times daily for 12 days. This drug kills the microfilariae but not the adult worms. Several courses of the drug may be necessary. Antibiotics may be necessary to control secondary infection.

B. General Measures

Prompt removal of recently infected patients from the endemic area almost always results in regression of the symptoms and signs in early cases.

C. Surgical Measures

Elephantiasis of the external genitalia may require surgical excision.

D. Treatment of Chyluria

Mild cases require no therapy. Spontaneous cure occurs in 50% of cases. If nutrition is impaired, the lymphatic channels may be sealed off by irrigating the renal pelvis with 2% silver nitrate solution. Should this fail, renal decapsulation and resection of the renal lymphatics should be performed (Okamoto and Ohi, 1983).

Prognosis

If exposure has been limited, resolution of the disease is spontaneous and the prognosis is excellent. Frequent reinfection may lead to elephantiasis of the scrotum or chyluria.

ECHINOCOCCOSIS (HYDATID DISEASE)

Involvement of the urogenital organs by hydatid disease is relatively rare in the United States. It is common in Australia, New Zealand, South America, Africa, Asia, the Middle East, and Europe. Livestock are the intermediate hosts. Canines, especially dogs, are the final hosts.

Etiology

The adult tapeworm (*Echinococcus*) inhabits the intestinal tracts of carnivorous animals. Its eggs pass out with the feces and may be ingested by such animals as sheep, cattle, pigs, and occasionally humans. Larvae from these eggs pass through the intestinal wall of the various intermediate hosts and are disseminated throughout the body. In humans, the liver is principally involved, but about 3% of infected humans develop echinococcosis of the kidney.

If a cyst of the liver should rupture into the peritoneal cavity, the scoleces (tapeworm heads) may directly invade the retrovesical tissues, thus leading to the development of cysts in this area.

Clinical Findings

If renal hydatid disease is closed (not communicating with the pelvis), there may be no symptoms until a mass is found. With communicating disease, there may be symptoms of cystitis, and renal colic may occur as cysts are passed from the kidney. X-ray films may show calcification in the wall of the cyst (Figure 14–5), and urograms often reveal changes typical of a space-occupying lesion. The cystic nature of the lesion may be demonstrated on sonograms and computed tomography scans. Calcification in the cyst wall may be noted. Scintillation scanning or angiography can also suggest the presence of a cyst. Serologic tests that should be done include immunoelectrophoresis and indirect hemagglutination. The Casoni intracutaneous procedure is unreliable.

Retroperitoneal (perivesical) cysts may cause symptoms of cystitis, or acute urinary retention may develop secondary to pressure. The presence of a suprapubic

Figure 14–5. Hydatid disease, right kidney. Plain film showing 2 calcified hydatid cysts.

mass may be the only finding. It may rupture into the bladder and cause hydatiduria, which establishes the diagnosis.

Treatment

Nephrectomy is generally the treatment of choice for renal hydatid disease. Aspiration of the cyst is unwise; leakage or rupture may occur. Retroperitoneal cysts are best treated by marsupialization and curettage.

Prognosis

Echinococcosis of the kidney usually has a good prognosis. The problem presented by perivesical cysts is more troublesome. After surgical intervention, drainage may be prolonged. It must be remembered, too, that involvement of other organs, especially the liver, is usually present.

REFERENCES

Tuberculosis

Abel BJ, Gow JG: Results of caecocystoplasty for tuberculous bladder contracture. Br J Urol 1978;50:511.

Carl P, Stark L: Indications for surgical management of genitourinary tuberculosis. World J Surg 1997;21:505.

Cos CR, Cockett ATK: Genitourinary tuberculosis revisited. Urology 1982;20:111.

Das KM, Indudhara R, Vaidyanathan S: Sonographic features of genitourinary tuberculosis. AJR 1992;158:327.

Ehrlich RM, Lattimer JK: Urogenital tuberculosis in children. J Urol 1971;105:461.

Gokalp A, Gultekin EY, Ozdamar S: Genito-urinary tuberculosis: A review of 83 cases. Br J Clin Pract 1990;44:599.

Gow JG: Genitourinary tuberculosis: A 7-year review. Br J Urol 1979;51:239.

Gow JG: The management of genitourinary tuberculosis. In: Hendry WF (editor): *Recent Advances in Urology/Andrology*, 3rd ed., p. 91. Churchill Livingstone, 1981.

Hamrick-Turner J, Abbitt PL, Ros PR: Tuberculosis of the lower genitourinary tract: Findings on sonography and MR. (Letter.) AJR 1992;158:919.

Lenk S, Schroeder J: Genitourinary tuberculosis. Curr Opin Urol 2001;11:93.

Management of extra-pulmonary tuberculosis. Drug Ther Bull 1991;29:26.

Mehta JB et al: Epidemiology of extrapulmonary tuberculosis: A comparative analysis with pre-AIDS era. Chest 1991; 99:1134.

Poulios C, Malovrouvas D: Progress in the approach of tuberculosis of the genitourinary tract: Remarks on a decade's experience over cases. Acta Urol Belg 1990;58:101.

Skoutelis A et al: Serious complications of tuberculous epididymitis. Infection 2000;28:193.

Tikkakoski T et al: Tuberculosis of the lower genitourinary tract: Ultrasonography as an aid to diagnosis and treatment. J Clin Ultrasound 1993;21:269.

Valentini AL, Summaria V, Marano P: Diagnostic imaging of genitourinary tuberculosis. Rays 1998;23:126.

Amicrobic (Abacterial) Cystitis

Hohlbrugger G, Riedl C: Non-bacterial cystitis. Curr Opin Urol 2000;10:371.

Holm-Bentzen M et al: A prospective double-blind clinically controlled multicenter trial of sodium pentosanpolysulfate in the treatment of interstitial cystitis and related painful bladder disease. J Urol 1987;138:503.

Jensen H, Nielsen K, Frimodt-Moller C: Abacterial cystitis in urinary incontinent females. Urol Int 1990;45:20.

Morgan MG et al: Controversies in the laboratory diagnosis of community-acquired urinary tract infection. Eur J Clin Microbiol Infect Dis 1993;12:491.

Theoharides TC, Sant GR: New agents for the medical treatment of interstitial cystitis. Expert Opin Investig Drugs 2001; 10:521.

Genitourinary Candidiasis

Graybill JR et al: Ketoconazole therapy for fungal urinary tract infections. J Urol 1983;129:68.

Priestley CJ et al: What is normal vaginal flora? Genitourin Med 1997;73:23.

Rivera L, Bellotti MG, Malighetti V: Morphotypes of *Candida albicans* and their associations with underlying diseases and source of samples. New Microbiol 1996;19:335.

Rodgers CA, Beardall AJ: Recurrent vulvovaginal candidiasis: Why does it occur? Int J STD AIDS 1999;10:435.

Sandin KJ et al: Candida pyelonephritis complicating traumatic C5 quadriplegia: Diagnosis and management. Arch Phys Med Rehab 1991;72:243.

Wise GJ, Talluri GS, Marella VK: Fungal infections of the genitourinary system: Manifestations, diagnosis, and treatment. Urol Clin North Am 1999;26:701.

Wise GJ et al: Miconazole: A cost-effective antifungal genitourinary irrigant. J Urol 1987;138:1413.

Woolley PD, Higgins SP: Comparison of clotrimazole, fluconazole and itraconazole in vaginal candidiasis. Br J Clin Pract 1995; 49:65.

Actinomycosis

Jani AN, Casibang V, Mufarrij WA: Disseminated actinomycosis presenting as a testicular mass: A case report. J Urol 1990; 143:1012.

Lee YC et al: Computed tomography guided core needle biopsy diagnosis of pelvic actinomycosis. Gynecol Oncol 2000;79:318.

Lippes J: Pelvic actinomycosis: A review and preliminary look at prevalence. Am J Obstet Gynecol 1999;180(Pt 1):265.

Pollock PG et al: Rapid diagnosis of actinomycosis by thin-needle aspiration biopsy. Am J Clin Pathol 1978;70:27.

Smego RA Jr et al: Actinomycosis. Clin Infect Dis 1998;26:1255.

Schistosomiasis (Bilharziasis)

Abdel-Halim RE: Ileal loop replacement and restoration of kidney function in extensive bilharziasis of the ureter. Br J Urol 1980;52:280.

Al Ghorab MM: Radiological manifestations of genitourinary bilharziasis. Clin Radiol 1968;19:100.

Al Ghorab MM, El-Badawi AA, Effat H: Vesico-ureteric reflux in urinary bilharziasis: A clinico-radiological study. Clin Radiol 1966;17:41.

Badawi AF et al: Role of schistosomiasis in human bladder cancer: Evidence of association, aetiological factors, and basic mechanisms of carcinogenesis. Eur J Cancer Prev 1995;4:45.

Barrou B et al: Results of renal transplantation in patients with Schistosoma infection. J Urol 1997;157:1232.

Bazeed MA, Nabeeh A, Atwan N: Xanthogranulomatous pyelonephritis in bilharzial patients: A report of 25 cases. J Urol 1989;141:261.

El-Feky HM et al: Histopathological study of the bilharzial affection on the bladder and ureter. J Egypt Soc Parasitol 1992; 22:71.

Ghoneim MA: Bilharziasis of the genitourinary tract. BJU Int 2002;89 (Suppl 1):22.

Hanafy MH, Youssef TK, Saad MS: Radiographic aspects of (bilharzial) schistosomal ureter. Urology 1975;6:118.

Helling-Giese G et al: Schistosomiasis in women: Manifestations in the upper reproductive tract. Acta Trop 1996;62:225.

Ibrahim A et al: Bilharzial vesicoureteric reflux and bladder neck stenosis: Fact or fiction? Br J Urol 1991;68:582.

Johansson SL, Cohen SM: Epidemiology and etiology of bladder cancer. Semin Surg Oncol 1997;13:291.

Mostafa MH, Sheweita SA, O'Connor PJ: Relationship between schistosomiasis and bladder cancer. Clin Microbiol Rev 1999; 12:97.

Naude JH: Reconstructive urology in the tropical and developing world: A personal perspective. BJU Int 2002;89 (Suppl 1):31.

Patil KP et al: Specific investigations in chronic urinary bilharziasis. Urology 1992;40:117.

Sato K et al: Efficacy of metrifonate in a highly endemic area of urinary schistosomiasis in Kenya. Am J Trop Med Hyg 1988; 38:81.

Sharfi AR, Rayis AB: The continuing challenge of bilharzial ureteric stricture. Scand J Urol Nephrol 1989;23:123.

Shokeir AA: Renal transplantation: The impact of schistosomiasis. BJU Int 2001;88:915.

Stock JA, Scherz HC, Kaplan GW: Urinary schistosomiasis in childhood. Urology 1994;44:305.

Filariasis

Brunkwall J et al: Chyluria treated with renal autotransplantation: A case report. J Urol 1990;143:793.

DeVries CR: The role of the urologist in the treatment and elimination of lymphatic filariasis worldwide. BJU Int 2002; 89(Suppl 1):37.

Kohli V, Gulati S, Kumar L: Filarial chyluria. Indian Pediatr 1994; 31:451.

Okamoto K, Ohi Y: Recent distribution and treatment of filarial chyluria in Japan. J Urol 1983;129:64.

Pool MO et al: Bilateral excision of perinephric fat and fascia (Gerota's fasciectomy) in the treatment of intractable chyluria. J Urol 1991;146:1374.

Punekar SV et al: Surgical disconnection of lymphorenal communication for chyluria: A 15-year experience. Br J Urol 1997; 80:858.

Taylor MJ, Hoerauf A: A new approach to the treatment of filariasis. Curr Opin Infect Dis 2001;14:727.

Xu YM et al: Microsurgical treatment of chyluria: A preliminary report. J Urol 1991;145:1184.

Yagi S et al: Endoscopic treatment of refractory filarial chyluria: A preliminary report. J Urol 1998;159:1615.

Onchocerciasis

Kumate J: Infectious diseases in the 21st century. Arch Med Res 1997;28:155.

Ottesen EA: Immune responsiveness and the pathogenesis of human onchocerciasis. J Infect Dis 1995;171:659.

Van Laethem Y, Lopes C: Treatment of onchocerciasis. Drugs 1996;52:861.

Echinococcosis (Hydatid Disease)

Cirenei A: Histopathology, clinical findings and treatment of renal hydatidosis. Ann Ital Chir 1997;68:275.

Martorana G, Giberi C, Pescatore D: Giant echinococcal cyst of the kidney associated with hypertension evaluated by computerized tomography. J Urol 1981;126:99.

Migaleddu V et al: Imaging of renal hydatid cysts. AJR 1997; 169:1339.

Pasaoglu E et al: Hydatid cysts of the kidney, seminal vesicle and gluteus muscle. Australas Radiol 1997;41:297.

Ranzini AC et al: Ultrasonographic diagnosis of pelvic echinococcosis: Case report and review of the literature. J Ultrasound Med 2002;21:207.

Yeniyol CO, Minareci S, Ayder AR: Primary cyst hydatid of adrenal: A case report. Int Urol Nephrol 2000;32:227.

Sexually Transmitted Diseases

15

John N. Krieger, MD

The usual approach to sexually transmitted diseases (STDs) considers the causative agents, emphasizing different classes, genera, species, and microbiological characteristics. This fits with most medical school curricula since the causative agents span the full spectrum of medical microbiology (viruses, bacteria, protozoa, ectoparasites, etc). This classical approach may prove difficult in clinical practice, where many different types of agents must be considered in the differential diagnosis of an individual patient.

This chapter takes a very selective and practical approach. Because patients present with symptoms and signs that may be caused by pathogens from different microbiological classes, we will emphasize diagnosis and treatment of clinical syndromes in contrast to traditional teaching (Table 15–1). This is a large subject with much active research and a huge literature. We stress the most important conditions encountered in urology: urethritis, epididymitis, genital ulcers, genital warts, plus a brief consideration of human immunodeficiency virus (HIV) infection.

URETHRITIS & CERVICITIS

Urethritis in Men

Urethritis, or urethral inflammation, is often caused by infection. Characteristically, patients complain of urethral discharge and dysuria. On examination the discharge may be purulent or mucopurulent. Asymptomatic infections are common (McCormack and Rein, 1990; Krieger, 1996; Centers for Disease Control and Prevention, 1998). The most important pathogens are bacteria, *Neisseria gonorrhoeae,* and *Chlamydia trachomatis.*

Testing is recommended to document a specific disease because both of these infections are reportable to health departments, and because specific diagnosis may improve compliance and partner notification (Centers for Disease Control and Prevention, 1998). The traditional diagnostic algorithm includes microscopic examination of the Gram-stained urethral smear for gram-negative intracellular diplococci and culture for *N gonorrhoeae.* New nucleic acid amplification tests have proved accurate for detection of *N gonorrhoeae* and *C trachomatis* in first-void urine in high-risk populations (Mahony et al, 2001). If diagnostic testing is unavailable, patients should be treated empirically for both infections (Centers for Disease Control and Prevention, 1998).

Complications of urethritis in men include epididymitis (see below), disseminated gonococcal infection, and Reiter's syndrome (McCormack and Rein, 1990; Krieger, 1996; Mead, 1990). Complications of urethritis in female sexual partners include pelvic inflammatory disease, ectopic pregnancy, and infertility (Centers for Disease Control and Prevention, 1998; Rein, 1996). Complications in children include neonatal pneumonia and ophthalmia neonatorum (Centers for Disease Control and Prevention, 1998).

A. ETIOLOGY

Gonorrhea is diagnosed when *N gonorrhoeae* is detected by Gram stain, culture, or nucleic acid amplification testing. Nongonococcal urethritis (NGU) is diagnosed when gram-negative intracellular organisms cannot be diagnosed on microscopic examination. *C trachomatis,* the most common infectious cause of NGU, is responsible for 23–55% of cases in reported series, but the proportion of cases is substantially lower in urological practice. The prevalence of chlamydial infection differs by age group, with a lower prevalence among older men. In addition, the proportion of NGU caused by *C trachomatis* has been declining. Documentation of chlamydial NGU is important because this diagnosis supports partner referral, evaluation, and treatment (Centers for Disease Control and Prevention, 1998).

The etiology of most cases of nonchlamydial NGU is unknown. The genital mycoplasmas, *Ureaplasma urealyticum* and perhaps *Mycoplasma genitalium* or *Mycoplasma hominis,* are implicated in 20–30% of cases in some series (Krieger, 1996; Horner et al, 2001; Totten et al, 2001). Specific diagnostic tests for these organisms are not indicated routinely. *Trichomonas vaginalis,* a protozoan parasite, and herpes simplex virus (HSV) may also cause NGU (Joyner et al, 2000; Madeb et al, 2000). Testing and treatment for these organisms should be considered in situations where NGU is unresponsive to treatment (McCormack and Rein, 1990; Centers for Disease Control and Prevention, 1998).

B. DOCUMENT URETHRITIS

It is important to document the presence of urethritis because some patients have symptoms in the absence of

Table 15–1. Sexually transmitted disease (STD) syndromes.[a]

Urethritis and cervicitis[b]	Nongonococcal urethritis
	Gonococcal infection
	Chlamydial infection
	Mucopurulent cervicitis
Epididymitis[b]	
Genital ulcers[b]	Genital herpes simplex
	virus (HSV)
	Syphilis
	Chancroid
	Lymphogranuloma
	venereum (LGV)
	Granuloma inguinale
	(donovanosis)
Human papillomavirus	Genital warts
(HPV) infections[b]	Subclinical genital HPV
HIV infection[b]	
Vaginal discharge	Trichomoniasis
	Vulvovaginal candidiasis
	Bacterial vaginosis
Pelvic inflammatory disease	
Ectoparasitic infections	Pediculosis pubis
	Scabies
Vaccine-preventable STDs	Hepatitis A
	Hepatitis B
Proctitis, proctocolitis,	
and enteritis	
Sexual assault and STDs	

[a]According to Centers for Disease Control and Prevention: 2002 Sexually Transmitted Disease Treatment Guideline. MMWR 2002;51:1.
[b]Considered in this chapter.

inflammation. Urethritis may be documented by the presence of any of the following clinical signs: mucopurulent urethral discharge on physical examination, ≥ 5 leukocytes per oil immersion microscopic field of the Gram-stained urethral secretions, a positive leukocyte esterase test on first void-urine, or ≥ 10 leukocytes per high-power microscopic field of the first-void urine (Krieger, 1996; Centers for Disease Control and Prevention, 1998). The Gram stain is the preferred diagnostic test for documenting urethritis and for evaluating presence or absence of gonococcal infection because it is highly sensitive and specific.

If none of the criteria for urethritis are met, then treatment should be deferred. The patient should be tested for both *N gonorrhoeae* and *C trachomatis* and followed up closely in the event of a positive test result.

Empiric treatment of symptoms without documenting the presence of urethritis is recommended only if the patient is at high risk for infection and is unlikely to return for follow-up. Empiric treatment should be appropriate for both gonococcal and chlamydial infection. Sex partners should be referred for appropriate evaluation and treatment.

C. TREATMENT OF GONOCOCCAL INFECTIONS

There are an estimated 600,000 new gonococcal infections per year in the United States. In men, most infections cause symptoms that cause the patient to seek treatment soon enough to prevent serious sequelae. However, this may not be soon enough to prevent transmission of infection to sex partners. In contrast, many gonococcal (and also chlamydial) infections in women do not cause recognizable symptoms until the patient presents with complications, such as pelvic inflammatory disease. Symptomatic and asymptomatic pelvic inflammatory disease both result in tubal scarring, increased rates of ectopic pregnancy, and infertility.

Dual therapy is recommended for both gonococcal and chlamydial infection because patients are often coinfected with both pathogens (Krieger, 1996; Centers for Disease Control and Prevention, 1998). Some authorities feel that routine use of dual therapy has led to substantial decreases in the prevalence of gonorrhea. Since most gonococci in the United States are susceptible to doxycycline and azithromycin, cotreatment may also limit development of antimicrobial-resistant *N gonorrhoeae*. Quinolone-resistant *N gonorrhoeae* have been reported from many geographic areas, and such infections are becoming widespread in parts of Asia (Rahman et al, 2001; Tompkins and Zenilman, 2001; Trees et al, 2001). To date, however, the prevalence of quinolone-resistance has been exceedingly low in the United States. Although resistant strains will continue to be imported into the United States, quinolones can still be recommended for treatment. Table 15–2 summarizes recommended treatment regimens for uncomplicated gonococcal infections, where the recommended treatments reliably cure ≥ 97% of infections (Centers for Disease Control and Prevention, 1998). Pharyngeal infections are more difficult to treat, and few regimens reliably cure > 90% of infections. Patients who cannot tolerate cephalosporins or quinolones should be treated with spectinomycin (2 g as a single intramuscular dose). However, this regimen is only 52% effective for pharyngeal infections.

Routine test-of-cure cultures are no longer recommended for patients treated with the recommended regimens. Such patients should refer their sex partners for evaluation and treatment. However, patients should be reevaluated if their symptoms persistent after therapy. Any gonococci that persist should be evaluated for antimicrobial susceptibility. However, infections identi-

Table 15–2. Urethritis, cervicitis, and related infections: Recommended treatment regimens[a].

Gonococcal infections
  Uncomplicated urethral, cervical, and rectal infections
    Cefixime, 400 mg as a single oral dose; or ceftriaxone, 125 mg as a single IM dose; or ciprofloxacin, 500 mg as a single oral dose; or ofloxacin, 400 mg as a single oral dose, or levofloxacin, 250 mg as a single oral dose, plus azithromycin, 1 g as a single oral dose; or doxycycline, 100 mg orally twice a day for 7 days
  Uncomplicated pharyngeal infections
    Ceftriaxone, 125 mg as a single IM dose; or ciprofloxacin, 500 mg as a single oral dose; or ofloxacin, 400 mg as a single oral dose, plus azithromycin, 1 g as a single oral dose; or doxycycline, 100 mg orally twice a day for 7 days
Nongonococcal urethritis (chlamydial infections)
  Azithromycin, 1 g as a single oral dose; or doxycycline, 100 mg orally twice a day for 7 days
Recurrent and persistent urethritis
  Metronidazole, 2 g as a single oral dose, plus erythromycin base, 500 mg orally 4 times a day for 7 days; or erythromycin ethylsuccinate, 800 mg orally 4 times a day for 7 days

---

[a]According to Centers for Disease Control and Prevention: 2002 Sexually Transmitted Disease Treatment Guidelines. MMWR 2002;51:1.

fied after treatment are usually reinfections rather than treatment failures. Persistent inflammation may be caused by *C trachomatis* or other organisms.

A few patients have complications such as disseminated gonococcal infection, perihepatitis, meningitis, or endocarditis. These infections result from gonococcal bacteremia. Disseminated gonococcal infection often causes petechial or pustular skin lesions, asymmetrical arthralgias, tenosynovitis, or septic arthritis. Occasionally patients have perihepatitis, and rare patients have endocarditis or meningitis. *N gonorrhoeae* strains that cause disseminated infection tend to cause minimal genital tract inflammation. The recommended treatment is ceftriaxone (1 g intramuscularly or intravenously every 24 h for disseminated infection or 1 g intravenously every 12 h for meningitis or endocarditis).

D. Treatment of Nongonococcal Urethritis (NGU)

Treatment should be initiated as soon as possible after diagnosis (Table 15–2). Single-dose regimens are preferred because these treatments offer the advantages of improved compliance and directly observed therapy (Centers for Disease Control and Prevention, 1998). The recommended treatments employ either azithromycin or doxycycline. Alternative choices for patients who are allergic or cannot tolerate these drugs include a 7-day course of either erythromycin or ofloxacin. Routine follow-up and repeat testing are no longer recommended for patients taking the recommended regimens. However, patients should return for reevaluation if symptoms persist or recur after completion of treatment. The presence of symptoms alone without documentation of signs or laboratory findings of inflammation is not sufficient for re-treatment. Patients should

refer their sex partners for appropriate evaluation and treatment.

E. Treatment of Recurrent and Persistent Urethritis

Objective signs of urethritis should be documented before prescribing a repeat course of empirical therapy (Krieger, 1996; Centers for Disease Control and Prevention, 1998). Men with persistent or recurrent urethritis should be re-treated with the initial regimen if they did not comply with treatment or if they were reexposed to an untreated sex partner. Other patients should have a wet mount and urethral culture for *T vaginalis*. For patients who were compliant with the initial regimen and who were not reexposed, the regimen in Table 15–2 should be used. This provides treatment for both *T vaginalis* and the genital mycoplasmas.

Mucopurulent Cervicitis in Women

Mucopurulent cervicitis holds many parallels to urethritis in men (Centers for Disease Control and Prevention, 1998; Mead, 1990; Rein, 1990). Characteristically, patients have a purulent or mucopurulent endocervical exudate visible in the endocervical canal or on an endocervical swab sample. Easily induced endocervical bleeding is also common, as is an increased number of polymorphonuclear cells on the Gram-stained endocervical secretions. Patients may present with abnormal vaginal discharge or abnormal vaginal bleeding, for example, after intercourse, but many are asymptomatic.

As is the case with urethritis in men, *N gonorrhoeae* and *C trachomatis* are the most important infectious causes of mucopurulent cervicitis. However, neither pathogen may be identified in many women. Treatment should be guided by the results of testing for gonococcal and chlamydial infection, unless the patient is considered unlikely to return for follow-up. In such cases, empirical therapy should be given for both *C trachomatis* and *N gonorrhoeae*.

EPIDIDYMITIS

Epididymitis is caused by sexually transmitted pathogens or by organisms causing urinary tract infection (Krieger, 1996; Centers for Disease Control and Prevention, 1998; Krieger, 1990). Among sexually active men < 35 years old, most cases of epididymitis are caused by sexually transmitted pathogens, particularly *C trachomatis* and *N gonorrhoeae*. Epididymitis may also be caused by *E coli* among men who are the insertive partners during anal intercourse. Sexually transmitted epididymitis is usually associated with urethritis, which is often asymptomatic. Patients with uncomplicated sexually transmitted epididymitis do not require thorough evaluation for anatomic abnormalities.

Most cases of epididymitis in men older than 35 years are associated with urinary tract infection. The most common pathogens are Gram-negative enteric bacteria. Epididymitis associated with urinary infection is more common among men who have anatomic abnormalities or those who have recently had urinary tract instrumentation. Therefore, evaluation of genitourinary tract anatomy is indicated for men with epididymitis associated with urinary tract infection.

Epididymitis is typically associated with unilateral hemiscrotal pain and tenderness. An inflammatory hydrocele and palpable swelling of the epididymis are characteristic. Diagnostic recommendations include a Gram-stained smear for evaluation of urethritis and for presumptive identification of gonococcal infection, diagnostic testing for *N gonorrhoeae* and *C trachomatis*, urine Gram stain and culture, syphilis serology and HIV testing (if sexually transmitted epididymitis is likely).

Treatment

Outpatient management is appropriate for most patients with epididymitis. Hospitalization should be considered when severe pain suggests other possible diagnoses, such as testicular torsion, testicular infarction, or testicular abscess; when patients are febrile; or when noncompliance with medication regimens is likely (Krieger, 1996; Centers for Disease Control and Prevention, 1998; Krieger, 1990). Empiric antimicrobial regimens are summarized in Table 15–3. Adjunctive measures include bed rest, scrotal elevation, and analgesics until fever and local inflammation subside.

Table 15–3. Epididymitis: Recommended treatment regimens[a]

Gonococcal or chlamydial infection likely
Ceftriaxone, 250 mg in a single IM dose, plus doxycyline, 100 mg orally twice a day for 10 days
Enteric infection likely
Ofloxacin, 300 mg orally twice a day for 10 days, or levofloxacin, 500 mg orally once a day for 10 days

[a]According to Centers for Disease Control and Prevention: 2002 Sexually Transmitted Disease Treatment Guidelines. MMWR 2002;51:1.

Routine follow-up is recommended. Failure to respond within 3 days requires reevaluation of both the diagnosis and treatment. Swelling and tenderness that persist after completion of antimicrobial therapy should be reevaluated to consider possible testicular tumor, abscess, infarction, tuberculosis, fungal epididymitis, or collagen-vascular disorders (Skoutelis et al, 2000; Kaklamani et al, 2000; Giannopoulos et al, 2001; de Vries et al, 2001). HIV-infected patients with epididymitis should receive the same initial therapy as HIV-negative men. However, fungal, atypical mycobacteria, and other opportunistic infections are more likely than in nonimmunosuppressed patients.

GENITAL ULCER DISEASES

In the United States, genital herpes (HSV) is the most common cause of genital ulcers. Other important considerations are syphilis and chancroid. In contrast, lymphogranuloma venereum and granuloma inguinale (donovanosis) are uncommon causes of genital ulcers in this country. Each of these ulcerative STDs is associated with a 2- to 5-fold increased risk of HIV transmission.

Diagnostic Testing

Diagnosis based solely on the history and physical findings is often inaccurate (Centers for Disease Control and Prevention, 1998). Patients may be infected with more than one agent simultaneously. Ideally, evaluation of patients with genital ulcers should include testing for the most common causes: HSV, syphilis, and chancroid. These tests include a culture or antigen test for HSV, a darkfield examination or direct immunofluorescence test for *Treponema pallidum* (syphilis), and a culture for *Haemophilus ducreyi* (chancroid). In the future, improved molecular detection tests may become available commercially for these organisms. After thorough diagnostic evaluation, 25% of patients with genital ulcers do not have a laboratory-confirmed diagnosis. HIV testing also should be recommended for patients who have genital ulcers (see below).

Often patients must be treated before test results become available. In this situation, treatment is recommended for both syphilis and chancroid.

Genital Herpes Virus (HSV) Infection

Genital HSV is an incurable and recurrent viral infection. Characteristic genital lesions start as painful papules or vesicles. Often the genital lesions have evolved into pustules or ulcers when the patient is seen in the office. With primary genital herpes, the ulcerative lesions persist for 4–15 days until crusting or reepithelization or both occur. Pain, itching, vaginal or urethral discharge, and tender inguinal adenopathy are the predominant local symptoms. Primary HSV infection is associated with a high frequency and prolonged duration of systemic and local symptoms. Fever, headache, malaise, and myalgias are common. The clinical symptoms of pain and irritation from genital lesions gradually increase over the first 6–7 days, reach maximum intensity between days 7 and 11 of disease, and then recede gradually during the second or third week.

In contrast to first episodes, recurrent HSV infection is characterized by symptoms, signs, and anatomic sites localized to the genital region. Local symptoms, such as pain and itching, are mild compared with the symptoms of initial infection, and the duration of the usual episode ranges from 8 to 12 days or less.

Two HSV serotypes cause genital ulcers, HSV-1 and HSV-2. Both viruses infect the genital tract. Studies suggest that 5–30% of first-episode cases of genital HSV infection are caused by HSV-1. However, recurrences of HSV-1 infection are substantially less likely than recurrences of HSV-2. Therefore, HSV-2 cases accumulate in the population of patients with recurrent genital lesions. Typing the infecting strain has prognostic importance and is useful for patient counseling. However, most commercially available antibody tests are not accurate enough to distinguish HSV-1 from HSV-2 infection. Better assays should become available in the future.

Serologic studies suggest that 45 million people in the United States are infected with genital HSV-2. Most infections are mild or unrecognized. Therefore, most HIV-infected people do not receive this diagnosis. Such asymptomatic or mildly symptomatic persons shed virus intermittently in their genital tracts and can infect their sex partners. First-episode genital HSV infections are more likely to cause symptoms than recurrent infections. Occasional cases are severe enough to require hospitalization for complications such as dis-

seminated infection, pneumonitis, hepatitis, meningitis, or encephalitis.

TREATMENT

Systemic antiviral therapy results in partial control of symptoms and signs of genital HSV infection. Treatment does not cure the infection or change the frequency or severity of recurrences after discontinuation of treatment. Three antiviral drugs have proved beneficial in randomized clinical trials: acyclovir, valacyclovir, and famciclovir (Table 15–4). Topical treatment with acyclovir has proved substantially less effective than systemic treatment.

Patients with first clinical episodes of genital HSV should receive antiviral treatment to speed healing of genital lesions and shorten the duration of viral shedding. Patients should also be counseled about the natural history of genital herpes, the risks for sexual and perinatal transmission, and methods to reduce transmission. Patients with severe disease should receive intravenous treatment with acyclovir.

Most persons with first clinical episodes of genital HSV-2 experience recurrent episodes. Treatment can shorten the duration of lesions and decrease recurrences. Thus, many patients can benefit from antiviral therapy, and this option should be discussed. There are 2 approaches to antiviral therapy for recurrent HSV: episodic treatment and daily suppressive treatment. Episodic therapy is beneficial for many patients with occasional recurrences. Such therapy is started during the prodrome or first day of lesions. Thus, patients receiving episodic therapy should receive the medication or a prescription so that they may initiate treatment at the first symptom or sign of lesions. Traditionally, 5 days of treatment has been recommended for recurrent HSV (Table 15–4), but recent data suggest that shorter (3-day) courses may work equally well (Leone, Trottier, and Miller, 2002; Wald et al, 2002).

Daily suppressive therapy is useful for patients who experience frequent recurrences (6 or more per year). Therapy reduces the frequency of recurrences by > 75%. Such treatment has been shown to be safe and effective for as long as 6 years with acyclovir and for as long as 1 year with both valacyclovir and famciclovir. Daily therapy does not appear to be associated with clinically significant HSV-drug resistance. After 1 year, discontinuation of treatment should be considered, since the frequency of recurrences often decreases with time.

Syphilis

Syphilis may be the deepest and darkest subject in all of infectious diseases. This complex illness is caused by *T*

Table 15–4. Genital ulcers: Recommended treatment regimens.[a]

Genital herpes
  First episode
    Acyclovir, 400 mg orally 3 times a day for 7–10 days; or acyclovir, 200 mg orally 5 times a day for 7–10 days; or famciclovir, 250 mg orally 3 times a day for 7–10 days; or valacyclovir, 1 g orally twice a day for 7–10 days
  Severe disease
    Acyclovir, 5–10 mg/kg body weight IV every 8 h for 2–7 days or until clinical resolution
  Recurrent episodes
  Episodic recurrences
    Acyclovir, 400 mg orally 3 times a day for 5 days; or acyclovir, 200 mg orally 5 times a day for 5 days; or acyclovir, 800 mg orally twice a day for 5 days; or famciclovir, 125 mg orally twice a day for 5 days; or valacyclovir, 500 mg orally twice a day for 3–5 days, or valacyclovir 1 g orally once a day for 5 days
  Daily suppressive therapy
    Acyclovir, 400 mg orally twice a day; or famciclovir, 250 mg orally twice a day; or valacyclovir, 250 mg orally twice a day; or valacyclovir, 500 mg orally twice a day; or valacyclovir, 1 g orally once a day
Syphilis
  Primary and secondary
    Benzathine penicillin G, 2.4 million units IM as a single dose
  Tertiary (except neurosyphilis)
    Benzathine penicillin G, 2.4 million units IM weekly for 3 weeks
  Neurosyphilis
    Aqueous crystalline penicillin G, 3–4 million units IV every 4 hours for 10–14 days; or procaine penicillin, 2.4 million units IM daily for 10–14 days, plus probenecid, 500 mg orally 4 times a day for 10–14 days
  Latent syphilis
    Early
        Benzathine penicillin G, 2.4 million units IM as a single dose
    Late or of unknown duration
        Benzathine penicillin G, 2.4 million units IM weekly for 3 weeks
Chancroid
    Azithromycin, 1 g as a single oral dose; or ceftriaxone, 250 mg as a single IM dose; or ciprofloxacin, 500 mg orally twice a day for 3 days; or erythromycin base, 500 mg orally 4 times a day for 7 days
Granuloma inguinale
    Trimethoprim-sulfamethoxazole, 1 double-strength tablet orally twice a day for a minimum of 3 weeks; or doxycycline, 100 mg orally twice a day for a minimum of 3 weeks
Lymphogranuloma venereum
    Doxycycline, 100 mg orally twice a day for 21 days

[a]According to Centers for Disease Control and Prevention: 2002 Sexually Transmitted Disease Treatment Guidelines. MMWR 2002; 51:1.

pallidum, a spirochete, and holds a special place in the history of medicine as "the great impostor" and "the great imitator." Sir William Osler in 1897 said, "Know syphilis in all its manifestations and relations, and all other things clinical will be added unto you."

Syphilis is a systemic disease. Patients may seek treatment for symptoms of signs of primary, secondary, or tertiary infection. Primary infection is characterized by an ulcer, or chancre, at the site of infection. Secondary manifestations include rash, mucocutaneous lesions, and adenopathy. Tertiary infection may present with cardiac, neurologic, ophthalmic, auditory, or gummatous lesions. In addition, syphilis may be diagnosed by serologic testing of asymptomatic patients; this is termed latent syphilis. Latent syphilis acquired within the preceding year is classified as early latent

syphilis. All other cases of latent syphilis are classified as late latent or syphilis of unknown duration.

Sexual transmission of syphilis occurs only when mucocutaneous lesions are present. These manifestations are uncommon after the first year of infection in untreated patients. However, all persons exposed to a person with syphilis should be evaluated clinically and by serologic testing.

Definitive diagnosis of early syphilis is done by darkfield examination or direct immunofluorescent antibody tests of lesion exudate. Presumptive diagnosis depends on serologic testing. Serologic tests are either nontreponemal, such as the Venereal Disease Research Laboratory (VDRL) and rapid plasma reagin (RPR) tests, or treponemal, such as the fluorescent treponemal antibody absorption (FTA-ABS) test and microagglutination assay for antibody to *T pallidum* (MHA-TP). Use of only one type of serologic test is considered insufficient for diagnosis. False-positive nontreponemal tests occur with a variety of medical conditions. Nontreponemal tests correlate with disease activity, with results reported quantitatively. In general, a 4-fold change in titer is considered significant. Most patients with reactive treponemal tests remain reactive for life. Treponemal test titers correlate poorly with disease activity. Thus, combination of both treponemal and nontreponemal tests is necessary for patient management.

Tremendous progress during the last decade has led to sequencing of the entire genome of *T pallidum* and to correlation of functional activities with this genetic information (Norris, Cox, and Weinstock, 2001). From an epidemiological perspective, the real news is that eradication of syphilis from the United States (Centers for Disease Control, 2001a and b) and from the world (Rompalo, 2001) has been established as an important public health goal.

TREATMENT

For more than 40 years penicillin has been the treatment of choice for syphilis (Table 15–4). Patients who are allergic to penicillin should receive a 2-week course of doxycycline (100 mg orally twice daily) or tetracycline (500 mg orally 4 times a day). Treatment results in healing of local lesions and prevents sexual transmission and late sequelae. Patients with syphilis should be tested for HIV infection. In areas with a high prevalence of HIV, this test should be repeated after 3 months if the initial HIV test is negative. Patients with syphilis and symptoms or signs of ophthalmic disease should have a slit-lamp examination and those with symptoms or signs of neurologic disease should have cerebrospinal fluid evaluation. Treatment failures occur with any regimen. Thus, serologic testing should be repeated 6 and 12 months after initial treatment.

Chancroid

Chancroid is an acute ulcerative disease, often associated with inguinal adenopathy ("bubo"). *H ducreyi,* a gram-negative facultative bacillus, is the causative agent. The infection is endemic in parts of the United States and the disease also occurs in outbreaks. It is estimated that 10% of patients with chancroid are coinfected with either *T pallidum* or HSV. Each of these infections is associated with an increased rate of HIV transmission.

Definitive diagnosis of chancroid requires identification of the causative bacteria, *H ducreyi,* on specialized culture media that are not widely available. In addition, these media have an estimated sensitivity < 80%. In practice, a probable diagnosis of chancroid may be based on the following: The patient has a painful genital ulcer; there is no evidence of *T pallidum* by darkfield examination or by a negative syphilis serologic testing at least 7 days before the onset of ulcers; an HSV test is negative; and the clinical appearance is typical. The combination of a painful genital ulcer and tender inguinal adenopathy suggests the diagnosis of chancroid. Unfortunately, this characteristic clinical appearance occurs in only one-third of cases. However, the combination of a painful genital ulcer and suppurative inguinal adenopathy is considered almost pathognomonic. The combination of a human model of infection with new molecular methods has resulted in improved understanding of *H ducreyi* genes and virulence factors (Bong et al, 2001; Gelfanova, Humphreys, and Spinola, 2001; Throm and Spinola, 2001; Young et al, 2001).

TREATMENT

Recommended antimicrobial regimens are summarized in Table 15–4. Appropriate treatment of chancroid cures the infection, resolves symptoms, and prevents transmission. Successful treatment results in dramatic resolution of ulcers and symptoms. However, scarring can continue in extensive cases despite successful treatment. Uncircumcised or HIV-infected patients may respond less well to treatment. Testing for HIV and syphilis is recommended at the time of diagnosis and again 3 months later, if the initial test results for syphilis or HIV were negative.

Follow-up evaluation is recommended after 3–7 days. If there is minimal or no clinical improvement, another diagnosis or the possibility of coinfection with another STD should be considered. A few *H ducreyi* strains are resistant to antimicrobial agents. Large ulcers or fluctuant lymphadenopathy may take > 2 weeks for resolution. Occasionally, patients require incision and drainage or needle aspiration of fluctuant inguinal nodes (Ernst, Marvez-Valls, and Martin, 1995).

Lymphogranuloma Venereum (LGV)

Lymphogranuloma venereum is caused by the invasive serovars of *C trachomatis* (L1, L2, and L3). The disease is a rare cause of genital ulcers in the United States.

Tender inguinal or femoral lymphadenopathy or both, often unilateral, is the characteristic clinical presentation in heterosexual men. Women and homosexual men may present with inflammatory involvement of perirectal and perianal lymphatics, strictures, fistulas, or proctocolitis. The self-limited genital ulcers have usually healed when most patients seek medical care. Usually, diagnosis is made by serologic testing plus exclusion of other causes of inguinal adenopathy or genital ulcers.

TREATMENT

Therapy causes microbiological cure and prevents ongoing tissue destruction (Table 15–4). Doxycycline is preferred. Erythromycin and azithromycin are alternatives. Prolonged therapy, for a minimum of 3 weeks, is necessary with each of these drugs. However, tissue reaction and scarring can progress after effective treatment. Inguinal adenopathy, known as "bubos," may require needle aspiration through intact skin or incision and drainage to prevent inguinal or femoral ulcerations. Patients should be followed up until clinical symptoms and signs are resolved.

Granuloma Inguinale (Donovanosis)

Granuloma inguinale is caused by *Calymmatobacterium granulomatis,* a gram-negative intracellular bacillus, that has many similarities to *Klebsiella* species (Kharsany et al, 1999; O'Farrell, 2001). This infection is rare in the United States. Granuloma inguinale is an important cause of genital ulcers in tropical and developing countries, particularly India, Papua New Guinea, central Australia, and southern Africa.

Clinically, granuloma inguinale presents with painless, progressive genital ulcers. The genital lesions are highly vascular, with a "beefy red" appearance. Patients seldom have inguinal adenopathy. The causative organism cannot be cultured on standard microbiologic media. Diagnosis requires visualization of dark-staining Donovan bodies on tissue crush preparations or biopsy specimens. Molecular diagnostic tests should be available in the near future (O'Farrell, 2001; Behets et al, 1999). Secondary bacterial infections may develop in the lesions. In addition, coinfection with other STD agents may occur.

TREATMENT

Effective treatment halts progressive tissue destruction (Table 15–4). Trimethoprim-sulfamethoxazole or doxycycline is recommended. Alternative drugs are ciprofloxacin or erythromycin. Azithromycin also appears promising (O'Farrell, 2001; Bowden and Savage, 1998). Prolonged duration of treatment is often necessary to facilitate granulation and reepithelization of the ulcers. Patients should be reevaluated after the first few days of treatment. Addition of an aminoglycoside, such as gentamicin, should be considered if lesions have not responded. Treatment should be continued until all lesions have healed. Relapse can occur 6–18 months after effective initial therapy.

Genital Warts

Genital warts are caused by human papillomavirus (HPV) infection. Of the more than 80 HPV genotypes, more than 20 infect the genital tract. Most of these genital HPV infections are asymptomatic, subclinical, or unrecognized. Depending on their size and anatomic locations, visible external warts can be painful, friable, pruritic, or all three. Most visible genital warts are caused by HPV types 6 or 11. These HPV types can also cause exophytic warts on the cervix and within the vagina, urethra, and anus. HPV types 6 and 11 are only rarely associated with development of invasive squamous cell carcinoma of the external genitalia.

HPV types 16, 18, 31, 33, and 35 are uncommon in visible, external genital warts. These HPV types are associated with cervical dysplasia, as well as vaginal, anal, and cervical squamous cell carcinoma. HPV types 16, 18, 31, 33, and 35 have also been associated with external genital intraepithelial neoplastic lesions, including squamous cell carcinoma, carcinoma in situ, bowenoid papulosis, erythroplasia of Queyrat, and Bowen disease. Patients with external genital warts can be infected simultaneously with multiple HPV types.

Most often, the diagnosis of genital warts can be made by inspection. Diagnosis can be confirmed by biopsy, if necessary, although biopsy is rarely necessary for diagnosis. Biopsy is indicated if the diagnosis is uncertain, if lesions do not respond to standard therapy, if the disease worsens during treatment, if the patient is immunocompromised, or if warts are pigmented, indurated, fixed, or ulcerated. Routine use of type-specific HPV nucleic acid tests is not indicated for diagnosis or management of visible genital warts.

TREATMENT

For visible genital warts, the primary goal of treatment is removal of symptomatic lesions. Treatment can induce wart-free periods in most patients. Genital warts are often asymptomatic, and clinical lesions may resolve spontaneously. Currently, there are no data indicating that available therapy can eradicate HPV infection or change the natural history of infection. In theory, removal of exophytic warts may decrease infectivity, but there is no evidence that treatment changes the risk for development of dysplastic or cancerous lesions in the patient or in sexual partners.

Treatment decisions should be guided by the provider's experience and patient preferences. None of the recommended therapies is superior or ideal for every case. Current treatments can be considered as patient-applied or provider-administered (Table 15–5). Most patients with visible warts have lesions that respond to most treatment modalities. Many patients require a course of therapy. In general, lesions on moist surfaces or in intertriginous areas respond better to topical treatments, such as trichloracetic acid, podophyllin, or imiquimod, than do warts on drier surfaces.

Table 15–5. External genital warts: Recommended treatment regimens.[a]

Patient-applied
Podofilox, 0.5% solution of gel to lesions twice a day for 3 days, followed by 4 days off therapy; repeat as needed for up to 4 cycles; or imiquimod, 5% cream to lesions at bedtime 3 times a week for up to 16 weeks; wash off after 6–10 h

Provider-administered
Cryotherapy with liquid nitrogen or cryoprobe; repeat as necessary every 1–2 weeks; or podophyllin resin, 10–25% in tincture of benzoin; repeat weekly as necessary; or trichlor/bichloracetic acid, 80–90%; apply until white "frosting"; repeat weekly as necessary; or surgical removal (claser surgery), or intralesional interferon

[a]According to Centers for Disease Control and Prevention: 2002 Sexually Transmitted Disease Treatment Guidelines. MMWR 2002;51:1.

Podofilox is an antimitotic drug that results in destruction of warts. Most patients experience pain or local irritation after treatment. Imiquimod is a topically active immune enhancer that stimulates production of cytokines, followed by local inflammation and resolution of warts (Moore et al, 2001; Fife et al, 2001). Effective use of cryotherapy requires training to avoid either overtreatment or undertreatment and poor results. Pain is common after application of the liquid nitrogen, followed by necrosis of the warts. Podophyllin resin contains several antimitotic compounds. Different resin preparations vary in the concentrations of active components and contaminants. Although both trichloroacetic acid and bichloroacetic acid are recommended and are used widely, these treatments are associated with several potential problems. The acid can spread rapidly if applied excessively, with damage to normal adjacent tissues. These solutions should be applied sparingly and allowed to dry before the patient stands. If the patient experiences excessive discomfort, the acid can be neutralized by using soap or sodium bicarbonate (baking soda). Recent data suggest that the treatment approach should be changed if a patient has not improved substantially after 3 provider-administered treatments or if warts do not resolve completely after 6 treatments.

Surgical removal offers the advantage of rendering the patient wart-free in a single visit. Several approaches are possible, including tangential scissor or shave excision, curettage, electrosurgery, or laser surgery. All of these methods require local anesthesia and are more time-consuming and expensive than the methods discussed in the previous paragraph. Surgical approaches are most useful for patients who have a large number or a large volume of genital warts, if the diagnosis is uncertain, or if patients have been unresponsive to other treatments. Patients should be warned that scarring, hypopigmentation, and hyperpigmentation are common after ablative therapies. Occasionally, patients have chronic pain after such treatment.

Recurrence of warts is common after all therapies, with most recurrences occurring within the first 3 months. Women should be counseled about the need for regular cervical cytologic screening. Examination of sex partners is unnecessary for management of external genital warts, because the role of reinfection is probably minimal. However, sex partners of patients with genital warts may benefit from evaluation for genital warts and other STDs.

Subclinical Genital HPV Infection

Subclinical HPV infection (without visible genital warts) is more common than visible genital lesions. Most cases are diagnosed indirectly by cervical cytology, colposcopy, or biopsy of genital skin, or by routine use of acetic acid soaks and examination with magnification for "acetowhite" areas. The consensus of expert opinion is to discourage routine examination for "acetowhiting." This test has poor specificity for HPV infection. In addition, the acetowhite test has many false-positive results in low-risk populations. Definitive diagnosis of subclinical HPV infection requires detection of HPV nucleic acid or capsid protein, but this test is not recommended outside of research settings.

Treatment of subclinical HPV infection is not recommended in the absence of dysplasia. Diagnosis is often questionable because many of the diagnostic tests (ie, cytology, acetowhiting, colposcopy) correlate poorly with detection of HPV DNA or RNA. Furthermore, no therapy has been proved to eradicate infection. HPV has been demonstrated in normal-appearing tissue adjacent to treated areas after aggressive surgical treatment.

HIV INFECTION: OVERVIEW OF DETECTION, INITIAL EVALUATION, & REFERRAL

Infection with HIV includes a wide clinical spectrum, ranging from asymptomatic infection to AIDS. The rate of clinical progression is highly variable. Some persons progress from HIV infection to AIDS within a few months; others remain asymptomatic for decades.

Overall, the median time from infection to AIDS is around 10 years. In general, adults with HIV infection remain asymptomatic for prolonged periods. However, HIV viral replication continues during all stages of infection, with substantial increases in the viral burden during later stages of infection, accompanied by marked deterioration in immune functions.

Increasing awareness of risk factors for HIV infection has led to increased testing and earlier diagnosis for many patients. The primary risk factors for HIV infection are sexual contact with an HIV-infected person and sharing injecting-drug equipment.

Early diagnosis is important because treatment can slow the decline in immune function. HIV-infected persons with evidence of immune dysfunction are at risk for preventable infections. Prophylactic treatment can substantially reduce the risk for pneumonia (*Pneumocystis carinii* and bacterial), toxoplasma encephalitis, and mycobacterial disease (tuberculosis and *Mycobacterium avium* complex). Early diagnosis also facilitates patient counseling, which may reduce transmission. In addition, early diagnosis facilitates planning for referral to a health care provider/facility experienced in care of HIV-infected persons.

Testing for HIV

Diagnostic testing for HIV should be offered to anyone at risk for infection, especially those seeking evaluation for STDs. Appropriate pre- and posttest counseling and informed consent should be included in the test procedure. Some states required documentation of informed consent.

Usually, HIV infection is documented using HIV-1 antibody tests. HIV antibodies are detected in > 95% of infected persons within 6 months of infection. In most laboratories, this is a 2-stage procedure beginning with a sensitive screening test, such as an enzyme immunoassay. Reactive screening test results are then confirmed by a supplemental test, such as the Western blot, or an immunofluorescence assay. Patients with positive results on both the screening and confirmatory tests are infected with HIV. Such infected persons can transmit HIV.

In the United States, almost all HIV infections are caused by HIV-1. Extremely rare cases are caused by a second virus, HIV-2. Thus, routine clinical testing for HIV-2 is not recommended. The only indications are in blood centers or for persons who have specific demographic or behavioral risk factors for HIV-2. These persons include those from countries where HIV-2 is endemic (West Africa, Angola, Mozambique, France, and Portugal) and their sex partners. The possibility of HIV-2 infection should also be considered in situations where there is clinical suspicion of HIV disease in the absence of a positive HIV-1 antibody test.

Acute Retroviral Syndrome

This syndrome occurs in many persons shortly after HIV infection, before antibody tests are positive. The syndrome is characterized by acute symptoms and signs, including fever, malaise, lymphadenopathy, and skin rash. Suspicion of acute retroviral syndrome should prompt nucleic acid testing to detect HIV. New data suggest that early initiation of treatment during this period can result in a lower HIV viral burden, delay HIV-related complications, and perhaps result in immune reconstitution.

Initial Management of HIV Infection

It is advisable to refer HIV-infected persons to a single clinical resource for comprehensive care. Because of the limited availability of these facilities, it is often advisable to initiate evaluation and provide access to psychosocial services while planning for referral and continuation of medical care. Thus, brief consideration of initial management is in order.

Recently diagnosed HIV infection may not have been acquired recently. Persons with newly diagnosed HIV infection can be at any of the clinical stages of infection. Thus, it is important to be alert for signs and symptoms that suggest advanced infection, such as fever, weight loss, diarrhea, oral candidiasis, cough, or shortness of breath. These findings suggest the need for urgent referral.

In nonemergent situations, the recommended evaluation of a person with a newly diagnosed HIV infection includes a detailed medical history that emphasizes sexual and substance abuse history, previous STDs, and specific HIV-related symptoms or diagnoses. The physical examination should include a pelvic examination in women, with Pap smear and testing for gonorrhea and chlamydial infection. Recommended blood work includes complete blood count with platelet count; chemistry profile; testing for toxoplasma antibody and hepatitis viral markers; syphilis serologic test, and a CD4+ T-lymphocyte count. Other evaluations should include a tuberculin skin test and chest X-ray. Finally, provision should be made for evaluation and management of sex and injecting-drug partners.

REFERENCES

Behets FM et al: Genital ulcers: Etiology, clinical diagnosis, and associated human immunodeficiency virus infection in Kingston, Jamaica. Clin Infect Dis 1999;28:1086.

Bong CT et al: DsrA-deficient mutant of *Haemophilus ducreyi* is impaired in its ability to infect human volunteers. Infect Immun 2001;69:1488.

Bowden FJ, Savage J: Azithromycin for the treatment of donovanosis. Sex Transm Infect 1998;74:78.

Centers for Disease Control: Congenital syphilis–United States, 2000. MMWR Morb Mortal Wkly Rep 2001a;50:573.

Centers for Disease Control: Primary and secondary syphilis—United States, 1999. MMWR Morb Mortal Wkly Rep 2001b;50:113.

Centers for Disease Control and Prevention: 1998 Guidelines for treatment of sexually transmitted diseases. MMWR 1998; 47:1.

de Vries M et al: Polyarteritis nodosa presenting as an acute bilateral epididymitis. Arch Intern Med 2001;161:1008.

Ernst AA, Marvez-Valls E, Martin DH: Incision and drainage versus aspiration of fluctuant buboes in the emergency department during an epidemic of chancroid. Sex Transm Dis 1995;22:217.

Fife KH et al: Treatment of external genital warts in men using 5% imiquimod cream applied three times a week, once daily, twice daily, or three times a day. Sex Transm Dis 2001; 28:226.

Gelfanova V, Humphreys TL, Spinola SM: Characterization of *Haemophilus ducreyi*-specific T-cell lines from lesions of experimentally infected human subjects. Infect Immun 2001; 69:4224.

Giannopoulos A et al: Epididymitis caused by *Candida glabrata:* A novel infection in diabetic patients? Diabetes Care 2001; 24:2003.

Horner P et al: Role of *Mycoplasma genitalium* and *Ureaplasma urealyticum* in acute and chronic nongonococcal urethritis. Clin Infect Dis 2001;32:995.

Joyner JL et al: Comparative prevalence of infection with *Trichomonas vaginalis* among men attending a sexually transmitted diseases clinic. Sex Transm Dis 2000;27:236.

Kaklamani VG et al: Recurrent epididymo-orchitis in patients with Behçet's disease. J Urol 2000;163:487.

Kharsany AB et al: Phylogenetic analysis of *Calymmatobacterium granulomatis* based on 16S rRNA gene sequences. J Med Microbiol 1999;48:841.

Krieger J: Prostatitis, epididymitis and orchitis. In: Mandell G, Bennett D, Dolin R (editors): *Mandell, Douglas, and Bennett's Principles and Practice of Infectious Diseases,* vol. 2, 4th ed, Chapter 91, pp. 1098–1102. Churchill Livingstone, 1990.

Krieger J: Urethritis: Etiology, diagnosis, treatment, and complications. In: Gillenwater J et al (editors): *Adult and Pediatric Urology,* vol. 2, Chapter 38, pp. 1879–1918. Mosby, 1996.

Leone PA, Trottier S, Miller JM: Valacyclovir for episodic treatment of genital herpes: A shorter 3-day treatment course compared with 5-day treatment. Clin Infect Dis 2002; 34:958.

Madeb R et al: Need for diagnostic screening of herpes simplex virus in patients with nongonococcal urethritis. Clin Infect Dis 2000;30:982.

Mahony JB et al: Evaluation of the NucliSens Basic Kit for detection of *Chlamydia trachomatis* and *Neisseria gonorrhoeae* in genital tract specimens using nucleic acid sequence-based amplification of 16S rRNA. J Clin Microbiol 2001;39:1429.

McCormack W, Rein M: Urethritis. In: Mandell G, Bennett D, Dolin R (editors): *Mandell, Douglas, and Bennett's Principles and Practice of Infectious Diseases,* vol. 2, 4th ed, Chapter 88, pp. 1063–1073. Churchill Livingstone, 1990.

Mead P: Infections of the female pelvis. In: Mandell G, Bennett D, Dolin R (editors): *Mandell, Douglas, and Bennett's Principles and Practice of Infectious Diseases,* vol. 2, 4th ed, Chapter 90, pp. 1090–1097. Churchill Livingstone, 1990.

Moore RA et al: Imiquimod for the treatment of genital warts: A quantitative systematic review. BMC Infect Dis 2001;1:3.

Norris SJ, Cox DL, Weinstock GM: Biology of *Treponema pallidum:* Correlation of functional activities with genome sequence data. J Mol Microbiol Biotechnol 2001;3:37.

O'Farrell N: Donovanosis: An update. Int J STD AIDS 2001; 12:423.

Rahman M et al: Treatment failure with the use of ciprofloxacin for gonorrhea correlates with the prevalence of fluoroquinolone-resistant *Neisseria gonorrhoeae* strains in Bangladesh. Clin Infect Dis 2001;32:884.

Rein M: Genital skin and mucous membrane lesions. In: Mandell G, Bennett D, Dolin R (editors): *Mandell, Douglas, and Bennett's Principles and Practice of Infectious Diseases,* vol. 2, 4th ed, Chapter 87, pp. 1055–1062. Churchill Livingstone, 1990.

Rein M: Sexually transmitted diseases. In: Mandel J (editor): *Atlas of Infectious Diseases,* vol. 5. Churchill Livingstone, 1996.

Rompalo AM: Can syphilis be eradicated from the world? Curr Opin Infect Dis 2001;14:41.

Skoutelis A et al: Serious complications of tuberculous epididymitis. Infection 2000;28:193.

Throm RE, Spinola SM: Transcription of candidate virulence genes of *Haemophilus ducreyi* during infection of human volunteers. Infect Immun 2001;69:1483.

Tompkins JR, Zenilman JM: Quinolone resistance in *Neisseria gonorrhoeae.* Curr Infect Dis Rep 2001;3:156.

Totten PA et al: Association of *Mycoplasma genitalium* with nongonococcal urethritis in heterosexual men. J Infect Dis 2001; 183:269.

Trees DL et al: Molecular epidemiology of *Neisseria gonorrhoeae* exhibiting decreased susceptibility and resistance to ciprofloxacin in Hawaii, 1991–1999. Sex Transm Dis 2001; 28:309.

Wald A et al: Two-day regimen of acyclovir for treatment of recurrent genital herpes simplex virus type 2 infection. Clin Infect Dis 2002;34:944.

Young RS et al: Expression of cytolethal distending toxin and hemolysin is not required for pustule formation by *Haemophilus ducreyi* in human volunteers. Infect Immun 2001;69:1938.

Urinary Stone Disease

16

Marshall L. Stoller, MD

Urinary calculi are the third most common affliction of the urinary tract, exceeded only by urinary tract infections and pathologic conditions of the prostate. They are common in both animals and humans. The nomenclature associated with urinary stone disease arises from a variety of disciplines. Struvite stones, for example, composed of magnesium ammonium phosphate hexahydrate, are named in honor of H.C.G. von Struve (1772–1851), a Russian naturalist. Before the time of von Struve, the stones were referred to as guanite, because magnesium ammonium phosphate is prominent in bat droppings. Calcium oxalate dihydrate is frequently referred to as weddellite, because it was commonly found in floor samples collected from the Weddell Sea in Antarctica. The history of the nomenclature associated with urinary stone disease is as intriguing as that of the development of the interventional techniques used in their treatment.

Urinary stones have plagued humans since the earliest records of civilization. The etiology of stones remains speculative. If urinary constituents are similar from each kidney and if there is no evidence of obstruction, why do most stones present in a unilateral fashion? Why don't small stones pass uneventfully down the ureter early in their development? Why do some people form one large stone and others form multiple small calculi? There is much speculation concerning these and other questions.

Advances in the surgical treatment of urinary stones have outpaced our understanding of their etiology. As clinicians we are concerned with an expedient diagnosis and efficient treatment. Equally important is a thorough metabolic evaluation directing appropriate medical therapy and lifestyle changes to help reduce recurrent stone disease. Without such follow-up and medical intervention, stone recurrence rates can be as high as 50% within 5 years. Uric acid calculi can recur even more frequently. Physicians look forward to gaining a better understanding of this multifactorial disease process in hopes of developing more effective prophylaxis.

RENAL & URETERAL STONES

Etiology

Mineralization in all biologic systems has a common theme in that the crystals and matrix are intertwined.

Urinary stones are no exception; they are polycrystalline aggregates composed of varying amounts of crystalloid and organic matrix. Theories to explain urinary stone disease are incomplete.

Stone formation requires supersaturated urine. Supersaturation depends on urinary pH, ionic strength, solute concentration, and complexation. Urinary constituents may change dramatically during different physiologic states from a relatively acid urine in a first morning void to an alkaline tide noted after meals. Ionic strength is determined primarily by the relative concentration of monovalent ions. As ionic strength increases, the activity coefficient decreases. The activity coefficient reflects the availability of a particular ion.

The role of solute concentrations is clear: The greater the concentration of 2 ions, the more likely they are to precipitate. Low ion concentrations result in undersaturation and increased solubility. As ion concentrations increase, their activity product reaches a specific point termed the **solubility product** (K_{sp}). Concentrations above this point are metastable and are capable of initiating crystal growth and heterogeneous nucleation. As solutions become more concentrated, the activity product eventually reaches the formation product (K_{fp}). Supersaturation levels beyond this point are unstable, and spontaneous homogeneous nucleation may occur.

Multiplying 2 ion concentrations reveals the concentration product. The concentration products of most ions are greater than established solubility products. Other factors must play major roles in the development of urinary calculi, including complexation. Complexation influences the availability of specific ions. For instance, sodium complexes with oxalate and decreases its free ionic form, while sulfates can complex with calcium. Crystal formation is modified by a variety of other substances found in the urinary tract, including magnesium, citrate, pyrophosphate, and a variety of trace metals. These inhibitors may act at the active crystal growth sites or as inhibitors in solution (as with citrate).

The nucleation theory suggests that urinary stones originate from crystals or foreign bodies immersed in supersaturated urine. This theory is challenged by the same arguments that support it. Stones do not always form in patients who are hyperexcretors or who are at risk for dehydration. Additionally, many stone formers'

24-h urine collections are completely normal with respect to stone-forming ion concentrations.

The crystal inhibitor theory claims that calculi form owing to the absence or low concentration of natural stone inhibitors, including magnesium, citrate, pyrophosphate, and a variety of trace metals. This theory does not have absolute validity since many people lacking such inhibitors may never form stones, and others with an abundance of inhibitors may, paradoxically, form them.

A. Crystal Component

Stones are composed primarily of a crystalline component. Crystals of adequate size and transparency are easily identified under a polarizing microscope. X-ray diffraction is preferred to assess the geometry and architecture of calculi. A group of stones from the same geographic location or the same historical time period typically have crystalline constituents that are common.

Multiple steps are involved in crystal formation, including nucleation, growth, and aggregation. Nucleation initiates the stone process and may be induced by a variety of substances, including proteinaceous matrix, crystals, foreign bodies, and other particulate tissues. Heterogeneous nucleation (epitaxy), which requires less energy and may occur in less saturated urine, is a common theme in stone formation. It should be suspected whenever an oriented conglomerate is found. A crystal of one type thereby serves as a nidus for the nucleation of another type with a similar crystal lattice. This is frequently seen with uric acid crystals initiating calcium oxalate formation. It takes time for these early nidi to grow or aggregate to form a stone incapable of passing with ease through the urinary tract.

How these early crystalline structures are retained in the upper urinary tract without uneventful passage down the ureter is unknown. The theory of mass precipitation or intranephronic calculosis suggests that the distal tubules or collecting ducts, or both, become plugged with crystals, thereby establishing an environment of stasis, ripe for further stone growth. This explanation is unsatisfactory; tubules are conical in shape and enlarge as they enter the papilla, thereby reducing the possibility of ductal obstruction. Additionally, urine transit time from the glomerulus into the renal pelvis is only a few minutes, making crystal aggregation and growth within the uriniferous tubules unlikely.

The fixed particle theory postulates that formed crystals are somehow retained within cells or beneath tubular epithelium. Randall noted whitish-yellow precipitations of crystalline substances occurring on the tips of renal papillae as submucosal plaques. These can be appreciated during endoscopy of the upper urinary tract. Carr hypothesized that calculi form in obstructed lymphatics and then rupture into adjacent fornices of a calyx. Arguing against Carr's theory are the grossly visible early stone elements in areas remote from fornices.

B. Matrix Component

The amount of the noncrystalline, matrix component of urinary stones varies with stone type, commonly ranging from 2% to 10% by weight. It is composed predominantly of protein, with small amounts of hexose and hexosamine. An unusual type of stone called a matrix calculus can be associated with previous kidney surgery or chronic urinary tract infections and has a gelatinous texture (Figure 16–1). Histologic inspection reveals laminations with scant calcifications. On plain abdominal radiographs, matrix calculi are usually radiolucent and can be confused with other filling defects, including blood clots, upper-tract tumors, and fungal bezoars. Computed tomography (CT) reveals calcifications and can help to confirm the diagnosis. The role of matrix in the initiation of ordinary urinary stones as well as matrix stones is unknown. It may serve as a nidus for crystal aggregation or as a naturally occurring glue to adhere small crystal components and thereby hinder uneventful passage down the urinary tract. Alternatively, matrix may have an inhibitory role in stone formation or may be an innocent bystander, playing no active role in stone formation.

Urinary Ions

A. Calcium

Calcium is a major ion present in urinary crystals. Only 50% of plasma calcium is ionized and available for filtration at the glomerulus. Well over 95% of the calcium filtered at the glomerulus is reabsorbed at both the proximal and distal tubules and limited amounts in the collecting tube. Less than 2% is excreted in the

Figure 16–1. Gross picture of matrix calculus percutaneously extracted after extracorporeal shock wave lithotripsy failure.

urine. Diuretic medications may exert a hypocalciuric effect by further decreasing calcium excretion. Many factors influence the availability of calcium in solution, including complexation with citrate, phosphate, and sulfate. An increase in monosodium urates and a decrease in urinary pH further interfere with this complexation and therefore promote crystal aggregation.

B. OXALATE

Oxalate is a normal waste product of metabolism and is relatively insoluble. Normally, approximately 10–15% of oxalate found in the urine originates from the diet; the vast majority is a metabolic by-product. Most of the oxalate that enters the large bowel is consumed by bacterial decomposition. Diet, however, can have an impact on the amount of oxalate found in the urine. Once absorbed from the small bowel, oxalate is not metabolized and is excreted almost exclusively by the proximal tubule. The presence of calcium within the bowel lumen is an important factor influencing the amount of oxalate that is absorbed. The control of oxalate in the urine plays a pivotal role in the formation of calcium oxalate calculi. Normal excretion ranges from 20 to 45 mg/d and does not change significantly with age. Excretion is higher during the day when one eats. Small changes in oxalate levels in the urine can have a dramatic impact on the supersaturation of calcium oxalate. The principal precursors of oxalate are glycine and ascorbic acid; however, the impact of ingested vitamin C (< 2 g/day) is negligible.

Hyperoxaluria may develop in patients with bowel disorders, particularly inflammatory bowel disease, small-bowel resection, and bowel bypass. Renal calculi develop in 5–10% of patients with these conditions. Chronic diarrhea with fatty stools results in a saponification process. Intraluminal calcium binds to the fat, thereby becoming unavailable to bind to oxalate. The unbound oxalate is readily absorbed.

Excessive oxalate may occur secondary to the accidental or deliberate ingestion of ethylene glycol (partial oxidation to oxalate). This may result in diffuse and massive deposition of calcium oxalate crystals and may occasionally lead to renal failure.

C. PHOSPHATE

Phosphate is an important buffer and complexes with calcium in urine. It is a key component in calcium phosphate and magnesium ammonium phosphate stones. The excretion of urinary phosphate in normal adults is related to the amount of dietary phosphate (especially in meats, dairy products, and vegetables). The small amount of phosphate filtered by the glomerulus is predominantly reabsorbed in the proximal tubule. Parathyroid hormone inhibits this reabsorption. The predominant crystal found in those with hyperparathyroidism is phosphate, in the form of hydroxyapatite, amorphous calcium phosphate, and carbonate apatite.

D. URIC ACID

Uric acid is the by-product of purine metabolism. The pKa of uric acid is 5.75. Undissociated uric acid predominates with pH values less than this. Elevated pH values increase urate, which is soluble. Approximately 10% of the filtered uric acid finds its way into the urine. Other defects in purine metabolism may result in urinary stone disease. Rarely, a defect in xanthine oxidase results in increased levels of xanthine; the xanthine may precipitate in urine, resulting in stone formation. Unusual alterations in adenine metabolism may result in the production of 2,8-dihydroxyadeninuria, which is poorly soluble in urine and may develop into a urinary stone. This results from a deficiency of adenine phosphoribosyltransferase (APRT). Pure uric acid crystals and calculi are typically radiolucent in nature and may not be identified on plain abdominal films (Figure 16–2). They are visible on noncontrast CT images. Some uric acid calculi may be partially radiopaque, however, because of associated calcium deposits.

E. SODIUM

Although not identified as one of the major constituents of most urinary calculi, sodium plays an important role in regulating the crystallization of calcium salts in urine. Sodium is found in higher than expected concentrations in the core of renal calculi and may play

Figure 16–2. Radiolucent right staghorn renal calculus appreciated after percutaneous injection of radiocontrast material. This uric acid stone was effectively removed in a single percutaneous procedure. Postoperative urinary alkalinization has been effective prophylaxis.

a role in initiating crystal development and aggregation. High dietary sodium intake increases urinary calcium excretion. This reduces the ability of urine to inhibit calcium oxalate crystal agglomeration. These effects are thought to be due to a sodium-induced increase in bicarbonaturia and decrease in serum bicarbonate. Conversely, a reduction in dietary sodium helps to reduce recurrent calcium nephrolithiasis.

F. CITRATE

Citrate is a key factor affecting the development of calcium urinary stones. A deficiency commonly is associated with stone formation in those with chronic diarrhea or renal tubular acidosis type I (distal tubular defect) and in patients undergoing chronic thiazide therapy. Citrate plays a pivotal role in the citric acid cycle in renal cells. Metabolic stimuli that consume this product (as with intracellular metabolic acidosis due to fasting, hypokalemia, or hypomagnesemia) reduce the urinary excretion of citrate. Estrogen increases citrate excretion and may be a factor that decreases the incidence of stones in women, especially during pregnancy. Alkalosis also increases citrate excretion.

G. MAGNESIUM

Dietary magnesium deficiency is associated with an increased incidence of urinary stone disease. Magnesium is a component of struvite calculi. Experimentally, lack of dietary magnesium is associated with increased calcium oxalate stone formation and calcium oxalate crystalluria. The exact mechanism whereby magnesium exerts its effect is undefined. Dietary magnesium supplements do not protect against stone formation in normal people.

H. SULFATE

Urinary sulfates may help prevent urinary calculi. They can complex with calcium. These sulfates occur primarily as components of longer urinary proteins, such as chondroitin sulfate and heparin sulfate.

I. OTHER URINARY STONE INHIBITORS

Inhibitors of urinary stone formation other than citrate, magnesium, and sulfates have been identified. These consist predominantly of urinary proteins and other macromolecules such as glycosaminoglycans, pyrophosphates, and uropontin. Although citrate appears to be the most active inhibitory component in urine, these substances demonstrate a substantial role in preventing urine crystal formation. The N-terminal amino acid sequence and the acidic amino acid content of these protein inhibitors, especially their high aspartic acid content, appear to play pivotal inhibitory roles. Fluoride may be an inhibitor of urinary stone formation.

Stone Varieties

A. CALCIUM CALCULI

Calcifications can occur and accumulate in the collecting system, resulting in nephrolithiasis. Eighty to eighty-five percent of all urinary stones are calcareous.

Calcium nephrolithiasis is most commonly due to elevated urinary calcium, elevated urinary uric acid, elevated urinary oxalate, or a decreased level of urinary citrate. Hypercalciuira is found as a solitary defect in 12% of patients and in combination with other defects in an additional 18%. Hyperuricosuria is identified as a solitary defect in 8% of patients and associated with additional defects in 16%. Elevated urinary oxalate is found as a solitary finding in 5% of patients and as a combined defect in 16%. Finally, decreased urinary citrate is found as an isolated defect in 17% of patients and as a combined defect in an additional 10%. Approximately one-third of patients undergoing a full metabolic evaluation will find no identiable metabolic defect.

Symptoms are secondary to obstruction, with resultant pain, infection, nausea, and vomiting, and rarely culminate in renal failure. Asymptomatic hematuria or repetitive urinary tract infections recalcitrant to apparently appropriate antibiotics should lead one to suspect a urinary stone. Calcifications within the parenchyma of the kidney, known as nephrocalcinosis, rarely cause symptoms, however, and usually are not amenable to traditional therapies appropriate for urinary stone disease (Figure 16–3). Nephrocalcinosis is frequently encountered with renal tubular acidosis and hyperparathyroidism. Nephrolithiasis and nephrocalcinosis

Figure 16–3. Retrograde pyelogram demonstrating multiple punctate calcifications within the renal parenchyma establishing the diagnosis of nephrocalcinosis. Renal pelvis and infundibula are free of calculi.

frequently coexist. Most patients with nephrolithiasis, however, do not have obvious nephrocalcinosis.

Nephrocalcinosis may result from a variety of pathologic states. Ectatic collecting tubules, as seen with medullary sponge kidney, are common. This is frequently a bilateral process. Increased calcium absorption from the small bowel is common with sarcoidosis, milk-alkali syndrome, hyperparathyroidism, and excessive vitamin D intake. Disease processes resulting in bony destruction, including hyperparathyroidism, osteolytic lesions, and multiple myeloma, are a third mechanism. Finally, dystrophic calcifications forming on necrotic tissue may develop after a renal insult.

1. Absorptive hypercalciuric nephrolithiasis—Normal calcium intake averages approximately 900–1000 mg/d. Approximately one-third is absorbed by the small bowel, and of that portion approximately 150–200 mg is obligatorily excreted in the urine. A large reservoir of calcium remains in the bone. Most dietary calcium is excreted in the stool. Absorptive hypercalciuria is secondary to increased calcium absorption from the small bowel, predominantly from the jejunum. This results in an increased load of calcium filtered from the glomerulus. The result is suppression of parathyroid hormone, leading to decreased tubular reabsorption of calcium, culminating in hypercalciuria (> 4 mg/kg). This physiologic cascade is in response to the primary defect, an increased absorption of calcium from the small bowel.

Absorptive hypercalciuria can be subdivided into 3 types. Type I absorptive hypercalciuria is independent of diet and represents 15% of all calcareous calculi. There is an elevated urinary calcium level (> 150–200 mg/24 h) even during a calcium-restricted diet. Cellulose phosphate is an effective nonabsorbable exchange resin. This effectively binds the calcium in the gut, preventing bowel absorption. Cellulose phosphate has no impact on the calcium transport defect. Urinary calcium excretion returns to normal values with therapy.

Cellulose phosphate must be taken with meals to be available when calcium is ingested. A typical dose is 10–15 g orally in 3 divided doses and is well tolerated. This therapy is relatively contraindicated in postmenopausal women and in children during their active growth cycles. Inappropriate use may lead to a negative calcium balance and a secondary hyperparathyroid state. As with all stone formers, long-term follow-up is required. Cellulose phosphate may bind other cations besides calcium, including magnesium. Secondary hyperoxaluria may develop owing to decreased calcium in the gut. See the section on hyperoxaluria for a more detailed discussion.

Hydrochlorothiazides are an alternative treatment for type I absorptive hypercalciuria. Initially there is a reduction in renal excretion of calcium. The increased absorbed calcium is likely deposited in bone. Eventually the bone reservoir reaches its capacity and the drug becomes ineffective. Hydrochlorothiazides have limited long-term efficacy (approximately 3–5 years). These drugs have no effect on the defective bowel transport system. Hydrochlorothiazides may be alternated with cellulose phosphate as an effective treatment regimen.

Type II absorptive hypercalciuria is dietary dependent and is a common cause of urinary stone disease. There is no specific medical therapy. Calcium excretion returns to normal on a calcium-restricted diet. Patients should limit their calcium intake to 400–600 mg/d. Type II absorptive hypercalciuria is not as severe as type I.

Type III absorptive hypercalciuria is secondary to a phosphate renal leak and accounts for 5% of all urinary calculi. Decreased serum phosphate leads to an increase in 1,25-dihydroxyvitamin D synthesis. The physiologic cascade culminates in an increased absorption of phosphate and calcium from the small bowel and an increased renal excretion of calcium—hence its classification as absorptive hypercalciuria. Successful treatment replaces bioavailable phosphate. Orthophosphate (Neutra-Phos) inhibits vitamin D synthesis and is administered as 250 mg 3–4 times daily. It is best taken after meals and before bedtime. Orthophosphates do not alter intestinal calcium absorption.

2. Resorptive hypercalciuric nephrolithiasis—About half the patients with clinically obvious primary hyperparathyroidism present with nephrolithiasis. This group represents less than 5–10% of all patients with urinary stones. Patients with calcium phosphate stones, women with recurrent calcium stones, and those with both nephrocalcinosis and nephrolithiasis should be suspected of having hyperparathyroidism. Hypercalcemia is the most consistent sign of hyperparathyroidism.

Parathyroid hormone results in a cascade of events starting with an increase in urinary phosphorus and a decrease in plasma phosphorus, followed by an increase in plasma calcium and a decrease in urinary calcium. Its action on the kidney and on the bone are independent of each other. Ultimately renal damage is secondary to the hypercalcemia. It limits the concentrating ability of the kidney and impairs the kidney's ability to acidify urine. Surgical removal of the offending parathyroid adenoma is the only effective way of treating this disease. Attempts at medical management are futile.

3. Renal induced hypercalciuric nephrolithiasis—Hypercalciuria of renal origin is due to an intrinsic renal tubular defect in calcium excretion. This creates a physiologically vicious cycle. Excessive urinary calcium excretion results in a relative decrease in serum calcium, which leads to a secondarily increased parathyroid hormone level that mobilizes calcium from the bone and increases calcium absorption from the gut. This step completes the pathologic cycle by delivering increased levels of calcium back to the kidney, whereby the renal tubules excrete large amounts of calcium. These patients have an elevated fasting urinary calcium level, normal serum calcium level, and an elevated parathyroid hormone level.

Renal hypercalciuria is effectively treated with hydrochlorothiazides. Unlike their role in type I absorptive hypercalciuria, in this setting hydrochlorothiazides have a durable long-term effect. As a diuretic, they decrease the circulating blood volume and subsequently stimulate proximal tubular absorption of calcium as well as other constituents. They also increase reabsorption at the distal tubule. Both mechanisms correct the secondary hyperparathyroid state.

Hypercalciuric states may result in elevated parathyroid levels. To differentiate primary from secondary hyperparathyroidism in patients with urinary stone disease, one can prescribe a hydrochlorothiazide challenge of 50 mg twice a day for approximately 10 days. Patients with secondary hyperparathyroidism will have normal serum parathyroid levels, while those with primary hyperparathyroism will continue to have elevated serum values.

4. Hyperuricosuric calcium nephrolithiasis—Hyperuricosuric calcium nephrolithiasis is due to either an excessive dietary intake of purines or an increase in endogenous uric acid production. In both situations there is an increase in urinary monosodium urates. Monosodium urates absorb and adsorb urinary stone inhibitors and facilitate heterogeneous nucleation.

Patients have elevated urinary uric acid levels (> 600 mg/24 h in women and > 750 mg/24 h in men) and consistently have a urinary pH > 5.5. The urinary pH helps to differentiate hyperuricosuric calcium from hyperuricosuric uric acid stone formation.

Patients with excessive purine intake can be effectively treated by changing their diet to one with low purines. Those with excessive endogenous uric acid production can be successfully treated with allopurinol. Allopurinol is a xanthine oxidase inhibitor. Allopurinol reduces uric acid synthesis and renal excretion of uric acid. It also inhibits uric acid–calcium oxalate crystallization. Allopurinol has many potential side effects, including a variety of skin rashes and liver toxicity, and should be administered with careful monitoring (300 mg daily). Potassium citrate is an alternative treatment, especially when associated with hypocitraturia.

5. Hyperoxaluric calcium nephrolithiasis—Hyperoxaluric calcium nephrolithiasis is secondary to increased urinary oxalate levels (> 40 mg/24 h). It is frequently found in patients with inflammatory bowel disease or other chronic diarrheal states that result in severe dehydration. It is rarely associated with excessive oxalate intake, as seen in poisoning with ethylene glycol or endogenous overproduction.

Chronic diarrheal states alter oxalate metabolism. Malabsorption leads to increased luminal fat and bile. Intraluminal calcium readily binds to fat, resulting in a saponification process. Urinary calcium levels are usually low (< 100 mg/24 h). The intraluminal gut calcium that normally would have bound to oxalate is decreased. The unbound oxalate is readily absorbed and is unaffected by the usual metabolic inhibitors of energy-dependent pumps. Bile salts may increase the passive bowel absorption of oxalate. A small increase in oxalate absorption and subsequent urinary excretion dramatically increases the formation product of calcium-oxalate. This increases the potential for heterogeneous nucleation and crystal growth in this metastable environment. All patients with increased urinary excretion of oxalate do not form calcium oxalate calculi. Other factors must be contributory, therefore, including dehydration, hypocitraturia (associated with an acidosis), decreased excretion of urinary inhibitors including magnesium, and protein malabsorption.

Enteric hyperoxaluric calcium nephrolithiasis is successfully treated with oral calcium supplementation. The calcium binds to the intraluminal oxalate and limits its absorption. It must be given with meals when the oxalate is present. Other oral cations are effective, including magnesium supplements. An alternative therapy includes a diet limited to medium-chain fatty acids and triglycerides; however, it is poorly tolerated by patients. Equally difficult is an attempt to alter oxalate intake. Unless large amounts of specific oxalate-rich foods can be excluded, an alternative diet may result in *increased* oxalate levels.

Primary hyperoxaluria is a rare hereditary disease. It is associated with calcium oxalate renal calculi, nephrocalcinosis, and other distant deposits of oxalate, culminating in progressive renal failure and eventual death. Type I is associated with an enzyme deficiency of 2-oxoglutarate:glyoxylate carboligase, resulting in elevated urinary levels of glycolic acid and oxalic acid. Type II has increased excretory levels of L-glyceric acid rather than elevated levels of glycolic acid. It is associated with a D-glycerate dehydrogenase enzyme deficiency. This ultimately results in the accumulation of hydroxypyruvate, which is eventually converted to oxalate. Oxalate crystal deposits develop rapidly in transplanted kidneys. Combined liver and renal transplantation has cured this previously fatal rare disease.

6. Hypocitraturic calcium nephrolithiasis—Citrate is an important inhibitor of urinary stone disease. Increased metabolic demands on the mitochondria of renal cells decrease the excretion of citrate. Such conditions include intracellular metabolic acidosis, hypokalemia (as with thiazide therapy), fasting, hypomagnesemia, androgens, gluconeogenesis, and an acid-ash diet. Citrate may be consumed in the urine by bacteria during a urinary tract infection. The cause of hypocitraturia may be unknown in some cases. In contrast, alkalosis, alkaline-ash diet, estrogen, and vitamin D increase urinary citrate levels.

Citrate has its action in solution. It complexes with calcium, thereby decreasing the ionic calcium concentration and thus the activity product and thereby decreasing the energy for crystallization. Citrate decreases agglomeration, spontaneous nucleation, and crystal growth of calcium oxalate. Citrate also decreases calcium oxalate calculi by decreasing monosodium urates that can absorb inhibitors and facilitate heterogeneous nucleation.

Hypocitraturic (< 320 mg/24 h) calcium nephrolithiasis is associated commonly with renal tubular acidosis type I (distal tubule) (Figure 16–4), thiazide therapy (accompanied by potassium wastage), and chronic diarrhea. Treatment is successful with potassium citrate supplementation. Routine dosage is 20–30 mEq 2–3 times daily and is usually well tolerated. Six to 8 glasses of lemonade can increase urinary citrate excretion by approximately 150 mg/24 h and thus either limit or eliminate the need for pharmacologic citrate supplementation.

B. NONCALCIUM CALCULI

1. Struvite—Struvite stones are composed of magnesium, ammonium, and phosphate (MAP). They are found most commonly in women and may recur rapidly. They frequently present as renal staghorn calculi and rarely present as ureteral stones except after surgical intervention (Figure 16–5). Struvite stones are

Figure 16–4. Scout abdominal radiograph demonstrating bilateral, multiple renal calculi in a patient with renal tubular acidosis, type I.

Figure 16–5. Scout abdominal radiograph demonstrating large bilateral struvite staghorn calculi. Patient was treated for many years with numerous antibiotics for recurrent urinary tract infections. Only after this radiograph were calculi identified and removed and the infections resolved.

infection stones associated with urea-splitting organisms, including *Proteus, Pseudomonas, Providencia, Klebsiella, Staphylococci,* and *Mycoplasma.* The high ammonium concentration derived from the urea-splitting organisms results in an alkaline urinary pH. The urinary pH of a patient with a MAP stone rarely is below 7.2 (normal urinary pH is 5.85). It is only at this elevated urinary pH (> 7.19) that MAP crystals precipitate. MAP crystals are soluble in the normal urinary pH range of 5–7. Preoperative bladder cultures do not necessarily reflect the bacteriologic composition found in calculi. Foreign bodies and neurogenic bladders may predispose patients to urinary infections and subsequent struvite stone formation. Massive diuresis does not prevent struvite calculi. Women with recurrent infections despite apparently appropriate antibiotic therapy should be evaluated for struvite calculi with a conventional kidney-ureter-bladder (KUB) film or renal ultrasound, or both. It is impossible to sterilize such calculi with antibiotics. Culture-specific antibiotics can reduce urease levels by 99% and help reduce stone recurrence. Stone removal is therapeutic.

Long-term management is optimized with the removal of all foreign bodies, including catheters of all varieties. A short ileal loop helps decrease the risk of stones in those with supravesical urinary diversion. All stone fragments should be removed with or without the aid of follow-up irrigations. Hemiacidrin (Renacidin) irrigations should be used with caution if at all. Rapid magnesium toxicity can result in death even with a low-pressure irrigation setup (< 20 cm water pressure), negative daily urine cultures, and no evidence of upper-tract extravasation. Acetohydroxamic acid inhibits the action of bacterial urease, thereby reducing the urinary pH and decreasing the likelihood of precipitation. Most patients have a difficult time tolerating this medication.

2. Uric acid—Uric acid stones compose less than 5% of all urinary calculi and are usually found in men. Patients with gout, myeloproliferative diseases, or rapid weight loss, and those treated for malignant conditions with cytotoxic drugs have a high incidence of uric acid lithiasis. Most patients with uric acid calculi, however, do not have hyperuricemia. Elevated uric acid levels are frequently due to dehydration and excessive purine intake. Patients present with a urinary pH consistently < 5.5, in contrast to patients with hyperuricosuric calcium nephrolithiasis, who have a urinary pH > 5.5. As the urinary pH increases above the dissociation constant pKa of 5.75, it dissociates into a relatively soluble urate ion. Treatment is centered on maintaining a urine volume > 2 L/d and a urinary pH > 6.0. Reducing dietary purines or the administration of allopurinol also helps reduce uric acid excretion. Alkalinization (with oral sodium bicarbonate, potassium bicarbonate, potassium citrate, or intravenous 1/6 normal sodium lactate) may dissolve calculi and is dependent on the stone surface area. Stone fragments after lithotripsy have a dramatically increased surface area and will dissolve more rapidly. Dissolution proceeds at approximately 1 cm of stone (as seen on KUB) per month, with compliant alkalinization.

3. Cystine—Cystine lithiasis is secondary to an inborn error of metabolism resulting in abnormal intestinal (small bowel) mucosal absorption and renal tubular absorption of dibasic amino acids, including cystine, ornithine, lysine, and arginine. The genetic defects associated with cystinuria have now been mapped to chromosome 2p.16 and more recently to 19q13.1. Cystine lithiasis is the only clinical manifestation of this defect. Classic cystinuria is inherited in an autosomal recessive fashion. Homozygous expression has a prevalence of 1:20,000, while the heterozygous expression is 1:2000. It represents 1–2% of all urinary stones, with a peak incidence in the second or third decade. Homozygous cystinurics excrete more than 250 mg/d, resulting in constant supersaturation. Heterozygous patients usually excrete 100–150 mg/d. Unaffected patients typically excrete less than 40 mg/d. Approximately 400 mg/L of cystine can remain in solution at a urinary pH of 7.0. As the urinary pH increases above 7.0, the amount of soluble cystine increases exponentially.

The solubility of cystine is pH-dependent, with a pK of approximately 8.1. There is no difference in the solubility curves in normal versus cystinuric patients. There is no known inhibitor for cystine calculi, and cystine stone formation is completely dependent on excessive cystine excretion. Cystine stones are frequently associated with calcium calculi and their related metabolic abnormalities. They may present as single, multiple, or staghorn stones. The diagnosis is suspected in patients with a family history of urinary stones and the radiographic appearance of a faintly opaque, ground-glass, smooth-edged stone (Figure 16–6). Urinalysis frequently reveals hexagonal crystals. Stone analysis confirms the diagnosis. Quantitative urinary cystine evaluation helps confirm the diagnosis and differentiate heterozygous from homozygous states. It is also important to titrate medical therapy.

Medical therapy includes high fluid intake (> 3 L/d) and urinary alkalinization. Patients should monitor their pH with nitrazine indicator paper and keep their pH

Figure 16–6. Scout radiograph demonstrating a right cystine calculus. Note ground-glass appearance with smooth edges.

values above 7.5. It is difficult or impossible to maintain levels higher than 8.0. A low-methionine (precursor to cystine) diet has limited impact, as most of the cystine is endogenous and most of the ingested methionine is incorporated into protein. Glutamine, ascorbic acid, and captopril are effective in some patients. Penicillamine can reduce urinary cystine levels. It complexes with the amino acid, and this complex is dramatically more soluble. Treatment should be titrated with quantitative urinary cystine values. Many patients poorly tolerate penicillamine, reporting skin rashes (discrete or confluent macules with occasional itching), loss of taste, nausea, vomiting, and anorexia. It may inhibit pyridoxine, which should be supplemented during treatment (50 mg/d). Mercaptopropionylglycine (Thiola), 300–1200 mg in divided doses, forms a soluble complex with cystine and can reduce stone formation. Side effects and frequent dosing decrease patient compliance rates. It is better tolerated than penicillamine and is now the first drug of choice in these difficult cases.

Surgical treatment is similar to that for other stones except that most stones are recalcitrant to extracorporeal shock wave lithotripsy (ESWL). One should have a low threshold to proceed with percutaneous stone extraction in symptomatic patients. Two populations of cystine stones have been described, including the rough and smooth varieties, and may reflect subpopulations: those that are effectively treated with ESWL and those that require more invasive therapy. Despite optimum medical therapy, a high stone recurrence rate frequently frustrates both patient and physician. Minimally invasive techniques and optimum medical therapy are paramount.

4. Xanthine—Xanthine stones are secondary to a congenital deficiency of xanthine oxidase. This enzyme normally catalyzes the oxidation of hypoxanthine to xanthine and of xanthine to uric acid. It is of interest that allopurinol, used to treat hyperuricosuric calcium nephrolithiasis and uric acid lithiasis, produces iatrogenic xanthinuria. Blood and urine levels of uric acid are lowered, and hypoxanthine and xanthine levels are increased; however, there are no case reports of xanthine stone formation resulting from allopurinol treatment. It is unlikely that allopurinol completely inhibits xanthine oxidase. Urinary stones develop in approximately 25% of patients with a xanthine oxidase deficiency. The stones are radiolucent and are tannish-yellow in color. Treatment should be directed by symptoms and evidence of renal obstruction. High fluid intake and urinary alkalinization are required for prophylaxis. If stones recur, a trial of allopurinol and a purine-restricted diet is appropriate.

5. Indinavir—Protease inhibitors are a popular and effective treatment in patients with acquired immunodeficiency syndrome. Indinavir is the most common protease inhibitor that results in radiolucent stones in up to 6% of patients who are prescribed this medication. Indinavir calculi are the only urinary stones to be radiolucent on noncontrast CT scans. They may be associated with calcium components and in these situations will be visible on noncontrast CT images. Temporary cessation of the medication with intravenous hydration frequently allows these stones to pass. The stones are tannish-red and usually fall apart during basket extraction.

6. Rare—Silicate stones are very rare and are usually associated with long-term use of antacids containing silica. Surgical treatment is similar to that of other calculi.

Triamterene stones are radiolucent and have been identified with an increased frequency. They are associated with antihypertensive medications containing triamterene, such as Dyazide. Discontinuing the medication eliminates stone recurrences. Other medications that may become stone constituents include glafenine and antrafenine.

Rarely, patients arrive at an emergency room at an odd hour feigning signs and symptoms of passing a urinary stone in hopes of obtaining pain medications. They may add blood to their urine and give a believable story of a severe allergy to intravenous contrast medium. Occasionally, patients present a fake urinary stone, with specks of paint or other obvious curiosities. Such patients have Munchausen syndrome, and the diagnosis is difficult and made by exclusion.

Symptoms & Signs at Presentation

Upper-tract urinary stones usually eventually cause pain. The character of the pain depends on the location. Calculi small enough to venture down the ureter usually have difficulty passing through the ureteropelvic junction, over the iliac vessels, or entering the bladder at the ureterovesical junction (Figure 16–7).

A. Pain

Renal colic and noncolicky renal pain are the 2 types of pain originating from the kidney. Renal colic usually is caused by stretching of the collecting system or ureter, while noncolicky renal pain is caused by distention of the renal capsule. These symptoms may overlap, making a clinical differentiation difficult or impossible. Urinary obstruction is the main mechanism responsible for renal colic. This may be mimicked by the pain a patient experiences when a retrograde ureteropyelogram is performed under local anesthesia, with excessive pressure resulting in overdistention of the collecting system. This pain is due to a direct increase in intraluminal pressure, stretching nerve endings.

Renal colic does not always wax and wane or come in waves like intestinal or biliary colic but may be rela-

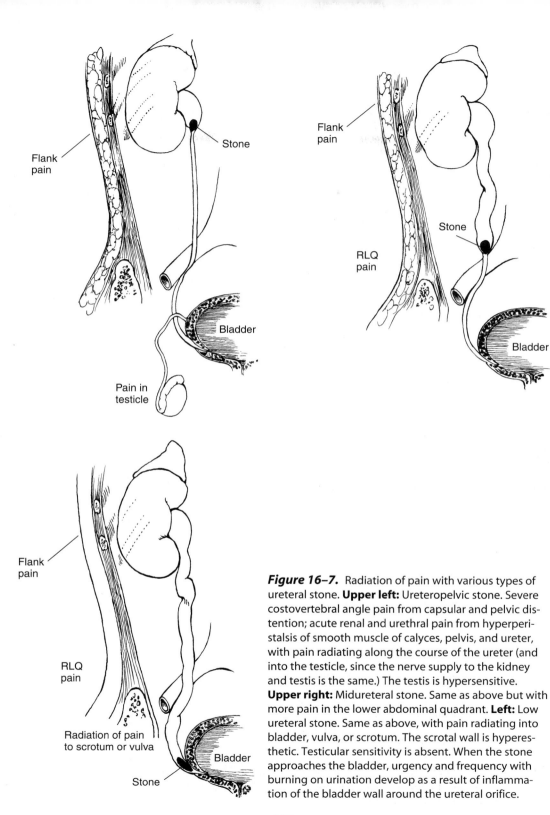

Figure 16–7. Radiation of pain with various types of ureteral stone. **Upper left:** Ureteropelvic stone. Severe costovertebral angle pain from capsular and pelvic distention; acute renal and urethral pain from hyperperistalsis of smooth muscle of calyces, pelvis, and ureter, with pain radiating along the course of the ureter (and into the testicle, since the nerve supply to the kidney and testis is the same.) The testis is hypersensitive. **Upper right:** Midureteral stone. Same as above but with more pain in the lower abdominal quadrant. **Left:** Low ureteral stone. Same as above, with pain radiating into bladder, vulva, or scrotum. The scrotal wall is hyperesthetic. Testicular sensitivity is absent. When the stone approaches the bladder, urgency and frequency with burning on urination develop as a result of inflammation of the bladder wall around the ureteral orifice.

tively constant. Renal colic implies an intraluminal origin. Patients with renal calculi have pain primarily due to urinary obstruction.

Local mechanisms such as inflammation, edema, hyperperistalsis, and mucosal irritation may contribute to the perception of pain in patients with renal calculi. In the ureter, however, local pain is referred to the distribution of the ilioinguinal nerve and the genital branch of the genitofemoral nerve, whereas pain from obstruction is referred to the same areas as for collecting system calculi (flank and costovertebral angle), thereby allowing discrimination.

The vast majority of urinary stones present with the acute onset of pain due to acute obstruction and distention of the upper urinary tract. The severity and location of the pain can vary from patient to patient due to stone size, stone location, degree of obstruction, acuity of obstruction, and variation in individual anatomy (intrarenal versus extrarenal pelvis, for example). The stone burden does not correlate with the severity of the symptoms. Small ureteral stones frequently present with severe pain, while large staghorn calculi may present with a dull ache or flank discomfort.

The pain frequently is abrupt in onset and severe and may awaken a patient from sleep. The severity of the pain is worsened by the unexpected nature of its onset. Patients frequently move constantly into unusual positions in an attempt to relieve the pain. This movement is in contrast to the lack of movement of someone with peritoneal signs; such a patient lies in a stationary position.

The symptoms of acute renal colic depend on the location of the calculus; several regions may be involved: renal calyx, renal pelvis, upper and mid ureter, and distal ureter. An orderly progression of symptoms as a stone moves down the urinary tract is the exception.

1. Renal calyx—Stones or other objects in calyces or caliceal diverticula may cause obstruction and renal colic. In general, nonobstructing stones cause pain only periodically, owing to intermittent obstruction. The pain is a deep, dull ache in the flank or back that can vary in intensity from severe to mild. The pain may be exacerbated after consumption of large amounts of fluid. Radiographic imaging may not reveal evidence of obstruction despite the patient's complaints of intermittent symptoms. It remains unclear how much of this pain is related to local mucosal irritation with activation of chemoreceptors. The presence of infection or inflammation in the calyx or diverticulum (milk of calcium, for example) in addition to obstruction may contribute to pain perception. Caliceal calculi occasionally result in spontaneous perforation with urinoma, fistula, or abscess formation.

Caliceal calculi are frequently small and numerous and appear to be able to pass spontaneously. Long-term retention against the flow of urine and against the forces of gravity and antegrade peristalsis suggests a significant element of obstruction. Effective long-term treatment requires stone extraction and elimination of the obstructive component.

Pain relief has been reported in many patients following ESWL for small symptomatic caliceal calculi. Thus, if a patient continues to complain of pain in the face of a small caliceal calculus, ESWL treatment may be justified for both diagnosis and treatment. Percutaneous, retrograde, and laparoscopic techniques have been successful in the management of calculi in calyces or caliceal diverticula.

2. Renal pelvis—Stones in the renal pelvis > 1 cm in diameter commonly obstruct the ureteropelvic junction, generally causing severe pain in the costovertebral angle, just lateral to the sacrospinalis muscle and just below the 12th rib. This pain may vary from dull to excruciatingly sharp and is usually constant, boring, and difficult to ignore. It often radiates to the flank and also anteriorly to the upper ipsilateral abdominal quadrant. It may be confused with biliary colic or cholecystitis if on the right side and with gastritis, acute pancreatitis, or peptic ulcer disease if on the left, especially if the patient has associated anorexia, nausea, or emesis. Acquired or congenital ureteropelvic junction obstruction may cause a similar constellation of symptoms. Symptoms frequently occur on an intermittent basis following a drinking binge or consumption of large quantities of fluid.

Partial or complete staghorn calculi that are present in the renal pelvis are not necessarily obstructive. In the absence of obstruction, these patients often have surprisingly few symptoms such as flank or back pain. Recurrent urinary tract infections frequently culminate in radiographic evaluation with the discovery of a staghorn calculus. If untreated, these "silent" staghorn calculi can often lead to significant morbidity, including renal deterioration, infectious complications, or both.

3. Upper and mid ureter—Stones or other objects in the upper or mid ureter often cause severe, sharp back (costovertebral angle) or flank pain. The pain may be more severe and intermittent if the stone is progressing down the ureter and causing intermittent obstruction. A stone that becomes lodged at a particular site may cause less pain, especially if it is only partially obstructive. Stationary calculi that result in high-grade but constant obstruction may allow autoregulatory reflexes and pyelovenous and pyelolymphatic backflow to decompress the upper tract, with diminution in intraluminal pressure gradually easing the pain. Pain associated with ureteral calculi often projects to corresponding dermatomal and spinal nerve root innervation regions. The pain of upper ureteral stones thus radiates to the lumbar region and flank. Midureteral calculi tend to cause pain that radiates caudally and anteriorly toward the mid and lower abdomen in a curved, bandlike fashion. This band initially parallels the lower costal margin but deviates caudad toward the bony pelvis and inguinal ligament. The pain may mimic acute appendicitis if on the right or acute diverticulitis if on the left side, especially if concurrent gastrointestinal symptoms are present.

4. Distal ureter—Calculi in the lower ureter often cause pain that radiates to the groin or testicle in males and the labia majora in females. This referred pain is often generated from the ilioinguinal or genital branch of the genitofemoral nerves. Diagnosis may be confused with testicular torsion or epididymitis. Stones in the intramural ureter may mimic cystitis, urethritis, or prostatitis by causing suprapubic pain, urinary frequency and urgency, dysuria, stranguria, or gross hematuria. Bowel symptoms are not uncommon. In women the diagnosis may be confused with menstrual pain, pelvic inflammatory disease, and ruptured or twisted ovarian cysts. Strictures of the distal ureter from radiation, operative injury, or previous endoscopic procedures can present with similar symptoms. This pain pattern is likely due to the similar innervation of the intramural ureter and bladder.

B. Hematuria

A complete urinalysis helps to confirm the diagnosis of a urinary stone by assessing for hematuria and crystalluria and documenting urinary pH. Patients frequently admit to intermittent gross hematuria or occasional tea-colored urine (old blood). Most patients will have at least microhematuria. Rarely (in 10–15% of cases), complete ureteral obstruction presents without microhematuria.

C. Infection

Magnesium ammonium phosphate (struvite) stones are synonymous with infection stones. They are commonly associated with *Proteus, Pseudomonas, Providencia, Klebsiella,* and *Staphylococcus* infections. They are rarely if ever associated with *Escherichia coli* infections. Calcium phosphate stones are the second variety of stones associated with infections. Calcium phosphate stones with a urine pH < 6.6 are frequently referred to as brushite stones, whereas infectious apatite stones have a urinary pH > 6.6. Rarely, matrix stones with minimal crystalline components are associated with urinary tract infections. All stones, however, may be associated with infections secondary to obstruction and stasis proximal

to the offending calculus. Culture-directed antibiotics should be administered before elective intervention.

Infection may be a contributing factor to pain perception. Uropathogenic bacteria may alter ureteral peristalsis by the production of exotoxins and endotoxins. Local inflammation from infection can lead to chemoreceptor activation and perception of local pain with its corresponding referral pattern.

1. Pyonephrosis—Obstructive calculi may culminate in the development of pyonephrosis. Unlike pyelonephritis, pyonephrosis implies gross pus in an obstructed collecting system. It is an extreme form of infected hydronephrosis. Presentation is variable and may range from asymptomatic bacteriuria to florid urosepsis. Bladder urine cultures may be negative. Radiographic investigations are frequently nondiagnostic. Renal ultrasonography may be misguiding because of the nonspecific and variable appearance of pyonephrosis. Renal urine aspiration is the only way to make the definitive diagnosis. If the condition is noted at the time of a percutaneous nephrolithotomy, the procedure should be postponed to allow for adequate percutaneous drainage and treatment with appropriate intravenous antibiotics (Figure 16–8). If unrecognized and untreated, pyonephrosis may develop into a renocutaneous fistula.

2. Xanthogranulomatous pyelonephritis—Xanthogranulomatous pyelonephritis is associated with upper-tract obstruction and infection. One-third of patients present with calculi; two-thirds present with flank pain, fever, and chills. Fifty percent present with persistent bacteriuria. Urinalysis usually shows numerous red and white cells. This condition is a common imitator of other pathologic states of the kidney. It usually presents

Figure 16–8. Bilateral renal calculi seen on scout radiograph with numerous bilateral percutaneous nephrostomy tubes to drain severe bilateral pyonephrosis.

in a unilateral fashion. Open surgical procedures, such as a simple nephrectomy for minimal or nonrenal function, can be challenging owing to marked and extensive reactive tissues.

D. Associated Fever

The association of urinary stones with fever is a relative medical emergency. Signs of clinical sepsis are variable and include fever, tachycardia, hypotension, and cutaneous vasodilation. Costovertebral angle tenderness may be marked with acute upper-tract obstruction; however, it cannot be relied on to be present in instances of long-term obstruction. In such instances a mass may be palpable resulting from a grossly hydronephrotic kidney. Fever associated with urinary tract obstruction requires prompt decompression. This may be accomplished with a retrograde catheter (double-J, or an externalized variety to serve as a port for selective urine collections, injection of contrast material, or both). If retrograde manipulations are unsuccessful, insertion of a percutaneous nephrostomy tube is required.

E. Nausea and Vomiting

Upper-tract obstruction is frequently associated with nausea and vomiting. Intravenous fluids are required to restore a euvolemic state. Intravenous fluids should not be used to force a diuresis in an attempt to push a ureteral stone down the ureter. Effective ureteral peristalsis requires coaptation of the ureteral walls and is most effective in a euvolemic state.

Special Situations

A. Renal Transplantation

Urinary stones associated with renal transplantation are rare. Perirenal nerves are severed at the time of renal harvesting. Classic renal colic is not found in these patients. The patients usually are admitted with the presumptive diagnosis of graft rejection. Only after appropriate radiographic and ultrasonic evaluation is the correct diagnosis made (Figure 16–9).

B. Pregnancy

Renal colic is the most common nonobstetric cause of acute abdominal pain during pregnancy (Figure 16–10). Despite marked hypercalciuria associated with pregnancy, calculi are relatively rare, with an incidence approximating 1:1500 pregnancies. Women with known urinary stone disease do not have an increased risk of stones during pregnancy. The increased filtered load of calcium, uric acid, and sodium from the 25–50% increase in glomerular filtration rate associated with pregnancy has been thought to be a responsible factor in stone development.

Figure 16–9. Scout abdominal radiograph demonstrating renal calculus in a renal transplant in the right iliac fossa. Note native renal vasculature with marked calcifications secondary to malignant diabetes mellitus.

The fetus demands special considerations regarding the potential dangers of radiation exposure (especially during the first trimester), medications, anesthesia, and surgical intervention. About 90% of symptomatic calculi present during the second and third trimesters. Initial investigations can be undertaken with renal ultrasonography and limited abdominal x-rays with appropriate shielding. Treatment requires balancing the safety of the fetus with the health of the mother. Temporizing measures to relieve upper-tract obstruction with a double-J ureteral stent or a percutaneous nephrostomy tube can be performed under local anesthesia. Treatment usually can be delayed until after delivery.

C. Dysmorphia

Patients with severe skeletal dysmorphia that is either congenital (spina bifida, myelomeningocele, cerebral palsy) or acquired (arthritis, traumatic spinal cord injuries) and concurrent urinary calculi represent a unique clinical situation requiring special considerations (Figure 16–11). These skeletal abnormalities may preclude appropriate positioning for ESWL or percutaneous approaches. Calculi on the concave side in a patient with severe scoliosis may eliminate percutaneous

Figure 16–11. Scout abdominal radiograph demonstrating a right renal calculus (arrow) in a patient with severe kyphoscoliosis. Respiratory compromise limited patient positioning for surgery.

Figure 16–10. Scout radiograph demonstrating left renal calculus with double-J ureteral stent in place. Skeletal fetal structures can be appreciated in this pregnant patient.

puncture access between the rib and the posterosuperior iliac spine. Retrograde manipulations may need to be performed with flexible endoscopes due to marked contractures, making conventional dorsal lithotomy positioning impossible. Many such patients have undergone supravesical urinary diversion, so that retrograde access may be limited. Risks that need to be addressed include hypercalciuria associated with immobilization, relative dehydration due to patients' or attendants' attempts to reduce urinary output into external collecting devices, and the potential inability to drink without assistance. A full metabolic evaluation is even more important because these social and physical restrictions may be difficult or impossible to remedy.

D. Obesity

Obesity is a risk factor for the development of urinary calculi. Surgical bypass procedures can cause hyperoxaluria. Massive weight gain or loss also may precipitate stone development. Obesity limits diagnostic and treatment options. A large pannus may limit the physical examination and misguide incisions. Ultrasound examination is hindered by the attenuation of ultrasound beams. Computed tomography, magnetic resonance imaging, fluoroscopy tables, and lithotripters all have weight limitations, and patients weighing more than 300 pounds may be unsuited for diagnosis and treatment with these resources. Standard lithotripters have focal lengths less than 15 cm between the energy source and the F2 target, frequently making treatment of obese patients impossible. A large anterior pannus limits prone positioning on lithotripters. Standard Amplatz nephrostomy sheaths may not be long enough to enter the collecting system. Such sheaths may need to be advanced well below the skin. A preplaced heavy suture eases removal of such sheaths.

Risks of anesthesia are increased and special high-pressure respirators may be required if patients are placed in a prone position for a percutaneous procedure. Careful positioning for open procedures helps to reduce the likelihood of crush injuries and associated rhabdomyolysis. These patients are at increased risk of anesthetic complications. Postoperative prophylaxis for thromboembolic complications should be considered.

E. Medullary Sponge Kidney

Medullary sponge kidney is a common condition characterized by tubular ectasia associated with parenchymal cysts and clefts that predispose to nephrolithiasis in 50% of affected patients. It is most often an asymptomatic condition; however it may present with renal colic, hematuria, or urinary tract infection. It is a radiographic diagnosis. The condition can involve select papillae or, more frequently, can be global. A full metabolic evaluation helps direct appropriate medical therapy.

F. RENAL TUBULAR ACIDOSIS

There are 3 main types of renal tubular acidosis: types I, II, and IV. Type I is associated with renal calculi.

Patients with type I renal tubular acidosis present with persistent acidemia with a low serum bicarbonate value unexplained by hyperventilation or known renal failure. The diagnosis should be suspected in those with a known family history, severe hypocitraturia, nephrocalcinosis, medullary sponge kidney, or a fasting urine pH > 6.0 in the absence of infection. Patients usually present with nephrolithiasis (calcium phosphate), nephrocalcinosis, or osteomalacia (or a combination). This disease can be acquired as an adult or inherited with an autosomal dominant pattern. The diagnosis is confirmed by assessing the patient's response to an acid load. This is frequently produced by a rapid oral ammonium chloride load (0.1 g/kg over 1 h). The dose can be given before bedtime in the evening; the patient is instructed to fast until a second morning voided urine sample and a serum bicarbonate level are obtained. A normal person responds by eliminating the acid load in the urine, resulting in a urinary pH below 5.3. Those who do not respond in this fashion can be said to have type I renal tubular acidosis. Additionally, the diagnosis should be challenged in those with normal citrate values. Treatment is centered on base replacement with potassium citrate or potassium bicarbonate solutions. Urinary citrate levels can be used to monitor effective treatment.

G. ASSOCIATED TUMORS

Squamous cell carcinoma of the upper urinary tract is uncommon but has been associated with calculi in more than 50% of cases. Chronic irritation from calculi or infection may be contributory factors. Upper-tract calculi may predispose patients to transitional cell carcinoma.

H. PEDIATRIC PATIENTS

Urinary calculi are unusual in children. A full and thorough metabolic evaluation should be undertaken. Stone analysis is particularly helpful in directing these investigations. Children born prematurely and given furosemide while in the neonatal intensive care unit are at increased risk of developing urinary stone disease. Treatment may be limited by endoscope size. Preliminary data show no change in renal growth after ESWL.

I. CALICEAL DIVERTICULA

Pyelocaliceal diverticula are cystic urine-containing eventrations of the upper tract lying within the renal parenchyma; they communicate through a narrow channel into the main collecting system (Figure 16–12). These diverticula occur in approximately 0.2–0.5% of the population and are congenital in origin; up to 40% are associated with calculi. Type I diverticula are the most common and are closely related to minor calyces. Type II have a direct communication with the renal pelvis and tend to be larger and symptomatic. Caliceal diverticuli are usually asymptomatic, but patients may complain of flank pain or recurrent urinary tract infections. Frequently many small calculi, rather than a solitary stone, are found in these obstructed cavities. When intervention was required in the past, treatment was with nephrectomy, heminephrectomy, or open surgical unroofing. Less invasive means are used today. Communications with the collecting system are commonly pinpoint and may be difficult to locate through a retrograde approach. Retrograde access into superior pole diverticula has been successful. Surprisingly, treatment may be successful with ESWL if stone fragments are small enough to pass uneventfully. More commonly, percutaneous access and, more recently, laparoscopic means are used with success. Dilation of the caliceal neck, direct cauterization or sclerosis of the caliceal epithelium, or direct cauterization and sclerosis of the caliceal epithelium can help reduce stone recurrence rates.

J. RENAL MALFORMATIONS

Anatomic renal variants such as ectopic kidneys, including the horseshoe kidney, predispose to renal cal-

Figure 16–12. Intravenous pyelogram demonstrating symptomatic right calyceal diverticula with numerous small calculi.

culi due to impaired urinary drainage. Pain symptoms appear to be no different from those reported in patients with normally positioned kidneys. Radiographic diagnosis may be difficult due to the unexpected location of the ureters and kidneys (Figure 16–13). If calculi can be targeted with ESWL, most stone fragments pass surprisingly uneventfully. Large stone burdens should be approached percutaneously as in normally positioned kidneys. Severe outlet obstruction should be corrected with open surgery, and concurrent calculi can be removed at the same setting. Aberrant vasculature should be appreciated before percutaneous and open procedures are undertaken.

Evaluation

A. DIFFERENTIAL DIAGNOSIS

Urinary stones can mimic other retroperitoneal and peritoneal pathologic states. A full differential diagnosis of the acute abdomen should be made, including acute appendicitis, ectopic and unrecognized pregnancies, ovarian pathologic conditions including twisted ovarian cysts, diverticular disease, bowel obstruction, biliary stones with and without obstruction, peptic ulcer dis-

Figure 16–13. Scout abdominal radiograph demonstrating horseshoe kidney with lateral ureteral deviation and double-J ureteral stent. Extraosseous calcifications are left lower calyceal stones.

ease, acute renal artery embolism, and abdominal aortic aneurysm—to mention a few. Peritoneal signs should be sought during physical examination.

B. HISTORY

A proper evaluation requires a thorough medical history. The nature of the pain should be evaluated, including its onset; character; potential radiation; activities that exacerbate or ease the pain; associated nausea, vomiting, or gross hematuria; and a history of similar pain. Patients with previous stones frequently have had similar types of pain in the past, but not always.

C. RISK FACTORS

1. Crystalluria—Crystalluria is a risk factor for stones. Stone formers, especially those with calcium oxalate stones, frequently excrete more calcium oxalate crystals, and those crystals are larger than normal > 12 μm). The rate of stone formation is proportional to the percentage of large crystals and crystal aggregates. Crystal production is determined by the saturation of each salt and the urinary concentration of inhibitors and promoters. Urine samples should be fresh; they should be centrifuged and examined immediately for optimum results. Cystine crystals are hexagonal; struvite stones appear as coffin lids; brushite ($CaHPO_4$) stones are splinterlike and may aggregate with a spokelike center; calcium apatite—$(Ca)_5(PO_4)_3(OH)$—and uric acid crystals appear as amorphous powder because the crystals are so small; calcium oxalate dihydrate stones are bipyramids; and calcium oxalate monohydrate stones are small biconcave ovals that may appear as a dumbbell. Cystine and struvite crystals are always abnormal and require further investigations. Other crystals are frequently found in normal urinalyses.

2. Socioeconomic factors—Renal stones are more common in affluent, industrialized countries. Immigrants from less industrialized nations gradually increase their stone incidence and eventually match that of the indigenous population. Use of soft water does not decrease the incidence of urinary stones.

3. Diet—Diet may have a significant impact on the incidence of urinary stones. As per capita income increases the average diet changes, with an increase in saturated and unsaturated fatty acids, an increase in animal protein and sugar, and a decrease in dietary fiber, vegetable protein, and unrefined carbohydrates. A less energy-dense diet may decrease the incidence of stones. This fact has been documented during war years when diets containing minimal fat and protein resulted in a decreased incidence of stones. Vegetarians may have a decreased incidence of urinary stones. High sodium intake is associated with increased urinary sodium, calcium, and pH, and a decreased excretion of citrate; this increases the likelihood of calcium salt crystallization because the urinary saturation of monosodium urate and calcium phosphate (brushite) is increased. Fluid intake and urine output may have an effect on urinary stone disease. The average daily urinary output in stone formers is 1.6 L/d.

4. Occupation—Occupation can have an impact on the incidence of urinary stones. Physicians and other white-collar workers have an increased incidence of stones compared with manual laborers. This finding may be related to differences in diet but also may be related to physical activity; physical activity may agitate urine and dislodge crystal aggregates. Individuals exposed to high temperatures may develop higher concentrations of solutes owing to dehydration, which may have an impact on the incidence of stones.

5. Climate—Individuals living in hot climates are prone to dehydration, which results in an increased incidence of urinary stones, especially uric acid calculi. Although heat may cause a higher fluid intake, sweat loss results in lowered voided volumes. Hot climates usually expose people to more ultraviolet light, increasing vitamin D_3 production. Increased calcium and oxalate excretion has been correlated with increased exposure time to sunlight. This factor has more impact on light-skinned people and may help explain why African Americans in the United States have a decreased stone incidence.

6. Family history—A family history of urinary stones is associated with an increased incidence of renal calculi. A patient with stones is twice as likely as a stone-free cohort to have at least one first-degree relative with renal stones (30% versus 15%). Those with a family history of stones have an increased incidence of multiple and early recurrences. Spouses of patients with calcium oxalate stones have an increased incidence of stones; this may be related to environmental or dietary factors.

7. Medications—A thorough history of medications taken may provide valuable insight into the cause of urinary calculi. The antihypertensive medication triamterene is found as a component of several medications, including Dyazide, and has been associated with urinary calculi with increasing frequency. Long-term use of antacids containing silica has been associated with the development of silicate stones. Carbonic anhydrase inhibitors may be associated with urinary stone disease (10–20% incidence). The long-term effect of sodium- and calcium-containing medications on the development of renal calculi is not known. Protease inhibitors in immunocompromised patients are associated with radiolucent calculi.

D. Physical Examination

A detailed physical examination is an essential component of the evaluation of any patient suspected of having a urinary calculus. The patient presenting with acute renal colic typically is in severe pain, often attempting to find relief in multiple, frequently bizarre, positions. This fact helps differentiate patients with this condition from those with peritonitis, who are afraid to move. Systemic components of renal colic may be obvious, with tachycardia, sweating, and nausea often prominent. Costovertebral angle tenderness may be apparent. An abdominal mass may be palpable in patients with long-standing obstructive urinary calculi and severe hydronephrosis.

Fever, hypotension, and cutaneous vasodilation may be apparent in patients with urosepsis. In such instances there is an urgent need for decompression of the obstructed urinary tract, massive intravenous fluid resuscitation, and intravenous antibiotics. Occasionally, intensive care support is needed.

A thorough abdominal examination should exclude other causes of abdominal pain. Abdominal tumors, abdominal aortic aneurysms, herniated lumbar disks, and pregnancy may mimic renal colic. Referred pain may be similar owing to common afferent neural pathways. Intestinal ileus may be associated with renal colic or other intraperitoneal or retroperitoneal processes. Bladder palpation should be performed because urinary retention may present with pain similar to renal colic. Incarcerated inguinal hernias, epididymitis, orchitis, and female pelvic pathologic states may mimic urinary stone disease. A rectal examination helps exclude other pathologic conditions.

E. Radiologic Investigations

1. Computed tomography—Noncontrast spiral CT scans are now the imaging modality of choice in patients presenting with acute renal colic. It is rapid and is now less expensive than an intravenous pyelogram (IVP). It images other peritoneal and retroperitoneal structures and helps when the diagnosis is uncertain. It does not depend on an experienced radiologic technician to obtain appropriate oblique views when there is confusion with overlying bowel gas in a nonprepped abdomen. There is no need for intravenous contrast. Distal ureteral calculi can be confused with phleboliths. These images do not give anatomic details as seen on an IVP (for example, a bifid collecting system) that may be important in planning intervention. If intravenous contrast material is used during the study, a KUB film can give additional helpful information. Uric acid stones are visualized no differently from calcium oxalate stones. Matrix calculi have adequate amounts of calcium to be visualized easily by CT.

2. Intravenous pyelography—An intravenous pyelogram (IVP) can document simultaneously nephrolithiasis and upper-tract anatomy. Extraosseous calcifications on radiographs may be erroneously assumed to be urinary tract calculi (Figure 16–14). Oblique views easily differentiate gallstones from right renal calculi. Static hard-copy films can be interpreted by most clinicians. Anecdotally, small ureteral stones have passed spontaneously during such studies. An inadequate bowel preparation, associated ileus and swallowed air, and lack of available technicians may result in a less than ideal study when obtained during acute renal colic. A delayed, planned IVP may result in a superior study.

Acute forniceal rupture is not uncommonly associated with a highly obstructive ureteral calculus. It may result in dramatic radiographs but is of no clinical significance, and no intervention is required. The rupture may be precipitated by the osmotic diuresis of the intravenous contrast agent based solely on radiographs.

Figure 16–14. Scout abdominal radiograph demonstrating large extraosseous calcification that represents a uterine fibroid. This easily could be confused with a large bladder calculus.

3. Tomography—Renal tomography is useful to identify calculi in the kidney when oblique views are not helpful. It visualizes the kidney in a coronal plane at a set distance from the top of the x-ray table. This study may help identify poorly opacified calculi, especially when interfering abdominal gas or morbid obesity make KUB films suboptimal.

4. KUB films and directed ultrasonography—A KUB film and renal ultrasound may be as effective as an IVP in establishing a diagnosis. The ultrasound examination should be directed by notation of suspicious areas seen on a KUB film; it is, however, operator-dependent. The distal ureter is easily visualized through the acoustic window of a full bladder. Edema and small calculi missed on an IVP can be appreciated with such studies.

5. Retrograde pyelography—Retrograde pyelography occasionally is required to delineate upper-tract anatomy and localize small or radiolucent offending calculi. Bulb ureterograms frequently leak contrast material back into the bladder, resulting in a suboptimal study. Advancing an angiographic exchange catheter with or without the aid of a guidewire 3–4 cm into the ureter is an alternative technique. Intermittent fluoroscopic images direct appropriate injection volumes and help reduce the likelihood of pyelolymphatic, pyelosinus, and pyelovenous reflux.

6. Magnetic resonance imaging—Magnetic resonance imaging is a poor study to document urinary stone disease.

7. Nuclear scintigraphy—Nuclear scintigraphic imaging of stones has recently been appreciated. Bisphosphonate markers can identify even small calculi that are difficult to appreciate on a conventional KUB film (Figure 16–15). Differential radioactive uptake dependent on stone composition appreciated during in vitro studies cannot be appreciated on in vivo studies. Nuclear scintigraphy cannot delineate upper-tract anatomy in sufficient detail to help direct a therapeutic plan.

Intervention

A. CONSERVATIVE OBSERVATION

Most ureteral calculi pass and do not require intervention. Spontaneous passage depends on stone size, shape, location, and associated ureteral edema (which is likely to depend on the length of time that a stone has not progressed). Ureteral calculi 4–5 mm in size have a 40–50% chance of spontaneous passage. In contrast, calculi > 6 mm have a less than 5% chance of spontaneous passage. This does not mean that a 1-cm stone will not pass or that a 1- to 2-mm stone will always pass uneventfully.

A

B

C

Figure 16–15. **A:** Scout abdominal radiograph demonstrating large left staghorn renal calculus. **B:** Nuclear scintigraphic evaluation of renal calculi. Posterior view demonstrating uptake on large left staghorn calculus after furosemide (lasix) diuresis. Note right kidney with uptake in lower pole. **C:** Follow-up tomogram confirms calculus (arrow) in right lower pole missed on initial radiograph.

The vast majority of stones that pass do so within a 6-week period after the onset of symptoms. Ureteral calculi discovered in the distal ureter at the time of presentation have a 50% chance of spontaneous passage, in contrast to a 25% and 10% chance in the mid and proximal ureter, respectively.

B. Dissolution Agents

The effectiveness of dissolution agents depends on stone surface area, stone type, volume of irrigant, and mode of delivery. Oral alkalinizing agents include sodium or potassium bicarbonate and potassium citrate. Extra care should be employed in patients susceptible to congestive heart failure or renal failure. Citrate is metabolized to bicarbonate and comes in a variety of preparations. Polycitra contains potassium and sodium citrate and citric acid. Bictra contains only sodium citrate and citric acid. Food does not alter the effectiveness of these agents. Alternatively, orange juice alkalinizes urine. Intravenous alkalinization is effective with 1/6 molar sodium lactate.

Intrarenal alkalinization may be performed successfully under a low-pressure system (< 25 cm water pressure). This may be achieved through a percutaneous nephrostomy tube or an externalized retrograde catheter. A manometer, similar to those used for central venous pressure monitoring, is cheap, available, and practical. Agents include sodium bicarbonate, 2–4 ampules in 1 L of normal saline, producing a urinary pH between 7.5 and 9.0. Tromethamine-E and tromethamine can produce urinary pHs of 8.0–10.5 and are especially effective with pH-sensitive calculi as in uric acid and cystine lithiasis.

Cystine calculi can be dissolved with a variety of thiols, including D-penicillamine (0.5% solution), N-acetylcysteine (2–5% solution), and alpha-mercapto-propionylglycine (Thiola) (5% solution).

Struvite stone dissolution requires acidification and may be achieved successfully with Suby's G solution and hemiacidrin (Renacidin). Urinary pH may get down to 4.0. Hemiacidrin must be used with sterile urine and careful monitoring of serum magnesium levels is required. The Food and Drug Administration has not approved hemiacidrin for upper-tract irrigations, and thus appropriate informed consent is required.

C. Relief of Obstruction

Urinary stone disease may result in significant morbidity and possible mortality in the presence of obstruction, especially with concurrent infection. A patient with obstructive urinary calculi with fever and infected urine requires emergent drainage. Retrograde pyelography to define upper-tract anatomy is logically followed by retrograde placement of a double-J ureteral stent. On occasion such catheters are unable to bypass the offending calculus or may perforate the ureter. In such situations one must be prepared to place a percutaneous nephrostomy tube.

D. Extracorporeal Shock Wave Lithotripsy

Extracorporeal shock wave lithotripsy has revolutionized the treatment of urinary stones. The concept of using shock waves to fragment stones was noted in the 1950s in Russia. However, it was during the investigation of pitting on supersonic aircraft that Dornier, a German aircraft corporation, rediscovered that shock waves originating from passing debris in the atmosphere can crack something that is hard. It was the ingenious application of a model developed in hopes of understanding such shock waves that extracorporeal (outside the body) shock wave lithotripsy (ESWL) emerged. The first clinical application with successful fragmentation of renal calculi was in 1980. The HM-1 (Human Model-1) lithotriptor underwent modifications in 1982 leading to the HM-2 and, finally, to the widespread application of the HM-3 in 1983 (Figure 16–16). Since then, thousands of lithotriptors have been put into use around the world, with millions of patients successfully treated.

All require an energy source to create the shock wave, a coupling mechanism to transfer the energy from outside to inside the body, and either fluoroscopic or ultrasonic modes, or both, to identify and position the calculi at a focus of converging shock waves. They differ in generated pain and anesthetic or anesthesiologist requirements, consumable components, size, mobility, cost, and durability. Focal peak pressures (400–1500 bar), focal dimensions (6 × 28 mm to 50 × 15 mm), modular design, utilization to help increase mobility of frozen joints, varied distances (12–17.0 cm) between focus 1 (the shock wave source) and focus 2 (the target), and purchase price differentiate the various machines available today.

1. Shock wave physics—In contrast to the familiar ultrasonic wave with sinusoidal characteristics and longitudinal mechanical properties, acoustic shock waves are unharmonic and have nonlinear pressure characteristics. There is a steep rise in pressure amplitude that results in compressive forces (Figure 16–17). There are 2 basic types of shock wave sources, supersonic and finite amplitude emitters.

Supersonic emitters release energy in a confined space, thereby producing an expanding plasma and an acoustic shock wave. Such shock waves occur in nature—the familiar thunderstorm with lightning (an electrical discharge) followed by thunder (an acoustic sonic boom) is an analogous situation. Under controlled conditions, such an acoustic shock wave can successfully fragment calculi. The initial compression wave travels faster than the speed of sound in water and rapidly slows down to that speed. The traveling pressure wave is reduced in a nonlinear fashion. Medical applications have focused such waves to concentrate energy on a calculus (Figure 16–18).

Finite amplitude emitters, in contrast to point source energy systems, create pulsed acoustic shock waves by displacing a surface activated by electrical discharge. There are 2 major types of finite amplitude emitters, piezoceramic and electromagnetic. The piezoceramic variety results in a shock wave after an electrical discharge causes the ceramic component to elongate in such a manner that the surface is displaced and an

Figure 16–16. Diagrammatic representation of a Dornier HM-3 lithotriptor.

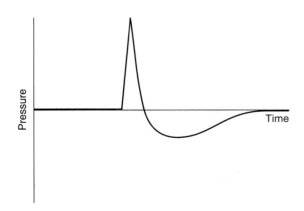

Figure 16–17. Shock wave. Vertical axis represents pressure and horizontal axis represents time.

acoustic pulse is generated. Thousands of such components placed on the concave side of a spheric surface directed toward a focus result in high stress, strain, and cavitation pressures (Figure 16–19). Electromagnetic systems are similar in concept to a stereo speaker system. An electrical discharge to a slab, adjacent to an insulating foil, creates an electric current that repulses a metal membrane, displacing it and generating an acoustic pulse into an adjacent medium. These waves need to be focused toward the offending stone.

All shock waves, despite their source, are capable of fragmenting stones when focused. Fragmentation is achieved by erosion and shattering (Figure 16–20). Cavitational forces result in erosion at the entry and exit sites of the shock wave. Shattering results from energy absorption with stress, strain, and shear forces. Surrounding biologic tissues are resilient because they are not brittle nor are the shock waves focused on them.

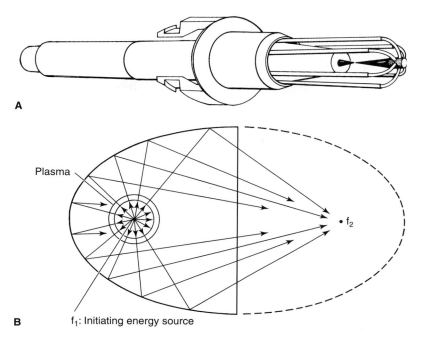

A

Plasma

f_1: Initiating energy source

$\bullet f_2$

B

Figure 16–18. **A:** Supersonic shock wave emission from a spark gap electrode. **B:** Reflecting the shock wave from focus 1 to focus 2 allows for stone fragmentation.

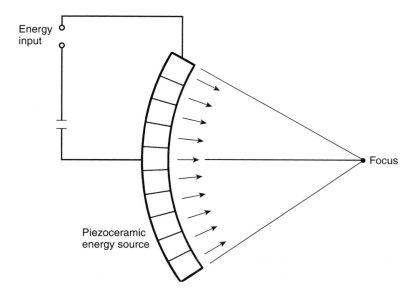

Energy input

Focus

Piezoceramic energy source

Figure 16–19. Piezoceramic finite amplitude emitter. Ceramic components are placed on the concave surface of a sphere and each component is directed to an identified focus.

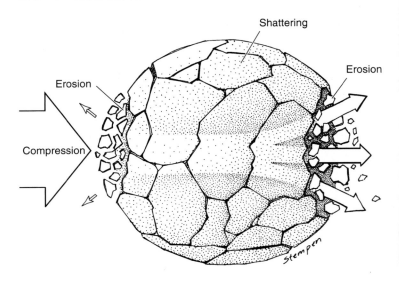

Figure 16-20. Incoming shock waves result in fragmentation from erosion and shattering.

2. Preoperative evaluation—Physical examination should be as thorough as in preparation for any other surgical procedure. Vital signs including blood pressure should be noted. Body habitus including any gross skeletal abnormalities, contractures, or excessive weight (> 300 lb) may severely limit or preclude ESWL. Borderline individuals require simulation before treatment. Pregnant women and patients with large abdominal aortic aneurysms or uncorrectable bleeding disorders should not be treated with ESWL. Individuals with cardiac pacemakers should be thoroughly evaluated by a cardiologist. If ESWL is contemplated, a cardiologist with thorough knowledge and with the ability to override the pacemaker should be present in the lithotripsy suite.

3. Intraoperative considerations—

a. Stone localization—Proper patient positioning is a prerequisite for successful lithotripsy. Palpating the patient's ribs and pelvic bony girdle can approximate appropriate positioning. Anterior located kidneys, medial oriented portions of a horseshoe kidney, or transplant kidneys are best treated in the prone position. Understanding positioning options with the various lithotriptors available today is required to optimize therapy.

Small or poorly calcified calculi can be difficult to image with fluoroscopy, irrespective of their location. Placing a ureteral catheter identifies known anatomy and supplies an injection port for radiocontrast agents. A poorly calcified caliceal calculus can be identified by injecting dilute contrast agents into the collecting system and then focusing on the appropriate calyx or filling defect. In patients who cannot have retrograde

stents placed, intravenous contrast agents may be used to help localize and thus focus on such stones.

b. Fluoroscopic imaging—The conditions for fluoroscopic imaging include appropriate collimation, dimmed room lighting, and adequate bowel preparation to decrease bothersome bowel gas and thus decrease radiation exposure and improve the quality of the fluoroscopic image. Intermittent fluoroscopy reveals movement of calculi with respiration and is helpful in locating and focusing on offending calculi.

c. Ultrasonic imaging—Ultrasound localization has the advantage of eliminating radiation exposure to the patient or lithotripsy team. There are 2 basic types: the coaxial unit, aligned with the shock wave generator, and the articulating arm unit with a mobile transducer. Ultrasound can easily identify radiolucent or small calculi that are difficult to visualize with fluoroscopy. However, ureteral or other medially located calculi may be difficult or impossible to identify, especially in nonobstructive collecting systems. Visualization may be difficult or impossible with obese patients. Proficiency in ultrasound localization and assessment of fragmentation has a longer learning curve than that of fluoroscopy. Ultrasound images may be confusing when multiple stones or stone fragments are present.

d. Coupling—Successful fragmentation requires effective coupling. Coupling devices should have properties similar to those of human skin. Optimal systems should prevent pain, ecchymoses, hematomas, or skin breakdown. Interfaces between gas and tissue can result in tissue damage. Air bubbles entrapped by hair, by bandages from prior percutaneous procedures, or by inadequately degassed fluid, or air in coupling cushions can significantly impede directed shock waves and result in skin ecchymoses or breakdown. Despite adequate coupling, fragmentation may be inadequate owing to refraction and reflection of shock waves at tissue interfaces, especially with obese patients.

The water bath provides good coupling. Submersion of patients can result in profound hemodynamic changes including peripheral venous compression resulting in increased right atrial pressure, increased pulmonary capillary wedge pressure, and increased cardiac index. These hemodynamic changes should be appreciated and appropriate monitoring should be used in individuals with marginal cardiovascular reserve.

In contrast, water cushion coupling systems have decreased water demands. A coupling gel like those used with ultrasonography provides an excellent interface with skin. The volume of such water cushions can frequently be adjusted to help focus calculi when patients are either extremely thin (eg, children) or obese. Very small patients may require an interposed bag (1–3 L) of normal saline to help with coupling. Both water coupling systems require degassed water to decrease water bubbles.

e. Shock wave triggering—Triggering shock waves with the electrocardiogram was originally performed to decrease cardiac dysrhythmias. The lithotriptor would sense the large swing of the QRS complex and initiate the shock wave 20 ms later; this would decrease shock waves during the repolarization phase of the cardiac cycle (myocardium is most sensitive during this time). If cardiac dysrhythmias occur, interruption of the procedure frequently stops them. However, if they continue, standard medical therapy is effective. Conceptually, it makes more sense to trigger the shock waves in response to the respiratory cycle to optimize accurate focusing on the offending calculi that move with respiratory motion. Such systems are available. Many lithotriptors are now triggered without electrocardiogram gating and with unusual associated cardiac dysrhythmias. This can speed up therapy, especially in those with slow heart rates that are not amenable to pharmacologic manipulation.

f. Fragmentation—Safe shock wave dosage is unknown. Shock waves induce trauma, including intrarenal and perirenal hemorrhage and edema, and thus the minimal shocks needed to achieve fragmentation should be given. Casual overtreatment should be avoided since long-term complications are not yet known.

Determination of adequate fragmentation during treatment may be difficult. Initial sharp edges become fuzzy or blurred and have a shotgun-blast-like appearance. Stones that were initially visualized may disappear after successful fragmentation. Intermittent visualization ensures accurate focusing and assessment of progress and eventual termination of the procedure.

Bilateral nephrolithiasis may be treated in the same setting. One must first approach the side that is symptomatic or potentially more troublesome. If there is uncertainty concerning a large stone burden, one or more double-J catheters should be placed to decrease the likelihood of bilateral obstruction.

4. Postoperative care—Patients should be encouraged to maintain an active ambulatory status to facilitate stone passage. Gross hematuria should resolve during the first postoperative week. Fluid intake should be encouraged. Follow-up in approximately 2 weeks for discussion and evaluation of a KUB and renal ultrasonography will help assess success of fragmentation and passage of gravel. Patients may return to work as soon as they feel comfortable in doing so.

Abdominal pain may be related to the shock waves. Severe pain unresponsive to routine intravenous or oral medications should alert the physician for possible rare (0.66%) perirenal hematomas. In such a situation, CT should then be undertaken to stage the injury.

The potential association of ESWL with the development of hypertension has not been substantiated. Long-term data are still being collected.

Stone burden correlates with postoperative complications. Steinstrasse (stone street) or columnation of stone gravel in a ureter can be frustrating. It should be specifically ruled out when postoperative radiographs are evaluated. Asymptomatic individuals can be followed up with serial KUBs and ultrasonography. Severe pain or fever requires intervention. Percutaneous nephrostomy drainage is usually uncomplicated owing to the associated hydronephrosis. Decompressing the collecting system allows for effective coaptation of the ureteral walls and encourages resolution of the problem. It is only in the rare patient that steinstrasse does not resolve with the procedures outlined; such cases require retrograde endoscopic manipulations to relieve the obstructed stone fragments. Usually one finds one or two relatively large fragments that are obstructing. With their removal the columnation of fragments resolves.

Patients with large renal pelvic calculi (> 1.5 cm) have a stone-free rate at 3 months approximating 75%, in comparison with those with a similar stone in a lower calyx, which approximates only 50%. Patients with small renal pelvic stones (< 1.5 cm) have approximately a 90% stone-free rate in comparison to those with similar stones in a middle calyx (approximately 75%) or lower calyx (approximately 70%). Lower calyceal stone-free rates are increased with a small stone burden, a short and wide infundibulum, and a nonacute infundibulo-pelvic angle. Overall, approximately 75% of patients with renal calculi treated with ESWL become stone-free in 3 months. As stones increase in size, stone-free rates decrease, more so in the lower and middle calyces than in superior calyceal and renal pelvic locations.

E. Ureteroscopic Stone Extraction

Ureteroscopic stone extraction is highly efficacious for lower ureteral calculi. The use of small-caliber ureteroscopes and the advent of balloon dilation or ureteral access sheaths have increased stone-free rates dramatically. Even relatively large-caliber endoscopes without balloon dilation are effective in lower ureteral stone retrieval. Stone-free rates range from 66% to 100% and are dependent on stone burden and location, length of time the stone has been impacted, history of retroperitoneal surgery, and the experience of the operator. Complication rates range from 5% to 30%; the rates increase when manipulations venture into the proximal ureter. Ureteral stricture rates are less than 5%. Postoperative vesicoureteral reflux is extremely rare. Calculi that measure less than 8 mm are frequently removed intact. Round wire stone baskets can be torqued to help entrap stone or stone fragments. Flat wire baskets should be used with caution; if twisted, they can develop sharp, knifelike edges resulting in ureteral injury. Excessive force with any instrument in the ureter may result in ureteral injury.

A variety of lithotrites can be placed through an ureteroscope, including electrohydraulic; solid, and hollow-core ultrasonic probes; a variety of laser systems; and pneumatic systems such as the Swiss lithoclast. Electrohydraulic lithotrites have power settings as high as 120 V that result in a cavitation bubble, followed by collapse of this bubble causing subsequent shock waves. Care should be taken to keep the tip of the electrode away from surrounding tissue and the tip of the endoscope. Ultrasonic lithotrites have a piezoceramic energy source that converts electrical energy into ultrasonic waves in the range of 25,000 Hz. This vibratory action is effective in fragmenting calculi. Hollow probes can suction stone fragments and debris simultaneously. Laser systems are discussed elsewhere in this book. The electromechanical impactors are similar to jackhammers with a movable pistonlike tip that fragments calculi.

F. Percutaneous Nephrolithotomy

Percutaneous removal of renal and proximal ureteral calculi is the treatment of choice for large (> 2.5 cm) calculi, those resistant to ESWL, select lower pole calyceal stones with a narrow, long infundibulum and an acute infundibulo-pelvic angle, and instances with evidence of obstruction; the method can rapidly establish a stone-free status. Needle puncture is directed by fluoroscopy, ultrasound, or both, and is routinely placed from the posterior axillary line into a posterior inferior calyx. Superior caliceal puncture may be required, and in such situations care should be taken to avoid injury to the pleura, lungs, spleen, and liver. Tract dilation is performed by sequential plastic dilators (Amplatz system), telescoping metal dilators (Alken), or balloon dilation with a backloaded Amplatz sheath. Tracts placed during open renal procedures are frequently tortuous and suboptimal for subsequent endourologic procedures.

Percutaneous extraction of calculi requires patience and perseverance. Hard-copy radiographs help to confirm a stone-free status. Remaining calculi can be retrieved with the aid of flexible endoscopes, additional percutaneous puncture access, follow-up irrigations, ESWL, or additional percutaneous sessions. Realistic goals should be established. Patients should be informed that complex calculi frequently require numerous procedures.

Maintenance of body temperature with appropriate blankets during preoperative patient positioning and with warmed irrigation fluids helps to prevent bleeding diatheses associated with hypothermia. The average blood loss during a percutaneous nephrolithotomy is 2.0–2.8 g/dL of hemoglobin. Multiple percutaneous punctures and renal pelvic perforations are associated with a greater blood loss. Overall, such procedures are safe and effective and have a transfusion rate well below 10%.

G. Open Stone Surgery

Open stone surgery is the classic way to remove calculi. The morbidity of the incision, the possibility of retained stone fragments, and the ease and success of less invasive techniques have made these procedures relatively uncommon when instruments and surgical experience are available. It is mandatory to obtain a radiograph before the incision is made; calculi frequently move. A variety of incisions to access the kidney are available.

H. Pyelolithotomy

Pyelolithotomy is effective, especially with an extrarenal pelvis. A transverse pyelotomy is effective and does not require interruption of the renal arterial blood supply. Inspection with flexible endoscopes helps ensure a stone-free status. Multiple, small renal pelvic calculi and difficult-to-access caliceal calculi can be retrieved with the aid of a coagulum. Coagulum was initially produced from pooled human fibrinogen. The risks of hepatitis and other viral infections have made this method unacceptable. Cryoprecipitate can be obtained from rapid freezing of plasma. Autologous plasma may be used to decrease the incidence of bloodborne infections. The tensile strength of cryoprecipitate is approximately 10 times that of a blood clot. Injected into the renal pelvis, endogenous clotting factors result in a Jello-like coagulum of the collecting system. Small stones are entrapped and removed with the coagulum. A variety of Randall stone forceps help gain access into most of the collecting system.

I. ANATROPHIC NEPHROLITHOTOMY

Anatrophic nephrolithotomy is used with complex staghorn calculi. A complete staghorn calculus is a cast of the renal pelvis and calyces (Figure 16–21). A partial staghorn calculus involves the renal pelvis and extends into at least 2 infundibula. To gain access to the entire collecting system, a longitudinal incision is made on the convex surface of the kidney just posterior to the line of Brödel, taking advantage of the converging anterior and posterior renal blood supplies. Occlusion of the renal artery followed by renal cooling with slushed ice gives a relatively bloodless surgical field. A nerve hook is helpful to tease out calculi. Careful inspection of the entire collecting system helps remove all stones. Repair of narrowed infundibula helps reduce stone recurrence rates. The collecting system is closed followed by the renal capsule. Intraoperative placement of a nephrostomy tube for possible follow-up irrigations or endoscopic inspection or stone retrieval makes hemostasis difficult. Open stone surgery becomes progressively more difficult after the first procedure owing to reactive scar tissue.

J. RADIAL NEPHROTOMY

Radial nephrotomy gives access to limited calyces of the collecting system. An appropriate approach to localized calculi, it is frequently used in blown-out calyces with thin overlying parenchyma. Intraoperative ultrasound helps to localize the calyx and the calculi. Once the kidney has been opened, the introduction of air can make interpretation of subsequent ultrasound scans confusing. A shallow incision of the renal capsule can be followed by puncture into the collecting system. Brain retractors provide excellent exposure. Care should be taken not to force stones through narrow infundibula. Stones may be cut with heavy Mayo scissors, and remaining fragments can be retrieved. Inspection with flexible endoscopes is helpful. Intraoperative radiographs help document a stone-free status.

K. OTHER RENAL PROCEDURES

Partial nephrectomy is appropriate with a large stone burden in a renal pole with marked parenchymal thinning. Caution should be taken with a simple nephrectomy even with a normal contralateral kidney, as stones are frequently associated with a systemic metabolic defect that may recur in the contralateral kidney. What may seem prudent and simple today may be regretted tomorrow.

Other unusual procedures include ileal ureter substitution performed with the hope of decreasing pain with frequent stone passage. Autotransplantation with pyelocystostomy is another option for patients with rare malignant stone disease.

L. URETEROLITHOTOMY

Long-standing ureteral calculi—those inaccessible with endoscopy and those resistant to ESWL—can be extracted with a ureterolithotomy. Again, a preoperative radiograph documents stone location and directs an appropriate incision. The proximal ureter may be approached with a dorsal lumbotomy. An incision lateral to the sacrospinalis muscles allows medial retraction of the quadratus lumborum. The anterior fascicle of the dorsal lumbar fascia must be incised to gain proper exposure despite the appearance of potentially opening the peritoneum. Once the ureter is identified, a vessel loop or a Babcock clamp should be placed proximal to the stone to prevent frustrating stone migration. Extension of this incision is limited superiorly by the 12th rib and inferiorly by the iliac crest. A longitudinal incision over the stone with a hooked blade exposes the calculus. The nerve hook is excellent to help tease out the stone. A flank or anterior abdominal muscle splitting incision gives excellent exposure to mid and distal ureteral stones.

Prevention

In general, 50% of patients experience recurrent urinary stones within 5 years without prophylactic intervention. Appropriate education and preventive measures are best instituted with a motivated patient after spontaneous stone passage or surgical stone removal. Risk factors as described previously should be identified

Figure 16–21. Plain abdominal radiograph demonstrating complete staghorn calculus with renal pelvic extension into all infundibula and calyces.

and modified, if possible. Irrespective of the final metabolic evaluation and stone analysis, the patient's fluid intake should be about 1.6 L/24 h. Fluids should be encouraged during mealtime. Additionally, liquids should be increased approximately 2 h after meals. Water produced as a metabolic by-product reaches its nadir at this time, and thus the body is relatively dehydrated. Fluid ingestion also should be encouraged to force a nighttime diuresis adequate to awaken the patient to void. Awakening and ambulating to void limit urinary stasis and offer an opportunity to ingest additional fluids. These lifestyle changes are difficult to maintain and should be encouraged during subsequent office visits. Motivated patients who regularly return to a urinary stone clinic have a reduced stone recurrence rate that is probably due to increased compliance.

A. METABOLIC EVALUATION

A systematic metabolic evaluation should be instituted after a patient has recovered from urinary stone intervention or spontaneous stone passage. Stone analysis should be obtained to help direct the workup. An outpatient urine collection during typical activities and fluid intake helps unmask significant abnormalities. An initial 24-h urine collection for calcium stone formers should include tests for calcium, uric acid, oxalate, citrate, sodium, volume, and pH. An open dialog with local laboratories helps to standardize collection routines and determine whether an outside laboratory is preferred. Baseline serum levels for blood urea nitrogen, creatinine, calcium, phosphorous, and uric acid are appropriate.

Hypercalciuria is the most common abnormality. To differentiate among hypercalciuria types I, II, and III, a patient should be placed on a sodium- and calcium-restricted diet for a few days to a week. This is easily achieved (100 mEq/d) by eliminating table salt and reducing obviously salty foods. Calcium is restricted (400–500 mg) by excluding dairy products. A repeat 24-h urine collection is evaluated for calcium. A urinary calcium level < 250 mg/d confirms a diagnosis of dietary-dependent hypercalciuria, type II. Type I and type III hypercalciuria must be differentiated in patients with urinary calcium levels > 250 mg/d. A calcium binder such as cellulose phosphate is prescribed (5 g 3 times daily with meals) for a few days. This is followed by a repeat 24-h urine calcium level and parathyroid hormone blood value. Patients who have type I absorptive hypercalciuria have at least a 50% drop in urinary calcium levels and normal parathyroid hormone levels.

Hyperuricosuria, hyperoxaluria, and hypocitraturia calcium stone formers can be treated appropriately and followed with repeat 24-h urine collections. Many calcium stone formers have multiple defects; although one treatment may reverse one defect, it may exacerbate others. Subsequent 24-h urine collections are critical for effective long-term follow-up and stone prevention. Treatment of cystinuria should be titrated with repeat 24-h cystine levels. Repeat urine cultures should be obtained in patients with infectious calculi.

B. ORAL MEDICATIONS

1. Alkalinizing pH agents—Potassium citrate is an oral agent that elevates urinary pH effectively by 0.7–0.8 pH units. Typical dosing is 60 mEq in 3 or 4 divided doses daily. It is available in wax-matrix 10-mEq tablets, liquid preparations, and crystals that must be mixed with fluids. The effect is maintained over many years. Care should be taken in patients susceptible to hyperkalemia, those with renal failure, and those taking potassium-sparing diuretics. Although the medication is usually well tolerated, some patients may complain of abdominal discomfort, especially with tablet preparations. It is indicated in those with calcium oxalate calculi secondary to hypocitraturia (< 320 mg/d), including those with renal tubular acidosis. Potassium citrate also may be used effectively to treat uric acid lithiasis and nonsevere forms of hyperuricosuric calcium nephrolithiasis.

Sodium and potassium bicarbonate, orange juice, and lemonade are alternative alkalinizing agents. There are no effective long-term urinary acidifying agents.

2. Gastrointestinal absorption inhibitor—Cellulose phosphate binds calcium in the gut and thereby inhibits calcium absorption and urinary excretion. It is a popular drug in the treatment of absorptive hypercalciuria type I with recurrent calcium nephrolithiasis, although it only prevents new stone formation. Patients should have normal parathyroid hormone values, normal serum calcium and phosphate values, no evidence of bone disease, and evidence of increased intestinal calcium absorption. The drug decreases the urinary saturation of calcium phosphate and calcium oxalate. It may increase urinary oxalate and urinary phosphate levels. A typical starting dosage is 5 g 3 times daily with meals; the dosage may be titrated by following 24-h urinary calcium levels. Urinary magnesium, calcium, oxalate, and sodium levels and serum parathyroid hormone should be monitored 1–2 times yearly. Magnesium supplements are frequently required and should be taken at least 1 h before or after cellulose phosphate is taken. Cellulose phosphate is associated with a sodium load and should be used with caution in those with congestive heart failure. Gastrointestinal side effects are infrequent; they include dyspepsia and loose bowel movements.

Cellulose phosphate may be suboptimal treatment for postmenopausal women who are at risk for bone disease. An alternative treatment for such patients would be hydrochlorothiazides supplemented with potassium citrate to offset the potential hypokalemia and hypocitraturia.

3. Phosphate supplementation—Renal phosphate leak is best treated by replacing phosphate. Phosphate absorption may be inhibited in the presence of aluminum-, magnesium-, or calcium-containing antacids. This treatment should be used with caution in digitalized patients and in those with severe renal failure, Addison disease, or severe hepatic dysfunction. It is generally well tolerated. Dosing can begin with 250 mg 3–4 times daily and may be doubled depending on follow-up serum electrolyte, calcium, and phosphorus levels.

4. Diuretics—Thiazides can correct the renal calcium leak associated with renal hypercalciuria. This prevents a secondary hyperparathyroid state and its associated elevated vitamin D synthesis and intestinal calcium absorption. A rapid decrease in urinary calcium excretion is appreciated and is sustained long-term (> 10 years). A starting dose of 25 mg may be titrated based on urinary calcium levels. Side effects are usually well tolerated. Potassium levels should be monitored. Hypokalemia induces a hypocitraturic state; potassium replacement corrects the hypokalemia and its associated hypocitraturia.

Thiazides result in a transient decrease in urinary calcium excretion in absorptive hypercalciurics. Urinary calcium excretion rebounds to pretreatment values in 50% of such patients after 4–5 years of therapy. Dietary changes are not believed to be responsible for this phenomenon. Thiazides do not restore normal intestinal absorption of calcium.

5. Calcium supplementation—Enteric hyperoxaluric calcium nephrolithiasis is effectively treated with calcium supplements. Calcium gluconate and calcium citrate are better absorbed and are more effective in increasing serum calcium availability than are other forms of calcium. Calcium carbonate, calcium phosphate, and oyster shell are forms of calcium that are less efficiently absorbed; they remain in the intestinal lumen, available to bind oxalate, thus reducing its absorption. These less efficiently absorbed forms of calcium are optimal to treat enteric hyperoxaluric calcium nephrolithiasis and must be given with meals to be effective.

6. Uric acid-lowering medications—Allopurinol is used to treat hyperuricosuric calcium nephrolithiasis with or without hyperuricemia. Unlike uricosuric agents that reduce serum uric acid levels by increasing urinary uric acid excretion, allopurinol is a xanthine-oxidase inhibitor and reduces both serum and urinary levels of uric acid. It has no impact on the biosynthesis of purines; rather, it acts exclusively on purine catabolism. Elevated levels of xanthine and hypoxanthine in the urine secondary to allopurinol have not been associated with nephrolithiasis. Allopurinol is a potentially dangerous drug and should be discontinued at the first appearance of a skin rash, which infrequently may be fatal. Therapy can start at 300 mg per day. It is tolerated best when taken after meals.

7. Urease inhibitor—Acetohydroxamic acid is an effective adjunctive treatment in those with chronic urea-splitting urinary tract infections associated with struvite stones. Acetohydroxamic acid reversibly inhibits bacterial urease, decreasing urinary ammonia levels, and will subsequently acidify urine. It is best used as prophylaxis after removal of struvite stones. It also may be used after unsuccessful attempts at curative surgical removal of calculi or culture-specific antibiotic therapy. Patients with serum creatinine > 2.5 mg/dL are unable to achieve therapeutic urinary levels. Acetohydroxamic acid is not effective with non-urease-producing bacteria. Long-term data (> 7 years) are unavailable. A significant number of patients complain of side effects, including headaches that are usually short-lived and responsive to aspirin compounds. Other frequent complaints include nausea, vomiting, anorexia, nervousness, and depression. A typical dosing regimen is one 250 mg tablet 3 or 4 times daily (total dosage: 10–15 mg/kg/d).

8. Prevention of cystine calculi—Conservative measures, including massive fluid intake and urinary alkalinization, are frequently inadequate to control cystine stone formation. Penicillamine, the same drug that is used to chelate excess copper in the treatment of Wilson disease, undergoes a thiol-disulfide exchange with cystine. This reduces the amount of urinary cystine that is relatively insoluble. Cystine solubility is pH-dependent (pH 5.0: 150–300 mg/L; pH 7.0: 200–400 mg/L; pH 7.5: 220–500 mg/L). D-Penicillamine is associated with numerous and frequent side effects, including rashes and hematologic, renal, and hepatic abnormalities. An initial dosage of 250 mg daily in 3–4 divided doses may help reduce severe side effects. It may be increased gradually to 2 g/d. Dosage should be titrated with quantitative urinary cystine values. Penicillamine increases the requirement of pyridoxine (vitamin B_6), which should be supplemented with 25–50 mg/d.

Mercaptopropionylglycine (Thiola) is better tolerated by patients than is penicillamine. Mercaptopropionylglycine, a reducing agent, binds to the sulfide portion of cystine, forming a mixed disulfide (Thiola-cysteine) water-soluble compound. It may retard the rate of new stone formation. The dosage should be titrated with repeat 24-h urinary cystine values. An initial dosage may be 200–300 mg 3 times daily, either 1 h before or 2 h after each meal. Side effects are not infrequent and may include drug fever; nausea, vomiting, and gastrointestinal upset; rash, wrinkling, or friable skin; lupuslike symptoms, decreased taste perception; and a variety of hematologic disorders.

BLADDER STONES

Bladder calculi usually are a manifestation of an underlying pathologic condition, including voiding dysfunction or a foreign body. Voiding dysfunction may be due to a urethral stricture, benign prostatic hyperplasia, bladder neck contracture, or flaccid or spastic neurogenic bladder, all of which result in static urine. Foreign bodies such as Foley catheters and forgotten double-J ureteral catheters can serve as nidi for stones (Figure 16–22). Most bladder calculi are seen in men. In developing countries, they are frequently found in prepubescent boys. Stone analysis frequently reveals ammonium urate, uric acid, or calcium oxalate stones. A solitary bladder stone is the rule, but there are numerous stones in 25% of patients (Figure 16–23). Patients present with irritative voiding symptoms, intermittent urinary stream, urinary tract infections, hematuria, or pelvic pain. Physical examination is unrevealing. A large percentage of bladder stones are radiolucent (uric acid).

Ultrasound of the bladder identifies the stone with its characteristic shadowing. The stone moves with changing body position.

Stones within a ureterocoele do not move with body position (Figure 16–24) as seen on ultrasound examination. They frequently are nonobstructive. Endoscopic incision and stone removal rarely result in vesicoureteral reflux. The mode of stone removal for other bladder stones should be directed by the underlying cause.

Early instruments used to remove bladder calculi were both clever and bizarre. Simple mechanical crushing devices are still used today. Mechanical lithotrites should be used with caution to prevent bladder injury when the jaws are closed. Ensuring partially full bladder and endoscopic visualization of unrestricted lateral movement before forceful crushing of the stones helps reduce this troublesome complication. Cystolitholapaxy allows most stones to be broken and subsequently removed through a cystoscope. Electrohydraulic, ultrasonic, laser, and pneumatic lithotrites similar to those used through a nephroscope are effective. Cystolithotomy can be performed through a small abdominal incision.

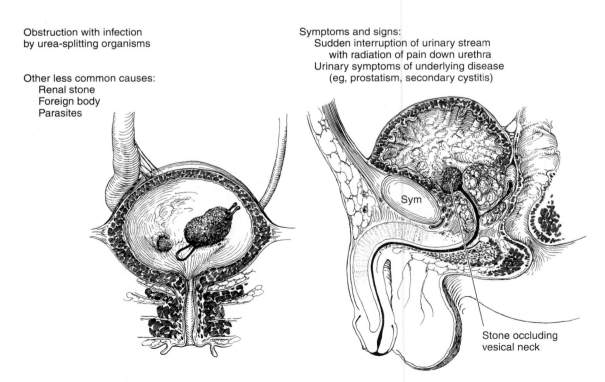

Obstruction with infection
by urea-splitting organisms

Other less common causes:
   Renal stone
   Foreign body
   Parasites

Symptoms and signs:
   Sudden interruption of urinary stream
     with radiation of pain down urethra
   Urinary symptoms of underlying disease
     (eg, prostatism, secondary cystitis)

Sym

Stone occluding
vesical neck

Figure 16–22. Genesis and symptoms and signs of vesical calculus.

A   B

Figure 16–23. **A:** Plain abdominal radiograph demonstrating 2 bladder calculi. **B:** Gross picture of removed bladder calculi. Note the characteristic shape of jack-stones typically composed of uric acid.

A   B

Figure 16–24. **A:** Scout abdominal radiograph demonstrating extraosseous calcification in the region of the bladder. **B:** Intravenous pyelogram demonstrates stone to be within a ureterocele.

PROSTATIC & SEMINAL VESICLE STONES

Prostatic calculi are found within the prostate gland per se and are found uncommonly within the prostatic urethra. They are thought to represent calcified corpora amylacea and are rarely found in boys. Usually small and numerous, they are noted to be tannish-gray in color during transurethral resection of the prostate. They are commonly located at the margin of the surgically resected adenoma and are composed of calcium phosphate. Although usually of no clinical significance, rarely they are associated with chronic prostatitis. Large prostatic calculi may be misinterpreted as a carcinoma. The prostate is usually mobile, however, and a radiograph or transrectal ultrasound helps to confirm the diagnosis.

Seminal vesicle stones are smooth and hard and are extremely rare. They may be associated with hematospermia. Physical examination reveals a stony hard gland, and when multiple stones are present, a crunching sensation may be noted. These stones occasionally are confused with tuberculosis of the seminal vesicle.

URETHRAL & PREPUCIAL STONES

Urethral calculi usually originate from the bladder and rarely from the upper tracts. Most ureteral stones that pass spontaneously into the bladder can pass through the urethra unimpeded. Urethral stones may develop secondary to urinary stasis, secondary to a urethral diverticulum, near urethral strictures, or at sites of previous surgery. Most urethral stones in men present in the prostatic or bulbar regions and are solitary. Patients with recurrent pendulous urethral calculi without evidence of other pathologic conditions should be suspected of self-introduction of such stones in an attempt to obtain pain medications or for attention, as seen in Munchausen syndrome.

Females rarely develop urethral calculi owing to their short urethra and a lower incidence of bladder calculi. Most urethral stones found in women are associated with urethral diverticula.

Symptoms are similar to bladder calculi—intermittent urinary stream, terminal hematuria, and infection. The stones may present with dribbling or during acute urinary retention. Pain may be severe and, in men, may radiate to the tip of the penis. The diagnosis may be confirmed by palpation, endoscopic visualization, or radiographic study.

Treatment should be directed by the underlying cause. Stones associated with a dense urethral stricture or complex diverticula can be removed during definitive open surgical repair. Small stones may be grasped successfully and removed intact. More frequently they need to be fragmented and removed. Long-standing, large impacted stones are best removed through a urethrotomy.

Preputial calculi are rare and usually occur in adults. They develop secondary to a severe obstructive phimosis. They may occur secondary to poor hygiene with inspissated smegma. Diagnosis is confirmed by palpation. Treating the underlying cause with a dorsal preputial slit or a formal circumcision prevents recurrent calculi.

REFERENCES

Ions In Urinary Stone Formation

Calcium

Ackermann D et al: Influence of calcium content in mineral water on chemistry and crystallization conditions in urine of calcium stone formers. Eur Urol 1988;14:305.

Breslau NA et al: Relationship of animal protein-rich diet to kidney stone formation and calcium metabolism. J Clin Endocrinol Metab 1988;66:140.

Fellstrom B et al: Dietary habits in renal stone patients compared with healthy subjects. Br J Urol 1989;63:575.

Fuss M et al: Calcitonin secretion in idiopathic renal stone formers. J Bone Miner Res 1991;6:35.

Fuss M et al: Low calcium diet in idiopathic urolithiasis: A risk factor for osteopenia as great as in primary hyperparathyroidism. Br J Urol 1990;65:560.

Gentle DL et al: Geriatric nephrolithiasis. J Urol 1997;158:2221.

Harvey JA, Pak CY: Gouty diathesis and sarcoidosis in patient with recurrent calcium nephrolithiasis. J Urol 1988;139:1287.

Iguchi M et al: Glucose metabolism in renal stone patients. Urol Int 1993;51:185.

Jabbour N et al: The natural history of renal stone disease after parathyroidectomy for primary hyperparathyroidism. Surg Gynecol Obstet 1991;172:25.

Jahnen A et al: Dietary fibre: The effectiveness of a high bran intake in reducing renal calcium excretion. Urol Res 1992;20:3.

Jarrar K et al: Relationship between 1,25-dihydroxyvitamin-D, calcium and uric acid in urinary stone formers. Urol Int 1996;56:16.

Langley SE, Fry CH: The influence of pH on urinary ionized [Ca2+]: Differences between urinary tract stone formers and normal subjects. Br J Urol 1997;79:8.

Litin RB, Diessner GR, Keating FR: Urinary excretion of calcium in patients with renal lithiasis. J Urol 1961;86:17.

Menon M: Value of repeated analyses of 24-hour urine in recurrent calcium urolithiasis. J Urol 1995;153:555.

Milosevic D et al: Determination of urine saturation with computer program EQUIL 2 as a method for estimation of the risk of urolithiasis. J Chem Inf Comput Sci 1998;38:646.

Parivar F, Low RK, Stoller ML: The influence of diet on urinary stone disease. J Urol 1996;155:432.

Preminger GM, Sakhaee K, Pak CY: Alkali action on the urinary crystallization of calcium salts: Contrasting responses to sodium citrate and potassium citrate. J Urol 1988;139:240.

Tiselius HG: Metabolic evaluation of patients with stone disease. Urol Int 1997;59:131.

Trinchieri A et al: The influence of diet on urinary risk factors for stones in healthy subjects and idiopathic renal calcium stone formers. Br J Urol 1991;67:230.

Urivetzky M et al: Urinary excretion of oxalate by patients with renal hypercalciuric stone disease: Effect of chronic treatment with hydrochlorothiazide. Urology 1991;37:327.

Oxalate

Bataille P et al: Diet, vitamin D and vertebral mineral density in hypercalciuric calcium stone formers. Kidney Int 1991; 39:1193.

Brown JM et al: The variability and dietary dependence of urinary oxalate excretion in recurrent calcium stone formers. Ann Clin Biochem 1987;24:385.

Grases F, Sohnel O: Mechanism of oxalocalcic renal calculi generation. Int Urol Nephrol 1993;25:209.

Hatch M: Oxalate status in stone-formers: Two distinct hyperoxaluric entities. Urol Res 1993;21:55.

Kohri K, Garside J, Blacklock NJ: The role of magnesium in calcium oxalate urolithiasis. Br J Urol 1988;61:107.

Koide T et al: Promotive effect of urine from patients with primary hyperparathyroidism on calcium oxalate crystal aggregation in an in vitro whole urine system. J Urol 1988;140:1571.

Kok DJ et al: The effects of dietary excesses in animal protein and in sodium on the composition and the crystallization kinetics of calcium oxalate monohydrate in urines of healthy men. J Clin Endocrinol Metab 1990;71:861.

Laminski NA et al: Hyperoxaluria in patients with recurrent calcium oxalate calculi: Dietary and other risk factors. Br J Urol 1991;68:454.

Lanzalaco AC et al: The influence of urinary macromolecules on calcium oxalate monohydrate crystal growth. J Urol 1988; 139:190.

Nakada T et al: Effect of high-calcium diet on urinary oxalate excretion in urinary stone formers. Eur Urol 1988;15:264.

Ryall RL: The scientific basis of calcium oxalate urolithiasis: Predilection and precipitation, promotion and proscription. World J Urol 1993;11:59.

Ryall RL et al: Urinary risk factors in calcium oxalate stone disease: Comparison of men and women. Br J Urol 1987;60:480.

Tiselius HG: Standardized estimate of the ion activity product of calcium oxalate in urine from renal stone formers. Eur Urol 1989;16:48.

Williams HE, Wandzilak TR: Oxalate synthesis, transport and the hyperoxaluric syndromes. J Urol 1989;141:742.

Phosphate

Gault MH et al: Bacteriology of urinary tract stones. J Urol 1995; 153:1164.

Kohri K et al: Relationship between metabolic acidosis and calcium phosphate urinary stone formation in women. Int Urol Nephrol 1991;23:307.

Lingeman JE, Siegel YI, Steele B: Metabolic evaluation of infected renal lithiasis: Clinical relevance. J Endourol 1995;9:51.

Ohman S, Larsson L, Tiselius HG: Clinical significance of phosphate in calcium oxalate renal stones. Ann Clin Biochem 1992;29:59.

Schwille PO et al: Urinary phosphate excretion in the pathophysiology of idiopathic recurrent calcium urolithiasis: Hormonal interactions and lipid metabolism. Urol Res 1997;25:417.

Tiselius HG, Larsson L: Calcium phosphate: An important crystal phase in patients with recurrent calcium stone formation? Urol Res 1993;21:175.

Tozuka K et al: Study of calcium phosphate crystalluria. J Urol 1987;138:326.

Uric Acid

Asplin JR: Uric acid stones. Semin Nephrol 1996;16:412.

Fukushima T et al: Prophylaxis of uric acid stone in patients with inflammatory bowel disease following extensive colonic resection. Gastroenterol Jpn 1991;26:430.

Gutman AB, Yu TF: Uric acid nephrolithiasis. Am J Med 1968; 45:756.

Jarrar K et al: Relationship between 1,25-dihydroxyvitamin-D, calcium and uric acid in urinary stone formers. Urol Int 1996; 56:16.

Stoller ML: Gout and stones or stones and gout? J Urol 1995; 154:1670.

Teichman JM et al: Holmium:YAG lithotripsy: Photothermal mechanism converts uric acid calculi to cyanide. J Urol 1998; 160:320.

Yu TF: Urolithiasis in hyperuricemia and gout. J Urol 1981; 126:424.

Cystine

Chow GK, Streem SB: Contemporary urological intervention for cystinuric patients: Immediate and long-term impact and implications. J Urol 1998;160:341, 344.

Gupta M, Bolton DM, Stoller ML: Etiology and management of cystine lithiasis. Urology 1995;45:344.

Katz G et al: Place of extracorporeal shock-wave lithotripsy (ESWL) in management of cystine calculi. Urology 1990; 36:124.

Sakhaee K, Poindexter JR, Pak CY: The spectrum of metabolic abnormalities in patients with cystine nephrolithiasis. J Urol 1989;141:819.

Stoller ML et al: Acalculous cystinuria. J Endourol 1997;11:235.

Xanthine

Badertscher E et al: Xanthine calculi presenting at 1 month of age. Eur J Pediatr 1993;152:252.

Kario K, Matsuo T, Tankawa H: Xanthine urolithiasis: Ultrastructure analysis of renal and bladder calculi. Int Urol Nephrol 1991;23:317.

Triamterene

Dooley DP, Callsen ME, Geiling JA: Triamterene nephrolithiasis. Milit Med 1989;154:126.

Silicate

Lee MH et al: Silica stone—Development due to long time oral trisilicate intake. Scand J Urol Nephrol 1993;27:267.

Matrix Urinary Calculi

Binette JP, Binette MB: The matrix of urinary tract stones: Protein composition, antigenicity, and ultrastructure. Scanning Microsc 1991;5:1029.

Iwata H et al: The organic matrix of urinary uric acid crystals. J Urol 1988;139:607.

Urinary Stone Inhibitors

Citrate

Alvarez Arroyo MV, Traba ML, Rapado A: Hypocitraturia as a pathogenic risk factor in the mixed (calcium oxalate/uric acid) renal stones. Urol Int 1992;48:342.

Alvarez-Arroyo MV et al: Role of citric acid in primary hyperparathyroidism with renal lithiasis. Urol Res 1992;20:88.

Coe FL, Nakagawa Y, Parks JH: Inhibitors within the nephron. Am J Kidney Dis 1991;17:407.

Grases F et al: Evolution of lithogenic urinary parameters with a low dose potassium citrate treatment. Int Urol Nephrol 1998;30:1.

Hojgaard I, Tiselius HG: The effects of citrate and urinary macromolecules on the aggregation of hydroxyapatite crystals in solutions with a composition similar to that in the distal tubule. Urol Res 1998;26:89.

Mandel NS, Mandel GS, Hasegawa AT: The effect of some urinary stone inhibitors on membrane interaction potentials of stone crystals. J Urol 1987;138:557.

Pak CY: Citrate and renal calculi: New insights and future directions. Am J Kidney Dis 1991;17:420.

Pak CY: Southwestern Internal Medicine Conference: Medical management of nephrolithiasis—a new, simplified approach for general practice. Am J Med Sci 1997;313:215.

Sakhaee K et al: Alkali absorption and citrate excretion in calcium nephrolithiasis. J Bone Miner Res 1993;8:789.

Seltzer MA et al: Dietary manipulation with lemonade to treat hypocitraturic calcium nephrolithiasis. J Urol 1996;156:907.

Singh RK et al: Circadian periodicity of urinary inhibitor of calcium oxalate crystallization in healthy Indians and renal stone formers. Eur Urol 1993;24:387.

Orthophosphates & Pyrophosphates

Schwille PO et al: Urinary pyrophosphate in patients with recurrent calcium urolithiasis and in healthy controls: A re-evaluation. J Urol 1988;140:239.

Wolf JS, Stoller ML: Inhibition of calculi fragment growth by metal bisphosphonate complexes demonstrated with a new assay measuring the surface activity of urolithiasis inhibitors. J Urol 1994;152:1609.

Urinary Proteins

Baggio B et al: Correction of erythrocyte abnormalities in idiopathic calcium-oxalate nephrolithiasis and reduction of urinary oxalate by oral glycosaminoglycans. Lancet 1991; 338:403.

Buck AC, Davies RL, Harrison T: The protective role of eicosapentaenoic acid (EPA) in the pathogenesis of nephrolithiasis. J Urol 1991;146:188.

Edyvane KA et al: Macromolecules inhibit calcium oxalate crystal growth and aggregation in whole human urine. Clin Chim Acta 1987;167:329.

Hesse A, Wuzel H, Vahlensieck W: Significance of glycosaminoglycans for the formation of calcium oxalate stones. Am J Kidney Dis 1991;17:414.

Khan SR: Interactions between stone-forming calcific crystals and macromolecules. Urol Int 1997;59:59.

Singhal GD et al: Urinary mucoprotein in pediatric urolithiasis. J Pediatr Surg 1987;22:218.

Winter P et al: Extracorporeal shock wave lithotripsy and glycosaminoglycans in urine. Int Urol Nephrol 1998;30:113.

Trace Elements

Gentle DL et al: Protease inhibitor-induced urolithiasis. Urology 1997;50:508.

Komleh K et al: Zinc, copper and manganese in serum, urine and stones. Int Urol Nephrol 1990;22:113.

Li LC et al: Inhibitory effect of fluoride on renal stone formation in rats. Urol Int 1992;48:336.

Puche RC et al: Increased fractional excretion of sulphate in stone formers. Br J Urol 1993;71:523.

Su CJ et al: Effect of magnesium on calcium oxalate urolithiasis. J Urol 1991;145:1092.

Wandt MA, Underhill LG: Covariance biplot analysis of trace element concentrations in urinary stones. Br J Urol 1988; 61:474.

2,8-Dihydroxyadenine Urolithiasis

Fye KH et al: Adenine phosphoribosyltransferase deficiency with renal deposition of 2,8-dihydroxyadenine leading to nephrolithiasis and chronic renal failure. Arch Int Med 1993; 153:767.

Hesse A et al: 2,8-Dihydroxyadeninuria: Laboratory diagnosis and therapy control. Urol Int 1988;43:174.

Kamatani N et al: Identification of a compound heterozygote for adenine phosphoribosyltransferase deficiency (APRT*J/APART*Q0) leading to 2,8-dihydroxyadenine urolithiasis. Hum Gen 1990;85:500.

Renal Tubular Acidosis

Buckalew VM Jr: Nephrolithiasis in renal tubular acidosis. J Urol 1989;141:731.

Caruana RJ, Buckalew VM Jr: The syndrome of distal (type 1) renal tubular acidosis: Clinical and laboratory findings in 58 cases. Medicine 1988;67:84.

Homayoon K: Spontaneous steinstrasse due to renal tubular acidosis. Br J Urol 1996;77:610.

Osther PJ et al: Pathophysiology of incomplete renal tubular acidosis in recurrent renal stone formers: Evidence of disturbed calcium, bone and citrate metabolism. Urol Res 1993;21:169.

Schneeberger W, Hesse A, Vahlensieck W: Recurrent nephrolithiasis in renal tubular acidosis: Metabolic profiles, therapy and course. Urol Res 1992;20:98.

Singh PP et al: A study of recurrent stone formers with special reference to renal tubular acidosis. Urol Res 1995;23:201.

Urinary Stone Disease In Uncommon Situations

Spinal Cord Dysfunction

Hall MK et al: Renal calculi in spinal cord–injured patient: Association with reflux, bladder stones, and Foley catheter drainage. Urology 1989;34:126.

Nath M, Wheeler JS Jr, Walter JS: Urologic aspects of traumatic central cord syndrome. J Am Paraplegia Soc 1993;16(3):160.

Vaidyanathan S et al: Recurrent bilateral renal calculi in a tetraplegic patient. Spinal Cord 1998;36:454.

Wan J et al: Urinary tract status of patients with neurogenic dysfunction presenting with upper tract stone disease. J Urol 1992;148:1126.

Pregnancy

Denstedt JD, Razvi H: Management of urinary calculi during pregnancy. J Urol 1992;148:1072, 1074.

Erturk E, Ptak AM, Monaghan J: Fertility measures in women after extracorporeal shockwave lithotripsy of distal ureteral stones. J Endourol 1997;11:315.

Gorton E, Whitfield HN: Renal calculi in pregnancy. Br J Urol 1997;80:(Suppl 1):4.

Shokeir AA, Mutabagani H: Rigid ureteroscopy in pregnant women. Br J Urol 1998;81:678.

Strothers L, Lee LM: Renal colic in pregnancy. J Urol 1992; 148:1383.

Renal Transplantation

Benoit G et al: Treatment of kidney graft lithiasis. Transplantation Proc 1995;27:1743.

Caldwell TC, Burns JR: Current operative management of urinary calculi after renal transplantation. J Urol 1988;140:1360.

Cho DK et al: Urinary calculi in renal transplant recipients. Transplantation 1988;45:899.

Dumoulin G et al: Lack of increased urinary calcium-oxalate supersaturation in long-term kidney transplant recipients. Kidney Int 1997;51:804.

Makisalo H et al: Urological complications after 2084 consecutive kidney transplantations. Transplantation Proc 1997;29:152.

Obesity

Hofmann R, Stoller ML: Endoscopic and open stone surgery in morbidly obese patients. J Urol 1992;148:1108.

Anatomic Renal Anomalies

Baskin LS, Floth A, Stoller ML: The horseshoe kidney: Therapeutic considerations with urolithiasis. J Endourol 1989;(3):51.

Cussenot O et al: Anatomical bases of percutaneous surgery for calculi in horseshoe kidney. Surg Radiol Anat 1992;14:209.

Locke DR et al: Extracorporeal shock-wave lithotripsy in horseshoe kidneys. Urology 1990;35:407.

Torres VE et al: Renal stone disease in autosomal dominant polycystic kidney disease. Am J Kidney Dis 1993;22:513.

Pediatrics

MacDonald I, Azmy AF: Recurrent and residual renal calculi in children. Br J Urol 1988;61:395.

Perrone HC et al: Urolithiasis in childhood: Metabolic evaluation. Pediatr Nephrol 1992;6:54.

Caliceal Diverticulae

Ellis JH et al: Stones and infection in renal caliceal diverticula: Treatment with percutaneous procedures. AJR 1991; 156:995.

Lang EK: Percutaneous infundibuloplasty: Management of calyceal diverticula and infundibular stenosis. Radiology 1991; 181:871.

Tumors

Mhiri MN et al: Association between squamous cell carcinoma of the renal pelvis and calculi. Br J Urol 1989;64:201.

Medical Therapy

Burns JR, Cargill JG III: Kinetics of dissolution of calcium oxalate calculi with calcium-chelating irrigating solutions. J Urol 1987;137:530.

Hymes LC, Warshaw BL: Thiazide diuretics for the treatment of children with idiopathic hypercalciuria and hematuria. J Urol 1987;138:1217.

Insogna KL et al: Trichlormethiazide and oral phosphate therapy in patients with absorptive hypercalciuria. J Urol 1989;141:269.

Mitwalli A et al: Control of hyperoxaluria with large doses of pyridoxine in patients with kidney stones. Int Urol Nephrol 1988;20:353.

Pak CY: Prevention and treatment of kidney stones: Role of medical prevention. J Urol 1989;141:798.

Preminger GM: The metabolic evaluation of patients with recurrent nephrolithiasis: A review of comprehensive and simplified approaches. J Urol 1989;141:760.

Stegmayr B et al: Urinary tract calculi dissolved by means of Renacidin: An experimental study. Scand J Urol Nephrol 1990;24:215.

Surgical Therapy

Assimos DG et al: A comparison of anatrophic nephrolithotomy and percutaneous nephrolithotomy with and without extracorporeal shock wave lithotripsy for management of patients with staghorn calculi. J Urol 1991;145:710.

Extracorporeal Shock Wave Lithotripsy

Barcena M et al: EMLA cream for renal extracorporeal shock wave lithotripsy in ambulatory patients. Eur J Anaesthesiol 1996;13:373.

Baskin LS, Floth A, Stoller ML: Monitored anesthesia care with the standard Dornier HM3 lithotriptor. J Endourol 1990;4:49.

Chaussy CG et al: First clinical experience with extracorporeally induced destruction of kidney stones by shock waves. J Urol 1982;127:417.

Drach GW et al: Report of the United States cooperative study of extracorporeal shock wave lithotripsy. J Urol 1986;135:1127.

Dretler SP: Stone fragility: A new therapeutic distinction. In: Lingeman JE, Newman DM (editors): *Shock Wave Lithotripsy: State of the Art.* Plenum Press, 1988.

Elbahnasy AM et al: Lower caliceal stone clearance after shock wave lithotripsy or ureteroscopy: The impact of lower pole radiographic anatomy. J Urol 1998;159:676.

Gleeson MJ, Shabsigh R, Griffith DP: Outcome of extracorporeal shock wave lithotripsy in patients with multiple renal calculi based on stone burden and location. J Endourol 1988;2:145.

Heine G: Physical aspects of shock-wave treatment. In: Gravenstein JS, Peter K (editors): *Extracorporeal Shock Wave Lithotripsy for Renal Stone Disease.* Butterworths, 1986.

Jewett MA et al: A randomized controlled trial to assess the incidence of new onset hypertension in patients after shock wave lithotripsy for asymptomatic renal calculi. J Urol 1998; 160:1241.

Kamihira O et al: Long-term stone recurrence rate after extracorporeal shock wave lithotripsy. J Urol 1996;156:1267.

Kaude JV et al: Renal morphology and function immediately after extracorporeal shock wave lithotripsy. AJR 1985;145:305.

Lingeman JE, Woods JR, Toth PD: Blood pressure changes following extracorporeal shock wave lithotripsy and other forms of treatment for nephrolithiasis. JAMA 1990;263:1789.

Lingeman JE et al: Shock wave lithotripsy with the Dornier MFL 5000 lithotriptor using an external fixed rate signal. J Urol 1995;154:951.

Low RL et al: Outcome assessment of double-J stents during extracorporeal shock wave lithotripsy of small, solitary renal calculi. J Endourol 1996;10:341.

Politis G, Griffith DP: ESWL: Stone-free efficacy based on stone size and location. World J Urol 1987;5:255.

Sen S et al: Effect of extracorporeal shock wave lithotripsy on glomerular and tubular functions. Int Urol Nephrol 1996; 28:309.

Stoller ML, Litt L, Salazar RG: Severe hemorrhage after extracorporeal shock-wave lithotripsy. Ann Intern Med 1989;111:612.

Streem SB, Yost A, Mascha E: Clinical implications of clinically insignificant stone fragments after extracorporeal shock wave lithotripsy. J Urol 1996;155:1186.

Percutaneous Nephrostolithotomy

Candela J et al: "Tubeless" percutaneous surgery: A new advance in the technique of percutaneous renal surgery. Tech Urol 1997;3:6.

Knoll LD et al: Long-term followup in patients with cystine urinary calculi treated by percutaneous ultrasonic lithotripsy. J Urol 1988;140:246.

Lam HS et al: Staghorn calculi: Analysis of treatment results between initial percutaneous nephrostolithotomy and extracorporeal shock wave lithotripsy monotherapy with reference to surface area. J Urol 1992;147:1219.

Lingeman JE et al: Comparison of results and morbidity of percutaneous nephrostolithotomy and extracorporeal shock wave lithotripsy. J Urol 1987;138:485.

Meretyk S et al: Complete staghorn calculi: Random prospective comparison between extracorporeal shock wave lithotripsy monotherapy and combined with percutaneous nephrostolithotomy. J Urol 1997;157:780.

Streem SB: Long-term incidence and risk factors for recurrent stones following percutaneous nephrostolithotomy or percutaneous nephrostolithotomy/extracorporeal shock wave lithotripsy for infection related calculi. J Urol 1995;153:584.

Ureteroscopy

Bagley DH: Removal of upper urinary tract calculi with flexible ureteropyeloscopy. Urology 1990;35:412.

Seeger AR, Rittenberg MH, Bagley DH: Ureteropyeloscopic removal of ureteral calculi. J Urol 1988;139:1180.

Stoller ML et al: Ureteroscopy without routine balloon dilatation: An outcome assessment. J Urol 1992;147:1238.

Injuries to the Genitourinary Tract   17

Jack W. McAninch, MD

EMERGENCY DIAGNOSIS & MANAGEMENT

About 10% of all injuries seen in the emergency room involve the genitourinary system to some extent. Many of them are subtle and difficult to define and require great diagnostic expertise. Early diagnosis is essential to prevent serious complications.

Initial assessment should include control of hemorrhage and shock along with resuscitation as required. Resuscitation may require intravenous lines and a urethral catheter in seriously injured patients. In men, before the catheter is inserted, the urethral meatus should be examined carefully for the presence of blood.

The history should include a detailed description of the accident. In cases involving gunshot wounds, the type and caliber of the weapon should be determined, since high-velocity projectiles cause much more extensive damage.

The abdomen and genitalia should be examined for evidence of contusions or subcutaneous hematomas, which might indicate deeper injuries to the retroperitoneum and pelvic structures. Fractures of the lower ribs are often associated with renal injuries, and pelvic fractures often accompany bladder and urethral injuries. Diffuse abdominal tenderness is consistent with perforated bowel, free intraperitoneal blood or urine, or retroperitoneal hematoma.

Patients who do not have life-threatening injuries and whose blood pressure is stable can undergo more deliberate radiographic studies. This provides more definitive staging of the injury.

Special Examinations (Figures 17–1 through 17–3)

When genitourinary tract injury is suspected on the basis of the history and physical examination, additional studies are required to establish its extent.

A. CATHETERIZATION AND ASSESSMENT OF INJURY

Assessment of the injury should be done in an orderly fashion so that accurate and complete information is obtained. This process of defining the extent of injury is termed **staging.** The algorithms (Figures 17–1 through 17–3) outline the staging process for urogenital trauma.

1. Catheterization—Blood at the urethral meatus in men indicates urethral injury; catheterization should not be attempted if blood is present, but retrograde urethrography should be done immediately. If no blood is present at the meatus, a urethral catheter can be carefully passed to the bladder to recover urine; microscopic or gross hematuria indicates urinary system injury. If catheterization is traumatic despite the greatest care, the significance of hematuria cannot be determined, and other studies must be done to investigate the possibility of urinary system injury.

2. Computed tomography (CT)—Abdominal CT with contrast media is the best imaging study to detect and stage renal and retroperitoneal injuries. It can define the size and extent of the retroperitoneal hematoma, renal lacerations, urinary extravasation, and renal arterial and venous injuries; additionally, it can detect intra-abdominal injuries (liver, spleen, pancreas, bowel). Spiral CT scanning, now common, is very rapid, but it may not detect renal parenchymal lacerations, urinary extravasation, or ureteral and renal pelvic injuries. We recommend repeat scanning 10 min after the initial study to aid the diagnosis of these conditions.

3. Retrograde cystography—Filling of the bladder with contrast material is essential to establish whether bladder perforations exist. At least 300 mL of contrast medium should be instilled for full vesical distention. A film should be obtained with the bladder filled and a second one after the bladder has emptied itself by gravity drainage. These 2 films establish the degree of bladder injury as well as the size of the surrounding pelvic hematomas.

Cystography with CT is excellent for establishing bladder injury. At the time of scanning, this likewise must be done with retrograde filling of the bladder with 300 mL of contrast media to ensure adequate distention to detect injury.

4. Urethrography—A small (12F) catheter can be inserted into the urethral meatus and 3 mL of water placed in the balloon to hold the catheter in position. After retrograde injection of 20 mL of water-soluble contrast material, the urethra will be clearly outlined on film, and extravasation in the deep bulbar area in case of straddle injury—or free extravasation into the

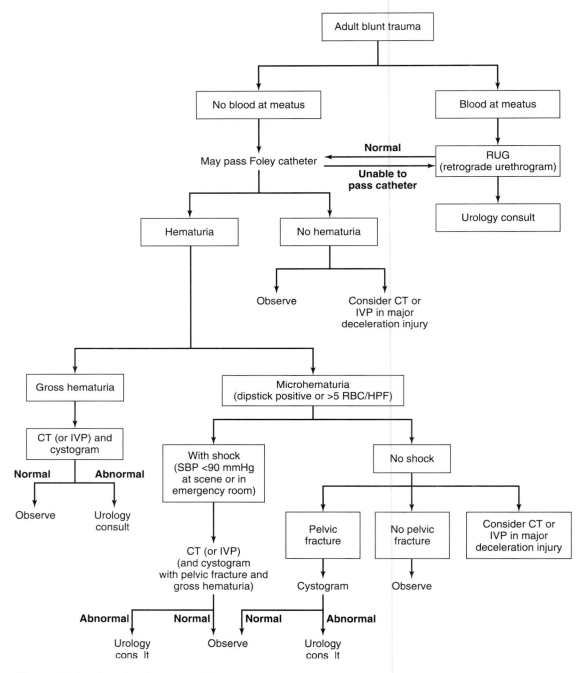

Figure 17–1. Algorithm for staging blunt trauma in adults.

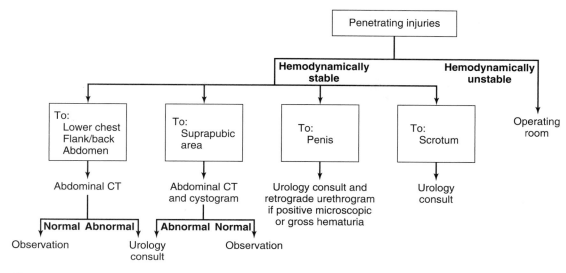

Figure 17–2. Algorithm for staging penetrating trauma in adults.

retropubic space in case of prostatomembranous disruption—will be visualized.

5. Arteriography—Arteriography may help define renal parenchymal and renal vascular injuries. It is also useful in the detection of persistent bleeding from pelvic fractures for purposes of embolization with Gelfoam or autologous clot.

6. Intravenous urography—Intravenous urography can be used to detect renal and ureteral injury. This is best done with high-dose bolus injection of contrast media (2.0 mL/kg) followed by appropriate films.

B. CYSTOSCOPY AND RETROGRADE UROGRAPHY

Cystoscopy and retrograde urography may be useful to detect ureteral injury, but are seldom necessary, since information can be obtained by less invasive techniques.

C. ABDOMINAL SONOGRAPHY

Abdominal sonography has not been shown to add substantial information during initial evaluation of severe abdominal trauma.

INJURIES TO THE KIDNEY

Renal injuries are the most common injuries of the urinary system. The kidney is well protected by heavy lumbar muscles, vertebral bodies, ribs, and the viscera anteriorly. Fractured ribs and transverse vertebral proc-

esses may penetrate the renal parenchyma or vasculature. Most injuries occur from automobile accidents or sporting mishaps, chiefly in men and boys. Kidneys with existing pathologic conditions such as hydronephrosis or malignant tumors are more readily ruptured from mild trauma.

Etiology (Figure 17–4)

Blunt trauma directly to the abdomen, flank, or back is the most common mechanism, accounting for 80–85% of all renal injuries. Trauma may result from motor vehicle accidents, fights, falls, and contact sports. Vehicle collisions at high speed may result in major renal trauma from rapid deceleration and cause major vascular injury. Gunshot and knife wounds cause most penetrating injuries to the kidney; any such wound in the flank area should be regarded as a cause of renal injury until proved otherwise. Associated abdominal visceral injuries are present in 80% of renal penetrating wounds.

Pathology & Classification (Figure 17–5)

A. EARLY PATHOLOGIC FINDINGS

Lacerations from blunt trauma usually occur in the transverse plane of the kidney. The mechanism of injury is thought to be force transmitted from the center of the impact to the renal parenchyma. In injuries from rapid deceleration, the kidney moves upward or downward, causing sudden stretch on the renal pedicle and

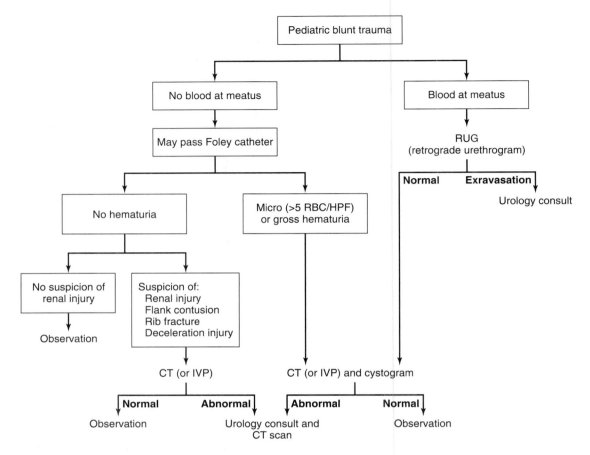

Figure 17–3. Algorithm for staging blunt trauma in children.

sometimes complete or partial avulsion. Acute thrombosis of the renal artery may be caused by an intimal tear from rapid deceleration injuries owing to the sudden stretch.

Pathologic classification of renal injuries is as follows:

Grade 1 (the most common)—Renal contusion or bruising of the renal parenchyma. Microscopic hematuria is common, but gross hematuria can occur rarely.

Grade 2—Renal parenchymal laceration into the renal cortex. Perirenal hematoma is usually small.

Grade 3—Renal parenchymal laceration extending through the cortex and into the renal medulla. Bleeding can be significant in the presence of large retroperitoneal hematoma.

Grade 4—Renal parenchymal laceration extending into the renal collecting system; also, main renal artery thrombosis from blunt trauma, segmental renal vein, or both; or artery injury with contained bleeding.

Grade 5—Multiple Grade 4 parenchymal lacerations, renal pedicle avulsion, or both; main renal vein or artery injury from penetrating trauma.

B. LATE PATHOLOGIC FINDINGS (FIGURE 17–6):

1. Urinoma—Deep lacerations that are not repaired may result in persistent urinary extravasation and late complications of a large perinephric renal mass and, eventually, hydronephrosis and abscess formation.

2. Hydronephrosis—Large hematomas in the retroperitoneum and associated urinary extravasation may result in perinephric fibrosis engulfing the ureteropelvic junction, causing hydronephrosis. Follow-up excretory urography is indicated in all cases of major renal trauma.

3. Arteriovenous fistula—Arteriovenous fistulas may occur after penetrating injuries but are not common.

Figure 17–4. Mechanisms of renal injury. **Left:** Direct blow to abdomen. Smaller drawing shows force of blow radiating from the renal hilum. **Right:** Falling on buttocks from a height (contrecoup of kidney). Smaller drawing shows direction of force exerted on the kidney from above. Tear of renal pedicle.

4. Renal vascular hypertension—The blood flow in tissue rendered nonviable by injury is compromised; this results in renal vascular hypertension in less than 1% of cases. Fibrosis from surrounding trauma has also been reported to constrict the renal artery and cause renal hypertension.

Clinical Findings & Indications for Studies

Microscopic or gross hematuria following trauma to the abdomen indicates injury to the urinary tract. It bears repeating that stab or gunshot wounds to the flank area should alert the physician to possible renal injury whether or not hematuria is present. Some cases of renal vascular injury are not associated with hematuria. These cases are almost always due to rapid deceleration accidents and are an indication for imaging studies.

The degree of renal injury does not correspond to the degree of hematuria, since gross hematuria may occur in minor renal trauma and only mild hematuria in major trauma. However, not all adult patients sustaining blunt trauma require full imaging evaluation of the kidney (Figure 17–1). Miller and McAninch (1995) made the following recommendations based on findings in over 1800 blunt renal trauma injuries: Patients with gross hematuria or microscopic hematuria with

shock (systolic blood pressure < 90 mm Hg) should undergo radiographic assessment; patients with microscopic hematuria without shock need not. However, should physical examination or associated injuries prompt reasonable suspicion of a renal injury, renal imaging should be undertaken. This is especially true of patients with rapid deceleration trauma, who may have renal injury without the presence of hematuria.

A. SYMPTOMS

There is usually visible evidence of abdominal trauma. Pain may be localized to one flank area or over the abdomen. Associated injuries such as ruptured abdominal viscera or multiple pelvic fractures also cause acute abdominal pain and may obscure the presence of renal injury. Catheterization usually reveals hematuria. Retroperitoneal bleeding may cause abdominal distention, ileus, and nausea and vomiting.

B. SIGNS

Initially, shock or signs of a large loss of blood from heavy retroperitoneal bleeding may be noted. Ecchymosis in the flank or upper quadrants of the abdomen is often noted. Lower rib fractures are frequently found. Diffuse abdominal tenderness may be found on palpation; an "acute abdomen" usually indicates free blood

Figure 17–5. Classification of renal injuries. Grades I and II are minor. Grades III, IV, and V are major. **A:** Grade I—microscopic or gross hematuria; normal findings on radiographic studies; contusion or contained subcapsular hematoma without parenchymal laceration. **B:** Grade II—nonexpanding, confined perirenal hematoma or cortical laceration less than 1 cm deep without urinary extravasation. **C:** Grade III—parenchymal laceration extending less than 1 cm into the cortex without urinary extravasation. **D:** Grade IV—parenchymal laceration extending through the corticomedullary junction and into the collecting system. A laceration at a segmental vessel may also be present.

Figure 17–5. E: Grade IV—thrombosis of a segmental renal artery without a parenchymal laceration. Note the corresponding parenchymal ischemia. **F:** Grade V—thrombosis of the main renal artery. The inset shows the intimal tear and distal thrombosis. **G:** Grade V—multiple major lacerations, resulting in a "shattered" kidney. **H:** Grade V—avulsion of the main renal artery or vein or both.

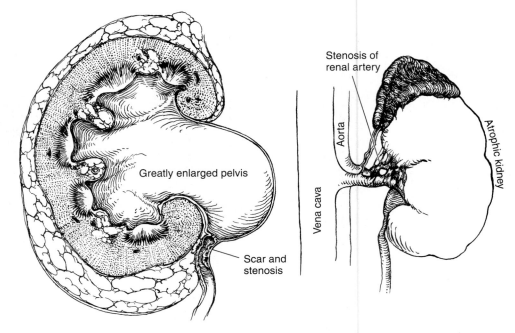

Figure 17–6. Late pathologic findings in renal trauma. **Left:** Ureteropelvic stenosis with hydronephrosis secondary to fibrosis from extravasation of blood and urine. **Right:** Atrophy of kidney caused by injury (stenosis) of arterial blood supply.

in the peritoneal cavity. A palpable mass may represent a large retroperitoneal hematoma or perhaps urinary extravasation. If the retroperitoneum has been torn, free blood may be noted in the peritoneal cavity but no palpable mass will be evident. The abdomen may be distended and bowel sounds absent.

C. Laboratory Findings

Microscopic or gross hematuria is usually present. The hematocrit may be normal initially, but a drop may be found when serial studies are done. This finding represents persistent retroperitoneal bleeding and development of a large retroperitoneal hematoma. Persistent bleeding may necessitate operation.

D. Staging and X-Ray Findings

Staging of renal injuries allows a systematic approach to these problems (Figures 17–1 through 17–3). Adequate studies help define the extent of injury and dictate appropriate management. For example, blunt trauma to the abdomen associated with gross hematuria and a normal urogram requires no additional renal studies; however, nonvisualization of the kidney requires immediate arteriography or CT scan to determine whether renal vascular injury exists. Ultrasonography and retro-

grade urography are of little use initially in the evaluation of renal injuries.

Staging begins with an abdominal CT scan, the most direct and effective means of staging renal injuries. This noninvasive technique clearly defines parenchymal lacerations and urinary extravasation, shows the extent of the retroperitoneal hematoma, identifies nonviable tissue, and outlines injuries to surrounding organs such as the pancreas, spleen, liver, and bowel (Figure 17–7). (If CT is not available, an intravenous pyelogram can be obtained [Figure 17–8] .)

Arteriography defines major arterial and parenchymal injuries when previous studies have not fully done so. Arterial thrombosis and avulsion of the renal pedicle are best diagnosed by arteriography and are likely when the kidney is not visualized on imaging studies (Figure 17–9). The major causes of nonvisualization on an excretory urogram are total pedicle avulsion, arterial thrombosis, severe contusion causing vascular spasm, and absence of the kidney (either congenital or from operation).

Radionuclide renal scans have been used in staging renal trauma. However, in emergency management, this technique is less sensitive than arteriography or CT.

Figure 17–7. Computed tomography scan of right kidney following knife stab wound. Laceration with urine extravasation is seen. Large right retroperitoneal hematoma is present.

Figure 17–9. Arteriogram following blunt abdominal trauma shows typical findings of acute renal artery thrombosis (arrow) of left kidney.

Differential Diagnosis

Trauma to the abdomen and flank areas is not always associated with renal injury. In such cases, there is no hematuria, and the results of imaging studies are normal.

Complications

A. EARLY COMPLICATIONS

Hemorrhage is perhaps the most important immediate complication of renal injury. Heavy retroperitoneal bleeding may result in rapid exsanguination. Patients must be observed closely, with careful monitoring of blood pressure and hematocrit. Complete staging must be done early (Figures 17–1 through 17–3). The size and expansion of palpable masses must be carefully monitored. Bleeding ceases spontaneously in 80–85% of cases. Persistent retroperitoneal bleeding or heavy gross hematuria may require early operation.

Urinary extravasation from renal fracture may show as an expanding mass (urinoma) in the retroperitoneum. These collections are prone to abscess formation and sepsis. A resolving retroperitoneal hematoma may cause slight fever (38.3 °C [101 °F]), but higher temperatures suggest infection. A perinephric abscess may form, resulting in abdominal tenderness and flank pain.

B. LATE COMPLICATIONS

Hypertension, hydronephrosis, arteriovenous fistula, calculus formation, and pyelonephritis are important late complications. Careful monitoring of blood pressure for several months is necessary to watch for hypertension. At 3–6 months, a follow-up excretory urogram

Figure 17–8. Blunt renal trauma to left kidney demonstrating extravasation (at arrow) on intravenous urogram.

or CT scan should be obtained to be certain that perinephric scarring has not caused hydronephrosis or vascular compromise; renal atrophy may occur from vascular compromise and is detected by follow-up urography. Heavy late bleeding may occur 1–4 weeks after injury.

Treatment

A. EMERGENCY MEASURES

The objectives of early management are prompt treatment of shock and hemorrhage, complete resuscitation, and evaluation of associated injuries.

B. SURGICAL MEASURES

1. Blunt injuries—Minor renal injuries from blunt trauma account for 85% of cases and do not usually require operation. Bleeding stops spontaneously with bed rest and hydration. Cases in which operation is indicated include those associated with persistent retroperitoneal bleeding, urinary extravasation, evidence of nonviable renal parenchyma, and renal pedicle injuries (less than 5% of all renal injuries). Aggressive preoperative staging allows complete definition of injury before operation.

2. Penetrating injuries—Penetrating injuries should be surgically explored. A rare exception to this rule is when staging has been complete and only minor parenchymal injury, with no urinary extravasation, is noted. In 80% of cases of penetrating injury, associated organ injury requires operation; thus, renal exploration is only an extension of this procedure.

C. TREATMENT OF COMPLICATIONS

Retroperitoneal urinoma or perinephric abscess demands prompt surgical drainage. Malignant hypertension requires vascular repair or nephrectomy. Hydronephrosis may require surgical correction or nephrectomy.

Prognosis

With careful follow-up, most renal injuries have an excellent prognosis, with spontaneous healing and return of renal function. Follow-up excretory urography and monitoring of blood pressure ensure detection and appropriate management of late hydronephrosis and hypertension.

INJURIES TO THE URETER

Ureteral injury is rare but may occur, usually during the course of a difficult pelvic surgical procedure or as a result of gunshot wounds. Rapid deceleration accidents may avulse the ureter from the renal pelvis. Endoscopic basket manipulation of ureteral calculi may result in injury.

Etiology

Large pelvic masses (benign or malignant) may displace the ureter laterally and engulf it in reactive fibrosis. This may lead to ureteral injury during dissection, since the organ is anatomically malpositioned. Inflammatory pelvic disorders may involve the ureter in a similar way. Extensive carcinoma of the colon may invade areas outside the colon wall and directly involve the ureter; thus, resection of the ureter may be required along with resection of the tumor mass. Devascularization may occur with extensive pelvic lymph node dissections or after radiation therapy to the pelvis for pelvic cancer. In these situations, ureteral fibrosis and subsequent stricture formation may develop along with ureteral fistulas.

Endoscopic manipulation of a ureteral calculus with a stone basket or ureteroscope may result in ureteral perforation or avulsion.

Pathogenesis & Pathology

The ureter may be inadvertently ligated and cut during difficult pelvic surgery. In such cases, sepsis and severe renal damage usually occur postoperatively. If a partially divided ureter is unrecognized at operation, urinary extravasation and subsequent buildup of a large urinoma will ensue, which usually leads to ureterovaginal or ureterocutaneous fistula formation. Intraperitoneal extravasation of urine can also occur, causing ileus and peritonitis. After partial transection of the ureter, some degree of stenosis and reactive fibrosis develops, with concomitant mild to moderate hydronephrosis.

Clinical Findings

A. SYMPTOMS

If the ureter has been completely or partially ligated during operation, the postoperative course is usually marked by fever of 38.3–38.8 °C (101–102 °F) as well as flank and lower quadrant pain. Such patients often experience paralytic ileus with nausea and vomiting. If ureterovaginal or cutaneous fistula develops, it usually does so within the first 10 postoperative days.

Ureteral injuries from external violence should be suspected in patients who have sustained stab or gunshot wounds to the retroperitoneum. The mid portion of the ureter seems to be the most common site of penetrating injury. There are usually associated vascular and other abdominal visceral injuries.

B. SIGNS

The acute hydronephrosis of a totally ligated ureter results in severe flank pain and abdominal pain with nausea and vomiting early in the postoperative course and with associated ileus. Signs and symptoms of acute peritonitis may be present if there is urinary extravasation into the peritoneal cavity. Watery discharge from the wound or vagina may be identified as urine by determining the creatinine concentration of a small sample—urine has many times the creatinine concentration found in serum—and by intravenous injection of 10 mL of indigo carmine, which will appear in the urine as dark blue.

C. Laboratory Findings

Ureteral injury from external violence is manifested by microscopic hematuria in 90% of cases. Urinalysis and other laboratory studies are of little use in diagnosis when injury has occurred from other causes.

D. Imaging Findings

Diagnosis is by excretory urography. A plain film of the abdomen may demonstrate a large area of increased density in the pelvis or in an area of retroperitoneum where injury is suspected. After injection of contrast material, delayed excretion is noted with hydronephrosis. Partial transection of the ureter results in more rapid excretion, but persistent hydronephrosis is usually present, and contrast extravasation at the site of injury is noted on delayed films (Figure 17–10).

In acute injury from external violence, the excretory urogram usually appears normal, with very mild fullness down to the point of extravasation at the ureteral transection.

Retrograde ureterography demonstrates the exact site of obstruction or extravasation.

E. Ultrasonography

Ultrasonography outlines hydroureter or urinary extravasation as it develops into a urinoma and is perhaps the best means of ruling out ureteral injury in the early postoperative period.

F. Radionuclide Scanning

Radionuclide scanning demonstrates delayed excretion on the injured side, with evidence of increasing counts owing to accumulation of urine in the renal pelvis. Its great benefit, however, is in the assessment of renal function after surgical correction.

Differential Diagnosis

Postoperative bowel obstruction and peritonitis may cause symptoms similar to those of acute ureteral obstruction from injury. Fever, "acute abdomen," and associated nausea and vomiting following difficult pelvic surgery are definite indications for screening sonography or excretory urography to establish whether ureteral injury has occurred.

Deep wound infection must be considered postoperatively in patients with fever, ileus, and localized tenderness. The same findings are consistent with urinary extravasation and urinoma formation.

Acute pyelonephritis in the early postoperative period may also result in findings similar to those of ureteral injury. Sonography shows normal results, and urography shows no evidence of obstruction.

Complications

Ureteral injury may be complicated by stricture formation with resulting hydronephrosis in the area of injury. Chronic urinary extravasation from unrecognized injury may lead to formation of a large retroperitoneal urinoma. Pyelonephritis from hydronephrosis and urinary infection may require prompt proximal drainage.

Treatment

Prompt treatment of ureteral injuries is required. The best opportunity for successful repair is in the operating room when the injury occurs. If the injury is not recognized until 7–10 days after the event and no infection, abscess, or other complications exist, immediate reexploration and repair are indicated. Proximal urinary drainage by percutaneous nephrostomy or formal nephrostomy should be considered if the injury is recognized

Figure 17–10. Stab wound of right ureter shows extravasation (at arrow) on intravenous urogram.

late or if the patient has significant complications that make immediate reconstruction unsatisfactory. The goals of ureteral repair are to achieve complete debridement, a tension-free spatulated anastomosis, watertight closure, ureteral stenting (in selected cases), and retroperitoneal drainage.

A. Lower Ureteral Injuries

Injuries to the lower third of the ureter allow several options in management. The procedure of choice is reimplantation into the bladder combined with a psoas-hitch procedure to minimize tension on the ureteral anastomosis. An antireflux procedure should be done when possible. Primary ureteroureterostomy can be used in lower-third injuries when the ureter has been ligated without transection. The ureter is usually long enough for this type of anastomosis. A bladder tube flap can be used when the ureter is shorter.

Transureteroureterostomy may be used in lower-third injuries if extensive urinoma and pelvic infection have developed. This procedure allows anastomosis and reconstruction in an area away from the pathologic processes.

B. Midureteral Injuries

Midureteral injuries usually result from external violence and are best repaired by primary ureteroureterostomy or transureteroureterostomy.

C. Upper Ureteral Injuries

Injuries to the upper third of the ureter are best managed by primary ureteroureterostomy. If there is extensive loss of the ureter, autotransplantation of the kidney can be done as well as bowel replacement of the ureter.

D. Stenting

Most anastomoses after repair of ureteral injury should be stented. The preferred technique is to insert a silicone internal stent through the anastomosis before closure. These stents have a J memory curve on each end to prevent their migration in the postoperative period. After 3–4 weeks of healing, stents can be endoscopically removed from the bladder. The advantages of internal stenting are maintenance of a straight ureter with a constant caliber during early healing, the presence of a conduit for urine during healing, prevention of urinary extravasation, maintenance of urinary diversion, and easy removal.

Prognosis

The prognosis for ureteral injury is excellent if the diagnosis is made early and prompt corrective surgery is done. Delay in diagnosis worsens the prognosis because of infection, hydronephrosis, abscess, and fistula formation.

INJURIES TO THE BLADDER

Bladder injuries occur most often from external force and are often associated with pelvic fractures. (About 15% of all pelvic fractures are associated with concomitant bladder or urethral injuries.) Iatrogenic injury may result from gynecologic and other extensive pelvic procedures as well as from hernia repairs and transurethral operations.

Pathogenesis & Pathology (Figure 17–11)

The bony pelvis protects the urinary bladder very well. When the pelvis is fractured by blunt trauma, fragments from the fracture site may perforate the bladder. These perforations usually result in extraperitoneal rupture. If the urine is infected, extraperitoneal bladder perforations may result in deep pelvic abscess and severe pelvic inflammation.

When the bladder is filled to near capacity, a direct blow to the lower abdomen may result in bladder disruption. This type of disruption ordinarily is intraperitoneal. Since the reflection of the pelvic peritoneum

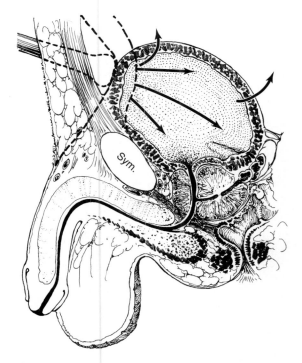

Figure 17–11. Mechanism of vesical injury. A direct blow over the full bladder causes increased intravesical pressure. If the bladder ruptures, it will usually rupture into the peritoneal cavity.

covers the dome of the bladder, a linear laceration will allow urine to flow into the abdominal cavity. If the diagnosis is not established immediately and if the urine is sterile, no symptoms may be noted for several days. If the urine is infected, immediate peritonitis and acute abdomen will develop.

Clinical Findings

Pelvic fracture accompanies bladder rupture in 90% of cases. The diagnosis of pelvic fracture can be made initially in the emergency room by lateral compression on the bony pelvis, since the fracture site will show crepitus and be painful to the touch.

A. Symptoms

There is usually a history of lower abdominal trauma. Blunt injury is the usual cause. Patients ordinarily are unable to urinate, but when spontaneous voiding occurs, gross hematuria is usually present. Most patients complain of pelvic or lower abdominal pain.

B. Signs

Heavy bleeding associated with pelvic fracture may result in hemorrhagic shock, usually from venous disruption of pelvic vessels. Evidence of external injury from a gunshot or stab wound in the lower abdomen should make one suspect bladder injury, manifested by marked tenderness of the suprapubic area and lower abdomen. An acute abdomen may occur with intraperitoneal bladder rupture. On rectal examination, landmarks may be indistinct because of a large pelvic hematoma.

C. Laboratory Findings

Catheterization usually is required in patients with pelvic trauma but not if bloody urethral discharge is noted. Bloody urethral discharge indicates urethral injury, and a urethrogram is necessary before catheterization (Figures 17–1 through 17–3). When catheterization is done, gross or, less commonly, microscopic hematuria is usually present. Urine taken from the bladder at the initial catheterization should be cultured to determine whether infection is present.

D. X-Ray Findings

A plain abdominal film generally demonstrates pelvic fractures. There may be haziness over the lower abdomen from blood and urine extravasation. A CT scan should be obtained to establish whether kidney and ureteral injuries are present.

Bladder disruption is shown on cystography. The bladder should be filled with 300 mL of contrast material and a plain film of the lower abdomen obtained. Contrast medium should be allowed to drain out completely, and a second film of the abdomen should be

obtained. The drainage film is extremely important, because it demonstrates areas of extraperitoneal extravasation of blood and urine that may not appear on the filling film (Figure 17–12). With intraperitoneal extravasation, free contrast medium is visualized in the abdomen, highlighting bowel loops (Figure 17–13).

CT cystography is an excellent method for detecting bladder rupture; however, retrograde filling of the bladder with 300 mL of contrast medium is necessary to distend the bladder completely. Incomplete distention with consequent missed diagnosis of bladder rupture often occurs when the urethral catheter is clamped during standard abdominal CT scan with intravenous contrast injection.

Complications

A pelvic abscess may develop from extraperitoneal bladder rupture; if the urine becomes infected, the pelvic hematoma becomes infected too.

Intraperitoneal bladder rupture with extravasation of urine into the abdominal cavity causes delayed peritonitis.

Partial incontinence may result from bladder injury when the laceration extends into the bladder neck. Meticulous repair may ensure normal urinary control.

Treatment

A. Emergency Measures

Shock and hemorrhage should be treated.

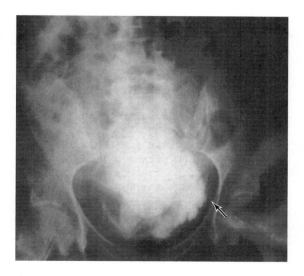

Figure 17–12. Extraperitoneal bladder rupture. Extravasation (at arrow) seen outside the bladder in the pelvis on cystogram.

Figure 17–13. Intraperitoneal bladder rupture. Cystogram shows contrast surrounding loops of bowel.

B. SURGICAL MEASURES

A lower midline abdominal incision should be made. As the bladder is approached in the midline, a pelvic hematoma, which is usually lateral, should be avoided. Entering the pelvic hematoma can result in increased bleeding from release of tamponade and in infection of the hematoma, with subsequent pelvic abscess. The bladder should be opened in the midline and carefully inspected. After repair, a suprapubic cystostomy tube is usually left in place to ensure complete urinary drainage and control of bleeding.

1. Extraperitoneal bladder rupture—Extraperitoneal bladder rupture can be successfully managed with urethral catheter drainage only. (Typically 10 days will provide adequate healing time.) Large blood clots in the bladder or injuries involving the bladder neck should be managed surgically.

As the bladder is opened in the midline, it should be carefully inspected and lacerations closed from within. Polyglycolic acid or chromic absorbable sutures should be used.

Extraperitoneal bladder lacerations occasionally extend into the bladder neck and should be repaired meticulously. Fine absorbable sutures should be used to ensure complete reconstruction so that the patient will have urinary control after injury. Such injuries are best managed with indwelling urethral catheterization and suprapubic diversion.

2. Intraperitoneal rupture—Intraperitoneal bladder ruptures should be repaired via a transperitoneal approach after careful transvesical inspection and closure

of any other perforations. The peritoneum must be closed carefully over the area of injury. The bladder is then closed in separate layers by absorbable suture. All extravasated fluid from the peritoneal cavity should be removed before closure. At the time of closure, care should be taken that the suprapubic cystostomy is in the extraperitoneal position.

3. Pelvic fracture—Stable fracture of the pubic rami is usually present. In such cases, the patient can be ambulatory within 4–5 days without damage or difficulty. Unstable pelvic fractures requiring external fixation have a more protracted course.

4. Pelvic hematoma—There may be heavy uncontrolled bleeding from rupture of pelvic vessels even if the hematoma has not been entered at operation. At exploration and bladder repair, packing the pelvis with laparotomy tapes often controls the problem. If bleeding persists, it may be necessary to leave the tapes in place for 24 h and operate again to remove them. Embolization of pelvic vessels with Gelfoam or skeletal muscle under angiographic control is useful in controlling persistent pelvic bleeding.

Prognosis

With appropriate treatment, the prognosis is excellent. The suprapubic cystostomy tube can be removed within 10 days, and the patient can usually void normally. Patients with lacerations extending into the bladder neck area may be temporarily incontinent, but full control is usually regained. At the time of discharge, urine culture should be performed to determine whether catheter-associated infection requires further treatment.

INJURIES TO THE URETHRA

Urethral injuries are uncommon and occur most often in men, usually associated with pelvic fractures or straddle-type falls. They are rare in women.

Various parts of the urethra may be lacerated, transected, or contused. Management varies according to the level of injury. The urethra can be separated into 2 broad anatomic divisions: the posterior urethra, consisting of the prostatic and membranous portions, and the anterior urethra, consisting of the bulbous and pendulous portions.

INJURIES TO THE POSTERIOR URETHRA
Etiology (Figure 17–14)

The membranous urethra passes through the pelvic floor and voluntary urinary sphincter and is the portion of the posterior urethra most likely to be injured. When

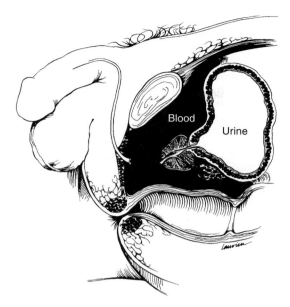

Figure 17–14. Injury to the posterior (membranous) urethra. The prostate has been avulsed from the membranous urethra secondary to fracture of the pelvis. Extravasation occurs above the triangular ligament and is periprostatic and perivesical.

pelvic fractures occur from blunt trauma, the membranous urethra is sheared from the prostatic apex at the prostatomembranous junction. The urethra can be transected by the same mechanism at the interior surface of the membranous urethra.

Clinical Findings

A. SYMPTOMS

Patients usually complain of lower abdominal pain and inability to urinate. A history of crushing injury to the pelvis is usually obtained.

B. SIGNS

Blood at the urethral meatus is the single most important sign of urethral injury. The importance of this finding cannot be overemphasized, because an attempt to pass a urethral catheter may result in infection of the periprostatic and perivesical hematoma and conversion of an incomplete laceration to a complete one. The presence of blood at the external urethral meatus indicates that immediate urethrography is necessary to establish the diagnosis.

Suprapubic tenderness and the presence of pelvic fracture are noted on physical examination. A large developing pelvic hematoma may be palpated. Perineal or suprapubic contusions are often noted. Rectal examination may reveal a large pelvic hematoma with the prostate displaced superiorly. Rectal examination can be misleading, however, because a tense pelvic hematoma may resemble the prostate on palpation. Superior displacement of the prostate does not occur if the puboprostatic ligaments remain intact. Partial disruption of the membranous urethra (currently 10% of cases) is not accompanied by prostatic displacement.

C. X-RAY FINDINGS

Fractures of the bony pelvis are usually present. A urethrogram (using 20–30 mL of water-soluble contrast material) shows the site of extravasation at the prostatomembranous junction. Ordinarily, there is free extravasation of contrast material into the perivesical space (Figure 17–15). Incomplete prostatomembranous disruption is seen as minor extravasation, with a portion of contrast material passing into the prostatic urethra and bladder.

D. INSTRUMENTAL EXAMINATION

The only instrumentation involved should be for urethrography. Catheterization or urethroscopy should not be done, because these procedures pose an increased risk of hematoma, infection, and further damage to partial urethral disruptions.

Differential Diagnosis

Bladder rupture may be associated with posterior urethral injuries in approximately 20% of cases. Cystography cannot be done preoperatively, since a urethral catheter should not be passed. Careful evaluation of the bladder at operation is necessary.

Figure 17–15. Ruptured prostatomembranous urethra shows free extravasation on urethrogram. No contrast medium is seen entering the prostatic urethra.

Complications

Stricture, impotence, and incontinence as complications of prostatomembranous disruption are among the most severe and debilitating mishaps that result from trauma to the urinary system. Stricture following primary repair and anastomosis occurs in about 50% of cases. If the preferred suprapubic cystostomy approach with delayed repair is used, the incidence of stricture can be reduced to about 5%.

The incidence of impotence after primary repair is 30–80% (mean, about 50%). This figure can be reduced to 30–35% by suprapubic drainage with delayed urethral reconstruction.

Incontinence in primary reanastomosis is noted in one-third of patients. Delayed reconstruction reduces the incidence to less than 5%.

Treatment

A. EMERGENCY MEASURES

Shock and hemorrhage should be treated.

B. SURGICAL MEASURES

Urethral catheterization should be avoided.

1. Immediate management—Initial management should consist of suprapubic cystostomy to provide urinary drainage. A midline lower abdominal incision should be made, with care being taken to avoid the large pelvic hematoma. The bladder and prostate are usually elevated superiorly by large periprostatic and perivesical hematomas. The bladder often is distended by a large volume of urine accumulated during the period of resuscitation and operative preparation. The urine is often clear and free of blood, but gross hematuria may be present. The bladder should be opened in the midline and carefully inspected for lacerations. If a laceration is present, the bladder should be closed with absorbable suture material and a cystostomy tube inserted for urinary drainage. This approach involves no urethral instrumentation or manipulation. The suprapubic cystostomy is maintained in place for about 3 months. This allows resolution of the pelvic hematoma, and the prostate and bladder will slowly return to their anatomic positions.

Incomplete laceration of the posterior urethra heals spontaneously, and the suprapubic cystostomy can be removed within 2–3 weeks. The cystostomy tube should not be removed before voiding cystourethrography shows that no extravasation persists.

2. Delayed urethral reconstruction—Reconstruction of the urethra after prostatic disruption can be undertaken within 3 months, assuming there is no pelvic abscess or other evidence of persistent pelvic infection.

Before reconstruction, a combined cystogram and urethrogram should be done to determine the exact length of the resulting urethral stricture. This stricture usually is 1–2 cm long and situated immediately posterior to the pubic bone. The preferred approach is a single-stage reconstruction of the urethral rupture defect with direct excision of the strictured area and anastomosis of the bulbous urethra directly to the apex of the prostate. A 16F silicone urethral catheter should be left in place along with a suprapubic cystostomy. Catheters are removed within a month, and the patient is then able to void (Figure 17–16).

3. Immediate urethral realignment—Some surgeons prefer to realign the urethra immediately. Persistent bleeding and surrounding hematoma create technical problems. The incidence of stricture, impotence, and incontinence appears to be higher than with immediate cystostomy and delayed reconstruction. However, several authors have reported success with immediate urethral realignment.

C. GENERAL MEASURES

After delayed reconstruction by a perineal approach, patients are allowed ambulation on the first postoperative day and usually can be discharged within 3 days.

D. TREATMENT OF COMPLICATIONS

Approximately 1 month after the delayed reconstruction, the urethral catheter can be removed and a voiding cystogram obtained through the suprapubic cys-

Figure 17–16. Delayed repair of urethral injury. Normal voiding urethrogram after transpubic repair of stricture following prostatomembranous urethral disruption. Arrow indicates area of repair.

tostomy tube. If the cystogram shows a patent area of reconstruction free of extravasation, the suprapubic catheter can be removed; if there is extravasation or stricture, suprapubic cystostomy should be maintained. A follow-up urethrogram should be obtained within 2 months to watch for stricture development.

Stricture, if present (< 5%), is usually very short, and urethrotomy under direct vision offers easy and rapid cure.

The patient may be impotent for several months after delayed repair. Impotence is permanent in about 10% of patients. Implantation of a penile prosthesis is indicated if impotence is still present 2 years after reconstruction (see Chapter 37).

Incontinence after posterior urethral rupture and delayed repair is rare (< 2%) and is usually related to the extent of injury rather than to the repair.

Prognosis

If complications can be avoided, the prognosis is excellent. Urinary infections ultimately resolve with appropriate management.

INJURIES TO THE ANTERIOR URETHRA

Etiology (Figure 17–17)

The anterior urethra is the portion distal to the urogenital diaphragm. Straddle injury may cause laceration or contusion of the urethra. Self-instrumentation or iatrogenic instrumentation may cause partial disruption.

Pathogenesis & Pathology

A. CONTUSION

Contusion of the urethra is a sign of crush injury without urethral disruption. Perineal hematoma usually resolves without complications.

B. LACERATION

A severe straddle injury may result in laceration of part of the urethral wall, allowing extravasation of urine. If the extravasation is unrecognized, it may extend into the scrotum, along the penile shaft, and up to the abdominal wall. It is limited only by Colles' fascia and often results in sepsis, infection, and serious morbidity.

Clinical Findings

A. SYMPTOMS

There is usually a history of a fall, and in some cases a history of instrumentation. Bleeding from the urethra is usually present. There is local pain into the perineum and sometimes massive perineal hematoma. If voiding has occurred and extravasation is noted, sudden swelling in the area will be present. If diagnosis has been delayed, sepsis and severe infection may be present.

B. SIGNS

The perineum is very tender, and a mass may be found. Rectal examination reveals a normal prostate. The patient usually has a desire to void, but voiding should not be allowed until assessment of the urethra is complete. No attempt should be made to pass a urethral

Figure 17–17. Injury to the bulbous urethra. **Left:** Mechanism: Usually a perineal blow or fall astride an object; crushing of urethra against inferior edge of pubic symphysis. **Right:** Extravasation of blood and urine enclosed within Colles' fascia (see Figure 1–9).

catheter, but if the patient's bladder is overdistended, percutaneous suprapubic cystostomy can be done as a temporary procedure.

When presentation of such injuries is delayed, there is massive urinary extravasation and infection in the perineum and the scrotum. The lower abdominal wall may also be involved. The skin is usually swollen and discolored.

C. LABORATORY FINDINGS

Blood loss is not usually excessive, particularly if secondary injury has occurred. The white count may be elevated with infection.

D. X-RAY FINDINGS

A urethrogram, with instillation of 15–20 mL of water-soluble contrast material, demonstrates extravasation and the location of injury (Figure 17–18). A contused urethra shows no evidence of extravasation.

Complications

Heavy bleeding from the corpus spongiosum injury may occur in the perineum as well as through the urethral meatus. Pressure applied to the perineum over the site of the injury usually controls bleeding. If hemorrhage cannot be controlled, immediate operation is required.

The complications of urinary extravasation are chiefly sepsis and infection. Aggressive debridement and drainage are required if there is infection.

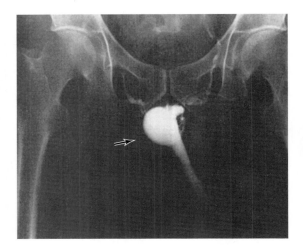

Figure 17–18. Ruptured bulbar (anterior) urethra following straddle injury. Extravasation (at arrow) on urethrogram.

Stricture at the site of injury is a common complication, but surgical reconstruction may not be required unless the stricture significantly reduces urinary flow rates.

Treatment

A. GENERAL MEASURES

Major blood loss usually does not occur from straddle injury. If heavy bleeding does occur, local pressure for control, followed by resuscitation, is required.

B. SPECIFIC MEASURES:

1. Urethral contusion—The patient with urethral contusion shows no evidence of extravasation, and the urethra remains intact. After urethrography, the patient is allowed to void; and if the voiding occurs normally, without pain or bleeding, no additional treatment is necessary. If bleeding persists, urethral catheter drainage can be done.

2. Urethral lacerations—Instrumentation of the urethra following urethrography should be avoided. A small midline incision in the suprapubic area readily exposes the dome of the bladder so that a suprapubic cystostomy tube can be inserted, allowing complete urinary diversion while the urethral laceration heals. Percutaneous cystostomy may also be used in such injuries. If only minor extravasation is noted on the urethrogram, a voiding study can be performed within 7 days after suprapubic catheter drainage to search for extravasation. In more extensive injuries, one should wait 2–3 weeks before doing a voiding study through the suprapubic catheter. Healing at the site of injury may result in stricture formation. Most of these strictures are not severe and do not require surgical reconstruction. The suprapubic cystostomy catheter may be removed if no extravasation is documented. Follow-up with documentation of urinary flow rates will show whether there is urethral obstruction from stricture.

3. Urethral laceration with extensive urinary extravasation—After major laceration, urinary extravasation may involve the perineum, scrotum, and lower abdomen. Drainage of these areas is indicated. Suprapubic cystostomy for urinary diversion is required. Infection and abscess formation are common and require antibiotic therapy.

4. Immediate repair—Immediate repair of urethral lacerations can be performed, but the procedure is difficult and the incidence of associated stricture is high.

C. TREATMENT OF COMPLICATIONS

Strictures at the site of injury may be extensive and require delayed reconstruction.

Prognosis

Urethral stricture is a major complication but in most cases does not require surgical reconstruction. If, when stricture resolves, urinary flow rates are poor and urinary infection and urethral fistula are present, reconstruction is required.

INJURIES TO THE PENIS

Disruption of the tunica albuginea of the penis (penile fracture) can occur during sexual intercourse. At presentation, the patient has penile pain and hematoma. This injury should be surgically corrected.

Gangrene and urethral injury may be caused by obstructing rings placed around the base of the penis. These objects must be removed without causing further damage. Penile amputation is seen occasionally, and in a few patients, the penis can be surgically replaced successfully by microsurgical techniques.

Total avulsion of the penile skin occurs from machinery injuries. Immediate debridement and skin grafting are usually successful in salvage.

Injuries to the penis should suggest possible urethral damage, which should be investigated by urethrography.

INJURIES TO THE SCROTUM

Superficial lacerations of the scrotum may be debrided and closed primarily. Blunt trauma may cause local hematoma and ecchymosis, but these injuries resolve without difficulty. One must be certain that testicular rupture has not occurred.

Total avulsion of the scrotal skin may be caused by machinery accidents or other major trauma. The testes and spermatic cords are usually intact. It is important to provide coverage for these structures: this is best done by immediate surgical debridement and by placing the testes and spermatic cords in the subcutaneous tissues of the upper thighs. Later reconstruction of the scrotum can be done with a skin graft or thigh flap.

INJURIES TO THE TESTIS

Blunt trauma to the testis causes severe pain and, often, nausea and vomiting. Lower abdominal tenderness may be present. A hematoma may surround the testis and make delineation of its margin difficult. Ultrasonography can be used as an aid to better define the organ. If rupture has occurred, the sonogram will delineate the injury, which should be surgically repaired.

REFERENCES

Emergency Diagnosis & Management

Cunningham MA et al: Does free fluid on abdominal computed tomographic scan after blunt trauma require laparotomy? J Trauma 1998;44:599.

Franko ER, Ivatury RR, Schwalb DM: Combined penetrating rectal and genitourinary injuries: A challenge in management. J Trauma 1993;34:347.

Goldman HB, Idom CB Jr, Dmochowski RR: Traumatic injuries of the female external genitalia and their association with urological injuries. J Urol 1998;159:956.

Knudson MM et al: Hematuria as a predictor of abdominal injury after blunt trauma. Am J Surg 1992;164:482, 485.

Perez-Brayfield MR et al: Blunt traumatic hematuria in children: Is a simplified algorithm justified? J Urol 2002;167:2543.

Injuries To The Kidney

Armenakas NA, Duckett CP, McAninch JW: Indications for nonoperative management of renal stab wounds. J Urol 1999;161:768.

Bretan PN Jr et al: Computerized tomographic staging of renal trauma: 85 consecutive cases. J Urol 1986; 136:561.

Carroll PR et al: Renovascular trauma: Risk assessment, surgical management, and outcome. J Trauma 1990;30:547.

Cass AS: Renovascular injuries from external trauma: Diagnosis, treatment, and outcome. Urol Clin North Am 1989; 16:213.

Husmann DA et al: Major renal lacerations with a devitalized fragment following blunt abdominal trauma: A comparison between nonoperative (expectant) versus surgical management. J Urol 1993;150:1774.

Knudson MM et al: Outcome after major renovascular injuries: A Western Trauma Association multicenter report. J Trauma 2000;49:1116.

McAninch JW, Carroll PR: Renal exploration after trauma: Indications and reconstructive techniques. Urol Clin North Am 1989;16:203.

McAninch JW et al: Renal gunshot wounds: Methods of salvage and reconstruction. J Trauma 1993;35:279, 283.

McAninch JW et al: Renal reconstruction after injury. J Urol 1991;145:932.

Miller KS, McAninch JW: Radiographic assessment of renal trauma: Our 15-year experience. J Urol 1995;154:352.

Montgomery RC, Richardson JD, Harty JI: Posttraumatic renovascular hypertension after occult renal injury. J Trauma 1998;45:106.

Moore EE et al: Organ injury scaling: Spleen, liver, and kidney. J Trauma 1989;29:1664.

Morey AF et al: Single shot intraoperative excretory urography for the immediate evaluation of renal trauma. J Urol 1999;161:1088.

Safir MH, McAninch JW: Management of complex violent trauma to the upper urinary tract. Trauma 1999;1:323.

Santucci RA, McAninch JW: Grade IV renal injuries: Evaluation, treatment and outcome. World J Surg 2001;25:1562.

Santucci RA et al: Validation of the American Association for the Surgery of Trauma organ injury severity scale for the kidney. J Trauma 2001;50:195.

Wessells H et al: Criteria for nonoperative treatment of significant penetrating renal lacerations. J Urol 1996;157:24.

Injuries To the Ureter

Perez-Brayfield MR et al: Gunshot wounds to the ureter: A 40-year experience at Grady Memorial Hospital. J Urol 2001;166:119.

Presti JC Jr, Carroll PR, McAninch JW: Ureteral and renal pelvic injuries from external trauma: Diagnosis and management. J Trauma 1989;29:370.

Injuries To the Bladder

Deck AJ et al: Computerized tomography cystography for the diagnosis of traumatic bladder rupture. J Urol 2000;164:43.

Santucci RA, McAninch JW: Bladder injuries: Evaluation and management. Braz J Urol 2000;26:408.

Injuries To the Urethra

Andrich DE, Mundy AR: The nature of urethral injury in cases of pelvic fracture urethral trauma. J Urol 2001;165:1492.

Koraitim MM: Pelvic fracture urethral injuries: The unresolved controversy. J Urol 1999;161:1433.

Morey AF, McAninch JW: Reconstruction of posterior urethral disruption injuries: Outcome analysis in 82 patients. J Urol 1997;157:506.

Podesta ML, Jordan GH: Pelvic fracture urethral injuries in girls. J Urol 2001;165:1660.

Injuries To the Penis

Gomes CM et al: Genital trauma due to animal bites. J Urol 2001;165:80.

Gomez RG, Castanheira AC, McAninch JW: Gunshot wounds to the male external genitalia. J Urol 1993;150:1147.

Mydlo JH: Surgeon experience with penile fracture. J Urol 2001;166:526.

Zargooshi J: Penile fracture in Kermanshah, Iran: Report of 172 cases. J Urol 2000;164:364.

Injuries To the Scrotum

Aboseif S, Gomez R, McAninch JW: Genital self-mutilation. J Urol 1993;150:1143.

McAninch JW: Management of genital skin loss. Urol Clin North Am 1989;16:387.

Immunology & Immunotherapy of Urologic Cancers

Eric J. Small, MD

Both experimental and naturally occurring tumors are capable of stimulating a specific antitumor immune response. This observation suggests that there are foreign proteins (antigens) on tumor cells that classically have been described as resulting in humoral and cellular immune responses. However, experimental models suggest that a T-cell (cell-mediated) response may be more important in the killing of tumor cells than a B-cell (humoral) response.

A detailed description of the components of the immune system is beyond the scope of this chapter, but certain features of the immune system as they pertain to diagnostic and therapeutic issues will be reviewed.

Tumor Antigens

Tumor antigens can be divided into tumor-specific antigens and tumor-associated antigens. Tumor-specific antigens are not found on normal tissue, and they permit the host to recognize a tumor as foreign. Tumor-specific antigens have been shown to exist in oncogenesis models utilizing chemical, physical, and viral carcinogens but appear to be less common in models of spontaneous tumor development.

The identification of tumor-specific antigens led to the theory of immune surveillance, which suggests that the immune system is continuously trolling for foreign (tumor-specific) antigens. This theory is supported by the observation that at least some cancers are more common in immune-suppressed patients such as transplant patients or human immunodeficiency virus-infected individuals. However, many cancers are not overrepresented in these patient populations. Furthermore, spontaneous tumor models, which more closely resemble human carcinogenesis, appear to have a less extensive repertoire of tumor-specific antigens but instead have been found to express many tumor-associated antigens.

Tumor-associated antigens are found on normal cells but either become less prevalent in normal tissue after embryogenesis (eg, alpha-fetoprotein [AFP]) or remain present on normal tissue but are overexpressed on cancer cells (eg, prostate-specific antigen [PSA]). In either case, the more ubiquitous nature of these antigens appears to cause reduced immune reactivity (also known as tolerance) to the specific antigen. The mechanisms of tolerance are complex and may be due in part to the absence of other required costimulatory molecules (such as B7, a molecule required for T-cell stimulation).

The development of monoclonal (hybridoma) technology has allowed the development of many antibodies against many tumor-associated antigens and has provided insight into the regulation and expression of these antigens. The re-expression or upregulation of these tumor-associated antigens during carcinogenesis may lead to immune response (or loss of tolerance). Many novel therapeutic approaches have sought to break this tolerance, and approaches to enhance a patient's immune response will be discussed.

Humoral Immunity

Many monoclonal antibodies have been developed against a variety of tumor-associated antigens. Oncofetal antigens such as AFP and beta-human chorionic gonadotropin (β-hCG) are important markers in germ cell tumors. β-hCG is also expressed in a small percentage of patients with bladder carcinoma. Growth factor receptors constitute another group of tumor-associated antigens that show promise as therapeutic targets as well as prognostic factors. For example, the receptor for fibroblastic growth factor appears to be expressed on prostate cancer cells, and therapies against growth factors such as fibroblastic growth factor, platelet-derived growth factor, and vascular endothelial growth factor are under investigation. The growth factor receptor HER2-neu has proved to be a strong predictive and prognostic marker, as well as a therapeutic target in breast cancer, and its utility in several urologic cancers is currently being evaluated.

Antibodies in Cancer Diagnosis & Detection

A. PROSTATE CANCER

Immunoassays are used to test both body fluids and tissues for the presence of tumor-associated antigens. In the urologic cancers, the most obvious example is the development of monoclonal antibodies against PSA.

The utility and limitations of PSA are described elsewhere in this volume. Other antigens that have been tested in prostate cancer include prostatic acid phosphatase, which has largely been replaced by PSA in screening programs and in patients with low tumor burden. Prostatic acid phosphatase may be of some use in detecting or following up bone metastases and as a predictive marker of response to therapy for metastatic disease, both hormone-sensitive and -insensitive. More recently, antibodies to prostate-specific membrane antigen (PSMA) have been used, primarily for immunohistochemistry.

B. RENAL CELL CARCINOMA

Unfortunately, there are as yet no well-established antigens (or antibodies) that can be used to reliably evaluate and monitor renal cell carcinoma, although a variety of target antigens are being evaluated.

C. BLADDER CANCER

Two oncofetal antigens, β-hCG and carcinoembryonic antigen, are expressed by a minority (20% or less) of transitional cell carcinomas. These markers are not routinely used, but in diagnostic dilemmas, measurement of serum levels of β-hCG or staining of tissue for this antigen may be useful.

D. GERM CELL TUMORS

As described in Chapter 23, antibodies to hCG and AFP are routinely used to detect shed antigen from germ cell tumors in the bloodstream. These antigens can also be detected on tissue samples in the setting of some diagnostic dilemmas. Although the use of serum markers in germ cell tumors is reviewed elsewhere, it is worth noting that the presence of the oncofetoprotein AFP, either in serum or on tissue specimens, is pathognomonic for a nonseminomatous germ cell tumor, regardless of results of routine pathologic evaluation. In addition to their diagnostic utility, AFP and hCG can be used as markers of response to therapy and as predictive factors of outcome. For example, the international germ cell tumor risk classification schema for patients with metastatic disease relies heavily on AFP and hCG levels as well as levels of a nonspecific marker, lactate dehydrogenase, to assign patients with nonseminomatous germ cell tumors to one of 3 risk levels. Thus, patients can be classified as low-risk (92% 5-year survival) only if AFP is < 1000 ng/mL and hCG is < 5000 IU/L (with other criteria evaluating extent and location of tumor). By contrast, AFP > 1000 and < 10,000 or hCG > 5000 and < 50,000 immediately places a patient in an intermediate risk category (80% 5-year survival), and AFP > 10,000 and hCG > 50,000 has an ominous prognosis (48% 5-year survival).

E. RADIOIMMUNODETECTION

A growing field is the use of monoclonal antibodies for radioimmunodetection. Monoclonal antibodies to a specific antigen are radiolabeled, and the preferential binding of the monoclonal antibody to tumor cells can be exploited. Theoretically, such an approach could be used for the presurgical evaluation of disease, postsurgical evaluation for minimal residual disease, confirmation of cancer identified by other imaging modalities, and detection of recurrent disease. Unfortunately, these potential uses have not been successfully developed in the urologic cancers, with one possible exception. There are several potential impediments to successful tumor radioimmunodetection. These include dilution of antibody in the bloodstream; metabolism of the antibody; nonspecific binding in liver, reticuloendothelial system, bone marrow, and elsewhere; binding of antibody by circulating or shed antigen; and the development of neutralizing human antimouse antibodies.

The only radioimmunodetection system for urologic cancers at this time is ^{111}In-capromab pendetide, a murine monoclonal antibody to PSMA. Its use has been hampered by a fairly laborious administration process, tremendous operator dependence in interpretation of scans, and a less than satisfactory positive predictive value.

Immunotherapy With Monoclonal Antibodies

Immunotherapy with monoclonal antibodies alone ("naked antibodies") has been fairly extensively evaluated. The use of monoclonal antibodies against tumor-associated antigens has met with only limited success in patients with solid tumors. In lymphoproliferative disorders such as leukemia and lymphoma, some antibodies to tumor-associated surface antigens appear to result in tumor cell death. The mechanism for these effects is certainly multifactorial but may in part be mediated by resultant complement fixation.

Direct antiproliferative effects of antibodies on cancer cells can be achieved by antibodies against functionally important antigens. Thus, the inhibition of growth factors and growth factor receptors and the activation or inhibition of signal transducing molecules are attractive therapeutic targets. As noted above, an anti-HER2-neu antibody has been shown to have activity in breast cancer. The utility of this antibody to treat transitional cell cancer is being investigated. In the urologic cancers, although no approved monoclonal antibody therapy exists, trials of antibodies against growth factors, vascular endothelial growth factor (an angiogenic molecule), and signal transduction molecules are being undertaken. In addition to the problems cited above in the discussion on radioimmunodetection, with the administration of any monoclonal antibody, one additional reason that naked antibody therapy could prove unsuccessful is that antigenic heterogeneity may result in only a small percentage of cancer cells being recognized, resulting in incomplete cell killing.

An alternative approach to naked antibodies is to conjugate any of a variety of cytotoxic agents to an antibody. The advantage of this approach is a "bystander effect," making it unnecessary to use an antibody that binds each and every cell. This can be achieved in several ways. The most straightforward is to use the monoclonal antibody as a means of providing some targeting specificity for the cytotoxic agent used. Cytotoxic agents used include radioisotopes, chemotherapy, and toxins such as ricin. Other means of providing some specificity is to bind a prodrug (with an antibody) to the tumor site and then to activate the bound prodrug. (Conversely, a nontoxic prodrug administered systemically could be activated in situ by the addition of an activating enzyme bound to a localizing antibody.) Finally, targeting with bispecific antibodies (eg, to antigen and to an effector T cell, or to antigen and toxin) has been undertaken. These approaches have all been tested in prostate cancer, but all remain investigational at this point. Considerable difficulties remain with nonspecific binding and the development of human antimouse antibodies. Humanization of antibodies largely prevents the development of human antimouse antibodies and allows repetitive dosing.

Cell-Mediated Immunity

There is considerable evidence, both clinical and preclinical, that tumor-associated antigens can elicit a cell-mediated immune response. In some models, when carcinogen-induced tumors in mice are resected and the mouse is reinoculated with tumor cells, the tumor fails to regrow, suggesting the development of immunity to specific antigens. Specific antigens that are rejected in immunized hosts are termed transplantation antigens. The specificity of tumor rejection has since been demonstrated to reside in T lymphocytes (at a minimum). Lymphocytes of cancer patients can sometimes be stimulated in vitro to recognize specific tumor-associated antigens and consequently demonstrate properties of cytolytic T lymphocytes. Unfortunately, the phenomenon of tumor rejection is by no means universal, either in the laboratory or clinically, and it is unusual to detect cytolytic-T-lymphocyte activity against many tumor-associated antigens.

Nevertheless, several clinical scenarios suggest that cell-mediated antitumor responses exist. These observations have promoted a broad search for the means of enhancing patients' immune responses to tumor-associated antigens. Renal cell carcinoma (RCC) is in many ways the prototypical immune-mediated tumor and, along with melanoma, has until recently been the primary target of immune manipulations. A dramatic example of such an immune-mediated response is the phenomenon of spontaneous regression of metastatic RCC deposits after nephrectomy. Although classically this has been described in less than 1% of patients, recent data suggest that the spontaneous regression rate may be somewhat higher. The impact of tumor debulking may also explain why a subset of RCC patients with lymph node or renal vein involvement who undergo resection are seemingly cured. The exact mechanism of this phenomenon is not well understood but may involve elimination of inhibitors of cell-mediated immunity. Indeed, tumor-infiltrating lymphocytes in RCC have been shown to exhibit mutant or faulty T-cell-receptor components, and it is not unreasonable to speculate that involvement in the tumor milieu in some fashion results in "deactivation" of such lymphocytes.

Immunotherapy Involving Cell-Mediated Immunity

Additional evidence of cell-mediated immunity playing a role in tumor rejection lies in the results of a variety of immunotherapeutic interventions. Immunotherapy can be broadly classified as active or passive. This classification refers to the role the host's immune system plays. Thus, the passive transfer of preformed antibodies is contrasted with a vaccination program in which the host's immune system must be capable of mounting an immune response. Adoptive therapy refers to a middle ground in which efforts are made to reconstitute, modify, or bolster one of the effector cells involved ex vivo, followed by reinfusion into the patient, where the rest of the immune cascade must then be recruited.

Active Immunotherapy: Vaccination

Vaccine therapy is a type of active specific immunotherapy. This approach remains experimental, and, although occasional dramatic responses are seen, consistent efficacy is elusive. Autologous vaccination programs (the vaccination of patients with their own tumor cells) have been extensively explored. The advantage of autologous vaccination is that the vaccine bears the antigens of the patient's tumor, although the distinct disadvantage is that not every patient has tumor available for vaccine preparation, and the preparation of each vaccine is tremendously labor-intensive. By contrast, allogeneic vaccination (the use of a generic vaccine or antigen) has the benefit of mass production and ease of use, and the identification of specific tumor rejection antigens allows specific antigenic targeting. However, this approach runs the risk of a more narrow shared antigenic spectrum with the patient's tumor. Both autologous and allogeneic vaccination strategies are under evaluation, both in RCC and prostate cancer.

Several means exist to undertake vaccination. The simplest is to use intact but inactivated tumor cells. Inactivation can be achieved with ultraviolet radiation, external beam (photon) radiation, or freeze-thawing. Crude extracts of cells can also be used. The advantage of using cell extracts is that inactivation is not necessary and small particles and proteins that might be more easily phagocytosed are available. One can also enhance the immunogenicity of inoculated cells by growing the cells in cytokines, coinjecting with cytokines (nonspecific active immunotherapy, described below), or transfecting these cells with the genes for immune stimulatory cytokines or the costimulatory molecule B7. An example of an active immunotherapy trial in a urologic cancer is a current clinical trial under way that uses prostate cancer cell lines transfected with the GM-CSF gene for vaccination in patients with prostate cancer. Purified protein or peptides represent a second potential vaccination schema. In prostate cancer, trials of vaccination with PSMA and PSA are under way. A third way of undertaking specific vaccination is to attempt to bypass the antigen-presenting function of the immune system and to directly stimulate professional antigen-presenting cells, such as dendritic cells, ex vivo. These cells can be stimulated by pulsing them with protein or peptides of interest or by transfecting them with a gene encoding the antigenic peptide of interest before reinfusion. Early trials of antigen-pulsed dendritic cells in prostate cancer (the antigens used have included PSMA and PAP) have demonstrated preliminary activity. Confirmatory trials are ongoing.

Nonspecific Active Immunotherapy: Cytokines & Biologic Response Modifiers

BCG (bacillus Calmette-Guérin) is a live attenuated form of tubercle bacillus that appears to have local activity against some tumors but has been largely disappointing as systemic therapy. The utility of BCG in the treatment of superficial bladder cancer is well described and is beyond the scope of this chapter. The mechanism by which BCG can elicit a local immune response in the uroepithelium and thereby exhibit impressive anticancer activity is not well delineated. However, possible mechanisms of action include macrophage activation, lymphocyte activation, recruitment of dendritic cells, and natural killer cells. It is intriguing that this is strictly a local phenomenon and that BCG has no role in the treatment of muscle-invasive or metastatic disease.

Interleukin-2 (IL-2) is a naturally occurring cytokine that has multiple immunoregulatory properties. The observation that exogenously administered IL-2 could result in tumor regression in patients with RCC and melanoma was the first unequivocal indication that cancer regression could be mediated by immune manipulations. IL-2 stimulates lymphocyte proliferation, enhances cytolytic-T-cell activity, induces natural killer cell activity, and induces interferon-gamma and tumor necrosis factor production. IL-2 has no direct cytotoxicity, but when administered endogenously will activate effector cells of the host immune system, including lymphocytes, natural killer cells, lymphokine-activated killer cells, and tumor-infiltrating lymphocytes. As noted above, in many ways RCC is the prototypical immunologically reactive cancer. The details of immunotherapy for RCC are beyond the scope of this chapter. Nevertheless, in brief, IL-2 has been administered in RCC in several different schemas, including high-dose intravenous bolus (IL-2 is FDA-approved with this schedule), continuous intravenous infusion, and at lower doses subcutaneously. The high-dose regimens must be administered on an inpatient basis and are characterized by significant, albeit manageable, toxicities, including fever; malaise; vascular leak syndrome; hypotension; and cardiac, renal, and hepatic dysfunction. Subcutaneous IL-2 is self-administered by patients in the outpatient setting, and while clearly less toxic, still has associated malaise and constitutional symptoms. The optimal dosing regimen is not well established, and overall response proportions rarely exceed 20%. Durable complete responses of 5–8% have been reported with some of the high-dose regimens. IL-2 has also been combined with other active agents such as interferon-alpha and chemotherapy, although it is not clear if these combinations provide additional benefit.

Interferon-alpha is a naturally occurring cytokine that has direct cytotoxic and possibly antiproliferative properties, but also has immunoregulatory properties. It enhances major histocompatibility complex expression, thereby potentially increasing the efficiency of antigen processing and recognition. Interferon-alpha has anticancer activity in both RCC and superficial bladder cancer. Its primary toxicity is fever, malaise, and constitutional symptoms, although at higher doses it can result in bone marrow toxicity, central nervous system toxicity, and hepatic toxicity. In RCC, as a single agent, interferon-alpha can result in clinical responses in up to 20% of patients. In contradistinction to IL-2 as a single agent, durable complete responses are quite rare. Nevertheless, in randomized trials, interferon-alpha appears to confer a modest survival advantage over other agents now known to be largely inactive. Interferon-alpha is also used as an intravesicle treatment in superficial bladder cancer, where it has established activity, and is not infrequently used as second-line therapy after BCG (see Chapter 19).

Adoptive Immunotherapy

Adoptive immunotherapy is the transfer of cellular products (effector cells) to the host or patient in an effort to develop an immune response. The use of adoptive immunotherapy was prompted by the observation that T cells derived from patients with melanoma or RCC had the ability to recognize antigens on the primary tumor. Thus, it was hoped that these cells could be harvested, activated ex vivo, and then reinfused into patients. Lymphokine-activated killer cells and tumor-infiltrating lymphocytes have been used to treat patients with metastatic RCC in the investigational setting, frequently along with IL-2. However, randomized trials comparing IL-2 alone with IL-2 plus cellular products have failed to demonstrate an improvement in response proportions or survival. Chapter 21 gives specific details of immunotherapy in RCC.

REFERENCES

Agarwala SS, Kirkwood JM: Interferons in the treatment of solid tumors. Oncology 1994;51:129.

Anichini A, Fossati G, Parmiani G: Clonal analysis of the cytolytic T-cell response to human tumors. Immunol Today 1987;8:385.

Berd D: Cancer vaccines: Reborn or just recycled? Semin Oncol 1998;25:605.

Berd D, Maguire HC Jr, Mastrangelo MJ: Induction of cell-mediated immunity to autologous melanoma cells and regression of metastases after treatment with a melanoma cell vaccine preceded by cyclophosphamide. Cancer Res 1986;46:2572.

Berd D et al: Treatment of metastatic melanoma with an autologous tumor-cell vaccine: Clinical and immunologic results in 64 patients. J Clin Oncol 1990;11:1858.

Bukowski RM: Natural history and therapy of metastatic renal cell carcinoma: The role of interleukin-2. Cancer 1997;80:1198.

Fyfe G et al: Results of treatment of 255 patients with metastatic RCC who received high-dose recombinant interleukin-2 therapy. J Clin Oncol 1995;13:688.

Gitlitz BJ, Belldegrun A, Figlin R: Immunotherapy and gene therapy. Semin Urol Oncol 1996;14:237.

Goedegebuure PS, Eberlen TJ: Vaccine trials for the clinician: Prospects for viral and non-viral vectors. Oncologist 1997;2:300.

Hewitt H, Blake E, Walder A: A critique of the evidence for active host defense against cancer based on personal studies of 27 murine tumors of spontaneous origin. Br J Cancer 1976;33:241.

Hoover HC Jr et al: Adjuvant active specific immunotherapy for human colorectal cancer: 6.5-year median follow-up of a phase III prospectively randomized trial. J Clin Oncol 1993;11:390.

Hsu FJ, Engleman EG, Levy R: Dendritic cells and their application in immunotherapeutic approaches to cancer therapy. PPO Updates 1997;11:1.

International Germ Cell Cancer Collaborative Group: International germ cell consensus classification: A prognostic factor-based staging system for metastatic germ cell cancers. J Clin Oncol 1997;15:594.

Lamm DL: Long-term results of intravesical therapy for superficial bladder cancer. Urol Clin North Am 1992;19:573.

Morales A, Nickel JC: Immunotherapy for superficial bladder cancer. Urol Clin North Am 1992;19:549.

Morton DL et al: Prolongation of survival in metastatic after active specific immunotherapy with a new polyvalent melanoma vaccine. Ann Surg 1992;216:463.

Osanto S: Vaccine trials for the clinician: Prospects for tumor antigens. Oncologist 1997;2:284.

Rini BI, Small EJ: Immunotherapy for prostate cancer. Current Oncol Rep 2001;3:418.

Rosenberg SA et al: Treatment of 283 consecutive patients with metastatic melanoma or renal cell cancer using high-dose bolus interleukin-2. JAMA 1994;271:907.

Rosenberg SA et al: Use of tumor-infiltrating lymphocytes and interleukin-2 in the immunotherapy of patients with metastatic melanoma. N Engl J Med 1988;319:1676.

Schlag P et al: Active specific immunotherapy with Newcastle-disease-virus-modified autologous tumor cells following resection of liver metastases in colorectal cancer. Cancer Immunol Immunother 1992;35:325.

Shepard HM et al: Monoclonal antibody therapy of human cancer: Taking the HER2 protooncogene to the clinic. J Clin Immunol 1991;11:117.

Simons JW, Mikhak B: Ex vivo gene therapy using cytokine-transduced tumor vaccines: Molecular and clinical pharmacology. Semin Oncol 1998;25:661.

Texter JH Jr, Neal CE: The role of monoclonal antibody in the management of prostate adenocarcinoma. J Urol 1998;160:2393.

Vanky F, Klein E: Specificity of auto-tumor cytotoxicity exerted by fresh, activated and propagated human T lymphocytes. Int J Cancer 1982;29:547.

Velders MP, Schreiber H, Kast WM: Active immunization against cancer cells: Impediments and advances. Semin Oncol 1998;25:697.

Chemotherapy of Urologic Tumors 19

Eric J. Small, MD

The use of chemotherapy and biologic therapy in the treatment of malignant tumors of the genitourinary system serves as a paradigm for a multidisciplinary approach to cancer. The careful integration of surgical and chemotherapeutic treatments has resulted in impressive advances in the management of urologic cancer. By definition, surgical interventions are directed at local management of urologic tumors, whereas chemotherapy and biologic therapy are systemic in nature. Although there is no question that there are times in the natural history of genitourinary tumor when only one therapeutic method is required, a multidisciplinary approach is always called for. This chapter details the importance of a joint surgical-medical approach to patients with urologic cancer. A practicing urologist should collaborate closely with an oncologist and should feel comfortable speaking with patients about the uses, risks, and benefits of chemotherapy.

PRINCIPLES OF SYSTEMIC THERAPY

A. CLINICAL USES OF CHEMOTHERAPY AND IMMUNOTHERAPY

Systemic therapy is indicated in the treatment of disseminated cancer when either cure or palliation is the goal. Additionally, chemotherapy may be used as part of a multimodality treatment plan in an effort to improve both local and distant control of the tumor. An understanding of the goals and limitations of systemic therapy in each of these settings is essential to its effective use.

1. Curative intent of metastatic disease—In considering the role of potentially curative chemotherapy or biologic therapy in patients with metastatic disease, several factors must be taken into account. The first is the responsiveness of the tumor. Responsiveness is generally defined by the observed partial, complete, and overall responses. It is important to note that a complete response implies complete resolution of abnormal serum tumor markers, if any, and complete radiographic resolution of any abnormalities. This makes the assessment of neoplasms with frequent bony metastases such as prostate cancer, renal cell carcinoma, and transitional cell carcinoma (TCC) difficult, as a persistently abnormal bone scan does not necessarily imply residual cancer. Patients in whom the only site of disease is bone generally must be considered nonassessable

by conventional measures, and if available, intermediate markers of response (such as prostate-specific antigen) are required.

If cure is the intent with systemic therapy, the relevant response criterion to consider is the percentage of patients achieving a complete response. This number is less than 10% in patients with metastatic renal cell carcinoma and hormone-refractory prostate cancer, 25% or less in patients with metastatic TCC, and up to 80% in patients with metastatic germ cell malignancies. Under some circumstances, however (for example, in post-chemotherapy residual masses in patients with germ cell carcinoma), an apparent partial response can be converted into a complete response with judicious resection (see section A. 3.)

The second feature to consider in treating patients with potentially curative systemic therapy is the anticipated toxicity of such therapy. In general, higher levels of toxicity are acceptable if a cure can be achieved, although care must be exercised to avoid a "cure worse than the disease." This is particularly true in the case of fairly toxic therapies such as interleukin-2 (IL-2) or bone marrow transplantation. These treatments can result in apparent cures of approximately 10% and 20%, respectively, of patients with metastatic renal cell carcinoma or refractory germ cell tumors (GCTs). Patients undergoing these rigorous therapies must be carefully selected and must be as fully informed as possible about potential toxicities.

2. Treatment of patients with incurable metastatic cancer—When the goal of systemic therapy is palliation of symptoms rather than cure, the toxicity of the treatment to be offered must be balanced against the cancer-related symptoms the patient is experiencing, and in general, more toxic therapies are not indicated. Nonetheless, the potential capabilities of systemic therapy must be understood because even in otherwise incurable disease there may be a role for systemic therapy if there is a likelihood that the patient's life can be prolonged with its use.

3. Systemic therapy used in conjunction with surgery: adjuvant and neoadjuvant therapy—Systemic therapy administered after a patient has been rendered free of disease surgically is termed **adjuvant therapy.** Several important criteria must be met if adjuvant therapy is to be used outside of a research setting. First, an assessment must be undertaken of known risk factors predictive of relapse or development of distant metastases. Patients at low risk of relapse generally should not receive adjuvant therapy because they are unlikely to derive a benefit and will be unnecessarily exposed to the toxicity of therapy. Second, the proposed therapy must have been shown to decrease the rate of relapse and increase the disease-free interval (and, it is hoped, survival) in a randomized, phase III trial. Finally, because patients who are being treated with adjuvant therapy are free of disease and presumably asymptomatic, toxicity must be kept at a minimum. This opens the way to a tailored approach in which patients with high-risk disease, as determined by pathologic review of the surgical specimen, are treated in order to decrease the risk of micrometastatic disease.

In contrast, neoadjuvant therapy is administered before definitive surgical resection. Here, the potential advantages include early therapy of micrometastatic disease and tumor debulking to allow a more complete resection. Patients with known metastatic disease generally do not exhibit high enough response rates to systemic therapy to warrant surgery following chemotherapy, with the clear exception of patients with GCTs. Whether or not patients with metastatic renal cell carcinoma who exhibit a partial response to systemic therapy may benefit from resection of residual masses is not known. As with adjuvant therapy, the proposed therapy must have been demonstrated to impact favorably on rate of relapse, disease-free interval, and survival in a randomized phase III trial.

B. Chemotherapeutic Agents and Their Toxicity

The usefulness of antineoplastic agents lies in their therapeutic index, or preferential toxicity to malignant cells over normal, nonmalignant cells. The mechanism of action of most chemotherapeutic drugs is based on their toxicity to rapidly dividing cells. Thus, in general, malignancies that have relatively rapid growth, such as GCTs, are relatively chemosensitive, whereas slower-growing neoplasms such as prostate cancer and renal cell carcinoma are less sensitive. Toxicity from chemotherapeutic agents is seen primarily in normal, nonmalignant cells that are also rapidly dividing, such as hematopoietic cells in the bone marrow, gastrointestinal mucosa, and hair follicles, and is manifested in cytopenias, mucositis, and alopecia. Other common toxicities observed with agents frequently used in the treatment of genitourinary malignancies include nephrotoxicity, neurotoxicity, hemorrhagic cystitis, pulmonary fibrosis, and cardiotoxicity. Table 19–1 summarizes the spectrum of activity and primary toxicities of commonly used chemotherapeutic agents.

The development of chemotherapy drug resistance remains an important clinical problem in the field of oncology. Malignant cells develop resistance in a variety of ways, including the induction of transport pumps, which actively pump the drug out of the cell, and through increased activity of enzymes necessary to inactivate the particular chemotherapeutic agent. Although there are several experimental methods of circumventing these mechanisms of drug resistance, one practical approach to this problem is the use of multiagent chemotherapy. Increased tumor cell killing is achieved by exposing neoplastic cells to multiple agents with different mechanisms of action. Furthermore, this approach allows the selection of agents with nonoverlapping toxicity profiles.

The use of increased dose intensity (higher doses of a drug administered over the same time period) as a means of overcoming drug resistance remains experimental in urologic malignancies, with one clear exception. A subset of patients with chemotherapy-refractory GCTs appears to be curable with high-dose chemotherapy and autologous bone marrow transplant support (see the section Germ Cell Malignancies, following).

C. Biologic Agents and Their Toxicity

Whereas chemotherapy is based on direct cytotoxicity, biologic therapy can be broadly considered to consist of treatment with agents that augment or diminish biologic phenomena normally observed in malignant cells. For the purposes of this chapter, two types of biologic therapy are considered: immunotherapy and growth-factor-related therapy. Immunotherapy is an important component of the therapy of urologic malignancies, particularly of superficial bladder carcinoma and renal cell carcinoma. Immunotherapy is designed to either elicit or augment an immune response in the patient in order to stop tumor growth or enhance tumor killing. In contrast to chemotherapy, the target of immunotherapy is not necessarily rapidly dividing cells but rather cells that can be recognized as foreign by the host. Most immunotherapeutic agents that are currently in use are fairly nonspecific. This is reflected in systemic toxicity in the form of constitutional symptoms such as fever, malaise, fatigue, myalgias, and arthralgias, as well as cutaneous toxicity. In very high doses (of IL-2, for example), toxicity may include severe vascular leak syndrome with hypotension, pulmonary edema, and renal insufficiency.

Specific biologic agents used in the therapy of urologic malignancies include bacillus Calmette-Guérin (BCG), interferon-alpha, and IL-2. The use of BCG for the treatment of superficial bladder cancer is based on the premise that local BCG instillation will result in a local immune response causing tumor cell kill. Interferons and interleukins are cytokines that are normally produced in the body as mediators of immune response. The exogenous administration of these agents

Table 19–1. Commonly used antineoplastic agents in urologic oncology, and their toxicity.

Agent	Activity	Common Toxicities
Cisplatin	Bladder cancer, germ cell tumors, prostate cancer	Renal insufficiency, peripheral neuropathy, auditory toxicity, myelosuppression[a]
Carboplatin	Bladder cancer, germ cell tumors	Myelosuppression
Bleomycin	Germ cell tumors	Fever, chills, pulmonary fibrosis
Doxorubicin	Bladder cancer, prostate cancer	Myelosuppression, mucositis, cardiomyopathy
Etoposide (VP-16)	Germ cell tumors, prostate cancer[b]	Myelosuppression
5-Fluorouracil	Renal cell carcinoma, bladder cancer, prostate cancer	Mucositis, diarrhea, myelosuppression
Floxuridine (FUdR)	Renal cell carcinoma	Mucositis, diarrhea
Methotrexate	Germ cell tumors, bladder cancer	Mucositis, myelosuppression, renal toxicity
Ifosfamide	Germ cell tumors	Myelosuppression, neurologic (CNS) toxicity, cystitis
Vinblastine	Renal cell carcinoma, bladder cancer, germ cell tumors, prostate cancer[b]	Peripheral, autonomic neuropathy; myelosuppression
Estramustine	Prostate cancer	Nausea, thromboembolic events
Paclitaxel (Taxol)	Bladder cancer, germ cell tumors, prostate cancer[b]	Myelosuppression, neuropathy
Docetaxel (Taxotere)	Bladder cancer, germ cell tumors, prostate cancer[b]	Myelosuppression, neuropathy
Gemcitabine (Gemzar)	Bladder cancer	Myelosuppression
Interferon-alpha	Renal cell carcinoma	Flulike symptoms, myelosuppression
Interleukin-2	Renal cell carcinoma	Flulike symptoms, hypotension, renal toxicity, hepatic toxicity, neurologic (CNS) toxicity, respiratory distress, dermatologic symptoms, sepsis

[a]Because of recent advances in the treatment of chemotherapy-induced nausea and vomiting, even the most emetogenic agents, such as cisplatin, have virtually no associated nausea and vomiting.
[b]In combination with estramustine.

can result in an enhanced immune response and tumor regression. Direct cytotoxicity or antiproliferative effects also appear to be mechanisms by which interferon-alpha, in particular, is active. Table 19–1 summarizes the spectrum of activity and primary toxicities of commonly used immunotherapeutic agents. Experimental immunologic approaches being evaluated include the development of vaccines for renal cell carcinoma and prostate cancer.

Growth factor manipulation is a novel and exciting element of antineoplastic therapy. The use of exogenous growth factors such as granulocyte colony-stimulating factor, granulocyte-macrophage colony-stimulating factor, thrombopoietin, and erythropoietin, which are normally involved in hematopoiesis, has allowed more dose-intensive therapy to be delivered. When bone marrow suppression occurs as a consequence of therapy, use of these agents has the potential for abrogating toxicity.

D. Unique Features of Genitourinary Malignancies

The systemic therapy of urologic malignancies offers unique challenges to the practitioner. Renal insuffi-

ciency due to obstructive uropathy from local extension of the tumor or postsurgical or postradiotherapy changes is not infrequent and may alter antineoplastic drug clearance. In patients with renal cell carcinoma, previous nephrectomy also may impact on drug clearance. Furthermore, the common use of the nephrotoxic chemotherapeutic agent cisplatin in the treatment of urologic malignancies (most prominently, in bladder and testicular neoplasms) may further diminish renal function. Careful attention must be paid, therefore, to renal function throughout the course of systemic therapy, with appropriate dose adjustments made. Dosing adjustments also must be considered in patients who have undergone cystectomy because ileal conduits or neobladders have the capacity to resorb chemotherapeutic agents that are excreted in the urine in active form (most notably, methotrexate).

Frequent local extension in the pelvis presents additional unique problems. Patients with previous pelvic radiotherapy have markedly diminished bone marrow reserves, which may limit the use of myelosuppressive drugs. Furthermore, local pelvic relapses have the potential to be symptomatic and painful. Particularly in patients who have already received radiotherapy, systemic therapy may be important for palliation.

GERM CELL MALIGNANCIES

A. OVERVIEW

The evolution of therapy for germ cell tumors (GCTs) has been deliberate and thoughtful, and has resulted in cures of 80–85% of men with GCTs, serving as a model for the treatment of curable cancers. Nonetheless, challenges in the management of GCTs remain. Because of their young age, patients who have been cured are at risk of delayed, treatment-induced toxicity. Furthermore, an 80–85% cure rate also implies that 15–20% of patients with GCTs will not be cured and ultimately will succumb to their disease. An understanding of staging and risk assessment is crucial if (1) patients with good risk features are not to be overtreated and exposed to undue toxic risks, and (2) patients with poor risk features are to receive adequate (curative) therapy.

The most common multiagent chemotherapy regimen for the treatment of GCTs is a 3-drug combination consisting of cisplatin, etoposide, and bleomycin (PEB). The treatment is repeated every 21 days. One cycle consists of cisplatin 20 mg/m^2 IV d 1–5, etoposide 100 mg/m^2 IV d 1–5, and bleomycin, 30 units IV, d 2, 9, and 16. Frequently the first 5 days of treatment require hospitalization. The deletion of bleomycin from this regimen results in the PE regimen.

B. USE OF CHEMOTHERAPY FOR PATIENTS WITH STAGE I AND II DISEASE

The standard of care for patients with stage I GCTs remains orchiectomy followed by retroperitoneal lymphadenectomy (nonseminoma), radiation therapy (seminoma), or in selected patients, careful surveillance. The use of chemotherapy in stage I GCTs in lieu of lymphadenectomy or irradiation remains investigational despite encouraging early results.

Patients with stage II nonseminomatous microscopic disease identified at lymphadenectomy (stage IIA) or patients with low-volume clinical stage II disease (stage IIB) who have undergone retroperitoneal lymphadenectomy may benefit from 2 cycles of adjuvant PE or PEB chemotherapy. The use of adjuvant therapy results in a 96% long-term disease-free survival. Although the relapse rate for patients who do not receive adjuvant therapy approaches 40%, the vast majority of relapsing patients can also be cured with either 3 or 4 cycles of chemotherapy, yielding an identical long-term survival rate. The decision about adjuvant chemotherapy after lymphadenectomy must be individualized. Patients at high risk for relapse may choose to undergo 2 cycles of chemotherapy at that point in order to avoid the possibility of 3–4 cycles in the future.

C. USE OF CHEMOTHERAPY IN PATIENTS WITH ADVANCED DISEASE

Patients with advanced GCTs should be treated with systemic therapy after completion of their orchiectomy. This group includes some stage IIB nonseminomatous tumors and all stage IIC or higher tumors, both seminomas and nonseminomas. A variety of chemotherapy regimens will result in approximately 80% of patients with advanced GCTs achieving a complete response and 70% achieving long-term apparent cures (good prognosis). By the same token, however, 20–30% of patients have a poor prognosis and will still ultimately die of their disease. Studies of pretreatment clinical characteristics have sought to identify prognostic features that can be prospectively used to segregate this diverse group of advanced GCTs patients into poor- and good-prognostic subsets.

A common classification system has been developed by the International Germ Cell Cancer Collaborative Group (IGCCC). In this system, good- and intermediate-prognosis patients with nonseminomatous GCTs have a testis or retroperitoneal primary tumor, no nonpulmonary visceral metastases, and low serum tumor markers. Intermediate-prognosis patients are the same as good-prognosis patients but have intermediate serum tumor markers. Poor-prognosis patients have a mediastinal primary tumor or nonpulmonary visceral metastases (liver, bone, brain) or high levels of serum tumor markers. Five-year overall survival for the good-, intermediate-, and poor-prognosis categories with current regimens is 92%, 80%, and 48%, respectively. By definition, seminomas are never in the poor-prognosis category. Seminomas are segregated into good-prognosis cases (any primary site, but no nonpulmonary visceral metastases), with an 86% 5-year survival, and intermediate-prognosis cases (any primary site but with the presence of nonpulmonary visceral metastases), with a 72% 5-year survival.

Because it is not likely that the extraordinarily high cure rate for good-prognosis patients can be improved upon, most efforts in the treatment of these patients have been aimed at optimizing treatment with less toxic regimens that will have equal efficacy. Trials evaluating (1) the elimination of bleomycin, (2) a reduction in the number of chemotherapy cycles administered, or (3) the substitution of carboplatin for cisplatin have been undertaken.

The outlook for poor-prognosis patients is grim, with only 38–62% of patients achieving a complete response. Thus, whereas the major concern in good-prognosis patients has been the reduction of toxicity, the major objective of clinical investigation in poor-prognosis patients has been to improve efficacy, with less concern for reducing toxicity. Clinical trials in poor-prognosis patients have by and large relied on one or both of two approaches. The first has been to exploit agents that have been demonstrated to be efficacious in the salvage setting, and the second has been to evaluate the role of dose escalation.

There is a lack of consensus regarding the optimal management of high-risk GCTs. Every effort should be made to enroll and treat patients with poor-prognosis GCTs in clinical trials.

Currently acceptable regimens for good-prognosis patients are fairly well defined and include 3 cycles of PEB or 4 cycles of PE; in contrast, optimal therapy for poor-prognosis patients continues to be investigated; 4 cycles of PEB are used in many centers.

D. ADJUNCTIVE SURGERY AND "SALVAGE" THERAPY

Postchemotherapy adjunctive surgery must be integrated into the treatment plan of patients with advanced GCTs. Between 10% and 20% of patients with nonseminomatous tumors have residual masses after systemic therapy, and up to 80% of patients with seminomas have residual radiographic abnormalities. The role of adjunctive surgery in patients with GCTs with postchemotherapy residual masses has been reviewed. Except in rare circumstances, adjunctive surgery is not indicated in the presence of persistently elevated serum tumor markers. Adjunctive surgery usually can be undertaken safely within 1–2 months of completion of chemotherapy. It must be noted, however, that all patients who have received bleomycin, whether or not there is clinical evidence of pulmonary fibrosis, are at risk of development of oxygen-related pulmonary toxicity. The anesthesiologist must be made aware of the patient's previous exposure to bleomycin and every effort taken to maintain the FiO_2 as low as possible throughout the surgical procedure. Patients who are found to have active carcinoma in their resected specimens are frequently treated with further "salvage" chemotherapy, generally with a different regimen, although compelling evidence supporting this procedure is still forthcoming. Patients who appear to benefit from postsurgical chemotherapy are patients with incomplete resections, patients whose resected specimen contains more than 10% viable cancer cells, and patients who were in the IGCCCG high-risk group prior to beginning frontline chemotherapy.

Although approximately 80% of patients with GCTs can currently be cured with platinum-based therapy, 20% ultimately die of their disease, either because a complete response is not achieved with induction therapy or because they relapse after becoming disease-free with primary therapy. Before the initiation of salvage therapy, the diagnosis of relapsed or primary, refractory GCTs must be clearly established. In particular, falsely elevated human chorionic gonadotropin or alpha-fetoprotein values and false-positive radiographic studies of the chest due to previous bleomycin use must

be ruled out. Persistent or slowly growing masses, particularly in the absence of serologic progression, may represent benign teratoma. Therapies based on ifosfamide, paclitaxel, or high-dose chemotherapy with autologous bone marrow transplant provide a salvage rate of approximately 25% in patients with relapsed or refractory GCTs.

ADVANCED TRANSITIONAL CELL CARCINOMA OF THE UROEPITHELIUM

A. NONMETASTATIC DISEASE

The development of effective chemotherapy regimens for the treatment of metastatic TCC has resulted in more widespread use of these regimens in combination with other modes for the treatment of locally advanced but nonmetastatic disease. In bulky inoperable invasive bladder tumors (T3b, T4, N+), chemotherapy has been used as a means of cytoreduction in order to make surgery possible. Chemotherapy before surgery, termed **neoadjuvant therapy,** has also been used in muscle-invasive cancers that *are* resectable, in an effort to treat micrometastatic disease before cystectomy. It must be borne in mind that the pathologic complete response rate in the bladder after neoadjuvant chemotherapy is probably in the 30–40% range; therefore, definitive surgical resection after chemotherapy is usually required. A European trial has failed to show an advantage of neoadjuvant therapy. Results of a major US intergroup trial are anticipated in the near future.

Other investigators believe that adjuvant therapy administered *after* radical cystectomy should be the means of treating patients with invasive bladder cancer at risk for relapse. Adjuvant trials generally have been used to treat only patients found to have pathologic T3 and T4 lesions. Several small randomized trials have shown a benefit to various adjuvant chemotherapy regimens; a large randomized multi-institution trial remains to be done.

Chemotherapy in combination with radiation therapy has been advocated by some as a bladder-preserving approach for muscle-invasive tumors. Patients are usually treated with 2 cycles of chemotherapy, followed by radiation therapy and concomitant cisplatin as a radiosensitizer. If follow-up cystoscopy reveals no cancer, consolidative multiagent systemic chemotherapy is administered. This approach appears to be particularly useful for smaller, lower-stage tumors. Although longer follow-up is required, it appears that approximately 30–50% of patients can attain long-term disease-free status with a functional bladder with this approach.

B. METASTATIC DISEASE

The development of successful therapy of metastatic bladder TCC has been based on the use of cisplatin.

Until recently, two common cisplatin-based regimens have been in wide use: (1) cisplatin, methotrexate, and vinblastine (CMV) and (2) the same drugs in a slightly different schedule and dose along with doxorubicin (Adriamycin), in a regimen known as MVAC. These regimens result in overall response rates of approximately 50–60% and complete remission rates in the 20–35% range. Median overall survival for patients with metastatic disease treated with these regimens is in the 8- to 14-month range. Despite early promise, however, long-term survival after MVAC or CMV remains in the single digits. Both CMV and MVAC are intensive regimens, with myelosuppression occurring commonly. The use of hematopoietic growth factors has made it easier to administer full doses on schedule, although this improvement in dose intensity does not appear to translate into a clinical benefit.

More recently, the combination of gemcitabine and cisplatin has been compared to MVAC. This new regimen is far less toxic, is better tolerated, and appears to be equivalent in efficacy to MVAC. As a consequence, gemcitabine/cisplatin can be considered the new standard of care for the treatment of advanced TCC. For patients with impaired renal function, agents such as carboplatin and paclitaxel have been utilized.

RENAL CELL CARCINOMA

The treatment of metastatic renal cell carcinoma remains largely unsatisfactory. The general lack of active agents and the excessive toxicity of many of the agents that exhibit some activity have contributed to the absence of adjuvant or neoadjuvant trials. The only such trials used adjuvant interferon-alpha for patients considered at high risk for relapse after nephrectomy and failed to show an advantage of the adjuvant therapy. Prenephrectomy systemic therapy remains experimental and cannot be advocated at this time. In contrast, nephrectomy prior to systemic therapy is recommended, particularly in patients in whom the bulk of disease is in the renal mass, and who have a good performance status.

Metastatic renal cell carcinoma is relatively resistant to chemotherapy. The fluoropyrimidines (floxuridine, 5-fluorouracil, capecitabine) have modest activity, as does gemcitabine, with response proportions of 10–15% reported. Renal cell carcinoma is one of very few neoplasms that clearly are responsive to biologic response modifiers. Interferon-alpha has limited but reproducible activity in renal cell carcinoma. Although initial response rates of 30% were reported, more recent large studies have suggested a response rate of less than 15% to single-agent interferon-alpha. Furthermore, considerable toxicities consisting of fever, chills, myalgias, and malaise are common, even though tolerance

to some of these side effects may be developed over several months. The toxicities associated with interferon-alpha must be weighed against the potential benefits of the drug.

IL-2 has been extensively studied in patients with metastatic renal cell carcinoma. The activity of IL-2 is mediated in part by its activation and promotion of growth of T cells, B cells, and natural killer cells. IL-2 has been studied in combination with a variety of other modes of immunotherapy, including use of lymphokine-activated killer (LAK) cells or tumor-infiltrating lymphocytes, but the efficacy of these combinations is not superior to that of IL-2 alone. Responses to high-dose IL-2 are observed in 15–25% of patients. Additionally, a unique feature of IL-2 is the 8–10% durable complete remission rate. These remissions may translate into cure for a highly selected group of patients. The toxicity of IL-2 therapy is substantial and requires careful screening of potential candidates to minimize the incidence of fatal toxicity. Fever, chills, hypotension, and capillary leak syndrome occur with therapy with high-dose IL-2. Treatment frequently requires the use of an intensive care unit because hypotension is severe, often requiring pressor support. Patients with brain or spinal cord metastases should not be treated with IL-2 because of peritumoral edema, and patients with renal, pulmonary, or coronary artery disease are ineligible because of the risks of azotemia, respiratory distress, and myocardial ischemia, respectively. Patients who have been treated with IL-2 have an increased risk of infection, particularly staphylococcal infections.

Although the toxicities of IL-2 are considerable, selected patients may be cured with this form of immunotherapy. The use of low-dose subcutaneous injections of IL-2 has been explored, and several trials have reported encouraging results. Combination regimens such as (1) IL-2 plus interferon-alpha or (2) 5-fluorouracil or FUdR plus interferon-alpha or IL-2 also show some promise. Other biologic response modifiers that may be less toxic than IL-2, including autolymphocyte therapy and vaccines, are currently being tested.

HORMONE-REFRACTORY PROSTATE CANCER

The systemic therapy of patients with metastatic prostate cancer in whom hormonal therapy has failed has been disappointing. It must be pointed out that 15–30% of patients who have had progressive disease despite therapy with combined androgen blockade have a fall in prostate-specific antigen (PSA) when their antiandrogen is discontinued. This maneuver is mandated, therefore, before initiating other systemic therapy. Furthermore, second-line hormonal maneuvers such as adrenal androgen deprivation with ketoconazole clearly have activity and, particularly in asymptomatic patients, should be considered. As noted previously, the evaluation of responses in patients with bone disease only is difficult at best. The use of the PSA in this setting has been fairly extensively evaluated, and it appears to be a reasonable intermediate endpoint. Thus, a brisk and significant (> 50%) fall in PSA appears to be predictive of longer survival for the patient. Despite this fact, it must be borne in mind that the median survival after the diagnosis of hormone-refractory prostate cancer (HRPC) is 12–20 months, and no agent or combination of agents has yet been shown to have an impact on overall survival. HRPC remains incurable.

Several agents or combinations of agents show promise in the therapy of HRPC. Not only can a significant decline in PSA be demonstrated in some patients, but also objective responses in patients with soft-tissue disease have been observed. Furthermore, considerable palliation of pain is often possible with chemotherapy in patients in whom narcotics or corticosteroids have failed and irradiation is not an option.

Mitoxantrone is approved in combination with prednisone for the treatment of progressive, symptomatic HRPC. Twenty-nine percent of those treated with the combination experienced decreased pain, compared with 12% receiving prednisone alone. In addition, there were greater improvements in quality-of-life measures. The toxicity of the treatment was mild in both groups; fewer than 2% of patients had infectious episodes. Median survival for both groups was approximately 1 year. Mitoxantrone has modest albeit definable activity in HRPC, although it probably does not significantly prolong survival.

Estramustine is an oral drug originally developed to target hormonally responsive cancers. However, more recent laboratory studies suggest that estramustine probably affects the function of microtubules, structural nuclear proteins, and the nuclear matrix. Because of its effects on microtubules, estramustine has been investigated in combination with other antimicrotubule agents such as vinblastine, etoposide, and the taxanes. Many of these studies have reported PSA response rates of 60% to 70% (nearly twice that seen with mitoxantrone), objective responses of 25% to 50%, and acceptable toxicity. Fatigue, mild myelosuppression, and dose-dependent reversible peripheral neuropathy have been noted. Based on these data, the standard of care for HRPC patients requiring chemotherapy has become an estramustine/taxane combination. Mitoxantrone or prednisone is frequently used as second-line chemotherapy.

The above observations suggest that chemotherapy has a palliative role to play in the management of some patients with HRPC. Patients with adequate bone marrow function and performance status but a significant tumor burden or rapidly progressive disease are candidates for cytotoxic treatment, although currently available data do not identify one regimen as superior. Future randomized studies will be necessary to compare these various treatment programs and to determine if improvements in survival can be obtained in addition to symptomatic benefit. Because no therapy has a proven survival advantage, all patients with HRPC should be considered candidates for appropriate clinical trials.

REFERENCES

Bajorin DF, Bosl GJ: Bleomycin in germ cell tumor therapy: Not all regimens are created equal. (Editorial.) J Clin Oncol 1997; 15:1717.

Beyer J et al: High-dose chemotherapy as salvage treatment in germ cell tumors: A multivariate analysis of prognostic factors. J Clin Oncol 1996;14:2638.

Beyer J et al: Long term survival of patients with recurrent or refractory germ cell tumors after high dose chemotherapy. Cancer 1997;79:161.

Garrow GC, Johnson DH: Treatment of "good risk" metastatic testicular cancer. Semin Oncol 1992;19:159.

Harker WG et al: Cisplatin, methotrexate, and vinblastine (CMV): An effective chemotherapy regimen for metastatic transitional cell carcinoma of the urinary tract: A Northern California Oncology Group study. J Clin Oncol 1985;3:1463.

International Germ Cell Cancer Collaborative Group: International Germ Cell Consensus Classification: A prognostic factor-based staging system for metastatic germ cell cancers. J Clin Oncol 1997;15:594.

Kelly WK et al: Prostate-specific antigen as a measure of disease outcome in metastatic hormone-refractory prostate cancer. J Clin Oncol 1993;11:1566.

Oh WK, Kantoff PW: Management of hormone refractory prostate cancer: Current standards and future prospects. J Urol 1998; 160:1220.

Parkinson DR, Sznol M: High-dose interleukin-2 in the therapy of metastatic renal cell carcinoma. Semin Oncol 1995;22:61.

Pont J et al: Adjuvant chemotherapy for high-risk clinical stage I nonseminomatous testicular germ cell cancer: Long-term results of a prospective trial. J Clin Oncol 1996;14:441.

Savarese D et al: Phase II study of docetaxel, estramustine, and low-dose hydrocortisone in men with hormone refractory prostate cancer: A final report of CALGB 9780. J Clin Oncol 2002; 19:2509.

Small EJ, Srinivas S: The antiandrogen withdrawal syndrome: Experience in a large cohort of unselected patients with advanced prostate cancer. Cancer 1995;76:1428.

Small EJ, Vogelzang NJ: Second-line hormonal therapy for advanced prostate cancer: A shifting paradigm. J Clin Oncol 1997;15:382.

Stadler WM, Vogelzang NJ: Low-dose interleukin-2 in the treatment of metastatic renal cell carcinoma. Semin Oncol 1995; 22:67.

Sternberg SN et al: Methotrexate, vinblastine, doxorubicin, and cisplatin for advanced transitional cell carcinoma of the urothelium: Efficacy and patterns of response and relapse. Cancer 1989;64:2448.

Tannock I et al: Chemotherapy with mitoxantrone plus prednisone or prednisone alone for symptomatic hormone-resistant prostate cancer: A Canadian randomized study with palliative end points. J Clin Oncol 1996;14:1756.

Vaughn DJ et al: Paclitaxel plus carboplatin in advanced carcinoma of the urothelium: An active and tolerable outpatient regimen. J Clin Oncol 1998;16:255.

Williams SD et al: Immediate adjuvant chemotherapy versus observation with treatment at relapse in pathologic stage II testicular cancer. N Engl J Med 1987;317:1433.

Williams SD et al: Treatment of disseminated germ cell tumors with cisplatin, bleomycin, and either vinblastine or etoposide. N Engl J Med 1987;316:1435.

Yagoda A, Abi-Rached B, Petrylak D: Chemotherapy for advanced renal cell carcinoma: 1983–1993. Semin Oncol 1995;22:42.

Urothelial Carcinoma: Cancers of the Bladder, Ureter, & Renal Pelvis

20

Gary D. Grossfeld, MD, & Peter R. Carroll, MD

BLADDER CARCINOMAS

Incidence

Bladder cancer is the second most common cancer of the genitourinary tract. It accounts for 7% of new cancer cases in men and 2% of new cancer cases in women. The incidence is higher in whites than in African Americans, and there is a positive social class gradient for bladder cancer in both sexes. The average age at diagnosis is 65 years. At that time, approximately 85% of bladder cancers are localized to the bladder; 15% have spread to regional lymph nodes or distant sites.

Risk Factors & Pathogenesis

Cigarette smoking accounts for 50% of cases in men and 31% in women (Wynder and Goldsmith, 1977). In general, smokers have approximately a 2-fold increased risk of bladder cancer than nonsmokers, and the association appears to be dose-related (Thompson and Fair, 1990; Mommsen and Aagaard, 1983). The causative agents are thought to be alpha- and beta-naphthylamine, which are secreted into the urine of smokers.

Occupational exposure accounts for 15–35% of cases in men and 1–6% in women (Matanoski and Elliott, 1981). Workers in the chemical, dye, rubber, petroleum, leather, and printing industries are at increased risk. Specific occupational carcinogens include benzidine, beta-naphthylamine, and 4-aminobiphenyl, and the latency period between exposure and tumor development may be prolonged. Patients who have received cyclophosphamide (Cytoxan) for the management of various malignant diseases are also at increased risk (Fairchild et al, 1979). Ingestion of artificial sweeteners has been proposed to be a risk factor, but several studies have failed to confirm any association (Howe et al, 1977; Najem et al, 1982; Elcock and Morgan, 1993). Physical trauma to the urothelium induced by infection, instrumentation, and calculi increases the risk of malignancy (Hicks, 1982).

The exact genetic events leading to the development of bladder cancer are unknown, but they are likely to be multiple and may involve the activation of oncogenes and inactivation or loss of tumor suppressor genes (Olumi et al, 1990). Loss of genetic material on chromosome 9 appears to be a consistent finding in patients with both low-grade, low-stage and high-grade, high-stage disease (Tsai et al, 1990; Miyao et al, 1993), which suggests that this may be an early event in bladder cancer development. Loss of chromosome 9 in multiple tumors from an individual patient supports the concept that genetic changes in bladder cancer represent a "field defect" that may occur throughout the urothelium. Additional genetic changes have been described that are specific for invasive bladder tumors. Chromosome 11p, which contains the c-Ha-ras proto-oncogene, is deleted in approximately 40% of bladder cancers (Olumi et al, 1990). Increased expression of the c-Ha-ras protein product, p21, has been detected in dysplastic and high-grade tumors but not in low-grade bladder cancers. Deletions of chromosome 17p have also been detected in over 60% of all invasive bladder cancers, but 17p deletions have not been described in superficial tumors. This finding is noteworthy because the p53 tumor suppressor gene maps to chromosome 17p. p53 alterations represent the most commonly identified genetic abnormality in human cancers, making deletion of this chromosome an important finding in muscle invasive bladder cancer.

Staging

The initial staging system for bladder cancer was proposed by Jewett and Strong (1946) and was later modified by Marshall (1952). Currently, the most commonly used staging system allows for a precise and simultaneous description of the primary tumor stage (T stage), the status of lymph nodes (N stage), and metastatic sites (M stage) (American Joint Committee on Cancer, 1997). The 2 staging systems are compared in Figure 20–1. Although either provides a reasonable estimate of a given tumor's biologic potential and the need for and type of treatment, significant staging errors exist when one compares the clinical stage (that based on physical examination and imaging) with the pathologic stage (that based on removal of the bladder and regional lymph nodes). Overstaging is relatively uncommon, but clinical understaging may occur in up to 53% of patients (Skinner, 1977; Skinner, 1982; Dutta et al, 2001).

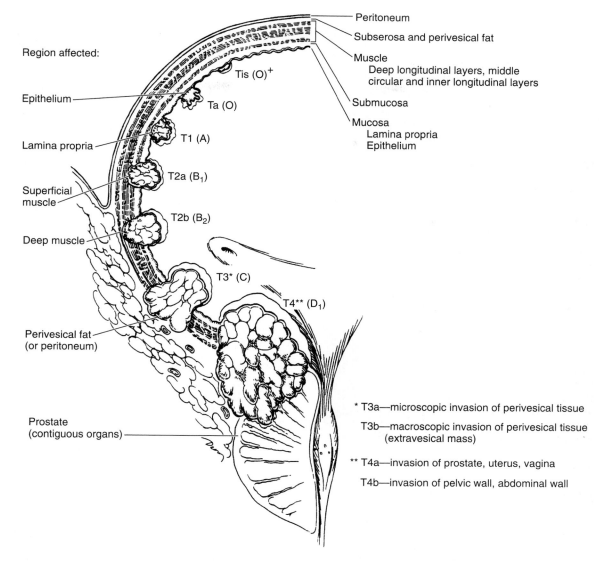

Figure 20–1. Staging of bladder cancer.

Histopathology

Ninety-eight percent of all bladder cancers are epithelial malignancies, with most being transitional cell carcinomas.

A. NORMAL UROTHELIUM

The normal urothelium is composed of 3–7 layers of transitional cell epithelium resting on a basement membrane composed of extracellular matrix (collagen, adhesive glycoproteins, glycosaminoglycans) (Figure 20–2A). The epithelial cells vary in appearance: The basal cells are actively proliferating cells resting on the basement membrane; the luminal cells, perhaps the most important feature of a normal bladder epithelium, are larger umbrella-like cells that are bound together by tight junctions. Beyond the basement membrane is loose connective tissue, the lamina propria, in which occasionally smooth-muscle fibers can be identified. These fibers should be distinguished from deeper, more extensive muscle elements defining the true muscularis propria. The muscle wall of the bladder is composed of

A

B

C

Figure 20–2. **A:** Normal urothelium (125×). **B:** Moderately well-differentiated, papillary bladder cancer (60×). **C:** Carcinoma in situ (200×).

muscle bundles coursing in multiple directions. As these converge near the bladder neck, 3 layers can be recognized: inner and outer longitudinally oriented layers and a middle, circularly oriented layer.

B. PAPILLOMA

The World Health Organization recognizes a papilloma as a papillary tumor with a fine fibrovascular stalk supporting an epithelial layer of transitional cells with normal thickness and cytology (Epstein et al, 1998). Papillomas are a rare benign condition usually occurring in younger patients.

C. TRANSITIONAL CELL CARCINOMA

Approximately 90% of all bladder cancers are transitional cell carcinomas. These tumors most commonly appear as papillary, exophytic lesions (Figure 20–2B); less commonly, they may be sessile or ulcerated. Whereas the former group are usually superficial in nature, sessile growths are often invasive. The World Health Organization has proposed that transitional cell carcinomas be divided into 3 categories on the basis of urothelial architecture, cell size, nuclear size and shape, the presence or absence of nucleoli, hyperchromatism, and the number of mitoses present (Epstein et al, 1998).

Carcinoma in situ (CIS) is recognizable as flat, anaplastic epithelium. The urothelium lacks the normal cellular polarity, and cells contain large, irregular hyperchromatic nuclei with prominent nucleoli (Figure 20–2C). Carcinoma in situ may occur either close to or remote from an exophytic lesion or, rarely, it may occur as focal or diffuse lesions in a patient without macroscopic tumors. It has a variable natural history, but many cases progress to invasive disease. In addition, exophytic lesions occurring with CIS are more likely to recur and invade than those without CIS.

The frequency of tumor invasion, recurrence, and progression is strongly correlated with tumor grade (Lutzeyer, Rubben, and Dahm, 1982; Torti et al, 1987): Progression is noted infrequently in patients with papillary urothelial neoplasm of low malignant potential, in less than 5% of patients with low-grade papillary urothelial carcinoma, and in 15–40% of patients with high-grade papillary urothelial carcinoma (Epstein et al, 1998).

D. NONTRANSITIONAL CELL CARCINOMAS

1. Adenocarcinoma—Adenocarcinomas account for less than 2% of all bladder cancers. Primary adenocarcinomas of the bladder may be preceded by cystitis and metaplasia. Histologically, adenocarcinomas are mucussecreting and may have glandular, colloid, or signetring patterns. Whereas primary adenocarcinomas often arise along the floor of the bladder, adenocarcinomas arising from the urachus occur at the dome. Both tumor types are often localized at the time of diagnosis, but muscle invasion is usually present. Five-year survival is usually less than 40%, despite aggressive surgical management (Kramer et al, 1979; Malek, Rosen, and O'Dea, 1983; Abenoza, Manivel, and Fraley, 1987; Bernstein et al, 1988).

2. Squamous cell carcinoma—Squamous cell carcinoma accounts for between 5% and 10% of all bladder cancers in the United States and is often associated here with a history of chronic infection, vesical calculi, or chronic catheter use. It may also be associated with bilharzial infection owing to *Schistosoma haematobium,* because squamous cell carcinoma accounts for approximately 60% of all bladder cancers in Egypt, parts of Africa, and the Middle East, where this infection is prevalent (El-Bolkainy et al, 1981). These tumors are often nodular and invasive at the time of diagnosis. Histologically they appear as poorly differentiated neoplasms composed of polygonal cells with characteristic intercellular bridges. Keratinizing epithelium is present, although often in small amounts.

3. Undifferentiated carcinomas—Undifferentiated bladder carcinomas, which are rare (accounting for less than 2%), have no mature epithelial elements. A small-cell type has been described that histologically resembles similar lesions of the lung (Mills et al, 1987).

4. Mixed carcinoma—Mixed carcinomas constitute 4–6% of all bladder cancers and are composed of a combination of transitional, glandular, squamous, or undifferentiated patterns. The most common type comprises transitional and squamous cell elements (Murphy, 1989). Most mixed carcinomas are large and infiltrating at the time of diagnosis.

E. RARE EPITHELIAL AND NONEPITHELIAL CANCERS

Rare epithelial carcinomas identified in the bladder include villous adenomas, carcinoid tumors, carcinosarcomas, and melanomas. Rare nonepithelial cancers of the urinary bladder include pheochromocytomas, lymphomas, choriocarcinomas, and various mesenchymal tumors (hemangioma, osteogenic sarcoma, and myosarcoma) (Murphy, 1989). Cancers of the prostate, cervix, and rectum may involve the bladder by direct extension. The most common tumors metastatic to the bladder include (in order of incidence) melanoma, lymphoma, stomach, breast, kidney, and lung (Murphy, 1989; Goldstein, 1967).

Clinical Findings

A. SYMPTOMS

Hematuria is the presenting symptom in 85–90% of patients with bladder cancer. It may be gross or microscopic, intermittent rather than constant. In a smaller percentage of patients, it is accompanied by symptoms of vesical irritability: frequency, urgency, and dysuria. Irritative voiding symptoms seem to be more common in patients with diffuse CIS (Farrow et al, 1977). Symptoms of advanced disease include bone pain from bone metastases or flank pain from retroperitoneal metastases or ureteral obstruction.

B. SIGNS

Most patients with bladder cancer have no pertinent physical signs, owing to the superficial nature of their disease. However, patients with large-volume or invasive tumors may be found to have bladder wall thickening or a palpable mass—findings that may be detected on a careful bimanual examination under anesthesia. Masses palpable before transurethral resection but not identifiable thereafter are most often either very large superficial lesions or tumors that have penetrated the more superficial layers of the bladder wall (ie, T2). Those that remain palpable are often locally extensive (≥ T3a). Tumors that are movable anteroposteriorly are classified as a lower stage than T3b, whereas those that are fixed or are invading contiguous organs (rectum, prostate, vagina) are considered to be stage T4.

Hepatomegaly and supraclavicular lymphadenopathy are signs of metastatic disease. Lymphedema from occlusive pelvic lymphadenopathy may be seen occasionally.

C. LABORATORY FINDINGS

1. Routine testing—The most common laboratory abnormality is hematuria. It may be accompanied by pyuria, which on occasion may result from concomitant urinary tract infection. Azotemia may be noted in patients with ureteral occlusion owing to the primary bladder tumor or lymphadenopathy. Anemia may be a presenting symptom owing to chronic blood loss, or replacement of the bone marrow with metastatic disease.

2. Urinary cytology—Exfoliated cells from both normal and neoplastic urothelium can be readily identified in voided urine. Larger quantities of cells can be obtained by gently irrigating the bladder with isotonic saline solution through a catheter or cystoscope. Examination of cytologic specimens obtained in either fashion allows for tumor detection either at the time of initial presentation or during follow-up. Cytologic examination of exfoliated cells may be especially useful in screening high-risk populations and assessing response to treatment. Detection rates vary depending on the adequacy of the specimen and the grade and volume of the tumor.

Cytologic preparations are made by fixing exfoliated cells, placing them on glass slides, and staining them.

High-grade and infiltrating carcinomas are commonly detected, but low-grade or superficial carcinomas may be missed.

3. Other markers—The sensitivity of voided urine cytologic tests depends on a variety of factors, including the number of urine specimens examined, the stage and grade of the bladder tumor, and the expertise of the cytopathologist. Consequently, newer tests that are also performed on voided urine specimens are currently being developed and validated to determine their ability to reliably predict the presence of bladder cancer. These tests include, but are not limited to, the BTA test (Bard Urological, Covington, GA), the BTA stat test (Bard Diagnostic Sciences, Inc, Redmond, WA), the BTA TRAK assay (Bard Diagnostic Sciences, Inc), determination of urinary nuclear matrix protein (NMP22; Matritech Inc, Newton, MA), quantification of urinary fibrinogen/fibrin degradation products (AuraTek FDP; PerImmune Inc, Rockville, MD), identification of the Lewis X antigen on exfoliated urothelial cells, and the determination of telomerase activity in exfoliated cells. Several studies have examined the performance of these voided urinary markers for the detection and follow-up of patients with bladder cancer (summarized in Grossfeld and Carroll, 1998; Grossfeld et al, 2001; Konety and Getzenberg, 2001) (Table 20–1).

Most of the studies performed to date have evaluated these voided markers in patients with known bladder cancer, either primary or recurrent, and have compared the results with those obtained in a control group without bladder cancer. Although these tests may, in many clinical situations, complement traditional evaluation and surveillance techniques, more information on their performance is needed before they are performed routinely. Such exfoliated markers, if they prove to be both specific and sensitive, may play an important role in the initial evaluation and follow-up of patients with bladder cancer.

In addition to enhancing the detection of bladder cancer, such tests may give important information on the natural history of the bladder cancer detected. For example, loss of blood group antigens may correlate with bladder cancer stage and risk of progression. Fradet and colleagues (1990) identified a set of bladder carcinoma cell antigens detected by monoclonal antibodies whose expression correlates not only with tumor stage but also with progression rates.

D. Imaging

Although bladder cancers may be detected by various imaging techniques, their presence is confirmed by cystoscopy and biopsy. Imaging is therefore used to evaluate the upper urinary tract and, when infiltrating bladder tumors are detected, to assess the depth of muscle wall infiltration and the presence of regional or distant metastases (See and Fuller, 1992). Intravenous urography remains one of the most common imaging tests for the evaluation of hematuria. Bladder tumors may be recognized as pedunculated, radiolucent filling defects projecting into the lumen (Figure 20–3); nonpapillary, infiltrating tumors may result in fixation or flattening

Table 20–1. Exfoliated markers for the detection of bladder cancer.

Marker	Sensitivity (%)	Specificity (%)	PPV (%)	NPV (%)
Cytology	35–61	93–100	–	–
BTA	28–100	40–96	33–80	52–94
NMP22	47–100	61–99	29–65	60–100
BTA stat	57–83	33–95	20–56	70–95
BTA TRAK	62–78	51–98	62	73
Lewis X antigen	80–97	73–86	72–81	83–98
Telomerase	62–80	60–99	84	89
FDP	33–83	66–91	79	78
Cytoberatin 20	91	85	95	76
Quantiant	45–59	71–93	–	–
Hyaluronic acid	92	93	–	–
Hyaluronidase	100	89	–	–
BLCA-4	96	100	–	–
Flow cytometry	45–72	80–87	–	–

FDP, fibrinogen/fibrin degradation products; PPV, positive predictive value; NPV, negative predictive value.

Figure 20–3. Image of the urinary bladder obtained on an intravenous urogram. The filling defect represents a papillary bladder cancer.

of the bladder wall. Hydronephrosis from ureteral obstruction is usually associated with deeply infiltrating lesions and poor outcome after treatment (Haleblian et al, 1998).

Superficial (Ta, Tis) bladder cancers staged with a properly performed transurethral resection and examination under anesthesia do not require additional imaging of the bladder or pelvic organs. However, higher-stage lesions are often understaged, and the addition of imaging may be useful. Both computed tomography and magnetic resonance imaging (Figure 20–4) have been used to characterize the extent of bladder wall invasion and detect enlarged pelvic lymph nodes, with overall staging accuracy ranging from 40% to 85% for computed tomography and from 50% to 90% for magnetic resonance imaging (Amendola et al, 1986; Koss et al, 1981; Fisher, Hricak, and Tanagho, 1985; Husband

et al, 1989; Wood et al, 1988). Both techniques rely on size criteria for the detection of lymphadenopathy: Lymph nodes larger than 1 cm are thought to be suggestive of metastases; unfortunately, small-volume pelvic lymph node metastases are often missed. Because invasive bladder cancers may metastasize to the lung or bones, staging of advanced lesions is completed with chest x-ray and radionuclide bone scan.

E. CYSTOURETHROSCOPY AND TUMOR RESECTION

The diagnosis and initial staging of bladder cancer is made by cystoscopy and transurethral resection. Cystoscopy can be done with either flexible or rigid instruments, although the former may be associated with less discomfort. For either, topical anesthetic solutions are injected directly into the urethra. Superficial, low-grade tumors usually appear as single or multiple papillary

A **B**

Figure 20–4. MRI scan of invasive bladder carcinoma: **Left:** T1-weighted image; **Right:** T2-weighted image. Bladder wall invasion is best assessed on T2-weighted images because of heightened contrast between tumor (asterisks) and detrusor muscle along with ability to detect interruption of the thin high-intensity line representing normal bladder wall. The heterogeneous appearance of the prostate (arrow) on the T2-weighted image owes to benign prostatic hypertrophy, confirmed at cystectomy.

lesions; most measure less than 3 cm in diameter. Higher-grade lesions are larger and sessile. Carcinoma in situ may appear as flat areas of erythema and mucosal irregularity.

Once a tumor is visualized or suspected, the patient is scheduled for examination under anesthesia and transurethral resection or biopsy of the suspicious lesion. The objectives are tumor diagnosis, assessment of the degree of bladder wall invasion (staging), and complete excision of the low-stage lesions amenable to such treatment.

Patients are placed in the lithotomy position. A careful bimanual examination is performed. The presence, position, and size of any masses are noted, along with any degree of fixation to contiguous structures. Cystoscopy is repeated with a lens that permits complete visualization of the entire bladder surface. A resectoscope is then placed into the bladder, and visible tumors are removed by electrocautery. Suspicious areas may have biopsies done with cup biopsy forceps and the areas may be cauterized with an electrode. Some clinicians routinely perform random bladder biopsies of normal-appearing urothelium both close to and remote from the tumor. Although detection of dysplasia or CIS occurs in up to 65% of selected patients, probably less than 15% of all patients with initial bladder tumors have such lesions (Althausen, Prout, and Dal, 1976; Wolf and Hojgaard, 1983). Those who do are at a greater risk of both recurrence and progression to a higher stage.

Natural History & Selection of Treatment

A. Standard Histopathological Assessment

The natural history of bladder cancers is defined by 2 separate but related processes: tumor recurrence and progression. Progression, including metastasis, represents the greater biologic risk. However, recurrence, even without progression, represents substantial patient morbidity in that it requires periodic reevaluation (cytology, cystoscopy, etc), repeat endoscopic ablation, and often intravesical chemotherapy (which may be costly, uncomfortable, and associated with complications). Treatment decisions are made after tumor staging has been completed. Such decisions are based variously on tumor stage (TNM), grade, size, multiplicity, and recurrence pattern (Table 20–2).

At initial presentation, approximately 50–70% of bladder tumors are superficial—stage Tis or Ta (Cutler, Heney, and Friedell, 1982). Invasion into the lamina propria or muscle wall is identified in a smaller number of patients, approximately 28% and 24%, respectively; regional or distant metastases are found in approximately 15%. Unfortunately, 80% of patients with invasive or metastatic disease have no previous history of bladder cancer (Brawn, 1982; Kaye and Lange, 1982). Bladder carcinomas also may be stratified at the time of initial presentation on the basis of grade: Approximately 43% of tumors are classified as grade I; 25% as grade II; and 32% as grade III (Gilbert et al, 1978).

Table 20–2. Initial treatment options for bladder cancers.

Cancer Stage	Initial Treatment Options
Tis	Complete TUR followed by intravesical BCG
Ta (single, low-to-moderate grade, not recurrent)	Complete TUR
Ta (large, multiple, high-grade, or recurrent)	Complete TUR followed by intravesical chemo- or immunotherapy
T1	Complete TUR followed by intravesical chemo- or immunotherapy
T2–T4	Radical cystectomy
	Neoadjuvant chemotherapy followed by radical cystectomy
	Radical cystectomy followed by adjuvant chemotherapy
	Neoadjuvant chemotherapy followed by concomitant chemotherapy and irradiation
Any T, N+, M+	Systemic chemotherapy followed by selective surgery or irradiation

TUR, transurethral resection.

There are strong correlations between tumor grade and stage and tumor recurrence, progression, and survival (Frazier et al, 1993). Patients with low-stage, low-grade disease have a low risk (< 5%) of progression to invasive disease, while as many as 40% of patients with low-stage but high-grade disease will progress with extended follow-up (Herr, 2000). Disease-free survival is excellent for patients with superficial disease (PO, PI, PIS, 80–88%). However, it falls for patients with P2 (53–80%), P3 (39–68%), and P4 (25–40%) tumors (Stein et al, 2001; Frazier et al, 1993; Thrasher et al, 1994)—owing to the greater likelihood of metastasis in tumors of higher stage. Whereas lymph node metastases are uncommon (5%) in tumors of low stage, they are increasingly more common in higher-stage tumors: 10–30% for P3A, 31–46% for P3B, and 35–64% for P4 (Stein et al, 2001; Frazier et al, 1993). In patients with organ-confined disease, the presence of pelvic lymph node metastases appears to be the most important prognostic factor (Vieweg et al, 1999).

Although metastasis is less common with superficial bladder cancers, such tumors may progress; most recur and require additional treatment. Stratification of superficial disease into different grades and stages (Ta and T1) is of clinical benefit, because progression and recurrence are related to both. Tumor progression occurs in less than 6% of patients with Ta disease, but in up to

53% of those with T1 disease, with or without concomitant CIS (Heney et al, 1983; Pauwels et al, 1988; Abel et al, 1988; Cookson et al, 1997). It occurs in 10–20% of patients with grade I tumors, 19–37% with grade II tumors, and 33–64% with grade III tumors (Torti et al, 1987; Lutzeyer, Rubben, and Dahm, 1982).

Tumor recurrence is related to history of disease and grade, number, and size of the tumor. It is more common in the first 12 months after diagnosis (but can become manifest many years later), and patients with one recurrence are more likely to have another. Patients with T1, multiple (> 4), large (> 5), or high-grade tumors are at greater risk, as are those with either CIS or severe dysplasia in normal-appearing urothelium remote from the tumor site (Heney et al, 1983; Wolf, Olsen, and Hojgaard, 1985).

B. MOLECULAR MARKERS

Conventional histopathologic analysis of bladder tumors, including determination of tumor grade and stage, may not reliably predict the behavior of many bladder cancers. Assessment of molecular markers of disease, most often with immunohistochemical methods, may complement traditional assessment of cancer stage and grade and better predict outcome. Some markers may be assessed in biopsy specimens, whereas others may be prognostic only when evaluating cystectomy specimens.

Tumor growth and metastasis require the growth of new blood vessels, a process called angiogenesis. New vessel growth is tightly regulated by both angiogenic stimulators, such as the fibroblastic growth factors and vascular endothelial growth factor, and by angiogenic inhibitors, such as thrombospondin-1 and angiostatin. Immunohistochemical methods have been developed for quantification of angiogenesis in a given tumor by measuring microvessel density. Microvessel density is a useful prognostic indicator for a variety of human malignancies, including bladder cancer. In bladder cancer, microvessel density has been associated with lymph node metastases, disease progression, and overall survival in patients with invasive bladder cancer treated with radical cystectomy (Dickinson et al, 1994; Jaeger et al, 1995; Bochner et al, 1997). Furthermore, immunohistochemical expression of thrombospondin-1 has been reported to be significantly associated with both tumor recurrence and overall survival (Grossfeld et al, 1997).

Normal cellular proliferation is the result of an orderly progression through the cell cycle, whereas malignancy is characterized by uncontrolled cell growth. Cell cycle–associated protein complexes composed of cyclins and cyclin-dependent kinases tightly regulate this progression. These protein complexes phosphorylate key proteins involved in cell cycle transition points, including the protein encoded by the retinoblastoma (pRB) and p53 genes. Loss of cell cycle control may be an early step in the development of carcinogenesis. The most extensively characterized molecular marker in patients with invasive bladder cancer is p53 expression. The p53 gene is a tumor suppressor gene that plays a key role in the regulation of the cell cycle. When DNA damage occurs, the level of p53 protein increases, causing cell cycle arrest and repair of DNA. Mutations in the p53 gene result in the production of an abnormal protein product, allowing cells with damaged DNA to continue through the cell cycle. The altered p53 protein has a prolonged half-life compared with the wild-type protein, allowing for its detection by immunohistochemical techniques. Increased p53 immunoreactivity has been found in high-grade and high-stage bladder cancers, and it is associated with disease progression and decreased overall and disease-specific survival. Patients with altered p53 expression (indicating possible mutation of the p53 gene) appear to have an increased risk for disease recurrence and a decreased overall survival when compared with patients with normal p53 expression (Esrig et al, 1995). Cancers that are p53 positive are associated with recurrence rates of 62% for pT1, 56% for pT2, and 80% for P3a, compared with 7%, 12%, and 11%, respectively, for cancers without p53 reactivity. This information has recently led to a clinical trial in which patients are assigned to adjuvant treatment after radical cystectomy based on the p53 status of their tumor. Assessment of p21, another cell cycle protein, may complement knowledge gained from assessment of p53 expression (Stein et al, 1998).

The retinoblastoma (Rb) gene, a tumor suppressor gene, is expressed in several human tumors, including transitional cell carcinoma of the bladder. Rb alteration, as determined by immunohistochemical methods, is associated with high-grade, high-stage bladder cancers. In addition, Rb alteration appears to be significantly associated with decreased overall survival in such patients (Cordon-Cardo et al, 1992; Logothetis et al, 1992). Studies in which both p53 and Rb have been examined in patients with invasive bladder cancer suggest that bladder tumors with alterations in both genes have a poorer prognosis and decreased overall survival when compared with tumors with wild-type p53 and Rb. Tumors with an alteration of only one of these genes behave in an intermediate fashion.

Assessment of other markers that may correlate with outcome in patients with bladder cancer includes that of tumor growth fraction (proliferative index) and cellular adhesion molecule expression (E-cadherin) (Okamura et al, 1990; Lipponen and Eskelinen, 1995).

C. Treatment Selection

Patients with superficial bladder cancers can be treated with transurethral resection followed by selective intravesical chemotherapy or immunotherapy. Patients with initial low-grade, small tumors are at low risk of progression and may be treated by transurethral resection alone followed by surveillance. Patients with T1, high-grade, multiple, large, recurrent tumors or those associated with CIS in remote bladder biopsies are at a higher risk of progression and recurrence and should be considered candidates for intravesical chemotherapy or immunotherapy after complete and careful transurethral resection. Management of T1 tumors is somewhat controversial; some clinicians advise radical cystectomy, especially for grade III lesions, which are associated with a high rate of progression. However, progression rates can be reduced by intravesical chemotherapy (Herr et al, 1989; Cookson and Sarosdy, 1992). Recurrence of T1 disease after a trial of intravesical therapy warrants more aggressive therapy (Herr, 1991; Herr and Sogani, 2001).

Patients with more invasive, but still localized, tumors (T2, T3) are candidates for more aggressive local treatment, including partial or radical cystectomy, or a combination of either irradiation or surgery and systemic chemotherapy. It has been suggested that selected patients with stage T2 disease may be treated adequately with transurethral resection alone. However, this mode of treatment leaves residual disease in most patients (Henry et al, 1988; Herr, 1987; Solsona et al, 1998). Superficial ductal or acinar in situ carcinoma of the prostatic urethra, not invading the basement membrane or prostatic stroma, may be treated with transurethral resection and intravesical chemotherapy or immunotherapy rather than cystectomy (Bretton et al, 1989). However, patients with more extensive involvement of the prostatic urethra by transitional cell carcinoma, or recurrence after conservative therapy, require more aggressive therapy (Schellhammer, Bean, and Whitmore, 1977). Patients with unresectable local tumors (T4B) are candidates for systemic chemotherapy, followed by surgery (or possibly irradiation). Patients with either local or distant metastases should receive systemic chemotherapy followed by the selective use of either irradiation or surgery, depending on the response.

Treatment

A. Intravesical Chemotherapy

In most patients with superficial bladder cancer, tumors recur. Because a certain percentage of these are of higher stage or grade, attempts to reduce recurrence should be undertaken.

Immunotherapeutic or chemotherapeutic agents can be instilled into the bladder directly via catheter, thereby avoiding the morbidity of systemic administration in most cases. Intravesical therapy can have a prophylactic or therapeutic objective, either to reduce recurrence in patients whose tumors have been completely resected or to eradicate existing disease in patients whose superficial tumors are so extensive that complete transurethral resection is not possible. Therefore, intravesical chemotherapy or immunotherapy may be delivered in 3 different fashions to achieve individual goals (Table 20–3). Considerable experience has been gained, but comparison of different agents is difficult owing to the paucity of randomized trials and variations in dose, contact time, patient population, and intervals between treatments. Most agents are administered weekly for 6 weeks. Maintenance therapy (ie, monthly or bimonthly intravesical therapy) may decrease recurrence rates further. Although local toxicity is relatively common—primarily irritative voiding symptoms—systemic toxicity is rare because of the limited absorption of drugs across the lumen of the bladder. Severe systemic complications can be avoided by not administering intravesical chemotherapy in patients with gross hematuria. Efficacy may be improved by increasing contact time and drug concentration (ie, by restricting fluid intake before administration, asking the patient to lie in different positions during treatment, avoiding instillation of air during drug administration, and requiring the patient to avoid urinating for 1–2 h thereafter). The most common agents in the United States are mitomycin C, thiotepa, doxorubicin, and bacillus Calmette-Guérin. Patients in whom treatment with one agent fails may respond to another.

1. Mitomycin C—Mitomycin C is an antitumor, antibiotic, alkylating agent that inhibits DNA synthesis. With a molecular weight of 329, systemic absorption is minimal. Between 39% and 78% of patients with residual tumor experience a complete response to intravesical mitomycin C (Kowalkowski and Lamm, 1988), and recurrence is reduced in 2–33% after complete transurethral resection (Herr, Laudone, and Whitmore, 1987). Side effects are noted in 10–43% of patients and consist largely of irritative voiding symptoms including urinary frequency, urgency, and dysuria (Soloway, 1989). Unique to this drug is the appearance of a rash on the palms and genitalia in approximately 6% of patients, but this effect can be alleviated if patients wash their hands and genitalia at the time of voiding after intravesical administration.

2. Thiotepa—Thiotepa is an alkylating agent with a molecular weight of 189. Although various doses have been used, 30 mg weekly seems to be sufficient. Up to 55% of patients respond completely. Most series show significantly lower recurrence rates in patients taking thiotepa than in those taking a placebo (Herr, Laudone, and Whitmore, 1987; Kowalkowski and Lamm, 1988; Prout et al, 1983). Cystitis is not uncommon after instillation but is usually mild and self-limited. Myelosuppression manifested as leukopenia and thrombocytopenia occurs in up to 9% of patients owing to systemic absorption. A complete blood count should be obtained in all patients before successive instillations.

3. Doxorubicin—Doxorubicin is an intercalating agent of high molecular weight (580). Complete response rates vary among series, with a mean of 38% (Kowalkowski and Lamm, 1988). As a prophylactic agent, the benefit of intravesical administration of this drug ranges from 10% to 23% (Herr, Laudone, and Whitmore, 1987). Cystitis is not uncommon, but systemic toxicity is rare.

4. Bacillus Calmette-Guérin (BCG)—Bacillus Calmette-Guérin (BCG) is an attenuated strain of *Mycobacterium bovis*. Many different strains of BCG exist, and the marketed preparations vary in the number, pathogenicity, viability, and immunogenicity of organisms (Catalona and Ratliff, 1990). The exact mechanism by which BCG exerts its antitumor effect is unknown, but it seems to be immunologically mediated. Mucosal ulceration and granuloma formation are commonly seen after intravesical instillation. Activated helper T lymphocytes can be identified in the granulomas, and interleukin-2 reportedly can be detected in the urine of treated patients (Haaf, Catalona, and Ratliff, 1986). Bacillus Calmette-Guérin has been shown to be very effective both therapeutically and prophylactically. It appears to be the most efficacious intravesical agent for the management of CIS. Complete responses are recorded in 36–71% of patients with residual carcinoma (Herr, Laudone, and Whitmore, 1987; Catalona and Ratliff, 1990). Recurrence rates are

Table 20–3. Delivery of intravesical chemotherapy or immunotherapy.

Use	Timing	Goal
Adjunctive	At TUR	Prevent implantation
Prophylactic	After complete TUR	Prevent or delay recurrence or progression
Therapeutic	After incomplete TUR	Cure residual disease

TUR, transurethral resection.

reduced substantially in patients treated after endoscopic resection (11–27% versus a 70% recurrence after endoscopic resection alone) (Catalona and Ratliff, 1990; Herr, Laudone, Whitmore, 1987; Camacho et al, 1980; Herr et al, 1985; Lamm, 1985). Bacillus Calmette-Guérin has been shown to be superior to intravesical chemotherapy in preventing recurrence in patients with high-risk superficial bladder cancer (Lamm et al, 1991). Although BCG appears to be effective in delaying progression of high-risk superficial bladder cancer, 40–50% of these patients will experience disease progression with extended follow-up and many patients will ultimately require cystectomy (Cookson et al, 1997; Herr et al, 1995; Davis et al, 2002). The optimal schedule of intravesical BCG is not known with certainty; the most commonly recommended induction regimen is BCG weekly for 6 weeks followed by a period of 6 weeks where no BCG is given. At 12 weeks, if no cancer is identified, BCG is given weekly for 3 weeks. Continuous administration of BCG for more than 6 weeks may be immunosuppressive. Maintenance therapy at 3- to 6-month intervals should be considered in high-risk patients (Lamm et al, 2000). Combining dermal scarification with intravesical instillation appears to result in no enhanced benefit (Badalament et al, 1987; Hudson et al, 1987). Side effects of intravesical BCG administration are relatively common, although severe complications are uncommon. Most patients experience some degree of urinary frequency and urgency. Hemorrhagic cystitis occurs in approximately 7% of patients, and evidence of distant infection is found in less than 2%. Patients with mild systemic or moderate local symptoms should be treated with isoniazid (300 mg daily), and the dosage of BCG should be reduced. Isoniazid is continued while symptoms persist and restarted 1 day before the next instillation.

Patients with severe systemic symptoms should have instillations stopped. Patients with prolonged high fever (> 103 °F), symptomatic granulomatous prostatitis, or evidence of systemic infection require treatment with isoniazid and rifampin (600 mg daily). Patients with signs and symptoms of BCG sepsis (eg, high fever, chills, confusion, hypotension, respiratory failure, jaundice) should be treated with isoniazid, rifampin, and ethambutol (1200 mg). The addition of cycloserine (500 mg twice daily) or prednisolone (40 mg daily) increases survival rates (Lamm, 1992).

5. New intravesical agents and approaches—The rate of metachronous tumor recurrence is high compared with that of low-grade cancers occurring in other organs (eg, nasopharynx, colon). Recurrence of superficial bladder cancer is related to cancer stage, grade and number of tumors, associated dysplasia, and DNA content. Recurrent tumors may be due to regrowth of previously re-

sected cancers, growth of new cancers at remote sites, or implantation and subsequent proliferation of cells released into the bladder at the time of endoscopic treatment of the original tumor. Several investigators have studied the efficacy of single-dose therapy delivered at the time of complete transurethral resection (Tolley et al, 1988; Oosterlinck et al, 1993; Rajala et al, 1999). Such therapy has been shown to decrease recurrence rates, probably by decreasing the risk of tumor cell implantation at the time of initial cancer resection. Trials of interferon-alpha, bropirimine (an oral immunomodulator), and valrubicin (an anthracycline derivative) suggest that these agents, either alone or perhaps in combination with other agents, may be effective in either high-risk patients or those who fail to respond to first-line therapy (Belldegrun et al, 1998; Sarosdy et al, 1998; Steinberg et al, 2000). Preliminary studies suggest that low-dose BCG, in combination with interferon, may be successful in 50–60% of patients with high-risk superficial bladder cancer who have failed BCG therapy alone (O'Donnell, Krohn, and DeWolf, 2001). Given the relatively easy accessibility of bladder cancer cells to direct application of therapeutic agents, such cancers may be ideal targets for genetic manipulation (Miyake et al, 1998).

B. Surgery

1. Transurethral resection—Transurethral resection is the initial form of treatment for all bladder cancers. It allows a reasonably accurate estimate of tumor stage and grade and the need for additional treatment. Patients with single, low-grade, noninvasive tumors may be treated with transurethral resection alone; those with superficial disease but high-risk features should be treated with transurethral resection followed by selective use of intravesical therapy, as described above. Transurethral resection alone has rarely been used in the management of patients with invasive bladder cancer because of a high likelihood of recurrence and progression. Such an approach has been used infrequently for carefully selected patients with comorbid medical conditions and either no residual disease or minimal disease only at restaging transurethral resection of bladder tumor (Herr, 1987; Solsona et al, 1998). Careful follow-up of patients with superficial bladder cancers is mandatory because disease will recur in 30–80% of patients, depending on cancer grade, tumor stage, and number of tumors. Disease status at 3 months after initial resection is an important predictor of the risk of subsequent recurrence and progression (Holmang and Johansson, 2002; Solsona et al, 2000). All patients who undergo transurethral resection should undergo cystoscopy at 3 months. For patients who presented initially with solitary, low-grade lesions and who are free of recurrence at 3 months, repeat cystoscopy at 1 year is suggested. Patients who presented initially with multiple or higher-grade lesions (or both) and those who have recurrences at 3 months require more careful surveillance. In such patients, cystoscopy at 3-month intervals is necessary. Although periodic cystoscopy is suggested for all patients with a history of bladder cancer, the risk of recurrence decreases as the tumor-free interval increases. After 5 years without recurrence, the risk of recurrence has been estimated to be 22%; the rate is 2% for 10 years (Morris et al, 1995).

2. Partial cystectomy—Patients with solitary, infiltrating tumors (T1–T3) localized along the posterior lateral wall or dome of the bladder are candidates for partial cystectomy, as are patients with cancers in a diverticulum. Disease remote from the primary tumor must be excluded by random bladder biopsies preoperatively. Few patients with invasive transitional cell carcinomas are candidates (Utz et al, 1973). To minimize tumor implantation resulting from contamination of the wound with cancer cells at the time of surgery, short-course, limited-dose (1000–1600 cGy) irradiation can be used, and an intravesical chemotherapeutic agent can be instilled preoperatively (Ojeda and Johnson, 1983; Van der Werf-Messing, 1969). Although survival rates of well-selected patients may approach those for patients with similar-stage tumors treated by radical cystectomy, local recurrences are common (Whitmore, 1983; Cummings et al, 1978; Merrell, Brown, and Rose, 1979; Schoborg, Sapolsky, and Lewis, 1979; Sweeney et al, 1992). Given current techniques of bladder replacement surgery, partial cystectomy is rarely indicated in the management of patients with invasive bladder cancer.

3. Radical cystectomy—Radical cystectomy implies removal of the anterior pelvic organs: in men, the bladder with its surrounding fat and peritoneal attachments, the prostate, and the seminal vesicles; in women, the bladder and surrounding fat and peritoneal attachments, cervix, uterus, anterior vaginal vault, urethra, and ovaries. This remains the "gold standard" of treatment for patients with muscle invasive bladder cancer. Disease-free survival 5 years after surgery is based on tumor stage: 88% for patients with P0, Pa, or PIS disease; 80% for patients with P1 disease; 81% for patients with P2 disease; 68% for patients with P3a and 47% for those with P3b disease; and 44% for patients with P4a disease (Stein et al, 2001). Recurrences after surgery usually occur within the first 3 years. Local pelvic recurrence rates are low (7–10%); most patients who fail therapy have distant disease recurrence.

The risk of urethral tumor occurrence or recurrence in men who undergo radical cystectomy is 6.1–10.6%. Risk factors for urethral tumor involvement in men include infiltration of the prostatic stroma or prostatic urethra with cancer or CIS. Patients with these risk factors are candidates for urethrectomy either at the time of radical cystectomy or as a separate procedure (Zabbo and Montie, 1984; Schellhammer and Whitmore, 1976). Although prostatic urethral disease is a risk factor for urethral recurrence, recent evidence suggests that urethrectomy may be omitted and orthotopic urinary diversion performed safely in men with only proximal prostatic urethral involvement and a negative urethral margin at radical cystectomy (Iselin et al, 1997).

Urethrectomy was once routinely performed in all women undergoing radical cystectomy. However, recent clinical experience suggests that bladder replacement may be an acceptable procedure in women as well as men. Women with bladder cancer who have a clear urethral margin at the time of cystectomy are candidates for this procedure. Approximately 66% of women undergoing radical cystectomy for the management of bladder cancer fall into this group (Stein et al, 1995; Stenzl et al, 1995; Stein et al, 1998).

A bilateral pelvic lymph node dissection is usually performed simultaneously with radical cystectomy. Lymph node metastases are identified in approximately 20–35% of patients (Lieskovsky, Aherling, and Skinner, 1988; Stein et al, 2001)—an incidence that reflects the inability of any imaging mode to identify consistently small-volume lymph node metastases preoperatively. Patients with lymph node metastases have a poorer prognosis. However, some patients (10–33%) with limited disease in regional lymph nodes may be cured by radical cystectomy and lymphadenectomy (Lerner et al, 1993; Vieweg et al, 1999; Stein et al, 2001). Patients with fewer than 5 positive lymph nodes and organ-confined disease in the primary tumor tend to have a better prognosis than patients with more extensive disease. These patients may also benefit from adjuvant chemotherapy (see section D, below).

Urinary diversion may be accomplished using a variety of techniques. Methods have been developed that allow construction of reservoirs that are continent and do not require the patient to wear an external appliance for collection of urine (see Chapter 24).

C. RADIOTHERAPY

External beam irradiation (5000–7000 cGy), delivered in fractions over a 5- to 8-week period, is an alternative to radical cystectomy in patients with deeply infiltrating bladder cancers. Treatment is generally well tolerated, but approximately 15% of patients may have significant bowel, bladder, or rectal complications. Five-year survival rates for stages T2 and T3 disease range from 18% to 41% (Timmer, Hartliff, and Hooijkaas, 1985; Goffinet et al, 1975; Corcoran et al, 1985; Miller, 1977; Woon et al, 1985; Quilty and Duncan, 1986; Rider and Evans, 1976; Cummings et al, 1976). Unfortunately, local recurrence is common, occurring in approximately 33–68% of patients. Consequently, radiation as monotherapy is usually offered only to those patients who are poor surgical candidates due to advanced age or significant comorbid medical problems.

D. CHEMOTHERAPY

Approximately 15% of patients who present with bladder cancer are found to have regional or distant metastases; approximately 30–40% of patients with invasive disease develop distant metastases despite radical cystectomy or definitive radiotherapy. Without treatment, survival is limited. Early results with single chemotherapeutic agents and, more recently, combinations of drugs have shown that a significant number of patients with metastatic bladder cancer respond partially or completely (Scher and Sternberg, 1985). The single most active agent is cisplatin, which, when used alone, produces responses in approximately 30% of patients (Yagoda, 1983). Other effective agents include methotrexate, doxorubicin, vinblastine, cyclophosphamide, and 5-fluorouracil. Response rates improve when active agents are combined. Methotrexate, vinblastine, doxorubicin, and cisplatin (MVAC) has been the most commonly used regimen for patients with advanced bladder cancer (Sternberg et al, 1988; Tannock et al, 1989). Approximately 13–35% of patients receiving such regimens attain a complete response. However, the median survival time is approximately 1 year, and the sustained survival rate is 20–25%. Treatment with MVAC is associated with substantial toxicity, including a toxic death rate of 3–4%.

Other newer agents demonstrating activity in this disease include ifosfamide, gemcitabine, paclitaxel, and gallium nitrate (Fagbemi and Stadler, 1998). A recent study demonstrated similar overall survival, time to treatment failure, and response rate for patients treated with MVAC and those treated with the newer combination of gemcitabine and cisplatin (von der Maase et al, 2000). The advantage of gemcitabine and cisplatin over MVAC is significantly lower toxicity and improved tolerability.

E. COMBINATION THERAPY

Once it became apparent that patients with metastatic bladder cancer could benefit from combination chemotherapy, investigators began treating patients with locally invasive (T2–T4), but not metastatic, cancer similarly. Chemotherapy can be given before planned radical cystectomy (neoadjuvant) in an attempt to decrease recurrence rates and, in selected cases, allow for bladder preservation. Approximately 22–43% of patients achieve a complete response to chemotherapy alone (Scher, 1990; Scher et al, 1988). However, additional treatment is still indicated because a substantial number of patients believed to be free of tumors after chemotherapy alone are found to have infiltrating disease at the time of

surgery (Scher et al, 1989). Preliminary results from a recent randomized trial suggest that neoadjuvant chemotherapy followed by surgery may improve results when compared with surgery alone for patients with invasive disease. Alternatively, adjuvant chemotherapy may be offered to selected patients after radical cystectomy because of an increased risk of recurrence due to the presence of locally advanced disease (ie, P3, P4, or N+) (Skinner et al, 1991; Logothetis et al, 1988; Scher, 1990; Stockle et al, 1992; Stockle et al, 1995; Freiha et al, 1996). These studies suggest that patients initially managed with radical cystectomy who are found to be at an increased risk of systemic relapse due to the presence of lymph node metastases or regionally advanced disease are candidates for adjuvant chemotherapy.

Owing to high local and systemic failure rates after definitive irradiation, several investigators have explored the possibility of combining irradiation with systemic chemotherapy to decrease recurrence rates, improve patient survival, and allow bladder preservation. Trials of single-agent chemotherapy and irradiation have shown better local response rates than are found in historical series of irradiation alone (Shipley et al, 1984; Jakse, Fritsch, and Frommhold, 1985; Pearson and Raghaven, 1985).

More recently, investigators have treated patients with invasive bladder cancer with complete transurethral resection and intravenously administered combination chemotherapy followed by concomitant chemotherapy and radiation (Given et al, 1995; Chauvet et al, 1996; Shipley et al, 1997; Zietman et al, 1997; Cervek et al, 1998; Kachnic et al, 1997; Tester et al, 1996; Serretta et al, 1998). Early cystectomy is offered to those who do not tolerate chemotherapy, radiation, or both owing to toxicity and those whose cancers fail to respond to such therapy. Complete response rates to chemoradiation may be as high as 50–70% initially, with 5-year overall survival rates approaching 50–60%. However, local recurrence is common, exceeding 50% in many of these studies. Owing to invasive local recurrences, only 18–44% of patients may be alive with an intact bladder 5 years after chemoradiation. Predictors of poor outcome after combined chemoradiation for invasive bladder cancer include hydronephrosis at presentation, advanced clinical tumor stage, inability to complete the entire treatment protocol, and poor performance status. A recent study has suggested that chemoradiation may also be inappropriate for patients with bladder tumors that are p53-positive (Herr et al, 1999).

Systemic chemotherapy for locally invasive, but not metastatic, bladder cancer should not yet be considered standard therapy. The durability of the response, ultimate survival rates, and optimal candidates for the treatment regimens described will be determined only after completion of randomized studies.

URETERAL & RENAL PELVIC CANCERS

Incidence

Carcinomas of the renal pelvis and ureter are rare, accounting for only 4% of all urothelial cancers. The ratio of bladder–renal pelvic–ureteral carcinomas is approximately 51:3:1 (Williams and Mitchell, 1973). The mean age at diagnosis is 65 years, and the male-female ratio is 2–4:1 (Babaian and Johnson, 1980; Hawtrey, 1971). Urothelial cancer often presents as a widespread urothelial abnormality: Patients with a single upper-tract carcinoma are at risk of developing bladder carcinomas (30–50%) and contralateral upper-tract carcinoma (2–4%). Conversely, patients with primary bladder cancer are at low risk (< 2%) of developing upper urinary tract cancers (Oldbring et al, 1989). However, patients with multiple, recurrent superficial and in situ bladder cancers that are successfully treated by transurethral resection and BCG are at a substantial, lifelong risk of development of upper-tract cancers (Herr, 1998). The cumulative risks of such cancers have been estimated to be 10% at 5 years of follow-up, 26% at 5–10 years, and 34% at > 10 years.

Etiology

As with bladder carcinoma, smoking and exposure to certain industrial dyes or solvents are associated with an increased risk of upper urinary tract transitional cell carcinomas (Shinka et al, 1988). However, these tumors also occur with increased frequency in patients with a long history of excessive analgesic intake, those with Balkan nephropathy, and those exposed to Thorotrast, a contrast agent previously used for retrograde pyelography. Patients with carcinomas associated with analgesic abuse are more likely to be women, have higher-stage disease, and be younger than others (Taylor, 1972; Mahoney et al, 1977). All the major constituents of the analgesic compounds consumed (acetaminophen, aspirin, caffeine, and phenacetin) may be associated with an increased risk of upper urinary tract cancer (Ross et al, 1989; Jensen et al, 1989). Balkan nephropathy is an interstitial inflammatory disease of the kidneys that affects Yugoslavians, Rumanians, Bulgarians, and Greeks (Markovic, 1972); associated upper-tract carcinomas are generally superficial and more likely to be bilateral. The exact mechanism of tumor induction in these patients remains unknown.

Pathology

The mucosal lining of the renal pelvis and ureter is similar to that of the urinary bladder, being composed of transitional cell epithelium. Thus, most renal pelvic and ureteral cancers (90% and 97%, respectively) are transitional cell carcinomas. Grading is similar to that for bladder carcinomas. Papillomas account for approximately 15–20% of cases (Grabstald, Whitmore, and Melamed, 1971; Bennington and Beckwith, 1975). They are isolated in just over 50% of patients and multiple in the rest, and in approximately 25% of patients with isolated papillomas and 50% of patients with multiple papillomas, carcinomas eventually develop. Among patients with carcinomas of the ureter, multicentricity approaches 50% (Bennington and Beckwith, 1975). There is a relationship between tumor grade and the likelihood of urothelial abnormalities elsewhere: Low-grade cancers are associated with a low incidence of urothelial atypia or CIS in remote sites; however, these abnormalities are common with high-grade neoplasms (McCarron, Chasko, and Bray, 1982). Most upper urinary tract transitional cell carcinomas are localized at the time of diagnosis; the most common metastatic sites include regional lymph nodes, bone, and lung (Abeshouse, 1956).

Squamous carcinomas account for approximately 10% of renal pelvic cancers and are much rarer in the ureter. Most carcinomas are usually sessile and infiltrating at the time of diagnosis. Such tumors are commonly identified in patients with a history of chronic inflammation from infection or calculous disease. Adenocarcinomas are very rare tumors of the upper urinary tract and, like squamous carcinomas, tend to be far advanced at the time of diagnosis.

Mesodermal tumors of the renal pelvis and ureter are quite rare. Benign tumors include fibroepithelial polyps (the most common), leiomyomas, and angiomas. Fibroepithelial polyps occur most commonly in young adults and are characterized radiographically by a long, slender, and polyploid filling defect within the collecting system. The most common malignant mesodermal tumors are leiomyosarcomas. The ureter and renal pelvis may be invaded by cancers of contiguous structures, such as primary renal, ovarian, or cervical carcinomas. True metastases to the ureter are rare. The most common metastatic tumors include those of stomach, prostate, kidney, and breast as well as lymphomas (Bennington and Beckwith, 1975).

Staging & Natural History

Staging of both renal pelvic and ureteral carcinomas (Table 20–4) is based on an accurate assessment of the degree of tumor infiltration and parallels the staging system developed for bladder cancer (Batata et al, 1975; Grabstald, Whitmore, and Melamed, 1971; American Joint Committee on Cancer, 1997). Tumor stage and grade correlate with survival (Cummings et al, 1975; Batata et al, 1975; Batata and Grabstald, 1976; Bloom, Vidone, and Lytton, 1970; Reitelman et al, 1987).

Table 20–4. Staging of ureteral and renal pelvic carcinoma.

	System	
	Batata[a]	**TNM**[b]
Confined to mucosa	O	Ta, Tis
Invasion of lamina propria	A	T1
Invasion of muscularis	B	T2
Extension through muscularis into fat or renal parenchyma	C	T3
Spread to adjacent organs	D	T4
Lymph node metastases	D	N+
Metastases	D	M+

[a]Drawn from Batata et al, 1975.
[b]Drawn from American Joint Committee on Cancer, 1997.

Low-grade and low-stage cancers of the renal pelvis and ureter are associated with survival rates between 60% and 90%, compared with 0% and 33% for tumors of higher grade or those that have penetrated deep into or through the renal pelvic or ureteral wall (Hall et al, 1998). The latter figures reflect a high likelihood of regional or distant metastases—40% and 75% in patients with stages B and C (T2–T4) cancers, respectively.

Clinical Findings

A. SYMPTOMS AND SIGNS

Gross hematuria is noted in 70–90% of patients. Flank pain, present in 8–50%, is the result of ureteral obstruction from blood clots or tumor fragments, renal pelvic or ureteral obstruction by the tumor itself, or regional invasion by the tumor. Irritative voiding symptoms are present in approximately 5–10% of patients. Constitutional symptoms of anorexia, weight loss, and lethargy are uncommon and are usually associated with metastatic disease. A flank mass owing to hydronephrosis or a large tumor is detected in approximately 10–20% (Geerdsen, 1979), and flank tenderness may be elicited as well. Supraclavicular or inguinal adenopathy or hepatomegaly may be identified in a small percentage of patients with metastatic disease.

B. LABORATORY FINDINGS

Hematuria is identified in most patients but may be intermittent. Elevated liver function levels due to liver metastases are noted in a few patients. Pyuria and bacteriuria may be identified in patients with concomitant urinary tract infection from obstruction and urinary stasis.

As with bladder cancers, upper urinary tract cancers may be identified by examining exfoliated cells in the urinary sediment. In addition, specimens may be ob-

tained directly with a ureteral catheter or by passing a small brush through the lumen of an open-ended catheter (Gill, Lu, and Thomsen, 1973; Blute, Gittes, and Gittes, 1981; Dodd et al, 1997). Detection depends on the grade of the tumor and the adequacy of the specimen obtained: 20–30% of low-grade cancers may be detected by cytologic testing compared with more than 60% of higher-grade lesions (McCarron, Mullis, and Vaughn, 1983); using barbotage or a ureteral brush increases diagnostic accuracy (Zincke et al, 1976). The utility of the newer voided markers, such as the BTA stat test (Bard Diagnostic Sciences, Inc, Redmond, WA), in detecting upper-tract urothelial cancers has not yet been determined (Zimmerman et al, 1998).

C. IMAGING

Findings on intravenous urography in patients with upper urinary tract cancers are usually abnormal. The most common abnormalities identified include an intraluminal filling defect, unilateral nonvisualization of the collecting system, and hydronephrosis (Williams and Mitchell, 1973; Batata et al, 1975; Almgard, Freedman, and Ljungqvist, 1973). Ureteral and renal pelvic tumors must be differentiated from nonopaque calculi, blood clots, papillary necrosis, and inflammatory lesions such as ureteritis cystica, fungus infections, or tuberculosis. The intravenous urography is often indeterminate, requiring retrograde pyelography for more accurate visualization of collecting-system abnormalities and simultaneous collection of cytologic specimens. Contrast material is injected into the ureteral orifice with a bulb or acorn-tip catheter. Intraluminal filling defects may then be identified in the ureter or renal pelvis (Figure 20–5). Ureteral tumors are often characterized by dilation of the ureter distal to the lesion, creating the appearance of a "goblet." Nonopaque ureteral calculi appear as a narrowing of the ureter distal to the calculus. A ureteral catheter passed up the ureter may coil distal to a ureteral tumor (Bergman's sign) (Bergman, Friedenberg, and Sayegh, 1961). Ultrasonography, computed tomography, and magnetic resonance imaging frequently identify soft-tissue abnormalities of the renal pelvis but may fail to identify ureteral filling defects directly, although they may show hydronephrosis (Figure 20–6). All 3 imaging techniques differentiate blood clot and tumor from nonopaque calculi. In addition, computed tomography and magnetic resonance imaging allow simultaneous examination of abdominal and retroperitoneal structures for signs of regional (lymph node) or more distant metastases.

D. URETEROPYELOSCOPY

The use of rigid and flexible ureteropyeloscopes has allowed direct visualization of upper urinary tract abnor-

Figure 20–5. Filling defect representing a transitional cell carcinoma (arrow) on retrograde pyelography.

malities. These instruments are passed transurethrally through the ureteral orifice; in addition, they (and the similarly constructed but larger nephroscopes), can be passed percutaneously into renal calyces and the pelvis directly. The latter instrument carries with it the theoretic possibility of tumor spillage along the percutaneous tract. Indications for ureteroscopy include evaluation of

filling defects within the upper urinary tract and after positive results on cytologic study or after noting unilateral gross hematuria in the absence of a filling defect. Ureteroscopy is also performed as a surveillance procedure in patients who have undergone conservative surgery for removal of a ureteral or renal pelvic tumor. Visualization, biopsy, and, on occasion, complete tumor resection, fulguration, or laser vaporization of the tumor are possible endoscopically. Detection of renal pelvic and ureteral tumors with these methods seems to be superior to that from conventional methods (Blute et al, 1989).

Treatment

Treatment of renal pelvic and ureteral tumors should be based primarily on grade, stage, position, and multiplicity. Renal function and anatomy should be assessed. The standard therapy for both tumor types has been nephroureterectomy owing to the possibility of multifocal disease within the ipsilateral collecting system. This procedure may be performed using either an open or laparoscopic approach (Landman et al, 2002; Jarrett et al, 2001). When the operation is performed for proximal ureteral or renal pelvic cancers, the entire distal ureter with a small cuff of bladder needs to be removed to avoid recurrence within this segment (Strong et al, 1976; Reitelman et al, 1987). Tumors of the distal ureter may be treated with distal ureterectomy and ureteral reimplantation into the bladder if no proximal defects suggestive of cancer have been noted (Babaian and Johnson, 1980).

Indications for more conservative surgery, including open or endoscopic excision, are not well defined. Absolute indications for renal-sparing procedures include

Figure 20–6. Computed tomography scan showing the presence of a renal pelvic tumor (arrow).

tumor within the collecting system of a single kidney and bilateral urothelial tumors of the upper urinary tract or in patients with 2 kidneys but marginal renal function. In patients with 2 functioning kidneys, endoscopic excision alone should be considered only for low-grade and noninvasive tumors. One must realize that endoscopic examination may fail to detect the degree of infiltration adequately and therefore may understage some tumors. Limited experience with endoscopic resection, fulguration, or vaporization suggests that the procedure is safe in properly selected patients (Blute et al, 1989). However, recurrences have been noted in 15–80% of patients treated with open or endoscopic excision (Maier et al, 1990; Blute et al, 1989; Orihuela and Smith, 1988; Keeley et al, 1997; Stoller et al, 1997). Recurrence may be avoided by treating with instillation of immunotherapeutic or chemotherapeutic agents such as BCG or mitomycin C (Orihuela and Smith, 1988; Keeley and Bagley, 1997; Studer et al, 1989). These agents can be delivered to the upper urinary tract through single or double-J ureteral catheters (Patel and Fuchs, 1998). If patients are treated conservatively, it has been suggested that routine follow-up should include routine endoscopic surveillance because imaging alone may be inadequate for detecting recurrence (Chen et al, 2000).

Radiotherapy plays a limited role in upper urinary tract cancers. Although controversial, postoperative irradiation is believed by some investigators to decrease recurrence rates and improve survival in patients with deeply infiltrating cancers (Brookland and Richter, 1985; Batata et al, 1975). Patients with metastatic, transitional cell cancers of the upper urinary tract should receive cisplatin-based chemotherapeutic regimens as described for patients with metastatic bladder cancers.

Future Directions

Urothelial cancers represent a spectrum of disease defined by various recurrence and progression rates. A greater understanding of tumor induction and progression may allow the clinician to select treatments more wisely. Further development of biologic markers such as tumor proliferation or antigen expression may permit a better estimate of the biologic potential of individual tumors. More refined imaging techniques, perhaps with monoclonal antibodies, would allow clinicians to identify more advanced disease earlier and thereby select treatment strategies better. An assessment of the true benefit, if any, of either neoadjuvant or adjuvant chemotherapy awaits completion of large clinical trials. New agents for the management of most patients with metastatic disease who do not respond to conventional chemotherapy need to be developed. Mechanisms of drug resistance and the means to circumvent them need to be investigated.

REFERENCES

Bladder Carcinomas

Abel PD, Hall RR, Williams G: Should pT1 transitional cell cancers of the bladder still be classified as superficial? Br J Urol 1988;62:235.

Abenoza P, Manivel C, Fraley EE: Primary adenocarcinoma of urinary bladder. Urology 1987;29:2.

Althausen AF, Prout GR, Dal JJ: Non-invasive papillary carcinoma of the bladder associated with carcinoma-in-situ. J Urol 1976; 116:575.

Amendola MA et al: Staging of bladder carcinoma: MRI-CT surgical correlation. AJR 1986;146:1179.

American Joint Committee on Cancer: *Cancer Staging Manual.* Lippincott, 1997.

Badalament RA et al: A prospective randomized trial of maintenance versus non-maintenance intravesical bacillus Calmette-Guérin therapy of superficial bladder cancer. J Clin Oncol 1987;55:441.

Belldegrun A et al: Superficial bladder cancer: The role of interferon-alpha. J Urol 1998;159:1793.

Bernstein SA et al: Primary signet-ring cell carcinoma of urinary bladder. Urology 1988;31:432.

Bochner BH et al: Relationship of tumor angiogenesis and nuclear p53 accumulation in invasive bladder cancer. Clin Cancer Res 1997;3:1615.

Brawn PN: The origin of invasive carcinoma of the bladder. Cancer 1982;50:515.

Bretton PR et al: Intravesical bacillus Calmette-Guérin therapy for in situ transitional cell carcinoma involving the prostatic urethra. J Urol 1989;141:853.

Camacho F et al: Treatment of superficial bladder cancer with intravesical BCG. Proc Am Soc Clin Oncol 1980;21:359.

Catalona WJ, Ratliff TL: Bacillus Calmette-Guérin and superficial bladder cancer. Surg Annu 1990;22:363.

Cervek J et al: Invasive bladder cancer: Our experience with bladder sparing approach. Int J Radiat Oncol Biol Phys 1998; 41:273.

Chauvet B et al: Concurrent cisplatin and radiotherapy for patients with muscle invasive bladder cancer who are not candidates for radical cystectomy. J Urol 1996;156:1258.

Cookson MS, Sarosdy M: Management of stage T1 bladder cancer with intravesical bacillus Calmette-Guérin therapy. J Urol 1992;148:797.

Cookson MS et al: The treated natural history of high-risk superficial bladder cancer: 15-year outcome. J Urol 1997;158:62.

Corcoran MO et al: Invasive bladder cancer treated by radical external radiotherapy. Br J Urol 1985;57:40.

Cordon-Cardo C et al: Altered expression of the retinoblastoma gene product: Prognostic indicator in bladder cancer. J Natl Cancer Inst 1992;84:1251.

Cummings KB et al: Observations on definitive cobalt radiation for cure in bladder carcinoma: 15 year followup. J Urol 1976; 115:152.

Cummings KB et al: Segmental resection in the management of bladder carcinoma. J Urol 1978;118:56.

Cutler SJ, Heney NM, Friedell GH: Longitudinal study of patients with bladder cancer: Factors associated with disease recurrence and progression. In: Bonney WW, Prout GR (editors): *Bladder Cancer*, AUA Monographs. Williams & Wilkins, 1982.

Davis JW et al: Superficial bladder carcinoma treated with Bacillus Calmette-Guerin: Progression-free and disease specific survival with minimum 10 year followup. J Urol 2002;167:494.

Dickinson AJ et al: Quantification of angiogenesis as an independent predictor of prognosis in invasive bladder carcinomas. Br J Urol 1994;74:762.

Dutta SC et al: Clinical under staging of high risk nonmuscle invasive urothelial carcinoma treated with radical cystectomy. J Urol 2001;166:490.

El-Bolkainy MN et al: The impact of schistosomiasis on the pathology of bladder carcinoma. Cancer 1981;48:2643.

Elcock M, Morgan RW: Update on artificial sweeteners and bladder cancer. Regul Toxicol Pharmacol 1993;17:35.

Epstein JI et al: The World Health Organization/International Society of Urological Pathology consensus classification of urothelial (transitional cell) neoplasms of the urinary bladder. Amer J Surg Pathol 1998;22:1435.

Esrig D et al: Prognostic importance of p53 and Rb alterations in transitional cell carcinoma of the bladder. J Urol 1995;153(Pt 2):362A.

Fagbemi S, Stadler W: New chemotherapy regimens for advanced bladder cancer. Semin Urol Oncol 1998;16:23.

Fairchild WV et al: The incidence of bladder cancer after cyclophosphamide therapy. J Urol 1979;122:163.

Farrow GM et al: Clinical observations in 69 cases of in situ carcinoma of the urinary bladder. Cancer Res 1977;37:2794.

Fisher MR, Hricak H, Tanagho EA: Urinary bladder MR imaging. 2. Neoplasm. Radiology 1985;157:471.

Fradet Y et al: Clinical cancer progression in urinary bladder tumors evaluated by multiparameter flow cytometry with monoclonal antibodies. Laval University Urology Group. Cancer Res 1990;50:432.

Frazier HA et al: The value of pathologic factors in predicting cancer-specific survival among patients treated with radical cystectomy for transitional cell carcinoma of the bladder and prostate. Cancer 1993;71:3993.

Freiha F et al: A randomized trial of radical cystectomy versus radical cystectomy plus cisplatin, vinblastine, and methotrexate chemotherapy for muscle invasive bladder cancer [see comments]. J Urol 1996;155:495.

Gilbert HA et al: The natural history of papillary transitional cell carcinoma of the bladder and its treatment in an unselected population on the basis of histologic grading. J Urol 1978;119:488.

Given RW et al: Bladder-sparing multimodality treatment of muscle-invasive bladder cancer: A five-year follow-up. Urology 1995;46:499.

Goffinet DR et al: Bladder cancer: Results of radiation therapy in 384 patients. Radiology 1975;117:149.

Goldstein AG: Metastatic carcinoma to the bladder. J Urol 1967; 98:209.

Grossfeld GD, Carroll PR: Evaluation of asymptomatic microscopic hematuria. Urol Clin N Amer 1998;25:661.

Grossfeld GD et al: Evaluation of asymptomatic microscopic hematuria in adults (Part II): American Urological Association Best Practice Policy. Urology 2001;57:604.

Grossfeld GD et al: Thrombospondin-1 expression in bladder cancer: Association with p53 alterations, tumor angiogenesis, and tumor progression. J Natl Cancer Inst 1997;89:219.

Haaf EO, Catalona WJ, Ratliff TL: Detection of interleukin 2 in urine of patients with superficial bladder tumors after treatment with intravesical BCG. J Urol 1986;136:970.

Haleblian GE et al: Hydronephrosis as a prognostic indicator in bladder cancer patients. J Urol 1998;160:2011.

Heney NM et al: Superficial bladder cancer: Progression and recurrence. J Urol 1983;130:1083.

Henry K et al: Comparison of transurethral resection to radical therapies for stage B bladder tumors. J Urol 1988;140:964.

Herr HW: Conservative management of muscle infiltrating bladder cancer: Prospective experience. J Urol 1987;138:1162.

Herr HW: Progression of stage T1 bladder tumors after intravesical bacillus Calmette-Guérin. J Urol 1991;145:40.

Herr HW: Tumor progression and survival of patients with high grade, noninvasive papillary (TaG3) bladder tumors: 15-year outcome. J Urol 2000;163:60.

Herr HW, Sogani PC: Does early cystectomy improve the survival of patients with high risk superficial bladder tumors? J Urol 2001;166:1296.

Herr HW, Laudone VP, Whitmore WF: An overview of intravesical therapy for superficial bladder tumors. J Urol 1987; 138:1363.

Herr HW et al: Can p53 help select patients with invasive bladder cancer for bladder preservation? J Urol 1999;161:20.

Herr HW et al: Experience with intravesical bacillus Calmette-Guérin therapy of superficial bladder tumors. Urology 1985; 25:119.

Herr HW et al: Intravesical bacillus Calmette-Guerin therapy prevents tumor progression and death from superficial bladder cancer: Ten-year follow-up of a prospective randomized trial. J Clin Oncol 1995;13:1404.

Herr HW et al: Superficial bladder cancer treated with bacillus Calmette-Guérin: A multivariate analysis of factors affecting tumor progression. J Urol 1989;141:22.

Hicks RM: Promotion in bladder cancer. Carcinogenesis 1982; 7:139.

Holmang S, Johansson SL: Stage Ta–T1 bladder cancer: The relationship between findings at first followup cystoscopy and subsequent recurrence and progression. J Urol 2002; 167:1634.

Howe GR et al: Artificial sweeteners and bladder cancer. Lancet 1977;2:578.

Hudson MA et al: Single course versus maintenance bacillus Calmette-Guérin therapy for superficial bladder tumours: A prospective randomized trial. J Urol 1987;138:295.

Husband JES et al: Bladder cancer: Staging with CT and MR imaging. Radiology 1989;173:435.

Iselin C et al: Does prostate transitional cell carcinoma preclude orthotopic bladder reconstruction after radical cystoprostatectomy for bladder cancer? J Urol 1997;158:2123.

Jaeger TM et al: Tumor angiogenesis correlates with lymph node metastases in invasive bladder cancer. J Urol 1995;154:69.

Jakse G, Fritsch E, Frommhold H: Combination of chemotherapy and irradiation for non-resectable bladder carcinoma. World J Urol 1985;3:121.

Jewett HJ, Strong GH: Infiltrating carcinoma of the bladder: Relation of the depth of penetration of the bladder wall to incidence of local extension and metastasis. J Urol 1946;55:366.

Kachnic LA et al: Bladder preservation by combined modality therapy for invasive bladder cancer. J Clin Oncol 1997;15:1022.

Kaye KW, Lange PH: Mode of presentation of invasive bladder cancer: Reassessment of the problem. J Urol 1982;128:31.

Konety BR, Getzenberg RH: Urine based markers of urological malignancy. J Urol 2001;165:600.

Koss JC et al: CT staging of bladder carcinoma. AJR 1981; 137:359.

Kowalkowski TS, Lamm DL: Intravesical chemotherapy of superficial bladder cancer. In: Resnick M (editor): *Current Trends in Urology*. Williams & Wilkins, 1988.

Kramer SA et al: Primary non-urachal adenocarcinoma of the bladder. J Urol 1979;121:278.

Lamm DL: Bacillus Calmette-Guérin immunotherapy for bladder cancer. J Urol 1985;134:40.

Lamm DL: Complications of bacillus Calmette-Guérin immunotherapy. Urol Clin North Am 1992;19:565.

Lamm DL et al: A randomized trial of intravesical doxorubicin and immunotherapy with bacillus Calmette-Guérin for transitional cell carcinoma of the bladder. N Engl J Med 1991; 325:1205.

Lamm DL et al: Maintenance bacillus Calmette-Guérin immunotherapy for recurrent Ta, T1 and carcinoma in situ transitional cell carcinoma of the bladder: A randomized Southwest Oncology Group study. J Urol 2000;163:1124.

Lerner SP et al: The rationale for en bloc pelvic lymph node dissection for bladder cancer patients with nodal metastases: Long-term results. J Urol 1993;149:758.

Lieskovsky G, Aherling T, Skinner DG: Diagnosis and staging of bladder cancer. In: Skinner DR, Lieskovsky G (editors): *Diagnosis and Management of Genitourinary Cancer*. Saunders, 1988.

Lipponen PK, Eskelinen MJ: Reduced expression of E-cadherin is related to invasive disease and frequent recurrence in bladder cancer. J Cancer Res Clin Oncol 1995;121:303.

Logothetis CJ et al: Adjuvant cyclophosphamide, doxorubicin, and cisplatin chemotherapy for bladder cancer: An update. J Clin Oncol 1988;6:1590.

Logothetis CJ et al: Altered expression of retinoblastoma protein and known prognostic variables in locally advanced bladder cancer. J Natl Cancer Inst 1992;84:1256.

Lutzeyer W, Rubben H, Dahm H: Prognostic parameters in superficial bladder cancer: An analysis of 315 cases. J Urol 1982; 127:250.

Malek RS, Rosen JS, O'Dea MJ: Adenocarcinoma of bladder. Urology 1983;21:357.

Marshall VF: The relation of the preoperative estimate to the pathologic demonstration of the extent of vesical neoplasms. J Urol 1952;68:714.

Matanoski GM, Elliott EA: Bladder cancer epidemiology. Epidemiol Rev 1981;3:203.

Merrell RW, Brown HE, Rose JF: Bladder carcinoma treated by partial cystectomy: A review of 54 cases. J Urol 1979; 122:471.

Miller LS: Bladder cancer: Superiority of preoperative irradiation and cystectomy in clinical stages B2 and C. Cancer 1977; 39(Suppl):973.

Mills SE et al: Small cell undifferentiated carcinoma of the urinary bladder. Am J Surg Pathol 1987;79:728.

Miyake H et al: Enhancement of chemosensitivity in human bladder cancer cells by adenoviral-mediated p53 gene transfer. Anticancer Res 1998;18:3087.

Miyao N et al: Role of chromosome 9 in human bladder cancer. Cancer Res 1993;53:4066.

Mommsen S, Aagaard J: Tobacco as a risk factor in bladder cancer. Carcinogenesis 1983;4:335.

Morris S et al: Superficial bladder cancer: How long should a tumor-free patient have check cystoscopies? Br J Urol 1995; 75:193.

Murphy WM: Diseases of the urinary bladder, urethra, ureters, and renal pelvis. In: Murphy WM (editor): *Urological Pathology*. Saunders, 1989.

Najem GR et al: Life time occupation, smoking, caffeine, saccharine, hair dyes, and bladder carcinogenesis. Int J Epidemiol 1982;11:212.

O'Donnell MA, Krohn J, DeWolf WC: Salvage intravesical therapy with interferon-alpha 2B plus low dose bacillus Calmette-Guérin is effective in patients with superficial bladder cancer in whom bacillus Calmette-Guérin alone previously failed. J Urol 2001;166:1300.

Ojeda L, Johnson DE: Partial cystectomy: Can it be incorporated into an integrated therapy program? Urology 1983;22:115.

Okamura K et al: Growth fractions of transitional cell carcinomas of the bladder defined by the monoclonal antibody Ki-67. J Urol 1990;144:875.

Olumi AF et al: Molecular analysis of human bladder cancer. Semin Urol 1990;8:270.

Oosterlinck W et al: A prospective European Organization for Research and Treatment of Cancer Genitourinary Group Randomized trial comparing transurethral resection followed by a single intravesical instillation of epirubicin or water in single stage Ta, T1 papillary carcinoma of the bladder. J Urol 1993;149:749.

Pauwels RPE et al: Grading in superficial bladder cancer. 1. Morphological criteria. Br J Urol 1988;61:129.

Pearson BS, Raghaven D: First line intravenous cisplatin for deeply invasive bladder cancer: Update on 70 cases. Br J Urol 1985; 57:690.

Prout GR et al: Long-term fate of 90 patients with superficial bladder cancer randomly assigned to receive or not to receive thiotepa. J Urol 1983;130:677.

Quilty PM, Duncan W: Primary radical radiotherapy for T3 transitional cell cancer of the bladder: Analysis of survival and control. Int J Radiat Oncol Biol Phys 1986;12:853.

Rajala P et al: Transurethral resection with perioperative instillation of interferon-alpha or epirubicin for the prophylaxis of recurrent primary superficial bladder cancer: A prospective randomized multicenter study–Finnbladder III. J Urol 1999; 161:1133.

Rider WD, Evans DH: Radiotherapy in the treatment of recurrent bladder cancer. Br J Urol 1976;48:595.

Ruppert JM, Tokino K, Sidransky D: Evidence for two bladder cancer suppressor loci on human chromosome 9. Cancer Res 1993;53:5093.

Sarosdy M et al: Oral bropirimine immunotherapy of bladder carcinoma in situ after prior intravesical bacille Calmette-Guérin. Urology 1998;51:226.

Schellhammer PF, Whitmore WF: Transitional cell carcinoma of the urethra in men having cystectomy for bladder cancer. J Urol 1976;115:56.

Schellhammer PF, Bean MA, Whitmore WF: Prostatic involvement by transitional cell carcinoma: Pathogenesis patterns and prognosis. J Urol 1977;118:399.

Scher HI: Neoadjuvant therapy of invasive bladder tumors. In: Williams R, Carroll PR (editors): *Treatment Perspectives in Urologic Oncology.* Pergamon Press, 1990.

Scher HI, Sternberg CN: Chemotherapy of urologic malignancies. Semin Urol 1985;3:239.

Scher HI et al: Neoadjuvant chemotherapy for invasive bladder cancer: Experience with the M-VAC regimen. Br J Urol 1989;64:250.

Scher HI et al: Neoadjuvant M-VAC (methotrexate, vinblastine, doxorubicin and cisplatin) effect on the primary bladder lesion. J Urol 1988;139:470.

Schoborg TW, Sapolsky JL, Lewis CW: Carcinoma of the bladder treated by segmental resection. J Urol 1979;122:473.

See WA, Fuller JR: Staging of advanced bladder cancer: Current concepts and pitfalls. Urol Clin North Am 1992;19:663.

Serretta V et al: Urinary NMP22 for the detection of recurrence after transurethral resection of transitional cell carcinoma of the bladder: Experience in 137 patients. Urology 1998;52:793.

Shipley WU et al: Cisplatin and full dose irradiation for patients with invasive bladder carcinoma: A preliminary report of tolerance and local response. J Urol 1984;132:899.

Shipley WU et al: Invasive bladder cancer: Treatment strategies using transurethral surgery, chemotherapy and radiation therapy with selection for bladder conservation. Int J Radiat Oncol Biol Phys 1997;39:937.

Skinner DG: Current state of classification and staging of bladder cancer. Cancer Res 1977;37:2838.

Skinner DG: Management of invasive bladder cancer: A meticulous lymph node dissection can make a difference. J Urol 1982;128:34.

Skinner DG et al: The role of adjuvant chemotherapy following cystectomy for invasive bladder cancer: A prospective comparative trial. J Urol 1991;145:459.

Soloway MS: Diagnosis and management of superficial bladder cancer. Semin Surg Oncol 1989;5:247.

Solsona E et al: Feasibility of transurethral resection for muscle infiltrating carcinoma of the bladder: Long-term followup of a prospective study. J Urol 1998;159:95.

Solsona E et al: The 3-month clinical response to intravesical therapy as a predictive factor for progression in patients with high risk superficial bladder cancer. J Urol 2000;164:685.

Stein JP et al: Effect of p21WAF1/CIP1 expression on tumor progression in bladder cancer. J Natl Cancer Inst 1998a;90:1072.

Stein JP et al: Indications for lower urinary tract reconstruction in women after cystectomy for bladder cancer: A pathological review of female cystectomy specimens. J Urol 1995; 154:1329.

Stein JP et al: Prospective pathologic analysis of female cystectomy specimens: Risk factors for orthotopic diversion in women. Urology 1998b;51:951.

Stein JP et al: Radical cystectomy in the treatment of invasive bladder cancer: Long-term results in 1,054 patients. J Clin Oncol 2001;19:666.

Steinberg G et al: Efficacy and safety of Valrubicin for the treatment of bacillus Calmette-Guérin refractory carcinoma in situ of the bladder. J Urol 2000;163:761.

Stenzl A et al: The risk of urethral tumors in female bladder cancer: Can the urethra be used for orthotopic reconstruction of the lower urinary tract? J Urol 1995;153(3 Pt 2):950.

Sternberg CN et al: M-VAC (methotrexate vinblastine doxorubicin and cisplatin) for advanced transitional cell carcinoma of the urothelium. J Urol 1988;139:461.

Stockle M et al: Adjuvant polychemotherapy of nonorgan-confined bladder cancer after radical cystectomy revisited: Long-term results of a controlled prospective study and further clinical experience. J Urol 1995;153:47.

Stockle M et al: Advanced bladder cancer (stages pT3b, pT4a, pN1 and pN2): Improved survival after radical cystectomy and 3 adjuvant cycles of chemotherapy. Results of a controlled prospective trial. J Urol 1992;148:302.

Sweeney P et al: Partial cystectomy. Urol Clin North Am 1992; 19:701.

Tannock I et al: M-VAC (methotrexate vinblastine doxorubicin and cisplatin) chemotherapy for transitional cell carcinoma: The Princess Margaret Hospital experience. J Urol 1989; 142:289.

Tester W et al: Neoadjuvant combined modality program with selective organ preservation for invasive bladder cancer: Results of Radiation Therapy Oncology Group phase II trial 8802. J Clin Oncol 1996;14:119.

Thompson I, Fair W: Occupational and environmental factors in bladder cancer. In: Chisolm GD, Fair WR (editors): *Scientific Foundations of Urology,* 2nd ed. Heinemann Medical Books, 1990.

Thrasher JB et al: Clinical variables which serve as predictors of cancer-specific survival among patients treated with radical cystectomy for transitional cell carcinoma of the bladder and prostate. Cancer 1994;73:1708.

Timmer PR, Hartliff HA, Hooijkaas JAP: Bladder cancer: Pattern of recurrence in 142 patients. Int J Radiat Oncol Biol Phys 1985;11:899.

Tolley D et al: Effect of mitomycin C on recurrence of newly diagnosed superficial bladder cancer: Interim report from the Medical Research Council Subgroup on Superficial Bladder Cancer. Br Med J 1988;296:1759.

Torti FM et al: Superficial bladder cancer: The primacy of grade in the development of invasive disease. J Clin Oncol 1987; 5:125.

Tsai YC et al: Allelic losses of chromosomes 9, 11, and 17 in human bladder cancer. Cancer Res 1990;50:44.

Utz DC et al: A clinicopathologic evaluation of partial cystectomy for carcinoma of the urinary bladder. Cancer 1973;32:1075.

Van der Werf–Messing B: Carcinoma of the bladder treated by suprapubic radium implants. Eur J Cancer 1969;5:27.

Vieweg J et al: Impact of primary stage on survival in patients with lymph node positive bladder cancer. J Urol 1999;161:72.

Von der Maase H et al: Gemcitabine and cisplatin versus methotrexate, vinblastine, doxorubicin and cisplatin in advanced or metastatic bladder cancer: Results of a large, randomized, multinational, multicenter phase III study. J Clin Oncol 2000;17:3068.

Wallace DM, Bloom HJG: The management of deeply infiltrating (T3) bladder carcinoma: Controlled trial of radical radiotherapy versus preoperative radiotherapy and radical cystectomy. Br J Urol 1976;48:587.

Whitmore WF: Management of invasive bladder neoplasms. Semin Urol 1983;1:34.

Wolf H, Hojgaard K: Prognostic factors in local surgical treatment of invasive bladder cancer with special reference to the presence of urothelial dysplasia. Cancer 1983;51:1710.

Wolf H, Olsen PR, Hojgaard K: Urothelial dysplasia concomitant with bladder tumours: A determinant for future new occurrences in patients treated by full course radiotherapy. Lancet 1985;I:1005.

Wood DP et al: The role of magnetic resonance imaging in the staging of bladder carcinoma. J Urol 1988;140:741.

Woon SY et al: Bladder carcinoma: Experience with radical and preoperative radiotherapy in 421 patients. Cancer 1985; 56:1293.

Wynder EL, Goldsmith K: The epidemiology of bladder cancer: A second look. Cancer 1977;40:1246.

Yagoda A: Chemotherapy for advanced urothelial cancer. Semin Urol 1983;1:60.

Zabbo A, Montie JE: Management of the urethra in men undergoing radical cystectomy for bladder cancer. J Urol 1984; 131:267.

Zietman A et al: The case for radiotherapy with or without chemotherapy in high-risk superficial and muscle-invading bladder cancer. Semin Urol Oncol 1997;15:161.

Ureteral & Renal Pelvic Cancers

Abeshouse BS: Primary benign and malignant tumors of the ureter: A review of the literature and report of one benign and 12 malignant tumors. Am J Surg 1956;91: 237.

Almgard LE, Freedman D, Ljungqvist A: Carcinoma of the ureter with special reference to malignancy grading and prognosis. Scand J Urol Nephrol 1973;7:165.

American Joint Committee on Cancer: *Cancer Staging Manual.* Lippincott, 1997.

Babaian RJ, Johnson DE: Primary carcinoma of the ureter. J Urol 1980;123:357.

Batata M, Grabstald H: Upper urinary tract urothelial tumors. Urol Clin North Am 1976;3:79.

Batata MA et al: Primary carcinoma of the ureter: A prognostic study. Cancer 1975;35:1626.

Bennington J, Beckwith JB: Tumors of the renal pelvis and ureter. In: *Atlas of Tumor Pathology.* Armed Forces Institute of Pathology, Fasc 12, 1975.

Bergman H, Friedenberg RM, Sayegh V: New roentgenologic signs of carcinoma of the ureter. Am J Roentgenol 1961;86:707.

Bloom NA, Vidone RA, Lytton B: Primary carcinoma of the ureter: A report of 102 new cases. J Urol 1970;103:590.

Blute ML et al: Impact of endourology on diagnosis and management of upper urinary tract urothelial cancer. J Urol 1989; 141:1298.

Blute RD, Gittes RR, Gittes RF: Renal brush biopsy: Survey of indications, techniques, and results. J Urol 1981;126:146.

Brookland RK, Richter MP: The postoperative irradiation of transitional cell carcinoma of the renal pelvis and ureter. J Urol 1985;133:952.

Chen GL, El-Gabry EA, Bagley DH: Surveillance of upper tract transitional cell carcinoma: The role of ureteroscopy, retrograde pyelography, cytology and urinalysis. J Urol 2000; 164:1901.

Cummings KB et al: Renal pelvic tumors. J Urol 1975;113:158.

Dodd L et al: Endoscopic brush cytology of the upper urinary tract: Evaluation of its efficacy and potential limitations in diagnosis. Acta Cytol 1997;41:377.

Geerdsen J: Tumours of the renal pelvis and ureter: Symptomatology, diagnosis, treatment, and prognosis. Scand J Urol Nephrol 1979;13:287.

Gill WB, Lu CT, Thomsen S: Retrograde brushing: A new technique for obtaining histologic and cytologic material from ureteral renal pelvic and renal caliceal lesions. J Urol 1973; 109:573.

Grabstald H, Whitmore WF, Melamed MR: Renal pelvic tumors. JAMA 1971;218:845.

Hall M et al: Prognostic factors, recurrence, and survival in transitional cell carcinoma of the upper urinary tract: A 30-year experience in 252 patients. Urology 1998;52:594.

Hawtrey CE: Fifty-two cases of primary ureteral carcinoma: A clinical-pathologic study. J Urol 1971;105:188.

Herr H: Long-term results of BCG therapy: Concern about upper tract tumors. Semin Urol Oncol 1998;16:13.

Jarrett TW et al: Laparoscopic nephroureterectomy for the treatment of transitional cell carcinoma of the upper urinary tract. Urology 2001;57:448.

Jensen OM et al: The Copenhagen case-control study of renal pelvis and ureter cancer: Role of analgesics. Int J Cancer 1989;44:965.

Keeley F et al: Ureteroscopic treatment and surveillance of upper urinary tract transitional cell carcinoma. J Urol 1997; 157:1560.

Keeley FX, Bagley DH: Adjuvant mitomycin C following endoscopic treatment of upper tract transitional cell carcinoma. J Urol 1997;158:2074.

Landman J et al: Comparison of hand assisted and standard laparoscopic radical nephroureterectomy for the management of localized transitional cell carcinoma. J Urol 2002;167:2387.

Mahoney JF et al: Analgesic abuse renal parenchymal disease and carcinoma of the kidney or ureter. Aust NZ J Med 1977; 7:463.

Maier U et al: Organ-preserving surgery in patients with urothelial tumors of the upper urinary tract. Eur Urol 1990;1 8:197.

Markovic B: Endemic nephritis and urinary tract cancer in Yugoslavia, Bulgaria and Romania. J Urol 1972;107:212.

McCarron JP, Chasko SB, Bray GF: Systematic mapping of nephroureterectomy specimens removed for urothelial cancer: Pathological findings and clinical correlations. J Urol 1982; 128:243.

McCarron JP, Mullis C, Vaughn ED: Tumors of the renal pelvis and ureter: Current concepts and management. Semin Urol 1983;1:75.

Oldbring J et al: Carcinoma of the renal pelvis and ureter following bladder carcinoma: Frequency risk factors and clinicopathological findings. J Urol 1989;141:1311.

Orihuela E, Smith AD: Percutaneous treatment of transitional cell carcinoma of the upper urinary tract. Urol Clin North Am 1988;15:425.

Patel A, Fuchs G: New techniques for the administration of topical adjuvant therapy after endoscopic ablation of upper urinary tract transitional cell carcinoma. J Urol 1998;159:71.

Reitelman C et al: Prognostic variables in patients with transitional cell carcinoma of the renal pelvis and proximal ureter. J Urol 1987;138:1144.

Ross RK et al: Analgesics, cigarette smoking, and other risk factors for cancer of the renal pelvis and ureter. Cancer Res 1989; 49:1045.

Shinka T et al: Occurrence of uroepithelial tumors of the upper urinary tract after the initial diagnosis of bladder cancer. J Urol 1988;140:745.

Stoller M et al: Endoscopic management of upper tract urothelial tumors. Tech Urol 1997;3:152.

Strong DW et al: The ureteral stump after nephroureterectomy. J Urol 1976;115:654.

Studer UE et al: Percutaneous bacillus Calmette-Guérin perfusion of the upper urinary tract for carcinoma in situ. J Urol 1989;142:975.

Taylor JS: Carcinoma of the urinary tract and analgesic abuse. Med J Aust 1972;1:407.

Williams CB, Mitchell JP: Carcinoma of the ureter: A review of 54 cases. Br J Urol 1973;45:377.

Zimmerman R et al: Utility of the Bard BTA test in detecting upper urinary tract transitional cell carcinoma. Urology 1998;51:956.

Zincke H et al: Significance of urinary cytology in the early detection of transitional cell cancer of the upper urinary tract. J Urol 1976;116:781.

Badrinath R. Konety, MD, Robert Dreicer, MD, MS, FACP, & Richard D. Williams, MD

BENIGN TUMORS

With the liberal use of computed tomography (CT) scans and magnetic resonance imaging (MRI), benign renal masses are being detected more frequently.

Benign renal tumors include adenoma, oncocytoma, angiomyolipoma, leiomyoma, lipoma, hemangioma, and juxtaglomerular tumors.

Renal Adenomas

The adenoma is the most common benign renal parenchymal lesion (Williams, 1992). These are small, well-differentiated glandular tumors of the renal cortex. They are typically asymptomatic and usually identified incidentally. At autopsy, 7–22% of patients are found to have a renal adenoma (Bonsib, 1985). Despite the classification of adenoma as a benign tumor, no clinical, histologic, or immunohistochemical criteria differentiate renal adenoma from renal carcinoma. Previously, all renal tumors less than 3 cm were considered adenomas. However, even such small tumors can metastasize and are now classified as renal cell carcinoma (RCC). Adenomas of any size should be treated as a fortuitous finding representative of an early renal cancer, and the patient should be evaluated and treated appropriately.

Renal Oncocytoma

Renal oncocytoma has a spectrum of behavior ranging from benign to malignant. Composed of large epithelial cells with finely granular eosinophilic cytoplasm (oncocytes), oncocytomas occur in various organs and organ systems including adrenal, salivary, thyroid, and parathyroid glands as well as the kidney (Hamperl, 1962). An estimated 3–5% of renal tumors are oncocytomas, accounting for approximately 500 cases per year (Lieber and Tsukamoto, 1986). Men are affected twice as often as women.

Renal oncocytomas generally occur within a well-defined fibrous capsule, with tumor tissue rarely penetrating the renal capsule, pelvis, collecting system, or perinephric fat. On cut section, the surface of the tumor is usually tan or light brown with a central stellate scar, but necrosis typical of renal adenocarcinoma is absent. The tumors are usually solitary and unilateral,

although several bilateral cases and multiple oncocytomas occurring simultaneously (**oncocytomatosis**) have been reported (Tickoo et al, 1999).

Oncocytomas can also be associated with benign tumors of hair follicles (**fibrofolliculomas**), colon polyps/tumors, and pulmonary cysts as part of the Birt-Hogg-Dubé syndrome (Toro et al, 1999). Histologically, well-differentiated oncocytomas are made up of large, uniform cells containing an intensely eosinophilic cytoplasm, which on ultrastructural studies is found to be packed with mitochondria. Mitotic activity is absent, and nuclear pleomorphism is uncommon (Figure 21–1). The cellular origin of renal oncocytes has not been fully elucidated, although some early evidence suggested that oncocytes resemble proximal convoluted tubular cells (Merino and Librelsi, 1982). Recent findings suggest their origin may be a precursor stem cell (Cohen, McCue, and Derose, 1988) or the intercalated cells of the collecting ducts (Storkel et al, 1989).

The diagnosis of oncocytoma is predominantly pathologic because there are no reliable distinguishing clinical characteristics. Gross hematuria and flank pain occur in less than 20% of patients (Lieber and Tsukamoto, 1986). No characteristic features of the tumors appear on CT, ultrasound (US), intravenous urography (IVU), or MRI. Ambos et al (1978) and Weiner and Bernstein (1977) have described angiographic features of oncocytomas, including the "spoke-wheel" appearance of tumor arterioles, the "lucent rim sign" of the capsule, and a homogeneous capillary nephrogram phase. Unfortunately, these findings are not invariable (Older et al, 1978), and similar findings have been reported in patients with RCC (Maatman et al, 1984).

High-grade oncocytomas may be intermixed with elements of RCC (Davis et al, 1991) and can be found as coexisting lesions within the same or opposite kidney (Licht et al, 1993). The role of fine-needle aspiration in the preoperative diagnosis of oncocytomas remains controversial and limited, due to lack of characteristic features that distinguish oncocytoma from RCC.

Angiomyolipoma (Renal Hamartoma)

Angiomyolipoma is a rare benign tumor of the kidney seen in 2 distinct clinical populations. Angiomyolipomas are found in approximately 45–80% of patients

Figure 21–1. Histologic section of a grade I (benign) renal oncocytoma (original magnification, × 100).

with tuberous sclerosis and are typically bilateral and asymptomatic. Tuberous sclerosis is a familial inherited disorder comprising adenoma sebaceum, mental retardation, and epilepsy. In patients without tuberous sclerosis, renal angiomyolipomas can be unilateral and tend to be larger than those associated with tuberous sclerosis (Anderson and Hatcher, 1990). There is no known histologic difference between the lesions seen in these 2 populations. As many as 25% of cases can present with spontaneous rupture and subsequent hemorrhage into the retroperitoneum (Wong, McGeorge, and Clark, 1981).

Angiomyolipomas are unencapsulated yellow-to-gray lesions, typically round to oval, that elevate the renal capsule, producing a bulging smooth or irregular mass. They are characterized by 3 major histologic components: mature fat cells, smooth muscle, and blood vessels. Renal hamartomas may extend to perirenal or renal sinus fat and involve regional lymphatics (Busch, Bark, and Clyde, 1976) and other visceral organs (Ditonno et al, 1992). The presence of renal hamartomas in extrarenal sites is a manifestation of multicentricity rather than metastatic potential, because only one well-documented case of malignant transformation of angiomyolipoma has been reported (Lowe et al, 1992).

Patients with a rare condition termed **lymphangioleiomyomatosis** may have multiple renal and hepatic angiomyolipomata, multiple pulmonary cysts, enlarged abdominal lymph nodes, and lymphangiomyomas (Avila et al, 2000; Urban et al, 1999). The diagnosis of renal angiomyolipoma has evolved with the widespread use of US and CT. Arteriography can reveal neovascularity similar to that of renal cancer and therefore is not helpful in differential diagnosis. Ultrasonography and

CT are frequently diagnostic in lesions with high fat content. Fat visualized on US appears as very high intensity echoes. Fat imaged by CT has a negative density −20 to −80 Hounsfield units), which is pathognomonic for angiomyolipomas when observed in the kidney (Figure 21–2) (Pitts et al, 1980). The role of MRI as a diagnostic tool has been investigated; as in CT, the high fat content makes this lesion suitable for MRI diagnosis (Uhlenbrock, Fischer, and Beyer, 1988); however, because the presence of bleeding in any renal tumor can mimic the typical pattern of angiomyolipoma, MRI should not be considered the diagnostic method of choice.

The management of angiomyolipomas historically has been correlated with symptoms. Steiner and colleagues (1993) reported a long-term follow-up study of 35 patients with angiomyolipomas. They proposed that patients with isolated lesions less than 4 cm be followed up with yearly CT or US. Patients with asymptomatic or mildly symptomatic lesions greater than 4 cm should be followed up with semiannual US. Patients with lesions greater than 4 cm with moderate or severe symptoms (bleeding or pain) should undergo renal-sparing surgery or renal arterial embolization. Given the difference in the natural history of angiomyolipomas in patients with tuberous sclerosis, Steiner et al advocate prophylactic intervention in patients with lesions greater than 4 cm irrespective of symptoms, with close follow-up of smaller lesions.

Other Rare Benign Renal Tumors

Several other benign renal tumors are quite rare, including leiomyomas, hemangiomas, lipomas, and juxtaglomerular cell tumors. With the exception of juxtaglomerular tumors, there are no features that

Figure 21–2. Computed tomogram of an angiomyolipoma (arrows).

unequivocally establish the diagnosis before surgery; therefore, the pathologist most often provides the diagnosis after nephrectomy.

Leiomyomas are rare small tumors typically found in smooth–muscle-containing areas of the kidney including the renal capsule and renal pelvis. Two groups of renal leiomyomas have been described (Steiner et al, 1990). The more common group comprises cortical tumors that are less than 2 cm and may be multiple. These tumors are typically found at autopsy and are not clinically significant. A larger, commonly solitary leiomyoma has been described, which may cause symptoms and is confirmed pathologically after nephrectomy.

Hemangiomas are small vascular tumors occurring in the kidney with a frequency second only to that in the liver among visceral organs (White and Braunstein, 1946). Multiple lesions in one kidney occur in approximately 12% of cases; however, they are rarely bilateral. They can occasionally be the elusive source of hematuria in an otherwise well-evaluated patient. The diagnosis may be determined by angiography or by direct visualization by endoscopy (Ekelund and Gothlin, 1975).

Renal lipomas are very uncommon deposits of mature adipose cells without evident mitosis that arise from the renal capsule or perirenal tissue. They are seen primarily in middle-aged females and, owing to the characteristic CT differentiation of fat, are best detected radiographically on CT scanning.

The **juxtaglomerular cell tumor** is the most clinically significant member of this subgroup of rare benign tumors because it causes significant hypertension that can be cured by surgical treatment. It is a very rare lesion, with about 40 reported cases (Ducret et al, 1991). The tumors originate from the pericytes of afferent arterioles in the juxtaglomerular apparatus and can be shown to contain renin secretory granules. They are typically encapsulated and located in the cortical area. The diagnosis is suspected when there is secondary hyperaldosteronism and is confirmed by selected renal vein sampling for renin (Bonnin et al, 1977). Although complete nephrectomy was advocated in the past, several recent reports indicate that partial nephrectomy can be equally effective (Haab et al, 1995).

ADENOCARCINOMA OF THE KIDNEY (RENAL CELL CARCINOMA)

In the United States in 2002, an estimated 31,800 new cases of adenocarcinoma of the kidney are expected to be diagnosed, and 11,600 deaths will occur from this disease (Jemal et al, 2002). Renal cell carcinoma (RCC) accounts for roughly 2.5% of adult cancers and constitutes approximately 85% of all primary malignant renal tumors. There appears to be an increase in the incidence of all stages of RCC over the past few decades (Chow et al, 1999; Hock, Lynch, and Balaji, 2002). RCC occurs most commonly in the fifth to sixth decade and has a male-female ratio of 2:1. The incidence of renal cancer may vary based on race, with black men demonstrating a higher incidence than in men of all other races. Black men may also have a higher likelihood of a subsequent RCC in the contralateral kidney (Rabbani et al, 2002). Asians appear to have the lowest incidence of RCC (Miller, 1996).

Multiple terms have been used to describe renal adenocarcinoma, including hypernephroma, Grawitz tumor, clear cell carcinoma, and alveolar carcinoma.

Etiology

The cause of renal adenocarcinoma is unknown. Occupational exposures, chromosomal aberrations, and tumor suppressor genes have been implicated. Cigarette smoking is the only risk factor consistently linked to RCC by both epidemiologic case-control and cohort studies (La Vecchia et al, 1990), with most investigations demonstrating at least a 2-fold increase in risk for the development of RCC in smokers (Yu et al, 1986). Exposure to asbestos, solvents, and cadmium has also been associated with an increased incidence of RCC (Mandel et al, 1995).

RCC occurs in two forms, inherited and sporadic. In 1979, Cohen and colleagues described a pedigree with hereditary RCC in which the pattern of inheritance was consistent with an autosomal dominant gene with a balanced reciprocal translocation between the short arm of chromosome 3 and the long arm of chromosome 8. Subsequent work has documented that both the hereditary and sporadic forms of RCC are associated with structural changes in chromosome 3 (Kovacs et al, 1988; Erlandsson, 1998).

Two other hereditary forms of RCC have been described. **Von Hippel-Lindau disease** is a familial cancer syndrome in which affected individuals have a predisposition to have tumors develop in multiple organs, including cerebellar hemangioblastoma, retinal angiomata, and bilateral clear cell RCC. In 1993, Latif and colleagues identified the von Hippel-Lindau gene, leading to the detection of a germ line mutation in approximately 75% of families affected by von Hippel-Lindau disease (Chen et al, 1995).

Hereditary papillary renal carcinoma was described in 1994 and is characterized by a predisposition to develop multiple bilateral renal tumors with a papillary histologic appearance (Zbar et al, 1994). In contrast to von Hippel-Lindau patients, the major neoplastic manifestations appear to be confined to the kidney.

Acquired cystic disease of the kidneys is a well-recognized entity of multiple bilateral cysts in the native kidneys of uremic patients (Reichard, Roubidoux, and Dunnick, 1998). The risk of developing RCC has been estimated to be greater than 30 times higher in patients receiving dialysis who have cystic changes in their kidney than in the general population (Brennan et al, 1991). Several series reported in the literature suggest that RCC occurs in 3–9% of patients with acquired cystic disease of the kidneys (Gardner and Evan, 1984; Gulanikar et al, 1998). Most RCC cases have been described in patients undergoing hemodialysis, but RCC has been reported in association with peritoneal dialysis (Smith et al, 1987) and successful renal transplants (Vaziri et al, 1984) and in patients with long-term renal insufficiency not requiring dialysis (Bretan et al, 1986; Fallon and Williams, 1989).

Pathology

RCC originates from the proximal renal tubular epithelium, as evidenced by electron microscopy (Makay, Ordonez, and Khoursland, 1987) and immunohistochemical analysis (Holthöfer, 1990). These tumors occur with equal frequency in either kidney and are randomly distributed in the upper and lower poles. RCCs originate in the cortex and tend to grow out into perinephric tissue, causing the characteristic bulge or mass effect that aids in their detection by diagnostic imaging studies. Grossly, the tumor is characteristically yellow to orange because of the abundance of lipids, particularly in the clear cell type. RCCs do not have true capsules but may have a pseudocapsule of compressed renal parenchyma, fibrous tissue, and inflammatory cells.

Histologically, RCC is most often a mixed adenocarcinoma containing clear cells, granular cells, and, occasionally, sarcomatoid-appearing cells. There has recently been a reclassification of the subtypes of RCC based on morphology and cytogenetic characteristics. Most RCCs are classified into 1 of the following histologic subtypes: conventional clear cell, papillary (chromophilic), chromophobe, collecting duct, neuroendocrine, and unclassified (Mostofi and Davis, 1998). Benign renal tumors are papillary adenoma, renal oncocytoma, and metanephric adenoma. Clear cells are rounded or polygonal with abundant cytoplasm, which contains cholesterol, triglycerides, glycogen, and lipids (Figure 21–3).

The cells present in the papillary (chromophilic) type contain less glycogen and lipids, and electron microscopy reveals that the granular cytoplasm contains many mitochondria and cytosomes. Chromophobe-type carcinomas contain large polygonal cells with distinct cell borders and reticulated cytoplasm, which can stain diffusely with Hale's colloidal iron (Theones et al, 1988). Oncocytic RCC or oncocytomas tend to have

Figure 21–3. Photomicrograph of clear cell renal adenocarcinoma (original magnification, × 125).

cytoplasm packed with mitochondria, giving it a granular appearance. Collecting duct tumors tend to have irregular borders and a basophilic cytoplasm with extensive anaplasia and are likely to invade blood vessels and cause infarction of tissue. Sarcomatoid cells are spindle-shaped and form sheets or bundles. This cell type rarely occurs as a pure form and is most commonly a small component of either the clear cell or papillary cell type (or both).

Pathogenesis

RCCs are vascular tumors that tend to spread either by direct invasion through the renal capsule into perinephric fat and adjacent visceral structures or by direct extension into the renal vein. Approximately 25–30% of patients have evidence of metastatic disease at presentation (Waters and Ritchie, 1979). The most common site of distant metastases is the lung. However, liver, bone (osteolytic), ipsilateral adjacent lymph nodes, adrenal gland, brain, the opposite kidney, and subcutaneous tissue are frequent sites of disease spread.

Tumor Staging & Grading

A. TUMOR STAGING

The ultimate goal of staging is to select appropriate therapy and obtain prognostic information. Appropriate studies for a complete clinical staging evaluation include history and physical examination, complete blood count, serum chemistries (renal and hepatic function), urinalysis, chest x-ray (chest CT scan for an equivocal exam), CT scan of abdomen and pelvis, and a radionuclide bone scan (with x-rays of abnormal areas).

Owing to the lack of useful diagnostic studies and effective therapy for metastatic disease, early staging systems were primarily geared toward evaluation of operative findings for prognostic information. Flocks and Kadesky (1958) proposed a staging system based on gross physical characteristics of the tumor. Robson (1963) proposed modifications to the Flocks and Kadesky staging scheme, taking into account the degree of vascular involvement.

Stage I:—Tumor is confined within the kidney parenchyma (no involvement of perinephric fat, renal vein, or regional lymph nodes).

Stage II:—Tumor involves the perinephric fat but is confined within Gerota's fascia (including the adrenal).

Stage IIIA:—Tumor involves the main renal vein or inferior vena cava.

Stage IIIB:—Tumor involves regional lymph nodes.

Stage IIIC:—Tumor involves both local vessels and regional lymph nodes.

Stage IVA:—Tumor involves adjacent organs other than the adrenal (colon, pancreas, etc).

Stage IVB:—Distant metastases.

Although the Robson system is easy to use, long-term evaluation of patients, especially those with stage III disease, has determined that it does not relate directly to prognosis. Patients with renal vein (or proximal vena cava) involvement (stage IIIA), but without disease extension into perinephric fat and lymph nodes, have survival rates comparable to those of patients with disease confined to the kidney (stages I and II) (Siminovitch, Montie, and Straffon, 1983).

The Tumor-Node-Metastasis (TNM) system more accurately classifies the extent of tumor involvement and is more commonly used. The TNM classification system for RCC was redefined and simplified in 1997 (Sobin and Wittekind) (Table 21–1).

B. Tumor Grading

Fuhrman grading has become commonly used by pathologists in North America (Fuhrman, Lasky, and Limas, 1982; Goldstein, 1997). The system uses 4 grades based on nuclear size and irregularity and nucleolar prominence. The system is most effective in predicting metastasis (50% of high-grade tumors within 5 years). When high-grade, predominantly granular tumors are corrected for grade and stage, there is no apparent difference between clear cell and granular cell tumor prognosis (McNichols, Segura, and DeWeerd,

Table 21–1. TNM classification system for renal cell carcinoma.[a]

Classification	Definition
T—Primary tumor	
TX	Primary tumor cannot be assessed.
T0	No evidence of primary tumor.
T1	Tumor 7.0 cm or less limited to the kidney.
T2	Tumor more than 7.0 cm limited to the kidney.
T3	Tumor extends into major veins or invades adrenal gland or perinephric tissues but not beyond Gerota's fascia.
T3a	Tumor invades adrenal gland or perinephric tissues but not beyond Gerota's fascia.
T3b	Tumor grossly extends into renal vein(s) or vena cava.
T3c	Tumor grossly extends into vena cava above diaphragm.
T4	Tumor invades beyond Gerota's fascia.
N—Regional lymph nodes	
NX	Regional lymph nodes cannot be assessed.
N0	No regional lymph node metastasis.
N1	Metastasis in a single regional lymph node 2 cm or less.
N2	Metastasis in more than a single regional lymph node.
M—Distant metastases	
MX	Distant metastasis cannot be assessed.
M0	No distant metastasis.
M1	Distant metastasis.

[a]All sizes measured in greatest dimension.

1981). However, patients presenting with advanced disease do poorly irrespective of tumor grade. Until effective adjuvant therapy is available, grading early-stage tumors will continue to have minimal clinical utility.

Clinical Findings

A. SYMPTOMS AND SIGNS

The classically described triad of gross hematuria, flank pain, and a palpable mass occurs in only 10–15% of patients and is frequently a manifestation of advanced disease. Sixty percent of patients present with gross or microscopic hematuria. Pain, an abdominal mass, or both are seen in approximately 40% of patients (Skinner et al, 1971). Symptoms secondary to metastatic disease, such as dyspnea and cough, seizure and headache, or bone pain from lung, brain, and bone metastases, respectively, lead to a diagnosis in up to 30% of patients. With the routine use of CT scanning, renal tumors are increasingly detected incidentally; therefore, older literature describing RCC presentation may no longer be accurate.

B. PARANEOPLASTIC SYNDROMES

RCC is associated with a wide spectrum of paraneoplastic syndromes including erythrocytosis, hypercalcemia, hypertension, and nonmetastatic hepatic dysfunction. Overall, these manifestations can occur in 10–40% of patients with RCC.

RCC is the most common cause of paraneoplastic erythrocytosis, which is reported to occur in 3–10% of patients with this tumor (Sufrin et al, 1989). In patients with RCC, the elevated erythrocyte mass is physiologically inappropriate and may result either from enhanced production of erythropoietin from the tumor or as a consequence of regional renal hypoxia promoting erythropoietin production from nonneoplastic renal tissue (Hocking, 1987).

Hypercalcemia has been reported to occur in up to 20% of patients with RCC (Muggia, 1990). Hypercalcemia may be due to production of a parathyroid hormone–related peptide that mimics the function of parathyroid hormone (Strewler et al, 1987) or other humoral factors such as osteoclast-activating factor, tumor necrosis factor, and transforming growth factor-alpha (Muggia, 1990).

Hypertension associated with RCC has been reported in up to 40% of patients (Sufrin et al, 1989), and renin production by the neoplasm has been documented in 37%. The excess renin and hypertension associated with RCC are typically refractory to antihypertensive therapy but may respond after nephrectomy (Gold et al, 1996).

In 1961, Stauffer described a reversible syndrome of hepatic dysfunction in the absence of hepatic metastases associated with RCC. Hepatic function abnormalities include elevation of alkaline phosphatase and bilirubin, hypoalbuminemia, prolonged prothrombin time, and hypergammaglobulinemia. Stauffer syndrome tends to occur in association with fever, fatigue, and weight loss and typically resolves after nephrectomy. The reported incidence of Stauffer syndrome varies from 3% to 20% (Gold et al, 1996). It may be due to overproduction of granulocyte-macrophage colony stimulating factor by the tumor (Chang et al, 1992).

RCC is known to produce a multitude of other biologically active products that result in clinically significant syndromes, including adrenocorticotropic hormone (Cushing syndrome), enteroglucagon (protein enteropathy), prolactin (galactorrhea), insulin (hypoglycemia), and gonadotropins (gynecomastia and decreased libido; or hirsutism, amenorrhea, and male pattern balding) (Sufrin, Golio, and Murphy, 1986).

A paraneoplastic syndrome present at the time of disease diagnosis does not in and of itself confer a poor prognosis. However, patients whose paraneoplastic metabolic disturbances fail to normalize after nephrectomy (suggesting the presence of clinically undetectable metastatic disease) have very poor prognoses (Hanash, 1982; Robson, 1982).

C. LABORATORY FINDINGS

In addition to the laboratory abnormalities associated with the various RCC paraneoplastic syndromes, anemia, hematuria, and an elevated sedimentation rate are frequently observed.

Anemia occurs in about 30% of RCC patients. The anemia typically is not secondary to blood loss or hemolysis and is commonly normochromic. The serum iron and total iron-binding capacity are usually low, as in the anemia of chronic disease. Iron therapy is usually ineffective; however, surgical removal of early-stage tumors usually leads to physiologic correction of the anemia. The potential role of recombinant erythropoietin for patients with unresectable disease represents a potential, but untested, option.

Gross or microscopic hematuria can be seen in up to 60% of patients presenting with RCC. An elevated erythrocyte sedimentation rate is also commonly seen, with a reported incidence as high as 75%. These findings are nonspecific, and normal findings do not rule out a diagnosis of RCC.

D. X-RAY FINDINGS

Although many radiologic techniques are available to aid in the detection and diagnosis of renal masses, CT scanning remains the primary technique with which others must be compared. Other radiologic techniques used include US, MRI, and arteriography. In this era of cost containment, selecting the appropriate studies for an efficient, cost-effective evaluation is mandatory.

The most appropriate diagnostic method is to some extent dictated by the clinical presentation. Patients presenting with microscopic hematuria should have IVU as their initial radiologic evaluation; however, patients with a suspicious renal mass found during either a US evaluation or IVU for other indications would best be evaluated with CT scanning.

E. Intravenous Urography

When used alone, IVU is only 75% accurate, and additional studies are needed for confirmation. Calcification overlying the renal shadow is an important diagnostic finding because its presence significantly increases the probability of cancer (Daniel et al, 1972).

F. Ultrasonography

US examination is a noninvasive, relatively inexpensive technique able to further delineate a renal mass seen on IVU. It is approximately 98% accurate in defining simple cysts. Strict ultrasonographic criteria for a simple cyst include through transmission, a well-circumscribed mass without internal echoes, and adequate visualization of a strong posterior wall (Figure 21–4). Extension

of tumor thrombus into the inferior vena cava can also be determined by ultrasonography.

G. CT Scanning

CT scanning has been shown to be more sensitive than US or IVU for renal cancer detection (Warshauer et al, 1988). A typical finding of RCC on CT is a mass that becomes enhanced with the use of intravenous contrast media. In general, RCC exhibits an overall decreased density in Hounsfield units compared with normal renal parenchyma but shows a heterogeneous pattern of enhancement or increased attenuation (slightly decreased from the surrounding parenchyma) when contrast is used (Figure 21–5) (Kosko, Lipuma, and Resnick, 1984). In addition to defining the primary lesion, CT scanning is also the method of choice in staging the patient by visualizing the renal hilum, perinephric space, renal vein and vena cava, adrenals, regional lymphatics, and adjacent organs. In patients with equivocal chest x-ray findings, a CT scan of the chest is indicated. Patients who present with symptoms consistent with brain metastases should be evaluated with either CT or MRI. Spiral CT with 3-dimensional reconstruction has become useful for evaluating tumors before nephron-sparing surgery to delineate the 3-dimensional extent of the tumor and precisely outline the vasculature, which can aid the surgeon in preventing positive surgical margins (Holmes et al, 1997).

A

B

Figure 21–4. **A:** Ultrasound image of a simple renal cyst showing renal parenchyma (long arrows), cyst wall (arrowheads), and a strong posterior wall (short arrows). **B:** Ultrasound image of a solid renal mass (arrows).

Figure 21–5. Computed tomogram (contrast enhancement) of a renal cell carcinoma (arrows).

Figure 21–6. Right renal angiogram showing typical neovascularity (arrows) in a large lower pole renal cell cancer.

H. RENAL ANGIOGRAPHY

With the widespread availability of CT scanners, the role of renal angiography in the diagnostic evaluation of RCC has markedly diminished and is now very limited. Angiography is capable of demonstrating neovascularity and arteriovenous fistulas as well as renal vein and vena caval tumor involvement, but it is of limited usefulness in the approximately 10% of patients whose tumors are not hypervascular (Figure 21–6). In addition, angiography is invasive and carries a small but real risk of complications, including hemorrhage, pseudoaneurysm formation at the puncture site, arterial emboli, and contrast-related nephrotoxicity. Furthermore, renal angiography is relatively expensive and may require hospitalization. There remain a very few specific clinical situations in which angiography may be useful; for example, guiding the operative approach in a patient with an RCC in a solitary kidney when attempting to perform a partial nephrectomy may be indicated. However, CT angiography or MR angiography can give better information with less risk to the patient.

I. RADIONUCLIDE IMAGING

Determination of metastases to bones is most accurate by radionuclide bone scan, although the study is nonspecific and requires confirmation with bone x-rays of identified abnormalities to verify the presence of the typical osteolytic lesions. There is evidence that patients without bone pain and with a normal alkaline phosphatase level have a very low incidence of bone metastases (Henriksson et al, 1992), and thus a routine bone scan is not necessary in such patients.

J. MAGNETIC RESONANCE IMAGING

MRI is equivalent to CT for staging of RCC (Hricak et al, 1988). Its primary advantage is in the evaluation of patients with suspected vascular extension (Figure 21–7). Prospective trials have demonstrated that MRI is superior to CT in assessing inferior vena caval involvement (Kabala et al, 1991) and is at least as accurate as venacavography (Horan et al, 1989). In contrast to both CT and cavography, MRI evaluation does not require either iodinated contrast material or ionizing radiation. Recent studies using MRI angiography with gadolinium or CT angiography have improved vascular evaluation of renal neoplasms (Bluemke and Chambers, 1995). MR angiography can also be used to delineate the vascular supply before planned nephron-sparing surgery.

K. POSITRON EMISSION TOMOGRAPHY (PET)

This technique allows the measurement of systemically administered biochemical agents such as 18-fluoro-2-deoxyglucose (FDG), which can accumulate in the kidney. Although FDG-PET scanning can yield

Figure 21–7. Transaxial magnetic resonance image (T2) of a renal cell carcinoma (long arrows) with vena caval tumor thrombus (short arrows).

false-positive results in some patients with RCC (Bachor et al, 1996), it may be useful in monitoring response to systemic therapy in those with metastatic disease (Hoh, Seltzer, and Franklin, 1998). FDG-PET may also be more accurate than routine CT scanning in detecting disease recurrence or progression, which may alter treatment decisions in up to 50% of cases (Ramdave et al, 2001). However, further studies are required before it can be widely used for routine staging of RCC.

L. FINE-NEEDLE ASPIRATION

Fine-needle aspiration has a limited role in the evaluation of RCC. Patients with radiologic findings consistent with RCC require definitive surgical management. Fine-needle aspiration of renal lesions is the diagnostic approach of choice in those patients with clinically apparent metastatic disease who may be candidates for nonsurgical therapy. Other settings in which fine-needle aspiration may be appropriate include establishing a diagnosis in patients who are not surgical candidates, differentiating a primary RCC from a renal metastasis in patients with known primary cancers of nonrenal origin, and evaluating some radiographically indeterminate lesions (Renshaw, Granter, and Cibas, 1997). Rare reports of seeding of the needle tract have been reported.

M. INSTRUMENTAL AND CYTOLOGIC EXAMINATION

Patients presenting with hematuria should be evaluated with cystoscopy. Blood effluxing from the ureteral orifice identifies the origin of bleeding from the upper tract. Most renal pelvis tumors can be distinguished radiographically from RCC; however, endoscopic evaluation of the bladder, ureters, and renal pelvis is occasionally helpful in making a diagnosis. Additionally, although urine cytologic study is rarely helpful in the diagnosis of RCC, cytologic study of urine with renal pelvis washing is frequently diagnostic in renal pelvis tumors.

N. TUMOR MARKERS

As noted previously, RCC is associated with numerous biologically active substances. However, at present there are no clinically relevant tumor markers to aid in screening, diagnosis, or evaluating response to therapy.

Differential Diagnosis

When a patient presents with clinical findings consistent with metastatic disease and is found to have a renal mass, a diagnosis of RCC can be straightforward. Most patients present with a renal mass discovered after an evaluation of hematuria or pain or as an incidental finding during an imaging workup of an unrelated problem. The differential diagnosis of RCC includes other solid renal lesions. The great majority of renal masses are simple cysts. Once the diagnosis of a cyst is confirmed by US, no additional evaluation is required if the patient is asymptomatic. Equivocal findings or the presence of calcification within the mass warrant further evaluation by CT. A wide variety of pathologic entities appear as solid masses on CT scans, and differentiation of benign from malignant lesions is frequently difficult. Findings on CT scan that suggest malignancy include amputation of a portion of the collecting system, presence of calcification, a poorly defined interface between the renal parenchyma and the lesion, invasion into perinephric fat or adjacent structures, and the presence of abnormal periaortic adenopathy or distant metastatic disease (Kosko, Lipuma, and Resnick, 1984).

Some characteristic lesions can be defined using CT criteria in combination with clinical findings. Angiomyolipomas (with large fat components) can easily be identified by the low-attenuation areas classically produced by substantial fat content. A renal abscess may be strongly suspected in a patient presenting with fever, flank pain, pyuria, and leukocytosis, and an early needle aspiration and culture should be performed. Other benign renal masses (in addition to those previously described) include granulomas and arteriovenous malformations. Renal lymphoma (both Hodgkin's disease and non-Hodgkin's disease), transitional cell carcinoma of the renal pelvis, adrenal cancer, and metastatic disease are additional diagnostic possibilities that may be suspected based on CT and clinical findings.

Treatment

A. SPECIFIC MEASURES

1. Localized disease—Surgical removal of the early-stage lesion remains the only potentially curative therapy available for RCC patients. Appropriate therapy depends almost entirely on the stage of tumor at presentation and therefore requires a thorough staging evaluation. The prognoses of patients with stages I, II, and IIIA (renal vein only) are very similar after surgical removal of the kidney and enveloping fascia are accomplished (Skinner, Vermillion, and Colvin, 1972).

Radical nephrectomy is the primary treatment for localized RCC. Its goal is to achieve the removal of tumor and to take a wide margin of normal tissue. Radical nephrectomy (Robson, 1963) entails en bloc removal of the kidney and its enveloping fascia (Gerota's) including the ipsilateral adrenal, proximal one-half of the ureter, and lymph nodes up to the area of transection of the renal vessels (Figure 21–8).

Various incisions provide optimal access for the radical nephrectomy, including an anterior subcostal (unilateral chevron) or thoracoabdominal incision, and, oc-casionally, a midline incision or the classic flank incision (Droller, 1992).

The likelihood of local recurrence after radical nephrectomy is 2–3% (Itano et al, 2000; Konety et al, submitted 2002). Repeat resection of isolated local recurrence can be curative and yield a survival benefit (Itano et al, 2000; Tanguay et al, 1996). The role of regional lymphadenectomy in RCC remains controversial. Between 18% and 33% of patients undergoing radical nephrectomy with lymph node dissection for RCC have metastatic disease identified (Skinner, Lieskovsky, and Pritchett, 1988). Although several retrospective studies (Thrasher and Paulson, 1993) and a prospective, nonrandomized study (Herrlinger et al, 1991) suggest that regional lymphadenectomy can improve survival in patients with Robson stages I and II RCCs, this subject remains highly controversial. In a randomized study conducted in patients with localized RCC, lymphadenectomy did not appear to increase morbidity significantly, but its benefit was questionable (Blom et al, 1999). Removal of the adrenal is unnecessary if the tumor is not in the upper pole, because adrenal involvement is uncommon in this instance.

Preoperative renal artery embolization (angioinfarction) has been used as a surgical adjunct to facilitate radical nephrectomy, purportedly by decreasing operative blood loss and by causing edema in tissue planes (McLean and Meranze, 1985). Reported complications of embolization include migration of coils or balloons to the opposite kidney or distant sites, damage to the contralateral kidney by excessive use of contrast material during the procedure, and ischemic injury to the lower limbs or bowel from an overflow of the embolization agent. The postinfarction syndrome is characterized by flank pain, fever, and leukocytosis typically lasting an average of 3 days.

Because there is no conclusive evidence that preoperative embolization actually decreases blood loss or facilitates surgery, its use should be limited to patients with very large tumors in which the renal artery may be difficult to reach early in the procedure. Additionally, this technique may be useful to palliate patients with nonresectable tumors and significant symptoms such as hemorrhage, flank pain, or paraneoplastic syndromes.

Radiation therapy has been advocated as a neoadjuvant (preoperative) or adjuvant method to radical nephrectomy, but there has been controversy over its effectiveness (Rafla, 1970; van der Werf-Messing, 1973; Juusela, 1977). There is no evidence that postsurgical radiation therapy to the renal bed, whether or not residual tumor is present, contributes to prolonged survival.

RCC may invade renal vascular spaces and produce tumor thrombi extending into renal veins, inferior vena

Figure 21–8. Boundaries of a left radical nephrectomy. Dotted line represents both the surgical margin and Gerota's fascia.

cava, hepatic veins, and, occasionally, the right atrium. Between 5% and 10% of patients presenting with RCC have some degree of vena caval involvement (Figure 21–9) (Skinner, Lieskovsky, and Pritchett, 1988). As previously described, patients presenting with involvement of the renal vein and vena cava below the hepatic veins (stage IIIA or T3aN0M0) but without evidence of regional or distant metastases have a prognosis similar to patients with stage II (T2) disease when treated by radical excision. The surgical approach to the removal of caval thrombi depends entirely on the level of cephalad extension. In general, these thrombi do not invade the wall of the cava and therefore can be removed without resection of the caval wall. For tumor thrombi that have reached the level of the right atrium, the use of cardiopulmonary bypass is typically required.

Laparoscopic radical nephrectomy and even partial nephrectomy has been accomplished successfully and safely in several hundred patients. Laparoscopic radical nephrectomy is being used increasingly for patients with localized renal tumors that are not amenable to a partial nephrectomy. This approach results in quicker recovery with efficacy comparable to that of open radical nephrectomy (Portis et al, 2002; Gill et al, 2001).

The approach to the patient with either bilateral RCC or disease in a solitary kidney differs from the standard approach of radical nephrectomy. Bilateral RCC occurs with a frequency as high as 3% (Smith, 1986). Radical nephrectomy in these patients or in

those with solitary kidneys obviously commits patients to long-term dialysis or renal transplantation and the morbidities of these conditions. Staging these patients is essentially the same as previously outlined, with the notable exception that either MR or CT angiography is often used to assess the extent of tumor within the kidney and the renal artery anatomy. Surgical alternatives to radical nephrectomy include open or laparoscopic partial nephrectomy, ex vivo partial nephrectomy (bench surgery followed by autotransplantation) (Novick, Stewart, and Straffon, 1980), and enucleation of multiple lesions (Marshall et al, 1986). Given the lack of effective adjuvant therapy and the risk of inadequate excision and subsequent recurrence from various renal-sparing approaches, partial nephrectomy with an adequate parenchymal margin remains the preferred treatment.

Partial nephrectomy and wedge resection with an adequate margin of normal parenchyma is increasingly being used as primary surgical therapy for patients with tumors less than 4 cm in size, even in the presence of a normal contralateral kidney. Local recurrence of tumor in the same kidney ranges from 0% to 10%, and it is between 0% and 3% for tumors less than 4 cm in size (Uzzo and Novick, 2001; Morgan and Zincke, 1990; Hafez, Novick, and Campbell, 1997). In patients with multiple small tumors, such as those with von Hippel-Lindau disease, enucleation of the tumor(s) is also an acceptable approach. Long-term follow-up demonstrates that partial nephrectomy has a similar outcome as radical nephrectomy (Herr, 1999). It is now considered the approach of choice in patients with small (< 4 cm), incidentally discovered renal tumors that are peripherally located.

Additional therapeutic approaches being explored for the treatment of small, incidentally discovered renal lesions include the use of cryoablation, high-intensity focused US, and radiofrequency ablation (Murphy and Gill, 2001). Cryoablation with liquid nitrogen or argon gas, either percutaneously using MRI guidance or via laparoscopic probes, has proved to be feasible and effective in selected patients (Shingleton and Sewell, 2002; Gill et al, 2000). Radiofrequency ablation has also been accomplished via the percutaneous approach with minimal morbidity in small groups of patients (Pavlovich et al, 2002). These approaches are particularly attractive in patients with multiple small lesions or older individuals with many comorbidities. The long-term effectiveness of these emerging technologies remains to be determined.

Observation as treatment should also be mentioned for small (< 3.0 cm) lesions, particularly in elderly patients. One recent study noted a growth rate of 0–1.3 cm per year in 40 patients followed up for a mean of 3.5 years (Bosniak, 1995), indicating that with careful

Figure 21–9. Coronal magnetic resonance image (T1) of a large vena caval tumor thrombus (long arrows) in a patient with renal cell carcinoma. Thrombus extends just to entrance of hepatic veins (short arrows).

follow-up, watchful waiting may be appropriate in selected patients.

2. Disseminated disease—Approximately 30% of patients with RCC will present with advanced disease. Metastatic RCC has a natural history that is typically aggressive and rapidly progressive, with 5-year survival rates typically less than 10% (Motzer et al, 1996). Infrequently, the disease may have a more protracted course. The biological diversity of RCC is illustrated by the 6.6% response rate (including 3% complete responders) in the placebo arm of a recently completed phase III trial of interferon-gamma in advanced RCC (Gleave et al, 1998).

a. Surgery—The role of radical nephrectomy in the management of patients with advanced disease has recently been reevaluated based on the results of randomized clinical trials. Historically, radical nephrectomy was primarily used as a palliative procedure in the setting of metastatic disease for managing patients with severe hemorrhage or unremitting pain. Over the past 20 years, retrospective observations of the potential for nephrectomy to improve response rates of patients receiving biologic response modifier therapy prompted a prospective evaluation of this effect. The Southwest Oncology Group performed a randomized phase III trial, randomizing patients with advanced RCC to nephrectomy followed by interferon-alpha 2b versus interferon alone. Two hundred forty-one evaluable patients were enrolled. The median survival of patients undergoing nephrectomy followed by interferon was 11.1 months, compared to 8.1 months in those receiving only interferon ($P = 0.05$) (Flanigan et al, 2001). A similar, smaller, randomized trial conducted in Europe demonstrated similar findings (Mickisch et al, 2001). These 2 studies have prompted a shift in the standard of care for patients with metastatic RCC and good performance status who desire systemic biologic therapy to include an upfront nephrectomy.

Patients presenting with a solitary metastatic site (synchronous metastases) that is amenable to surgical resection may be candidates for combined nephrectomy and removal of the metastatic foci. In carefully selected patients, 5-year survival has approached 30% in some series (O'Dea et al, 1978; Toho and Whitmore, 1975).

The important role of surgical resection of solitary brain metastases has been highlighted by several randomized trials demonstrating an improvement in survival in patients with solitary brain metastases who undergo both surgical resection and whole-brain radiotherapy compared with patients who receive only radiation therapy (Patchell et al, 1990; Vecht et al, 1993).

b. Radiation therapy—Radiation therapy is an important method in the palliation of patients with metastatic RCC. Despite the belief that RCC is a relatively radioresistant tumor, effective palliation of metastatic disease to the brain, bone, and lungs is reported in up to two-thirds of patients (Fossa, Kjolseth, and Lund, 1982; Onufrey and Mohiuddin, 1985).

c. Hormonal therapy—There are numerous uncontrolled trials of progestational, androgenic, and antiestrogenic agents in the literature, with responses ranging from 0% to 33% (Bono, 1986). More recent studies in large numbers of patients have shown response rates of 1–2%, with responses typically being partial and of brief duration (Kjaer, 1988).

d. Chemotherapy— RCC is among the most chemotherapy-resistant epithelial cancers. The mechanism of drug resistance is complex and may in part be a consequence of the presence of the multidrug resistance–associated P-glycoprotein (Mickisch et al, 1990). A review of over 4000 RCC patients treated in 83 phase II trials over a 10-year span demonstrated only a 6% overall response rate (Yagoda et al, 1995).

e. Biologic response modifiers—The use of metastatic RCC as a model for the investigation of various biologic response modifiers is a consequence of both the lack of effective therapy and the long-recognized biologic "eccentricities" of this tumor. Spontaneous regression of metastatic RCC is a well-recognized, albeit rare, event (Kavoussi et al, 1986; Vogelzang et al, 1992). Although no specific evidence exists, many believe this phenomenon to be immunologically mediated.

Studies using partially purified human leukocyte interferon in renal cancer were first reported in 1983, with subsequent studies using human lymphoblastoid interferon and, more recently, recombinant interferon-alpha. Recombinant interferon-alpha used in various dose and schedules has demonstrated reproducible overall response rates of 10–15% in advanced renal cancer (Pastore et al, 2001). A modest impact on survival has been demonstrated in some randomized trials of interferon-alpha. The Medical Research Council compared interferon-alpha to medroxyprogesterone acetate and demonstrated a 2.5-month median survival improvement for patients receiving interferon-alpha (Medical Research Council Renal Cancer Collaborators, 1999). Other large randomized studies have failed to demonstrate a survival advantage of interferon-alpha compared to other biologic response modifiers (Negrier et al, 1998; Motzer et al, 2000). Interferon-alpha is commonly administered 3–5 days per week as a subcutaneous injection. Patients most likely to have a clinical benefit from interferon therapy are those who have minimal tumor burden (ie, primary kidney tumor removed), lung or nodal metastases only, and an excellent performance status. Given the modest activity of inter-

feron in patients with advanced disease, trials of interferon administered in the adjuvant setting to patients at
high risk of recurrence have been conducted but have
not demonstrated clinical benefit (Trump et al, 1996;
Pizzocaro et al, 2001). The experience with beta and
gamma interferons has been less extensive. In 1989,
Aulitzky and colleagues reported a 30% response rate in
a trial of low-dose interferon-gamma (Aulitzky et al,
1989). Unfortunately, subsequent trials, including a
phase III trial, have demonstrated response rates of less
than 10% (Gleave et al, 1998).

Interleukin-2 (IL-2), a T-cell growth factor, was first
identified in 1976. Recombinant IL-2 is the only agent
approved by the US Food and Drug Administration for
patients with advanced renal carcinoma. Despite initial
reports of response rates (complete and partial) of 30%,
subsequent experience suggests that the overall response
rates of IL-2 is in the 15% range. Although most patients do not benefit from IL-2 therapy, a subset of responding patients do very well, with 10–20% alive 5–10
years after therapy (Gitlitz et al, 2001). Controversy persists regarding the optimal dose and schedule for IL-2
administration, with early comparisons demonstrating
similar response rates for the high- and low-dose schedules. A recent preliminary report from the Cytokine
Working Group suggests a higher overall response rate
favoring high-dose IL-2 (McDermott et al, 2001). The
wide variability in response rates to IL-2 is likely a function of patient selection. Fyfe and colleagues (1995) reported a retrospective evaluation of 255 patients treated
with high-dose IL-2 and found that an Eastern Cooperative Oncology Group performance score of 0 was a significant predictor of clinical response.

Randomized trials comparing interferon-alpha, IL-
2, and IL-2 plus interferon-alpha have demonstrated
higher objective response rates to the combination therapy, with no difference in survival and significantly
higher toxicity associated with the combination (Negrier et al, 1998). Biochemotherapy regimens have been
evaluated, with a recent phase III trial demonstrating
no advantage to the combination of IL-2, interferon-
alpha, and fluorouracil versus IL-2 and interferon (Negrier et al, 2000).

B. FOLLOW-UP CARE

There is no universal agreement on the frequency or
studies required in the follow-up care of patients with
RCC. A stage-specific follow-up schedule is recommended for patients who have undergone radical or
partial nephrectomy (Levy et al, 1998; Hafez, Novick,
and Campbell, 1998). Patients with stage T1 disease
need less stringent follow-up, with yearly chest x-rays
and liver and renal function tests. Those with stage T2
or T3 disease require more frequent follow-up of at
least 3-month or 6-month intervals in the early postop-

erative period. Repeat CT scans of the abdomen should
also be obtained, especially in those who have undergone partial nephrectomy, to rule out local recurrence.
Patients with metastatic disease who are not undergoing therapy need continued follow-up to provide appropriate supportive care.

Prognosis

The prognosis of patients is most clearly related to the
stage of disease at presentation. Recent studies report 5-
year survival rates for patients with stage I disease in the
91–100% range, with rates of 74–96% for stage II and
59–70% for stage III. Patients presenting with metastatic disease have a poorer prognosis, with only a
16–32% 5-year survival rate.

NEPHROBLASTOMA (WILMS TUMOR)

Nephroblastoma, also known as Wilms tumor, is the
most common solid renal tumor of childhood, accounting for roughly 5% of childhood cancers. Between 450
and 500 new cases are reported annually. The peak age
for presentation is during the third year of life, and
there is no sex predilection. The disease is seen worldwide with a similar age of onset and sex distribution.
Tumors are commonly unicentric, but they occur in either kidney with equal frequency. In 5% of cases the
tumors are bilateral.

Wilms tumor occurs in familial and nonfamilial
forms. The National Wilms' Tumor Study (NWTS)
group documented the occurrence of a familial Wilms
tumor in approximately 1% of cases (Breslow and
Beckwith, 1982). Although a relatively rare neoplasm,
Wilms tumor has become a very important model for
the study of tumorigenesis and has become a prototypical neoplasm for collaborative clinical trials, with approximately 85% of all new cases diagnosed in North
America enrolled in NWTS group protocols (Beckwith,
1997). Approximately 10% of patients with Wilms tumors have recognized congenital malformations.
Among the more common disorders associated with
Wilms tumor are the overgrowth syndromes, such as
Beckwith-Wiedemann syndrome and isolated hemihypertrophy, and nonovergrowth disorders, such as isolated aniridia and trisomy 18 (Weiner, Coppes, and
Ritchey, 1998). Genitourinary abnormalities such as
hypospadias, cryptorchidism, and renal fusion are
found in 4.5–7.5% of patients with unilateral Wilms
tumor and in up to 13.4% of those with bilateral
disease (Breslow et al, 1993).

Etiology

In 1972 Knudson and Strong proposed a two-hit hypothesis to explain the earlier age of onset and bilateral

presentation in children with a familial history of Wilms tumor. In this hypothesis, the pathogenesis of the sporadic form of Wilms tumor results from two postzygotic mutations in a single cell. In contrast, the familial form of the disease arises after one prezygotic mutation and a subsequent postzygotic event. Karyotypic analyses of Wilms tumor patients with various congenital malformations and loss of heterozygosity studies helped identify a region on the short arm of chromosome 11 (11p13) (Riccardi et al, 1978; Huff, 1994). This work ultimately led to the identification of a gene associated with Wilms tumor development (WT1), which maps to chromosome 11p13 (Coppes, Haber, and Grundy, 1994). Although alterations in this gene have been associated with Wilms tumor and genitourinary abnormalities, only 5–10% of sporadic Wilms tumors have been demonstrated to have WT1 mutations (Varanasi et al, 1994). Genetic linkage studies of families with an inherited susceptibility to Wilms tumors suggest that other Wilms tumor genes exist (Weiner, Coppes, and Ritchey, 1998).

Pathogenesis & Pathology

In 1990 Beckwith and colleagues proposed a simplified nomenclature and classification of Wilms tumor precursor lesions known as nephrogenic rests (NR). Two distinct categories of NR were identified and designated as perilobar NR and intralobar NR. One concept of Wilms tumor development proposed that some NR remain dormant for many years, with some undergoing involution and sclerosis and others giving rise to Wilms tumors (Beckwith, Kiviat, and Bonadio, 1990; Beckwith, 1997). The typical Wilms tumor consists of blastemal, epithelial, and stromal elements in varying proportions (Figure 21–10). Tumors composed of blastema and stroma or blastema alone have been described.

The NWTS correlated pathologic specimens with clinical outcome and divided various histologic features into favorable and unfavorable prognostic groups. The unfavorable subgroup includes tumors that contain focal or diffuse elements of anaplastic cells or two other neoplastic entities considered not to be Wilms tumor variants, clear cell sarcoma of the kidney and rhabdoid tumor of the kidney (Beckwith and Palmer, 1978; Beckwith, 1997). Favorable histology tumors comprise all Wilms tumors without anaplasia. Anaplastic tumors are characterized by extreme nuclear atypia, hyperdiploidy, and numerous complex translocations.

Grossly, Wilms tumors are generally large, multilobulated, and gray or tan in color with focal areas of hemorrhage and necrosis. A fibrous pseudocapsule is occasionally seen.

Tumor dissemination can occur by direct extension through the renal capsule, hematogenously via the renal

Figure 21–10. Wilms tumor with characteristic tubular/glomeruloid structures and blastema (original magnification, × 40).

vein and vena cava, or via lymphatic spread. Metastatic disease is present at diagnosis in 10–15% of patients, with the lungs (85–95%) and liver (10–15%) the most common sites of involvement. Regional lymphatics are involved in as many as 25% of patients. Metastases to liver, bone, and brain are uncommon.

Tumor Staging

The NWTS staging system is most widely used and is based on surgical and pathologic findings. The original classification was used in the first and second NWTS trials and was modified for NWTS III (D'Angio et al, 1989).

Stage I:—Tumor limited to kidney and completely excised. The surface of the renal capsule is intact. Tumor was not ruptured before or during removal. There is no residual tumor apparent beyond the margins of resection.

Stage II:—Tumor extends beyond the kidney but is completely removed. There is regional extension of the tumor, ie, penetration through the outer surface of the renal capsule into perirenal soft tissues. Vessels outside the kidney substance are infiltrated or contain tumor thrombus. The tumor may have been biopsied or there has been local spillage of tumor confined to the flank. There is no residual tumor apparent at or beyond the margins of excision.

Stage III:—Residual nonhematogenous tumor confined to abdomen. Any one or more of the following occur: a. Lymph nodes on biopsy are found to be involved in the hilus, the periaortic chains, or beyond. b. There has been diffuse peritoneal contamination by tumor, such as spillage of tumor beyond the flank before or during surgery, or by tumor growth that has penetrated through the peritoneal surface. c. Implants are found on the peritoneal surfaces. d. The tumor extends beyond the surgical margins either microscopically or grossly. e. The tumor is not completely resectable because of local infiltration into vital structures. f. Tumor spill not confined to the flank occurred either before or during surgery.

Stage IV:—Hematogenous metastases. Deposits beyond stage III, eg, lung, liver, bone, and brain.

Stage V:—Bilateral renal involvement at diagnosis. An attempt should be made to stage each side according to the previously given criteria on the basis of extent of disease before biopsy.

Clinical Findings

A. Symptoms and Signs

The diagnosis of Wilms tumor is most commonly made after the discovery of an asymptomatic mass by a family member or a physician during a routine physical examination. Common symptoms at presentation include abdominal pain and distention, anorexia, nausea and vomiting, fever, and hematuria. The most common sign is an abdominal mass. Hypertension is seen in 25–60% of cases and is caused by elevated renin levels (D'Angio et al, 1982; Pizzo et al, 1989).

B. Laboratory Analysis

Urinalysis may show evidence of hematuria, and anemia may be present, particularly in patients with evidence of subcapsular hemorrhage. Patients with liver metastases may have abnormal serum chemistries.

C. X-Ray Imaging

Historically, IVU was the initial diagnostic study of choice to assess a suspected renal mass, but it has been replaced by newer modalities. Chest x-ray remains the initial examination of choice to evaluate for the presence of lung metastases.

Renal arteriography is typically indicated only in the patients with bilateral Wilms tumors or an involved horseshoe kidney. Chest x-ray remains the initial examination of choice for detection of metastatic disease. The role of a chest CT scan is controversial, and it is probably not indicated for routine use in low-risk patients; however, when done concomitantly with an abdominal CT, chest CT may provide clinically useful information in high-risk patients.

D. Ultrasonography, CT Scanning, and MRI

Ultrasonography is the current initial study of choice to evaluate palpable abdominal masses because it is accurate, does not require sedation, and is both widely available and cost-effective (Babyn et al, 1995).

CT of the abdomen is performed with suspected Wilms tumor and can be useful in providing information regarding tumor extension, the status of the contralateral kidney, and the presence of regional adenopathy. CT scanning remains an imperfect technique with a relatively high false-positive rate for hepatic invasion in right-sided tumors, and 7% of cases of surgically confirmed synchronous bilateral Wilms tumors were missed by preoperative CT imaging in the NWTS IV (Ritchey et al, 1995).

If pulmonary metastases are seen on chest x-ray, CT of the chest will not alter current therapy. However, the need for chest CT imaging in patients with negative results of chest x-ray remains controversial, because it is not clear whether those lesions detected by CT alone require more aggressive treatment (Weiner, Coppes, and Ritchey, 1998).

MRI can provide important information in defining the extent of tumor into the inferior vena cava, including those with intracardiac extension. It is limited in that there is no bowel contrast agent, and its use in children requires sedation (Babyn et al, 1995).

E. Radionuclide Imaging

Radionuclide bone scanning is rarely indicated. Abdominal CT scans essentially have taken the place of liver-spleen imaging.

F. Needle Biopsy

Preoperative biopsy is indicated routinely only in tumors deemed too large for safe primary surgical resection and for which preoperative chemotherapy or radiation therapy is planned.

Differential Diagnosis

The differential diagnosis of a flank mass in a child includes hydronephrosis, cystic kidneys, intrarenal neuroblastoma, mesoblastic nephroma, and various very rare sarcomas.

Ultrasonography can confirm the presence of hydronephrosis and evaluate for the presence of cystic kidneys. Neuroblastoma, while pathologically distinct from Wilms tumor, frequently presents in the abdomen as a mass arising from the adrenal glands or paraspinal ganglion. Neuroblastomas are radiographically indistinguishable from Wilms tumors, but there are several features that may aid in the differentiation. In contrast to Wilms tumors, which are typically confined to one side of the abdomen, neuroblastomas usually cross the midline. Wilms tumors are intrarenal masses and rarely cause a change in the axis of the kidney, while neuroblastomas may cause an outward and downward displacement of the kidney (drooping lily). Children with neuroblastomas are more likely to present with metastatic disease, and these tumors have a higher frequency of calcification observed radiographically. In addition, neuroblastomas may produce various tumor markers including vanillylmandelic acid and other catecholamines that are not seen in patients with Wilms tumor (Pizzo et al, 1989).

Mesoblastic nephromas are benign hamartomas and cannot be preoperatively distinguished from Wilms tumors. They are most commonly seen in the neonatal period and are typically identified by surgical pathology after nephrectomy. The tumor can occur in adults (Truong et al, 1998).

Treatment

The goal of therapy is to provide the highest possible cure rate with the lowest treatment-related morbidity. Significant improvements in survival rates for children with Wilms tumor have been achieved by an improved understanding of the disease and a multimodality approach to therapy, advocated by the NWTS, that incorporates surgery, radiation therapy, and chemotherapy.

A. Surgical Measures

For patients with unilateral kidney involvement whose tumors are deemed surgically resectable (tumors not crossing the midline or involving adjacent visceral organs), radical nephrectomy via a transabdominal incision is the procedure of choice.

Retroperitoneal lymph node dissection is not of proven value and is not recommended. However, biopsy of regional lymphatics (renal hilum and paraaortic nodes) and careful examination of the opposite kidney and the remainder of the abdomen provide crucial data for staging and prognosis. Tumor extending into the vena cava should be removed unless there is evidence of total obstruction. A major point of emphasis during surgical extirpation is to avoid spillage because there is evidence that this increases abdominal recurrence of disease (Shamberger et al, 1999; Ross and Kay, 1999).

A child with bilateral Wilms tumor, like an adult with bilateral RCC, requires an individualized approach. Patients with favorable histology tumors can frequently be managed with preoperative chemotherapy followed by renal-sparing surgery (Kumar, Fitzgerald, and Breatnach, 1998). In patients for whom preoperative chemotherapy is planned, a biopsy for diagnosis and staging is indicated (Blute et al, 1987). In some centers, needle aspiration biopsy has proved to be a reli-

able diagnostic tool when evaluated by experienced pathologists (Hanash, 1989). In patients with unfavorable histology tumors, the therapeutic approach consists of aggressive surgery followed by chemotherapy and radiation therapy.

B. Chemotherapy

Wilms tumor has been long recognized as a chemosensitive neoplasm. Consecutive multicenter randomized trials conducted by the National Wilms' Tumor Study Group (NWTSG) starting in the 1960s have carefully explored various treatment strategies to determine the role of various antineoplastics and the integration of surgery and radiotherapy, with the goal of optimizing response rates and cure while minimizing the toxicity of therapy. Current studies are focused on continued efforts to minimize toxicity (primarily by decreasing chemotherapy treatment duration and removing radiotherapy) in those favorable subgroups with impressive cure rates, and modifying efforts in poor-risk subgroups to improve response and survival.

Patients with stage I favorable or anaplastic histology and stage II favorable histology tumors undergo surgical resection and have adjuvant chemotherapy with vincristine and dactinomycin combinations without radiotherapy. Patients with stage III and IV favorable histology tumors undergo surgical resection and have adjuvant therapy with vincristine, dactinomycin, and doxorubicin, with adjuvant radiotherapy. Patients with stage II–IV anaplastic histology tumors receive therapy similar to that for advanced-stage favorable histology tumors (Green et al, 1998).

C. Radiation Therapy

Wilms tumor has long been recognized as a radiosensitive tumor. Despite the proven efficacy of radiation therapy in children, its use is complicated by its potential for growth disturbances and recognized cardiac, pulmonary, and hepatic toxicities. The development of effective chemotherapy combinations has practically replaced radiation therapy in the preoperative setting. The first and second NWTS trials demonstrated that postoperative radiotherapy was not required for patients with favorable histology stage I disease. NWTS III failed to show an advantage for postoperative radiotherapy in patients with favorable stage II disease and demonstrated that the relapse rate of patients with stage III disease was no different for patients receiving 1000 cGy compared with the traditional 2000 cGy (D'Angio et al, 1989). Postoperative radiation is recommended for patients with stage III or IV disease with favorable histology, stages II–IV with focal anaplasia and clear cell sarcoma, and all stages of rhabdoid tumor of the kidney (Weiner, Coppes, and Ritchey, 1998).

Prognosis

The multimodality approach to the treatment of children with Wilms tumors has significantly improved outcomes. The 4-year survival of patients with favorable histology Wilms tumor now approaches 90% (Weiner, Coppes, and Ritchey, 1998). The most important negative prognostic factors remain the unfavorable histologic subtypes (clear cell sarcoma, rhabdoid, and anaplastic tumors). Although the addition of doxorubicin in NWTS III significantly improved the 2-year survival rate for patients with clear cell sarcomas (61.5–90.3%), it did not affect the survival of children with rhabdoid tumors. Analysis of patients with bilateral Wilms tumors registered with NWTS II and III revealed a 3-year survival rate of 82% (Blute et al, 1987).

Future challenges include improvements in therapy for patients with anaplastic tumors (stages II–IV), clear cell sarcoma, and rhabdoid tumors, and efforts to improve outcomes in favorable histology tumors while decreasing both short-term and late toxicities.

SARCOMA OF THE KIDNEY

Primary sarcomas of the kidney are rare, with a reported incidence ranging from 1% to 3% of all malignant renal neoplasms (Vogelzang et al, 1993; Srinivas et al, 1984). Renal sarcomas are most commonly present in patients in the fifth decade of life, and there is a slight male predominance. Flank or abdominal pain and weight loss are the most frequent presenting symptoms. Primary renal sarcomas may be difficult to distinguish histologically from the sarcomatoid variant of renal carcinoma (Bonsib et al, 1987). Leiomyosarcomas compose approximately 50% of all renal sarcomas and occur with a female predominance of 2:1 (Loomis, 1972). The remaining 40–50% of renal sarcomas consist of fibrosarcomas, liposarcomas, and hemangiopericytomas. Extremely rare presentations of osteogenic sarcoma (Micolonghi et al, 1984) and malignant schwannomas (Farrow et al, 1968) have been reported. Renal sarcomas are typically of renal capsular origin. They present with symptoms analogous to those of other renal masses and tend to exhibit aggressive local spread with distant metastases to lung and liver as late findings.

Radical nephrectomy for localized disease is the only effective therapy. Adjuvant radiotherapy has been demonstrated to decrease the incidence of local recurrence in patients with resectable retroperitoneal sarcomas; however, there is no improvement in overall survival (Kinsella et al, 1988). Various chemotherapeutic agents, including doxorubicin, dacarbazine, and ifosfamide, have activity in the treatment of metastatic disease, but responses are typically partial and of brief duration.

SECONDARY RENAL TUMORS

The kidney is a frequent site for metastatic spread of both solid and hematologic tumors. Wagle, Moore, and Murphy (1975) surveyed 4413 autopsies at a major cancer center and found 81 (18%) cases of secondary carcinoma of the kidney (hematologic tumors were excluded). The most frequent primary site of cancer was lung (20%), followed by breast (12%), stomach (11%), and renal (9%). The authors noted that metastases to the renal parenchyma typically demonstrated capsular and stromal invasion with sparing of the renal pelvis and that bilateral secondary renal involvement was found in approximately 50% of cases.

Albuminuria and hematuria are relatively common findings in patients with secondary renal metastases; however, pain and renal insufficiency are rare (Wagle, Moore, and Murphy, 1975; Olsson, Moyer, and Laferte, 1971). Secondary metastatic disease to the kidneys tends to be a late event, frequently in the setting of widely disseminated disease, which typically portends a poor prognosis. Therapy is dictated by the responsiveness of the primary neoplasm; that is, patients with breast and ovarian cancers for which there is effective therapy are more likely to respond than patients with primary lung or gastric cancers.

Autopsy series have reported clinically evident renal invasion by lymphoma to be 0.5–7%, with the rates of Hodgkin's and non-Hodgkin's lymphoma distributed equally (Goffinet et al, 1977; Weimar et al, 1981). Renal involvement is usually in the form of bilateral, multiple, discrete tumor nodules. Renal involvement by non-Hodgkin's lymphoma is typically characterized by diffuse, aggressive histologic findings (ie, diffuse large cell) in the setting of extensive disease. Therapy typically consists of combination chemotherapy, with the prognosis of patients similar to that of patients without renal involvement but with widely disseminated, aggressive lymphomas (Geffen et al, 1985).

REFERENCES

Ambos MA et al: Angiographic pattern in renal oncocytomas. Radiology 1978;129:615.

Anderson EE, Hatcher PA: Renal angiomyolipoma. Probl Urol 1990;4:230.

Aulitzky W et al: Successful treatment of metastatic renal cell carcinoma with a biologically active dose of recombinant interferon-gamma. J Clin Oncol 1989;7:1875.

Avila NA et al: Lymphangioleiomyomatosis: Abdominopelvic CT and US findings. Radiology 2000;216:147.

Babyn P et al: Imaging patients with Wilms' tumor. Hematol Oncol Clin North Am 1995;9:1217.

Bachor R et al: Positron emission tomography in the diagnosis of renal cell carcinoma. Urologe A 1996;35:146.

Beckwith JB: New developments in the pathology of Wilms' tumor. Cancer Invest 1997;15:153.

Beckwith JB: Wilms' tumor and other renal tumors of childhood: A selective review from the National Wilms' Tumor Study Pathology Center. Hum Pathol 1983;14:481.

Beckwith JB, Palmer NF: Histopathology and prognosis of Wilms' tumor: Results from the first National Wilms' Tumor Study. Cancer 1978;41:1937.

Beckwith JB, Kiviat NB, Bonadio JF: Nephrogenic rests, nephroblastomatosis, and the pathogenesis of Wilms' tumor. Pediatr Pathol 1990;10:1.

Blom JHM et al: Radical nephrectomy with and without lymph node dissection: Preliminary results of the EORTC randomized phase III protocol 30881. Eur Urol 1999;36:570.

Bluemke DA, Chambers TP: Spiral CT angiography: An alternative to conventional angiography. Radiology 1995;195:317.

Blute ML et al: Bilateral Wilms' tumor. J Urol 1987;138:968.

Bonnin JM et al: Hypertension due to a renin-secreting tumour localized by segmental renal vein sampling. Aust NZ J Med 1977;7:630.

Bono AV: Steroid hormones and hormonal treatment in renal cell carcinoma. In: deKernion JB, Pavone-Macaluso M (editors): *Tumors of the Kidney.* Williams & Wilkins, 1986.

Bonsib SM: Pathologic features of renal parenchymal tumors. In: Culp DA, Loening SA (editors): *Genitourinary Oncology.* Lea & Febiger, 1985.

Bonsib SM et al: Sarcomatoid renal tumors: Clinicopathologic correlation of three cases. Cancer 1987;59:527.

Bosniak MA: Observation of small incidentally detected renal masses. Semin Urol Oncol 1995;13:267.

Brennan JF et al: Acquired renal cystic disease: Implications for the urologist. Br J Urol 1991;67:342.

Breslow N et al: Epidemiology of Wilms' tumor. Med Ped Oncol 1993;21:172.

Breslow NE, Beckwith JB: Epidemiological features of Wilms' tumor: Results of the National Wilms' Tumor Study. J Natl Cancer Inst 1982;68:429.

Bretan PN Jr et al: Chronic renal failure: A significant risk factor in the development of acquired renal cysts and renal cell carcinoma: Case reports and a review of the literature. Cancer 1986;57:1971.

Busch FM, Bark CC, Clyde HR: Benign renal angiomyolipoma with regional lymph node involvement. J Urol 1976;116:715.

Chang SY et al: Inhibitory effects of suramin on a human renal cell carcinoma line causing hepatic dysfunction. J Urol 1992;147:1147.

Chen F et al: Germline mutations in the von Hippel-Lindau disease tumor suppressor gene: Correlation with phenotype. Hum Mutat 1995;5:66.

Chow WH et al: Rising incidence of renal cell cancer in the United States. JAMA 1999;281:1628.

Cohen AJ et al: Hereditary renal-cell carcinoma associated with a chromosomal translocation. N Engl J Med 1979;301:592.

Cohen C, McCue PA, Derose PB: Histogenesis of renal cell carcinoma and renal oncocytoma: An immunohistochemical study. Cancer 1988;62:1946.

Coppes MJ, Haber DA, Grundy PE: Genetic events in the development of Wilms' tumor. N Engl J Med 1994;331:586.

D'Angio GJ et al: Treatment of Wilms' tumor: Results of the Third National Wilms' Tumor Study. Cancer 1989;64:349.

D'Angio GJ et al: Wilms' tumor: Genetic aspects and etiology: A report of the National Wilms' Tumor Study (NWTS) Committee of the NWTS Group. In: Kuss R et al (editors): *Renal Tumors: Proceedings of the First International Symposium on Kidney Tumors.* Alan R. Liss, 1982.

Daniel WW et al: Calcified renal masses: A review of 10 years experience at Mayo Clinic. Radiology 1972;103:503.

Davis CJ et al: Renal oncocytoma. Clinicopathological study of 166 patients. J Urogen Pathol 1991;1:42.

Ditonno P et al: Extrarenal angiomyolipomas of the perinephric space. J Urol 1992;147:447.

Droller MJ: *Surgical Management of Urologic Disease: An Anatomic Approach.* Mosby–Year Book, 1992.

Ducret F, et al: Renin secreting tumors and severe hypertension: Apropos of a new case. Nephrologie 1991;12:17.

Ekelund L, Gothlin J: Renal hemangiomas: An analysis of 13 cases diagnosed by angiography. Am J Roentgenol Radium Ther Nucl Med 1975;125:788.

Erlandsson R: Molecular genetics of renal cell carcinoma. Cancer Genet Cytogenet 1998;104:1.

Fallon B, Williams RD: Renal cancer associated with acquired cystic disease of the kidney and chronic renal failure. Semin Urol 1989;4:228.

Farrow GW et al: Sarcomas and sarcomatoid and mixed malignant tumors of the kidney in adults (parts 1–3). Cancer 1968;22:545.

Flanigan RC et al: Nephrectomy followed by interferon alfa-2b compared with interferon alfa-2b alone for metastatic renal cell cancer. N Engl J Med 2001;345:1655.

Flocks RH, Kadesky MC: Malignant neoplasms of the kidney: An analysis of 353 patients followed 5 years or more. J Urol 1958;79:196.

Fossa SD, Kjolseth I, Lund G: Radiotherapy of metastasis from renal cancer. Eur Urol 1982;8:340.

Fuhrman SA, Lasky LC, Limas C: Prognostic significance of morphologic parameters in renal cell carcinoma. Am J Surg Pathol 1982;6:655.

Fyfe G et al: Results of treatment of 255 patients with metastatic renal cell carcinoma who received high-dose recombinant interleukin-2 therapy. J Clin Oncol 1995;13:688.

Gardner KD, Evan AP: Cystic kidneys: An enigma evolves. Am J Kidney Dis 1984;3:403.

Geffen DB et al: Renal involvement in diffuse aggressive lymphomas: Results of treatment with combination chemotherapy. J Clin Oncol 1985;3:646.

Gill IS et al: Laparoscopic radical nephrectomy in 100 patients. Cancer 2001;92:1843.

Gill IS et al: Laparoscopic renal cryoablation in 32 patients. Urology 2000;56:748.

Gitlitz BJ et al: Treatment of metastatic renal cell carcinoma with high-dose bolus interleukin-2 in a non-intensive care unit: An analysis of 124 consecutively treated patients. Cancer J 2001;7:112.

Gleave ME et al: Interferon gamma-1b compared with placebo in metastatic renal cell carcinoma. N Engl J Med 1998; 338:1265.

Goffinet DR et al: Clinical and surgical (laparotomy) evaluation of patients with non-Hodgkin's lymphomas. Cancer Treat Rep 1977;61:981.

Gold PJ et al: Paraneoplastic manifestations of renal cell carcinoma. Semin Urol Oncol 1996;14:216.

Goldstein NS: The current state of renal cell carcinoma grading. Cancer 1997;80:977.

Green DM et al: Effect of duration of treatment outcome and cost of treatment for Wilms' tumor: A report from the National Wilms' Tumor Study Group. J Clin Oncol 1998;16:3744.

Gulanikar AC et al: Prospective pretransplant ultrasound screening in 206 patients for acquired renal cysts and renal cell carcinoma. Transplantation 1998;66:1669.

Haab F et al: Renin secreting tumors: Diagnosis, conservative surgical approach and long-term results. J Urol 1995;153:1781.

Hafez KS, Novick AC, Campbell SC: Patterns of tumor recurrence and guidelines for followup following nephron-sparing surgery for sporadic renal cell carcinoma. J Urol 1997;157: 2067.

Hamperl H: Benign and malignant oncocytoma. Cancer 1962; 15:1019.

Hanash KA: The nonmetastatic hepatic dysfunction syndrome associated with renal cell carcinoma (hypernephroma): Stauffer's syndrome. Prog Clin Biol Res 1982;100:301.

Hanash KA: Recent advances in the surgical treatment of bilateral Wilms' tumor. In: Murphy GP, Khoury S (editors): *Therapeutic Progress in Urological Cancers.* Alan R. Liss, 1989.

Henriksson C et al: Skeletal metastases in 102 patients evaluated before surgery for renal cell carcinoma. Scand J Urol Nephrol 1992;26:363.

Herr HW: Partial nephrectomy for unilateral renal carcinoma and a normal contralateral kidney: 10-year followup. J Urol 1999; 161:33.

Herrlinger A et al: What are the benefits of extended dissection of the regional lymph nodes in the therapy of renal cell carcinoma? J Urol 1991;146:1224.

Hock LM, Lynch J, Balaji KC: Increasing incidence of all stages of kidney cancer in the last 2 decades in the United States: An analysis of Surveillance, Epidemiology and End Results Program data. J Urol 2002;167:57.

Hocking WG: Hematologic abnormalities in patients with renal diseases. Hematol Oncol Clin North Am 1987;1:229.

Hoh CK, Seltzer MA, Franklin J: Positron emission tomography in urologic oncology. J Urol 1998;159:347.

Holmes NM et al: Renal imaging with spiral CT scan: Clinical applications. Tech Urol 1997;3:202.

Holthöfer H: Immunohistology of renal cell carcinoma. Eur Urol 1990;18(Suppl):15.

Horan JJ et al: The detection of renal cell carcinoma extension into the renal vein and inferior vena cava: A prospective comparison of venacavography and MRI. J Urol 1989;142:943.

Hricak H et al: Detection and staging of renal neoplasms: A reassessment of MR imaging. Radiology 1988;166:643.

Huff V: Inheritance and functionality of Wilms' tumor genes. Cancer Bull 1994;46:254.

Itano NB et al: Outcome of isolated renal cell carcinoma fossa recurrence after nephrectomy. J Urol 2000;164:322.

Jemal A et al: Cancer statistics, 2002. CA: Cancer J Clin 2002; 52:23.

Juusela H et al: Preoperative irradiation in the treatment of renal cell carcinoma. Scand J Urol Nephrol 1977;11:277.

Kabala JE et al: Magnetic resonance imaging in the staging of renal cell carcinoma. Br J Radiol 1991;64:683.

Kavoussi LR et al: Regression of metastatic renal cell carcinoma: A case report and literature review. J Urol 1986;125:1005.

Kinsella TJ et al: Preliminary results of a randomized study of adjuvant radiation therapy in resectable adult retroperitoneal soft-tissue sarcomas. J Clin Oncol 1988;6:18.

Kjaer M: The role of medroxyprogesterone acetate (MPA) in the treatment of renal adenocarcinoma. Cancer Treat Rev 1988; 15:195.

Knudson AG Jr, Strong LC: Mutation and cancer: A model for Wilms' tumor of the kidney. J Natl Cancer Inst 1972;48:313.

Kosko JW, Lipuma JP, Resnick MI: Radiological evaluation of renal mass. In: Javadpour N (editor): *Cancer of the Kidney.* Thieme-Stratton, 1984.

Kovacs G et al: Consistent chromosome 3p deletion and loss of heterozygosity in renal cell carcinoma. Proc Natl Acad Sci U S A 1988;85:1571.

Kumar R, Fitzgerald R, Breatnach F: Conservative surgical management of bilateral Wilms' tumor: Results of the United Kingdom Children's Cancer Study Group. J Urol 1998; 160:1450.

Latif F et al: Identification of the von Hippel-Lindau disease tumor suppressor gene. Science 1993;260:1317.

La Vecchia C et al: Smoking and renal cell carcinoma. Cancer Res 1990;50:5231.

Levy DA et al: Stage specific guidelines for surveillance after radical nephrectomy for local renal cell carcinoma. J Urol 1998; 159:1163.

Licht MR et al: Renal oncocytoma: Clinical and biological correlates. J Urol 1993;150:1380.

Lieber MM, Tsukamoto T: Renal oncocytoma. In: deKernion JB, Pavone-Macaluso M (editors): *Tumors of the Kidney.* Williams & Wilkins, 1986.

Loomis RC: Primary leiomyosarcoma of the kidney: Report of a case and a review of the literature. J Urol 1972;107:557.

Lowe BA et al: Malignant transformation of angiomyolipoma. J Urol 1992;147:1356.

Maatman TJ et al: Renal oncocytoma: A diagnostic and therapeutic dilemma. J Urol 1984;132:878.

Makay B, Ordonez NG, Khousrsland J: The ultrastructure and immunocytochemistry of renal cell carcinoma. Ultrastruct Pathol 1987;11:483.

Mandel JS et al: International renal cell cancer study. IV. Occupation. Int J Cancer 1995;61:601.

Marshall FF et al: The feasibility of surgical enucleation for renal cell carcinoma. J Urol 1986;135:231.

McDermott D et al: A randomized phase III trial of high-dose interleukin-2 versus subcutaneous IL2/interferon in patients with metastatic renal cell carcinoma. Proc Amer Soc Clin Oncol 2001;20 (abst 685):172a.

McLean GK, Meranze SG: Embolization techniques in the urinary tract. Urol Clin North Am 1985;12:743.

McNichols DW, Segura JW, DeWeerd JH: Renal cell carcinoma: Long term survival and late recurrence. J Urol 1981;126:17.

Medical Research Council Renal Cancer Collaborators: Interferon-α and survival in metastatic renal carcinoma: Early results of a randomised controlled trial. Lancet 1999;353:14.

Merino MJ, Librelsi VA: Oncocytomas of the kidney. Cancer 1982;50:1952.

Mickisch G et al: P-170 glycoprotein glutathione and associated enzymes in relation to chemoresistance of primary human renal cell carcinomas. Urol Int 1990;45:170.

Mickisch G et al: Radical nephrectomy plus interferon-alfa-based immunotherapy compared with interferon-alfa alone in metastatic renal-cell carcinoma: A randomised trial. Lancet 2001;358:966.

Micolonghi TS et al: Primary osteogenic sarcoma of the kidney. J Urol 1984;131:1164.

Miller BA: Racial/Ethnic Patterns of Cancer in the United States, 1988–1992. NIH Pub. No. 96-4104. National Cancer Institute, 1996.

Morgan WR, Zincke H: Progression and survival after renal-conserving surgery for renal cell carcinoma: Experience in 104 patients and extended followup. J Urol 1990;144:852.

Mostofi FK, Davis CJ Jr: *Histologic Typing of Kidney Tumors.* Springer-Verlag, 1998.

Motzer RJ et al: Renal-cell carcinoma. N Engl J Med 1996;335: 865.

Motzer RJ et al: Phase III trial of interferon alfa-2a with or without 13-*cis*-retinoic acid for patients with advanced renal cell carcinoma. J Clin Oncol 2000;18:2972.

Muggia FM: Overview of cancer-related hypercalcemia: Epidemiology and etiology. Semin Oncol 1990;17:3.

Murphy DP, Gill IS: Energy based renal tumor ablation: A review. Semin Urol Oncol 2001;19:133.

Negrier S et al: Recombinant human interleukin-2, recombinant human interferon alfa-2a, or both in metastatic renal cell carcinoma. N Engl J Med 1998;338:1272.

Negrier S et al: Treatment of patients with metastatic renal carcinoma with a combination of subcutaneous interleukin-2 and interferon alfa with or without fluorouracil. J Clin Oncol 2000;18:4009.

Novick AC, Stewart BH, Straffon RA: Extracorporeal renal surgery and autotransplantation: Indications, techniques and results. J Urol 1980;123:806.

O'Dea MJ et al: The therapy of renal cell carcinoma with solitary metastasis. J Urol 1978;120:540.

Older RA et al: Spoke-wheel angiographic pattern in renal masses: Nonspecificity. Radiology 1978;128:836.

Olsson CA, Moyer JD, Laferte RO: Pulmonary cancer metastatic to the kidneys: A common renal neoplasm. J Urol 1971; 105:492.

Onufrey V, Mohiuddin M: Radiation therapy in the treatment of metastatic renal cell carcinoma. Int J Radiat Oncol Biol Phys 1985;11:2007.

Pastore RD et al: Renal cell carcinoma and interferon at the millennium. Cancer Invest 2001;19:281.

Patchell RA et al: A randomized trial of surgery in the treatment of single metastases to the brain. N Engl J Med 1990;322:494.

Pavlovich CP et al: Percutaneous radio frequency ablation of small renal tumors: Initial results. J Urol 2002;167:10.

Pitts WR et al: Ultrasonography, computed tomography and pathology of angiomyolipoma of the kidney: Solution to a diagnostic dilemma. J Urol 1980;124:907.

Pizzo PA et al: Solid tumors of childhood. In: DeVita VT Jr, Hellman S, Rosenberg SA (editors): *Cancer Principles and Practice of Oncology.* Lippincott, 1989.

Pizzocaro G et al: Interferon adjuvant to radical nephrectomy in Robson stages II and III renal cell carcinoma: A multicentric randomized study. J Clin Oncol 2001;9:425.

Portis AJ et al: Long-term followup after laparoscopic radical nephrectomy. J Urol 2002;167:1257.

Rabbani F et al: Temporal change in risk of metachronous contralateral renal cell carcinoma: Influence of tumor characteristics and demographic factors. J Clin Oncol 2002;20:2370.

Rafla S: Renal cell carcinoma: Natural history and results of treatment. Cancer 1970;25:26.

Ramdave S et al: Clinical role of F-18-fluorodeoxyglucose positron emission tomography for detection and management of renal cell carcinoma. J Urol 2001;166:825.

Reichard EAP, Roubidoux MA, Dunnick NR: Renal neoplasms in patients with renal cystic disease. Abdom Imaging 1998; 23:237.

Renshaw AA, Granter SR, Cibas ES: Fine-needle aspiration of the adult kidney. Cancer (Cancer Cytopathol) 1997;81:71.

Riccardi VM et al: Chromosomal imbalance in the Aniridia-Wilms' tumor association: 11p interstitial deletion. Pediatrics 1978; 61:604.

Ritchey ML et al: Accuracy of current imaging modalities in the diagnosis of synchronous bilateral Wilms tumor: A report from the National Wilms' Tumor Study Group. Cancer 1995; 75:600.

Robson CJ: The natural history of renal cell carcinoma. Prog Clin Biol Res 1982;100:447.

Robson CJ: Radical nephrectomy for renal cell carcinoma. J Urol 1963;89:37.

Robson CJ, Churchill BM, Anderson W: The results of radical nephrectomy for renal cell carcinoma. J Urol 1969;101:297.

Ross JH, Kay R: Surgical considerations for patients with Wilms' tumor. Semin Urol Oncol 1999;17:33.

Shamberger RC et al: Surgery-related factors and local recurrence of Wilms' tumor in National Wilms' Tumor Study 4. Ann Surg 1999;229:292.

Shingleton WB, Sewell PE: Percutaneous renal cryoablation of renal tumors in patients with Von-Hippel-Lindau disease. J Urol 2002;167:1268.

Siminovitch JMP, Montie JE, Straffon RA: Prognostic indicators in renal adenocarcinoma. J Urol 1983;130:20.

Skinner DG, Lieskovsky G, Pritchett TR: Technique of radical nephrectomy. In: Skinner DG, Lieskovsky G (editors): *Genitourinary Cancer.* Saunders, 1988.

Skinner DG, Vermillion CD, Colvin RB: The surgical management of renal cell carcinoma. J Urol 1972; 107:705.

Skinner DG et al: Diagnosis and management of renal cell carcinoma: A clinical and pathologic study of 309 cases. Cancer 1971;28:1165.

Smith JW et al: Acquired renal cystic disease: Two cases of associated adenocarcinoma and a renal ultrasound survey of a peritoneal dialysis population. Am J Kidney Dis 1987;10:41.

Smith RB: The treatment of bilateral renal cell carcinoma or renal cell carcinoma in the solitary kidney. In: deKernion JB, Pavone-Macaluso M (editors): *Tumors of the Kidney.* Williams & Wilkins, 1986.

Sobin LH, Wittekind C for the International Union Against Cancer: *TNM Classification of Malignant Tumors,* 5th ed. John Wiley & Sons, 1997.

Srinivas V et al: Sarcomas of the kidney. J Urol 1984;32:13.

Stauffer MH: Nephrogenic hepatosplenomegaly. (Abstract.) Gastroenterology 1961;40:694.

Steiner MS et al: Leiomyoma of the kidney: Presentation of 4 new cases and the role of computerized tomography. J Urol 1990; 143:994.

Steiner MS et al: The natural history of renal angiomyolipoma. J Urol 1993;150:1782.

Storkel S et al: The human chromophobe cell renal carcinoma: Its probable relation to intercalated cells of the collecting duct. Virchows Arch [B] 1989;56:237.

Strewler GJ et al: Parathyroid hormone–like protein from human renal carcinoma cells: Structural and functional homology with parathyroid hormone. J Clin Invest 1987;80:1803.

Sufrin G, Golio A, Murphy GP: Serologic markers, paraneoplastic syndromes, and ectopic hormone production in renal adenocarcinoma. In: deKernion JB, Pavone-Macaluso M (editors): *Tumors of the Kidney.* Williams & Wilkins, 1986.

Sufrin G et al: Paraneoplastic and serologic syndromes of renal adenocarcinoma. Semin Urol 1989;7:158.

Tanguay S et al: Therapy of locally recurrent renal cell carcinoma after nephrectomy. J Urol 1996;155:26.

Theones W et al: Chromophobe cell carcinoma and its variants: A report on 32 cases. J Pathol 1988;155:277.

Thrasher JB, Paulson DF: Prognostic factors in renal cancer. Urol Clin North Am 1993;20:247.

Tickoo SK et al: Renal oncocytosis: A morphologic study of fourteen cases. Am J Surg Pathol 1999;23:1094.

Toho BM, Whitmore WE Jr: Solitary metastases from renal cell carcinoma. J Urol 1975;114:836.

Toro JR et al: Birt-Hogg-Dubé syndrome: A novel marker of kidney neoplasia. Arch Dermatol 1999;135:1195.

Trump DL et al: Randomized controlled trial of adjuvant therapy with lymphoblastoid interferon in resected, high-risk renal cell carcinoma. (Abstract.) Proc Am Soc Clin Oncol 1996; 15:648.

Truong LD et al: Adult mesoblastic nephroma: Expansion of the morphologic spectrum and review of literature. Am J Surg Pathol 1998;22:827.

Uhlenbrock D, Fischer C, Beyer HK: Angiomyolipoma of the kidney: Comparison between magnetic resonance imaging, computed tomography, and ultrasonography for diagnosis. Acta Radiol 1988;29:523.

Urban T et al: Pulmonary lymphangioleiomyomatosis: A study of 69 patients. Medicine 1999;78:321.

Uzzo RG, Novick AC: Nephron sparing surgery for renal tumors: Indications, techniques and outcomes. J Urol 2001;161:6.

van der Werf-Messing B: Carcinoma of the kidney. Cancer 1973; 32:1056.

Varanasi R et al: Fine structure analysis of the WT1 gene in sporadic Wilms' tumors. Proc Natl Acad Sci USA 1994;91:3554.

Vaziri ND et al: Acquired renal cystic disease in renal transplant recipients. Nephron 1984;37:203.

Vecht CJ et al: Treatment of single brain metastases: Radiotherapy alone or combined with neurosurgery? Ann Neurol 1993; 33:583.

Vogelzang NJ et al: Primary renal sarcoma in adults. Cancer 1993; 71:804.

Vogelzang NJ et al: Spontaneous regression of histologically proved pulmonary metastases from renal cell carcinoma: A case with 5-year followup. J Urol 1992;148:1247.

Wagle DG, Moore RH, Murphy GP: Secondary carcinomas of the kidney. J Urol 1975;114:30.

Warshauer DM et al: Detection of renal masses: Sensitivities and specificities of excretory urography/linear tomography, US and CT. Radiology 1988;169:363.

Waters WB, Richie JP: Aggressive surgical approach to renal cell carcinoma: Review of 130 cases. J Urol 1979;122:306.

Weimar G et al: Urogenital involvement by malignant lymphomas. J Urol 1981;125:230.

Weiner JS, Coppes MJ, Ritchey ML: Current concepts in the biology and management of Wilms' tumor. J Urol 1998;159: 1316.

Weiner SN, Bernstein RG: Renal oncocytoma: Angiographic features of two cases. Radiology 1977;125: 633.

White EW, Braunstein LE: Cavernous hemangioma: A renal vascular tumor requiring nephrectomy, an unusual entity. J Urol 1946;56:183.

Williams RD: Tumors of the kidney, ureter and bladder. In: Wyngaarden JB, Smith LH, Bennett JC (editors): *Cecil's Textbook of Medicine.* Saunders, 1992.

Wong AL, McGeorge A, Clark AH: Renal angiomyolipoma: A review of the literature and a report of 4 cases. Br J Urol 1981; 53:406.

Yagoda A et al: Chemotherapy for advanced renal cell carcinoma: 1983–1993. Semin Oncol 1995;22:42.

Yu MC et al: Cigarette smoking, obesity, diuretic use and coffee consumption as risk factors for renal cell carcinoma. J Natl Cancer Inst 1986;77:351.

Zbar B et al: Hereditary papillary renal cell carcinoma. J Urol 1994; 151:561.

Neoplasms of the Prostate Gland

22

Joseph C. Presti, Jr, MD

The prostate gland is the male organ most commonly afflicted with either benign or malignant neoplasms. It comprises the most proximal aspect of the urethra. Anatomically it resides in the true pelvis, separated from the pubic symphysis anteriorly by the retropubic space (space of Retzius). The posterior surface of the prostate is separated from the rectal ampulla by Denonvilliers' fascia. The base of the prostate is continuous with the bladder neck, and the apex of the prostate rests on the upper surface of the urogenital diaphragm. Laterally, the prostate is related to the levator ani musculature. Its arterial blood supply is derived from branches of the internal iliac artery (inferior vesical and middle rectal arteries). Venous drainage is via the dorsal venous complex, which receives the deep dorsal vein of the penis and vesical branches before draining into the internal iliac veins. Innervation is from the pelvic plexus. The normal prostate measures 3–4 cm at the base, 4–6 cm in cephalocaudad, and 2–3 cm in anteroposterior dimensions.

McNeal has popularized the concept of zonal anatomy of the prostate. Three distinct zones have been identified (Figure 22–1). The **peripheral zone** accounts for 70% of the volume of the young adult prostate, the **central zone** accounts for 25%, and the **transition zone** accounts for 5%. These anatomic zones have distinct ductal systems but, more important, are differentially afflicted with neoplastic processes. Sixty to 70 percent of carcinomas of the prostate (CaP) originate in the peripheral zone, 10–20% in the transition zone, and 5–10% in the central zone (McNeal et al, 1988). Benign prostatic hyperplasia uniformly originates in the transition zone (Figure 22–2).

BENIGN PROSTATIC HYPERPLASIA (BPH)

Incidence & Epidemiology

BPH is the most common benign tumor in men, and its incidence is age-related. The prevalence of histologic BPH in autopsy studies rises from approximately 20% in men aged 41–50, to 50% in men aged 51–60, and to over 90% in men older than 80. Although clinical evidence of disease occurs less commonly, symptoms of prostatic obstruction are also age-related. At age 55, approximately 25% of men report obstructive voiding symptoms. At age 75, 50% of men complain of a decrease in the force and caliber of their urinary stream.

Risk factors for the development of BPH are poorly understood. Some studies have suggested a genetic predisposition, and some have noted racial differences. Approximately 50% of men under the age of 60 who undergo surgery for BPH may have a heritable form of the disease. This form is most likely an autosomal dominant trait, and first-degree male relatives of such patients carry an increased relative risk of approximately 4-fold.

Etiology

The etiology of BPH is not completely understood, but it seems to be multifactorial and endocrine controlled. The prostate is composed of both stromal and epithelial elements, and each, either alone or in combination, can give rise to hyperplastic nodules and the symptoms associated with BPH. Each element may be targeted in medical management schemes.

Observations and clinical studies in men have clearly demonstrated that BPH is under endocrine control. Castration results in the regression of established BPH and improvement in urinary symptoms. Additional investigations have demonstrated a positive correlation between levels of free testosterone and estrogen and the volume of BPH. The latter may suggest that the association between aging and BPH might result from the increased estrogen levels of aging causing induction of the androgen receptor, which thereby sensitizes the prostate to free testosterone. However, no studies to date have been able to demonstrate elevated estrogen receptor levels in human BPH.

Pathology

As discussed above, BPH develops in the transition zone. It is truly a hyperplastic process resulting from an increase in cell number. Microscopic evaluation reveals a nodular growth pattern that is composed of varying amounts of stroma and epithelium. Stroma is composed of varying amounts of collagen and smooth muscle. The differential representation of the histologic components of BPH explains, in part, the potential responsiveness to medical therapy. Thus alpha-blocker therapy may result in excellent responses in patients with BPH that has a significant component of smooth

367

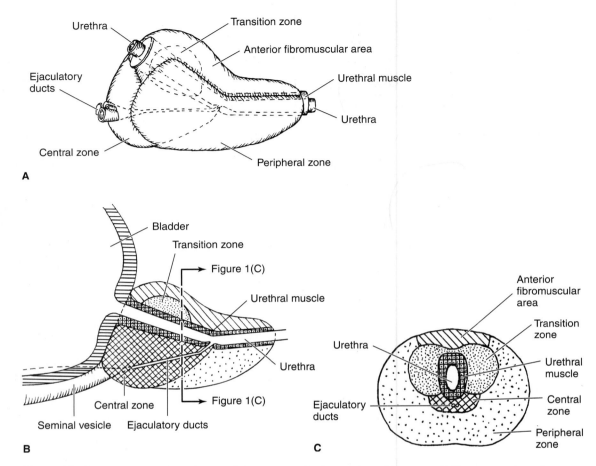

Figure 22–1. **A:** Schematic lateral view of the prostate. **B:** Cut section of the same. **C:** Transverse view of area shown in **B.**

muscle, while those with BPH predominantly composed of epithelium might respond better to 5α-reductase inhibitors. Patients with significant components of collagen in the stroma may not respond to either form of medical therapy. Unfortunately, one cannot reliably predict responsiveness to a specific therapy (see below).

As BPH nodules in the transition zone enlarge, they compress the outer zones of the prostate, resulting in the formation of a so-called surgical capsule. This boundary separates the transition zone from the peripheral zone and serves as a cleavage plane for open enucleation of the prostate during open simple prostatectomies performed for BPH.

Pathophysiology

One can relate the symptoms of BPH to either the obstructive component of the prostate or the secondary response of the bladder to the outlet resistance. The obstructive component can be subdivided into the mechanical and the dynamic obstruction.

As prostatic enlargement occurs, mechanical obstruction may result from intrusion into the urethral lumen or bladder neck, leading to a higher bladder outlet resistance. Prior to the zonal classification of the prostate, urologists often referred to the "3 lobes" of the prostate, namely, the median and the two lateral lobes. Prostatic size on digital rectal examination (DRE) correlates poorly with symptoms, in part because the median lobe is not readily palpable.

The dynamic component of prostatic obstruction explains the variable nature of the symptoms experienced by patients. The prostatic stroma, composed of smooth muscle and collagen, is rich in adrenergic nerve supply. The level of autonomic stimulation thus sets a tone to the prostatic urethra. Use of alpha-blocker ther-

Figure 22–2. Whole mount of prostate at level of midprostatic urethra. Note verumontanum (V) and areas of prostate cancer (CAP) in peripheral zone and areas of benign prostatic hyperplasia (BPH) in transition zone.

apy decreases this tone, resulting in a decrease in outlet resistance.

The irritative voiding complaints (see below) of BPH result from the secondary response of the bladder to the increased outlet resistance. Bladder outlet obstruction leads to detrusor muscle hypertrophy and hyperplasia as well as collagen deposition. Although the latter is most likely responsible for a decrease in bladder compliance, detrusor instability is also a factor. On gross inspection, thickened detrusor muscle bundles are seen as trabeculation on cystoscopic examination. If left unchecked, mucosal herniation between detrusor muscle bundles ensues, causing diverticula formation (so-called false diverticula composed of only mucosa and serosa).

Clinical Findings

A. Symptoms

As discussed above, the symptoms of BPH can be divided into obstructive and irritative complaints. Obstructive symptoms include hesitancy, decreased force and caliber of stream, sensation of incomplete bladder emptying, double voiding (urinating a second time within 2 h of the previous void), straining to urinate, and post-void dribbling. Irritative symptoms include urgency, frequency, and nocturia.

The self-administered questionnaire developed by the American Urological Association (AUA) is both valid and reliable in identifying the need to treat patients and in monitoring their response to therapy. The AUA Symptom Score questionnaire (Table 22–1) is perhaps the single most important tool used in the evaluation of patients with BPH and is recommended for all patients before the initiation of therapy. This assessment focuses on 7 items that ask patients to quantify the severity of their obstructive or irritative complaints on a scale of 0–5. Thus, the score can range from 0 to 35. A symptom score of 0–7 is considered mild, 8–19 is considered moderate, and 20–35 is considered severe. The relative distribution of scores for BPH patients and control subjects is, respectively, 20% and 83% in those with mild scores, 57% and 15% in those with moderate scores, and 23% and 2% in those with severe scores (McConnell et al, 1994).

A detailed history focusing on the urinary tract excludes other possible causes of symptoms that may not result from the prostate, such as urinary tract infection, neurogenic bladder, urethral stricture, or prostate cancer.

B. Signs

A physical examination, DRE, and focused neurologic examination are performed on all patients. The size and consistency of the prostate is noted, even though prostate size, as determined by DRE, does not correlate with severity of symptoms or degree of obstruction. BPH usually results in a smooth, firm, elastic enlargement of the prostate. Induration, if detected, must alert the physician to the possibility of cancer and the need for further evaluation (ie, prostate-specific antigen [PSA], transrectal ultrasound, and biopsy).

C. Laboratory Findings

A urinalysis to exclude infection or hematuria and serum creatinine measurement to assess renal function are required. Renal insufficiency may be observed in 10% of patients with prostatism and warrants upper-tract imaging. Patients with renal insufficiency are at an increased risk of developing postoperative complications following surgical intervention for BPH. Serum PSA is considered optional, but most physicians will include it in the initial evaluation. PSA, compared with DRE alone, certainly increases the ability to detect CaP, but because there is much overlap between levels seen in BPH and CaP, its use remains controversial (see Screening for CaP).

D. Imaging

Upper-tract imaging (intravenous pyelogram or renal ultrasound) is recommended only in the presence of concomitant urinary tract disease or complications from BPH (eg, hematuria, urinary tract infection, renal insufficiency, history of stone disease).

Table 22–1. Questionnaire for American Urological Association Symptom Score.

URINARY SYMPTOMS (SYMPTOM SCORE CRITERIA)	AUA Score					
	Not at all	Less than 1 time in 5	Less than half the time	About half the time	More than half the time	Almost always
1. Incomplete emptying Over the past month, how often have you had a sensation of not emptying your bladder completely after you finished urinating?	0	1	2	3	4	5
2. Frequency Over the past month, how often have you had to urinate again less than two hours after you finished urinating?	0	1	2	3	4	5
3. Intermittency Over the past month, how often have you found you stopped and started again several times when you urinate?	0	1	2	3	4	5
4. Urgency Over the past month, how often have you found it difficult to postpone urination?	0	1	2	3	4	5
5. Weak stream Over the past month, how often have you had a weak urinary stream?	0	1	2	3	4	5
6. Straining Over the past month, how often have you had to push or strain to begin urination?	0	1	2	3	4	5
	None	1 time	2 times	3 times	4 times	5 or more times
7. Nocturia Over the past month, how many times did you most typically get up to urinate from the time you went to bed at night until the time you got up in the morning?	0	1	2	3	4	5

AUA Symptom Score = sum of questions A1 to A7

QUALITY OF LIFE DUE TO URINARY PROBLEMS

	Delighted	Pleased	Mostly satisfied	Mixed—about equally satisfied and un-satisfied	Mostly dis-satisfied	Unhappy	Terrible
If you were to spend the rest of your life with your urinary condition just the way it is now, how would you feel about that?	0	1	2	3	4	5	6

Source: McConnell JD: *Benign Prostatic Hyperplasia; Diagnosis and Treatment.* Clinical Practice Guideline No. 8. AHCPR Publication No. 94-0582. Rockville, MD: Agency for Health Care Policy and Research, Public Health Serivce, US Department of Health and Human Services, 1994.

E. CYSTOSCOPY

Cystoscopy is not recommended to determine the need for treatment but may assist in choosing the surgical approach in patients opting for invasive therapy.

F. ADDITIONAL TESTS

Cystometrograms and urodynamic profiles are reserved for patients with suspected neurologic disease or those who have failed prostate surgery. Measurement of flow rate, determination of post-void residual urine, and pressure-flow studies are considered optional.

Differential Diagnosis

Other obstructive conditions of the lower urinary tract, such as urethral stricture, bladder neck contracture, bladder stone, or CaP, must be entertained when evaluating men with presumptive BPH. A history of previous urethral instrumentation, urethritis, or trauma should be elucidated to exclude urethral stricture or bladder neck contracture. Hematuria and pain are commonly associated with bladder stones. CaP may be detected by abnormalities on the DRE or an elevated PSA (see below).

A urinary tract infection, which can mimic the irritative symptoms of BPH, can be readily identified by urinalysis and culture; however, a urinary tract infection can also be a complication of BPH. Although irritative voiding complaints are also associated with carcinoma of the bladder, especially carcinoma in situ, the urinalysis usually shows evidence of hematuria. Likewise, patients with neurogenic bladder disorders may have many of the signs and symptoms of BPH, but a history of neurologic disease, stroke, diabetes mellitus, or back injury may be present as well. In addition, examination may show diminished perineal or lower extremity sensation or alterations in rectal sphincter tone or the bulbocavernosus reflex. Simultaneous alterations in bowel function (constipation) might also alert one to the possibility of a neurologic origin.

Treatment

After patients have been evaluated, they should be informed of the various therapeutic options for BPH. It is advisable for patients to consult with their physicians to make an educated decision on the basis of the relative efficacy and side effects of the treatment options.

Specific treatment recommendations can be offered for certain groups of patients. For those with mild symptoms (symptom score 0–7), watchful waiting only is advised. On the other end of the therapeutic spectrum, absolute surgical indications include refractory urinary retention (failing at least one attempt at catheter removal), recurrent urinary tract infection from BPH, recurrent gross hematuria from BPH, bladder stones from BPH, renal insufficiency from BPH, or large bladder diverticula (McConnell et al, 1994).

A. WATCHFUL WAITING

Very few studies on the natural history of BPH have been reported. The risk of progression or complications is uncertain. However, in men with symptomatic BPH, it is clear that progression is not inevitable and that some men undergo spontaneous improvement or resolution of their symptoms.

Retrospective studies on the natural history of BPH are inherently subject to bias, related to patient selection and the type and extent of follow-up. Very few prospective studies addressing the natural history of BPH have been reported. Recently, a large randomized study compared finasteride with placebo in men with moderately to severely symptomatic BPH and enlarged prostates on DRE (McConnell et al, 1998). Patients in the placebo arm of the study had a 7% risk of developing urinary retention over 4 years.

As mentioned above, watchful waiting is the appropriate management of men with mild symptom scores (0–7). Men with moderate or severe symptoms can also be managed in this fashion if they so choose. Neither the optimal interval for follow-up nor specific endpoints for intervention have been defined.

B. MEDICAL THERAPY

1. Alpha blockers—The human prostate and bladder base contains alpha-1-adrenoreceptors, and the prostate shows a contractile response to corresponding agonists. The contractile properties of the prostate and bladder neck seem to be mediated primarily by the subtype α_1a receptors. Alpha blockade has been shown to result in both objective and subjective degrees of improvement in the symptoms and signs of BPH in some patients. Alpha blockers can be classified according to their receptor selectivity as well as their half-life (Table 22–2).

Phenoxybenzamine and prazosin have comparable efficacy with respect to symptomatic relief, but the higher side-effect profile of phenoxybenzamine, associated with its lack of alpha-receptor specificity, precludes its use in BPH patients. Dose titration is necessary with prazosin, with typical therapy started at 1 mg at bedtime for 3 nights, then increased to 1 mg twice a day, which is titrated up to 2 mg twice a day if necessary. At higher doses, little additional symptomatic improvement is observed and side-effect profiles worsen. Typical side effects include orthostatic hypotension, dizziness, tiredness, retrograde ejaculation, rhinitis, and headache.

Long-acting alpha blockers make once-a-day dosing possible, but dose titration is still necessary. Terazosin is

Table 22–2. Classification of medical therapy and recommended dosage in BPH.

Classification	Oral Dosage
Alpha blockers	
Nonselective	
Phenoxybenzamine	10 mg twice a day
Alpha-1, short-acting	
Prazosin	2 mg twice a day
Alpha-1, long-acting	
Terazosin	5 or 10 mg daily
Doxazosin	4 or 8 mg daily
Alpha-1a selective	
Tamsulosin	0.4 or 0.8 mg daily
5α-reductase inhibitors	
Finasteride	5 mg daily

initiated at 1 mg daily for 3 days and increased to 2 mg daily for 11 days and then to 5 mg per day. Dosage can be escalated to 10 mg daily if necessary. Therapy with doxazosin is started at 1 mg daily for 7 days and increased to 2 mg daily for 7 days, and then to 4 mg daily. Dosage can be escalated to 8 mg daily if necessary. Side effects are similar to those described for prazosin.

The most recent advance in alpha-blocker therapy is related to the identification of subtypes of alpha-1-receptors. Selective blockade of the α_1a receptors, which are localized in the prostate and bladder neck, results in fewer systemic side effects (orthostatic hypotension, dizziness, tiredness, rhinitis, and headache), thus obviating the need for dose titration. Tamsulosin is initiated at 0.4 mg daily and can be increased to 0.8 mg daily if necessary.

Several randomized, double-blind, placebo-controlled trials, individually comparing terazosin, doxazosin, or tamsulosin with placebo, have demonstrated the safety and efficacy of all of these agents. Comparative trials of various alpha blockers are ongoing.

2. 5α-Reductase inhibitors—Finasteride is a 5α-reductase inhibitor that blocks the conversion of testosterone to dihydrotestosterone. This drug affects the epithelial component of the prostate, resulting in a reduction in the size of the gland and improvement in symptoms. Six months of therapy are required to see the maximum effects on prostate size (20% reduction) and symptomatic improvement.

Several randomized, double-blind, placebo-controlled trials have compared finasteride with placebo. Efficacy, safety, and durability are well established. However, symptomatic improvement is seen only in men with enlarged prostates (> 40 cm^3). Side effects include decreased libido, decreased ejaculate volume, and impotence. Serum PSA is reduced by approximately 50% in patients being treated with finasteride, but individual values may vary, thus complicating cancer detection.

A recent report suggests that finasteride therapy may decrease the incidence of urinary retention and the need for surgical intervention in men with enlarged prostates and moderate to severe symptoms (McConnell et al, 1998). However, optimal identification of appropriate patients for prophylactic therapy remains to be determined.

3. Combination therapy—The first randomized, double-blind, placebo-controlled study investigating combination alpha-blocker and 5α-reductase inhibitor therapy was recently reported (Lepor et al, 1996). This was a four-arm Veterans Administration Cooperative Trial comparing placebo, finasteride alone, terazosin alone, and combination finasteride and terazosin. Over 1200 patients participated, and significant decreases in symptom score and increases in urinary flow rates were seen only in the arms containing terazosin. However, one must note that enlarged prostates were not an entry criterion; in fact, prostate size in this study was much smaller than that in previous controlled trials using finasteride (32 versus 52 cm^3). Additional combination therapy trials are ongoing.

4. Phytotherapy—Phytotherapy refers to the use of plants or plant extracts for medicinal purposes. The use of phytotherapy in BPH has been popular in Europe for years, and its use in the United States is growing as a result of patient-driven enthusiasm. Several plant extracts have been popularized, including the saw palmetto berry, the bark of *Pygeum africanum,* the roots of *Echinacea purpurea* and *Hypoxis rooperi,* pollen extract, and the leaves of the trembling poplar. The mechanisms of action of these phytotherapies are unknown, and the efficacy and safety of these agents have not been tested in multicenter, randomized, double-blind, placebo-controlled studies.

C. CONVENTIONAL SURGICAL THERAPY

1. Transurethral resection of the prostate (TURP)—Ninety-five percent of simple prostatectomies can be done endoscopically. Most of these procedures involve the use of a spinal anesthetic and require a 1- to 2-day hospital stay. Symptom score and flow rate improvement with TURP is superior to that of any minimally invasive therapy. The length of hospital stay of patients undergoing TURP, however, is greater. Much controversy revolves around possible higher rates of morbidity and mortality associated with TURP in comparison with those of open surgery, but the higher rates observed in one study were probably related to more significant comorbidities in the TURP patients than in the patients undergoing open surgery. Several other studies could not confirm the difference in mortality when results were controlled for age and comorbidities. Risks of TURP include retrograde ejaculation (75%), impotence (5–10%), and incontinence (< 1%). Complications include bleeding, urethral stricture or bladder neck contracture, perforation of the prostate capsule with extravasation, and if severe, TUR syndrome resulting from a hypervolemic, hyponatremic state due to absorption of the hypotonic irrigating solution. Clinical manifestations of the TUR syndrome include nausea, vomiting, confusion, hypertension, bradycardia, and visual disturbances. The risk of the TUR syndrome increases with resection times over 90 min. Treatment includes diuresis and, in severe cases, hypertonic saline administration.

2. Transurethral incision of the prostate—Men with moderate to severe symptoms and a small prostate often have posterior commissure hyperplasia (elevated bladder neck). These patients will often benefit from an incision of the prostate. This procedure is more rapid and less morbid than TURP. Outcomes in well-selected patients are comparable, although a lower rate of retrograde ejaculation with transurethral incision has been reported (25%). The technique involves two incisions using the Collins knife at the 5 and 7 o'clock positions. The incisions are started just distal to the ureteral orifices and are extended outward to the verumontanum.

3. Open simple prostatectomy—When the prostate is too large to be removed endoscopically, an open enucleation is necessary. What constitutes "too large" is subjective and will vary depending upon the surgeon's experience with TURP. Glands over 100 g are usually considered for open enucleation. Open prostatectomy may also be initiated when concomitant bladder diverticulum or a bladder stone is present or if dorsal lithotomy positioning is not possible.

Open prostatectomies can be done with either a suprapubic or retropubic approach. A **simple suprapubic prostatectomy** is performed transvesically and is the operation of choice in dealing with concomitant bladder pathology. After the bladder is opened, a semicircular incision is made in the bladder mucosa, distal to the trigone. The dissection plane is initiated sharply, and then blunt dissection with the finger is performed to remove the adenoma. The apical dissection should be done sharply to avoid injury to the distal sphincteric mechanism. After the adenoma is removed, hemostasis is attained with suture ligatures, and both a urethral and a suprapubic catheter are inserted before closure.

In a **simple retropubic prostatectomy,** the bladder is not entered. Rather, a transverse incision is made in the surgical capsule of the prostate, and the adenoma is enucleated as described above. Only a urethral catheter is needed at the end of the procedure.

D. MINIMALLY INVASIVE THERAPY

1. Laser therapy—Many different techniques of laser surgery for the prostate have been described. Two main energy sources of lasers have been utilized—Nd:YAG and holmium:YAG.

Several different **coagulation necrosis** techniques have been described. Transurethral laser-induced prostatectomy (TULIP) is done with transrectal ultrasound guidance. The TULIP device is placed in the urethra, and transrectal ultrasound is used to direct the device as it is slowly pulled from the bladder neck to the apex. The depth of treatment is monitored with ultrasound.

Most urologists prefer to use visually directed laser techniques. **Visual coagulative necrosis** techniques have been popularized by Kabalin. Under cystoscopic control, the laser fiber is pulled through the prostate at several designated areas, depending upon the size and configuration of the prostate. Four quadrant and sextant approaches have been described for lateral lobes, with additional treatments directed at enlarged median lobes. Coagulative techniques do not create an immediate visual defect in the prostatic urethra, but rather tissue is sloughed over the course of several weeks and up to 3 months following the procedure.

Visual contact ablative techniques are more time-consuming procedures because the fiber is placed in direct contact with the prostate tissue, which is vaporized. An immediate defect is obtained in the prostatic urethra, similar to that seen during TURP.

Interstitial laser therapy places fibers directly into the prostate, usually under cystoscopic control. At each puncture, the laser is fired, resulting in submucosal coagulative necrosis. This technique may result in fewer irritative voiding symptoms, because the urethral mucosa is spared and prostate tissue is resorbed by the body rather than sloughed.

Advantages of laser surgery include (1) minimal blood loss, (2) rare instances of TUR syndrome, (3) ability to treat patients receiving anticoagulation therapy, and (4) ability to be done as an outpatient procedure. Disadvantages include (1) lack of availability of tissue for pathologic examination, (2) longer postoperative catheterization time, (3) more irritative voiding complaints, and (4) high cost of laser fibers and generators.

Large-scale, multicenter, randomized studies with long-term follow-up are needed to compare laser prostate surgery with TURP and other forms of minimally invasive surgery.

2. Transurethral electrovaporization of the prostate—Transurethral electrovaporization uses the standard resectoscope but replaces a conventional loop with a variation of a grooved rollerball. High current densities cause heat vaporization of tissue, resulting in a cavity in the prostatic urethra. Because the device requires slower sweeping speeds over the prostatic urethra, and the depth of vaporization is approximately one-third of a standard loop, the procedure usually takes longer than a standard TURP. Long-term comparative data are needed.

3. Hyperthermia—Microwave hyperthermia is most commonly delivered with a transurethral catheter. Some devices cool the urethral mucosa to decrease the risk of injury. However, if temperatures do not exceed 45 °C, cooling is unnecessary. Improvement in symptom score and flow rate is obtained, but as with laser surgery, large-scale, randomized studies with long-term follow-up are needed to assess durability and cost-effectiveness.

4. Transurethral needle ablation of the prostate—Transurethral needle ablation uses a specially designed urethral catheter that is passed into the urethra. Interstitial radiofrequency needles are then deployed from the tip of the catheter, piercing the mucosa of the prostatic urethra. The use of radio frequencies to heat the tissue results in a coagulative necrosis. This technique is not adequate treatment for bladder neck and median lobe enlargement. Subjective and objective improvement in voiding occurs, but as mentioned above, comparative long-term randomized studies are lacking.

5. High-intensity focused ultrasound—High-intensity focused ultrasound is another means of performing thermal tissue ablation. A specially designed, dual-function ultrasound probe is placed in the rectum. This probe allows transrectal imaging of the prostate and also delivers short bursts of high-intensity focused ultrasound energy, which heats the prostate tissue and results in coagulative necrosis. Bladder neck and median lobe enlargement are not adequately treated with this technique. Although ongoing clinical trials demonstrate some improvement in symptom score and flow rate, the durability of response is unknown.

6. Intraurethral stents—Intraurethral stents are devices that are endoscopically placed in the prostatic fossa and are designed to keep the prostatic urethra patent. They are usually covered by urothelium within 4–6 months after insertion. These devices are typically used for patients with limited life expectancy who are not deemed to be appropriate candidates for surgery or anesthesia. With the advent of other minimally invasive techniques requiring minimal anesthesia (conscious sedation or prostatic blocks), their application has become more limited.

7. Transurethral balloon dilation of the prostate—Balloon dilation of the prostate is performed with specially designed catheters that enable dilation of the prostatic fossa alone or the prostatic fossa and bladder neck. The technique is most effective in small prostates (< 40 cm^3). Although it may result in improvement in symptom score and flow rates, the effects are transient and the technique is rarely used today.

CARCINOMA OF THE PROSTATE (CaP)

Incidence & Epidemiology

Prostate cancer is the most common cancer diagnosed and is the second leading cause of cancer death in American men. Of all cancers, the prevalence of CaP increases the most rapidly with age. However, unlike most cancers, which have a peak age of incidence, the incidence of CaP continues to increase with advancing age. The lifetime risk of a 50-year-old man for latent CaP (detected as an incidental finding at autopsy, not related to the cause of death) is 40%; for clinically apparent CaP, 9.5%; and for death from CaP, 2.9%. Thus, many prostate cancers are indolent and inconsequential to the patient while others are virulent, and if detected too late or left untreated, they result in a patient's death. This broad spectrum of biological activity can make decision making for individual patients difficult.

Several risk factors for prostate cancer have been identified. As discussed above, increasing age heightens the risk for CaP. Which of the factors associated with the aging process are responsible for this observation is unknown. The probability of CaP developing in a man under the age of 40 is 1 in 10,000; for men 40–59 it is 1 in 103, and for men 60–79 it is 1 in 8. African Americans are at a higher risk for CaP than whites. In addition, African American men tend to present at a later stage of disease than whites. Controversial data have been reported suggesting that mortality from this disease may also be higher for African Americans. A positive family history of CaP also increases the relative risk for CaP. The age of disease onset in the family member with the diagnosis of CaP affects a patient's relative risk. If the age of onset is 70, the relative risk is increased 4-fold; if the age of onset is 60, the relative risk is increased 5-fold; and if the age of onset is 50, the relative risk is increased 7-fold. High dietary fat intake increases the relative risk for CaP by almost a factor of 2. Another exposure that may increase the risk for CaP involves cadmium, which is found in cigarette smoke, alkaline batteries, and in the welding industry. Previous vasectomy has been suggested as a factor that heightens the risk for CaP, but these data are controversial.

Etiology

The specific molecular mechanisms involved in the development and progression of CaP are an area of intense interest in the laboratory. The gene responsible for familial CaP resides on chromosome 1. Several regions of the human genome have been identified as possible areas that harbor tumor suppressor genes that may be involved in CaP. The regions most commonly identified are chromosomes 8p, 10q, 13q, 16q, 17p, and 18q.

Pathology

Over 95% of the cancers of the prostate are adenocarcinomas. Of the other 5%, 90% are transitional cell carcinomas, and the remaining cancers are neuroendocrine ("small cell") carcinomas or sarcomas. This discussion will address only adenocarcinomas.

The cytologic characteristics of CaP include hyperchromatic, enlarged nuclei with prominent nucleoli. Cytoplasm is often abundant; thus, nuclear-to-cytoplasmic ratios are not often helpful in making a diagnosis of CaP, unlike their usefulness in diagnosing many other neoplasms. Cytoplasm is often slightly blue-tinged or basophilic, which may assist in the diagnosis. The diagnosis of CaP is truly an architectural one. The basal cell layer is absent in CaP, although it is present in normal glands, BPH glands, and the precursor lesions of CaP. If the diagnosis of CaP is in question, high-molecular-weight keratin immunohistochemical staining is useful, as it preferentially stains basal cells. Absence of staining is thus consistent with CaP.

Prostatic intraepithelial neoplasia (PIN) is the precursor to invasive CaP. The critical distinguishing feature of invasive CaP is that the basal cell layer of the glandular architecture is absent. While PIN has the cytologic characteristics of CaP, the basal cell layer is present. PIN is usually classified into two categories, high grade (HGPIN) and low grade (LGPIN). The clinical importance of this distinction is that, when detected on prostate needle biopsy, HGPIN is usually associated with invasive CaP in approximately 50–80% of cases, whereas LGPIN is associated with invasive CaP only about 20% of the time. Thus, if a patient has needle biopsies showing only HGPIN, a repeat biopsy is critical to exclude the possibility of having missed an invasive cancer.

Sixty to 70 percent of cases of CaP originate in the peripheral zone, while 10–20% originate in the transition zone and 5–10% in the central zone. Radical prostatectomy series often demonstrate multifocal cancers within the prostate, with some variation in tumor grade.

Grading & Staging

The Gleason grading system is the most commonly employed grading system in the United States. It is truly a system that relies upon the low-power appearance of the glandular architecture under the microscope. In assigning a grade to a given tumor, pathologists assign a primary grade to the pattern of cancer that is most commonly observed and a secondary grade to the second most commonly observed pattern in the specimen. Grades range from 1 to 5. If the entire specimen has only one pattern present, then both the primary and secondary grade are reported as the same grade. The **Gleason score** or **Gleason sum** is obtained by adding the primary and secondary grades together. As Gleason grades range from 1 to 5, Gleason scores or sums thus range from 2 to 10. Well-differentiated tumors have a Gleason sum of 2–4; moderately differentiated tumors have a Gleason sum of 5–6; and poorly differentiated tumors have a Gleason sum of 8–10. Historically, tumors having a Gleason sum of 7 have sometimes been grouped with the moderately differentiated tumors and at other times with the poorly differentiated tumors. One point that needs to be clarified is that the primary Gleason grade is perhaps the most important with respect to placing patients in prognostic groups. This is most important in assessing patients with a Gleason sum of 7. Patients with a Gleason sum of 7 who have a primary Gleason grade of 4 (4 + 3) tend to have a worse prognosis than those who have a primary Gleason grade of 3 (3 + 4). Many clinical series have failed to distinguish between these two populations and, therefore, caution must be exercised in reviewing these series.

Gleason grades 1 and 2 are characterized by small, uniformly shaped glands, closely packed, with little intervening stroma. Gleason grade 3 is characterized by variable-sized glands that percolate between normal stroma. A variant of Gleason grade 3 is referred to as a cribriform pattern. Here a small mass of cells is perforated by several gland lumens with no intervening stroma. This results in a cookie-cutter-like appearance of cell nests. The border of these cribriform glands is smooth. Gleason grade 4 has several histologic appearances. The characteristic observation common to all Gleason grade 4 patterns is **incomplete gland formation.** Sometimes glands appear fused, sharing a common cell border. At other times sheets of cell nests are seen or long cords of cells are observed. Cribriform glands can also occur in Gleason grade 4, but the cell masses are large and borders tend to appear ragged, with infiltrating fingerlike projections. Gleason grade 5 usually has single infiltrating cells, with no gland formation or lumen appearance. Comedocarcinoma is an unusual variant of Gleason grade 5 carcinoma that has the appearance of cribriform glands with central areas of necrosis.

The TNM staging system for CaP is presented in Table 22–3 (American Joint Committee on Cancer, 1997). Note that with respect to the primary tumor categorization (T stage), the clinical staging system uses results of the DRE and transrectal ultrasound (TRUS), but not the results of the biopsy. Some examples to illustrate this staging system follow. If a patient has a palpable abnormality on one side of the prostate, even though biopsies demonstrate bilateral disease, his clinical stage remains T2a. If a patient has a normal DRE, with TRUS demonstrating a lesion on one side and a biopsy confirming cancer, his clinical stage is also T2a (using results of DRE and TRUS). A T1c cancer must have *both* a normal DRE and a normal TRUS.

Another popular staging system from a historical perspective is the Whitmore-Jewett staging system. One modification of this system is presented in Table 22–4 to assist the reader in the review of older published series. This system predates the use of TRUS and thus does not incorporate its findings.

Patterns of Progression

The pattern of CaP progression has been well defined. The likelihood of local extension outside the prostate (extracapsular extension) or seminal vesicle invasion and distant metastases increases with increasing tumor volume and more poorly differentiated cancers. Small and well-differentiated cancers (grades 1 and 2) are usually confined to the prostate, whereas large-volume (> 4 cm^3) or poorly differentiated (grades 4 and 5) cancers are more often locally extensive or metastatic to regional lymph nodes or bone. Penetration of the prostatic capsule by cancer is a common event and often occurs along perineural spaces. Seminal vesicle invasion is associated with a high likelihood of regional or distant disease. Locally advanced CaP may invade the bladder trigone, resulting in ureteral obstruction. Of note, rectal involvement is rare as Denonvilliers' fascia represents a strong barrier.

Lymphatic metastases are most often identified in the obturator lymph node chain. Other sites of nodal involvement include the common iliac, presacral, and periaortic lymph nodes. The axial skeleton is the most usual site of distant metastases, with the lumbar spine being most frequently implicated. The next most common sites in decreasing order are proximal femur, pelvis, thoracic spine, ribs, sternum, skull, and hu-

Table 22–3. TNM staging system for prostate cancer.

T—Primary tumor	
Tx	Cannot be assessed
T0	No evidence of primary tumor
Tis	Carcinoma in situ (PIN)
T1a	≤ 5% of tissue in resection for benign disease has cancer, normal DRE
T1b	> 5% of tissue in resection for benign disease has cancer, normal DRE
T1c	Detected from elevated PSA alone, normal DRE and TRUS
T2a	Tumor palpable by DRE or visible by TRUS on one side only, confined to prostate
T2b	Tumor palpable by DRE or visible by TRUS on both sides, confined to prostate
T3a	Extracapsular extension on one or both sides
T3b	Seminal vesicle involvement
T4	Tumor directly extends into bladder neck, sphincter, rectum, levator muscles, or into pelvic sidewall
N—Regional lymph nodes (obturator, internal iliac, external iliac, presacral lymph nodes)	
Nx	Cannot be assessed
N0	No regional lymph node metastasis
N1	Metastasis in a regional lymph node or nodes
M—Distant metastasis	
Mx	Cannot be assessed
M0	No distant metastasis
M1a	Distant metastasis in nonregional lymph nodes
M1b	Distant metastasis to bone
M1c	Distant metastasis to other sites

DRE, digital rectal examination; PIN, prostatic intraepithelial neoplasia; PSA, prostate-specific antigen; TRUS, transrectal ultrasound.
Source: American Joint Committee on Cancer: *Cancer Staging Manual,* 5th ed. Lippincott-Raven, 1997.

Table 22–4. Whitmore-Jewett staging system for prostate cancer.

A1	≤ 3 foci of carcinoma and ≤ 5% of tissue in resection for benign disease has cancer, Gleason sum < 7
A2	> 3 foci of carcinoma and > 5% of tissue in resection for benign disease has cancer, Gleason sum ≥ 7
B1	Palpable nodule ≤ 1.5 cm, confined to prostate
B2	Palpable nodule > 1.5 cm, confined to prostate
C1	Palpable extracapsular extension
C2	Palpable seminal vesicle involvement
D0	Clinically localized disease, with negative bone scan but elevated serum acid phosphatase
D1	Pelvic lymph node metastases
D2	Bone metastases
D3	Hormone-refractory prostate cancer

merus. The bone lesions of metastatic CaP are typically osteoblastic. Involvement of long bones can lead to pathologic fractures. Vertebral body involvement with significant tumor masses extending into the epidural space can result in cord compression. Visceral metastases most commonly involve the lung, liver, and adrenal gland. Central nervous system involvement is usually a result of direct extension from skull metastasis.

Clinical Findings

A. SYMPTOMS

Most patients with early-stage CaP are asymptomatic. The presence of symptoms often suggests locally advanced or metastatic disease. Obstructive or irritative voiding complaints can result from local growth of the tumor into the urethra or bladder neck or from its direct extension into the trigone of the bladder. Metastatic disease to the bones may cause bone pain. Metastatic disease to the vertebral column with impingement on the spinal cord may be associated with symptoms of cord compression, including paresthesias and weakness of the lower extremities and urinary or fecal incontinence.

B. SIGNS

A physical examination, including a DRE, is needed. Induration, if detected, must alert the physician to the possibility of cancer and the need for further evaluation (ie, PSA, TRUS, and biopsy). Locally advanced disease with bulky regional lymphadenopathy may lead to lymphedema of the lower extremities. Specific signs of cord compression relate to the level of the compression and may include weakness or spasticity of the lower extremities and a hyperreflexic bulbocavernosus reflex.

C. LABORATORY FINDINGS

Azotemia can result from bilateral ureteral obstruction either from direct extension into the trigone or from retroperitoneal adenopathy. Anemia may be present in metastatic disease. Alkaline phosphatase may be elevated in the presence of bone metastases. Serum acid phosphatase may be elevated with disease outside the confines of the prostate.

D. TUMOR MARKERS—PROSTATE-SPECIFIC ANTIGEN (PSA)

Serum PSA has revolutionized our ability to detect CaP. Current detection strategies include the efficient use of the combination of DRE, serum PSA, and TRUS with systematic biopsy. Unfortunately, PSA is not specific for CaP, as other factors such as BPH, urethral instrumentation, and infection can cause elevations of serum PSA. Although the last two factors can usually be clinically ascertained, distinguishing between elevations of serum PSA resulting from BPH and those related to CaP remains the most problematic.

Numerous strategies to refine PSA for cancer detection have been explored. Their common goal is to decrease the number of false-positive test results. This would increase the specificity and positive predictive value of the test and lead to fewer unnecessary biopsies, lower costs, and reduced morbidity of cancer detection. Attempts at refining PSA have included PSA velocity (change of PSA over time), PSA density (standardizing levels in relation to the size of the prostate), age-adjusted PSA reference ranges (accounting for age-dependent prostate growth and occult prostatic disease), and PSA forms (free versus protein-bound molecular forms of PSA).

1. PSA velocity—PSA velocity refers to the rate of change of serum PSA. A retrospective study has shown that men with prostate cancer have a more rapidly rising serum PSA in the years before diagnosis than do men without prostate cancer. Patients whose serum PSA increases by 0.75 ng/mL/y appear to be at an increased risk of harboring cancer. However, PSA velocity must be interpreted with caution. An elevated PSA velocity should be considered significant only when several serum PSA assays are carried out by the same laboratory over a period of at least 18 months.

2. PSA density—PSA levels are elevated approximately 0.12 ng/mL per gram of BPH tissue. Thus, patients with enlarged glands due to BPH may have elevated PSA levels. The ratio of PSA to gland volume is termed the PSA density. Some investigators advocate prostate biopsy only if the PSA density exceeds 0.1 or 0.15, while others have not found PSA density to be useful. Problems with this approach include the facts that (1) epithelial-stromal ratios vary from gland to gland and only the epithelium produces PSA, and (2) errors in calculating prostatic volume may approach 25%. The positive predictive value of PSA density is slightly higher than the use of a PSA level > 4 ng/mL in several series (30–40% vs. 20–30%).

3. Age-adjusted reference ranges for PSA—Age-adjusted PSA values for normal men are presented in Table 22–5 (Oesterling JE et al, 1993). It is thought that the rise in PSA with increasing age results from prostate gland growth from BPH, the higher incidence of subclinical prostatitis, and the growing prevalence of microscopic, clinically insignificant prostate cancers. Age-adjusted reference ranges increase the sensitivity in younger patients and increase the specificity in older patients. Concerns over the general applicability of these reference ranges have been raised because they were derived from US midwestern white men.

4. Racial variations in CaP detection—Although much evidence of racial variations in the incidence and mortality of CaP has been noted, little information is available on possible racial variations for cancer detection strategies. Recent reports have proposed different PSA density and age-specific reference ranges for African Americans and whites.

5. Molecular forms of PSA—The most recent refinement in PSA has been the recognition of the various molecular forms of PSA—free and protein-bound. Approximately 90% of the serum PSA is bound to alpha-1-antichymotrypsin, and lesser amounts are free or are

bound to alpha-2-macroglobulins. In the latter form, no epitopes to the antibodies used in the current assays are available, while PSA bound to alpha-1-antichymotrypsin may have 3 of its 5 epitopes masked. Early studies suggest that prostate cancer patients demonstrate a lower percentage of free PSA than do patients with benign disease. A large multicenter study has reported that in men with a normal DRE and a total PSA level between 4 and 10 ng/mL, a 25% free PSA cutoff would detect 95% of cancers while avoiding 20% of unnecessary biopsies. The cancers associated with greater than 25% free PSA were more prevalent in older patients and generally were less threatening in terms of tumor grade and volume (Catalona et al, 1998). Further validation studies with definition of optimal cutoff levels for different assays are needed, and issues such as possible racial variations in these levels must be addressed.

E. Prostate Biopsy

Systematic sextant prostate biopsy was the most commonly employed technique used in detecting CaP. Biopsies are usually obtained under TRUS guidance, from the apex, midsection, and base of each side of the prostate at the midsagittal line halfway between the lateral border and midline of the gland (Hodge et al, 1989). Information from sextant biopsies has mainly focused on cancer detection and has been underutilized for cancer staging. Several investigators have demonstrated some utility of systematic sextant biopsies in predicting extracapsular extension and risk of relapse following radical prostatectomy.

Refinement in systematic biopsy strategies to increase cancer detection rates is ongoing. It is clear that more extensive biopsy schemes that sample the lateral aspect of the prostate increase cancer detection (Eskew et al, 1997; Presti et al, 2000). Such extended biopsy schemes are critical in patients undergoing repeat biopsy (Chon et al, 2002).

F. Imaging

1. TRUS—TRUS is useful in performing prostatic biopsies and in providing some useful local staging information if cancer is detected. Almost all prostate needle biopsies are performed under TRUS guidance. This allows uniform spatial separation and sampling of the regions of the prostate and also makes lesion-directed biopsies possible. If visible, CaP tends to appear as a hypoechoic lesion in the peripheral zone.

TRUS provides more accurate local staging than does DRE. The sonographic criteria for extracapsular extension are bulging of the prostate contour or angulated appearance of the lateral margin. The criteria for seminal vesicle invasion are a posterior bulge at the base of the seminal vesicle or asymmetry in echogenicity of

Table 22–5. Age-adjusted reference ranges for PSA.

Age (y)	PSA Normal Ranges (ng/mL)
40–49	0–2.5
50–59	0–3.5
60–69	0–4.5
70–79	0–6.5

Data from Oesterling JE et al: Serum prostate-specific antigen in a community-based population of healthy men. Establishment of age-specific reference ranges. JAMA 1993; 270:860.

the seminal vesicle associated with hypoechoic areas at the base of the prostate.

TRUS also enables measurement of the prostate volume, which is needed in the calculation of PSA density. Typically, a prolate ellipsoid formula is used: $(\pi/6) \times$ (anterior-posterior diameter) $\times$ (transverse diameter) $\times$ (sagittal diameter). TRUS is also used in the performance of cryosurgery and brachytherapy (see below).

2. Endorectal magnetic resonance imaging—The reported staging accuracy of endorectal coil magnetic resonance imaging (MRI) varies from 51% to 92%. While rendering high image quality, the endorectal coil MRI appears to be operator dependent, requiring education and expertise. Costs associated with endorectal MRI are also high, and until this methodology demonstrates superiority in providing clinical information that alters patient management, its use should be limited. Attempts to identify patients who could potentially benefit from this imaging are ongoing.

3. Axial imaging (CT, MRI)—Cross-sectional imaging of the pelvis in patients with CaP is selectively performed to exclude lymph node metastases in high-risk patients who are thought to be candidates for definitive local therapy, whether it be surgery or irradiation. Both MRI and computed tomography (CT) are used for this purpose. Patients identified as having lymphadenopathy on imaging may undergo CT-guided fine-needle aspiration. If lymph node metastases are confirmed, such patients may be candidates for alternative treatment regimens. However, the incidence of lymph node metastases in contemporary radical prostatectomy series is low (< 10%). In addition, imaging is costly and its sensitivity is limited (30–40%). Various criteria can be used to identify patients for axial imaging, including negative bone scans and either T3 cancers or a PSA > 20 ng/mL and primary Gleason grade 4 or 5 cancers.

Analyses of several contemporary series of patients with clinically localized prostate cancer suggest that the risk of lymph node metastases is low and that its risk can be quantified on the basis of serum PSA, local tumor stage, and tumor grade. The serum concentration of PSA correlates well with cancer volume and stage. However, considerable overlap exists, making the use of serum PSA alone inaccurate for clinical staging in most patients. Use of serum PSA in conjunction with tumor grade and stage adds considerable sensitivity and specificity to the prediction of lymph node status compared with the use of PSA alone. Several investigators have published nomograms and probability curves that aid in predicting pathologic stage (Partin et al, 1997; Narayan et al, 1995; Bostwick et al, 1996).

4. Bone scan—When prostate cancer metastasizes, it most commonly does so to the bone. Soft tissue metastases (eg, lung and liver) are rare at the time of initial presentation. Although a bone scan has been considered a standard part of the initial evaluation of men with newly diagnosed prostate cancer, good evidence has been accumulated that it can be excluded in most of these men on the basis of serum PSA. Oesterling and colleagues have conducted studies to assess the ability of serum PSA to predict bone scan findings (Oesterling JE et al, 1993). On the basis of their results, bone scans can be omitted in patients with newly diagnosed, untreated prostate cancer who are asymptomatic and have serum PSA concentrations < 10 ng/mL.

G. Molecular Staging

Molecular staging refers to the detection of circulating prostate cells in the peripheral blood of men with CaP. The application of reverse transcription–polymerase chain reaction (RT-PCR) uses peripheral blood samples and attempts to identify the presence of the messenger RNA to PSA. If detected, this is indirect evidence of prostate cells in the peripheral circulation. However, the clinical significance of positive RT-PCR test results at the present time is unknown. Numerous tumor systems have been identified that shed tumor cells into the circulation, but this finding is not always indicative of metastatic disease or treatment failure. Further studies are needed before the widespread application of this methodology.

Differential Diagnosis

Not all patients with an elevated PSA concentration have CaP. Other factors that elevate serum PSA include BPH, urethral instrumentation, infection, prostatic infarction, or vigorous prostate massage. Induration of the prostate is associated not only with CaP, but also with chronic granulomatous prostatitis, previous TURP or needle biopsy, or prostatic calculi. Sclerotic lesions on plain x-ray films and elevated levels of alkaline phosphatase can be seen in Paget disease and can often be difficult to distinguish from metastatic CaP. In Paget disease, PSA levels are usually normal and x-ray findings demonstrate subperiosteal cortical thickening.

Screening for CaP

The case for CaP screening is supported by the following: The disease is burdensome in this country; PSA improves detection of clinically important tumors without significantly increasing the detection of unimportant tumors; most PSA-detected tumors are curable; prostate cancer mortality is declining in regions where screening occurs; and curative treatments are available. Although the benefit of screening was recently shown in one randomized Canadian study, several questions have been raised about the data analysis (Labrie et al, 1999). Two large randomized clinical trials to assess the benefit of screening are ongoing. In the Prostate, Lung, Colon and Ovarian Trial (PLCOT), 74,000 men have been randomized to annual DRE and PSA screening versus no screening. Results are anticipated in 2006. A larger trial involving 190,000 men in the European Randomized Study for Prostate Cancer Screening is anticipated to provide results in 2008. The efficacy of treatment is being examined in Scandinavia, where two randomized trials compare watchful waiting with radiation therapy or radical prostatectomy. A similar trial, Prostate Cancer Intervention Versus Observation Trial (PIVOT), is under way in the United States. Such trials, although imperfect, may give us the information we need before prostate cancer screening and treatment can be recommended with confidence.

In summary, many factors must be considered by both clinicians and their patients who are contemplating screening for prostate cancer. The information provided should attempt to answer such questions as the likelihood that an unscreened asymptomatic man will be adversely affected by prostate cancer in his lifetime, whether the screening test will lengthen or improve the quality of life, the chances of having a false-positive result and its consequences, the value of a normal result, and the recommendations of various experts. Based on available data, our bias has been that relatively young, healthy, asymptomatic men are encouraged to undergo screening. Screening is highly encouraged in certain populations with a higher disease prevalence or higher mortality rates, such as African American men or men with a significant family history of CaP. If CaP is detected, patients are carefully counseled regarding the benefits and risks of all treatment options, including watchful waiting. At the present time the data suggest that if screening is done, the combination of DRE and serum PSA is best.

Treatment

A. LOCALIZED DISEASE

1. General considerations—The optimal form of therapy for all stages of CaP remains a subject of great debate. Well-designed, randomized trials comparing various modalities for localized disease are lacking. Treatment dilemmas persist in the management of localized disease (T1 and T2) because of the uncertainty surrounding the relative efficacy of various modalities, including radical prostatectomy, radiation therapy, and surveillance. Currently, treatment decisions are based on the grade and stage of the tumor, the life expectancy of the patient, the ability of each therapy to ensure disease-free survival, its associated morbidity, and patient and physician preferences.

2. Watchful waiting—No randomized trial has demonstrated the therapeutic benefit of radical treatment for early-stage prostate cancer. Patients with prostate cancer are often older and may have concomitant illnesses. In addition, the small, well-differentiated prostate cancers commonly found in this population are often associated with very slow growth rates. Several studies have shown that surveillance alone may be an appropriate form of management for highly selected patients with prostate cancer (Table 22–6). However, most patients in such series are older and have very small, well-differentiated cancers. Even in such a selected population, cancer death rates approach 10%. In addition, end points for intervention in patients on surveillance regimens have not been defined.

3. Radical prostatectomy—The first radical perineal prostatectomy was performed by Hugh Hampton Young in 1904, and Millin first described the radical retropubic approach in 1945. However, the procedure remained unpopular because of frequent complications of incontinence and impotence. The rebirth of radical prostatectomy has resulted from a better understanding of the surgical anatomy of the pelvis. Description of the anatomy of the dorsal vein complex resulted in modifications in the surgical technique leading to reduced operative blood loss. In addition, improved visualization made possible a more precise apical dissection, allowing better reconstruction of the urinary tract and improved continence. Eversion of the bladder mucosa before anastomosis ensures a mucosa-to-mucosa apposition.

Table 22–6. Results of watchful waiting studies.

Study (year)	n	Follow-up (y)	Overall Mortality (%)	Disease-Specific Mortality (%)	CaP Progression (%)
Johansson et al (1992)	223	10.2	56	8	34
Whitmore, Warner, and Thompson (1991)	75	9.5	39	15	69
Hanash et al (1972)	179	15	55	45	NA
George (1988)	120	7	44	4	83
Madsen et al (1988)	50	10	52	6	18

Anatomic dissections have led to a better understanding of the prostate apex anatomy and its relationship to the distal urethral sphincteric mechanism. Description of the course of the cavernous nerves enabled modifications of the surgical technique, resulting in preservation of potency.

The prognosis of patients treated by radical prostatectomy correlates with the pathologic stage of the specimen. Distant metastasis is inevitable in patients with positive lymph nodes. A high percentage of patients with seminal vesical involvement at radical prostatectomy are destined to distant failure. Fortunately, the number of patients with these adverse prognostic factors undergoing surgery is decreasing because of better candidate selection based on appropriate use of preoperative clinical parameters. Several investigators have established nomograms to predict final pathologic stage at radical prostatectomy based on the serum PSA level, clinical DRE stage, and Gleason sum derived from the biopsy.

Patients with organ-confined cancer have 10-year disease-free survival ranging from 70% to 85% in several series. Those with focal extracapsular extension demonstrate 85% and 75% disease-free survival at 5 and 10 years, respectively. Patients with more extensive extracapsular extension demonstrate 70% and 40% disease-free survival at 5 and 10 years, respectively. High-grade tumors (Gleason sum > 7) have a higher risk of progression than do low-grade tumors. Disease-free survival at 10 years for patients with Gleason sum 2–6 tumors is in excess of 70%; for Gleason sum 7, 50%; and for Gleason sum > 8, 15%. Positive surgical margins significantly affect only tumors with extensive extracapsular extension.

The role of neoadjuvant hormonal therapy in men with localized CaP is currently being studied. Several investigators have reported a decrease in the number of positive surgical margins and the incidence of extracapsular extension. However, the largest randomized study to date demonstrated comparable serologic relapse rates at 4 years. Long-term data are still needed, and trials are ongoing.

The management of patients with positive surgical margins at radical prostatectomy remains controversial. Not all such patients relapse, but the identification of appropriate candidates for adjuvant radiation therapy remains problematic. A large multicenter randomized trial was recently closed to accrual to determine whether adjuvant radiation therapy in this setting is superior to radiation therapy at the time of relapse. Results of this study will not be available for several years.

Morbidity associated with radical prostatectomy can be significant and is in part related to the experience of the surgeon. Immediate intraoperative complications include blood loss, rectal injury, and ureteral injury.

Blood loss is more common with the retropubic approach than with the perineal approach because in the former, the dorsal venous complex must be divided. Rectal injury is rare with the retropubic approach and more common with the perineal approach but usually can be immediately repaired without long-term sequelae. Ureteral injury is exceedingly rare. Perioperative complications include deep venous thrombosis, pulmonary embolism, lymphocele formation, and wound infection. Late complications include urinary incontinence and impotence. Although total urinary incontinence tends to be rare (< 3%), stress urinary incontinence may be seen in up to 20% of patients. The return of continence after surgery is gradual, with 50% of patients continent at 3 months, 75% at 6 months, and the remainder at 9–12 months. Age is the single most important factor in the restoration of continence. Preservation of one or both neurovascular bundles may allow maintenance of erectile function in men who are potent and sexually active before the procedure. However, the nerve-sparing procedure should be used selectively, for extracapsular extension is a common finding in patients with presumed localized CaP. If extracapsular extension is present, preservation of the neurovascular bundle may increase the likelihood that the tumor will recur. Preservation of potency varies as a function of age, preoperative sexual function, and preservation of one or both neurovascular bundles. Reported rates of potency preservation vary from 40% to 82% in men under the age of 60 when both nerves are preserved and drops to 20–60% when only one nerve is preserved. For men between the ages of 60 and 69, comparable rates are 25–75% with bilateral nerve-sparing and 10–50% with unilateral nerve-sparing. Recovery of sexual function generally occurs within 6–12 months following surgery.

4. Radiation therapy—external beam therapy— Traditional external beam radiotherapy (XRT) techniques allow the safe delivery of 6500–7000 cGy to the prostate. Standard XRT techniques depend upon bony landmarks to define treatment borders or a single CT slice to define the target volume. These standard XRT techniques generally involve the use of open square or rectangular fields with minimal to no blocking and are characterized by the use of relatively small boost fields. Often, these XRT techniques fail to provide adequate coverage of the target volume in as many as 20–41% of patients with CaP irradiated.

Improved imaging and the use of 3-dimensional treatment planning software can now guarantee that the treatment field is accurately placed. This software can also allow higher doses of radiation to be given without exceeding the tolerances of surrounding normal tissues by causing the high-dose envelope of radiation to conform to the shape of the prostate. Conformal radiotherapy involves designing blocks from reconstructed CT images as viewed from the vantage point of the beam source. When viewed from the central axis, they are usually referred to as a "beam's-eye view." Computer-assisted beam's-eye views can be generated to design oblique and out-of-plane or noncoplanar beam arrangements. The approach is commonly referred to as 3-dimensional conformal radiotherapy. Additional benefits of this technique include the ability to calculate dose in 3 dimensions (to account more accurately for scattered radiation) and the ability to generate 3-dimensional dose displays and dose volume histograms. Three-dimensional dose displays allow so-called hot and cold spots (areas of overdosing and underdosing, respectively) to be recognized, while dose volume histograms allow different techniques to be compared and ranked for the relative sparing of surrounding normal tissues. Compared with standard XRT, considerably less normal tissue is irradiated because of the use of multiple complex fields.

Retrospective studies from several centers suggest that acute toxicity is reduced with the use of conformal radiotherapy compared with standard therapy. Possible improvement in PSA response rates has also been reported in several retrospective studies using 3-dimensional conformal radiotherapy. Although these results are encouraging, randomized trials and longer follow-up are required to determine if these improvements in PSA responses will translate into improved survival for these patients.

Readers are referred to Chapter 25 for a more detailed discussion of XRT in CaP.

5. Radiation therapy—brachytherapy—A resurgence in the interest in brachytherapy has occurred because of the technologic developments making it possible to place radioactive seeds under TRUS guidance. Previously, freehand seed placement techniques were used; however, very high failure rates were observed and the technique was virtually abandoned. Currently, with the use of computer software, one can preplan a precise dose of radiotherapy to be delivered by TRUS guidance.

Several investigators have reported their results using modern techniques. Data in men with low-volume, low-grade CaP are encouraging, but randomized studies comparing brachytherapy with other forms of radiotherapy are needed, as are studies assessing morbidity (impotence and urinary tract obstruction).

Readers are referred to Chapter 25 for a more detailed discussion of brachytherapy in CaP.

6. Cryosurgery—There has been a resurgence of interest in cryosurgery as a treatment for localized CaP in the past several years. This is due to an increased interest in less invasive forms of therapy for localized CaP as well as several recent technical innovations, including improved percutaneous techniques, expertise in TRUS, improved cryotechnology, and better understanding of cryobiology.

Freezing of the prostate is carried out by using a multiprobe cryosurgical device. Multiple hollow-core probes are placed percutaneously under TRUS guidance. Generally, 5 probes are placed: 2 anteromedially, 2 posterolaterally, and 1 posteriorly. Most surgeons routinely perform 2 freeze-thaw cycles in all patients, and if the iceball does not adequately extend to the apex of the prostate, the cryoprobes are pulled backwards into the apex and a third freeze-thaw cycle is undertaken. The temperature at the edge of the iceball is 0 to −2 °C, while actual cell destruction requires −25 to −50 °C. Therefore, actual tissue destruction occurs a few millimeters inside the iceball edge and cannot be monitored precisely by ultrasound imaging. Double freezing creates a larger tissue destruction area and theoretically brings the iceball edge and destruction zone edge closer together.

Studies to date indicate that, in the short term at least, cryosurgery can result in negative post-treatment prostatic biopsies and low or undetectable serum PSA levels. However, the morbidity of cryosurgery is significant and the long-term results are unknown. More recently, further refinement in the cryo technology has resulted in the development of smaller cryoprobes, which may result in a more controlled freezing. Currently, very few of these procedures are being performed, because other minimally invasive therapies are becoming more popular (brachytherapy).

B. LOCALLY ADVANCED DISEASE

1. Radiation therapy—Most patients with T3 CaP are, at the present time, treated with neoadjuvant hormonal therapy followed by XRT. This approach has proved to be superior to XRT alone in several randomized trials. One study reported on 456 evaluable patients, with high-volume T2, T3, and T4 patients randomized to receive 4 months of neoadjuvant complete androgen blockade with XRT (2 months before and 2 months during XRT) compared with XRT alone. The study demonstrated an improvement in local control and disease-free survival in the patients treated with neoadjuvant therapy (Pilepich et al, 2001). Another study reported on 401 evaluable patients with locally advanced CaP (predominantly T3) randomized to receive 3 years of androgen ablation therapy and XRT compared with XRT alone. This study also demonstrated improved survival in patients receiving combination therapy (Bolla et al, 1997). The optimal duration of hormonal therapy, both before and after radiation therapy, still needs to be defined.

C. Recurrent Disease

1. Following radical prostatectomy—The likelihood of recurrence following radical prostatectomy is related to cancer grade, pathologic stage, and the extent of extracapsular extension. Cancer recurrence is more common in those with positive surgical margins, established extracapsular extension, seminal vesicle invasion, and high-grade disease. For those patients in whom a detectable PSA level develops after radical prostatectomy, the site of recurrence (local versus distant) can be established with reasonable certainty based on the interval from surgery to the detectable PSA concentration, PSA doubling time, and selective use of imaging studies.

Patients with persistently detectable serum PSA levels immediately after surgery, those with PSA levels that become detectable in the early postoperative period, and those with serum PSA levels that double rapidly are more likely to have systemic relapse. Patients with initially undetectable serum PSA concentrations that become detectable a long time after radical prostatectomy, especially if PSA doubling times are prolonged, are more likely to have local recurrence (Pound et al, 1999).

2. Following radiation therapy—A rising PSA level following definitive radiotherapy is indicative of cancer recurrence. Biopsies of the prostate can identify local recurrences, while imaging with bone scans and possibly CT scans can identify distant recurrences. Irrespective of the site of recurrence, most patients receive androgen ablation therapy. While patients with clinical evidence of only local recurrence might be considered candidates for salvage radical prostatectomy or cryotherapy, morbidity remains high in this setting as well as subsequent clinical failure.

D. Metastatic Disease

1. Initial endocrine therapy—Since death due to CaP is almost invariably a result of failure to control metastatic disease, a great deal of research has concentrated on efforts to improve control of distant disease. It is well known that most prostatic carcinomas are hormone dependent and that approximately 70–80% of men with metastatic CaP respond to various forms of androgen deprivation. Testosterone, the major circulating androgen, is produced by the Leydig cells in the testes (95%), with a smaller amount being produced by peripheral conversion of other steroids. Although 98% of serum testosterone is protein bound, free testosterone enters prostate cells and is converted to DHT, the major intracellular androgen. DHT binds a cytoplasmic receptor protein and the complex moves to the cell nucleus, where it modulates transcription. Androgen deprivation may be induced at several levels along the pituitary-gonadal axis using a variety of methods or agents (Table 22–7). Use of a class of drugs (LHRH agonists) delivered as depot injections either monthly or, more recently, at 3-month or 4-month intervals has allowed induction of androgen deprivation without orchiectomy or administration of diethylstilbestrol. Currently, administration of LHRH agonists and orchiectomy are the most common forms of primary androgen blockade used. Because of its rapid onset of action, ketoconazole should be considered in patients with advanced prostate cancer who present with spinal cord compression or disseminated intravascular coagulation.

Table 22–7. Androgen ablation therapy for prostate cancer.

Level	Agent	Dose Route	Dose (mg)	Frequency
Pituitary				
	Diethylstilbestrol	Oral	1–3	Daily
	Goserelin	Subcutaneous	10.8	Every 3 months
	Goserelin	Subcutaneous	3.6	Every month
	Leuprolide	Intramuscular	22.5	Every 3 months
	Leuprolide	Intramuscular	7.5	Every month
Adrenal				
	Ketoconazole	Oral	400	Daily
	Aminoglutethimide	Oral	250	Four times a day
Testicle				
	Orchiectomy			
Prostate cell				
	Bicalutamide	Oral	50	Daily
	Flutamide	Oral	250	Three times a day
	Nilutamide	Oral	150	Daily

Although testosterone is the major circulating androgen, the adrenal gland secretes the androgens dehydroepiandrosterone, dehydroepiandrosterone sulfate, and androstenedione. Some investigators believe that suppressing both testicular and adrenal androgens (**complete androgen blockade**) allows for a better initial and a longer response compared with those methods that inhibit production of only testicular androgens. Complete androgen blockade can be achieved by combining an antiandrogen with the use of an LHRH agonist or orchiectomy. Antiandrogens appear to act by competitively binding the receptor for DHT, the intracellular androgen responsible for prostatic cell growth and development. When patients with metastatic prostate cancer are stratified with regard to extent of disease and performance status, those patients with limited disease and a good performance status who are treated with combined androgen blockade (an LHRH agonist and antiandrogen agent) seem to survive longer than those treated with an LHRH agonist alone (Crawford et al, 1989). However, another study comparing the use of an antiandrogen with and without an orchiectomy failed to demonstrate a survival difference between the two arms (Eisenberger et al, 1998). Ongoing trials are studying the use of intermittent androgen deprivation to determine whether this might result in a delay in the appearance of the hormone-refractory state.

The timing of initial endocrine therapy in CaP has been an area of great debate for many years. Data from the Veterans Administration Cooperative Studies from the 1960s did not demonstrate a clear survival advantage for early intervention with androgen ablation therapy in patients with advanced CaP. However, a randomized study from the Medical Research Council comparing early with delayed endocrine therapy in patients with advanced CaP demonstrated improved survival as well as lower complication rates (cord compression, ureteric obstruction, bladder outlet obstruction, and pathologic fractures) in patients treated with early endocrine therapy (Medical Research Council, 1997). In patients who undergo radical prostatectomy and are found to have microscopic lymph node involvement, early endocrine therapy has also resulted in a survival advantage (Messing et al, 1999).

2. Early manipulations for endocrine therapy failure—Patients receiving complete androgen blockade therapy who demonstrate a rise in serum PSA levels are currently managed by discontinuing the antiandrogen. Approximately 20–30% of such patients have a secondary PSA response. Responses are not just serologic, as regression of soft tissue disease has been reported. The pathophysiology underlying this secondary response, referred to as the antiandrogen withdrawal syndrome, is not understood. Some investigators have postulated that emergence of the hormone-refractory state results from mutations in the androgen receptor. Typically, antiandrogens competitively inhibit the androgen receptor, but it is possible that these agents actually stimulate a mutant androgen receptor. Removal of this stimulus (stopping the antiandrogen), thus leads to a secondary response.

Patients receiving monotherapy (LHRH agonist or orchiectomy) whose PSA level starts rising may respond to the addition of an antiandrogen. Response rates are approximately 20–30% in this setting.

3. Hormone-refractory disease—Readers are referred to Chapter 19 for a detailed discussion of the therapy for hormone-refractory disease.

REFERENCES

Prostate Gland

McNeal JE et al: Zonal distribution of prostatic adenocarcinoma. Am J Surg Pathol 1988;12:897.

Benign Prostatic Hyperplasia

Lepor H et al: The efficacy of terazosin, finasteride, or both in benign prostatic hyperplasia. Veterans Affairs Cooperative Studies Benign Prostatic Hyperplasia Study Group. N Engl J Med 1996;8:533.

McConnell JD et al: *Benign Prostatic Hyperplasia; Diagnosis and Treatment.* Clinical Practice Guideline No. 8. AHCPR Publication No. 94-0582. Rockville, MD: Agency for Health Care Policy and Research, Public Health Service, US Department of Health and Human Services, 1994.

McConnell JD et al: The effect of finasteride on the risk of acute urinary retention and the need for surgical treatment among men with benign prostatic hyperplasia. N Engl J Med 1998;338:557.

Carcinoma Of the Prostate

American Joint Committee on Cancer: *Cancer Staging Manual,* 5th ed. Lippincott-Raven, 1997.

Bolla M et al: Improved survival in patients with locally advanced prostate cancer treated with radiotherapy and goserelin. N Engl J Med 1997;337:295.

Bostwick DG et al: Prediction of capsular perforation and seminal vesicle invasion in prostate cancer. J Urol 1996;155:1361.

Catalona WJ et al: Use of the percentage of free prostate-specific antigen to enhance differentiation of prostate cancer from benign prostatic disease: A prospective multicenter clinical trial. JAMA 1998;279:1542.

Chon CH et al: Use of extended systematic sampling in patients with a prior negative prostate needle biopsy. J Urol 2002; 167:2457.

Crawford ED et al: A controlled trial of leuprolide with and without flutamide in prostatic carcinoma. N Engl J Med 1989; 321:419.

Eisenberger MA et al: Bilateral orchiectomy with or without flutamide for prostate cancer. N Engl J Med 1998;339:1036.

Eskew LA et al: Systematic 5 region prostate biopsy is superior to sextant method for diagnosing carcinoma of the prostate. J Urol 1997;157:199.

George NJR: Natural history of localized prostatic cancer managed by conservative therapy alone. Lancet 1988;(March 5):494.

Hanash KA et al: Carcinoma of the prostate: A 15 year follow-up. J Urol 1972;107:450.

Hodge KK et al: Random systematic versus directed ultrasound guided transrectal core biopsies of the prostate. J Urol 1989;142:71.

Johansson JE et al: High 10-year survival rate in patients with early, untreated prostatic cancer. JAMA 1992;267:2191.

Labrie F et al: Screening decreases prostate cancer death: First analysis of the 1988 Quebec prospective randomized controlled trial. Prostate 1999;38:83.

Madsen PO et al: Treatment of localized prostatic cancer: Radical prostatectomy versus placebo: A 15 year follow-up. Scand J Urol Nephrol Suppl 1988;110:95.

Medical Research Council Prostate Cancer Working Party Investigators Group: Immediate versus deferred treatment for advanced prostatic cancer: Initial results of the Medical Research Council trial. Br J Urol 1997;79:235.

Messing EM et al: Immediate hormonal therapy compared with observation after radical prostatectomy and pelvic lymphadenectomy in men with node positive prostate cancer. N Engl J Med 1999;341:1781.

Narayan P et al: The role of transrectal ultrasound-guided biopsy-based staging, preoperative serum prostate-specific antigen, and biopsy Gleason score in prediction of final pathologic diagnosis in prostate cancer. Urology 1995;46:205.

Oesterling J et al: The use of prostate-specific antigen in staging patients with newly diagnosed prostate cancer. JAMA 1993; 269:57.

Oesterling JE et al: Serum prostate-specific antigen in a community-based population of healthy men: Establishment of age-specific reference ranges. JAMA 1993;270:860.

Partin AW et al: Combination of prostate-specific antigen, clinical stage, and Gleason score to predict pathological stage of localized prostate cancer. JAMA 1997;277:1445.

Pilepich MV et al: Phase III radiation therapy oncology group (RTOG) trial 86-10 of androgen deprivation adjuvant to definitive radiotherapy in locally advanced carcinoma of the prostate. Int J Radiat Oncol Biol Phys 2001;50:1243.

Pound CR et al: Natural history of progression after PSA elevation following radical prostatectomy. JAMA 1999;281:1591.

Presti JC et al: The optimal systematic prostate biopsy scheme should include 8 rather than 6 biopsies: Results of a prospective clinical trial. J Urol 2000;163:163.

Whitmore WF, Warner JA, Thompson IM: Expectant management of localized prostatic cancer. Cancer 1991;67:1091.

Genital Tumors

23

Joseph C. Presti, Jr, MD

◼ TUMORS OF THE TESTIS

GERM CELL TUMORS OF THE TESTIS

Epidemiology & Risk Factors

Malignant tumors of the testis are rare, with approximately 2–3 new cases per 100,000 males reported in the United States each year. Of all primary testicular tumors, 90–95% are germ cell tumors (seminoma and nonseminoma), while the remainder are nongerminal neoplasms (Leydig cell, Sertoli cell, gonadoblastoma). The lifetime probability of developing testicular cancer is 0.2% for a white male in the United States. Survival of patients with testicular cancer has improved dramatically in recent years, reflecting the development and refinement of effective combination chemotherapy. Overall 5-year survival rates have increased from 78% in 1974–1976 to 91% in 1980–1985 ($P < .05$).

The incidence of testicular cancer shows marked variation among different countries, races, and socioeconomic classes. Scandinavian countries report up to 6.7 new cases per 100,000 males annually; Japan reports 0.8 per 100,000 males. In the United States, the incidence of testicular cancer in blacks is approximately one-fourth that in whites. Within a given race, individuals in the higher socioeconomic classes have approximately twice the incidence of those in the lower classes.

Testicular cancer is slightly more common on the right side than on the left, which parallels the increased incidence of cryptorchidism on the right side. Of primary testicular tumors, 1–2% are bilateral, and about 50% of these tumors occur in men with a history of unilateral or bilateral cryptorchidism. Primary bilateral tumors of the testis may happen synchronously or asynchronously but tend to be of the same histologic type. Seminoma is the most common germ cell tumor in bilateral *primary* testicular tumors, while malignant lymphoma is the most common bilateral tumor of the testis.

Although the cause of testicular cancer is unknown, both congenital and acquired factors have been associated with tumor development. The strongest association has been with the cryptorchid testis. Approximately 7–10% of testicular tumors develop in patients who have a history of cryptorchidism; seminoma is the most common form of tumor these patients have. However, 5–10% of testicular tumors occur in the contralateral, normally descended testis. The relative risk of malignancy is highest for the intra-abdominal testis (1 in 20) and is significantly lower for the inguinal testis (1 in 80). Placement of the cryptorchid testis into the scrotum (orchiopexy) does not alter the malignant potential of the cryptorchid testis; however, it does facilitate examination and tumor detection.

Exogenous estrogen administration to the mother during pregnancy has been associated with an increased relative risk for testicular tumors in the fetus, ranging from 2.8 to 5.3 over the expected incidence. Other acquired factors such as trauma and infection-related testicular atrophy have been associated with testicular tumors; however, a causal relationship has not been established.

Classification

Numerous classification systems have been proposed for germ cell tumors of the testis. Classification by histologic type proves to be the most useful with respect to treatment. The 2 major divisions are seminoma and nonseminomatous germ cell tumors (NSGCT), which include embryonal, teratoma, choriocarcinoma, and mixed tumors.

Tumorigenic Hypothesis for Germ Cell Tumor Development

During embryonal development, the totipotential germ cells can travel down normal differentiation pathways and become spermatocytes. However, if these totipotential germ cells travel down abnormal developmental pathways, seminoma or embryonal carcinomas (totipotential tumor cells) develop. If the embryonal cells undergo further differentiation along intraembryonic pathways, teratoma will result. If the embryonal cells undergo further differentiation along extraembryonic pathways, either choriocarcinoma or yolk sac tumors are formed (Figure 23–1). This model helps to explain why specific histologic patterns of testicular tumors produce certain tumor markers. Note that yolk sac tumors produce alpha-fetoprotein (AFP) just as the yolk sac produces AFP in normal development. Likewise,

Figure 23–1. Tumorigenic model for germ cell tumors of the testis.

choriocarcinoma produces human chorionic gonadotropin (hCG) just as the normal placenta produces hCG.

Pathology

A. SEMINOMA (35%)

Three histologic subtypes of pure seminoma have been described. However, stage for stage, there is no prognostic significance to any of these subtypes. Classic seminoma accounts for 85% of all seminomas and is most common in the fourth decade of life. Grossly, coalescing gray nodules are observed. Microscopically, monotonous sheets of large cells with clear cytoplasm and densely staining nuclei are seen. It is noteworthy that syncytiotrophoblastic elements are seen in approximately 10–15% of cases, an incidence that corresponds approximately to the incidence of hCG production in seminomas.

Anaplastic seminoma accounts for 5–10% of all seminomas. Diagnosis requires the presence of 3 or more mitoses per high-power field, and the cells demonstrate a higher degree of nuclear pleomorphism than the classic types. Anaplastic seminoma tends to present at a higher stage than the classic variety. When stage is taken into consideration, however, this subtype does not convey a worse prognosis.

Spermatocytic seminoma accounts for 5–10% of all seminomas. Microscopically, cells vary in size and are characterized by densely staining cytoplasm and round nuclei that contain condensed chromatin. More than half the patients with spermatocytic seminoma are over the age of 50.

B. EMBRYONAL CELL CARCINOMA (20%)

Two variants of embryonal cell carcinoma are common: the adult type and the infantile type, or yolk sac tumor (also called endodermal sinus tumor). Histologic structure of the adult variant demonstrates marked pleomorphism and indistinct cellular borders. Mitotic figures and giant cells are common. Cells may be arranged in sheets, cords, glands, or papillary structures. Extensive hemorrhage and necrosis may be observed grossly.

The infantile variant, or yolk sac tumor, is the most common testicular tumor of infants and children. When seen in adults, it usually occurs in mixed histologic types and possibly is responsible for AFP production in these tumors. Microscopically, cells demonstrate vacuolated cytoplasm secondary to fat and glycogen deposition and are arranged in a loose network with large intervening cystic spaces. Embryoid bodies are commonly seen and resemble 1- to 2-week-old embryos consisting of a cavity surrounded by syncytio- and cytotrophoblasts.

C. TERATOMA (5%)

Teratomas may be seen in both children and adults. They contain more than one germ cell layer in various stages of maturation and differentiation. Grossly, the tumor appears lobulated and contains variable-sized cysts filled with gelatinous or mucinous material. Mature teratoma may have elements resembling benign structures derived from ectoderm, mesoderm, and endoderm, while immature teratoma consists of undifferentiated primitive tissue. In contrast to its ovarian counterpart, the mature teratoma of the testis does not attain the same degree of differentiation as teratoma of the ovary. Microscopically, ectoderm may be represented by squamous epithelium or neural tissue; endoderm by intestinal, pancreatic, or respiratory tissue; and mesoderm by smooth or skeletal muscle, cartilage, or bone.

D. CHORIOCARCINOMA (< 1%)

Pure choriocarcinoma is rare. Lesions tend to be small within the testis and usually demonstrate central hemorrhage on gross inspection. Microscopically, syncytio- and cytotrophoblasts must be visualized. The syncytial elements are typically large, multinucleated cells with vacuolated, eosinophilic cytoplasm; the nuclei are large, hyperchromatic, and irregular. Cytotrophoblasts are uniform cells with distinct cell borders, clear cytoplasm, and a single nucleus.

Clinically, choriocarcinomas behave in an aggressive fashion characterized by early hematogenous spread. Paradoxically, small intratesticular lesions can be associated with widespread metastatic disease.

E. MIXED CELL TYPE (40%)

Within the category of mixed cell types, most (up to 25% of all testicular tumors) are teratocarcinomas, which are a combination of teratoma and embryonal cell carcinoma. Up to 6% of all testicular tumors are of the mixed cell type, with seminoma being one of the components. Treatment for these mixtures of seminoma and NSGCT is similar to that of NSGCT alone.

F. CARCINOMA IN SITU (CIS)

In a series of 250 patients with unilateral testicular cancer, Berthelsen et al (1982) demonstrated the presence of CIS in 13 (5.2%) of the contralateral testes. This is approximately twice the overall incidence of bilateral testicular cancer. The presence of contralateral atrophy or ultrasonographic microlithiasis in patients with testicular tumors warrants contralateral biopsy. If diagnosed, CIS is usually treated by external beam radiation therapy.

Patterns of Metastatic Spread

With the exception of choriocarcinoma, which demonstrates early hematogenous spread, germ cell tumors of the testis typically spread in a stepwise lymphatic fashion. Lymph nodes of the testis extend from T1 to L4 but are concentrated at the level of the renal hilum because of their common embryologic origin with the kidney. The primary landing site for the right testis is the interaortocaval area at the level of the right renal hilum. Stepwise spread, in order, is to the precaval, preaortic, paracaval, right common iliac, and right external iliac lymph nodes. The primary landing site for the left testis is the para-aortic area at the level of the left renal hilum. Stepwise spread, in order, is to the preaortic, left common iliac, and left external iliac lymph nodes. In the absence of disease on the left side, no crossover metastases to the right side have ever been identified. However, right-to-left crossover metastases are common. These observations have resulted in modified surgical dissections to preserve ejaculation in selected patients (see section on Treatment, following).

Certain factors may alter the primary drainage of a testis neoplasm. Invasion of the epididymis or spermatic cord may allow spread to the distal external iliac and obturator lymph nodes. Scrotal violation or invasion of the tunica albuginea may result in inguinal metastases.

Although the retroperitoneum is the most commonly involved site in metastatic disease, visceral metastases may be seen in advanced disease. The sites involved in decreasing frequency include lung, liver, brain, bone, kidney, adrenal, gastrointestinal tract, and spleen.

As mentioned previously, choriocarcinoma is the exception to the rule and is characterized by early hematogenous spread, especially to the lung. Choriocarcinoma also has a predilection for unusual sites of metastasis such as the spleen.

Clinical Staging

Many clinical staging systems have been proposed for testicular cancer. Most, however, are variations of the original system proposed by Boden and Gibb (1951). In this system, a stage A lesion was confined to the testis, stage B demonstrated regional lymph node spread, and stage C was spread beyond retroperitoneal lymph nodes. Numerous clinical staging systems have also been suggested for seminoma. A stage I lesion is confined to the testis. Stage II has retroperitoneal nodal involvement (IIA is < 2 cm, IIB is > 2 cm). Stage III has supradiaphragmatic nodal involvement or visceral involvement.

The TNM classification of the American Joint Committee (1996) has attempted to standardize clinical stages as in Table 23–1.

Clinical Findings

A. SYMPTOMS

The most common symptom of testicular cancer is a painless enlargement of the testis. Enlargement is usually gradual, and a sensation of testicular heaviness is not unusual. The typical delay in treatment from initial recognition of the lesion by the patient to definitive therapy (orchiectomy) ranges from 3 to 6 months. The length of delay correlates with the incidence of metas-

Table 23–1. TNM classification of tumors of the testis.

T—Primary tumor

TX:	Cannot be assessed.
T0:	No evidence of primary tumor.
Tis:	Intratubular cancer (CIS).
T1:	Limited to testis and epididymis, no vascular invasion.
T2:	Invades beyond tunica albuginea or has vascular invasion.
T3:	Invades spermatic cord.
T4:	Invades scrotum.

N—Regional lymph nodes

NX:	Cannot be assessed.
N0:	No regional lymph node metastasis.
N1:	Lymph node metastasis ≤ 2 cm and ≤ 5 lymph nodes.
N2:	Metastasis in > 5 nodes, nodal mass > 2 cm and < 5 cm.
N3:	Nodal mass > 5 cm.

M—Distant metastasis

MX:	Cannot be assessed.
M0:	No distant metastasis.
M1:	Distant metastasis present.

S—Serum tumor markers

SX:	Markers not available.
S0:	Marker levels within normal limits.
S1:	Lactic acid dehydrogenase (LDH) < 1.5 × normal and hCG < 5000 mIU/mL and AFP < 1000 ng/mL.
S2:	LDH 1.5–10 × normal or hCG 5000–50,000 mIU/mL or AFP 1000–10,000 ng/mL.
S3:	LDH > 10 × normal or hCG > 50,000 mIU/mL or AFP > 10,000 ng/mL.

Source: American Joint Committee on Cancer: *TNM Classification—Genitourinary Sites,* 1996.

tases. The importance of patient awareness and self-examination is apparent. Acute testicular pain is seen in approximately 10% of cases and may be the result of intratesticular hemorrhage or infarction.

Approximately 10% of patients present with symptoms related to metastatic disease. Back pain (retroperitoneal metastases involving nerve roots) is the most common symptom. Other symptoms include cough or dyspnea (pulmonary metastases); anorexia, nausea, or vomiting (retroduodenal metastases); bone pain (skeletal metastases); and lower extremity swelling (venacaval obstruction).

Approximately 10% of patients are asymptomatic at presentation, and the tumor may be detected incidentally following trauma, or it may be detected by the patient's sexual partner.

B. Signs

A testicular mass or diffuse enlargement is found in most cases. The mass is typically firm and nontender, and the epididymis should be easily separable from it. A hydrocele may accompany the testicular tumor and help to camouflage it. Transillumination of the scrotum can help to distinguish between these entities.

Palpation of the abdomen may reveal bulky retroperitoneal disease; assessment of supraclavicular, scalene, and inguinal nodes should be performed. Gynecomastia is present in 5% of all germ cell tumors but may be present in 30–50% of Sertoli and Leydig cell tumors. Its cause seems to be related to multiple complex hormonal interactions involving testosterone, estrone, estradiol, prolactin, and hCG. Hemoptysis may be seen in advanced pulmonary disease.

C. Laboratory Findings and Tumor Markers

Anemia may be detected in advanced disease. Liver function tests may be elevated in the presence of hepatic metastases. Renal function may be diminished (elevated serum creatinine) if ureteral obstruction secondary to bulky retroperitoneal disease is present. The assessment of renal function (creatinine clearance) is mandatory in patients with advanced disease who require chemotherapy.

Several biochemical markers are of importance in the diagnosis and management of testicular carcinoma, including AFP, hCG, and LDH. Alpha-fetoprotein is a glycoprotein with a molecular mass of 70,000 daltons and a half-life of 4–6 days. Although present in fetal serum in high levels, beyond the age of 1 year it is present only in trace amounts. While present to varying degrees in many NSGCTs (Table 23–2), it is never found in seminomas.

Human chorionic gonadotropin is a glycoprotein with a molecular mass of 38,000 daltons and a half-life of 24 h. It is composed of 2 subunits: alpha and beta. The alpha subunit is similar to the alpha subunits of luteinizing hormone (LH), follicle-stimulating hormone (FSH), and thyroid-stimulating hormone (TSH). The beta subunit conveys the activity to each of these

Table 23–2. Incidence of elevated tumor markers by histologic type in testis cancer.

	hCG (%)	AFP (%)
Seminoma	7	0
Teratoma	25	38
Teratocarcinoma	57	64
Embryonal	60	70
Choriocarcinoma	100	0

hormones and allows for a highly sensitive and specific radioimmunoassay in the determination of hCG levels. A normal man should not have significant levels of beta-hCG. While more commonly elevated in NS-GCTs, hCG levels may be elevated in up to 7% of seminomas.

Lactic acid dehydrogenase (LDH) is a cellular enzyme with a molecular mass of 134,000 daltons that has 5 isoenzymes; it is normally found in muscle (smooth, cardiac, skeletal), liver, kidney, and brain. Elevation of total serum LDH and in particular isoenzyme-I was shown to correlate with tumor burden in NSGCTs. LDH may also be elevated in seminoma.

Other markers have been described for testis cancer, including placental alkaline phosphatase (PLAP) and gamma-glutamyl transpeptidase (GGT). These markers, however, have not contributed as much to the management of patients as those mentioned previously.

D. Imaging

The primary testicular tumor can be rapidly and accurately assessed by scrotal ultrasonography. This technique can determine whether the mass is truly intratesticular, can be used to distinguish the tumor from epididymal pathology, and may also facilitate testicular examination in the presence of a hydrocele.

Once the diagnosis of testicular cancer has been established by inguinal orchiectomy, careful clinical staging of disease is mandatory. Chest radiographs (posteroanterior and lateral) and computed tomography (CT scan) of the abdomen and pelvis are used to assess the 2 most common sites of metastatic spread, namely, the lungs and retroperitoneum. The role of CT scanning of the chest remains controversial because of its decreased specificity. Of note is the fact that routine chest x-rays detect 85–90% of pulmonary metastases. Pedal lymphangiography (LAG) is rarely used owing to its invasiveness as well as low specificity, although it may be warranted in patients undergoing a surveillance protocol (see section on treatment).

Differential Diagnosis

An incorrect diagnosis is made at the initial examination in up to 25% of patients with testicular tumors and may result in delay in treatment or a suboptimal surgical approach (scrotal incision) for exploration. Epididymitis or epididymoorchitis is the most common misdiagnosis in patients with testis cancer. Early epididymitis should reveal an enlarged, tender epididymis that is clearly separable from the testis. In advanced stages, the inflammation may spread to the testis and result in an enlarged, tender, and indurated testis and epididymis. A history of acute onset of symptoms including fever, urethral discharge, and irritative voiding

symptoms may make the diagnosis of epididymitis more likely. Ultrasonography may identify the enlarged epididymis as the cause of the scrotal mass.

Hydrocele is the second most common misdiagnosis. Transillumination of the scrotum may readily distinguish between a translucent, fluid-filled hydrocele and a solid testicular tumor. Since 5–10% of testicular tumors may be associated with hydroceles, however, if the testis cannot be adequately examined a scrotal ultrasound examination is mandatory. Aspiration of the hydrocele should be avoided because positive cytologic results have been reported in hydroceles associated with testicular tumors.

Other diagnoses to be considered include spermatocele, a cystic mass most commonly found extending from the head of the epididymis; hematocele associated with trauma; granulomatous orchitis, most commonly resulting from tuberculosis and associated with beading of the vas deferens; and varicocele, which is engorgement of the pampiniform plexus of veins in the spermatic cord and should disappear when the patient is in the supine position.

Although most intratesticular masses are malignant, one benign lesion, an epidermoid cyst, may be seen on rare occasions. Usually these cysts are very small benign nodules located just underneath the tunica albuginea; however, on occasion they can be large. The diagnosis is usually made following inguinal orchiectomy; as frozen sections, the larger lesions are often difficult to distinguish from teratoma.

Treatment

Inguinal exploration with cross-clamping of the spermatic cord vasculature and delivery of the testis into the field is the mainstay of exploration for a possible testis tumor. If cancer cannot be excluded by examination of the testis, radical orchiectomy is warranted. Scrotal approaches and open testicular biopsies should be avoided. Further therapy depends on the histologic characteristics of the tumor as well as the clinical stage.

A. Low-Stage Seminoma (I, II-A)

Seminoma is exquisitely radiosensitive. Ninety-five percent of all stage I seminomas are cured with radical orchiectomy and retroperitoneal irradiation (usually 2500–3000 cGy). This low dose of radiation is usually well tolerated, with minimal, if any, gastrointestinal side effects.

Low-volume retroperitoneal disease also can be treated effectively with retroperitoneal irradiation with an average 5-year survival rate of 87%. Prophylactic mediastinal radiation is no longer employed because this may cause considerable myelosuppression and thus compromise the patient's ability to receive chemotherapy if required. Chemotherapy should be used as salvage therapy for patients who relapse following irradiation.

B. HIGH-STAGE SEMINOMA (II-B, III)

Patients with bulky seminoma and any seminoma associated with an elevated AFP should receive primary chemotherapy. Seminomas are also sensitive to platinum-based regimens, as are their NSGCT counterparts. Some of the successful regimens include cisplatin, etoposide, and bleomycin (PEB); vinblastine, cyclophosphamide, dactinomycin, bleomycin, and cisplatin (VAB-6); and cisplatin and etoposide. All seminomas receive low-risk chemotherapy regimens, which currently consist of cisplatin and etoposide (4 cycles) or 3 cycles of PEB.

Ninety percent of patients with stage III disease achieve a complete response with chemotherapy. Residual retroperitoneal masses following chemotherapy are often fibrosis (90%) unless the mass is well circumscribed and in excess of 3 cm, under which circumstances approximately 40% of patients harbor residual seminoma. In such cases surgical excision is warranted.

C. LOW-STAGE NONSEMINOMATOUS GERM CELL TUMORS

Standard treatment for stage A disease in the United States has included retroperitoneal lymph node dissection (RPLND). However, because three-fourths of patients with clinical stage A disease are cured by orchiectomy alone and the morbidity of RPLND is not negligible, other alternatives have been explored. These options include surveillance and modified RPLND.

Surveillance in stage A NSGCT was proposed because, as mentioned previously, 75% of patients with clinical stage A disease have, in fact, pathologic stage A disease. In addition, infertility related to disruption of sympathetic nerve fibers is common following RPLND. Clinical staging has been markedly improved in the presence of CT scanning and LAG. And finally, effective chemotherapy regimens have been developed for relapse. Patients are considered candidates for surveillance if the tumor is an NSGCT confined within the tunica albuginea, the tumor does not demonstrate vascular invasion, tumor markers normalize after orchiectomy, radiographic imaging shows no evidence of disease (chest x-ray [CXR], CT), and the patient is considered reliable.

Surveillance should be considered an active process on the part of both the physician and the patient. Patients are followed monthly for the first 2 years and bimonthly in the third year. Tumor markers are obtained at each visit, and CXR and CT scans are obtained every 3–4 months. Follow-up continues beyond the initial 3 years. Most relapses occur, however, within the first

8–10 months. With rare exceptions, patients who relapse can be cured by chemotherapy or surgery, or both.

Retroperitoneal lymph node dissection has been the preferred treatment of low-stage NSGCTs in the United States until recently. A thoracoabdominal or midline transabdominal approach may be used, and all nodal tissue between the ureters from the renal vessels to the bifurcation of the common iliac vessels is removed. Patients with negative nodes or N1 disease do not require adjuvant therapy, whereas the recommendation for those with N2 disease is to receive 2 cycles of chemotherapy because their relapse rate approaches 50%.

While effective in surgically staging and potentially curing a subset of patients, RPLND is associated with significant morbidity, especially with respect to fertility in young men. With a standard RPLND, sympathetic nerve fibers are disrupted, resulting in loss of seminal emission. Currently a modified RPLND has been developed that preserves ejaculation in up to 90% of patients. By modifying the dissection below the level of the inferior mesenteric artery to include only the nodal tissue ipsilateral to the tumor, important sympathetic fibers from the contralateral side are preserved, thus maintaining ejaculation.

D. HIGH-STAGE NONSEMINOMATOUS GERM CELL TUMORS

Patients with bulky retroperitoneal disease (> 3-cm nodes or 3 or more 1-cm cuts on CT scan) or metastatic NSGCT are treated with primary platinum-based combination chemotherapy following orchiectomy. If tumor markers normalize and a residual mass is apparent on imaging studies, resection of that mass is mandatory, because 20% of the time it will harbor residual cancer, 40% of the time it will be teratoma, and 40% of the time it will be fibrosis (Figure 23–2). In patients with residual cancer in the resected tissue, the histologic picture is usually embryonal cell carcinoma, but malignant teratoma is seen in less than 5% of cases. Malignant teratoma is unresponsive to chemotherapy, and only 15% of patients survive following surgical resection. If tumor markers fail to normalize following primary chemotherapy, salvage chemotherapy is required (cisplatin, etoposide, bleomycin, ifosfamide). Even if patients attain a complete response after chemotherapy (normal tumor markers, no mass on CT scan or CXR), some investigators advocate an RPLND because viable germ cell tumor may be seen in up to 10% of cases

Although the treatment plan described cures up to 70% of patients with high-volume disease, there are patients who fail to respond. Also, the potential complications from chemotherapy including sepsis, neuropathy, renal toxicity, and death must be considered. It is thus apparent that it is important to be able to discriminate between patients who are likely to respond to standard

Figure 23–2. **Upper:** Computed tomography scan of patient with bulky retroperitoneal mass after radical orchiectomy for embryonal carcinoma. **Lower:** Residual cystic mass after chemotherapy; it was resected and found to be teratoma.

chemotherapy (low risk) and those who may require more aggressive regimens (high risk). In a multivariant analysis only 3 parameters, the serum LDH, the serum hCG, and the total number of sites of metastasis provided unique information in predicting response to chemotherapy. The rate of decline of serum tumor markers during chemotherapy has also been used to predict response in patients with advanced disease.

Follow-up Care

All patients with testicular cancer require regular follow-up care. As discussed previously, patients on a surveillance protocol require vigorous follow-up. Those who have undergone surgery (RPLND) or radiotherapy are followed at 3-month intervals for the first 2 years, then every 6 months until 5 years, and then yearly. Follow-up visits should include careful examination of the remain-

ing testis, the abdomen, and the lymph node areas. Laboratory investigation should include AFP, hCG, and LDH levels. A CXR and an abdominal film (if an LAG was performed) should also be included at each visit. Abdominal CT scans are used less frequently as risk of relapse in the retroperitoneum is low following RPLND.

Prognosis

Survival in testicular cancer has improved dramatically over the past several years, reflecting the continuing improvement and refinement in combination chemotherapy.

For seminoma treated by orchiectomy and radiotherapy, the 5-year disease-free survival rate is 98% for stage I and 92–94% for stage II-A in several recent series. Higher-stage disease treated by orchiectomy and primary chemotherapy has a 5-year disease-free survival rate of 35–75%, yet the lower value comes from older series in which more crude chemotherapy regimens were employed.

Survival in patients with NSGCTs treated by orchiectomy and RPLND for stage A disease ranges from 96 to 100%. For low-volume stage B disease treated with chemotherapy plus surgery, greater than 90% 5-year disease-free survival rates are attainable. Patients with bulky retroperitoneal or disseminated disease treated with primary chemotherapy followed by surgery have a 5-year disease-free survival rate of 55–80%.

Currently much work is being done to stratify patients into "high-risk" and "low-risk" groups so that treatment regimens may be modified in order to increase survival and decrease morbidity.

NON–GERM CELL TUMORS OF THE TESTIS

Approximately 5–6% of all testis tumors are non–germ cell tumors of the testis. Three types will be considered, namely, Leydig cell tumors, Sertoli cell tumors, and gonadoblastomas.

1. Leydig Cell Tumors
Epidemiology & Pathology

Leydig cell tumors are the most common non–germ cell tumors of the testis and account for 1–3% of all testicular tumors. They follow a bimodal age distribution: the 5- to 9-year-old and the 25- to 35-year-old age groups. Twenty-five percent of these tumors occur in childhood. Bilaterality is seen in 5–10% of cases. The cause of these tumors is unknown; unlike germ cell tumors, there is no association with cryptorchidism.

Pathologic examination reveals a small, yellow, well-circumscribed lesion devoid of hemorrhage or necrosis.

Microscopically, hexagonally shaped cells with granular, eosinophilic cytoplasm containing lipid vacuoles are seen. Reinke crystals are fusiform-shaped cytoplasmic inclusions that are pathognomonic for Leydig cells.

Clinical Findings

Prepubertal children usually present with virilization, and tumors are benign. Adults are usually asymptomatic, although gynecomastia may be present in 20–25%. Ten percent of tumors in adults are malignant. Laboratory findings include elevated serum and urinary 17-ketosteroids as well as estrogens.

Treatment & Prognosis

Radical orchiectomy is the initial treatment for Leydig cell tumors. Clinical staging is similar to that for germ cell tumors, and levels of the 17-ketosteroids can be helpful in distinguishing between benign and malignant lesions. Elevations of 10–30 times normal are typical of malignancy. RPLND is recommended for malignant lesions. Because of the rarity of these lesions, the role of chemotherapy remains to be defined. Prognosis is excellent for benign lesions, while it remains poor for patients with disseminated disease.

2. Sertoli Cell Tumors

Epidemiology & Pathology

Sertoli cell tumors are exceedingly rare, composing less than 1% of all testicular tumors. A bimodal age distribution is seen: 1 year old or younger and the 20- to 45-year-old age group. Approximately 10% of the lesions are malignant. Gross examination reveals a yellow or gray-white lesion with cystic components. Benign lesions are well circumscribed, while malignant lesions show ill-defined borders. Microscopically, tumors appear heterogeneous with mixed amounts of epithelial and stromal components. Sertoli cells are columnar or hexagonal cells with a large nucleus and solitary nucleolus and contain vacuolated cytoplasm.

Clinical Findings

A testicular mass is the most common presentation. Virilization is often seen in children, and gynecomastia may be present in 30% of adults. Because of the rarity of these tumors, minimal endocrine data are available on these patients.

Treatment

Radical orchiectomy is the initial procedure of choice. In cases of malignancy, RPLND is indicated; however, the roles of chemotherapy and radiotherapy remain unclear.

3. Gonadoblastomas

Epidemiology & Pathology

Gonadoblastomas comprise 0.5% of all testicular tumors and are almost exclusively seen in patients with some form of gonadal dysgenesis. Most of these tumors occur in patients under 30 years of age, although the age distribution ranges from infancy to beyond 70 years.

Gross examination reveals a yellow or gray-white lesion that can vary in size from microscopic to greater than 20 cm and may exhibit calcifications. Microscopically, 3 cell types are seen: Sertoli cells, interstitial cells, and germ cells.

Clinical Findings

The clinical manifestations are predominantly related to the underlying gonadal dysgenesis and are discussed elsewhere in this book. It is noteworthy that four-fifths of patients with gonadoblastomas are phenotypic females. Males typically have cryptorchidism or hypospadias.

Treatment & Prognosis

Radical orchiectomy is the primary treatment of choice. In the presence of gonadal dysgenesis, a contralateral gonadectomy is recommended because the tumor tends to be bilateral in 50% of cases in this setting. Prognosis is excellent.

SECONDARY TUMORS OF THE TESTIS

Secondary tumors of the testis are rare. Three categories are considered: lymphoma, leukemia, and metastatic tumors.

1. Lymphoma

Epidemiology & Pathology

Lymphoma is the most common testicular tumor in a patient over the age of 50 and is the most common secondary neoplasm of the testis, accounting for 5% of all testicular tumors. It may be seen in 3 clinical settings: (1) late manifestation of widespread lymphoma; (2) initial presentation of clinically occult disease and (3) primary extranodal disease.

Gross examination reveals a bulging, gray or pink lesion with ill-defined margins. Hemorrhage and necrosis are common. Microscopically, diffuse histiocytic lymphoma is the most common type.

Clinical Findings

Painless enlargement of the testis is common. Generalized constitutional symptoms occur in one-fourth of patients. Bilateral testis involvement occurs in 50% of patients, usually asynchronously.

Treatment & Prognosis

Radical orchiectomy is indicated to make the diagnosis. Further staging and treatment should be handled in conjunction with the medical oncologist. Prognosis is related to the stage of disease. Some reports support adjuvant chemotherapy for primary testicular lymphoma, with improved survival rates of up to 93% after 44 months of follow-up.

2. Leukemic Infiltration Of the Testis

The testis is a common site of relapse for children with acute lymphocytic leukemia. Bilateral involvement may be present in one-half of cases. Testis biopsy rather than orchiectomy is the diagnostic procedure of choice. Bilateral testicular irradiation with 20 Gy and reinstitution of adjuvant chemotherapy constitute the treatment of choice. Prognosis remains guarded.

3. Metastatic Tumors

Metastasis to the testis is rare. These lesions are typically incidental findings at autopsy. The most common primary site is the prostate, followed by the lung, gastrointestinal tract, melanoma, and kidney. The typical pathologic finding is neoplastic cells in the interstitium with relative sparing of the seminiferous tubules.

■ EXTRAGONADAL GERM CELL TUMORS

Epidemiology & Pathology

Extragonadal germ cell tumors are rare, accounting for approximately 3% of all germ cell tumors. Debate continues over whether these lesions originate from "burned-out" testicular primaries or originate de novo. Most retroperitoneal tumors have their origin from a testicular primary, whereas mediastinal germ cell tumors are truly ectopic.

The most common sites of origin in decreasing order are mediastinum, retroperitoneum, sacrococcygeal area, and pineal gland. All germ cell types may

be observed. Seminoma composes more than half of the retroperitoneal and mediastinal tumors.

Clinical Findings

Clinical presentation depends on the site and volume of disease. Mediastinal lesions may present with pulmonary complaints. Retroperitoneal lesions may present with abdominal or back pain and a palpable mass. Sacrococcygeal tumors are most commonly seen in neonates and may present with a palpable mass and bowel or urinary obstruction. Pineal tumors may present with headache, visual or auditory complaints, or hypopituitarism.

Metastatic spread is to regional lymph nodes, lung, liver, bone, and brain. Metastatic workup is similar, therefore, to that of testicular germ cell tumors. A careful testicular examination is mandatory along with ultrasonography to exclude an occult testicular primary.

Treatment & Prognosis

Treatment of extragonadal germ cell tumors parallels that of testicular tumors. Low-volume seminoma can be managed with radiotherapy. High-volume seminoma should receive primary chemotherapy. Prognosis parallels that of testicular seminoma. Primary chemotherapy should be employed for nonseminomatous elements with surgical excision of residual masses; however, prognosis remains poor for these patients.

■ TUMORS OF THE EPIDIDYMIS, PARATESTICULAR TISSUES, & SPERMATIC CORD

Primary tumors of the epididymis are rare and are most commonly benign. Adenomatoid tumors of the epididymis are the most common and typically occur in the third and fourth decade of life. They are typically asymptomatic, solid lesions that arise from any portion of the epididymis.

Leiomyomas are the second most common tumor of the epididymis. These lesions tend to be painful and are often associated with a hydrocele.

Cystadenomas are benign lesions of the epididymis that are bilateral in 30% of cases and are frequently seen in association with von Hippel-Lindau disease. Histologically these lesions are difficult to distinguish from renal cell carcinoma. Malignant lesions of the epididymis are extremely rare. In general, an inguinal approach should be used, and if frozen section confirms a benign lesion, epididymectomy should be performed. If a malignant tumor is diagnosed, radical orchiectomy must be performed.

Tumors of the spermatic cord are typically benign. Lipomas of the cord account for most of these lesions. Of the malignant lesions, rhabdomyosarcoma is the most common, followed by leiomyosarcoma, fibrosarcoma, and liposarcoma.

Clinical diagnosis of tumors of the spermatic cord can be difficult. Differentiating between a hernia and a spermatic cord tumor may be possible only at exploration. In general, these lesions should be approached through an inguinal incision. The cord should be occluded at the internal ring and frozen sections obtained. If malignancy is diagnosed, attention should be directed toward performing wide local excision to avoid local recurrence. Staging of disease is similar to that of testicular tumors. For rhabdomyosarcoma, RPLND should be performed with adjuvant radiotherapy and chemotherapy. The value of RPLND for the other malignant spermatic cord tumors remains to be determined. Prognosis relates to the histologic status, stage, and site of disease.

TUMORS OF THE PENIS

Epidemiology & Risk Factors

Carcinoma of the penis accounts for less than 1% of cancers among males in the United States, with approximately 1–2 new cases being reported per 100,000 men. There is marked variation in incidence with geographic location. In areas such as Africa and regions of South America, penile carcinoma may compose 10–20% of all malignant lesions. Penile carcinoma occurs most commonly in the sixth decade of life, although rare case reports have included children.

The one etiologic factor most commonly associated with penile carcinoma is poor hygiene. The disease is virtually unheard of in males circumcised near birth. One theory postulates that smegma accumulation under the phimotic foreskin results in chronic inflammation leading to carcinoma. A viral cause has also been suggested as a result of the association of this tumor with cervical carcinoma.

Pathology

A. Precancerous Dermatologic Lesions

Leukoplakia is a rare condition that most commonly occurs in diabetic patients. A white plaque typically involving the meatus is seen. Histologic examination reveals acanthosis, hyperkeratosis, and parakeratosis. This

lesion may precede or occur simultaneously with penile carcinoma.

Balanitis xerotica obliterans is a white patch originating on the prepuce or glans and usually involving the meatus. The condition is most commonly observed in middle-aged diabetic patients. Microscopic examination reveals atrophic epidermis and abnormalities in collagen deposition.

Giant condylomata acuminata are cauliflowerlike lesions arising from the prepuce or glans. The cause is believed to be viral (human papillomavirus). These lesions may be difficult to distinguish from well-differentiated squamous cell carcinoma.

B. Carcinoma in Situ (Bowen Disease, Erythroplasia of Queyrat)

Bowen disease is a squamous cell carcinoma in situ typically involving the penile shaft. The lesion appears as a red plaque with encrustations.

Erythroplasia of Queyrat is a velvety, red lesion with ulcerations that usually involve the glans. Microscopic examination shows typical, hyperplastic cells in a disordered array with vacuolated cytoplasm and mitotic figures.

C. Invasive Carcinoma of the Penis

Squamous cell carcinoma composes most penile cancers. It most commonly originates on the glans, with the next most common sites, in order, being the prepuce and shaft. The appearance may be papillary or ulcerative.

Verrucous carcinoma is a variant of squamous cell carcinoma composing 5–16% of penile carcinomas. This lesion is papillary in appearance and on histologic examination is noted to have a well-demarcated deep margin unlike the infiltrating margin of the typical squamous cell carcinoma.

Patterns of Spread

Invasive carcinoma of the penis begins as an ulcerative or papillary lesion, which may gradually grow to involve the entire glans or shaft of the penis. Buck's fascia represents a barrier to corporal invasion and hematogenous spread. Primary dissemination is via lymphatic channels to the femoral and iliac nodes. The prepuce and shaft skin drain into the superficial inguinal nodes (superficial to fascia lata), while the glans and corporal bodies drain to both superficial and deep inguinal nodes (deep to fascia lata). There are many cross-communications, so that penile lymphatic drainage is bilateral to both inguinal areas. Drainage from the inguinal nodes is to the pelvic nodes. Involvement of the femoral nodes may result in skin necrosis and infection or femoral vessel erosion and hemorrhage. Distant metastases are clinically apparent in less than 10% of cases and may involve lung, liver, bone, or brain.

Tumor Staging

The staging system used most commonly in the United States was proposed by Jackson (1966), as follows: In stage I, the tumor is confined to the glans or prepuce. Stage II involves the penile shaft. Stage III has operable inguinal node metastasis. In stage IV, the tumor extends beyond the penile shaft, with inoperable inguinal or distant metastases.

The TNM classification of the American Joint Committee (1996) is given in Table 23–3.

Clinical Findings

A. Symptoms

The most common complaint at presentation is the lesion itself. It may appear as an area of induration or erythema, an ulceration, a small nodule, or an exophytic growth. Phimosis may obscure the lesion and result in a delay in seeking medical attention. In fact, 15–50% of patients delay for at least 1 year in seeking medical attention. Other symptoms include pain, discharge, irritative voiding symptoms, and bleeding.

Table 23–3. TNM classification of tumors of the penis.

T—Primary tumor	
TX:	Cannot be assessed.
T0:	No evidence of primary tumor.
Tis:	Carcinoma in situ.
Ta:	Noninvasive verrucous carcinoma.
T1:	Invades subepithelial connective tissue.
T2:	Invades corpus spongiosum or cavernosum.
T3:	Invades urethra or prostate.
T4:	Invades other adjacent structures.
N—Regional lymph nodes	
NX:	Cannot be assessed.
N0:	No regional lymph node metastasis.
N1:	Metastasis in single superficial inguinal node.
N2:	Metastasis in multiple or bilateral superficial inguinal nodes.
N3:	Metastasis in deep inguinal or pelvic nodes.
M—Distant metastasis	
MX:	Cannot be assessed.
M0:	No distant metastasis.
M1:	Distant metastasis present.

Source: American Joint Committee on Cancer: *TNM Classification—Genitourinary Sites,* 1996.

B. Signs

Lesions are typically confined to the penis at presentation. The primary lesion should be characterized with respect to size, location, and potential corporal body involvement. Careful palpation of the inguinal area is mandatory because more than 50% of patients present with enlarged inguinal nodes. This enlargement may be secondary to inflammation or metastatic spread.

C. Laboratory Findings

Laboratory evaluation is typically normal. Anemia and leukocytosis may be present in patients with long-standing disease or extensive local infection. Hypercalcemia in the absence of osseous metastases may be seen in 20% of patients and appears to correlate with volume of disease.

D. Imaging

Metastatic workup should include CXR, bone scan, and CT scan of the abdomen and pelvis. Disseminated disease is present in less than 10% of patients at presentation.

Differential Diagnosis

In addition to the dermatologic lesions discussed previously, carcinoma of the penis must be differentiated from several infectious lesions. Syphilitic chancre may present as a painless ulceration. Serologic and darkfield examination should establish the diagnosis. Chancroid typically appears as a painful ulceration of the penis. Selective cultures for *Haemophilus ducreyi* should identify the cause. Condylomata acuminata appear as exophytic, soft, "grape cluster" lesions anywhere on the penile shaft or glans. Biopsy can distinguish this lesion from carcinoma if any doubt exists.

Treatment

A. Primary Lesion

Biopsy of the primary lesion is mandatory to establish the diagnosis of malignancy. Treatment varies depending on the pathology as well as the location of the lesion.

Carcinoma in situ may be treated conservatively in reliable patients. Fluorouracil cream application or neodymium:YAG laser treatment is effective for CIS and is preserving of the penis. Patients must come for frequent follow-up examinations to monitor response.

The goal of treatment in invasive penile carcinoma is complete excision with adequate margins. For lesions involving the prepuce, this may be accomplished by simple circumcision. For lesions involving the glans or distal shaft, partial penectomy with a 2-cm margin to decrease local recurrence has traditionally been suggested. For lesions involving the proximal shaft or when partial penectomy results in a penile stump of insufficient length for sexual function or directing the urinary stream, total penectomy with perineal urethrostomy has been recommended. Less aggressive surgical resections such as Mohs micrographic surgery and local excisions directed at penile preservation are currently being studied (Mohs et al, 1985).

B. REGIONAL LYMPH NODES

As discussed previously, penile carcinoma spreads primarily to the inguinal lymph nodes. However, enlargement of inguinal nodes at presentation does not necessarily imply metastatic disease. In fact, up to 50% of the time this enlargement is caused by inflammation. Thus patients who present with enlarged inguinal nodes should undergo treatment of the primary lesion followed by a 4- to 6-week course of oral broad-spectrum antibiotics. Persistent adenopathy following antibiotic treatment should be considered to be metastatic disease, and sequential bilateral ilioinguinal node dissections should be performed. If lymphadenopathy resolves with antibiotics, observation in low-stage primary tumors (Tis, T1) is warranted. However, if lymphadenopathy resolves in higher-stage tumors, more limited lymph node samplings should be considered, such as the sentinel node biopsy described by Cabanas (1977) or a modified (limited) dissection as suggested by Catalona (1988) (Figure 23–3). If positive nodes are encountered, bilateral ilioinguinal node dissection should be performed. A decision tree for penile carcinoma is presented in Figure 23–4. Patients who initially have clinically negative nodes but in whom clinically palpable nodes later develop should undergo a unilateral ilioinguinal node dissection.

Patients who have inoperable disease and bulky inguinal metastases are treated with chemotherapy (cisplatin and 5-fluorouracil). In some cases regional radiotherapy can provide significant palliation by delaying ulceration and infectious complications and alleviating pain.

C. SYSTEMIC DISEASE

Four chemotherapeutic agents demonstrate activity against penile carcinoma: bleomycin, methotrexate, cisplatin, and 5-fluorouracil. However, no long-term responders have been reported. The rarity of the disease in the United States has resulted in limited clinical trials.

Prognosis

Survival in penile carcinoma correlates with the presence or absence of nodal disease. Five-year survival rates for patients with node-negative disease range from 65% to 90%. For patients with positive inguinal nodes, this rate decreases to 30–50% and with positive iliac nodes decreases to less than 20%. In the presence of soft-tissue or bony metastases, no 5-year survivors have been reported.

Figure 23–3. Comparison of limits of dissection of complete (dashed line) versus limited (solid line) inguinal lymphadenectomy.

Other Penile Tumors

Squamous cell carcinoma accounts for 98% of penile cancers. Sporadic cases of melanoma, basal cell carcinoma, and Paget disease have been reported. The incidence of Kaposi sarcoma of the penis is increasing with the increasing prevalence of the human immunodeficiency virus. It appears as a painful papule on the glans or shaft with bluish-purple discoloration. These lesions tend to be radiosensitive.

■ TUMORS OF THE SCROTUM

Tumors of the scrotal skin are rare. The most common benign lesion is a sebaceous cyst. Squamous cell carcinoma is the most common malignant tumor of the scrotum, although rare cases of melanoma, basal cell carcinoma, and Kaposi sarcoma have been reported. In the past, squamous cell carcinoma of the scrotum most commonly resulted from exposure to environmental

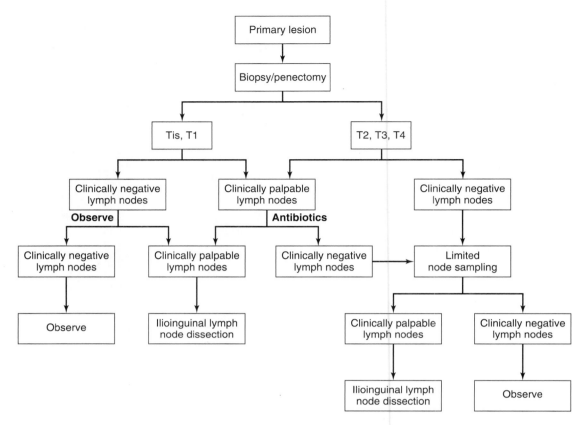

Figure 23–4. Management of penile carcinoma.

carcinogens including chimney soot, tars, paraffin, and some petroleum products. Today, most cases result from poor hygiene and chronic inflammation.

Biopsy of the scrotal lesion must be performed to establish a histologic diagnosis. Wide excision with a 2-cm margin should be performed for malignant tumors. Surrounding subcutaneous tissue should be excised with the primary tumor; however, resection of the scrotal contents is rarely necessary. Primary closure using the redundant scrotal skin is usually possible. The management of inguinal nodes should be similar to that of penile cancer.

Prognosis correlates with the presence or absence of nodal involvement. In the presence of inguinal node metastasis, the 5-year survival rate is approximately 25%; there are virtually no survivors if iliac nodes are involved.

REFERENCES

Tumors of the Testis

American Joint Committee on Cancer: *TNM Classification—Genitourinary Sites.* 1996.

Berthelsen JG et al: Screening for carcinoma in situ of the contralateral testis in patients with germinal testicular cancer. Br Med J 1982;285:1683.

Boden G, Gibb R: Radiotherapy and testicular neoplasms. Lancet 1951;2:1195.

Carroll PR, Presti JC Jr: Testis cancer. Urol Clin North Am 1998; 25(3). (Entire issue.)

Henderson BE, Ross RK, Pike MC: Epidemiology of testicular cancer. In: Skinner DG, Lieskovsky G (editors): *Diagnosis and Management of Genitourinary Cancer.* Saunders, 1988.

Sogani PC et al: Orchiectomy alone in treatment of clinical stage I nonseminomatous germ cell tumor of the testis. J Clin Oncol 1984;2:267.

Tumors of the Penis

American Joint Committee on Cancer: *TNM Classification—Genitourinary Sites.* 1996.

Cabanas RM: An approach for the treatment of penile carcinoma. Cancer 1977;39:456.

Catalona WJ: Modified inguinal lymphadenectomy for carcinoma of the penis with preservation of saphenous veins: Technique and preliminary results. J Urol 1988;140:306.

Jackson SM: The treatment of carcinoma of the penis. Br J Surg 1966;53:33.

Mohs FE et al: Microscopically controlled surgery in the treatment of carcinoma of the penis. J Urol 1985;133:961.

Urinary Diversion & Bladder Substitution

24

Peter R. Carroll, MD, Gary D. Grossfeld, MD, & Susan Barbour, RN, MS, CETN

Selected patients with lower urinary tract cancers or severe functional or anatomic abnormalities of the bladder may require urinary diversion. Although this can be accomplished by establishing direct contact between the urinary tract and the skin surface, it is most often performed by incorporating various intestinal segments into the urinary tract. Virtually every segment of the gastrointestinal tract has been used to create urinary reservoirs or conduits. No single technique is ideal for all patients and clinical situations. A decision is based on a patient's underlying disease and its method of treatment as well as on renal function, individual anatomy, and personal preference. An ideal method of urinary diversion would most closely approximate the normal bladder: it would be nonrefluxing, low pressure, continent, and nonabsorptive.

Individual methods of urinary diversion can be categorized in various ways, such as (1) by the segment of intestine used, and (2) by whether the method provides complete continence or simply acts as a conduit carrying urine from the renal pelvis or ureter to the skin, where the urine is collected in an appliance attached to the skin surface. Continent forms of urinary diversion can be categorized further according to whether they are attached to the urethra (ie, as a bladder substitute) or are placed in the abdomen and rely on another mechanism for continence (continent urinary reservoir).

Preoperative Counseling & Preparation

All candidates for urinary diversion or bladder substitution should undergo careful preoperative counseling and preparation, including a detailed discussion of the objectives and potential complications of each method. Any potential impact of a procedure on sexual function, body image, and lifestyle should be discussed. Overall satisfaction of most patients undergoing urinary diversion appears to be high (Dutta et al, 2002; Hara et al, 2002; Kitamura et al, 1999; Fujisawa et al, 2000a). However, because they allow freedom from an external appliance, continent forms of urinary diversion, especially bladder substitution, may be of great psychological and functional benefit to well-selected patients

(Okada et al, 1997; Bjerre, Johansen, and Steven, 1995).

A careful history taken from the patient should note any previous abdominal or pelvic surgery, irradiation, or systemic disease. A history of intestinal resection or irradiation, renal failure, diverticulitis, regional enteritis, or ulcerative colitis would be especially important to consider when selecting a method of urinary diversion or bladder substitution. A complete blood count and measurement of serum electrolytes, urea nitrogen, and creatinine should be performed. The upper urinary tract should be imaged with intravenous urography, ultrasound, or computed tomography to determine whether hydronephrosis, renal parenchymal scarring, or calculous disease exists. Contrast imaging of the small or large bowel or colonoscopy should be considered preoperatively for patients with a history of significant intestinal irradiation, occult bleeding, or other gastrointestinal diseases. Patients with benign bladder diseases—such as a reduced bladder capacity due to neurologic disorders or irradiation, bladder fistulas or interstitial cystitis—are occasionally considered candidates for urinary diversion or bladder substitution to manage urinary incontinence; however, with such patients, careful evaluation of bladder function and anatomy is required, as adequate urinary function can often be restored by urinary tract reconstruction, pharmacologic manipulation, or intermittent catheterization.

Patients undergo a standard mechanical and oral antibiotic bowel cleansing program beginning 1 or 2 days before surgery. Much of patients' dissatisfaction with urinary diversion can be attributed to poor stomal construction (Fitzgerald et al, 1997). The stoma site should be selected preoperatively and the patient evaluated in the lying, sitting, and standing positions. The most common site for stoma placement is along a line between the anterior superior iliac spine and umbilicus and at the lateral edge of the rectus abdominis muscle. The surface area should be flat and able to support an appliance. Bony prominences, fat folds, and scars should be avoided, as it is difficult to secure an appliance in these areas.

INTESTINAL CONDUIT URINARY DIVERSION

Ileal Conduit

Ureteroileal urinary diversion is the most common method of urinary diversion in the United States. The conduit is constructed using a segment of ileum approximately 15–20 cm proximal to the ileocecal valve (Figure 24–1). The length of the conduit varies depending on the habitus of the patient. As short a segment as possible, usually 18–20 cm, minimizes the absorptive surface of the bowel in contact with urine. Once the appropriate length of bowel is selected and isolated, the mesentery is divided proximally and distally and individual mesenteric blood vessels are ligated. The bowel is divided, thus isolating the segment selected for conduit construction. The continuity of the small intestine is reestablished, allowing for normal bowel function. The conduit is usually positioned in the right lower quadrant of the abdomen in an isoperistaltic direction. The base of the conduit is closed, and the ureters are reimplanted directly, creating a refluxing ureteroileal anastomosis. On occasion, ureteral stents (small-diameter, multichannel, silicone [Silastic] catheters) are placed through the ureteral anastomosis and conduit and into the renal pelvis to facilitate urinary drainage while the anastomosis is healing.

The preselected stoma site is identified and a small circle of skin and underlying fat excised. The fascia is incised in a cruciate fashion. The end of the conduit is brought through the lateral aspect of the rectus abdominis muscle and anchored to the fascia, and the stoma is then formed. The stoma should protrude, without tension, approximately 1–1.5 inches above the skin surface.

Jejunal Conduit

Jejunal conduit urinary diversion is used rarely, since many better alternatives are available. However, jejunal conduits have been used in cases in which there has been significant ileal and colonic disease caused by previous irradiation and inflammatory bowel disease or there has been loss of the middle and distal ureter. As is discussed later, electrolyte disturbances can occur after incorporation of intestinal segments into the urinary tract; these are more common when the jejunum is used for conduit construction. In approximately 40% of patients with jejunal urinary conduits, hyponatremic, hyperkalemic, hypochloremic metabolic acidosis and azotemia develop. The jejunum is unable to maintain large solute gradients, so large amounts of water and solute pass through the jejunal wall. Sodium and chloride are rapidly excreted into the conduit, and potassium is passively absorbed. Aldosterone is produced, resulting in reabsorption of hydrogen and excretion of potassium into the distal tubule of the kidney and consequent acidosis and movement of potassium from the body's intracellular stores. As water is lost into the conduit, extracellular fluid volume is reduced, as is the glomerular filtration rate. The renin-angiotensin system is activated, which further stimulates aldosterone secretion. Urea may be absorbed from the jejunal lumen, which (with dehydration) contributes to azotemia.

Colon Conduit

There are several advantages to using the large bowel in construction of urinary conduits: nonrefluxing ureterointestinal anastomoses are easily performed, possibly abrogating the deleterious effects of reflux on the upper urinary tracts (Richie and Skinner, 1975); stomal stenosis is uncommon because of the wide diameter of the large bowel; limited absorption of electrolytes occurs; and the blood supply to the transverse and sigmoid colon is abundant. Either the transverse or the sigmoid colon can be used, allowing for placement of the conduit high or low in the abdomen, depending on the integrity and condition of the ureters. Use of the transverse colon for conduit construction is especially well suited for patients who have received extensive pelvic irradiation or when the middle and distal ureters are absent.

The blood supply of the transverse colon is based on the middle colic artery. The greater omentum is separated from the superior surface of the transverse colon, and a segment of bowel, usually 15 cm in length, is selected for the conduit (Figure 24–2). Short mesenteric incisions are made, and the colon is divided proximally and distally. Once the conduit is isolated, bowel continuity is reestablished. The proximal end of the conduit is closed and fixed in the midline posteriorly. The ureters are brought through small incisions in the posterior peritoneum and reimplanted into the base of the conduit. The stoma may be positioned on either the patient's right or left side.

A sigmoid conduit is constructed in a similar manner. Great care should be taken to preserve the blood supply by carefully selecting a segment with a good blood supply and by making short mesenteric incisions. The conduit is positioned lateral to the reapproximated sigmoid colon. Ureteral reimplantation and stoma construction are completed.

The ureters can be reimplanted into the large intestine either in a way that prevents reflux or by anastomosis directly into the bowel. Ureteral reflux is prevented by constructing a short tunnel (approximately 2–3 cm in length) of bowel mucosa, through which the distal ureter runs. Frequently, this is accomplished by

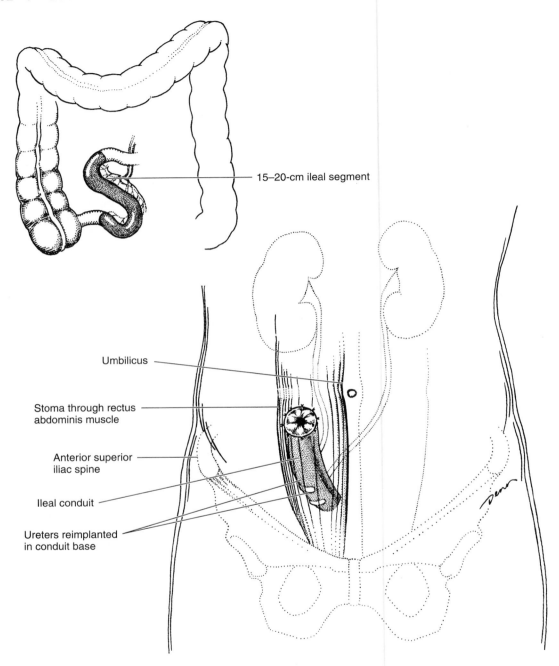

15–20-cm ileal segment

Umbilicus

Stoma through rectus
abdominis muscle

Anterior superior
iliac spine

Ileal conduit

Ureters reimplanted
in conduit base

Figure 24–1. Ileal conduit.

Figure 24–2. Transverse colon conduit.

incising the tenia of the large bowel for a distance of 3–4 cm. The incision is carried through the muscular fibers of the bowel wall, sparing the mucosa. A small elliptic segment of mucosa is removed, and a mucosa-to-mucosa anastomosis is performed between the ureter and the mucosa of the bowel. The muscularis of the tenia is reapproximated over the ureter to create the tunnel (Figure 24–3).

CONTINENT URINARY DIVERSION & BLADDER SUBSTITUTION

General Considerations

Various procedures have been developed for construction of bladder substitutes or continent urinary reservoirs that preclude the need for an external urine collection appliance. They offer psychological and functional advantages for selected patients who require urinary diversion. Such reservoirs or bladder substitutes are composed of 3 segments: ureterointestinal (afferent limb) anastomosis, the reservoir itself, and the conduit carrying the urine from the reservoir to the surface (efferent continence mechanism). Bladder substitutes rely on the intact urethra and sphincter to provide outlet resistance

and carry urine to the urethral meatus. In men and women whose urethra has cancer involvement or is not functional owing to benign diseases, an efferent continence mechanism can be constructed with the appendix or short segments of tapered, intussuscepted, or reimplanted intestine.

The decision to proceed with bladder replacement is dependent on the risk of urethral recurrence and the continence of the patient. Both men and women who have low risk of urethral recurrence and who have intact external urinary sphincters should be considered for bladder replacement rather than construction of a continent urinary reservoir. The risk of urethral occurrence or recurrence in men who undergo radical cystectomy is 6.1–10.6%. Carcinoma-in-situ and tumor multifocality appear to be risk factors for prostatic urethral tumor involvement in men with bladder cancer (Nixon et al, 2002). Although prostatic urethral disease is a risk factor for urethral recurrence, recent evidence suggests that orthotopic diversion may be considered in those with only proximal prostatic urethral involvement and negative urethral margins at cystectomy (Iselin et al, 1997). Urethral recurrence may actually be lower in those who undergo bladder substitution than in those who undergo either conduit urinary diversion or con-

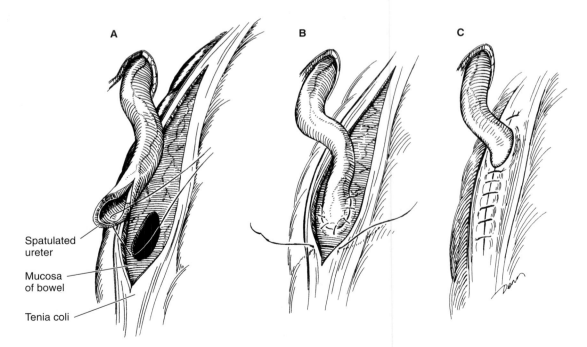

Spatulated ureter

Mucosa of bowel

Tenia coli

Figure 24–3. Creation of a submucosal tunnel in the wall of the colon to prevent ureteral reflux of urine. **A:** Incision in the tenia coli. **B:** Anastomosis of distal ureter to large intestine mucosa. **C:** Muscularis (tenia) approximated over ureter.

struction of a continent urinary reservoir and have their urethra left in place (Iselin et al, 1996). Although orthotopic bladder replacement was once reserved for men, recent clinical and laboratory experience suggests that it may be an acceptable procedure in women as well (Stein et al, 1997). Women with bladder cancer whose tumors are not located at the bladder neck and have a clear urethral margin at the time of cystectomy are candidates for this procedure. Approximately 66% of women undergoing radical cystectomy for the management of bladder cancer fall into this group (Stein et al, 1995, 1998a; Stenzl et al, 1995). Intraoperative inspection and frozen section assessment of the bladder neck limits the risk of urethral recurrence.

Although various segments of the gastrointestinal tract can be used, the principles for success are standard. The bowel segments should be opened and refashioned (detubularized) to interrupt the normal high-pressure contractions of the intact intestine (Hinman, 1988). A large radius is preferred, as this results in a reservoir with a larger geometric capacity and lower pressure. Continent reservoirs and bladder substitutes may be made of small intestine, large intestine, or a combination of both. Recently, there has been intense interest in bladder substitution and continent urinary diversion. Even though bladder substitution is perceived by some as a more complex procedure, prior studies have demonstrated complication and re-operation rates similar to those of ileal conduit urinary diversion in the hands of experienced surgeons (Gburek, Lieber, and Blute, 1998; Parekh et al, 2000). Long-term results of bladder replacement demonstrate excellent functional outcomes (Elmajian et al, 1996; Hautmann et al, 1999; Abol-Enein and Ghoneim, 2001; Steven and Poulsen, 2000; Stein et al, 1997; Stenzl et al, 2001). Daytime continence can be expected in 87–100% of men and 82–100% of women. Nighttime continence is achieved in 86–94% of men and 72–82% of women. Nearly all men are able to void to completion, while approximately 15–20% of women require intermittent catheterization to completely empty the neobladder. It is beyond the scope of this chapter to review all techniques and minor modifications; instead, the most common techniques and the general principles of continent diversion are reviewed.

Ureterosigmoidostomy

The first direct anastomosis of the ureters into the intact colon was performed by Smith in 1878 (Smith, 1879). Peritonitis (from fecal spillage) and pyelonephritis (resulting from ascending infection and stricturing of the ureteral anastomosis) led initially to very high surgical mortality rates. Recognizing that ascending infection from the rectum into the kidney was a major

problem, surgeons developed techniques to reimplant the ureters into the colon in an antirefluxing fashion. Since patients will retain large amounts of urine and fecal material simultaneously in the rectum, assurance of adequate rectal sphincter function is important preoperatively. Since ammonia may be absorbed across the bowel surface, patients with liver disease who may be at an increased risk of hyperammonemic encephalopathy should not undergo this procedure. Patients who have primary diseases of the colon or have received extensive pelvic irradiation should undergo alternative forms of diversion.

The ureters are identified at or below the common iliac arteries. The overlying peritoneum is incised and the ureters are mobilized carefully to preserve their blood supply. A site low in the sigmoid is selected for ureteral reimplantation. The ureters are reimplanted separately into the respective ipsilateral tenia coli, using the antirefluxing techniques described earlier. The peritoneum is sutured over the completed ureteral anastomosis (Figure 24–4).

One particularly worrisome complication of ureterosigmoidostomy is development of adenocarcinoma at the site where the ureters have been reimplanted into the large intestine. The incidence of this problem is uncertain, but there seems to be a several thousandfold increase in its incidence in patients who have undergone ureterosigmoidostomy over individuals who have not undergone this type of surgery. The

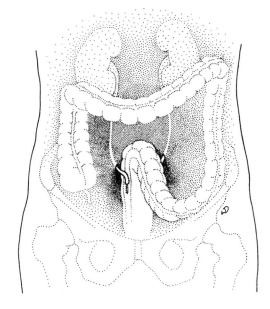

Figure 24–4. Ureterosigmoidostomy.

induction period varies but may be approximately 20 years; thus, the risk is especially high in young patients. Experimental studies have shown that the development of adenocarcinoma seems dependent on the presence of urine, feces, urothelium, and colonic epithelium in close approximation. All those who undergo ureterosigmoidostomy should be counseled to undergo yearly sigmoidoscopy starting 5 years after the procedure and at any time occult or gross gastrointestinal bleeding or a major change in bowel habits is noted.

Reservoirs Constructed of Small Intestine

Nils Kock was responsible for the early and ongoing development of a continent urinary reservoir fashioned entirely of small intestine (Kock et al, 1982; Nieh, 1997). Sixty to seventy centimeters of small intestine is selected for reservoir construction. The proximal and distal 15-cm segments are preserved for construction of nipple valves, allowing for antireflux ureteroileal anastomoses (inlet) and a continent, catheterizable abdominal stoma (outlet) (Figure 24–5). The middle 40 cm is opened along the antimesenteric border and folded into a U; the back wall is sutured together. The proximal and distal nipple valves are constructed by intussuscepting the bowel, stapling it in place, and further securing it with a mesh anchoring collar. This fixes the intussuscepted bowel segments in place and allows for high-pressure zones, which prevent ureteral reflux proximally and incontinence distally. The reservoir is closed by folding the middle segment and suturing it in place. The ureters are sutured to the proximal nipple valve. The distal nipple valve is brought to the skin as a "flush," catheterizable stoma. Revision of the nipple valve may be necessary in some patients to correct valve slippage or eversion. In men who have an intact urethra and external urinary sphincter, the distal nipple valve can be omitted and the reservoir attached directly to the urethra (Elmajian et al, 1996).

In an attempt to decrease the complication rate associated with the afferent intussuscepted antireflux nipple of the Kock ileal neobladder, Stein and colleagues (1998b) have described an innovative antireflux technique (Figure 24–6). This new reservoir, the T pouch, has several important advantages over the Kock ileal neobladder: (1) It requires a smaller segment of ileum to create the antireflux technique; (2) the serosal-lined antireflux mechanism eliminates the need for intussusception; (3) blood supply is better preserved; and (4) urine is not in contact with the implanted portion of the ileum.

Camey described a technique of bladder substitution whereby an intact segment of ileum was anastomosed directly to the urethra (Lilien and Camey, 1984). A 40-cm segment of ileum was isolated from the gastrointestinal tract, and its midpoint was anastomosed, without tension, directly to the urethra. The ureters were reimplanted into either end of the ileal segment in an antirefluxing fashion. However, failure to detubularize the ileal segment led to a high incidence of urinary incontinence compared with substitutes fashioned from detubularized small-bowel segments (Studer and Zingg, 1997; Hautmann et al, 1999). Forty- to sixty-centimeter segments of ileum can be detubularized and folded into U-, S-, or W-shaped reservoirs, which can be connected directly to the urethra (Figure 24–7). The ureters are reimplanted directly into the small bowel wall. They may be reimplanted in a fashion to prevent urinary reflux or in a simple end-to-side fashion. The larger diameter and lower pressure of these reservoirs compared with those of nondetubularized bowel have led to better continence rates.

Reservoirs Constructed of Large Intestine

Various investigators have described using segments of the large intestine alone or combinations of large- and small-bowel segments to fashion urinary reservoirs (Lampel et al, 1996; Bihrle, 1997). Bladder substitutes have been constructed using detubularized bowel segments from the ileocecal region or sigmoid colon. Use of the ascending colon and terminal ileum to construct continent urinary reservoirs has gained great popularity. Cecum and ascending colon are detubularized and refashioned or augmented with small intestine to provide for a spheric reservoir. The ureters are reimplanted in a nonrefluxing fashion (Figure 24–8). The reservoir can be anastomosed directly to the urethra. In women or in men who require a urethrectomy, a continent, catheterizable stoma can be fashioned of appendix or tapered terminal ileum (Figure 24–9).

Reservoirs Constructed of Stomach

The stomach may be used for bladder augmentation or substitution. It may have some advantages over intestinal segments: Its muscular elements make ureteral reimplantation easy; it secretes chloride and hydrogen ions and therefore may be especially well suited to those with renal insufficiency; it produces little mucus and may be associated with fewer infections. A wedge of stomach is harvested, and its blood supply is based on one gastroepiploic artery. When the gastric segment is anastomosed to the urethra, a tunnel may be fashioned to increase outlet resistance and aid in continence. Alternatively, a catheterizable stoma may be fashioned of appendix.

After either gastric bladder augmentation or reservoir construction, hematuria and dysuria may result from acid secretion. Treatment with either H_2 blockers

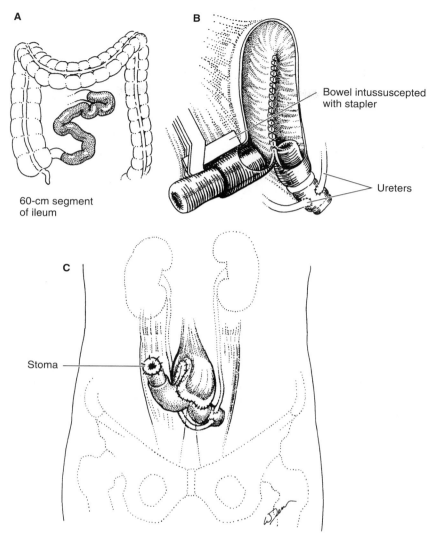

Figure 24–5. Kock Pouch urinary reservoir. **A:** 60 cm of small intestine selected. **B:** Afferent (nonrefluxing) limb for ureteral reimplantation and efferent limb for stoma fashioned using stapling devices. **C:** Completed reservoir.

or oral alkali may be necessary to buffer urine. Distention of the gastric segment with urine could increase serum gastrin levels. However, hypergastrinemia occurs rarely; furthermore, excluding the antrum in the gastric segment harvested decreases its likelihood further. Theoretically, in the native segment, decreased acid secretion and production of intrinsic factor could lead to protein maldigestion, iron-deficiency anemia, hypocalcemia, and vitamin B_{12} deficiency.

POSTOPERATIVE CARE

Postoperative care varies depending on the method of urinary diversion or bladder substitution. As with all patients who have undergone major abdominal surgery, early ambulation, use of intermittent compression stockings, and incentive spirometry may be used to prevent pulmonary emboli or respiratory complications. If a nasogastric tube is used, it is left in place until there

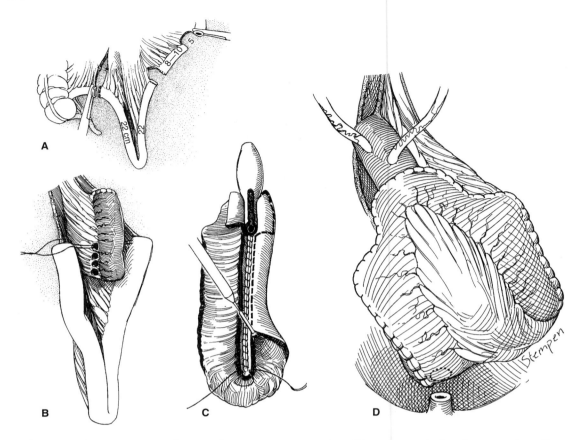

Figure 24–6. Construction of a T pouch. **A:** Two segments of small intestine are isolated; one portion will form the reservoir, and the smaller, more proximal portion will form the antireflux segment. **B:** The longer reservoir portion of the segments is folded into a V. The smaller, antireflux segment is fixed to the serosa of the reservoir portion. **C:** The antireflux segment has been opened and tapered with a stapling device. The ileal segments selected for the reservoir portion of the pouch are joined anteriorly and then opened, exposing the mucosa. As the opening reaches the ostium of the antireflux segment, the incisions are carried laterally and create wide flaps that can then be closed over the ostium to cover the tapered antireflux segment. **D:** The reservoir portion is closed.

are signs of intestinal peristalsis. Serum electrolytes and creatinine should be monitored postoperatively for the development of metabolic abnormalities. If ureteral stents have been placed, they are usually removed sometime after postoperative day 5; they may stay in place for up to 3 weeks in patients undergoing bladder replacement. Continent urinary reservoirs and bladder substitutes produce mucus. They should be irrigated regularly in the early postoperative period to prevent mucus accumulation. Mucus production decreases over time, and irrigation ultimately becomes unnecessary. Upper urinary tract surveillance for hydronephrosis should be performed on a regular basis using ultra-

sound, intravenous urography, or computed tomography. An initial assessment of the upper urinary tract is made in the early postoperative period; if upper urinary tract dilation is not found, the patient undergoes repeat imaging on a yearly basis.

COMPLICATIONS

Complications occurring after urinary diversion, bladder substitution, or continent urinary diversion are generally a product of surgical technique, the underlying disease process and its treatment, the age of the patient, and the length of follow-up (Carlin, Rutchik, and Resnick,

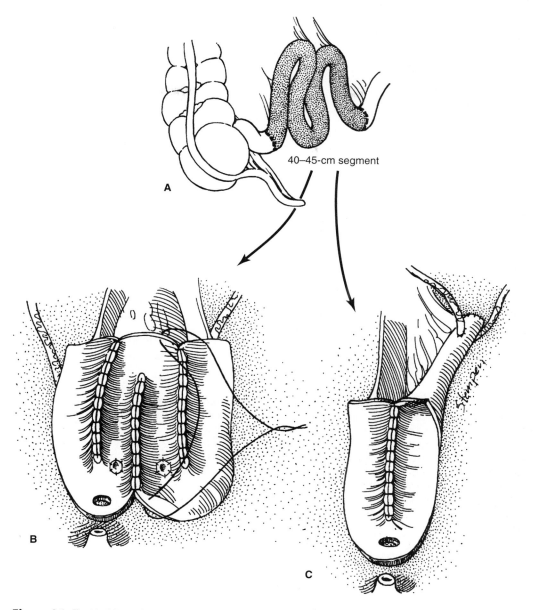

Figure 24–7. Bladder substitutes constructed entirely of small intestine. **A:** Forty to forty-five centimeters of small intestine is selected. **B:** Small intestine is opened and fashioned into a W. The
ureters are reimplanted into the second and third limbs of the reservoir, and the reservoir is attached to the urethra. **C:** Small intestine is folded into a J with the most proximal portion of the segment not opened. The ureters are reimplanted into the intact ileal segment of the reservoir, and the
reservoir is attached to the urethra.

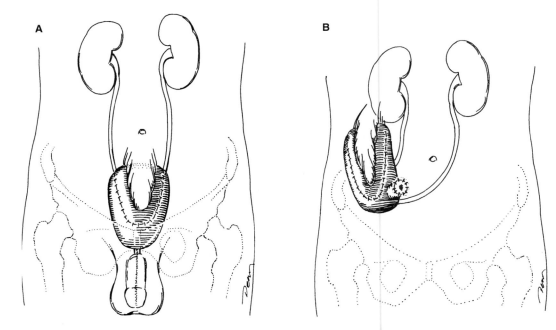

Figure 24–8. Use of the ileocecal segment to construct (**A**) a bladder substitute attached to the urethra or (**B**) a continent urinary reservoir placed in the abdomen using plicated terminal ileum as a stoma.

1997; Gburek et al, 1998). Early complications, which are uncommon (occurring in approximately 10% of patients), include excessive bleeding, intestinal obstruction, urinary extravasation, and infection. Late complications (10–20% of patients) include metabolic disorders, stomal stenosis, pyelonephritis, and calculi. Rarely, spontaneous neobladder rupture may occur presumably due to overdistension or blunt abdominal trauma (Nippgen et al, 2001). Such patients usually present with peritonitis and acute abdominal pain.

Metabolic & Nutritional Disorders

Fluid, electrolyte, nutrient, and waste product excretion or absorption normally occurs across the intestinal wall. The extent of absorption or excretion is dependent on the concentration of these substances in the lumen or blood and on which segment of bowel is in contact with them. Metabolic abnormalities may occur when intestinal segments are interposed into the urinary tract. As pointed out previously, use of the jejunum may result in hyponatremic, hypochloremic, hyperkalemic metabolic acidosis. This syndrome is often characterized clinically by nausea, vomiting, anorexia, and muscle weakness.

The pathogenesis and nature of metabolic abnormalities occurring after incorporation of the ileum or colon into the urinary tract differ from those associated with jejunal conduits. When such segments are used, sodium and chloride are absorbed across the bowel surface. Chloride is absorbed in slight excess of sodium, resulting in a net loss of bicarbonate into the bowel lumen. Preexisting renal failure contributes to the development and severity of the disorder, as does a large bowel surface area and long contact time. Hyperchloremic acidosis is more common in patients who undergo ureterosigmoidostomy than in patients who undergo simple conduit construction using either the ileum or the colon, because of the larger surface area and longer contact time with urine associated with ureterosigmoidostomies. Hyperchloremic metabolic acidosis may manifest clinically as weakness, anorexia, vomiting, Kussmaul breathing, and coma. One potential long-term complication of chronic acidosis may be decreased bone calcium content and osteomalacia (McDougal et al, 1988; Kawakita et al, 1996).

Because patients with gastric segments incorporated into the urinary tract may lose both hydrogen and chloride, they are at risk of dehydration and alkalosis if they have either diarrhea or vomiting. The resulting hyponatremic metabolic alkalosis requires treatment with intravenous salt replacement.

Bile salts are important for fat digestion and uptake of vitamins A and D. Bile salt metabolism may be al-

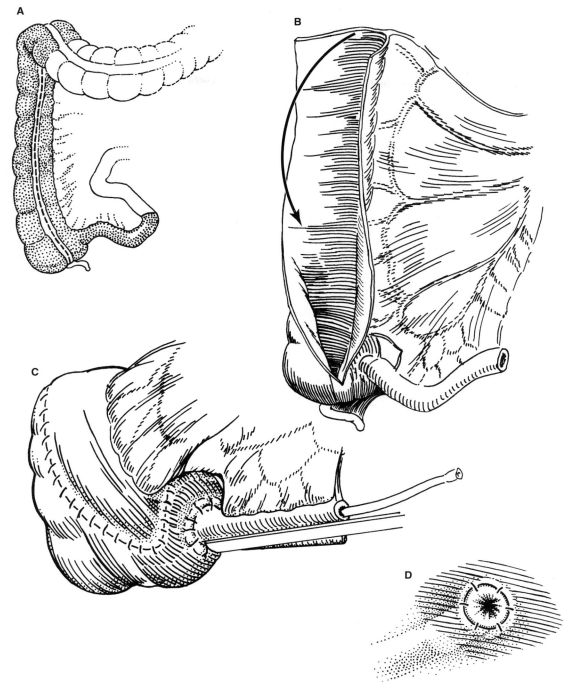

Figure 24–9. Continent urinary reservoir constructed from the ileocecal segment (**A**). **B:** Bowel detubularized. Stoma constructed by tapering the terminal ileum with intestinal stapling instrument (shown in **C**) or sutures. **D:** Completed stoma.

tered after ileal resection (Olofsson et al, 1998). Resection of small segments of the ileum may be associated with mild malabsorption and steatorrhea owing to increased concentrations of bile salts delivered to the colon. The increased concentration of such salts leads to decreased colonic absorption of water and electrolytes. Resection of large segments of ileum may reduce bile salt reabsorption to very low levels, leading to severe fat malabsorption. Bowel transit time may be reduced further by resection of the ileocecal valve. Cholestyramine may be used to treat secretory bile salt diarrhea. If diarrhea persists, addition of agents such as loperamide that decrease bowel motility and increase transit time may be effective. Cholelithiasis may be more common after ileal resections as well.

Vitamin B_{12} deficiency may occur as a result of either gastric or ileal resection (Terai et al, 1997; Fujisawa et al, 2000b). Because B_{12} stores are likely to last for years, B_{12} deficiency may not become apparent for several years after intestinal surgery. B_{12} deficiency results in megaloblastic anemia and peripheral nerve paresthesias. The levels of this vitamin should be assessed routinely in patients after ileal or gastric resection, and yearly replacement is necessary in those in whom deficiency is noted.

Stoma

A good deal of patients' dissatisfaction with urinary diversion can be attributed to stomal complications.

Stoma construction is especially important in procedures in which an appliance must be worn. Careful stomal construction as outlined earlier is essential (Fitzgerald et al, 1997). Stomal complications include stenosis, parastomal hernia formation, and various skin irritations or fungal infections. The likelihood of stomal stenosis increases with time. Stomal stenosis can lead to conduit elongation and upper-tract obstruction. This condition can be diagnosed relatively easily by catheterizing the stoma and measuring the residual urine volume. It is corrected by revision of the stoma.

Skin irritation or infections are most common in procedures in which an appliance is worn and there is prolonged contact of the skin with urine. Some patients' skin may be sensitive to adhesive agents.

Stomal or skin problems are minimized when the appliance or faceplate opening is cut to the proper size, preventing irritation of the stomal surface and prolonged skin contact with urine. The treatment of parastomal conditions is summarized in Table 24–1.

The most troublesome stomal complication of external urinary appliances is unexpected pouch leakage. This is often a result of improper application of the appliance but may be caused by poor stomal construction. With a properly constructed and located stoma, the choice of the appliance is relatively simple and is often determined by patient preference. Factors that must be taken into account when selecting an appliance include patient dexterity and preference, available resources, and stomal construction. Appliances constitute an ad-

Table 24–1. Common parastomal skin problems and their management.[a]

Problem	Cause	Management
Fungal infections—*Candida albicans* (Monilia)	Urine accumulating under barrier (seen more frequently with diabetes mellitus and concurrent antibiotic use)	• Apply nystatin (Mycostatin) powder • Dry skin thoroughly (use hair dryer) • Prevent leakage under water
Allergic contact dermatitis	Sensitivity to solvents, adhesives, detergents, wafers	• Identify irritant (skin patch test) and discontinue product • Apply hydrocortisone cream (avoid prolonged use) • Avoid solvents and soaps
Mechanical trauma	• Frequent or excessive pouch changing leading to skin stripping • Pressure from belts • Overuse of adhesive strips around the faceplate of barrier	• Minimize pouch changes • Encourage gentle skin care • Consider nonadhesive pouches (used with belt) • Minimize use of sealants and adhesives
Pseudoverrucous skin lesions	• Urine contact with skin over extended time	• Ensure that the barrier and pouch are the correct size

[a]The patient should see an enterostomal therapist nurse, if available.

hesive skin barrier that attaches to the skin and a pouch that collects urine. An opening is made in the middle of the skin barrier; this opening should be of a diameter just larger than the stoma to avoid erosion of the stoma or prolonged contact of the skin with urine.

Most patients favor using disposable urinary collection appliances, although reusable ones are available. Disposable, one-piece pouches are used once. Two-piece systems allow the patient to remove the pouch, leaving the skin barrier intact. Reusable appliances are composed of a rigid or semirigid faceplate secured to the skin with adhesive. A vinyl or rubber pouch is attached to the faceplate using an O ring. These pouches are reusable and last 1 or 6 months depending on whether they are composed of vinyl or rubber, respectively. A larger collection device is often attached to the pouch at night.

Pyelonephritis & Renal Deterioration

Pyelonephritis occurs in approximately 10% of patients who have undergone urinary diversion. Treatment is based on a properly collected urine sample for culture. A urine sample should not be collected from the pouch; rather, the pouch should be removed, the stoma cleansed with an antiseptic, and a catheter advanced gently through the stoma. If infection has occurred in a patient with a simple conduit, the volume of residual urine within the conduit should be recorded. Obstruction and stasis of urine within the reconstructed urinary tract are risk factors for the development of infection.

Although many patients with preexisting dilation of the upper urinary tract show improvement or resolution of the dilation after urinary diversion or bladder substitution, progressive renal deterioration as manifested by hydronephrosis or an increasing serum creatinine level(or both) occurs in a certain percentage of patients who undergo these procedures. The incidence of either complication increases after 10 years. Pyelographic evidence of upper urinary tract deterioration has been noted in up to 50% of patients who have undergone urinary diversion at an early age. Recurrent upper urinary tract infection and high-pressure ureteral reflux and obstruction, usually in combination, contribute to the likelihood of renal deterioration.

Calculi

Calculi occur in approximately 8% of patients who undergo urinary diversion or bladder substitution (Cohen and Streem, 1994; Terai et al, 1996). Such patients have several risk factors for the development of various calculi. Nonabsorbable staples, mesh, or suture material used to construct conduits or reservoirs may act as a nidus for stone formation. Colonization in either conduits or reservoirs is common, whereas symptomatic in-

fection is much rarer. Certain bacteria can contribute to stone formation; some bacteria commonly found in the urinary tract, including *Proteus, Klebsiella,* and *Pseudomonas* species, produce urease, a urea-splitting enzyme that contributes to the formation of ammonia and carbon dioxide. Hydrolysis of these products results in an alkaline urine supersaturated with magnesium ammonium phosphate, calcium phosphate, and carbonate apatite crystals. Management of such infection-related stones requires stone removal, resolution of infection, and, often, use of adjunctive agents to complete stone dissolution.

The likelihood of stone formation is increased by the development of systemic acidosis, as described previously (Terai et al, 1995). Prolonged contact of the urine with the intestinal surface facilitates the exchange of chloride for bicarbonate. Bicarbonate loss results in systemic acidosis and hypercalciuria. The combination of hypercalciuria and an alkaline urine predisposes a patient to the development of calcium calculi. In addition, the terminal ileum is responsible for bile salt absorption; if this portion of the intestine is used for conduit or bladder reservoir construction, excess bile salts in the intestine may bind calcium and result in increased absorption of oxalate, which may lead to the development of oxalate-containing calculi. Hypocitraturia may also be a risk factor for stone disease in patients undergoing bladder replacement (Osther, Poulsen, and Steven, 2000). Excess conduit length, urine stasis, and dehydration make the development of calculi more likely.

REFERENCES

General

Bjerre BD, Johansen C, Steven K: Health-related quality of life after cystectomy: Bladder substitution compared with ileal conduit diversion. A questionnaire survey. Br J Urol 1995; 75:200.

Carlin BI, Rutchik SD, Resnick MI: Comparison of the ileal conduit to the continent cutaneous diversion and orthotopic neobladder in patients undergoing cystectomy: A critical analysis and review of the literature. Semin Urol Oncol 1997; 15:189.

Dutta SC et al: Health related quality of life assessment after radical cystectomy: Comparison of ileal conduit with continent orthotopic neobladder. J Urol 2002;168:164.

Fitzgerald J et al: Stomal construction, complications, and reconstruction. Urol Clin North Am 1997;24:729.

Fujisawa M et al: Health-related quality of life with orthotopic neobladder versus ileal conduit according to the SF-36 survey. Urology 2000a;55:862.

Goldwasser B, Webster GD: Continent urinary diversion. J Urol 1985;134:227.

Hara I et al: Health-related quality of life after radical cystectomy for bladder cancer: A comparison of ileal conduit and orthotopic bladder replacement. BJU Int 2002;89:10.

King LR, Stone AR, Webster GD (editors): *Bladder Reconstruction and Continent Urinary Diversion.* Year Book, 1987.

Kitamura H et al: Quality of life in patients having an ileal conduit, continent reservoir, or orthotopic neobladder after cystectomy for bladder carcinoma. Int J Urol 1999;6:393.

Okada Y et al: Quality of life survey of urinary diversion patients: Comparison of continent urinary diversion versus ileal conduit. Int J Urol 1997;4:26.

Ileal Conduit

Bricker EM: Bladder substitution after pelvic evisceration. Surg Clin North Am 1950;30:1511.

Pitts WR, Muecke EC: A 20 year experience with ileal conduit: The fate of the kidneys. J Urol 1979;122:154.

Remigailo RV et al: Ileal conduit urinary diversion: Ten-year review. Urology 1976;7:343.

Schmidt JD et al: Complications, results, and problems of ileal diversions. J Urol 1973;109:210.

Schwarz GR, Jeffs RD: Ileal conduit urinary diversion in children: Computer analysis of followup from 2 to 16 years. J Urol 1975;114:285.

Shapiro SR, Lebowitz R, Colodny AH: Fate of 90 children with ileal conduit urinary diversion a decade later. J Urol 1975; 114:289.

Sullivan JW, Grabstald H, Whitmore WF: Complications of ureteroileal conduit with radical cystectomy: Review of 336 cases. J Urol 1980;124:797.

Jejunal Conduit

Golimbu M, Morales P: Jejunal conduits: Technique and complications. J Urol 1975;113:787.

Colon Conduit

Beckley S et al: Transverse colon conduit: A method of urinary diversion after pelvic irradiation. J Urol 1982;128:464.

Richie J, Skinner DG: Urinary diversion: The physiological rationale for nonrefluxing colonic conduits. Br J Urol 1975; 47:269.

Richie JP: Sigmoid conduit urinary diversion. Urol Clin North Am 1986;13:225.

Schmidt JA, Hawtry CE, Buschbaum HJ: Transverse colon conduit: A preferred method of urinary diversion for radiation-treated pelvic malignancies. J Urol 1975;113:08.

Wilbert DM, Hohenfellner R: Colonic conduit: Preoperative requirements, operative technique, postoperative management. World J Urol 1984;2:159.

Continent Urinary Diversion & Bladder Substitution

Abol-Enein H, Ghoneim MA: Functional results of orthotopic ileal neobladder with serous-lined extramural ureteral reimplantation: Experience with 450 patients. J Urol 2001;165:1427.

Bihrle R: The Indiana Pouch continent urinary reservoir. Urol Clin North Am 1997;24:773.

Carroll PR et al: Functional characteristics of the continent ileocecal urinary reservoir: Mechanisms of urinary continence. J Urol 1989;142:1032.

Elmajian D et al: The Kock ileal neobladder: Updated experience in 295 male patients. J Urol 1996;156:920.

Freeman JA et al: Urethral recurrence in patients with orthotopic ileal neobladders. J Urol 1996;156:1615.

Gburek BM, Lieber MM, Blute ML: Comparison of the Studer ileal neobladder and ileal conduit urinary diversion with respect to perioperative outcome and late complications. J Urol 1998;160:721.

Gilchrist RK, Merichs JW: Construction of a substitute bladder and urethra. Surg Clin North Am 1956;36:131.

Hautmann R et al: The ileal neobladder: Complications and functional results in 363 patients after 11 years of followup. J Urol 1999;161:422.

Hinman F Jr: Selection of intestinal segments for bladder substitution: Physical and physiological characteristics. J Urol 1988; 139:519.

Iselin C et al: Does prostate transitional cell carcinoma preclude orthotopic bladder reconstruction after radical cystoprostatectomy for bladder cancer? J Urol 1997;158:2123.

Kock NG et al: Urinary diversion via a continent ileal reservoir: Clinical results in 12 patients. J Urol 1982;128:469.

Lampel A et al: Continent diversion with the Mainz pouch. World J Urol 1996;14:85.

Lilien OM, Camey M: 25-year experience with replacement of the human bladder (Camey procedure). J Urol 1984;132:886.

Nieh P: The Kock Pouch urinary reservoir. Urol Clin North Am 1997;24:755.

Nixon et al: Carcinoma in situ and tumor multifocality predict the risk of prostatic urethral involvement at radical cystectomy in men with transitional cell carcinoma of the bladder. J Urol 2002;167:502.

Parekh DJ et al: Continent urinary reconstruction versus ileal conduit: A contemporary single-institution comparison of perioperative morbidity and mortality. Urology 2000;55:852.

Rowland RG et al: Indiana continent urinary reservoir. J Urol 1987;137:1136.

Skinner DG, Lieskovsky G, Boyd S: Continent urinary diversion. J Urol 1989;141:1323.

Stein JP et al: Indications for lower urinary tract reconstruction in women after cystectomy for bladder cancer: A pathological review of female cystectomy specimens [see comments]. J Urol 1995;154:1329.

Stein J et al: Orthotopic lower urinary tract reconstruction in women using the Kock ileal neobladder: Updated experience in 34 patients. J Urol 1997;158:400.

Stein J et al: Prospective pathologic analysis of female cystectomy specimens: Risk factors for orthotopic diversion in women. Urology 1998a;51:951.

Stein J et al: The T Pouch: An orthotopic ileal neobladder incorporating a serosal lined ileal antireflux technique. J Urol 1998b;159:1836.

Stenzl A et al: The risk of urethral tumors in female bladder cancer: Can the urethra be used for orthotopic reconstruction of the lower urinary tract? J Urol 1995;153(3 Pt 2):950.

Stenzl A et al: Urethra-sparing cystectomy and orthotopic urinary diversion in women with malignant pelvic tumors. Cancer 2001;92:1864.

Steven K, Poulsen AL: The orthotopic Kock ileal neobladder: Functional results, urodynamic features, complications, and survival in 166 men. J Urol 2000;164:288.

Studer U, Zingg E: Ileal orthotopic bladder substitutes. Urol Clin North Am 1997;24:781.

Ureterosigmoidostomy

Bristol JB, Williamson RCN: Ureterosigmoidostomy and colon carcinogenesis. Science 1981;214:851.

Crissey MM, Steele GD, Gittes RF: Rat model for carcinogenesis in ureterosigmoidostomy. Science 1980;207:1079.

Gittes RF: Carcinogenesis in ureterosigmoidostomy. Urol Clin North Am 1986;13:201.

Hinman F, Weyrauch HM Jr: A critical study of the different principles of surgery which have been used in uretero-intestinal implantation. Trans Am Assoc Genitourin Surg 1936;9:15.

Leadbetter WF, Clarke BG: Five years' experience with uretero-enterostomy by the "combined" technique. J Urol 1955;3:67.

Smith T: An account of an unsuccessful attempt to treat extroversion of the bladder by a new operation. St Barth Hosp Rep 1879;15:29.

Spirnak JP, Caldamone AA: Ureterosigmoidostomy. Urol Clin North Am 1986;13:285.

Gastric Bladder

Nguyen DH, Mitchell, ME: Gastric bladder reconstruction. Urol Clin North Am 1991;18:649.

Complications

Bloom DA, Grossman HB, Konnak JW: Stomal construction and reconstruction. Urol Clin North Am 1986;13:275.

Carlin BI, Rutchik SD, Resnick MI: Comparison of the ileal conduit to the continent cutaneous diversion and orthotopic neobladder in patients undergoing cystectomy: A critical analysis and review of the literature. Semin Urol Oncol 1997; 15:189.

Cohen T, Streem S: Minimally invasive endourologic management of calculi in continent urinary reservoirs. Urology 1994; 43:865.

Dretler SP: The pathogenesis of urinary tract calculi occurring after ileal conduit diversion: 1. Clinical study. 2. Conduit study. 3. Prevention. J Urol 1973;109:204.

Filmer RB, Spencer JR: Malignancies in bladder augmentation and intestinal conduits. J Urol 1990;143:671.

Fujisawa M et al: Long-term assessment of serum vitamin B_{12} concentrations in patients with various types of orthotopic intestinal neobladder. Urology 2000b;56:236.

Gburek B et al: Comparison of Studer ileal neobladder and ileal conduit urinary diversion with respect to perioperative outcome and late complications. J Urol 1998;160:721.

Hall MC, Koch MO, McDougal WS: Metabolic consequences of urinary diversion through intestinal segments. Urol Clin North Am 1991;18:25.

Kawakita M et al: Bone demineralization following urinary intestinal diversion assessed by urinary pyridium cross-links and dual energy x-ray absorptiometry. J Urol 1996;156:355.

Koch MO, McDougal WS: The pathophysiology of hyperchloremic metabolic acidosis after urinary diversion through intestinal segments. Surgery 1985;98:561.

Kosko JW, Kursh ED, Resnick MI: Metabolic complications of urologic intestinal substitutes. Urol Clin North Am 1986; 13:193.

Madsen PO: The etiology of hyperchloremic acidosis following ureterointestinal anastomosis: An experimental study. J Urol 1964;92:448.

McDougal WS et al: Boney demineralization following intestinal diversion. J Urol 1988;140:853.

Nippgen JBW et al: Spontaneous late rupture of orthotopic detubularized ileal neobladders: Report of five cases. Urology 2001;58:43.

Olofsson G et al: Bile acid malabsorption after continent urinary diversion with an ileal reservoir. J Urol 1998;160:724.

Osther PJ, Poulsen AL, Steven K: Stone risk after bladder substitution with the ileal-urethral Kock reservoir. Scand J Urol Nephrol 2000;34:257.

Stamey TA: The pathogenesis and implications of the electrolyte imbalance in ureterosigmoidostomy. Surg Gynecol Obstet 1956;103:736.

Stein R et al: Long-term metabolic effects in patients with urinary diversion. World J Urol 1998;16:292.

Steiner MS, Morton RA: Nutritional and gastrointestinal complications of the use of bowel segments in the lower urinary tract. Urol Clin North Am 1991;18:725.

Tanagho EA: A case against incorporation of bowel into the closed urinary system. J Urol 1975;113:796.

Terai A et al: Effect of urinary intestinal diversion on urinary risk factors for urolithiasis. J Urol 1995;153:37.

Terai A et al: Urinary calculi as a late complication of the Indiana continent urinary diversion: Comparison with the Kock pouch procedure. J Urol 1996;155:66.

Terai A et al: Vitamin B_{12} deficiency in patients with urinary intestinal diversion. Int J Urol 1997;4:21.

Ostomy Care

Borglund E, Nordstrom G, Nyman CR: Classification of peristomal skin changes in patients with urostomy. J Am Acad Dermatol 1988;19:623.

Fitzgerald J et al: Stomal construction, complications, and reconstruction. Urol Clin North Am 1997;24:729.

Johnson DE, Smith DB: Urinary diversions. In: Smith DB, Johnson DE (editors): *Ostomy Care and the Cancer Patient: Surgical and Clinical Considerations.* Grune & Stratton, 1986.

Maidl L: Stomal and peristomal skin complications with urostomies. Urol Nurs 1990;10:17.

Nordstrom GM, Borglund E, Nyman CR: Local status of the urinary stoma: The relationship to peristomal skin complications. Scand J Urol Nephrol 1990;24:117.

Tucker SB, Smith DB: Dermatologic conditions complicating ostomy care. In: Smith DB, Johnson DE (editors): *Ostomy Care and the Cancer Patient: Surgical and Clinical Considerations.* Grune & Stratton, 1986.

Radiotherapy of Urologic Tumors

25

Joycelyn L. Speight, MD, PhD, & Mack Roach III, MD

The primary management of genitourologic malignant diseases has been tied to the use of radiation for more than 100 years. In 1895 Roentgen described x-rays; by 1899 a patient with skin cancer was cured with radiation; and within 10 years, radiation was used to treat prostate cancer (Pasteau and Degrais, 1914). Radiotherapy became a mainstay of treatment for bladder and testicular cancers and later prostate cancer as supervoltage sources became available. Although chemotherapy and aggressive surgery have supplanted some of the uses of radiotherapy, radiation continues to play a major role in the management of carcinomas of the penis, urethra, prostate, and bladder. In this chapter we review general principles and the indications for using radiation as a component in the primary management of urologic malignant diseases. The role of radiation as an agent of palliation has been well documented elsewhere and is excluded from this review.

GENERAL PRINCIPLES OF RADIOTHERAPY

Mechanisms of Cytotoxicity

The effects of radiation on tumor and surrounding normal tissues are thought to be mediated primarily through the induction of unrepaired double-strand breaks in DNA. Excited electron species generated in the presence of oxygen form peroxide radicals, which fix chemical lesions and result in the generation of either repairable or nonrepairable DNA double-strand breaks. High linear energy transfer radiation (including neurons and heavy-charged particles) is associated with less DNA damage repair and directly induced DNA damage. Classically, the expression of radiation damage is not seen until the target cells enter mitosis. Differentiated normal tissues with low mitotic activity, such as the heart and spinal cord, tend to express the effects of radiation much later than cells from more kinetically active tissues, such as the epithelial cells lining the rectum, bladder, or urethra. However, differentiated normal tissues with low mitotic activity are more sensitive to the use of high dose per fraction or high linear energy transfer radiotherapy. In organs in which the functional stromal cells are postmitotic, such as muscle cells

and neurons, the damage is expressed by slowly dividing support cells such as endothelial cells.

In addition to the classic mechanism described above, radiation has been shown to induce programmed cell death (apoptosis). Androgen-independent human prostate cancer cells activate a genetic program of apoptotic cell death in response to exposure to ionizing radiation, in a dose-dependent fashion (Sklar, 1993). Results from animal models suggest that it is better to achieve maximal androgen suppression before starting radiation treatment (Zietman, 2000).

Radiation Sensitivity & Tolerance

Table 25–1 summarizes the classic radiation tolerances that have been assigned to the normal tissues of interest during conventional fractionated radiotherapy for tumors arising from the urinary tract. The term **conventional fractionation** generally refers to the delivery of single daily doses of from 180 cGy (1.8 Gy) to 200 cGy (2.0 Gy). The gray unit is equal to 100 rads. When used alone, cumulative doses of at least 65 Gy are necessary for local control of gross disease (adenocarcinomas, transitional cell carcinomas, and squamous carcinomas) arising from the prostate, bladder, urethra, or ureters. When used prophylactically for presumed microscopic disease (lymph nodes) or postoperatively, doses of 45–50 Gy are generally sufficient. For testicular seminomas, doses of 25 Gy are usually adequate.

Total dose, dose per fraction, and volume of normal tissue irradiated are the major risk factors for radiation-induced complications. The presence of several comorbid conditions such as previous surgery, diabetes, inflammatory bowel diseases, or old age is also associated with an increased risk of radiation-induced complications. Accurate estimates of the "true tolerance" of surrounding normal tissues have been hampered until recently by our inability to reconstruct the actual relationship between normal tissue doses and volumes in 3 dimensions. Early reports assumed that organ movement and day-to-day treatment setup error had an insignificant impact on the doses of radiation delivered to surrounding normal tissues. Recent studies have demonstrated that these assumptions are inaccurate and

Table 25–1. Whole-organ radiation tolerances for fractionated radiotherapy of urologic tumors.

Organ	TD5/5[a] (cGy)	TD5/50[b] (cGy)	Clinical End Point
Testes	100	200	Sterility
Kidney	2000	3000	Nephrosclerosis
Intestine	5000	6000	Ulcer
Colon	5500	6500	Ulcer
Bladder	6500	7500	Ulcer
Rectum	6000	8000	Ulcer
Urethra	6500	8000	Stricture

Modified from Rubin P, Constine LS, Nelson DF: Late effects of cancer treatment: Radiation and drug toxicity. In: Perez CA, Brady LW (editors): *Principles and Practice of Radiation Oncology*, 3rd ed. Lippincott-Raven, 1998.
[a]TD 5/5 = the dose associated with a 5% risk for the occurrence of the clinical end point noted at 5 years.
[b]TD 5/50 = the dose associated with a 50% risk for the occurrence of the clinical end point noted at 5 years.

probably result in an underestimate of the true tolerance of surrounding normal tissues to radiation (Langen and Jones, 2001).

Dose per Fraction Considerations

The impact of dose per fraction on chronic genitourinary toxicity is probably more critical than the total dose, volume, or time. The linear quadratic equation (L-Q equation) has been adopted by many clinical investigators as the most useful model for comparing various dose and fractionation schemes (Fowler et al, 2001). This equation can be written as follows:

$$\text{Effect} = E = n(\alpha d + \beta d), \text{ where}$$

$$d = \text{Dose per fraction}$$
$$\alpha = \text{Nonrepairable effects}$$
$$\beta = \text{Repairable effects}$$
$$n = \text{Number of identical fractions}$$

For comparing 2 different fractionation schemes, assuming a similar overall treatment time, the L-Q equation also can be written as follows:

$$D_2 / D_1 = (1 + d_1 \beta / \alpha) / (1 + d_2 \beta / \alpha)$$
$$D = \text{Total dose and } D_1 = n_1 d_1$$
$$d = \text{Dose} / \text{fraction}$$

For most clinical circumstances, it is assumed that the α/β ratio for late-reacting normal tissues such as the bladder or rectum is 3. For early-responding normal tissues and for tumor, it is assumed that the α/β ratio is 10.

Altered Fractionation Schedules

Radiobiologic modeling using the α/β ratios as described previously has been used to develop "altered fractionation schedules" to improve the therapeutic ratio between efficacy and toxicity. **Accelerated hyperfractionation** is the most frequently used altered fractionation schedule. With accelerated hyperfractionation, more than one treatment is given per day with a minimum of 6 h between treatments, using a decreased dose per fraction. Since most radiation-induced damage is repaired within 6 h, the use of multiple treatments per day in theory should allow greater doses of radiation to be given over a shorter period of time, reducing the opportunity for tumor repopulation. Using α/β modeling, the late effects predicted using 1.2 Gy fractions twice daily (separated by 6 h) to 69.6 Gy would be expected to be equivalent to those using conventional fractionation to 58 Gy. In contrast, early-responding tissues such as the epithelium of the bladder would be expected to respond as though they had been treated with a dose of 65 Gy using conventional fractionation. This model predicts an increase in acute effects, including tumor response, but a decrease in late effects, such as fibrosis.

Clinical use of hyperfractionation schemes in the management of urologic tumors has been limited. Preliminary results with hyperfractionation for prostate tumors have been mixed. Acceptable toxicity was reported among the first 20 patients treated with 1.3 Gy twice daily to 78 Gy (Forman et al, 1996). Because of practical considerations (such as time and cost), there appears to be more interest in hypofractionated regimens than in hyperfractionated ones.

Hypofractionation involves the use of larger than conventional fraction sizes. Such an approach results in nearly a 10% reduction in the total dose to the tumor without sparing late complications (assuming that the values chosen for the α/β ratio are correct for normal tissues and for tumors) (Fowler et al, 2001). Several recent investigators have argued that the α/β ratio for prostate cancer is much lower than previously thought and that this formed a strong rationale for the use of high dose rate (HDR) to treat prostate cancer (Brenner and Hall, 1999 #11; King and Fowler, 2001; Fowler et al, 2001). For patients being treated with external-beam radiotherapy, a growing number of investigators are studying the use of larger doses per fraction in an attempt to shorten overall time and cost (Pickett et al, 1999). Because of day-to-day setup variation, some type of monitoring will probably be required to ensure that this can be carried out safely.

Brachytherapy

The term **brachytherapy** refers to a treatment technique that places radioactive sources in close proximity to or directly into the tumor. Brachytherapy can be classified as either interstitial or intracavity. Interstitial brachytherapy involves the placement of radioactive needles, afterloaded needles or catheters, or radioactive seeds directly into the prostate, bladder, penis, or periurethral soft tissues. Intracavitary brachytherapy includes placement of radioactive catheters into a lumen or orifice such as in the urethra to treat urethral and penile tumors. Permanent implants involve the use of radioactive seeds that are left in the patient. Nowadays temporary implants generally involve the use of needles or catheters that act as conduits for delivering radiation from high-activity seeds attached to a long wire. Most modern temporary implants are delivered using high dose rate (HDR) brachytherapy systems to deliver moderately high doses of radiation over a relatively short period of time (minutes). HDR brachytherapy is usually delivered over 2 or more treatment sessions to reduce the risk of late complications. Low dose rate brachytherapy is usually delivered in a continuous fashion over days to weeks via temporary or permanent implants, respectively. Figure 25–1 depicts an example of a transrectal ultrasound–based iodine-125 permanent interstitial implant of the prostate. Figure 25–2 shows an example of intracavitary brachytherapy for a urethral tumor in a female patient.

SPECIFIC UROLOGIC SITES

Prostate Cancer

Many urologists are aware that the radical perineal prostatectomy (RPP) approach was first used to completely remove the prostate in the 1800s (Bilroth, 1869). Unfortunately, the first 2 patients so treated died in 14 months or less. Few urologists are aware that radiotherapy was first used to successfully treat prostate cancer 100 years ago and that it was not until 1949 that Memmelaar first reported the successful use of the retropubic approach— the radical retropubic prostatectomy (RRP)—for treatment of prostate cancer (Memmelaar, 1949; Reiner and Walsh, 1979). The basic RRP is very much unchanged since his description and is probably still the most common approach used today. In the 1950s and 1960s it was believed that radiotherapy provided comparable results with less morbidity. However, in 1979 Walsh and Donker demonstrated the potential value of the RRP to preserve nerves (Walsh and Donker, 1982). Radical perineal prostatectomies became less fashionable in the 1980s after Walsh and others reported improvements in the RRP that promised to reduce blood loss, minimize the risk of incontinence, and preserve potency (Reiner and Walsh, 1979). With this advancement the RRP became the surgical approach of choice in the eyes of most urologists.

Figure 25–1. Brachytherapy. Example of an ultrasound-guided permanent interstitial implant of the prostate.

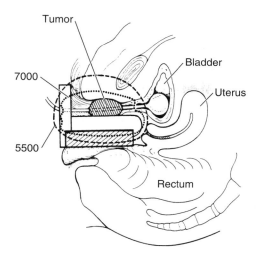

Figure 25–2. Example of intraluminal brachytherapy for urethral cancer. (Reproduced with permission from Sailer SL, Shipley WU, Wang CC: Carcinoma of the female urethra: A review of results with radiation therapy. J Urol 1988;140:1.)

A. CONVENTIONAL TREATMENT

Conventional external-beam radiotherapy (EBRT) has been used in the United States for treating prostate cancer for more than 35 years. From the late 1960s through the mid-1980s, definitive prostate radiation was delivered to the whole pelvis by using the "4-field box" technique, followed by a "cone down" prostate boost, popularized by Bagshaw and coworkers from Stanford University (Bagshaw et al, 1988). The placement of the treatment fields was based on bony anatomic landmarks. It is now known that this tech-

nique resulted in inadequate coverage of the target volume in nearly one-third of patients. Computed tomography has improved our ability to localize and reconstruct pelvic anatomy, allowing more accurate design of treatment portals.

Several retrospective and prospective studies support the efficacy of radiation therapy in the management of localized prostate cancer (Roach et al, 1999). Based on these studies, the local control rate following XRT has been estimated to be between 70% and 90%. The end points of these studies were based primarily on a clinical assessment of "local control." These end points are now known to underestimate the true incidence of local failures because of the presence of occult cancer in clinically controlled patients. Many patients whose disease was once thought to be controlled locally, according to physical examination, do in fact have persistent disease when assessed by prostate-specific antigen (PSA) or biopsy, or both (Crook et al, 2000). Although the post-treatment PSA is more sensitive, it is a less specific end point for treatment failure than is biopsy, because distant failures can contribute to a rising level. PSA has been long recognized as an acceptable end point for the assessment of disease status, but only recently has it been validated as a predictor of disease-specific survival (DSS) and overall survival (Roach et al, 2003b)

Table 25–2 summarizes patient characteristics and treatment outcomes for selected surgical and conventional radiotherapy series. It should be kept in mind, however, that in general patients treated with surgery tend to have lower Gleason scores and T stages, and many surgical series excluded lymph node-positive patients. When matched for pretreatment PSA, freedom from biochemical relapse at 5 years is not significantly different, suggesting similar efficacy for surgery and X-ray based radiotherapy (XRT) in the management of prostate cancer. There is a trend, however, for surgically

Table 25–2. Biochemical failure from selected surgical or radiotherapy series.

Pretreatment PSA	Surgical Aver. % (range)[a]	XRT Aver. % (range)[b]	Surgical b-NED 5 y[a]	XRT b-NED 5 y[b]	Comment
0–4	26 (15–43)	21 (11–33)	85–95	80–86	Patients treated with surgery usually were
4.1–10	41 (35–52)	30 (27–32)	55–93	42–67	not node-positive and tended to have
10–20	26 (16–32)	21 (18–22)	56	30–75	lower-grade and lower-stage tumors
> 20	13 (6–20)	35 (18–50)	—	45	than those treated with XRT.

Modified from Roach M, Wallner K: Prostate cancer. In: Leibel SA, Phillips TL (editors): *Textbook of Radiation Oncology.* Saunders, 1998.
β-NED, no evidence of disease based on biochemical failure; PSA, prostate-specific antigen; XRT, external-beam radiotherapy.
[a]Most series exclude node-positive patients and PSA failures > 0.2–0.6.
[b]Clinical staging includes only node-positive and T3–T4 patients and PSA failures > 1.0–4.0 or rising.

treated patients to have a slightly higher freedom from biochemical failure. This could be explained in part by the better parameters for surgical patients at the outset.

Table 25–3 summarizes some of the factors contributing to the risk of local failure following external-beam irradiation. Recent studies have demonstrated that traditional techniques were associated with inadequate coverage of the target volume in 20% to 41% of patients treated. Early series also routinely used total doses in the range of 65–70 Gy because it was believed that this dose was sufficient and close to the maximum dose allowable by the surrounding normal tissues. Another factor contributing to the data regarding biochemical relapse is that many of the patients had disease that was underestimated by physical examination, so they were incurable at the time of diagnosis.

An analysis of the long-term results from approximately 1500 men treated with XRT alone between 1980 and 1992 in one of 4 phase III randomized trials conducted by the Radiation Therapy Oncology Group (RTOG) has been completed (Roach, 2000a). In a multivariate analysis, Gleason score, clinical stage, and pathologic node status were correlated with overall survival and DSS. By combining patient groups with similar risk for DSS, 4 distinct prognostic subgroups have been defined with varying risk of death due to prostate cancer. Table 25–4 summarizes the estimated 5-, 10-, and 15-year DSS for each subgroup. These outcome data are likely to represent a worst-case scenario, since

the vast majority of these patients were treated before PSA screening. In addition, the patients for whom PSA levels were available had levels in the range of 20–30 ng/mL. Patients with lower PSAs treated with 3-D technology to higher doses are likely to do substantially better (Roach et al, 2003b).

The use of this risk stratification system to predict overall survival has been recently validated using contemporary patients (Roach et al, 2003a). Numerous other risk stratification schemes are currently in popular use by radiation oncologists in the management of prostate cancer (D'Amico et al, 2000; Kattan et al, 2001; Kattan et al, 2000; Ross and Scardino, 2001). Although these systems are more commonly used than the RTOG risk groups, in general to date they generally have not been shown to be predictive of overall survival or DSS (D'Amico, 2002). An additional benefit of the RTOG risk groups is their use in defining who and how long hormonal therapy should be used (Roach et al, 2000a).

Regarding **hormonal therapy and radiotherapy,** there currently exists no uniform consensus as to who should receive hormonal therapy and how long it should last. However, the best evidence suggests that low-risk patients do not benefit, intermediate-risk (T3 GS = 6 or T1–2 GS = 7) patients benefit from short-term hormonal therapy, and high-risk patients benefit from long-term hormonal therapy (Roach et al, 2000b). The standard for "short-term" hormonal therapy consists of combined androgen blockade using a luteinizing hormone-releasing hormone agent and an antiandrogen 2 months before (neoadjuvant) and 2 months during radiotherapy (Pilepich and Winter, 2001; Roach et al, 2000b; Roach et al, 2003b). Patients receiving hormonal therapy should probably also receive whole-pelvic radiotherapy. Patients with high-risk disease (T3 GS 7–10 or GS = 8–10) should receive neoadjuvant and concurrent hormonal therapy, but they should also receive long-term adjuvant hormonal therapy consisting of a luteinizing hormone-releasing hormone for 2–3 years (Roach et al, 2000; Bolla et al, 2002).

B. THREE-DIMENSIONAL CONFORMAL RADIOTHERAPY (3-DCRT) AND INTENSITY MODULATED RADIOTHERAPY (IMRT)

The technical problems mentioned in Table 25–3 have been addressed in several centers by the use of computed tomography–assisted localization and reconstruction of the pelvic anatomy. Beginning in the early 1990s, 3-DCRT began to be established as the new standard of care for treating clinically localized prostate cancer. This technology takes advantage of sophisticated imaging and computerized treatment planning software that allowed high-dose radiation to conform to

Table 25–3. Issues in risk of local failure following external-beam irradiation.

Explanations for the high local failure rate:
1. Inadequate target definitions.
   a. Field sizes too small or inferior border too high.
   b. Seminal vesicles not covered.
2. Inadequate doses of radiation.
   a. Doses limited by the belief that 65–70 Gy is sufficient for cure.
   b. Dose limited by technical difficulties and normal tissue tolerances.
3. Understanding of patients: patients with metastatic disease.

Solutions for the problems discussed:
1. Adequate target definitions: field designed conformally using 3-dimensional reconstructions of CT-based tumor volumes and urethrograms.
2. Adequate dose: higher doses of radiation to improve local control rate.
3. Better prestaging of patients: use of pretreatment PSA and Gleason score.

CT, computed tomography; PSA, prostate-specific antigen.

Table 25–4. Disease-specific survival by risk groups: Radiation Therapy Oncology Group randomized trials, radiotherapy alone (1975–1992).

Group[a]	Deaths/No.	5-Year (%)[b]	10-Year (%)[b]	15-Year (%)[b]
1	63/474	97 (95–99)	85 (81–89)	71 (61–81)
2	69/335	91 (88–94)	75 (69–81)	59 (49–69)
3	89/336	82 (78–86)	60 (52–68)	38 (21–55)
4	138/314	66 (60–72)	34 (26–42)	28 (19–37)

Modified from Roach M et al: Four prognostic groups predict long term survival from prostate cancer following radiotherapy alone in RT06 Clinical Trials. Int J Radiat Oncol Biol Phys 2000; 47(3):609.
[a]Group 1 had patients with a Gleason score (GS) = 2–5, any T stage, or T1–2Nx and GS = 6; group 2 had stage T3Nx, GS = 6, or any T stage, N+, GS = 6, or T1–2Nx, Gs = 7; group 3 had T3Nx, GS = 7, or any T stage, N+, GS = 7, or T1–2Nx, GS = 8–10; group 4 had T3Nx, GS = 8–10, or any T stage, N+, GS = 8–10.
[b]95% confidence intervals in parentheses.

the target volume with greater sparing of the surrounding normal tissues. Figure 25–3 is an example of the dose distribution associated with the use of several different types of IMRT. Figure 25–4A demonstrates a digitally reconstructed radiograph (DRR) from the treatment planning computed tomography and Figure 25–4B is a lateral port (treatment) film. The advantages provided by using improved imaging modality and treatment planning have resulted in the adoption of 3-DCRT by major centers as the new standard of care (Table 25–5) (Roach et al, 2000a). Because 3-DCRT

methods administer radiation to smaller volumes of normal tissue, they have the benefit of decreased side effects. This may in turn permit increased doses of radiation to be given and theoretically lead to improved local control.

In the mid 1990s, retrospective data from several centers suggested that PSA responses were improved with the use of higher doses of radiation in some subsets of patients. Early results from these studies suggest that 10% increases in dose may improve local control rates by as much as 20%. Based on these encouraging

A

B

Figure 25–3. Example of the dose distribution associated with the use of several different types of IMRT.

A   **B**

Figure 25–4. Example of a 7-field conformal external-beam irradiation technique for the treatment of prostate cancer. **A:** A digitally reconstructed radiograph (DRR) from the treatment planning CT. **B:** A lateral port (treatment) film.

Table 25–5. 3-DCRT and IMRT: Selected major prospective trials.

First Author (year)	Institution(s)	Type of Study	Conclusions
Dearnaley et al (1999)	United Kingdom, Medical Research Council	Prospective randomized phase III trial (n = 225)	Less late GI and GU toxicity with 3D compared to non-3D, but only 64 Gy delivered and 3D technology used for only a portion of the treatment.
Pollack et al (2002b)	MD Anderson	Prospective randomized phase III trial (n = 305) T1–3 randomized: 70 vs. 78 Gy	Patients with a PSA > 10 ng/mL benefited the most from the 78 Gy arm vs. 70 Gy (62% vs. 43%; $P = .01$). Rectal side effects were also greater with Grade 2 or higher toxicity rates at 6 years; rates were 12% and 26% for the 70 Gy and 78 Gy arms, respectively ($P = .001$).
Zelefsky et al (2002)	Memorial Sloan Kettering	Phase I–II including more (n = 772) patients treated with IMRT	After 81–86.4 Gy with IMRT, the 3-year risk of ≥ late Grade 2 rectal or urinary toxicity was 4% and 15%. The 3-year PSA relapse-free rates for low, intermediate, and high-risk patients were 92%, 86%, and 81%.
Ryu et al (2002)	RTOG (Radiation Therapy Oncology Group) Multi-institutional	Prospective phase I–II trial (n = 173)	Feasible to treat safely to higher than conventional dose of 79.2 Gy in a multi-institutional setting

3-DCRT, three-dimensional conformal radiotherapy; IMRT, Intensity Modulated Radiotherapy. From Roach M, HSU I-C: Fifteen year minimum follow-up of prostate brachytherapy series: Comparing the past with the present. Urology 2000; 56(3):439.

results, the RTOG A Large Phase I–II dose escalation study demonstrated that it was feasible in a multi-institutional environment to safely deliver higher than conventional doses without unacceptable toxicity (Ryu et al, 2002).

Although there appears to be no reduction in acute toxicity in patients treated with 3-DCRT compared to those receiving conventional radiotherapy, chronic rectal toxicity was reduced in patients treated with conformal radiotherapy and appears to be lower with 3-DCRT when the same dose is delivered (Dearnaley et al, 1999). When higher doses are given to the patients receiving 3-DCRT, late complications may be increased if the technique used is not sophisticated enough to compensate for the higher doses used (Pollack et al, 2002b). Biochemical failure rates appear to be improved, but no significant difference in local control or overall survival has been seen so far, although the follow-up is relatively short. A much larger phase III trial is being conducted by the RTOG (RTOG 0126) comparing results using 72.9or 83.2 Gy for "intermediate"-risk patients.

C. BRACHYTHERAPY

Alternative forms of radiation for the treatment of prostate cancer are growing in popularity. The most common of these alternative forms of radiation is brachytherapy. The major theoretic advantages with this form of radiation are the ability to deliver a very high dose of radiation to a localized area with a decreased number of treatment visits. The use of modern-era imaging techniques for visualizing the placement of radioactive seeds has obviated the need for open surgical procedures. Transrectal ultrasound–guided closed techniques are currently the standard. **Permanent implants** involve a lower dose rate of delivery but a higher total dose. **Temporary implants** generally involve a lower total dose but at a higher dose rate; hence the term "high dose rate" (HDR) brachytherapy. An example of an ultrasound-based iodine-125 permanent seed implant of the prostate, performed at our institution, is shown in Figure 25–1.

The failure rates reported in several older studies (done in the late 1960s and 1970s) suggested that the permanent implants are less effective than XRT. More recent series suggest that the results of permanent implants may be improved with the use of transrectal ultrasound, with long-term results equal to or better than other treatments (Blasko et al, 2002). Table 25–6 summarizes several studies that compared outcomes in patients treated with seed implants or XRT with or without radical prostatectomy. Four of the studies suggested that low-risk patients (stage ≤ T2a, PSA ≤ 10 ng/mL, GS ≤ 6) treated with seed implants had PSA outcomes

that were not statistically different from those treated with XRT. However, "intermediate"-risk and "high-risk" patients (PSA > 10, GS > 7) treated with radical prostatectomy or radiotherapy have better outcomes than those treated with implants alone (Seung et al, 1998; D'Amico et al, 1998; Brachman et al, 2000; Zelefsky et al, 1999). One study found that patients treated with seed implants fared better than those treated with XRT, but the patients treated with XRT in this series were high risk and received only 66 Gy.

At most centers, intermediate- and high-risk patients (groups 2, 3 and 4, Table 25–4) are treated with a combination of XRT and interstitial implant with or without hormonal therapy. Some clinicians routinely add XRT for all patients undergoing permanent seed implants (Critz et al, 2000). However, most brachytherapists agree that low-risk patients can be equally well treated without the additional cost or morbidity of EBRT (Potters et al, 2000; Robinson et al, 2002). Although proponents of prostate brachytherapy commonly believe that the morbidity associated with interstitial brachytherapy is less than that associated with 3-DCRT, most recent studies suggest that acute morbidity is greater with permanent implants, whereas long-term morbidity tends to be similar.

Temporary implants have the advantage of decreasing radiation exposure to hospital personnel and greater flexibility because of the ability to compensate for less than optimal needle placement. Temporary implants tend to be used for patients with more advanced disease in part because they are usually combined with EBRT and because HDR can be used to cover disease that is thought to be outside the gland. Iridium-192 is the only widely used isotope for temporary prostate implants. Based on the available data, in the hands of experts, it appears that HDR represents an excellent treatment option.

D. NEUTRONS, PROTONS, AND HEAVY-CHARGED PARTICLES

Eradication of tumor by radiation is believed to be dose dependent. Unfortunately, the dose beyond which no additional benefit is likely is unknown. 3-DCRT has 3 interrelated goals: (1) more accurate tumor targeting, (2) the safe delivery of higher doses of radiation to the tumor, and (3) diminishing of the normal tissue toxicity associated with high-dose radiation. Particle beam radiation is an alternative form of XRT. This class of radiation involves the use of heavy particles (eg, neutrons), charged particles (eg, protons), or heavy-charged particles (eg, neon). The theoretic advantage of proton-based radiotherapy is the potential for a more conformal dose distribution. The only prospective randomized trial completed to date showed a significant

Table 25–6. Selected series comparing permanent seed implants to conventional radiotherapy or surgery or both

First Author (year)	No. of Patients	Details	Conclusions
Seung (1998)	EBRT = 187	Patients treated with EBRT at UCSF who were candidates for BT compared to literature	Wide range of results overlapping with EBRT results
D'Amico (1998)	BT = 66, EBRT = 766, RT = 888	EBRT at Harvard vs Radical Retropubic Prostatectomy and BT at University of Penn	The outcome was similar for low risk, but intermediate and high-risk patients did worse with BT
King (1998)	BT = 63, EBRT = 85, RP = 73	Comparison of results from patients with T1/2 disease treated at Yale University	EBRT patients did the worse than RP or BT, but mean dose was only 66 Gy and higher risk than BT or RP patients
Beyer (2000)	BT = 695, EBRT = 1527	Retrospective study of large multi-physician practice.	Patients with GS > 7 or PSA > 10 ng/mL did significantly better with EBRT than BT
Krupski (2000)	BT = 70, EBRT + BT = 4, RP = 27	Retrospective quality of life survey.	Quality of life score worse in EBRT + BT patients; BT and RP were similar. Urinary symptoms score was worst with RP.
Brandeis (2000)	RP = 74, BT = 48	Compared HRQOL in men undergoing BT to RP and matched healthy controls.	Urinary leakage less in BT than in RP group but more irritative urinary symptoms and worse bowel function than controls. BT and EBRT worse in HRQOL domains than with BT alone.
Davis (2001)	BT = 122, EBRT = 188, RP = 220	Retrospective quality of life survey	HRQOL mostly unaffected by the treatment modality. EBRT had worse bowel "bothersomeness." RP had worse urinary and sexual function. Urinary symptoms score initially worse with BT but equal to other modalities after 12 months.
Lee (2001)	BT = 44, EBRT = 23, RP = 23	Prospective quality of life survey	HRQOL decreased in the first month after BT or RP but not after EBRT. No differences in the scores 12 months after treatment.

Modified from Roach M, HSU I-C: Fifteen year minimum follow-up of prostate brachytherapy series. Comparing the past with the present. Urology 2000; 56(3):439.

BT, permanent prostate brachytherapy; EBRT, external-beam radiotherapy; HRQOL, health-related quality of life; NSRP, nerve-sparing radical prostatectomy; PSA, prostate-specific antigen; RP, radical prostatectomy; UCSF, University of California, San Francisco.

improvement in local control in patients with high-grade tumors but no improvement in disease-free, relapse-free, or overall survival (Shipley et al, 1995). There was no benefit to other subsets of patients, and the 5-year actuarial rates of rectal bleeding were significantly higher ($P = .002$) with mixed beam treatment. Results from Loma Linda University Medical Center showed 4-year freedom from PSA relapse comparable to that for surgery and 3-DCRT (Slater et al, 1998).

The attractiveness of neutron-based radiotherapy relates to the relative lack of oxygen dependence. Heavy-charged particles are thought to have the advantages of both neutrons and protons. Early studies using this technology have been encouraging, but the series are small, follow-up is relatively short, and this equipment has limited availability. Longer follow-up studies will be required to assess the impact of these alternative types of radiation on long-term survival.

E. POSTOPERATIVE RADIOTHERAPY

The objective of postoperative radiotherapy is to improve local-regional control by eliminating microscopic residual tumor in the surgical bed, periprostatic tissues, and regional lymph nodes. As such, there are several indications for the use of adjuvant radiation, including (1) positive surgical margins, (2) seminal vesicle involvement, (3) lymph node involvement, (4) extracapsular extension, (5) increasing PSA, and (6) biopsy-proven recurrence. The presence of any of these variables is associated with a higher incidence of local recurrence. Adjuvant XRT appears to reduce the incidence of local recurrence in patients with postsurgical microscopic residual tumor after radical prostatectomy. Patients who are treated before clinically manifesting a local recurrence appear to have improved disease-free survival, time to distant metastasis, and freedom from biochemical relapse compared with patients undergoing salvage treatment (Nudell et al, 1999; Valicenti et al, 1999). Only 50% of such patients are successfully treated for biopsy-proven recurrence at 3 years (Rogers et al, 1998). Although definitive proof from a prospective randomized trial is lacking, it seems reasonable to assume that patients who have no other disease away from the pelvis would benefit from adjuvant treatment.

There is a common impression among some urologists that the risk of complications outweighs the benefits of adjuvant radiotherapy, but this impression is probably due to the consequence of older treatment techniques. More contemporary series suggest that, with modern equipment and 3-D planning, the incidence of complications is quite low.

F. COMPLICATIONS OF RADIOTHERAPY FOR PROSTATE CANCER

Most patients experience urinary frequency and dysuria during the course of their treatment. In patients receiving whole-pelvic irradiation, mild diarrhea may develop, but moderate to severe late complications are similar (Roach, 2003a). Mild, self-limited rectal bleeding occurs in approximately 10% of patients and is dose and volume related. Urinary incontinence is usually associated with a history of a prior transurethral resection of the prostate. Hematuria and ureteral strictures occur in less than 2% to 10% of patients and are usually mild and self-limited. Fecal incontinence is uncommon, but rectal urgency due to reduction in rectal distensibility may occur in 10% of patients (Litwin, 1994).

Loss of erectile function is the most worrisome, the most common, and the most permanent sequela of radiotherapy. Impotence is reported 35–40% of patients who were potent before treatment. Sexual dysfunction may be slightly lower after brachytherapy than after XRT (Robinson et al, 2002). However, most patients experience a decrease in the frequency and quality of intercourse, and most note a decrease in the volume of ejaculate. Potency diminishes further with time owing to aging and late radiation-induced normal tissue injury.

Acute urinary toxicity associated with brachytherapy is more common and longer lasting than that seen with 3-DCRT. The incidence of strictures is also higher. Acute obstruction occurs in 2–20% of patients. Although incontinence is quite uncommon following radiotherapy, it can occur in up to 50% of patients if they have had a previous transurethral resection of the prostate. The frequency of rectal toxicity following brachytherapy is generally believed to be less than that with external beam treatment 3-DCRT (Roach and Hsu, 2002).

Cancer of the Urinary Bladder

In 50% or more of cases, invasive bladder cancer is disseminated at diagnosis. Five-year survival rates up to 60% are reported for early invasive lesions (T1/T2a, N0); however, rates fall to ≤ 40% for more advanced tumors (T2b/T4,N+). Late systemic disease recurrence with or without local recurrence accounts for the decline in survival (Stein et al, 2001; Dalbagni et al, 2001). Following decades of unsuccessful single and bimodality treatments, contemporary management plans utilize combinations of cytotoxic chemotherapy, radiotherapy, and surgery in attempts to achieve organ preservation and improved survival.

A. RADIOTHERAPY MONOTHERAPY

Radical cystoprostatectomy remains the treatment standard for muscle invasive transitional cell carcinoma of the bladder in the United States. In contrast, radiotherapy is the more common primary treatment choice in Canada and Great Britain. Local control rates of up to 90% are achieved, though 5-year survival rates approximate 50% (Shipley et al, 1999; Geschwind et al, 2000; Parsons and Zlotecki, 1998). In the United States, definitive radiotherapy has been recommended for medically inoperable patients or patients deemed to be unsuitable for radical cystectomy due to disease extent. Radiotherapy yields poorer local control rates but comparable 5-year survival rates (average = 45%) when compared with cystectomy. Additionally, no significant difference in 5- and 10-year survival rates or rates of development of distant metastases is seen with delayed cystectomy performed as salvage versus immediate (primary) cystectomy (Horowich et al, 1995; Petrovich et al, 2001).

T stage, post–transurethral resection of bladder tumor disease residual, treatment duration, and complete tumor response to treatment are significant independent variables that predict for improved local control, disease free-survival, and survival with a functioning native bladder (Pollack and Zagars, 1996; Dunst et al, 2001). Hyperfractionated and accelerated fractionation schemes yield significant improvements in complete response rates and 5-year survival rates without significant increases in bowel toxicity (De Neve, Lybeert, and Goor, 1995; Hayter et al, 2000; Zeitman et al, 1998).

B. COMBINED-MODALITY THERAPY (PREOPERATIVE AND POSTOPERATIVE RADIOTHERAPY)

Randomized trials have not shown any disease-specific or overall survival benefits from precystectomy EBRT versus cystectomy alone (Cole et al,1995; Huncharek, Muscat, and Geschwind, 1998). Most studies, however, suffer from small sample sizes; compare pathologically and clinically staged patients, which leads to outcome bias favoring pathologically staged (cystectomy) patients; and utilize radiotherapy techniques that are inadequate by contemporary standards (Parsons and Zlotecki, 1998). Preoperative radiotherapy does result in significant T-stage and N-stage reduction in 75% and 50% of patients, respectively, and complete tumor response in 30–40% of patients on pathologic inspection of the surgical specimen at radical cystectomy. Postoperative radiotherapy is associated with unacceptably high complication rates with the administration of tumoricidal doses. The use of preoperative and postoperative radiotherapy results in improved 5-year survival rates but excessive small-bowel toxicity (Reisinger et al, 1992; Wijkstrom et al, 1998).

C. TRIMODALITY THERAPY: CONSERVATIVE SURGERY, CHEMOTHERAPY, AND RADIATION THERAPY

Multimodality therapy, which offers an attempt at organ preservation without compromising treatment outcomes, is the standard of care for many malignancies, including breast, esophageal, anorectal, and laryngeal cancer. The absence of inferior survival rates associated with delayed or salvage cystectomy made attempts at organ preservation for bladder cancer a reasonable endeavor. The approach of maximal transurethral resection of bladder tumors and induction chemoradiotherapy with consolidation chemoradiotherapy for complete responders yields long-term disease-free and overall survival rates and metastases-free survival rates equivalent to those achieved with "up-front" radical cystectomy: 40–63% at 5 years (Houssett et al, 1997; Nichols et al, 2000; Rodel et al, 2002; Shipley et al, 2003; Tester et al, 1996; Shipley et al, 1999; Zeitman and Shipley, 2000; Zeitman AL et al, 1998). Seventy to 80% of patients who are alive at 5 years after bladder-sparing treatment retain a well-functioning bladder. The incidence of cystectomy performed for bladder morbidity is extremely low (Zeitman et al, 2001).

Several cytotoxic agents have been evaluated for efficacy and safety when administered with radiotherapy. The timing of chemotherapy delivery has also been addressed. Combinations of cisplatin (CDDP)-based chemotherapy with 5-fluorouracil (5-FU), Taxol (paclitaxel), or gemcytabine (Gemzar) appear well suited for multimodality treatment for tolerability, radiosensitizing, and complementary cell-killing effects (Kaufman et al, 2000a, b; von der Maase et al, 2000). Randomized trials comparing neoadjuvant cytotoxic chemotherapy plus radiotherapy versus radiotherapy alone result in significant tumor downstaging but do not yield a survival benefit (Herr et al, 1998; Shipley et al, 1998; Zietman et al, 1998). Concurrent chemoradiation schedules offer the highest complete tumor response rates compared with sequential treatments.

In most patients who experience recurrence after bladder conservation, superficial disease in the region of previous cancer will develop. Superficial recurrences are successfully managed with TURBT and intravesical bacillus Calmette-Guérin, with success rates comparable to those achieved in de novo cases of Ta, Tis, or T1 tumors (Zeitman et al, 2001; Shipley et al, 1999; Dunst et al, 2001). Although no difference in overall survival is seen in patients in whom superficial relapse develops, the chance for 5-year survival with a native bladder is lower than for those in whom a recurrence does not develop. Invasive recurrences are managed with prompt cystectomy, without any compromise in survival.

Since only those patients who have a complete response to initial treatment are likely to experience sustained local control, careful patient selection based on prognostic factors is critical to achieve organ preservation without a compromise in survival.

D. BRACHYTHERAPY

Temporary interstitial brachytherapy, combined with EBRT, has been successfully used to treat patients with solitary muscle invasive lesions in some centers. However, in the absence of randomized prospective trials comparing treatment outcome and toxicity, EBRT cannot be considered a standard of care, and its use should probably be limited to centers with experienced and robust brachytherapy and multidisciplinary genitourinary oncology programs (Parsons and Zlotecki, 1998; Shipley et al, 1999; Wijnmaalen et al, 1997).

E. TREATMENT TOXICITY

Acute and chronic complications following combined-modality treatment for carcinoma of the urinary bladder are usually mild and managed symptomatically (Parsons and Zlotecki, 1998). Acute toxicities including enteritis and cystitis are common, occurring in 20–30% of patients. Chronic bladder discomfort or dysfunction occurs in approximately 10% of patients. With current radiotherapy techniques, symptomatic reduction of the bladder capacity is uncommon. Chronic, moderately severe rectal and small-bowel injuries are reported in 3–4% and 1–2%, respectively, of patients receiving high-dose radiotherapy (Parsons and Zlotecki, 1998). The mortality rate associated with radiotherapy is reported to be approximately 1%. More significant toxicity seems to stem from the combined use of cytotoxic chemotherapy and radiotherapy and predominantly affects the hematopoietic system.

Testicular Germ Cell Tumors (GCTs)

A. General Information

Testicular GCTs represent 1% of all malignancies occurring in men, with peak incidence of occurrence between the second and fourth decades of life (Greenlee et al, 2000; Parkin et al, 1992). Testicular GCTs are the most common tumors in men aged 15–35 and commonly present as a painless testicular mass or swelling. Men with a history of testicular maldescent have a 10–40 times greater risk of having cancer develop compared to men without this developmental history; both the ipsilateral and contralateral testes are at risk. Previous testicular cancer, vasectomy, hypospadias, hydrocele, immunosuppressed state, and horseshoe kidney are also associated with an increased risk of occurrence (Buetow, 1995; Liebovich et al, 1996). Additional associations with testicular GCTs have been noted for mumps orchitis, Kleinfelter syndrome, Down syndrome, and familial XY gonadal dysgenesis. Ninety percent of patients have been found to have isochrome of the short arm of chromosome 12, i(12p), and the presence of multiple copies has been correlated with a poorer prognosis (Sandberg et al, 1996; Atkin and

Baker, 1995). Seminoma accounts for 40% of testicular GCTs, occurs in slightly older men (median age, 33 years) than does nonseminoma testicular GCT, and is associated with elevations in serum β-hCG in 15% of cases. Nonseminoma GCTs (embryonal carcinoma, teratoma, choriocarcinoma, yolk sac tumor, and mixed GCT) comprise the remaining 60% of testicular tumors, peak at a slightly younger age (median age, 27 years), and are associated with elevations in β-hCG or alpha fetoprotein or both in 80% of cases.

B. Radiotherapy Treatment

Adjuvant radiotherapy has primarily been used in men with pure seminoma, to reduce the risk of local and regional recurrence in ipsilateral pelvic and para-aortic lymph nodes. Figures 25–5 and 25–6 show the incidence and location of nodal metastases in early-stage left- and right-sided testicular tumors.

1. Stage I (pT1–T3, N0, M0, S0) Seminoma— Equivalent disease-specific (97–99%) and overall survival rates have been demonstrated with postoperative surveillance and adjuvant radiotherapy, prompting the belief that surveillance is viable though a more costly treatment option (Sharda, Kinsella, and Eritter, 1996; Warde et al, 1997; Miki et al, 1998; Coleman et al, 1998). In most centers, however, postorchiectomy radiotherapy targeting the ipsilateral pelvic and para-aortic lymph nodes remains the standard of care. Because not

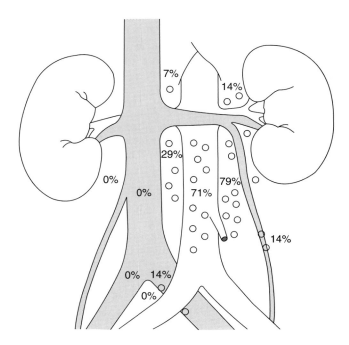

Figure 25–5. Incidence and location of lymph nodes at risk for an early-stage left-sided testicular seminoma. (Adapted from Donohue JP et al: Distribution of nodal nets in nonseminomatous testis cancer. J Urol 1982;126:315.)

Figure 25–6. Incidence and location of lymph nodes at risk for an early-stage right-sided testicular seminoma. (Adapted from Donohue JP et al: Distribution of nodal nets in nonseminomatous testis cancer. J Urol 1982;126:315.)

all patients elect to use or are suitable candidates for surveillance protocols, more recent interest has focused on tailoring radiotherapy treatment fields and using single-agent chemotherapy as a treatment alternative. The observation that most postorchiectomy relapses during surveillance occur in the para-aortic rather than the pelvic lymph nodes (84–89%) has led to treatment directed solely to the retroperitoneal nodes. With limited follow-up, survival rates appear equivalent to those achieved with the larger treatment volume. Pelvic surveillance should be included as part of this treatment plan (Fossa et al, 1999; Kiricuta, Sauer, and Bohndort, 1996; Logue et al, 2000; Sultanem et al, 1998). The objectives of limited-field irradiation are to minimize infertility, small-bowel toxicity, and the risk of secondary malignancy (Travis et al, 1997). Studies investigating adjuvant single-agent cisplatin (400 mg/m^2) have shown this approach to be well tolerated, with very low recurrence rates (Oliver et al, 1994; Dieckmann et al, 2000). The British Medical Research Council has an ongoing phase III trial comparing chemotherapy and para-aortic irradiation. Shorter overall treatment time and minimal gonadal morbidity are cited as advantages of this paradigm. Pathologic features associated with an increased risk of relapse must be considered when making treatment recommendations. They include anaplastic histology, tunicae invasion, lymphovascular invasion, extension beyond the rete testis, age ≤ 34 years at diagnosis, and tumor size > 6 cm (Warde et al, 1997; Warde and Gospodarowicz, 1998). Doses of 25 Gy are considered to be sufficient for the control of microscopic disease and yield cause-specific survival rates of 99–100% (Thomas, 1990). Higher doses are not associated with an increase in cause-specific survival but are associated with increased normal tissue toxicity. A summary of radiotherapy and management guidelines for testicular seminoma is shown in Table 25–7.

2. Stage II (pT1–3, N1–3, M0, S0-1) Seminoma— The use of adjuvant irradiation in stage II depends on the size of the retroperitoneal nodal disease. Patients with nodal masses ≤ 5 cm (IIA–IIB) receive radiotherapy to the para-aortic and ipsilateral pelvic lymph nodes, yielding cause-specific survival rates of 95–100%. Doses of 25 Gy to the pelvis and para-aortic nodes with a 10-Gy boost to the nodal masses are acceptable (Warde and Gospodarowicz, 1998). Patients with bulky retroperitoneal nodal disease (> 5 cm, IIC) have high rates of distant relapse. Adjuvant management consists of 4 cycles of cisplatin-containing multiagent chemotherapy, followed by observation for persistent nodal masses. Residual disease < 3 cm may be closely observed, treated with radiotherapy, or surgically resected. Masses ≥ 3 cm should be resected.

Radiotherapy plays no role in the management of stage III seminoma.

Radiotherapy has no established role in the management of any stage of nonseminoma testicular GCT

Table 25–7. Summary of radiotherapy guidelines for seminomas.

Stage	Post-XRT Relapses (%)	Recommended Volume Irradiated	Dose Recommended (Gy)
Stage I–IIA (< 2 cm)	2–4	Para-aortic and ipsilateral renal hilar nodes	25
Stage IIB (2–5 cm) (Nonpalpable)	4	Ipsilateral pelvic and para-aortic nodes	25–35
Stage IIC (5–10 cm)	10	(Chemotherapy alone)	25–35
Stage IID (> 10 cm)	50	(Chemotherapy alone)	

Modified and reproduced, with permission, from Rorth BJ et al and the Danish Testicular Cancer Group. Surveillance alone versus radiotherapy after orchiectomy for clinical stage I nonseminomatous testicular cancer. J Clin Oncol 1991; 9:1543. XRT, external-beam irradiation.

other than for palliation or the management of brain metastases (Thomas and Williams, 1998).

C. COMPLICATIONS OF RADIOTHERAPY

Acute sequelae of low-dose para-aortic irradiation are mild, consisting primarily of nausea, dry desquamation and erythema of the skin, and a transient reduction in spermatogenesis (Thomas and Williams, 1998). Late complications are uncommon, including temporary impairment of spermatogenesis (2–3 years), a small but measurable increase in the risk of secondary leukemia and solid tumors within the first 10 years after treatment, and an increased risk of gastrointestinal complications (Fossa et al, 1999; Thomas and Williams, 1998; Travis et al, 1997).

Carcinomas of the Kidney, Renal Pelvis, & Ureter

Surgery is the primary treatment for renal cell carcinoma. Two prospective randomized trials of postoperative radiotherapy did not demonstrate any survival advantage for patients treated with adjuvant radiation. It may be reasonable to use radiotherapy as the initial management in patients who have inoperable tumors or are unsuitable surgical candidates or for treatment of possible surgical margins. Several series suggest that radiotherapy is of value in the postoperative setting for carcinomas of the kidney, particularly when they are high grade and accompanied by invasion beyond the primary tumor into fat or nodes (Brookland and Richter, 1985; Babaian, Johnson, and Chan, 1980; Brady and Manning, 1981).

Retrospective data suggest that radiotherapy may increase local control when used in the adjuvant setting in patients with locally advanced (T3, T4) carcinoma of the renal pelvis or ureter or in lymph node-positive disease (Brookland and Richter, 1985).

Cancer of the Female Urethra

A. ANTERIOR URETHRA

Both EBRT and brachytherapy are comparable alternatives to surgical resection of early-stage urethral cancers. Early lesions in the distal one-third of the urethra may be treated with brachytherapy alone or with combined EBRT and interstitial implants. Radiation alone is associated with high local control rates, cure rates of 80–90%, and an overall 5-year survival in excess of 65%. For larger lesions, or lesions that extend into surrounding structures, preoperative EBRT radiation to the inguinal, external iliac, and hypogastric nodes is recommended (Grigsby, 1998b). Doses of 45–50 Gy are delivered to clinically uninvolved nodes, with an additional 10–15 Gy boost to any involved nodes. A total dose of 60–70 Gy is delivered to the tumor through reduced fields. An example of an intracavitary technique for a urethral tumor is shown in Figure 25–2.

B. POSTERIOR URETHRA

Lesions involving the posterior urethra often involve the bladder and have a high incidence of nodal involvement. Locally advanced tumors are managed with preoperative radiotherapy and exenteration. If feasible, early lesions are treated with resection and postoperative EBRT or EBRT alone. Local control rates of 20–30% and correspondingly low 5-year survival rates are noted (Grigsby, 1998b). Preoperative EBRT doses are typically in the range of 45–50 Gy. Definitive and postoperative doses deliver 45–50 Gy to the pelvis and clinically uninvolved nodes, with an additional 10–15 Gy boost to involved nodes. A total dose of 60 Gy is delivered to the entire surface of the vaginal mucosa and brachytherapy is employed to deliver a final tumor dose of 70–80 Gy (Grigsby, 1998a).

Urethral strictures are the most frequently reported complication. Urinary incontinence, cystitis, and vaginal atrophy and stenosis may occur. Fistulas and small-bowel obstruction due to radiation or tumor are uncommon.

Cancer of the Penis & Male Urethra

Surgery has been the primary management choice for penile cancer. Although quite effective, neither a partial nor a total penectomy is a desirable therapeutic choice. Because of the rarity of penile cancer, no randomized trials comparing various treatment options have been or are likely to be completed. High success rates achievable with surgical salvage have made attempts at organ preservation with the use of radiation alone possible. Similarly, the relative paucity of cases has precluded the development of standardized radiotherapy management; a minimum dose of 60–65 Gy is needed for control of the primary tumor. Careful patient selection is important, with optimal candidates described as having distal, well to moderately well-differentiated tumors that are ≤ 4 cm in diameter.

Both EBRT and interstitial brachytherapy may be used to treat penile lesions. If not previously performed, circumcision is required prior to radiotherapy treatment. Small superficial lesions of the glans and distal shaft may be treated with orthovoltage or low-energy electron beams. Larger, invasive lesions of the penis, penile urethra, and bulbous urethra are managed with EBRT alone or EBRT followed by an interstitial implant boost. Brachytherapy is required to achieve doses to the primary greater than 65 Gy. Prophylactic irradiation of the bilateral inguinal and pelvic lymph nodes to 45–50 Gy accompanies management of the primary for all but the most superficial lesions. Palpable and clinically suspicious nodes receive 65–70 Gy. Local failure rates of 15–37% have been reported (Chao and Perez, 1998; Sarin et al, 1997).

Lesions of the prostatic urethra are managed in a manner similar to that of prostate cancer.

Local failure rates of 15–37% are reported following radiation for penile cancer (Chao and Perez, 1998; Rozan et al, 1995; Sarin et al, 1997). The higher risk of systemic failure associated with urethral tumors results in 5-year survival rates of 55% and 15% for distal and proximal urethral tumors, respectively (Heysek et al, 1985). Neoadjuvant chemotherapy and radiotherapy, with surgery reserved for salvage, is one strategy for more advanced lesions (Husein, Benedetto, and Sridhar, 1990; Eisenberger, 1992).

Regarding **treatment toxicity,** acute, transient sequelae include brisk, moist desquamation of the skin of the penis, urinary frequency, urgency, dysuria, nocturia, and intermittent diarrhea. The risk of soft tissue necrosis, fibrosis, and paraphimosis are dose-limiting sequelae for penile irradiation. Urethral or meatal stricture or both are the most common complication of penile and urethral irradiation and are dose and technique dependent. Symptomatic strictures are managed with urethral dilation, with urethrotomy reserved for severe cases. Although sexual activity is almost uniformly interrupted during the course of treatment, most patients maintain full or slightly diminished potency after radiotherapy (Opjordsmoen and Fossa, 1994).

CONCLUSION

Table 25–8 provides a brief summary of the role for EBRT in the management of urologic malignancies. Despite the lack of scientifically rigorous studies, the available data suggest that a close working relationship between the urologist and the radiation oncologist is likely to ensure that patients with urologic tumors have the maximum probability of being rendered free of cancer.

Table 25–8. Summary of primary sites and roles for external-beam irradiation.

Primary Site	Definitive Irradiation Alone	Prophylactic Lymphatic Irradiation	Adjuvant Irradiation Following Surgery
Prostate	+++/++	+/–	+++ Positive margins following prostatectomy
Bladder	++	+	+/–
Kidney	–	+/–	+/–
Renal pelvis	–	+/–	+/–
Ureter	–	+/–	+/–
Testis seminoma	–	+++	
Testis non-seminoma	–	–	–
Penis	+++[a]	+/–	+++
Urethra (male)	+++[a]	+/–	++
Urethra (female)	+++[a]	+/–	++

+++ = Highly effective; ++ = effective; + = effective–marginally effective; +/– = unknown; – = not indicated.
[a]Refers to early lesions.

REFERENCES

General, Radiobiology, & Prostate Cancer

Bagshaw MA et al: Status of prostate cancer at Stanford University. NCI Monogr 1988;7:47.

Bedford JL et al: Optimization of coplanar six-field techniques for conformal radiotherapy of the prostate. Int J Radiat Oncol Biol Phys 2000;46(1):231.

Bilroth T: Carcinoma der Prostata. Chir Erfahrungen, Zurich, 1860–67. Archiv Fur Klinische Chirugie Bd 1869;X:548.

Blasko JC et al: Brachytherapy for carcinoma of the prostate: Techniques, patient selection, and clinical outcomes. Semin Radiat Oncol 2002;12(1):81.

Bolla M et al: Long-term results with immediate androgen suppression and external irradiation in patients with locally advanced prostate cancer (an EORTC study): A phase III randomised trial. Lancet 2002;360(9327):103.

Brachman DG et al: Failure-free survival following brachytherapy alone or external beam irradiation alone for T1–2 prostate tumors in 2222 patients: Results from a single practice. Int J Radiat Oncol Biol Phys 2000;48(1):111.

Brenner DJ, Hall EJ: Fractionation and protraction for radiotherapy of prostate carcinoma. Int J Radiat Oncol Biol Phys 1999;43(5number):1095.

Critz FA et al: Simultaneous irradiation for prostate cancer: Intermediate results with modern techniques. J Urol 2000;164(3 Pt 1):738, discussion 741.

Crook J et al: Postradiotherapy prostate biopsies: What do they really mean? Results for 498 patients. Int J Radiat Oncol Biol Phys 2000;48(2number):355.

D'Amico AV et al: Biochemical outcome after radical prostatectomy external beam radiation therapy or interstitial radiation therapy for clinically localized prostate cancer. JAMA 1998;280:969.

D'Amico AV et al: Clinical utility of the percentage of positive prostate biopsies in defining biochemical outcome after radical prostatectomy for patients with clinically localized prostate cancer. J Clin Oncol 2000;18(6):1164.

D'Amico AV et al: Determinants of prostate cancer-specific survival after radiation therapy for patients with clinically localized prostate cancer. J Clin Oncol 2002;20(23):4567.

Dearnaley DP et al: Comparison of radiation side-effects of conformal and conventional radiotherapy in prostate cancer: a randomised trial. Lancet 1999;353(9149):267.

Forman JD et al: Comparison of hyperfractionated conformal photon with conformal mixed neutron/photon irradiation in locally advanced prostate cancer. Bulletin du Cancer Radiotherapie 1996;83(Suppl 2):101.

Fowler J et al: Is alpha/beta for prostate tumors really low? Int J Radiat Oncol Biol Phys 2001;50(4):1021.

Kattan MW et al: Pretreatment nomogram for predicting freedom from recurrence after permanent prostate brachytherapy in prostate cancer. Urology 2001;58(3number):393.

Kattan MW et al: Pretreatment nomogram for predicting the outcome of three-dimensional conformal radiotherapy in prostate cancer. J Clin Oncol 2000;18(19number):3352.

King CR, Fowler JF: A simple analytic derivation suggests that prostate cancer alpha/beta ratio is low. Int J Radiat Oncol Biol Phys 2001;51(1number):213.

Kutcher GJ et al: Histogram reduction method for calculating complication probabilities for three-dimensional treatment planning evaluations. Int J Radiat Oncol Biol Phys 1991; 21(number):137.

Langen KM, Jones DT: Organ motion and its management. Int J Radiat Oncol Biol Phys (2001);50(1): 265.

Litwin MS: Measuring health related quality of life in men with prostate cancer. J Urol 1994;152(5 Pt 2):1882.

Memmelaar J: Total prostatovesiculectomy-retropubic approach. J Urol (1949);62:340.

Nudell DM et al: Radiotherapy after radical prostatectomy: treatment outcomes and failure patterns. Urology 1999;54 (6):1049.

Nutting CM et al: Potential improvements in the therapeutic ratio of prostate cancer irradiation: dose escalation of pathologically identified tumour nodules using intensity modulated radiotherapy. Br J Radiol 2002;75(890):151.

Parker CC et al: Pre-treatment nomogram for biochemical control after neoadjuvant androgen deprivation and radical radiotherapy for clinically localised prostate cancer. Br J Cancer 2002;86(5):686.

Pasteau O, Degrais P: The radium treatment of cancer of prostate. Arch Roentgen Ray 1914;18:396.

Pickett B et al: Static field intensity modulation to treat a dominant intra-prostatic lesion to 90 Gy compared to seven field 3-dimensional radiotherapy. Int J Radiat Oncol Biol Phys 1999; 44(4):921.

Pilepich MV et al: Phase III radiation therapy oncology group (RTOG) trial 86-10 of androgen deprivation adjuvant to definitive radiotherapy in locally advanced carcinoma of the prostate. Int J Radiat Oncol Biol Phys (2001;50(5):1243.

Pollack A et al: Preliminary results of a randomized radiotherapy dose-escalation study comparing 70 Gy with 78 Gy for prostate cancer. J Clin Oncol 2000;18(23):3904.

Pollack A et al: Prostate biopsy status and PSA nadir level as early surrogates for treatment failure: Analysis of a prostate cancer randomized radiation dose escalation trial. Int J Radiat Oncol Biol Phys 2002a;54(3):677.

Pollack A et al: Prostate cancer radiation dose response: Results of the M. D. Anderson phase III randomized trial. Int J Radiat Oncol Biol Phys 2002b;53(5):1097.

Potters L et al: Permanent source brachytherapy for prostate cancer. American College of Radiology. ACR Appropriateness Criteria. Radiology 2000;215(Suppl):1383.

Reiner WB, Walsh PC: An anatomical approach to the surgical management of the dorsal vein and Santorini's plexus during radical retropubic surgery. J Urol 1979;121:198.

Roach M, Hsu I-C: Fifteen year minimum followup of prostate brachytherapy series: Comparing the past with the present. Urology 2000;56(3):439.

Roach M et al: The "Critical Volume Tolerance Method" for estimating the limits of dose escalation during three-dimensional conformal radiotherapy for prostate cancer. Int J Radiat Oncol Biol Phys 1996;35:1019.

Roach M et al: Four Prognostic Groups Predict Long Term Survival From Prostate Cancer Following Radiotherapy Alone on Radiation Therapy Oncology Group Clinical Trials. Int J Radiat Oncol Biol Phys 2000a;47:609.

Roach M III et al: Long-term survival after radiotherapy alone: Radiation therapy oncology group prostate cancer trials. J Urol 1999;161(3):864.

Roach M et al: A phase III trial comparing whole pelvic versus prostate only radiotherapy and neoadjuvant concurrent versus adjuvant combined androgen suppression: Radiation Therapy Oncology Group (RTOG) (2003a);9413. J Clin Oncol (In Press).

Roach M et al: Predicting long term survival, and the need for hormonal therapy: A meta-analysis of RTOG prostate cancer trials. Int J Radiat Oncol Biol Phys (2000b);47:617.

Roach M et al: Serum prostate specific antigen (PSA) and survival following external beam radiotherapy for carcinoma of the prostate. Urology (2003b. (In Press).

Roach M III et al: Treatment planning for clinically localized prostate cancer. American College of Radiology. ACR Appropriateness Criteria. Radiology 2000c;215 Suppl:1441.

Robinson JW et al: Meta-analysis of rates of erectile function after treatment of localized prostate carcinoma. Int J Radiat Oncol Biol Phys 2002;54(4):1063.

Rogers R et al: Radiation therapy for the management of biopsy-proven, local recurrence following radical prostatectomy. J Urol 1998;160:1748.

Ross PL et al: A catalog of prostate cancer nomograms. J Urol 2001;165(5):1562.

Ryu JK et al: Interim report of toxicity from 3D conformal radiation therapy (3D-CRT) for prostate cancer on 3DOG/RTOG 9406, level III (79.2 Gy). Int J Radiat Oncol Biol Phys 2002;54(4):1036.

Seung KS et al: Candidates for prostate radioactive seed implantation treated by external beam radiotherapy. Cancer J Sci Am 1998 4(3):168.

Shipley WU et al: Advanced prostate cancer: The results of a randomized comparative trial of high dose irradiation boosting with conformal protons compared with conventional dose irradiation using photons alone. Int J Radiation Oncology Biol Phys 1995;32:3.

Sklar G: Combined antitumor effect of suramin plus irradiation in human prostate cancer cells: The role of apoptosis. J Urol 1993;150:1526.

Slater JD et al: Conformal proton therapy for prostate carcinoma. Int J Radiat Oncol Biol Phys 1998;42(2):299.

Storey MR et al: Complications from radiotherapy dose escalation in prostate cancer: Preliminary results of a randomized trial. Int J Radiat Oncol Biol Phys 2000;48(3):635.

Valicenti RK et al: The efficacy of early adjuvant radiation therapy for pT3N0 prostate cancer: A matched-pair analysis. International J Radiat Oncol Biol Phys 1999;45(1):53.

Walsh PC, Donker PJ: Impotence following radical prostatectomy: Insight into etiology and prevention. J Urol 1982;128:492.

Zelefsky MJ et al: Comparison of the 5-year outcome and morbidity of three-dimensional conformal radiotherapy versus transperineal permanent iodine-125 implantation for early stage prostate cancer. J Clin Oncol 1999;17:517.

Zelefsky MJ et al: High-dose intensity modulated radiation therapy for prostate cancer: Early toxicity and biochemical outcome in 772 patients. Int J Radiat Oncol Biol Phys 2002;53(5):1111.

Zietman AL: The case for neoadjuvant androgen suppression before radiation therapy. Mol Urol 2000;4(3):203; discussion 215.

Bladder Cancer

Cole DJ et al: Local control of muscle invasive bladder cancer: Preoperative radiotherapy and cystectomy versus cystectomy alone. Int J Radiat Oncol Biol Phys 1995;32:331.

Dalbagni G et al: Cystectomy for bladder cancer: A contemporary series. J Urol 2001;165:1111.

De Neve W, Lybeert ML, Goor C: Radiotherapy for T2 and T3 carcinoma of the bladder: The influence of overall treatment time. Radiother Oncol 1995;26:183.

Dunst J et al: Bladder preservation in muscle-invasive bladder cancer by conservative surgery and radiotherapy. Semin Surg Oncol 2001;20:24.

Geschwind JE et al: Radical cystectomy for invasive bladder cancer: Contemporary results and remaining controversies. Eur Urol 2000;38:121.

Hayter CR et al: The management and outcome of bladder carcinoma in Ontario 1982–1994. Cancer 2000;89(1):142.

Hayter CR et al: A population based study of the use and outcome of radical radiotherapy for invasive bladder cancer. Int J Radiat Oncol Biol Phys 1999;45:1239.

Herr HW et al: Neoadjuvant chemotherapy and bladder sparing surgery for invasive bladder cancer: 10 year outcome. J Clin Oncol 1998;16:1298.

Horowich A et al: Organ conservation in bladder cancer. Eur J Cancer Suppl 1995;31:208.

Housset M et al: Concomitant 5-fluorouracil, cisplatin and bifractionated split course radiation therapy for invasive bladder cancer. Proc Am Soc Clin Oncol 1997;16:319a.

Huncharek M, Muscat J, Geschwind JF: Planned preoperative radiation therapy in muscle invasive bladder cancer: Results of a meta-analysis. Anticancer Res 1998;18:1931.

Kaufman DS et al: Phase II trial of gemcytabine plus cisplatin in patients with metastatic urothelial cancer. J Clin Oncol 2000a;18:1921.

Kaufman DS et al: Gemcytabine and paclitaxel every two weeks: A multi-center phase II trial in locally advanced or metastatic urothelial cancer. Proc Am Soc Clin Oncol 2000b;19:1341 (abstr #1341).

Nichols RC et al: Radiation therapy and concomitant paclitaxel/carboplatin chemotherapy for muscle-invasive transitional cell carcinoma of the bladder: A well tolerated combination. Int J Cancer 2000;90:281.

Parsons JT, Zlotecki RA: Bladder. In: Perez CA, Brady LW (editors): *Principles and Practice of Radiation Oncology,* 3rd ed. Lippincott-Raven, 1998.

Petrovich Z et al: Radiotherapy for carcinoma of the bladder. Am J Clin Oncol 2001;24:1.

Pollack A, Zagars GZ: Radiotherapy for stage T3b transitional cell carcinoma of the bladder. Semin Urol Oncol 1996;14:86.

Reisinger SA et al: Combined pre and postoperative adjuvant radiation therapy for bladder cancer: A ten year experience. Int J Radiat Oncol Biol Phys 1992;24(3):463.

Rodal C et al: Combined modality treatment and selective organ preservation in invasive bladder cancer: Long-term results. J Clin Oncol 2002;20(4):3061.

Shipley WU et al: An update of combined modality therapy for patients with muscle invading bladder cancer using selective bladder preservation or cystectomy. J Urol 1999;162:445.

Shipley WU et al: Overview of bladder cancer trials in the Radiation Therapy Oncology Group. Cancer 2003;97(8 Suppl):2115.

Shipley WU et al: Phase III trial of neoadjuvant chemotherapy in patients with invasive bladder cancer treated with selective bladder preservation by combined radiation therapy and chemotherapy: Initial results of radiation therapy oncology group 89-03. J Clin Oncol 1998;16:3576.

Stein JP et al: Radical cystectomy in the treatment of invasive bladder cancer: Long-term results in 1054 patients. J Clin Oncol 2001;19:666.

Tester W et al: Neoadjuvant combined modality program with selective organ preservation for invasive bladder cancer: Results of Radiation Therapy Oncology Group phase II trial 8802. J Clin Oncol 1996;14:119.

Von der Maase H et al: Gemcytabine and cisplatin versus methotrexate, vinblastine, doxorubicin and cisplatin in advanced or metastatic bladder cancer: Results of a large randomized, multinational, multicenter, phase III study. J Clin Oncol 2000;18:3068.

Warde P, Gospodarowicz MK: New approaches in the use of radiation therapy in the treatment of infiltrative transitional-cell cancer of the bladder. World J Urol 1997;15:125.

Wijkstrom H et al: Evaluation of clinical staging before cystectomy transitional cell bladder carcinoma: A long-term follow-up of 276 consecutive patients Br J Urol 1998;81:686.

Wijnmaalen A et al: Muscle invading bladder cancer treated by transurethral resection followed by external beam radiation and interstitial iridium-192. Int J Rad Oncol Biol Phys 1997;39:1043.

Zeitman AL, Shipley WU: Organ-conserving approaches to muscle invading bladder cancer: Alternatives to the radical cystectomy in the new century. Ann Intern Med 2000;32:34.

Zietman A et al: A phase I/II trial of transurethral surgery combined with concurrent cisplatin, 5-fluorouracil and twice daily radiation followed by selective bladder preservation in operable patients with muscle invading bladder cancer. J Urol 1998;160:1673.

Zeitman AL et al: Selective bladder conservation using transurethral resection, chemotherapy and radiation: Management and consequences of Ta, T1 and Tis recurrence within the retained bladder. Urology 2001;58(3):380.

Testicular Cancer

Atkin N, Baker M: High chromosome numbers of testicular germ cell tumours. Cancer Genet Cytogenet 1995;88:90.

Buetow SA: Epidemiology of testicular cancer. Epidemiol Rev 1995;17:433.

Chao CK et al: Secondary malignancy among seminoma patients treated with adjuvant radiation therapy. Int J Radiat Oncol Biol Phys 1995;33:831.

Coia LR, Hanks GE: Complications from large field intermediate dose infradiaphragmatic radiation: An analysis of the Patterns of Care outcome studies for Hodgkin's disease and seminoma. Int J Radiat Oncol Biol Phys 1988;15:29.

Coleman JM et al: The management and clinical course of testicular seminoma: 15 years' experience at a single institution. Clin Oncol 1998;10:237.

Dieckmann KP et al: Adjuvant treatment of clinical stage I seminoma is a single course of carboplatin sufficient? Urology 2000;55(1):102.

Fossa SD et al: Optimal planning target volume for stage I testicular seminoma: A Medical Research Council randomized trial. J Clin Oncol 1999;17:1146.

Greenlee RT et al: Cancer Statistics, 2000. CA Cancer J Clin 2000;50:7.

Horowich A, Dearnaley DP: Treatment of seminoma. Semin Oncol 1992;19:171.

Kiricuta IC, Sauer J, Bohndort W: Omission of the pelvic irradiation in stage I testicular seminoma: A study of post-orchiectomy paraaortic radiotherapy. Int J Radiat Oncol Biol Phys 1996;35:293.

Lai PP et al: Radiation therapy for stage I and IIA testicular seminoma. Int J Radiat Oncol Biol Phys 1994;28:373.

Liebovich I et al: Malignant testicular neoplasms in immunosuppressed patients. J Urol 1996;155:1938.

Logue JP et al: Paraaortic radiation for stage I seminoma of the testis. Int J Radiat Oncol Biol Phys 2000;48(Suppl):208.

Miki T et al: Long-term results of adjuvant irradiation or surveillance for stage I testicular seminoma. Int J Urol 1998;5:357.

Oliver RTD et al: Pilot studies of 2 and 1 course carboplatin as adjuvant for stage I seminoma: Should it be tested in a randomized trial against radiotherapy? Int J Radiat Oncol Biol Phys 1994;29:3.

Parkin D et al: Cancer Incidence in five continents. Comparability and quality of data. IARC Sci Publ 1992;120:45.

Rorth BJ et al and the Danish Testicular Cancer Group: Surveillance alone versus radiotherapy after orchiectomy for clinical stage I nonseminomatous testicular cancer. J Clin Oncol 1991;9:1543.

Rorth M: Therapeutic alternatives in clinical stage I non-seminomatous disease. Semin Oncol 1992;19:190.

Sandberg AA et al: Reviews of chromosome studies in urologic tumors III. Cytogenetics and genes in testicular tumors. J Urol 1996;155:1531.

Shapiro E, Kinsella TI, Makuch RW: Effects of fractionated irradiation on endocrine aspects of testicular function. J Clin Oncol 1985;3:1232.

Sharda NN, Kinsella TI, Ritter MA: Adjuvant radiation versus observation: A cost analysis of alternate management schemes in early stage testicular seminoma. J Clin Oncol 1996;14:2933.

Sultanem K et al: Para-aortic irradiation only appears to be adequate treatment for patients with stage I seminoma of the testis. Int J Radiat Oncol Biol Phys 1998;40:455.

Thomas GM: Consensus statement on the investigation and management of testicular seminoma. In: Newling DW, Jones WG (editors): Prostate Cancer and Testicular Cancer (EORTC Genitourinary Group Monograph 7). Wiley-Liss, 1990.

Thomas GM: Controversies in the management of testicular seminoma. Cancer 1985;55:2298.

Thomas GM, Williams SD: Testis. In: Perez CA, Brady LW (editors): Principles and Practice of Radiation Oncology, 3rd ed. Lippincott-Raven, 1998.

Travis LB et al: Risk of second malignant neoplasms among long-term survivors of testicular cancer. J Natl Cancer Inst 1997;89(19):1429.

Warde P, Gospodarowicz M: Management of stage II seminoma. J Clin Oncol 1998;16:290.

Warde P et al: Prognostic factors for relapse in stage I testicular seminoma treated with surveillance. J Urol 1997;157:1705.

Zagars GK, Babaian RJ: The role of radiation in stage II testicular seminoma. Int J Radiat Oncol Biol Phys 1987;13:163.

Cancer of the Kidney, Renal Pelvis, & Ureter

Babaian RJ, Johnson DE, Chan RC: Combination nephroureterectomy and postoperative radiotherapy for infiltrative ureteral carcinoma. Int J Radiat Oncol Biol Phys 1980;6:1229.

Brady LW, Manning DM: The role of radiation therapy in primary carcinoma of the ureter. In: Berman H (editor): *The Ureter,* 2nd ed. Springer-Verlag, 1981.

Brookland RK, Richter MP: The postoperative irradiation of transitional cell carcinoma of the renal pelvis and ureter. J Urol 1985;133:952.

Michalski JM: Kidney, Renal pelvis and ureter. In: Perez CA, Brady LW (editors): *Principles and Practice of Radiation Oncology,* 3rd ed. Lippincott-Raven, 1998.

Cancer of the Female Urethra

Grigsby PW: Carcinoma of the urethra in women. Int J Radiat Oncol Biol Phys 1998a;41:535.

Grigsby PW: Female urethra. In: Perez CA, Brady LW (editors): *Principles and Practice of Radiation Oncology,* 3rd ed. Lippincott-Raven, 1998b.

Cancer of the Penis & Male Urethra

Chao KS, Perez CA: Penis and male urethra. In: Perez CA, Brady LW (editors): *Principles and Practice of Radiation Oncology,* 3rd ed. Lippincott-Raven, 1998.

Eisenberger MA: Chemotherapy for carcinomas of the penis and urethra. Urol Clin North Am 1992;2:333.

Heysek RV et al: Carcinoma of the male urethra. J Urol 1985;134:753.

Husein AM, Benedetto P, Sridhar KS: Chemotherapy with cisplatin and 5-fluorouracil for penile and urethral squamous cell carcinomas. Cancer 1990;65:433.

Kaushal V, Sharma SC: Carcinoma of the penis: A 12-year review. Acta Oncol 1987;26:413.

Krieg RM, Luk KH: Carcinoma of the penis: Review of cases treated by surgery and radiation therapy 1960–1970. Urology 1981;18:149.

Opjordsmoen S, Fossa SD: Quality of life in patients treated for penile cancer: A follow-up study. Br J Urol 1994;74(5):652.

Sagerman RH et al: External beam irradiation of carcinoma of the penis. Radiology 1984;152:183.

Sarin R et al: Treatment results and prognostic factors in 101 men treated for squamous cell carcinoma of the penis. Int J Radiat Oncol Biol Phys 1997;38(4):713.

Srinivas V, Khan SA: Male urethral cancer: A review. Int Urol Nephrol 1988;20:61.

Neuropathic Bladder Disorders

26

Emil A. Tanagho, MD, & Tom F. Lue, MD

The urinary bladder is probably the only visceral smooth-muscle organ that is under complete voluntary control from the cerebral cortex. Normal bladder function requires coordinated interaction of sensory and motor components of both the somatic and autonomic nervous systems. Because many levels of the nervous system are involved in the regulation of voiding function, neurologic diseases often cause changes in bladder function. Examples are multiple sclerosis, spinal cord injury, cerebrovascular disease, Parkinson disease, diabetes mellitus, meningomyelocele, and amyotrophic lateral sclerosis. Injury to the sacral roots or pelvic plexus from spinal surgery, herniation of an intervertebral disk, or pelvic surgery (hysterectomy, abdominoperineal resection) can also cause neuropathic bladder.

Significant bladder dysfunction may occur as a result of poor voiding habits in childhood or of degenerative changes in bladder muscle and nerve endings caused by aging, inflammation, or anxiety disorders. All the above conditions can disrupt efficient reflex coordination between sphincter and bladder, and with time, this leads to symptomatic dysfunction.

■ NORMAL VESICAL FUNCTION

ANATOMY & PHYSIOLOGY

The Bladder Unit

The bladder wall is composed of a syncytium of smooth-muscle fibers that run in various directions; near the internal meatus, however, 3 layers are distinguishable: a middle circular layer and inner and outer longitudinal layers. In females the outer layer extends down the entire length of the urethra, while in males it ends at the apex of the prostate. The muscle fibers become circular and spirally oriented around the urethra junction and thus function as part of the smooth-muscle sphincter. The middle circular layer ends at the internal meatus of the bladder and is most developed anteriorly. The inner layer remains longitudinally oriented and reaches the distal end of the urethra in females and the apex of the prostate in males. The convergence of these muscle fibers forms a thickened bladder neck, which functions as the internal sphincter.

The normal bladder is able to distend gradually to a capacity of 400–500 mL without appreciable increase in intravesical pressure. When the sensation of fullness is transmitted to the sacral cord, the motor arc of the reflex causes a powerful and sustained detrusor contraction and urination if voluntary control is lacking (as in infants). As myelinization of the central nervous system progresses, the young child is able to suppress the sacral reflex so that he or she can urinate when it is appropriate.

The functional features of the bladder include (1) a normal capacity of 400–500 mL, (2) a sensation of fullness, (3) the ability to accommodate various volumes without a change in intraluminal pressure, (4) the ability to initiate and sustain a contraction until the bladder is empty, and (5) voluntary initiation or inhibition of voiding despite the involuntary nature of the organ.

The Sphincteric Unit

In both males and females, there are 2 sphincteric elements: (1) an internal involuntary smooth-muscle sphincter at the bladder neck, and (2) an external voluntary striated-muscle sphincter from the prostate to the membranous urethra in males and at the mid urethra in females.

The bladder neck sphincter is a condensation of smooth muscle of the detrusor. This area is rich in sympathetic innervation. Active contraction of the bladder neck region occurs simultaneously with seminal emission, just before ejaculation. In the filling phase, the bladder neck remains closed to provide continence. It opens during both spontaneous contraction and contraction induced by stimulation of the pelvic nerve, indicating that it can be pulled open by contraction of the longitudinal muscles.

The external sphincter is composed of slow-twitch, small striated muscle fibers. This voluntary sphincter maintains a constant tonus and is the primary continence mechanism. While the resting tone is maintained by the slow-twitch intrinsic muscle, it can be voluntarily increased by contraction of the striated muscles of the pelvic floor (eg, levator ani), which contain both fast- and slow-twitch fibers. The levator muscles also contribute indirectly to continence through support of the bladder base. Weakness of the pelvic floor may impair the efficiency of the closure mechanism of the otherwise normal bladder and sphincter. During abdominal straining, the diaphragm and abdominal muscles contract, and the increased abdominal pressure is transmitted to add to the intravesical pressure. A reflex contraction of the pelvic musculature together with transmitted abdominal pressure helps to close the urethra and prevent stress incontinence.

Relaxation of the sphincter is mostly a voluntary act without which voiding is normally inhibited. Failure to initiate sphincteric relaxation is a mechanism of urinary retention often seen in children with dyssynergic voiding. In infancy, the detrusor behaves in an uninhibited fashion. As the central nervous system matures, children learn to suppress or enhance the micturition reflex through voluntary contraction or relaxation of the pelvic musculature.

The Ureterovesical Junction

The function of the ureterovesical junction is to prevent backflow of urine from the bladder to the upper urinary tract. Longitudinal muscle from the ureter contributes to the makeup of the trigone. Stretching of the trigone has an occlusive effect on the ureteral openings. During normal detrusor contraction, the increased pull on the ureters prevents reflux of urine. Conversely, the combination of detrusor hypertrophy and trigonal stretch owing to residual urine can significantly obstruct the flow of urine from the ureters into the bladder.

INNERVATION & NEUROPHYSIOLOGY

Nerve Supply

The lower urinary tract receives afferent and efferent innervation from both the autonomic and somatic nervous systems. The parasympathetic innervation originates in the second to fourth sacral segments. The cholinergic postganglionic fibers supply both the bladder and smooth muscle sphincter. The sympathetic nerves originate at T10–L2. The noradrenergic postganglionic fibers innervate the smooth muscles of the bladder base, internal sphincter, and proximal urethra. Somatic motor innervation originates in S2–3 and travels to the striated urethral sphincter via the pudendal nerve. Some motor neurons to the tonic small muscle fibers of the striated sphincter may also project through the pelvic nerve (Gosling and Dixon, 1990).

There are both somatic and visceral afferents from the bladder and urethra. The somatic afferent is carried by the pudendal nerve, while the visceral afferent projects through the sympathetic and parasympathetic nerves to their respective spinal areas.

The normal afferent pathway is mediated largely by A-delta fibers, which send information about the state of bladder fullness to the pontine micturition center.

After spinal disruption, a different type of afferent pathway emerges, mediated by capsaicin-sensitive C-fibers that drive a spinal segmental reflex pathway, causing neurogenic detrusor overactivity. The common sources of afferent information for either pathway are likely to be afferents from the urothelium, lamina propria, and afferents that originate in the bladder wall (Fowler, 2002). On the other hand, the thoracolumbar visceral afferents may transmit discomfort and pain (Janig and Koltzenburg, 1993).

The Micturition Reflex

Intact reflex pathways via the spinal cord and the pons are required for normal micturition. Afferents from the bladder are essential for the activation of the sacral center, which then causes detrusor contraction, bladder neck opening, and sphincteric relaxation. The pontine center, through its connection with the sacral center, may send either excitatory or inhibitory impulses to regulate the micturition reflex. Electrical or chemical stimulation of the neurons in the medial pontine micturition center generates contraction of the detrusor and relaxation of the external sphincter. Disruption of pontine control, as in upper spinal cord injury, leads to contraction of the detrusor without sphincteric relaxation (detrusor-sphincter dyssynergia).

In pathologic conditions affecting the urethra (eg, urethritis or prostatitis) or the bladder (eg, cystitis or obstructive hypertrophy), uninhibited detrusor contraction may occur because of facilitation of the micturition reflex (Figure 26–1).

The Storage Function

The external sphincter plays an important role in urine storage. The afferents from pelvic and pudendal nerves activate both the sacral and lateral pontine center; this enhances sphincteric contraction while suppressing the parasympathetic impulse to the detrusor. Voluntary tightening of the sphincter can also inhibit the urge to urinate. In addition, activation of sympathetic nerves increases urethral resistance and facilitates bladder storage (Figure 26–2).

Cerebral (Suprapontine) Control

Although micturition and urine storage are primarily functions of the autonomic nervous system, these are under voluntary control from suprapontine cerebral centers, so that other groups of muscles (arm, leg, hand, bulbocavernosus) can be integrated to assist in urination at the appropriate time and place. Cerebral lesions (eg, from tumor, Parkinson disease, vascular accident) are known to affect the perception of bladder sensation and result in voiding dysfunction.

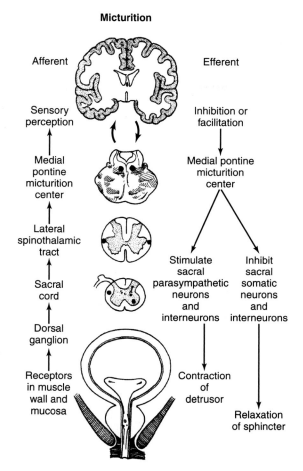

Figure 26–1. Afferent and efferent pathways and central nervous system centers involved in micturition.

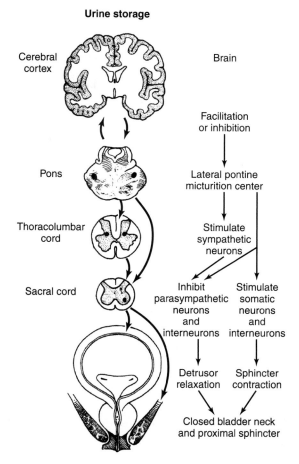

Figure 26–2. Pathways and central nervous system centers involved in urine storage.

Neurotransmitters & Receptors

In parasympathetic innervation, acetylcholine and nicotinic receptors mediate pre- to postganglionic transmission, while acetylcholine and M_2 muscarinic receptors mediate the postganglionic neuron–smooth muscle transmission. In some species, adenosine triphosphate (ATP) is released with acetylcholine and acts on purinoceptors (P_2) in the smooth-muscle cell. In sympathetic nerves, noradrenaline can act on the beta-2-adrenoreceptors to relax the detrusor or the alpha-1 receptors to contract the bladder neck and the external sphincter.

In addition, many neuropeptides, which usually colocalize with the classic transmitters, are also found in the genitourinary tract. Neuropeptide Y, encephalin, and vasoactive intestinal polypeptide (VIP) are found in cholinergic postganglionic neurons, while calcitonin gene-related peptide (CGRP), VIP, substance P, cholecystokinin, and encephalins are distributed in sacral visceral afferent fibers. These peptides are thought to be involved in modulation of efferent and afferent neurotransmissions.

URODYNAMIC STUDIES (See also Chapter 27)

Micturition

Urodynamic studies are techniques used to obtain graphic recordings of activity in the urinary bladder, urethral sphincter, and pelvic musculature. The 3 current methods involve use of gas or water to transfer pressure to a transducer housed near a polygraph or use of a transducer-tipped catheter to transfer pressure recordings directly to a polygraph. All the techniques have limitations, with gas being the least reliable of the three. Pressure recordings may be complemented by electromyography of the perineal musculature, ultrasound, or radiography (Figure 26–3).

Uroflowmetry

Uroflowmetry is the study of the flow of urine from the urethra. Uroflowmetry is best performed separately from all other tests and, whenever possible, as a standard office screening or monitoring procedure. The normal peak flow rate for males is 20–25 mL/s and for females 20–30 mL/s. Lower flow rates suggest outlet obstruction or a weak detrusor; higher flow rates suggest bladder spasticity or excessive use of abdominal muscles to assist voiding. Intermittent flow patterns generally reflect spasticity of the sphincter or straining to overcome resistance in the urethra.

Cystometry

Cystometry is the urodynamic evaluation of the reservoir function of the bladder. Cystometry is most informative when combined with studies of the external urethral sphincter and pelvic floor.

Normal bladder capacity is 400–500 mL. Bladder pressure during filling should remain low up to the point of voiding. The first desire to void is generally felt when the volume reaches 150–250 mL, but detrusor filling pressure should remain unchanged until there is a definite sense of fullness at 350–450 mL, the true capacity of the bladder. Detrusor contractions before this point are considered abnormal and the result of hyperreflexic or uninhibited behavior. Normal voiding pressures in the bladder should not rise above 30 cm of water pressure. With normal voiding there should not be any residual urine, and voiding should be accomplished without straining.

Urethral Pressure Recordings

Normal voiding requires a synergic action of the bladder (contraction) and urethra (relaxation). High pressures in the bladder during voiding reflect abnormal resistance in the urethral outlet. Increased outlet resistance can result from benign prostatic hypertrophy, urethral stricture, bladder neck contracture, or spasm of the external urethral sphincter. Low resistance in the urethral outlet generally reflects compromised function of the sphincter mechanism. Recording of urethral pressures with the bladder at rest as well as during contraction helps determine the presence of functional or anatomic disorders.

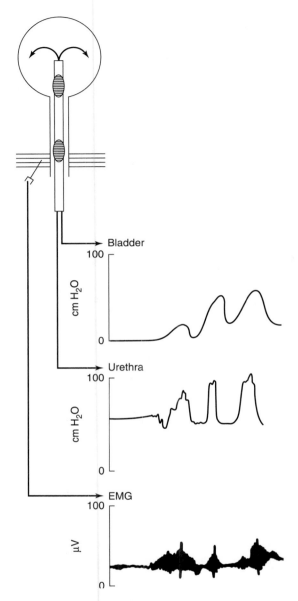

Figure 26–3. Simultaneous recording of bladder and urethral pressure as well as electromyographic recording of the external sphincter. Note the dyssynergic response. With bladder contraction there is increased activity in the external sphincter and pelvic floor, as recorded by the intraurethral pressure and electromyogram tracings.

Electromyography

With electromyography, the activity of the striated urethral muscles can be monitored without obstructing the urethral lumen. In the normal urethra, activity increases slightly as the bladder fills and falls precipitously just before voiding begins. Denervation results in an overall decrease in activity as well as production of denervation potentials. An overall increase in activity reflects a state of hyperreflexia. The technique provides a sensitive assessment of urethral and pelvic muscle behavior. The disadvantages of the technique are dependence on accurate needle position and a tendency to record artifacts.

■ ABNORMAL VESICAL FUNCTION

CLASSIFICATION OF NEUROPATHIC BLADDER

The traditional classification was according to neurologic deficit. Thus, the terms motor, spastic, upper motor neuron, reflexic, and uninhibited were used to describe dysfunction found with injury above the spinal cord micturition center. Coordination between the bladder and the sphincter was considered either balanced or unbalanced. The terms flaccid, atonic, areflexic, and sensory were used to describe loss of ability of the bladder to contract owing to injury of the pelvic nerves or the spinal micturition center. Dysfunction with both types of features was described as mixed.

Descriptions of neuromuscular dysfunction of the lower urinary tract should be individualized because no 2 neural injuries (no matter how similar) result in the same type of dysfunction. The standardization committee for the International Continence Society has attempted to create a functional classification that is easy to understand and provides a simple basis for therapy (Table 26–1).

1. Neuropathic Bladder Due To Lesions Above the Sacral Micturition Center

Most lesions above the level of the cord where the micturition center is located will cause bladder spasticity. Sacral reflex arcs remain intact, but loss of inhibition from higher centers results in spastic bladder and sphincter behavior on the segmental level. The degree of spasticity varies between the bladder and sphincter, from lesion to lesion, and from patient to patient with similar lesions. Common lesions found above the brain stem

Table 26–1. Various classifications of neuropathic bladder.

International Continence Society
  Detrusor: Normal (N), hyperreflexic (+), hyporeflexic (–)
  Striated sphincter: Normal (N), hyperactive (+), incompetent (–)
  Sensation: Normal (N), hypersensitive (+), hyposensitive (–)
Bors and Comarr
  Sensory neuron lesion
  Motor neuron lesion (balanced or unbalanced)
  Sensory-motor neuron lesion
    Upper motor neuron lesion
    Lower motor neuron lesion
    Mixed upper and lower motor neuron lesion
Nesbit, Lapides, and Baum
  Sensory neuron lesion
  Motor neuron lesion
  Unihibited bladder
  Reflex bladder
  Autonomous bladder
Krane
  Detrusor hyperreflexia
    Coordinated sphincters
    Striated muscle dyssynergia
    Smooth muscle dyssynergia
  Detrusor areflexia
    Coordinated sphincters
    Nonrelaxing striated sphincter
    Denervated striated sphincter
    Nonrelaxing smooth sphincter
Wain, Benson, and Raezer
  Failure to empty
  Failure to store

that affect voiding include dementia, vascular accidents, multiple sclerosis, tumors, and inflammatory disorders such as encephalitis or meningitis. These lesions can produce a wide range of functional changes, including precipitate urge, frequency, residual urine, retention of urine, recurrent urinary tract infections, and gross incontinence. Symptoms range from mild to disabling. Obviously, incontinence is especially troublesome. If the lesion is above the pontine micturition center, detrusor–striated sphincter dyssynergia usually does not occur. However, leakage may occur because the need to void cannot be felt or because the sphincter becomes more relaxed and can no longer inhibit spontaneous voiding. Lesions of the internal capsule include vascular accidents and Parkinson disease. Both spastic and semiflaccid voiding disorders are found with these lesions.

Spinal cord injury can be the result of trauma, herniated intervertebral disk, vascular lesions, multiple sclerosis, tumor, syringomyelia, or myelitis, or it may be iatrogenic. Traumatic spinal cord lesions are of greatest clinical concern. Partial or complete injuries may cause equally severe genitourinary dysfunction. Sphincter spasticity and voiding dyssynergia can lead to detrusor hypertrophy, high voiding pressures, ureteral reflux, or ureteral obstruction. With time, renal function may become compromised. If infection is combined with back pressure on the kidney, loss of renal function can be particularly rapid.

Spinal cord injuries at the cervical level are often associated with a condition known as autonomic dysreflexia. Because the lesions occur above the sympathetic outflow from the cord, hypertensive blood pressure fluctuations, bradycardia, and sweating can be triggered by insertion of a catheter, mild overdistention of the bladder with filling, or dyssynergic voiding.

In summary, the spastic neuropathic bladder is typified by (1) reduced capacity, (2) involuntary detrusor contractions, (3) high intravesical voiding pressures, (4) marked hypertrophy of the bladder wall, (5) spasticity of the pelvic striated muscle, and (6) autonomic dysreflexia in cervical cord lesions.

2. Neuropathic Bladder Due To Lesions at or Below the Sacral Micturition Center

Injury to the Detrusor Motor Nucleus

The most common cause of flaccid neuropathic bladder is injury to the spinal cord at the micturition center, S2–4. Other causes of anterior horn cell damage include infection due to poliovirus or herpes zoster and iatrogenic factors such as radiation or surgery. Herniated disks can injure the micturition center but more commonly affect the cauda equina or sacral nerve roots. Myelodysplasias could also be grouped here, but the mechanism is actually failure in the development or organization of the anterior horn cells. Lesions in this region of the cord are often incomplete, with the result commonly being a mixture of spastic behavior with weakened muscle contractility. Mild trabeculation of the bladder may occur. External sphincter and perineal muscle tone are diminished. Urinary incontinence usually does not occur in these cases because of the compensatory increase in bladder storage. Because pressure in the bladder is low, little outlet resistance is needed to provide continence. Evacuation of the bladder may be accomplished by straining, but with variable success.

Injury to the Afferent Feedback Pathways

Flaccid neuropathic bladder also results from a variety of neuropathies, including diabetes mellitus, tabes dorsalis, pernicious anemia, and posterior spinal cord lesions. Here the mechanism is not injury of the detrusor motor nucleus but a loss of sensory input to the detrusor nucleus or a change in motor behavior due to loss of neurotransmission in the dorsal horns of the cord. The end result is the same. Loss of perception of bladder filling permits overstretching of the detrusor. Atony of the detrusor results in weak, inefficient contractility. Capacity is increased and residual urine significant.

In summary, the flaccid neuropathic bladder is typified by (1) large capacity, (2) lack of voluntary detrusor contractions, (3) low intravesical pressure, (4) mild trabeculation (hypertrophy) of the bladder wall, and (5) decreased tone of the external sphincter.

Injury Causing Poor Detrusor Distensibility

Another cause of atonic neuropathic bladder is peripheral nerve injury. This category includes injury caused by radical surgical procedures such as low anterior resection of the colon or Wertheim hysterectomy. This type of dysfunction has been referred to as autonomous because the smooth muscle remains active but there is no central reflex to organize muscle activity. The end result is a bladder that stores poorly owing to failure to accommodate with filling. There is a rather steep pressure rise in the bladder with filling due to hypertonicity in the detrusor wall.

Radiation therapy can result in denervation of the detrusor or the sphincter. More commonly, it damages the detrusor, resulting in fibrosis and loss of distensibility. Other inflammatory causes of injury to the detrusor include chronic infection, interstitial cystitis, and carcinoma in situ. These lesions produce a fibrotic bladder wall that, for obvious reasons, distends poorly.

Selective Injury to the External Sphincter

Pelvic fracture often tears the nerves to the external sphincter. Selective denervation of the external sphincter muscle, with incontinence, can follow if the bladder neck is not sufficiently competent. Radical surgery in the perineum is highly unlikely to damage the motor innervation to the urethra, although sensory innervation of the external sphincter can be affected.

SPINAL SHOCK & RECOVERY OF VESICAL FUNCTION AFTER SPINAL CORD INJURY

Immediately following severe injury to the spinal cord or conus medullaris, regardless of level, there is a stage of flaccid paralysis, with numbness below the level of the injury. The smooth muscle of the detrusor and rectum is affected. The result is detrusor overfilling to the point of overflow incontinence and rectal impaction.

Spinal shock may last from a few weeks to 6 months (usually 2–3 months). Reflex response in striated muscle is usually present from the time of injury but is suppressed. With time, the reflex excitability of striated muscle progresses until a spastic state is achieved. Smooth muscle is much slower to develop this hyperreflex activity and, unlike striated muscle, loses spontaneous response after the injury. Urinary retention is the rule, therefore, in the early months following injury.

Urodynamic studies are indicated periodically to monitor the progressive return of reflex behavior. In the early recovery stages, a few weak contractions of the bladder may be found. Later, in injuries above the micturition center, more significant reflex activity will be found. Low pressure storage can be managed via intermittent catheterization. High pressure storage should be addressed early to avoid problems with the upper urinary tract.

A seldom used but valuable test is instillation of ice water. A strong detrusor contraction in response to filling with cold saline (3.3 °C [38 °F]) is one of the first indications of return of detrusor reflex activity. This test is of value in differentiating upper from lower motor neuron lesions early in the recovery phase.

Activity of the bladder after the spinal shock phase depends on the site of injury and extent of the neural lesion. With upper motor neuron (suprasegmental) lesions, there is obvious evidence of spasticity toward the end of the spinal shock phase (eg, spontaneous spasms in the extremities, spontaneous leakage of urine or stool, and, possibly, the return of some sensation). A plan of management can be made at this time. A few patients will retain the ability to empty the bladder reflexively by using trigger techniques, that is, by tapping or scratching the skin above the pubis or external genitalia. More often, detrusor hyperreflexia must be suppressed by anticholinergic medication to prevent incontinence. Evacuation of urine can then be accomplished by intermittent catheterization. Although incomplete lesions are more amenable to this approach than complete lesions, 70% of complete lesions ultimately can be managed using this program. Patients who cannot be managed in this way can be evaluated for sphincterotomy, dorsal rhizotomy, diversion, augmentation, or a pacemaker procedure.

In cases of lower motor neuron (segmental or infrasegmental) lesions, it is difficult to distinguish spinal shock from the end result of the injury. Spontaneous detrusor activity cannot be elicited on urodynamic evaluation. If the bladder is allowed to fill, overflow incontinence will occur. Striated muscle reflexes will be suppressed or absent. The bladder may be partially emptied by the Credé maneuver (ie, by manually pushing on the abdomen above the pubic symphysis) or, preferably, by intermittent catheterization.

DIAGNOSIS OF NEUROPATHIC BLADDER

The diagnosis of a neuropathic bladder disorder depends on a complete history and physical (including neurologic) examination, as well as use of radiologic studies (voiding cystourethrography, excretory urography, computed tomography scanning, magnetic resonance imaging, when necessary); urologic studies (cystoscopy, ultrasound); urodynamic studies (cystometry, urethral pressure recordings, uroflowmetry); and neurologic studies (electromyography, evoked potentials). Patients should be reevaluated often as recovery progresses.

1. Spastic Neuropathic Bladder

Spastic neuropathic bladder results from partial or extensive neural damage above the conus medullaris (T12). The bladder functions on the level of segmental reflexes, without efficient regulation from higher brain centers.

Clinical Findings

A. SYMPTOMS

The severity of symptoms depends on the site and extent of the lesion as well as the length of time from injury. Symptoms include involuntary urination, which is often frequent, spontaneous, scant, and triggered by spasms in the lower extremities. A true sensation of fullness is lacking, although vague lower abdominal sensations due to stretch of the overlying peritoneum may be felt. The major nonurologic symptoms are those of spastic paralysis and objective sensory deficits.

B. SIGNS

A complete neurologic examination is most important. The sensory level of the injury needs to be established, followed by assessment of the anal, bulbocavernosal, knee, ankle, and toe reflexes. These reflexes vary in degree of hyperreflexia on a scale of 1–4. Levator muscle tone and anal tone should be gauged separately, also on a scale of 1–4. Bladder volumes in established lesions are usually less than 300 mL (not infrequently, < 150 mL) and cannot be detected by abdominal percussion. Ultrasound can be a useful, rapid means of determining bladder capacity. Voiding often can be triggered by stimulation of the skin of the abdomen, thigh, or genitalia, often with spasm of the lower extremities.

With high thoracic and cervical lesions, distention of the bladder (due to a plugged catheter or during cystometry or cystoscopy) can trigger a series of responses, including hypertension, bradycardia, headache, piloerection, and sweating. This phenomenon is known as **autonomic dysreflexia.** It is triggered by pelvic autonomic afferent activity (overdistention of bowel or bladder, erection) and somatic afferent activity (ejaculation, spasm of lower extremities, insertion of a catheter, dilation of the external urethral sphincter). The headache can be severe and the hypertension life-threatening. Treatment must be immediate. Inserting a catheter and leaving the catheter on open drainage usually quickly reverses the dysreflexia.

C. Laboratory Findings

Virtually all patients experience one or more urinary tract infections during the recovery phase of spinal shock. This is due to the necessity of catheter drainage, either intermittent or continuous. Urinary stasis, prolonged immobilization, and urinary tract infections predispose to stone formation. Renal function may be normal or impaired, depending on the efficacy of treatment and the absence of complications (hydronephrosis, pyelonephritis, calculosis). Red blood cells (erythrocytes) in the urine may reflect a number of abnormalities. Uremia will result if complications are not addressed appropriately and the patient is not checked at regular intervals.

D. X-Ray Findings

Periodic excretory urograms and retrograde cystograms are essential because complications are common. A trabeculated bladder of small capacity is typical of this type of neuropathic dysfunction. The bladder neck may be dilated. The kidneys may show evidence of pyelonephritic scarring, hydronephrosis, or stone disease. The ureters may be dilated from obstruction or reflux. A voiding film often clearly outlines a narrowed zone created by the spastic sphincter but may also identify a strictured segment of the urethra. Most, if not all, of these features can be detected with ultrasound. Magnetic resonance imaging is especially useful for the sagittal view it offers of the bladder neck and posterior urethral zones.

E. Instrumental Examination

Cystoscopy and panendoscopy help assess the integrity of the urethra and identify stricture sites. The bladder shows variable degrees of trabeculation, occasionally with diverticula. Bladder capacity, stones, competency of the ureteral orifices, changes secondary to chronic infection or indwelling catheters, and the integrity of the bladder neck and external urethral sphincter can be assessed.

F. Urodynamic Studies

Combined recording of bladder and urethral sphincter activity during filling will reveal a low-volume bladder with spastic dyssynergy of the external sphincter (Figure 26–4). High voiding pressures in the bladder are not unusual. Ureteral reflux or obstruction is more likely if voiding pressures exceed 40 cm of water. A high resting pressure is noted in the external sphincter on the urethral pressure profile, and labile spastic behavior is noted during filling and voiding. Various auras replace a true sense of bladder filling, for example, sweating, vague abdominal discomfort, spasm of the lower extremities. Movement of a catheter in the urethra can trigger detrusor contraction and voiding.

2. Mildly Spastic Neuromuscular Dysfunction

Incomplete lesions of the cerebral cortex, pyramidal tracts, or spinal cord may weaken, but not abolish, cerebral restraint. The patient may have frequency and nocturia or urinary incontinence due to precipitous urge or voiding. Common causes include brain tumors, Parkinson disease, multiple sclerosis, dementias, cerebrovascular accidents, prolapsed disks, or partial spinal injury.

In many cases, the cause is unclear. The hyperreflexic behavior often seems to be associated with a peripheral abnormality (eg, prostatitis, benign prostatic hypertrophy, urethritis) or follows pelvic surgery (eg, anterior colporrhaphy, anteroposterior tumor resection). Symptoms are commonly associated with psychological factors.

Clinical Findings

A. Symptoms

Frequency, nocturia, and urgency are the principal symptoms. Hesitancy, intermittency, double voiding, and residual urine are also common. Incontinence may vary from pre- or postvoiding dribbling to complete

Figure 26–4. Spinal cord injury at T12. Simultaneous recording of intravesical and urethral pressure with bladder filling. Note the rise in intravesical pressure associated with unstable activity of the external sphincter, as reflected on the urethral pressure tracing.

voiding that the patient does not recognize or cannot inhibit once started.

B. SIGNS

The degree of voiding dysfunction does not parallel neurologic deficits. Slight physical disabilities can be associated with gross disturbances in bladder function, and the reverse is also true. However, it is always important to check lower extremity and perineal reflexes for evidence of hyperreflexia. Sensory or motor deficits may also be detected in the lumbar or sacral segments.

C. X-RAY FINDINGS

In the early stages, radiologically evident change is minimal for the most part in both the lower and upper urinary tracts. Low bladder volume and mild trabeculation of the bladder are usually evident.

D. INSTRUMENTAL EXAMINATION

Cystoscopy and urethroscopy are generally unremarkable. Mild detrusor and sphincter irritability and diminished capacity can be demonstrated.

E. URODYNAMIC STUDIES

The behavior patterns of the sphincter and bladder are similar to those of the previous group but on a milder scale. Uninhibited detrusor activity evident urodynamically may not be associated with the same symptom pattern on the clinical level. The patient occasionally perceives a sense of urgency and the need to void. However, these sensations may not be present, and the patient may complain of the actual leakage as the main inconvenience. Morphologic changes in the bladder are slight, with changes in the upper urinary tract occurring rarely and late because of lower pressures in the bladder.

3. Flaccid (Atonic) Bladder

Direct injury to the peripheral innervation of the bladder or sacral cord segments S2–4 results in flaccid paralysis of the urinary bladder. Characteristically, the capacity is large, intravesical pressure low, and involuntary contractions absent. Because smooth muscle is intrinsically active, fine trabeculations in the bladder may be seen. Common causes of this type of bladder behavior are trauma, tumors, tabes dorsalis, and congenital anomalies (eg, spina bifida, meningomyelocele).

Clinical Findings

A. SYMPTOMS

The patient experiences flaccid paralysis and loss of sensation affecting the muscles and dermatomes below the level of injury. The principal urinary symptom is retention with overflow incontinence. Male patients lose their erections. Surprisingly, despite weakness in the striated sphincter, neither bowel nor urinary incontinence is a major factor. Storage pressures within the bladder remain below the outlet resistance.

B. SIGNS

Neurologic changes are typically lower motor neuron. Extremity reflexes are hypoactive or absent. Sensation is diminished or absent. It is important to check sensation over the penis (S2) and perianal region (S2–3) for evidence of a mixed or partial injury. Anal tone (S2) should be compared with levator tone (S3–4), again for evidence of a mixed injury.

Similarly, sensation over the outside of the foot (S2), sole of the foot (S2–3), and large toe (S3) should be compared for evidence of mixed injury. Occasionally, extremity findings do not parallel those of the perineum, with the pattern being absent sensation and tone in the feet but partial tone or sensation in the perineum. This is especially true in patients who have spina bifida or meningomyelocele.

C. LABORATORY FINDINGS

Repeated urinalysis at regular intervals is no less important in this group than in others. Infection with white blood cells (leukocytes) and bacteria may occur because of the need for bladder catheterization. Advanced renal change is unusual because bladder storage is under low pressure, but chronic renal failure secondary to pyelonephritis, hydronephrosis, or calculus formation is still possible.

D. X-RAY FINDINGS

A plain film of the abdomen may reveal fracture of the lumbar spine or extensive spina bifida. Calcific shadows compatible with urinary stone may be seen. Excretory urograms should be performed initially to check for calculus, hydronephrosis, pyelonephritic scarring, or ureteral obstruction secondary to an overdistended bladder. A cystogram may detect morphologic changes in the detrusor (it is usually large and smooth-walled); vesicoureteral reflux may be present. Checks on the integrity of both the lower and upper urinary tracts can subsequently be made using ultrasound.

E. INSTRUMENTAL EXAMINATION

Visual inspection is performed to rule out pathologic changes (eg, bladder stones, urethral stricture, or ureteral reflux or obstruction).

Cystoscopy and urethroscopy performed some months or weeks after the injury will confirm the laxity and areflexia of the sphincter and pelvic floor; the bladder neck is usually funneled and open and the bladder should be large and smooth-walled. The integrity of the ureteral orifices should be normal. Fine trabeculation may be evident.

F. Urodynamic Studies

The urethral pressure profile reflects low smooth and striated sphincter tone. Bladder filling pressures are low; detrusor contractions are weak or absent; voiding is accomplished by straining or by the Credé maneuver, if at all; and there is a large volume of residual urine. Awareness of filling is markedly diminished and usually results from stretch on the peritoneum or abdominal distention.

G. Denervation Hypersensitivity

This test is classically performed by giving bethanechol chloride (Urecholine) 15 mg subcutaneously. A cystometrogram is performed after 20 min, and the results are compared with the findings obtained before the bethanechol was given. If the results are positive, a rise in filling pressure of more than 15 cm of water is noted, with a shift in the filling curve to the left; the same behavior in the bladder is noted only at a lower filling volume and slightly higher pressure. A finding of no change on filling reflects myogenic damage to the detrusor. A more physiologic way to perform the test is to fill the bladder to about half its capacity, administer urecholine, and monitor for change in storage pressure. The ice water test also checks for detrusor hypersensitivity.

Bethanechol does not facilitate a detrusor contraction; it can only increase tone in the detrusor wall, which in turn might trigger the voiding reflex. The test is not a check on the integrity of the voiding reflex but demonstrates denervation hypersensitivity in flaccid bladders and differentiates this condition from myogenic damage.

The test is not applicable in patients with reduced bladder capacity, decreased compliance (ie, sharp rise in detrusor filling pressure), or forceful contractions of the detrusor.

DIFFERENTIAL DIAGNOSIS OF NEUROPATHIC BLADDER

The diagnosis of neuropathic bladder is usually obvious from the history and physical examination. Neural impairment is evidenced by abnormal sacral reflex activity and decreased perineal sensation. Some disorders with which neuropathic bladder may be confused are cystitis, chronic urethritis, vesical irritation secondary to psychic disturbance, myogenic damage, interstitial cystitis, cystocele, and infravesical obstruction.

Cystitis

Inflammation of the bladder, both nonspecific and tuberculous, causes frequency of urination and urgency, even to the point of incontinence. Infections secondary to residual urine caused by neuropathic behavioral disturbance should be ruled out.

The urodynamics of the inflamed bladder are similar to those of the uninhibited neuropathic bladder. However, with inflammation, symptoms disappear after definitive antibiotic therapy, and the urodynamic behavior reverts to normal. If symptoms persist or infections return repeatedly, a neuropathic behavioral abnormality should be considered (eg, multiple sclerosis or even idiopathic detrusor-sphincter dysfunction).

Chronic Urethritis

Symptoms of frequency, nocturia, and burning on urination may be due to chronic inflammation of the urethra not necessarily associated with infection. The urodynamics will show an irritable urethral sphincter zone with labile, spastic tendencies. The cause is unknown.

Vesical Irritation Secondary to Psychic Disturbance

Anxious, tense individuals or those with pathologic psychological fixation on the perineum may present a long history of periodic bouts of urinary frequency or perineal or pelvic pain. The clinical picture and urodynamic findings are similar to those described previously for chronic urethritis. Often, however, if the patient's anxieties can be allayed, the symptoms subside. The underlying problem is one of excessive pelvic muscle tension and inefficient sphincter behavior. Some of the symptoms may improve with manual therapy of pelvic floor myofascial trigger points (Weiss, 2001).

Interstitial Cystitis

Interstitial cystitis is poorly understood chronic inflammation of the bladder. The typical patient is a woman over 40 years of age, with symptoms of frequency, nocturia, urgency, and suprapubic pain. The symptoms are brought on by bladder distention. Capacity is limited (often < 100 mL in the most symptomatic and disabled patients). Urinalysis is normal, and there is no residual urine. Urodynamic studies show a hypertonic, poorly compliant bladder. Distention of the bladder with cystoscopy produces bleeding from petechial hemorrhages and fissuring in the mucosa. The condition represents an end-stage inflammatory process of unknown cause in the detrusor.

Cystocele

Relaxation of the pelvic floor following childbirth may cause some frequency, nocturia, and stress incontinence. Residual urine may be present and predispose to infection. Loss of urine occurs with lifting, standing, or coughing.

Pelvic examination usually reveals relaxation of the anterior vaginal wall and descent of the urethra and bladder when the patient strains to void.

Bladder Outlet Obstruction

Urethral strictures, benign or malignant enlargement of the prostate gland, and congenital urethral valves all can produce significant obstruction of the urinary outlet. Hypertrophy (ie, trabeculation) of the detrusor develops, and residual urine can accumulate. Uninhibited detrusor activity is often found at this stage and resembles that of the spastic neuropathic bladder.

If decompensation occurs, the vesical wall becomes attenuated and atonic, and capacity may be markedly increased. Overflow incontinence may develop. The behavior of the bladder is similar to that of the flaccid neuropathic bladder.

If the difficulty is nonneuropathic, the anal sphincter tone is normal and the bulbocavernosus reflex intact. Peripheral sensation, voluntary muscle contraction, and limb reflexes should also be normal. Cystoscopy and urethroscopy reveal the local lesion causing obstruction. Once the obstruction is relieved, bladder function improves but may never return to normal.

TREATMENT OF NEUROPATHIC BLADDER

The treatment of any form of neuropathic bladder is guided by the need to restore low pressure activity to the bladder. In doing so, renal function is preserved, continence restored, and infection more readily controlled. Reflex evacuation may develop if detrusor integrity is protected and trigger techniques are practiced.

1. Spinal Shock

Following severe injury to the spinal cord, the bladder becomes atonic. With suprasegmental spinal injuries, the bladder gradually recovers its contractile capabilities within months. A spastic state evolves, the degree of which varies from patient to patient according to level of injury. Injuries to the sacral cord, if complete enough, may leave the bladder permanently flaccid. More often, however, these lesions are partial, and a mixed degree of detrusor-sphincter spasticity is found along with a variable degree of weakness.

During the spinal shock stage, some type of bladder drainage must be instituted immediately and maintained. Chronic overdistention can damage the detrusor smooth muscle and limit functional recovery of the bladder. Intermittent catheterization using strict aseptic technique has proved to be the best form of management. This avoids urinary tract infection as well as the complications of an indwelling catheter (eg, urethral stricture, abscess, erosions, stones).

If a Foley catheter becomes necessary, a few principles need to be followed. The catheter should not be larger than 16F and preferably should be made of silicon, and it should be taped to the abdomen. Taping the catheter to the leg puts unnecessary stress on the penoscrotal junction and bulbous urethra (ie, the curves in the urethra), and this can lead to stricture formation. The catheter should be changed with sterile procedure every 2–3 weeks.

Some urologists advocate the use of suprapubic cystostomy rather than a urethral catheter to avoid the risks associated with permanent indwelling catheters. Certainly, whenever catheter-related complications occur, the physician should not hesitate in resorting to cystostomy drainage.

Irrigation of the bladder with antibiotic solutions, use of systemic antibiotics, or covering the tip of the meatus with antibiotic creams does not significantly lower the long-term risk of bladder infection. Keeping the meatus lubricated does help avoid meatal stricturing, however.

As peripheral reflex excitability gradually returns, urodynamic evaluation should be performed. A cystogram is needed to rule out reflux. The urodynamic study should be repeated every 3 months as long as spasticity is improving and then annually to check for complications of the upper urinary tract.

To control infection, a fluid intake of at least 2–3 L/d should be maintained (100–200 mL/h) if at all possible. This reduces stasis and decreases the concentration of calcium in the urine. Renal and ureteral drainage are enhanced by moving the patient frequently, with ambulation in a wheelchair as soon as possible, and even by raising the head of the bed. These measures improve ureteral transport of urine, reduce stasis, and lower the risk of infection.

Additional measures aid in prophylaxis for calculus formation (eg, reduction of intake of calcium and oxalate and elimination of vitamin D in the diet).

2. Specific Types Of Neuropathic Bladder

Once a neuropathic voiding disorder is established, regardless of cause, the following steps should be taken to attain optimum function.

Spastic Neuropathic Bladder

A. PATIENT WITH REASONABLE BLADDER CAPACITY

To consider a bladder rehabilitated to a functional state, a patient should be able to go 2–3 h between voiding and not be incontinent during this interval.

Voiding is initiated using trigger techniques—tapping the abdomen suprapubically, tugging on the pubic hair, squeezing the penis, or scratching the skin of the lower abdomen, genitalia, or thighs. Patients can accomplish this on their own unless they are high quadriplegics with no upper limb function.

Some patients in this category can empty the bladder completely but are incontinent due to inconvenient triggering of the voiding reflex. They may be helped by low-dose anticholinergic medication or by neural stimulation.

B. Patient With Markedly Diminished Functional Vesical Capacity

If the functional capacity of the bladder is under 100 mL, involuntary voiding can occur as often as every 15 min. Satisfactory training of the bladder cannot be achieved, and alternative measures must be taken. First, the possibility that reduced functional bladder capacity is due to a large residual volume of urine must be ruled out. One of the following treatment regimens can then be administered.

1. A permanent indwelling catheter with or without anticholinergic medication.

2. A condom catheter and a leg bag in males if residual urine volumes are small and the patient does not have bladder pressures above 40 cm of water on urodynamic evaluation. If either of these parameters is found, the upper urinary tract is considered at risk from obstruction or reflux.

3. Performance of a sphincterotomy in males. It is possible to turn the bladder into a urinary conduit by surgically eliminating all outlet resistance from the bladder. This option should be used only when other options have failed, as it is irreversible. Patients having this procedure usually have more serious sequelae of a highly spastic bladder (ie, upper urinary tract dilatation, recurrent urinary tract infections, or marked autonomic dysreflexia).

4. Conversion of the spastic bladder to a flaccid bladder through sacral rhizotomy. Complete surgical section or percutaneous heat fulguration of the S3 and S4 roots is necessary. Chemical rhizotomy is unreliable, as spasticity usually returns after 6–9 months. These procedures may cause loss of reflex erections, and the decision to perform them should be weighed accordingly. They can relieve spasticity, lower intravesical pressures, increase bladder storage, and decrease the risk of damage to the upper urinary tract. The bladder would then be managed as a flaccid bladder (see below).

5. Neurostimulation of the sacral nerve roots to accomplish bladder evacuation (see section following).

6. Urinary diversion for irreversible, progressive upper urinary tract deterioration. A variety of procedures are available, including the standard ileal conduit, cutaneous ureterostomies, transureteroureterostomy, or nonrefluxing urinary reservoir (eg, Mainz pouch, Koch pouch, or one of several other continent diversions designed to protect the upper urinary tract and kidneys).

7. In females with a spastic bladder, one does not have the option of performing a sphincterotomy. If pharmacologic methods are unsuccessful, surgical conversion to a flaccid, low-pressure system or a urinary diversion should be considered.

C. Parasympatholytic Drugs

Because of the chronic nature of the neuropathic bladder, patients are not always willing to tolerate the side effects of parasympatholytic drugs. Several drugs in this category can be alternated to reduce the side effects of either drug. They also may be useful when given with skeletal muscle relaxants. Dosages must be individualized. Commonly used drugs and dosages are as follows: oxybutynin chloride (Ditropan), 5 mg 2–3 times daily; Ditropan XL, once daily; dicyclomine hydrochloride (Bentyl), 80 mg in 4 equally divided doses daily; methantheline bromide (Banthine), 50–100 mg every 6 h; and propantheline bromide (Pro-Banthine), 15 mg 30 min before meals and 30 mg at bedtime and Tolterodine (Detrol), 2 mg 2 times daily. These drugs may not be effective if incontinence is the result of uninhibited sphincter relaxation or compliance changes in the bladder wall.

D. Botulinum-A Toxin

Several centers have investigated injection of 85–300 Units of botulinum-A toxin into 30–40 sites in the detrusor muscle in both children and adults who have detrusor hyperreflexia. The early results are promising, as shown by a significant increase in bladder capacity and compliance as well as symptomatic improvement for several weeks after injection (Schulte-Baukloh, 2002).

E. Intravesical Instillation of Capsaicin or Resiniferatoxin

Capsaicin and resiniferatoxin are specific C-fiber afferent neurotoxins. After spinal cord injury, C-fiber afferents proliferate in the bladder mucosa and are involved in detrusor hyperreflexia. In a study of 24 spinal cord–injured patients with refractory detrusor hyperreflexia treated with a single dose of 2 mM capsaicin in 30 mL ethanol plus 70 mL of normal saline or 100 nM resiniferatoxin in 100 mL of normal saline, Cruz (1998) found no significant urodynamic or clinical improvement in the capsaicin arm at 30 and 60 days of follow-up. In the resiniferatoxin arm, the mean uninhibited detrusor contraction threshold plus or minus standard deviation increased from 176 ± 54 to 250 ± 107 mL at 30 days ($P < .05$) and to 275 ± 98 mL at 60 days ($P < .01$). Mean maximum bladder capacity increased from 196 ± 75 to 365 ± 113 mL at 30 days ($P < .001$) and to 357 ± 101 mL at 60 days ($P < .001$). Daily catheterizations and incontinent episodes were significantly decreased at 30 and 60 days of follow-up. Autonomic dysreflexia, limb spasms, suprapubic discomfort, and hematuria developed in most patients who received capsaicin but in none who received resiniferatoxin (Giannantoni et al, 2002).

F. Neurostimulation (Bladder Pacemaker)

Neuroprosthetics are becoming an established alternative to managing selective neuropathic bladder disorders. Patients are evaluated for a bladder pacemaker primarily by urodynamic monitoring of bladder and sphincter responses to trial stimulation of the various sacral nerve roots. Selective blocks are then prepared to the right and left pudendal nerves. If voiding is produced, patients are considered suitable for a neuroprosthesis. Other factors such as detrusor storage capability, sphincter competence, age, kidney function, and overall neurologic and psychological status are also taken into consideration.

Electrodes are implanted on the motor (ventral) nerve roots of those sacral nerves that will produce detrusor contraction on stimulation (always S3, occasionally S4). Steps are then taken to reduce sphincter hyperreflexia by selectively dividing the sensory (dorsal) component of these same sacral nerve roots and selective branches of the pudendal nerves. The electrodes are connected to a subcutaneous receiver that can be controlled from outside the body. Bladder or bowel evacuation or continence can then be controlled selectively by the external transmitter.

There are 3 overall goals in the management of the bladder in spastic upper motor neuron lesions—preservation of renal function, continence, and evacuation. The first 2 are accomplished by reducing intravesical pressures. This step protects the integrity of the upper urinary tract and restores continence by increasing storage capacity. Both can be achieved by combining neurostimulation of the sphincter with selective sacral neurotomies. This approach preserves sphincter integrity and avoids the need for drugs. Other options include complete bladder denervation or bladder augmentation.

The third goal, restoration of controlled evacuation, eliminates the need for catheters and associated risk of infection. This is the most difficult goal to achieve, and patients need to be carefully evaluated for their suitability.

Flaccid Neuropathic Bladder

If the neurologic lesion completely destroys the micturition center, volitional voiding cannot be accomplished without manual suprapubic pressure, that is, the Credé maneuver. Bladder evacuation can be accomplished by straining, using the abdominal and diaphragmatic muscles to raise intra-abdominal pressures. Partial injuries to the lower spinal cord (T10–11) result in a spastic bladder and a weak or weakly spastic sphincter. Incontinence can then result from spontaneous detrusor contraction.

A. Bladder Training and Care

In partial lower motor neuron injury, voiding should be tried every 2 h by the clock to avoid embarrassing leakage. This helps protect the bladder from overdistention due to a buildup of residual urine.

B. Intermittent Catheterization

Any patient with adequate bladder capacity can benefit from regular intermittent catheter drainage every 3–6 h. This technique eliminates residual urine, helps prevent infection, avoids incontinence, and protects against damage to the upper urinary tract. It simulates normal voiding and is easily learned and adapted by patients. It is an extremely satisfactory solution to the problems of the flaccid neuropathic bladder. A clean technique is used rather than the inconvenient, expensive, sterile technique. Urinary tract infections are infrequent, but if they occur, a prophylactic antibiotic can be given once daily. The method is contraindicated if ureteral reflux is present, unless the reflux is mild and the bladder emptied frequently.

C. Surgery

Transurethral resection is indicated for hypertrophy of the bladder neck or an enlarged prostate, either of which may cause obstruction of the bladder outlet and retention of residual urine. It also may be performed in some male patients to weaken the outlet resistance of the bladder to permit voiding by the Credé maneuver or abdominal straining.

Complete urinary incontinence due to sphincter incompetence can be managed by implanting an artificial sphincter. Bladder pressure should be low, however, for this to be successful. Bladder neck reconstruction also may be considered as a way to increase outlet resistance.

Incontinence in this group of patients can be treated with drugs or neurostimulation if it results from mild bladder spasticity.

D. Parasympathomimetic Drugs

The stable derivatives of acetylcholine are at times of value in assisting the evacuation of the bladder. Although they *do not* initiate or effect bladder contraction, they do provide increased bladder tonus. They may be helpful in symptomatic treatment of the milder types of flaccid neuropathic bladder. Drugs may be tried empirically, but usefulness is best gauged during urodynamic evaluation. If filling pressure or resting tonus is increased after bethanechol chloride (Urecholine) is administered, evacuation of the bladder through trigger reflexes or straining should be more effective. The drug then should be clinically helpful.

Bethanechol chloride is the drug of choice. It is given orally, 25–50 mg every 6–8 h. In special situations (eg, urodynamic study or immediately following operation), it may be given subcutaneously, 5–10 mg every 6–8 h.

Neuropathic Bladder Associated With Spina Bifida

Spina bifida is incomplete formation of the neural arch at various levels of the spine. The defect is recognized at birth and closed immediately to prevent infection. The scarring that results can entrap and tether nerves in the cauda equina. With failure of the neural arch to close, there is failure of anterior horn cell development and organization. The end result is a mixed type of neuropathic defect. Roughly two-thirds of patients have a spastic bladder with weakness in the feet and toes. About one-third have a flaccid bladder. Often, there is a greater degree of flaccidity in the pelvic floor than in the detrusor.

The goals of therapy are to control incontinence and preserve renal function.

A. Conservative Treatment

Clean intermittent catheterization is the best management. Parents can be taught to do this for the child, and eventually the child can take over this function. Frequency should be determined by the storage capacity of the bladder and the fluid intake, usually every 3–6 h. An anticholinergic drug may be required to mediate bladder spasticity and improve storage function in order to control incontinence.

1. Mild symptoms—If there is occasional dribbling or some residual urine associated with lack of desire to void, the patient should try to void every 2 h when awake. Manual suprapubic pressure enhances the efficiency of emptying. An external condom catheter or a small pad can be worn to protect against small-volume losses of urine.

2. More severe symptoms—If urinary incontinence is associated with residual urine or if ureteral reflux is found, the following steps should be taken:

a. Hypotonic bladder—If reflux has been demonstrated, intermittent self-catheterization 4–6 times a day may protect the upper urinary tract from deterioration and the consequences of pyelonephritis. Ureteral reimplantation can be considered for bilateral reflux or a transureteroureterostomy for single-sided reflux if all other considerations are favorable. Intermittent catheterization should then be reinstituted.

b. Hypertonic bladder—The problem with patients in this category is more serious because the bladder is spastic with reduced capacity and the sphincter is hypotonic. Virtually constant dribbling can result. The cystogram will reveal heavy trabeculation of the bladder, often with reflux and advanced hydroureteronephrosis. Anticholinergic medication should be given, and an indwelling catheter should be inserted for several months. Once upper urinary tract dilatation has improved and the bladder has been restored to a more spheric shape, intermittent catheterization may be reinstituted. With time and care, many of these children develop a more balanced type of bladder behavior. Continence may be gained without compromising the upper urinary tract.

Most of these patients will not require urinary diversion if they are carefully followed up and if the parents actively participate in their care.

B. Surgical Treatment

If the bladder is of the spastic type with diminished capacity, there are several surgical options short of actual urinary diversion. Sacral nerve block during urodynamic evaluation helps in determining whether sacral nerve root section would be beneficial. This helps in cases of spastic bladder but not in cases of poorly compliant, fibrotic bladder. Sectioning the S3 nerves reduces intravesical pressures, improves storage, and reduces the risk of reflux or obstruction of the ureters.

For the patient with a mildly spastic bladder and reasonable storage capacity (> 200 mL), urinary incontinence might be controlled via electrostimulation of the pelvic floor. Many of these patients have intact nerves to the sphincter. These can be stimulated to enhance sphincter tone and inhibit voiding. If the bladder has a limited capacity with poor compliance and poor contractility, augmentation cystoplasty followed by intermittent self-catheterization is the treatment of choice.

If the refluxing patient has recurrent fever (equivalent to pyelonephritis) despite the presence of an indwelling catheter or if incontinence cannot be controlled because of poor detrusor compliance, urinary diversion must be considered. Nonrefluxing continent reservoirs offer the most favorable long-term outlook for preservation of the upper urinary tract.

3. Control Of Urinary Incontinence

In the Hospital

Urinary incontinence is one of the most distressing aspects of neurovesical dysfunction, especially when the bladder has otherwise adequate function. The problem is minimized in men who are hospitalized because supervision is available, bathrooms are nearby, and a bedside urinal is always available. Women have a greater problem because they must use a bedpan or may require an indwelling catheter. Catheters have associated risks and do not always control leakage associated with spastic bladder. No simple, satisfactory solution to this problem has been devised for women.

After Discharge

After discharge from the hospital, most men with spastic bladders rely on a condom catheter for protection against leakage and for practical urine collection. The only exception is patients who are predictably dry between catheterizations. The condom catheter attaches to the penis without pressure and has a conduit to a leg bag. The adhesives are nonirritating and long-lasting. Problems involved in keeping these catheters in place are limited to noncircumcised patients and those with large suprapubic fat pads that shorten the length of the shaft of the penis. Circumcision or placement of a penile prosthesis will correct for these limitations.

Urethral compression by means of a Cunningham clamp is occasionally preferred by patients. This protects only against low-pressure leakage, however, and if it is applied too tightly, a urethral diverticulum may develop.

Other types of external collection devices are available (McGuire urinal, Texas catheter), but with advancements in adhesive glues for condom catheters and use of penile prostheses, the other methods are being used less frequently.

Neurostimulation

Extensive research continues to be conducted on methods of restoring complete voluntary control over the storage and evacuation functions of the bladder. Sacral and pudendal nerve anatomy has been determined, so that surgical exposure of these nerves and their branches is possible. An electrode can be placed for selective stimulation of the bladder, levator, and urethral or anal sphincters. A number of possibilities exist for neu-

rostimulation or rhizotomy, but only a few are practical. Urodynamic evaluation of bladder function following a nerve block or during neurostimulation can help determine the therapeutic value of these treatments.

Single or multiple electrodes can be placed on selected nerves and coupled to a subcutaneous receiver. The desired function (continence or evacuation) can be selected. Usually, one or the other is needed in any one patient. Much will change in this approach as technologic advances become adapted to the increased understanding of bladder physiology. Striking successes are also being seen with electroevacuation in highly selected patients.

COMPLICATIONS OF NEUROPATHIC BLADDER

The principal complications of the neuropathic bladder are recurrent urinary tract infection, hydronephrosis secondary to ureteral reflux or obstruction, and stone formation. The primary factors contributing to these complications are the presence of residual urine, sustained high intravesical pressures, and immobilization, respectively.

Incontinence in neuropathic disorders may be passive, as in flaccid lesions when outlet resistance is compromised, or may be the result of uninhibited detrusor contractions, as in spastic lesions.

Infection

Infection is virtually inevitable with the neuropathic bladder state. During the stage of spinal shock that follows cord injury, the bladder must be emptied by catheterization. Sterile intermittent catheterization is recommended at this stage, but for practical purposes or for the sake of convenience, a Foley catheter is often left indwelling. Chronic catheter drainage guarantees infection regardless of any preventive measures taken. Nevertheless, a recent clinical trial of colonization of the bladder with nonpathogenic *Escherichia coli* showed some promise; it significantly reduced the episodes of infection in a group of spinal cord injury patients with neurogenic bladder (Darouiche et al, 2001).

The upper urinary tract is usually protected from infection by the integrity of the ureterovesical junction. If this becomes incompetent, infected urine will reflux up to the kidneys. Decompensation of the ureterovesical junction results from the high intravesical pressures generated by the spastic bladder. It is most important that these cases be treated aggressively with an intensive program of self-catheterization and anticholinergic medication. The Credé maneuver should not be used.

A number of infective complications can result from the presence of a chronically indwelling Foley catheter. These include cystitis and periurethritis resulting from mechanical irritation. A periurethral abscess may follow, with formation of a fistula via eventual rupture of the abscess through the perineal skin. Drainage may also take place through the urethra, with the end result being a urethral diverticulum. Infection may travel up into the prostatic ducts (prostatitis) or seminal vesicles (seminal vesiculitis) and along the vas into the epididymis (epididymitis).

A. TREATMENT OF PYELONEPHRITIS

Episodic renal infection should be treated aggressively with appropriate antibiotics to prevent renal loss. The source and cause of infection should be eliminated if possible.

B. TREATMENT OF EPIDIDYMITIS

This condition is a complication of either dyssynergic voiding or an indwelling catheter. Treatment consists of appropriate antibiotics, bed rest, and scrotal elevation. The indwelling catheter should be removed or replaced with a suprapubic catheter. Preferred long-term management is to place the patient on an intermittent self-catheterization program. Rarely, ligation of the vas is required.

Hydronephrosis

Two mechanisms lead to back pressure on the kidney. Early, the effect of trigonal stretch secondary to residual urine and detrusor hypertonicity becomes compounded by evolving trigonal hypertrophy. The combination causes abnormal pull on the ureterovesical junction, with increased resistance to the passage of urine. A "functional" obstruction results, which leads to progressive ureteral dilatation and back pressure on the kidney. At this stage, this condition can be relieved by continuous catheter drainage or by combined intermittent catheter drainage and use of anticholinergics.

A delayed consequence of trigonal hypertrophy and detrusor spasticity is reflux due to decompensation of the ureterovesical junction. The causative factor appears to be a combination of high intravesical pressure and trabeculation of the bladder wall. The increased stiffness of the ureterovesical junction weakens its valvelike function, slowly eroding its ability to prevent reflux of urine during forceful bladder contractions.

When ureteral reflux is detected by cystography, previous methods of bladder care must be radically adjusted. An indwelling catheter may manage the problem temporarily. However, if the reflux persists after a reasonable period of drainage, antireflux surgery must

be considered. In addition, measures to reduce high intravesical pressure are needed (bladder augmentation, sacral rhizotomy, transurethral resection of the bladder outlet, or sphincterotomy). Progressive hydronephrosis may require nephrostomy. Urinary diversion is a last resort, which should be avoidable if the patient is followed up regularly.

Calculus

A number of factors contribute to stone formation in the bladder and kidneys. Bed rest and inactivity cause demineralization of the skeleton, mobilization of calcium, and subsequent hypercalciuria. Recumbency and inadequate fluid intake both contribute to urinary stasis, possibly with increased concentration of urinary calcium. Catheterization of the neurogenic bladder may introduce bacteria. Subsequent infection is usually due to a urea-splitting organism, which causes the urine to become alkaline, with reduced solubility of calcium and phosphate.

A. BLADDER STONES

Because these stones are usually soft, they can be crushed and will wash out through a cystoscope sheath. Occasionally, they are large and need to be removed via a suprapubic cystotomy.

B. URETERAL STONES

Virtually all ureteral stones can now be removed by antegrade or retrograde retrieval methods or by extracorporeal shock wave lithotripsy (ESWL).

C. RENAL STONES

In a patient with neurogenic bladder, kidney stones generally are the result of infection; if the infection is untreated, the stones become the source of persistent renal infection and eventual renal loss. Most of the stones in the renal pelvis can be removed by either a percutaneous endoscopic procedure or ESWL. Occasionally, a large staghorn stone may require open surgery.

Renal Amyloidosis

Secondary amyloidosis of the kidney is a common cause of death in patients with neuropathic bladder. It is a result of chronic debilitation in patients with difficult decubitus ulcers and poorly controlled infection. Fortunately, due to better medical care, this is an uncommon finding today.

Sexual Dysfunction

Men who have had traumatic cord or cauda equina lesions experience varying degrees of sexual dysfunction. Those with upper motor lesions fare well, with the majority having reflexogenic erectile capability. Dangerous elevations in blood pressure can occur with erections in patients with high thoracic or cervical lesions. Problems of quality of erection or premature detumescence are found with all levels of injury. Patients with lower motor lesions are, as a rule, impotent, unless the lesion is incomplete. There is a high degree of variability in the sexual capabilities of patients with all levels of spinal injury. Fortunately, sexual function can be restored to most patients by oral sildenafil, transurethral medications, a vacuum erection device, intracavernous injection, or a penile prosthesis.

Often, patients with spinal injury lose the ability to ejaculate even with preservation of functional erections. This is a result of lost coordination between reflexes normally synchronized through higher center regulation. Patients may have the capability to ejaculate after an erection but are either unable to trigger this sexual event or are unable to trigger it in proper sequence. Techniques using vibratory stimulation of the penis or transrectal electrical stimulation have been developed to accomplish semen collection in patients with "functional infertility."

Autonomic Dysreflexia

Autonomic dysreflexia is sympathetically mediated reflex behavior triggered by sacral afferent feedback to the spinal cord. The phenomenon is seen in patients with cord lesions above the sympathetic outflow from the cord. As a rule, it occurs in rather spastic lesions above T1 but on occasion in lesions of mild spasticity or those as low as T5. Symptoms include dramatic elevations in systolic or diastolic blood pressure (or both), increased pulse pressure, sweating, bradycardia, headache, and piloerection. Symptoms are brought on by overdistention of the bladder. Immediate catheterization is indicated and usually brings about prompt lowering of blood pressure. Oral nifedipine (20 mg) has been shown to alleviate this syndrome when given 30 min before cystoscopy (Dykstra, Sidi, and Anderson, 1987) or electroejaculation (Steinberger et al, 1990). The acute hemodynamic effect can be managed with a parenteral ganglionic blocking agent or alpha-adrenergic blockers (Barrett and Wein, 1987). Sphincterotomy and peripheral rhizotomy have been used by some to prevent recurring autonomic dysreflexia.

PROGNOSIS

The greater threat to the patient with a neuropathic bladder is progressive renal damage (pyelonephritis, calculosis, and hydronephrosis). Advances in the management of the neuropathic bladder, together with better follow-up of patients at regular intervals, have substantially improved the outlook for long-term survival.

REFERENCES

Andersson KE: The overactive bladder: Pharmacologic basis of drug treatment. Urology 1997;50(6A Suppl):74.

Artibani W: Diagnosis and significance of idiopathic overactive bladder. Urology 1997;50(6A Suppl):25.

Barrett D, Wein AJ: Voiding dysfunction: Diagnosis, classification and management. In: Gillenwater JY et al (editors): *Adult and Pediatric Urology.* Year Book Medical, 1987.

Bauer SB: Neurogenic bladder dysfunction. Pediatr Clin North Am 1987;34:1121.

Bosch J, Groen J: Sacral (S3) segmental nerve stimulation as a treatment for urge incontinence in patients with detrusor instability: Results of chronic electrical stimulation using an implantable neural prosthesis. J Urol 1995;154:504.

Brading AF: A myogenic basis for the overactive bladder. Urology 1997;50(6A Suppl):57.

Brindley GS: The sacral anterior root stimulator as a means of managing the bladder in patients with spinal cord lesions. Baillieres Clin Neurol 1995;4:1.

Buyse G et al: Intravesical oxybutynin for neurogenic bladder dysfunction: Less systemic side effects due to reduced first pass metabolism. J Urol 1998;160:892.

Churchill BM et al: Biological response of bladders rendered continent by insertion of artificial sphincter. J Urol 1987;138: 1116.

Crowe R, Burnstock G, Light JK: Adrenergic innervation of the striated muscle of the intrinsic external urethral sphincter from patients with lower motor spinal cord lesion. J Urol 1989;141:47.

Crowe R, Burnstock G, Light JK: Spinal cord lesions at different levels affect either the adrenergic or vasoactive intestinal polypeptide–immunoreactive nerves in the human urethra. J Urol 1988;140:1412.

Cruz F: Desensitization of bladder sensory fibers by the intravesical capsaicin or capsaicin analogs: A new strategy for treatment of urge incontinence in patients with spinal detrusor hyperreflexia or bladder hypersensitivity disorders. Int Urogynecol J Pelvic Floor Dysfunct 1998;9:214.

Darouiche RO et al: Pilot trial of bacterial interference for preventing urinary tract infection. Urology 2001;58:339.

De Groat WC: Anatomy of the central neural pathways controlling the lower urinary tract. Eur Urol 1998;34(Suppl 1):2.

De Groat WC: A neurologic basis for the overactive bladder. Urology 1997;50(6A Suppl):36.

Duel BP, Gonzalez R, Barthold JS: Alternative techniques for augmentation cystoplasty. J Urol 1998;159:998.

Dykstra D, Sidi AA, Anderson LL: The effect of nifedipine on cystoscopy induced autonomic hyperreflexia in patients with high spinal cord injuries. J Urol 1987;138:1155.

Dykstra DD et al: Effects of botulinum A toxin on detrusor-sphincter dyssynergia in spinal cord injury patients. J Urol 1988;139:919.

Fowler CJ: Bladder afferents and their role in the overactive bladder. Urology 2002;59(5 Suppl 1):37.

Fowler CJ: Investigation of the neurogenic bladder. J Neurol Neurosurg Psychiatry 1996;60:6.

Giannantoni A et al: Intravesical capsaicin versus resiniferatoxin in patients with detrusor hyperreflexia: A prospective randomized study. J Urol 2002;167:1710.

Gosling JA, Dixon JS: Anatomy of the bladder and urethra. In: Chisholm GP, Fair WR (editors): *Scientific Foundations of Urology.* Year Book Medical, 1990.

Gosling JA et al: Decrease in the autonomic innervation of human detrusor muscle in outflow obstruction. J Urol 1986;136: 501.

Hackler RH: A 25-year prospective mortality study in the spinal cord injured patient: Comparison with the long-term living paraplegic. J Urol 1977;117:486.

Hackler RH, Hall MK, Zampieri TA: Bladder hypocompliance in the spinal cord injury population. J Urol 1989;141:1390.

Jackson S: The patient with an overactive bladder—Symptoms and quality-of-life issues. Urology 1997;50(6A Suppl):18.

Janig W, Koltzenburg M: Pain arising from the urogenital tract. In: Maggi CA (editor): *Nervous Control of the Urogenital System.* Harwood Academic Publishers, 1993.

Jayanthi VR et al: The nonneurogenic bladder of early infancy. J Urol 1997;158(3 Pt 2):1281.

Joseph DB et al: Clean, intermittent catheterization of infants with neurogenic bladder. Pediatrics 1989;84:78.

Lepor H et al: Muscarinic cholinergic receptors in the normal and neurogenic human bladder. J Urol 1989;142:869.

Light JK, Beric A, Wise PG: Predictive criteria for failed sphincterotomy in spinal cord injury patients. J Urol 1987;138: 1201.

McGuire EJ, Cespedes RD, O'Connell HE: Leak-point pressures. Urol Clin North Am 1996;23:253.

McGuire EJ, Savastano JA: Long-term follow-up of spinal cord injury patients managed by intermittent catheterization. J Urol 1983;219:775.

McLorie GA et al: Determinants of hydronephrosis and renal injury in patients with myelomeningocele. J Urol 1988;140: 1289.

Mollard P, Mouriquand P, Joubert P: Urethral lengthening for neurogenic urinary incontinence (Kropp's procedure): Results of 16 cases. J Urol 1990;143:95.

Nickell K, Boone TB: Peripheral neuropathy and peripheral nerve injury. Urol Clin North Am 1996;23:491.

Rivas DA, Figueroa TE, Chancellor MB: Bladder autoaugmentation. Tech Urol 1995;1:181.

Rudy DC, Awad SA, Downie JW: External sphincter dyssynergia: An abnormal continence reflex. J Urol 1988;140:105.

Satoh K: Localization of the micturition center at dorsolateral pontine tegmentum of the rat. Neurosci Lett 1978;8:27.

Schmidt RA: Advances in genitourinary neurostimulation. Neurosurgery 1986;19:1041.

Schulte-Baukloh H et al: Efficacy of botulinum-a toxin in children with detrusor hyperreflexia due to myelomeningocele: preliminary results. Urology 2002;59:325.

Sidi AA, Reinberg Y, Gonzalez R: Comparison of artificial sphincter implantation and bladder neck reconstruction in patients with neurogenic urinary incontinence. J Urol 1987;138: 1120.

Smith AR, Hosker GL, Warrell DW: The role of partial denervation of the pelvic floor in the aetiology of genitourinary prolapse and stress incontinence of urine: A neurophysiological study. Br J Obstet Gynaecol 1989;96:24.

Steers WD, De Groat WC: Effect of bladder outlet obstruction on micturition reflex pathways in the rat. J Urol 1988;140:864.

Steinberger RE et al: Nifedipine pretreatment for autonomic dysreflexia during electroejaculation. Urology 1990;36:228.

Stone AR: Neurourologic evaluation and urologic management of spinal dysraphism. Neurosurg Clin North Am 1995;6:269.

Sullivan MP, Comiter CV, Yalla SV: Micturitional urethral pressure profilometry. Urol Clin North Am 1996;23:263.

Tanagho EA, Schmidt RA: Electrical stimulation in the clinical management of the neurogenic bladder. J Urol 1988;140: 1331.

Tanagho EA, Schmidt RA, Orvis BR: Neural stimulation for control of voiding dysfunction: A preliminary report in 22 patients with serious neuropathic voiding disorders. J Urol 1989;142:340.

Thomas TM, Karran OD, Meade TW: Management of urinary incontinence in patients with multiple sclerosis. J R Coll Gen Pract 1981;31:296.

Van Kerrebroeck PE: The role of electrical stimulation in voiding dysfunction. Eur Urol 1998;34(Suppl 1):27.

Vorstman B et al: Nerve crossover techniques for urinary bladder reinnervation: Animal and human cadaver studies. J Urol 1987;137:1043.

Watanabe T, Rivas DA, Chancellor MB: Urodynamics of spinal cord injury. Urol Clin North Am 1996;23:459.

Weiss JM: Pelvic floor myofascial trigger points: Manual therapy for interstitial cystitis and the urgency-frequency syndrome. J Urol 2001;166:2226.

Urodynamic Studies

Emil A. Tanagho, MD

Urodynamic study is an important part of the evaluation of patients with voiding dysfunctions—dysuria, urinary incontinence, neuropathic disorders, etc. Formerly, the examiner simply observed the act of voiding, noting the strength of the urinary stream and drawing inferences about the possibility of obstruction of the bladder outlet. In the 1950s, it became possible to observe the lower urinary tract by fluoroscopy during the act of voiding; and in the 1960s, the principles of hydrodynamics were applied to lower urinary tract physiology. The field of urodynamics now has clinical applications in evaluating voiding problems resulting from lower urinary tract disease.

The nomenclature of the tests used in urodynamic studies is not yet settled, and the meanings of urodynamic terms are sometimes overlapping or confusing. In spite of these difficulties, urodynamic tests are extremely valuable. Symptoms elicited by the history or by physical, endoscopic, or even radiographic examination often must be investigated further by urodynamic tests so that therapy can be devised that is based on an understanding of the altered physiology of the lower urinary tract.

As is true of many high-technology testing procedures (eg, electrocardiography, electroencephalography), urodynamic tests have the greatest clinical validity when their interpretation is left to the treating physician, who should either supervise the study or be responsible for correlating all of the findings with personal clinical observations.

FUNCTIONS RELEVANT TO URODYNAMICS & TESTS APPLICABLE TO EACH

Urodynamic study of the lower urinary tract can provide useful clinical information about the function of the urinary bladder, the sphincteric mechanism, and the voiding pattern itself.

Bladder function has been classically studied by cystography and fluoroscopy. Urodynamic studies use cystometry. Conventional radiographic studies and urodynamic studies can, of course, be usefully combined.

Sphincteric function depends on 2 elements: the smooth muscle sphincter and the voluntary sphincter. The activity of both elements can be recorded urody-

namically by pressure measurements; the activity of the voluntary sphincter also can be recorded by electromyography.

The act of voiding is a function of the interaction between bladder and sphincter, and the result is the **flow rate.** The flow rate is one major aspect of the total function of the lower urinary tract. It is generally recorded in milliliters per second as well as by total urine volume voided. The simultaneous recording of bladder activity (by intraluminal pressure measurements), sphincteric activity (by electromyography or pressure measurements), and flow rate reveals interrelationships among the 3 elements. Each measurement may give useful information about the normality or abnormality of one specific aspect of lower urinary tract function. A more complete picture is provided by integrating all 3 lower tract elements in a simultaneously recorded comparative manner. This comprehensive approach may involve synchronous recordings of variable pressures, flow rate, volume voided, and electrical activity of skeletal musculature around the urinary sphincter (electromyography), along with fluoroscopic imaging of the lower urinary tract. The multiple pressures to be recorded are quite variable and usually include intravesical pressure, intraurethral pressure at several levels, intra-abdominal pressure, and anal sphincteric pressure as a function of muscular activity of the pelvic floor.

The techniques of urodynamic study must be tailored to the needs of specific patients. Each method has advantages and limitations depending on the requirements of the study. In one patient, results of a single test might be sufficient to establish the diagnosis and suggest appropriate therapy; in another, many more studies might be necessary.

■ PHYSIOLOGIC & HYDRODYNAMIC CONSIDERATIONS

URINARY FLOW RATE

Because urinary flow rate is the product of detrusor action against outlet resistance, a variation from the normal flow rate might reflect dysfunction of either. The normal flow rate from a full bladder is about 20–25 mL/s in men and 25–30 mL/s in women. These variations are directly related to the volume voided and the person's age. Obstruction should be suspected in any adult voiding with a full bladder at a rate of less than 15 mL/s. A flow rate less than 10 mL/s is considered definite evidence of obstruction. Occasionally, one encounters "supervoiders" with flow rates far above the normal range. This may signify low outlet resistance but is of less concern clinically than obstruction.

Outlet Resistance

Outlet resistance is the primary determinant of flow rate and varies according to mechanical or functional factors. Functionally, outlet resistance is primarily related to sphincteric activity, which is controlled by both the smooth sphincter and the voluntary sphincter. The smooth sphincter is rarely overactive in women; we have never seen an example of it in any of our urodynamic evaluations. Overactivity of the smooth sphincter is rarely seen in men also but it may occur in association with hypertrophy of the bladder neck due to neurogenic dysfunction or distal obstruction. However, such cases must be critically evaluated before this conclusion is reached.

Increased voluntary sphincteric activity is not uncommon. It is often neglected as a primary underlying cause of increased sphincteric resistance. It is manifested either as lack of relaxation or as actual overactivity during voiding. The normal voluntary sphincter provides adequate resistance, along with the smooth sphincter, to prevent escape of urine from the bladder; if the voluntary sphincter does not relax during detrusor contraction, partial functional obstruction occurs. Overactivity of the sphincter, resulting in increased outlet resistance, is usually a neuropathic phenomenon. However, it can also be functional, resulting from irritative phenomena such as infection or other factors—chemical, bacterial, hormonal, or, even more commonly and often not appreciated, psychological.

Mechanical Factors

Mechanical factors resulting in obstruction to urine flow are the easiest to identify by conventional methods. In women, they may take the form of cystoceles, urethral kinks, or, most commonly, iatrogenic scarring, fibrosis, and compression from previous vaginal or periurethral operative procedures. Mechanical factors in men are well known to all urologists; the classic form is benign prostatic hypertrophy. Urethral stricture from various causes and posterior urethral valves are other common causes of urinary obstruction in men, and there are many others.

Normal voiding with a normal flow rate is the product of both detrusor activity and outlet resistance. A high intravesical pressure resulting from detrusor contraction is not necessary to initiate voiding, because outlet resistance has usually dropped to a minimum. Sphincteric relaxation usually precedes detrusor contraction by a few seconds, and when relaxation is maximal, detrusor activity starts and is sustained until the bladder is empty.

Variations in Normal Flow Rate

The sequence just described is not essential for normal flow rates. The flow rate may be normal in the absence of any detrusor contraction if sphincteric relaxation is assisted by increased intra-abdominal pressure from straining. Persons with weak outlet resistance and weak sphincteric control can achieve a normal flow rate by complete voluntary sphincteric relaxation without detrusor contraction or straining. A normal flow rate can be achieved in spite of increased sphincteric activity or lack of complete relaxation if detrusor contraction is increased to overcome outlet resistance.

Because a normal flow rate can be achieved in spite of abnormalities of one or more of the mechanisms involved, recording the flow rate alone does not provide insight into the precise mechanisms by which it occurs. Distinction between patterns of flow can be difficult. For practical purposes, if the flow rate is adequate and the recorded pattern and configuration of the flow curve are normal, these variations may not be clinically significant except in rare cases.

Nomenclature

The study of urinary flow rate itself is usually called **uroflowmetry.** The flow rate is generally identified as **maximum flow rate, average flow rate, flow time, maximum flow time** (the time elapsed before maximum flow rate is reached), and **total flow time** (the aggregate of flow time if the flow has been interrupted by periods of no voiding) (Figure 27–1). The **flow rate pattern** is characterized as continuous or intermittent, etc.

Pattern Measurement of Flow Rate

A normal flow pattern is represented by a bell-shaped curve (Figure 27–1). However, the curve is rarely completely smooth; it may vary within limits and still be normal. Flow rate can be determined by measuring a 5-s collection at the peak of flow and dividing the amount obtained by 5 to arrive at the average rate per second. This rough estimate is useful, especially if the flow rate is normal and the values are above 20 mL/s. Peak urine

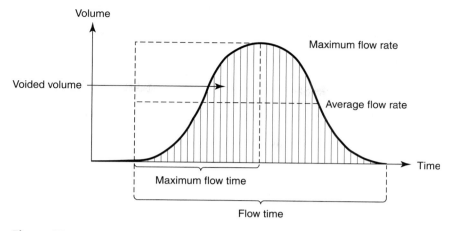

Figure 27–1. Uroflowmetry. Basic elements of maximum flow, average flow, total flow time, and total volume voided.

flow can also be measured quite easily with a peakometer—a device employing a color indicator strip that, when impregnated with urine, shows maximum flow rate by changes in color against a predetermined scale. The Drake uroflowmeter is a plastic container with several chambers into which the patient voids; the maximum flow rate is determined by noting how many chambers contain urine.

In modern practice, the flow rate is more often recorded electronically: The patient voids into a container on top of a measuring device that is connected to a transducer, the weight being converted to volume and recorded on a chart in milliliters per second. Figure 27–2 is an example of such a recording from a normal man. The general bell-shaped curve is quite clear, and the tracing shows all of the values discussed previously: total flow time, maximum flow time, maximum flow rate, average flow rate, and total volume voided. Occasional "supervoiders" can exceed the limits of the chart, but this is usually not of clinical concern (Figure 27–3). A possible variation in the bell appearance is seen in Figure 27–4.

The overall appearance of the flow curve may disclose unsuspected abnormalities. In Figure 27–5, for example, flow time is greatly prolonged. Maximum flow rate may not be low, but the average flow rate is very low—though the maximum flow rate is at one point within the normal range. Such fluctuation in flow rate is most commonly related to variations in voluntary sphincteric activity. In Figure 27–6, this pattern is extreme: Maximum flow rate never exceeds 15 mL/s, and average flow rate is about 10 mL/s, which is indicative of obstruction. (Again, this fluctuation in pattern probably reflects sphincteric hyperactivity.)

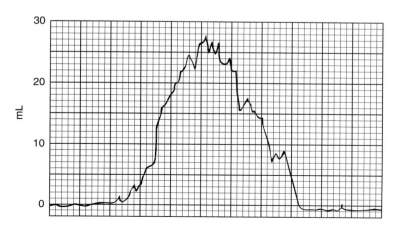

Figure 27–2. Classic normal flow rate, with peak of about 30 mL/s and average of about 20 mL/s. On the horizontal scale, one large square equals 5 s.

Figure 27–3. Flow rate of "supervoider." Maximum flow rate exceeds limits of chart. Tracing shows fast buildup and complete bladder emptying of large volume of urine in a very short period. On the horizontal scale, one large square equals 5 s.

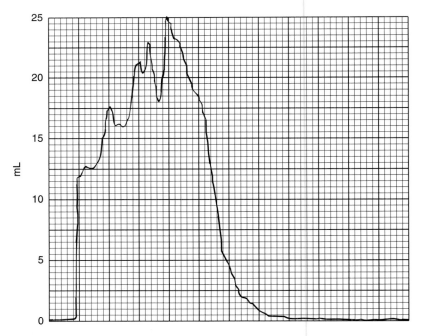

Figure 27–4. Normal flow rate with some variation in appearance of curve. Note rapid pressure rise but progressive increase to maximum, followed by a sharp drop. There is also fluctuation in ascending limb of tracing. On the horizontal scale, one large square equals 5 s.

Figure 27–5. Rather low flow rate (not exceeding 10 mL/s), yet at one point the peak reaches 27–32 mL/s. Note again fluctuation in flow. On the horizontal scale, one large square equals 5 s.

The flow rate pattern reveals a great deal about the forces involved. For example, if the patient is voiding without the aid of detrusor contractions—primarily by straining—this can be easily deduced from the pattern of the flow rate. Figure 27–7 shows an example of intermittent voiding, primarily by straining, with no detrusor activity and at a rate that sometimes does not reach the usual peaks. With experience, one becomes expert at detecting the mechanisms underlying abnormalities in flow rate. For example, in Figure 27–5, the maximum flow rate is in the normal range, the average flow rate is slightly low, and the curve has a general bell pattern, yet brief partial intermittent obstructions to flow can be readily interpreted as due to overactivity of the voluntary sphincter, a mild form of detrusor/sphincter dyssynergia (see discussion following).

Flow rates in mechanical obstruction are totally different, classically in the range of 5–6 mL/s; flow time is greatly prolonged, and there is sustained low flow with minimal variation (Figure 27–8). Figure 27–9 is a striking example of a curve for a patient with benign prostatic hypertrophy. No simultaneous studies are needed with such a pattern, since the pattern is obviously one of mechanical obstruction.

Reduced flow rate in the absence of mechanical obstruction is due to some impairment of sphincteric or detrusor activity. This is seen in a variety of conditions, for example, normal detrusor contraction with no associated sphincteric relaxation and normal detrusor contraction with sphincteric overactivity, which is more serious. These 2 entities are commonly referred to as **detrusor/sphincter dyssynergia.** If with detrusor contraction the sphincter does not relax and open up or (worse) if it becomes overactive, urine flow is obstructed (ie, flow rate is reduced and of abnormal pattern). Reduced flow rate may occur even with increased detrusor activity if the latter is not adequate to overcome sphincteric resistance.

So many variations are possible in the shape of the flow curve—no matter how accurately the flow is recorded or how often the study is repeated to confirm abnormal findings—that it is beneficial to relate it to simultaneous recordings, such as of bladder pressure, pelvic floor electromyography, urethral pressure profile, or simply cinefluoroscopy. Nevertheless, by itself it can be one of the most valuable urodynamic studies undertaken to evaluate a specific type of voiding dysfunction. Flowmetry not only is of diagnostic value but also is valuable in follow-up studies and in deciding on treatment. In some cases, however, flowmetry alone does not provide enough data about the abnormality in the voiding mechanism. More information must then be obtained by evaluation of bladder function.

BLADDER FUNCTION

The basic factors of normal bladder function are bladder capacity, accommodation, sensation, contractility, voluntary control, and response to drugs. All of them can be evaluated by cystometry. If all are within the normal range, bladder physiology can be assumed to be normal. Evaluation of every factor has its own implication and, before a definitive conclusion is reached, must be examined in the light of associated manifestations and findings.

Capacity, Accommodation, & Sensation

Cystometry can be done by either of 2 basic methods: (1) allowing physiologic filling of the bladder with secreted urine and continuously recording the intravesical pressure throughout a voiding cycle (starting the recording when the patient's bladder is empty and continuing it until the bladder has been filled—at which time the patient is asked to urinate—and voiding be-

Figure 27–6. Very low flow rate of short duration and small volume. Note that maximum flow is not above 15 mL/s; however, flow average is less than 10 mL/s, and flow is almost completely interrupted in the middle. On the horizontal scale, one large square equals 5 s.

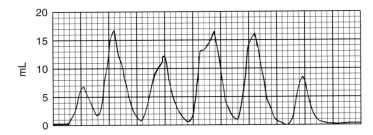

Figure 27–7. Classic flow rate due to abdominal straining with no detrusor activity. See effect of spurts of urine with complete interruption between them; patient cannot sustain increased intra-abdominal pressure. On the horizontal scale, one large square equals 5 s.

gins) or (2) by filling the bladder with water and recording the intravesical pressure against the volume of water introduced into the bladder.

With the first (physiologic filling) method, the assessment of bladder function is based on voided volume (assuming that the presence of residual urine has been ruled out). The second method permits accurate determination of the volume distending the bladder and of the pressures at each level of filling, yet it has inherent defects: fluid is introduced rather than naturally secreted, and bladder filling occurs more rapidly than it normally does.

The cystometrogram (Figure 27–10) is obtained during the phase of bladder filling; the volume of fluid in the bladder is plotted against the intravesical pressure to show bladder wall compliance to filling. The normal cystometric curve shows a fairly constant low intravesical pressure until the bladder nears capacity, then a moderate rise until capacity is reached, and then a sharp rise as voiding is initiated. Normally, the sensation of fullness is first perceived when the bladder contains 100–200 mL of fluid and strongly felt as the bladder nears capacity; the desire to void occurs when the bladder is full (normal capacity, 400–500 mL). However, the bladder has a power of accommodation, that is, it can maintain an almost constant intraluminal pressure throughout its filling phase regardless of the volume of fluid present, and this directly influences compliance. As the bladder progressively accommodates larger volumes with no change in intraluminal pressure, the

compliance values become higher (Compliance = Volume/Pressure) (Figure 27–10).

Contractility & Voluntary Control

The bladder normally shows no evidence of contractility or activity during the filling phase. However, once it is filled to capacity and the patient perceives the desire to urinate and consciously allows urination to proceed, strong bladder contractions occur and are sustained until the bladder is empty. The patient can of course consciously inhibit detrusor contraction. Both of these aspects of voluntary detrusor control must be assessed during cystometric study in order to rule out uninhibited bladder activity and to determine whether the patient can inhibit urination with a full bladder and initiate urination when asked to do so. The latter is occasionally difficult to verify clinically because of conscious inhibition by a patient who may be embarrassed by the unnatural circumstances.

Responses to Drugs

Drugs are being used with increasing frequency in the evaluation of detrusor function. They can help to diagnose underlying neuropathy and to determine whether drug treatment might be of value in individual cases. Study of the relationship of bladder capacity to intravesical pressure and bladder contractility gives a rough evaluation of the patient's bladder function. Low intravesical pressure with normal bladder capacity might

Figure 27–8. Flow rate in a case of urinary obstruction showing very low average flow rate (not above 5 or 6 mL/s). Prolonged duration of flow is associated with incomplete emptying. On the horizontal scale, one large square equals 5 s.

Figure 27–9. Classic low flow rate of bladder outlet obstruction (benign prostatic hypertrophy), markedly prolonged flow time, and fluctuation due to attempt at improving flow by increasing intra-abdominal pressure. On the horizontal scale, one large square equals 5 s.

not be significant, whereas low pressure with a very large capacity might imply sensory loss or a flaccid lower motor neuron lesion, a chronically distended bladder, or a large bladder due to myogenic damage. High pressure (usually associated with reduced capacity) that rises rapidly with bladder filling is most commonly due to inflammation, enuresis, or reduced bladder capacity. However, uninhibited bladder activity during this high-pressure filling phase might indicate neuropathic bladder or an upper motor neuron lesion.

The parasympathetic drug bethanechol chloride (Urecholine) is often used to assess bladder muscle function in patients with low bladder pressure associated with lack of detrusor contraction. No response to bethanechol suggests myogenic damage; a normal response indicates a bladder of large capacity with normal musculature; and an exaggerated response indicates a lower motor neuron lesion. The test has so many variables that it must be done meticulously to give reliable results.

Testing with anticholinergic drugs or muscle depressants may be helpful in the evaluation of uninhibited detrusor contraction or increased bladder tonus and

low compliance. The information thus obtained can be useful in choosing drugs for treatment.

Recording of Intravesical Pressure

Intravesical pressure can be measured directly from the vesical cavity, either by a suprapubic approach or via a transurethral catheter. The pressure inside the bladder is actually a function of both intra-abdominal and intravesical pressure. Thus, true detrusor pressure is the pressure recorded from the bladder cavity (intravesical pressure) minus intra-abdominal pressure. This point is important because variations in intra-abdominal pressure may alter the recorded intravesical pressure, and if the recorded intravesical pressure is mistakenly considered to reflect only detrusor pressure and not increased intra-abdominal pressure due to straining as well, erroneous conclusions may be reached.

In clinical practice, it is not necessary to measure intra-abdominal pressure, since abdominal wall contraction can be observed during the course of cystometry. A notation in the patient's chart serves to distin-

Figure 27–10. Cystometrogram of patient with normal bladder capacity. Note stable intravesical pressure during filling phase; slight rise at end of filling phase, indicating bladder capacity perceived as sense of fullness; and sharp rise at end (voiding contraction).

$$Compliance = \frac{\Delta V}{\Delta P}$$

guish true detrusor contraction from possible overlap or increase in intra-abdominal pressure. When necessary—that is, in case of uncertainty and in order to be absolutely accurate—intra-abdominal pressure should be recorded simultaneously with intravesical pressure, since there is no other way to determine the true detrusor pressure. Intra-abdominal pressure is usually recorded by a small balloon catheter inserted high in the rectum and connected to a separate transducer.

The most valuable part of the cystometric study is the determination of voiding activity or voiding contraction. The characteristics of intravesical pressure can be quite significant. Normally, voiding contractions are not high (20–40 cm of water); this magnitude of intravesical pressure is generally adequate to deliver a normal flow rate of 20–30 mL/s and completely empty the bladder if it is well sustained. A higher voiding pressure is indicative of possible increase in outlet resistance yet denotes an overactive, healthy detrusor musculature. Figure 27–11 shows a normal flow rate associated with

Figure 27–12. Recording of bladder pressure simultaneously with flow rate. Note slightly higher intravesical pressure with high flow rate, which, at its maximum, is that of a supervoider (see Figure 27–3). On the horizontal scale, one large square equals 5 s.

Figure 27–11. Simultaneous recording of voiding contraction and resulting flow rate. Note normal range of intravesical pressure during voiding phase as well as adequate normal flow rate (shown in Figure 27–4). On the horizontal scale, one large square equals 5 s.

normal detrusor contraction at a magnitude of 20 cm of water that is well sustained and of short duration and results in complete bladder emptying.

The quality of bladder pressure can also be informative, even without simultaneous recording of flow rate. In such cases, however, it is preferable to record flow rate under normal circumstances. A well-sustained detrusor contraction, high at initiation and sustained at normal values, is seen in Figure 27–12. In Figure 27–13, the voiding pressure is too high—there is an element of sphincteric dyssynergia triggering variations in voiding pressures and flow rate. Simultaneous recording of bladder and intra-abdominal pressures would provide more information. As suggested previously, recording the intravesical pressure alone does not give as much information as may be required, and increased intra-abdominal pressure might be mistaken for detrusor action. This situation is illustrated in Figure 27–14. The bladder pressure appears to indicate good detrusor

Figure 27–13. Simultaneous recording of flow rate and intra-abdominal pressure; intravesical pressure overlap in top recording. Note very high voiding pressure. However, flow rate is relatively low, with some interruption most likely due to sphincteric overactivity. On the horizontal scale, one large square equals 5 s.

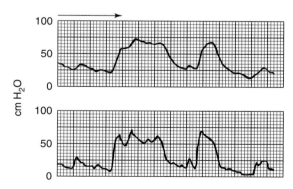

Figure 27–14. Simultaneous recording of intra-abdominal and intravesical pressures. If one considers only intravesical pressure (**upper recording**), one might assume adequate detrusor contraction. Comparison with intra-abdominal pressure (**lower recording**) shows that they are almost identical and that there is no detrusor contraction at all.

function; nevertheless, simultaneous recording of intra-abdominal pressure makes it clear that all of the apparent changes in vesical intraluminal pressure in fact represent variations in intra-abdominal pressure.

Figure 27–15 shows the 2 pressures recorded on the same chart, on the same channel, by having the writing pen share the time between 2 transducers—one recording intra-abdominal pressure; the other, intravesical pressure.

A. Pathologic Changes in Bladder Capacity

The bladder capacity is normally 400–500 mL, but it can be reduced or increased in a variety of disorders and lesions (Table 27–1). Some common causes of reduced bladder capacity are enuresis, urinary tract infection, contracted bladder, upper motor neuron lesion, and defunctionalized bladder. Reduced capacity also may occur in association with incontinence and in postsurgical bladder. Increased bladder capacity is not uncommon in women who have trained themselves to retain large volumes of urine. Bladder capacity is increased also in sensory neuropathic disorders, lower motor neuron lesions, and chronic obstruction from myogenic damage. It is important to relate bladder capacity to the intravesical pressure (Table 27–2). Slight variations in bladder capacity with no change in bladder pressure might be of less significance than the reverse. What is usually of greatest significance is the bladder with reduced capacity associated with normal pressure or, more important, with increased pressure, or the bladder with large capacity associated with decreased pressure.

B. Pathologic Changes in Accommodation

Accommodation reflects intravesical pressure in response to filling. In a bladder with normal power of accommodation—in which case the micturition center of the spinal cord is controlled by the central nervous system—intravesical pressure does not vary with progressive bladder filling until capacity is reached; in other

Figure 27–15. Simultaneous recording of 2 measurements—intravesical pressure (**top**) and intra-abdominal pressure (**bottom**)—on a single channel. The difference between the two can be clearly seen as pure detrusor contraction.

Table 27–1. Causes of reduced or increased bladder capacity. (Normal capacity in adults is 400–500 mL.)

Causes of reduced bladder capacity
    Enuresis or incontinence
    Bladder infections
    Bladder contracture due to fibrosis (from tuberculosis, interstitial cystitis, etc)
    Upper motor neuron lesions
    Defunctionalized bladder
    Postsurgical bladder
Causes of increased bladder capacity
    Sensory neuropathic disorders
    Lower motor neuron lesions
    Megacystis (congenital)
    Chronic urinary tract obstruction

words, when compliance is reduced, there will be a progressive increase in intravesical pressure and loss of accommodation. This usually occurs at smaller volumes and with reduced capacity. The patient being studied by cystometry can always note the presence or absence of a sensation of fullness. One normally does not sense volumes in the bladder but only changes in pressure.

C. PATHOLOGIC CHANGES IN SENSATION

A slight rise in intravesical pressure on cystometry signifies that the bladder is full to normal capacity and that the patient is perceiving it. This sign is usually absent in pure sensory neuropathy and in mixed sensory and motor loss. (Other sensations can be tested for in different ways; see Chapter 26.)

Table 27–2. Relationship between intravesical pressure and capacity in various diseases.

Low intravesical pressure
    Normal capacity
    Large capacity
        Sensory deficits (diabetes mellitus, tabes dorsalis)
        Flaccid lower motor neuron lesions
        Large bladder (due to repeated stretching)
High intravesical pressure
    Rapidly rising
        Reduced capacity
        Inflammation
        Enuresis
    Uninhibited contraction
        Uninhibited neurogenic bladder
        Upper motor neuron lesions

D. PATHOLOGIC CHANGES IN CONTRACTILITY

The bladder is normally capable of sustaining contraction until it is empty. Absence of residual urine after voiding usually denotes well-sustained contractions. Neuropathic dysfunction is usually associated with residual urine of variable amount depending on the type of dysfunction. Significant outlet resistance—mechanical or functional—is also a cause of residual urine.

Cystometric study may disclose complete absence of detrusor contractility due to motor or sensory deficits or conscious inhibition of detrusor activity (Table 27–3). Detrusor hyperactivity is shown as uninhibited activity, usually due to interruption of the neural connection between spinal cord centers and the higher midbrain and cortical centers.

An integrated picture of bladder capacity, intravesical pressure, and contractility is useful for general assessment of the basic physiologic mechanisms of the bladder. Low intravesical pressure in a patient with normal bladder capacity may have no clinical significance, whereas low pressure with a very large capacity may signify sensory loss or a flaccid lower motor neuron lesion, a chronically distended bladder, or a large bladder due to myogenic damage. High pressure (usually associated with reduced capacity) that rises rapidly with bladder filling is most commonly associated with inflammation, enuresis, or reduced bladder capacity. However, uninhibited activity during the interval of rising pressure that occurs with bladder filling may indicate a neurogenic bladder or an upper motor neuron lesion.

SPHINCTERIC FUNCTION

Urinary sphincteric function can be evaluated either by recording the electromyographic activity of the voluntary component of the sphincteric mechanism or by recording the activity of both smooth and voluntary

Table 27–3. Variations in detrusor contractility in various diseases.

Normal contractions
    Normal volume
    Well-sustained contractions
Absent or weak contractions
    Sensory neuropathic disorders
    Conscious inhibition of contractions
    Lower motor neuron lesions
Uninhibited contractions
    Upper motor neuron lesions
    Cerebrovascular lesions

components by measuring the intraurethral pressure of the sphincteric unit. The latter method is called **pressure profile measurement** (**profilometry**).

Profilometry

The urethral pressure profile is determined by recording the pressure in the urethra at every level of the sphincteric unit from the internal meatus to the end of the sphincteric segment. Water profilometry, which requires a flow rate of about 2 mL/min, gives fairly accurate results. It may be used for screening patients with incontinence or functional obstruction, but it is not very sensitive and only provides information about total urethral pressure. The membrane catheter and microtransducer techniques of profilometry described in the following sections provide much more accurate and detailed information.

A. MEMBRANE CATHETER TECHNIQUE

Membrane catheters used for recording pressure profiles usually have several channels, so that several measurements can be obtained simultaneously. My group's current membrane catheter has 4 lumens and an outside diameter of 7F. Two of the 4 lumens are open at the end, one for bladder filling and the other for recording bladder pressure; the other 2 lumens, which are situated 7 and 8 cm from the catheter tip, are covered by a thin membrane with a small chamber underneath (Figure 27–16). The space under the membrane and the lumen connected to it are filled with fluid, free of any gas, and connected to a pressure transducer. The pressure under this membrane should be zero at the level of the transducer so that it can register any pressure applied to the membrane whatever its level at any time. The catheter also has radiopaque markers at 1-cm intervals starting at the tip, with a heavier marker every 5 cm; it also has a special marker showing the site of each membrane. The markers permit fluoroscopic visualization of the catheter and the membrane levels during the entire study.

B. MICROTRANSDUCER TECHNIQUE

The results of microtransducer profilometry are as accurate as those obtained with the membrane catheter. Two microtransducers can be mounted on the same catheter, one at the tip for recording of bladder pressure and the other about 5–7 cm from the tip to record the urethral pressure profile as the catheter is gradually withdrawn from the bladder cavity to below the sphincteric segment.

Electromyographic Study of Sphincteric Function

Electromyography alone gives useful information about sphincteric function, but it is most valuable when done in conjunction with cystometry. There are several techniques for electromyographic studies of the urinary sphincter; either surface electrodes or needle electrodes are used. Surface electrode recordings can be obtained either from the lumen of the urethra in the region of the voluntary sphincter or, preferably, from the anal sphincter by using an anal plug electrode. Recording via needle electrodes can be obtained from the anal sphincter, from the bulk of the musculature of the pelvic floor, or from the external sphincter itself, though in the latter case the placement is difficult and the accuracy of the results is questionable.

Figure 27–16. Membrane catheter showing radiopaque markers. Note 2 membrane chambers for urethral pressure measurements and 4 separate channels— 2 channels for urethral pressure recording, one for bladder pressure recording, and one for bladder filling—each of which is connected to a separate ending. (Reproduced, with permission, from Tanagho EA, Jonas U: Membrane catheter: Effective for recording pressure in lower urinary tract. Urology 1977;10:173.)

Direct needle electromyography of the urethral sphincter provides the most accurate information. Because the technique is difficult, however, simpler approaches are generally used. The anal sphincter is readily accessible for electromyographic testing, and testing of any area of the pelvic floor musculature generally reflects the overall electrical activity of the pelvic floor, including the external sphincter. Electromyography is not simple, and the assistance of an experienced electromyographer is probably essential. Electromyographic study makes use of the electrical activity that is constantly present within the pelvic floor and external urinary sphincter at rest and that increases progressively with bladder filling. If the bladder contracts for voiding, electrical activity ceases completely, permitting free flow of urine, and is resumed at the termination of detrusor contraction to secure closure of the bladder outlet (Figure 27–17). Electromyography is important in showing this effect and, along with bladder pressure measurement, can pinpoint the exact time of detrusor contraction. Persistence of electromyographic activity during the phase of detrusor contraction for voiding—or, even worse, its overactivity during that phase—interferes with the voiding mechanism and leads to incoordination between detrusor and sphincter (**detrusor/ sphincter dyssynergia**). During the interval of detrusor contraction, increased electromyographic activity interferes with the free flow of urine, as can be shown by simultaneous recording of flow rate.

Electromyographic recording shows only the activity of the voluntary component of the urinary sphincteric mechanism and the overall activity of the pelvic floor. More information is gained when the electromyogram is recorded simultaneously with detrusor pressure or flow rate. However, this method gives no information about the smooth component of the urinary sphincter.

Pressure Measurement for Evaluation of Sphincteric Function

Perfusion profilometry, usually performed with the patient supine and with an empty bladder, provides a simple pressure profile that allows determination of the maximum pressure within the urethra. This is adequate for screening patients with incontinence or functional obstruction. However, in order to determine the maximum closure pressure (see section following), the bladder pressure must be recorded simultaneously with the urethral pressure profile. Such simultaneous recording is not possible with perfusion profilometry.

The membrane catheter and microtransducer techniques of profilometry, because they use multichannel recording, routinely provide much more detailed information; at least 4 distinct sets of measurements can be obtained from the simplest pressure profile made using the membrane catheter or microtransducer (Figure 27–18): (1) the maximum pressure exerted around the sphincteric segment, (2) the net closure pressure of the urethra, (3) the distribution of this closure pressure along the entire length of the sphincter, and (4) the exact functional length of the sphincteric unit and its relation to the anatomic length.

A. TOTAL PRESSURE

The urethral pressure profile recording shows the pressure directly recorded within the urethral lumen along the entire length of the urethra from internal to exter-

Figure 27–17. Simultaneous recording of bladder pressure, flow rate, and electromyography of anal sphincter. With rise in bladder pressure for voiding, start of flow rate has a smooth, continuous, bell-shaped curve. Note also complete absence of electromyographic activity of the anal sphincter throughout the voiding act. On the horizontal scale, one large square equals 5 s.

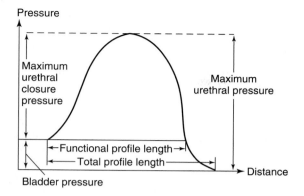

Figure 27–18. Urethral pressure profile and its components. Note functional length, anatomic length, and the shape of the profile, with maximum closure pressure in the middle segment of the urethra rather than at the level of the internal meatus. (Reproduced, with permission, from Bradley W: Cystometry and sphincter electromyography. Mayo Clin Proc 1976;329:335.)

nal meatus. From this measurement, the maximum pressure exerted around the sphincteric segment can be determined.

B. CLOSURE PRESSURE

The urethral closure pressure is the difference between intravesical pressure (bladder pressure) and urethral pressure, that is, the net closure pressure. The **maximum closure pressure** is the most important measurement in evaluating the activity of the sphincteric unit and its responses to various factors.

C. DISTRIBUTION OF CLOSURE PRESSURE

As the catheter is withdrawn down the urethra, the closure pressure at various levels along the entire length of the sphincteric segment is recorded.

D. FUNCTIONAL LENGTH OF SPHINCTERIC UNIT

The functional length of the sphincteric unit is the portion with positive closure pressure, that is, where urethral pressure is greater than bladder pressure. The distinction between anatomic length and functional length is important. Regardless of the anatomic length, the effectiveness of the urethral sphincter may be limited to a shorter segment. In women, the pressure is normally rather low at the level of the internal meatus but builds up gradually until it reaches its maximum in the mid urethra, where the voluntary sphincter is concentrated; it slowly drops until it is at its lowest at the external meatus. On the basis of these measurements, it

is clear that the anatomic and functional lengths of the normal urethra in women are about the same and that the maximum closure pressure is at about the center of the urethra—not at the level of the internal meatus. In men, the pressure profile is slightly different: the functional length is longer, and the maximum closure pressure builds up in the prostatic segment, reaches a peak in the membranous urethra, and drops as it reaches the level of the bulbous urethra (Figure 27–19). The entire functional length in men is about 6–7 cm; in women, it is about 4 cm.

Dynamic Changes in Pressure Profile

The usefulness of the pressure profile is enhanced if the examiner notes the sphincteric responses to various physiologic stimuli: (1) postural changes (supine, sitting, standing), (2) changes in intra-abdominal pressure (sharp increase with coughing; sustained increase with bearing down), (3) voluntary contractions of the pelvic floor musculature to assess activity of the voluntary sphincter, and (4) bladder filling. The latter test consists of making baseline recordings with both an empty bladder and a full bladder and comparing these recordings with recordings made under conditions of stress (coughing, bearing down) and during voluntary contraction with an empty bladder and a full bladder.

A simple pressure profile is informative but does not provide data that will delineate and identify specific sites of sphincteric dysfunction. The advantage of using a membrane catheter or microtransducer is that the pressure profile can be expanded by slowing the rate of withdrawal of the catheter and speeding up the motion of the recording paper. Since the catheter can be held at different levels for any length of time, other tests can be made and their effects monitored. Response to stress (particularly when standing), response to bladder distention, response to changes in position, the effects of drugs, and the effects of nerve stimulation can all be evaluated if needed. Bladder filling normally leads to increase in tonus of the sphincteric element, with some rise in closure pressure, especially when bladder filling approaches maximum capacity. Stress from coughing or straining also normally results in sustained or increased closure pressure (Figure 27–20). When the patient stands up, closure pressure is usually substantially increased (Figure 27–21). Testing for activity of the voluntary sphincter by the hold maneuver (asking the patient to actively contract the perineal muscles) produces a significant rise in urethral pressure (Figure 27–22). When the effects of all of these responses are recorded concomitantly with intravesical pressure, the data can be interrelated and the exact closure pressure at any given time can be ascertained.

Figure 27–19. Normal male urethral pressure profile showing progressive rise throughout prostatic segment and peak being reached in membranous urethra. (Reproduced, with permission, from Tanagho EA: Membrane and microtransducer catheters: Their effectiveness for profilometry of the lower urinary tract. Urol Clin North Am 1979;6:110.)

The response to stress with the patient standing usually should be recorded also. Especially in cases of stress incontinence, weakness of the sphincteric mechanism may not be apparent with the patient sitting or supine but becomes clear when the patient stands up.

The effectiveness of drugs in increasing or reducing the urethral pressure profile can be tested also. For example, phenoxybenzamine (Regitine) can be administered and the urethral pressure profile recorded; a drop in pressure indicates that alpha blockers may be an effective means of decreasing urethral resistance, with obvious implications for the management of urinary obstruction. Anticholinergic drugs such as propantheline bromide can be tested for possible use as detrusor depressants. Detrusor activity can be investigated by administering bethanechol chloride (Urecholine) and simultaneously recording bladder and urethral pressures.

Characteristics of Normal Pressure Profile (Figure 27–23)

The basic features of the ideal pressure profile are not easily defined. In women, the normal urethral pressure profile has a peak of 100–120 cm of water, and the closure pressure is in the range of 90–100 cm of water. Closure pressure is lowest at the level of the internal meatus, gradually builds up in the proximal 0.5 cm, and reaches its maximum about 1 cm below the internal meatus. It is sustained for another 2 cm and then starts to drop in the distal urethra. The functional length of a normal adult female urethra is about 4 cm. The response to stress with coughing and bearing down is sustained or augmented closure pressure. Standing up also increases this pressure, with maximum rise in the mid segment.

Pressure Profile in Pathologic Conditions

A. URINARY STRESS INCONTINENCE

The classic pressure changes noted in this type of incontinence are as follows:

1. Low urethral closure pressure.
2. Short urethral functional length at the expense of the proximal segment.

Figure 27–20. Simultaneous recording of intraurethral (U) and intravesical (B) pressures and their responses to coughing and bearing down. Rise in intravesical pressure as a result of increase in intraabdominal pressure is associated with simultaneous rise in intraurethral pressure, maintaining a constant closure pressure.

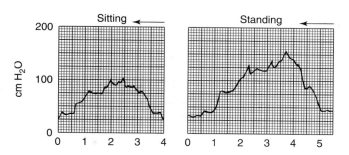

Figure 27–21. Urethral pressure profile of normal woman in sitting and standing positions. Note marked improvement in closure pressure (in both functional length and magnitude) when patient stands up. (Reproduced, with permission, from Tanagho EA: Urodynamics of female urinary incontinence with emphasis on stress incontinence. J Urol 1979;122:200.)

3. Weak responses to stress.
4. Loss of urethral closure pressure with bladder filling.
5. Fall in closure pressure on assuming the upright position.
6. Weak responses to stress in the upright position.

B. Urinary Urge Incontinence

The most pertinent pressure changes in urinary urge incontinence are normal or high closure pressures with normal responses to stress, normal responses to bladder filling, and normal responses when the patient stands up. Urge incontinence can result from any of the following mechanisms (Figure 27–24):

1. Detrusor hyperirritability, with active detrusor contractions overcoming urethral resistance and leading to urine leakage.
2. The exact reverse, that is, a constant detrusor pressure with no evidence of detrusor instability but with urethral instability in that urethral pressure becomes less than bladder pressure, so that urine leakage occurs without any detrusor contraction.
3. A combination of the 2 preceding mechanisms (the most common form), that is, some drop in closure pressure and some rise in bladder pressure. In such cases, the drop in urethral pressure is often the initiating factor.

C. Combination of Stress and Urge Incontinence

In this common clinical condition, profilometry is used to determine the magnitude of each component, that is, whether the incontinence is primarily urge, primarily stress, or both equally. As a guide to treatment, profilometric studies sometimes show that stress incontinence precipitates urge incontinence. The stress elements initiate urine leakage in the proximal urethra, exciting detrusor response and sphincteric relaxation and ending with complete urine leakage. Once the stress components are corrected, the urge element disappears. This combination cannot be detected clinically.

D. Postprostatectomy Incontinence

After prostatectomy, there is usually no positive pressure in the entire prostatic fossa, minimal closure pressure at the apex of the prostate, and normal or greater than normal pressure within the voluntary sphincteric segment of the membranous urethra. It is the functional length of the sphincteric segment above the genitourinary diaphragm that determines the degree of incontinence; the magnitude of closure pressure in the voluntary sphincteric segment has no bearing on the patient's symptoms. High pressure is almost always recorded within the voluntary sphincter despite the common belief that what someone termed "iatrogenically induced incontinence" is due to damage to the voluntary sphincter—which is definitely not the case.

Figure 27–22. Right: Urethral pressure profile in normal range. U, urethra; B, bladder. **Left:** Main point of effect of hold maneuver is significant increase in closure pressure of urethra (U) without change in bladder pressure (B)—act of voluntary sphincter.

Figure 27–23. Recording of normal female urethral pressure profile, showing basic features and actual values, including anatomic as well as functional length. U, urethra; B, bladder. (Reproduced, with permission, from Tanagho EA: Membrane and microtransducer catheters: Their effectiveness for profilometry of the lower urinary tract. Urol Clin North Am 1979;6:110.)

E. DETRUSOR/SPHINCTER DYSSYNERGIA

In this situation, findings of cystometric studies are normal at the filling phase, with possible closure pressure above average. However, the pathologic entity becomes clear when the patient attempts to void: Detrusor contraction is associated with a simultaneous increase in urethral closure pressure instead of a drop in pressure. This is a direct effect of overactivity of the voluntary component, leading to obstructive voiding or low flow rate and frequent interruption of voiding. This phenomenon is commonly seen in patients with supraspinal lesions. It can be encountered in several other conditions as well.

Value of Simultaneous Recordings

Measurement of each of the physiologic variables described previously gives useful clinical information. A

Figure 27–24. Three mechanisms of urinary urge incontinence. **Left:** Normal sphincter activity exceeded by hyperactive detrusor. **Center:** Normal detrusor, without any overactivity, yet unstable urethra with marked drop in urethral pressure leading to leakage. **Right:** Most common combination—some rise in intravesical pressure due to detrusor hyperirritability associated with drop in urethral pressure due to sphincteric relaxation. U, urethra; B, bladder.

rise in intravesical pressure has greater significance when related to intra-abdominal pressure. The urine flow rate is more significant if recorded in conjunction with the total volume voided as well as with evidence of detrusor contraction. The urethral pressure profile is more significant when related to bladder pressure and to variations in intra-abdominal pressure and voluntary muscular activity. And for greatest clinical usefulness, all data must be recorded simultaneously so that the investigator can analyze the activity involved in each sequence.

At a minimum, a proper urodynamic study should include recordings of intravesical pressure and intra-abdominal pressure (true detrusor pressure is intravesical pressure minus intra-abdominal pressure), urethral pressure or electromyography, flow rate, and, if possible, voided volume. For a complete study, the following are necessary: intra-abdominal pressure, intravesical pressure, urethral sphincteric pressure at various (usually 2) levels, flow rate, voided volume, anal sphincteric pressure (as a function of pelvic floor activity), and electromyography of the anal or urethral striated sphincter.

These physiologic data are recorded with the patient quiet as well as during activity (ie, voluntary increase in intra-abdominal pressure, changes in the state of bladder filling, voluntary contraction of perineal muscles, or—more comprehensively—an entire voiding act starting from an empty bladder; continuing through complete filling of the bladder, and initiation of voiding; and ending when the bladder is empty).

The data derived from urodynamic studies are descriptive of urinary tract function. Simultaneous visualization of the lower urinary tract as multiple recordings are made gives more precise information about the pathologic changes underlying the symptoms. By means of cinefluoroscopy, the examiner can observe the configuration of the bladder, bladder base, and bladder outlet during bladder filling (usually with radiopaque medium). The information obtained can then be correlated with the level of catheters, with pressure recordings, and with changes in pelvic floor support during voiding. Combined cinefluoroscopy and pressure measurements thus represent the ultimate in urodynamic studies.

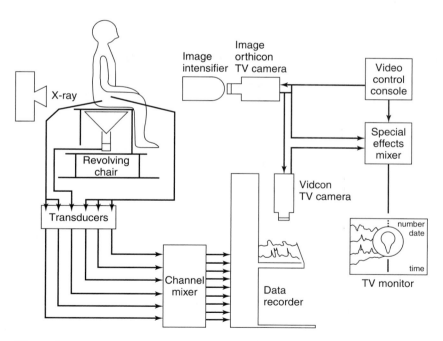

Figure 27–25. Urodynamic laboratory with specially designed toilet chair; patient sits between x-ray tube and image intensifier. A television camera records the fluoroscopic image, and a second camera picks up recordings from a polygraph machine to be projected onto one television monitor, photographed, and recorded on videotape.

A model of such a urodynamic laboratory has been developed at the University of California School of Medicine (San Francisco). As shown in Figure 27–25, the patient sits in a specially designed toilet chair over a device for collecting urine and measuring flow rate. The patient faces the x-ray tube that receives the image of the bladder and bladder outlet, which is projected on a fluoroscopic screen. The pressure-recording catheters are connected to a set of transducers that are in turn connected to a polygraph recording machine, on top of which a television camera is mounted. On a separate television monitor, the image of the pressure recording is combined with the image from the fluoroscopic monitor. A permanent record can be obtained on videotape or motion picture film.

REFERENCES

Urethra & Bladder

Abrams P: Lower urinary tract symptoms in women: Who to investigate and how. Br J Urol 1997;80(Suppl 1):43.

Abrams P: Managing lower urinary tract symptoms in older men. Br Med J 1995;310:1113.

Abrams P: Objective evaluation of bladder outlet obstruction. Br J Urol 1995;76(Suppl 1):11.

Artibani W: Diagnosis and significance of idiopathic overactive bladder. Urology 1997;50(6A Suppl):25.

Awad SA et al: Urethral pressure profile in female stress incontinence. J Urol 1978;120:475.

Bazeed MA et al: Histochemical study of urethral striated musculature in the dog. J Urol 1982;128:406.

Beck RP, McCormick S, Nordstrom L: Intraurethral-intravesical cough-pressure spike differences in 267 patients surgically cured of genuine stress incontinence of urine. Obstet Gynecol 1988;72:302.

Berger Y et al: Urodynamic findings in Parkinson's disease. J Urol 1987;138:836.

Bruschini H, Schmidt RA, Tanagho EA: Effect of urethral stretch on urethral pressure profile. Invest Urol 1977;15:107.

Bruskewitz R, Raz S: Urethral pressure profile using microtip catheter in females. Urology 1979;14:303.

Bump RC, Fantl JA, Hurt WG: Dynamic urethral pressure profilometry pressure transmission ratio determinations after continence surgery: Understanding the mechanism of success, failure, and complications. Obstet Gynecol 1988;72:870.

Cardenas DD et al: Residual urine volumes in patients with spinal cord injury: Measurement with a portable ultrasound instrument. Arch Phys Med Rehabil 1988; 69:514.

Coolsaet B: Bladder compliance and detrusor activity during the collection phase. Neurourol Urodynam 1985;4:263.

DeGroat WC: A neurologic basis for the overactive bladder. Urology 1997;50(6A Suppl):36.

Desai P: Bladder pressure studies combined with micturating cystourethrography. Radiography 1985;52:2.

Desmond AD, Ramayya GR: The adaptation of urethral pressure profiles to detect sphincter incompetence and sphincter obstruction using a microcomputer. J Urol 1987;137:457.

Dwyer PL, Rosamilia A: Evaluation and diagnosis of the overactive bladder. Clin Obstet Gynecol 2002;45:193.

Glen ES, Eadie A, Rowan D: Urethral closure pressure profile measurements in female urinary incontinence. Acta Urol Belg 1984;52:174.

Gosling JA et al: A comparative study of the human external sphincter and periurethral levator ani muscles. Br J Urol 1981; 53:35.

Graber P, Laurent G, Tanagho EA: Effect of abdominal pressure rise on the urethral profile: An experimental study on dogs. Invest Urol 1974;12:57.

Griffiths D: Clinical aspects of detrusor instability and the value of urodynamics: A review of the evidence. Eur Urol 1998; 34(Suppl 1):13.

Harvey MA, Versi E: Predictive value of clinical evaluation of stress urinary incontinence: A summary of the published literature. Int Urogynecol J Pelvic Floor Dysfunct 2001;12:31.

Henriksson L, Andersson K-E, Ulmsten U: The urethral pressure profiles in continent and stress-incontinent women. Scand J Urol Nephrol 1979;13:5.

Henriksson L, Aspelin P, Ulmsten U: Combined urethrocystometry and cinefluorography in continent and incontinent women. Radiology 1979;130:607.

Jepsen JV, Bruskewitz RC: Comprehensive patient evaluation for benign prostatic hyperplasia. Urology 1998;51(4A Suppl):13.

Jonas U, Klotter HJ: Study of three urethral pressure recording devices: Theoretical considerations. Urol Res 1978;6:119.

Kelly MJ, Roskamp D, Leach GE: Transurethral incision of the prostate: A preoperative and postoperative analysis of symptoms and urodynamic findings. J Urol 1989;142:1507.

Kim YH, Kattan MW, Boone TB: Bladder leak point pressure: The measure for sphincterotomy success in spinal cord injured patients with external detrusor-sphincter dyssynergia. J Urol 1998;159:493.

Koefoot RB Jr, Webster GD: Urodynamic evaluation in women with frequency, urgency symptoms. Urology 1983;21:648.

Koelbl H, Bernaschek G: A new method for sonographic urethrocystography and simultaneous pressure-flow measurements. Obstet Gynecol 1989;74:417.

Langer R et al: Detrusor instability following colposuspension for urinary stress incontinence. Br J Obstet Gynaecol 1988;95:607.

Lim CS, Abrams P: The Abrams-Griffiths nomogram. World J Urol 1995;13:34.

Lose G: Urethral pressure measurement. Acta Obstet Gynecol Scand Suppl 1997;166:39.

McGuire EJ: The role of urodynamic investigation in the assessment of benign prostatic hypertrophy. J Urol 1992;148:1133.

McGuire EJ, Cespedes RD, O'Connell HE: Leak-point pressures. Urol Clin North Am 1996;23:253.

Nørgaard JP et al: Standardization and definitions in lower urinary tract dysfunction in children. International Children's Continence Society. Br J Urol 1998;81(Suppl 3):1.

Ouslander J et al: Simple versus multichannel cystometry in the evaluation of bladder function in an incontinent geriatric population. J Urol 1988;140:1482.

Saxton HM: Urodynamics: The appropriate modality for the investigation of frequency, urgency, incontinence, and voiding difficulties. Radiology 1990;175:307.

Schafer W: Analysis of bladder-outlet function with the linearized passive urethral resistance relation, linPURR, and a disease-specific approach for grading obstruction: From complex to simple. World J Urol 1995;13:47.

Schafer W: Principles and clinical application of advanced urodynamic analysis of voiding function. Urol Clin North Am 1990;17:553.

Schmidt RA, Tanagho EA: Urethral syndrome or urinary tract infection? Urology 1981;18:424.

Schmidt RA, Witherow R, Tanagho EA: Recording urethral pressure profile. Urology 1977;10:390.

Schmidt RA et al: Urethral pressure profilometry with membrane catheter compared with perfusion catheter systems. Urol Int 1978;33:345.

Snyder JA, Lipsitz DU: Evaluation of female urinary incontinence. Urol Clin North Am 1991;18:197.

Sullivan MP, Comiter CV, Yalla SV: Micturitional urethral pressure profilometry. Urol Clin North Am 1996;23:263.

Tanagho EA: Interpretation of the physiology of micturition. In: Hinman F Jr (editor): Hydrodynamics. Thomas, 1971.

Tanagho EA: Membrane and microtransducer catheters: Their effectiveness for profilometry of the lower urinary tract. Urol Clin North Am 1979;6:110.

Tanagho EA: Neurophysiology of urinary incontinence. In: Cantor EB (editor): Female Urinary Stress Incontinence. Thomas, 1979.

Tanagho EA: Urodynamics of female urinary incontinence with emphasis on stress incontinence. J Urol 1979;122:200.

Tanagho EA: Vesicourethral dynamics. In: Lutzeyer W, Melchior H (editors): Urodynamics. Springer-Verlag, 1974.

Tanagho EA, Jones U: Membrane catheter: Effective for recording pressure in lower urinary tract. Urology 1977;10:173.

Tanagho EA, Meyers FH, Smith DR: Urethral resistance: Its components and implications. 2. Striated muscle component. Invest Urol 1969;7:136.

Tanagho EA, Miller ER: Functional considerations of urethral sphincteric dynamics. J Urol 1973;109:273.

Turner WH, Brading AF: Smooth muscle of the bladder in the normal and the diseased state: Pathophysiology, diagnosis and treatment. Pharmacol Ther 1997;75:77.

van Geelen JM et al: The clinical and urodynamic effects of anterior vaginal repair and Burch colposuspension. Am J Obstet Gynecol 1988;159:137.

Versi E: Discriminant analysis of urethral pressure profilometry data for the diagnosis of genuine stress incontinence. Br J Obstet Gynaecol 1990;97:251.

Woodside JR, McGuire EJ: A simple inexpensive urodynamic catheter. J Urol 1979;122:788.

Yalla SV et al: Striated sphincter participation in distal passive urinary continence mechanisms: Studies in male subjects deprived of proximal sphincter mechanism. J Urol 1979;122:655.

Urinary Flow

Bates CP, Whiteside CG, Turner-Warwick R: Synchronous cine-pressure-flow cystourethrography with special reference to stress and urge incontinence. Br J Urol 1970;42:714.

Gleason DM, Bottaccini MR: Urodynamic norms in female voiding. 2. Flow modulation zone and voiding dysfunction. J Urol 1982;127:495.

Griffiths D: Basics of pressure-flow studies. World J Urol 1995;13:30.

Griffiths DJ: Pressure-flow studies of micturition. Urol Clin North Am 1996;23:279.

Jensen KM-E, Jørgensen JB, Mogensen P: Relationship between uroflowmetry and prostatism. Proc Int Continence Soc 1985;15:134.

Jørgensen JB, Jensen KM: Uroflowmetry. Urol Clin North Am 1996;23:237.

Meyhoff HH, Gleason DM, Bottaccini MR: The effects of transurethral resection on the urodynamics of prostatism. J Urol 1989;142:785.

Nording J: A clinical view of pressure-flow studies. World J Urol 1995;13:70.

Siroky MB: Interpretation of urinary flow rates. Urol Clin North Am 1990;17:537.

Siroky MB, Olsson CA, Krane RJ: The flow rate nomogram. 2. Clinical correlation. J Urol 1980;23:208.

Stubbs AJ, Resnic MI: Office uroflowmetry using maximum flow rate purge meter. J Urol 1979;122:62.

Tanagho EA, McCurry E: Pressure and flow rate as related to lumen caliber and entrance configuration. J Urol 1971;105:583.

van Mastrigt R, Kranse M: Analysis of pressure-flow data in terms of computer-derived urethral resistance parameters. World J Urol 1995;13:40.

Electromyography

Colstrup H et al: Urethral sphincter EMG activity registered with surface electrodes in the vagina. Neurourol Urodynam 1985;4:15.

King DG, Teague CT: Choice of electrode in electromyography of external urethral and anal sphincter. J Urol 1980;124:75.

Koyanagi T et al: Experience with electromyography of the external urethral sphincter in spinal cord injury patients. J Urol 1982;127:272.

Nielsen KK et al: A comparative study of various electrodes in electromyography of the striated urethral and anal sphincter in children. Br J Urol 1985;57:557.

Siroky MB: Electromyography of the perineal floor. Urol Clin North Am 1996;23:299.

Urodynamic Testing

Barrent DM, Wein AJ: Flow evaluation and simultaneous external sphincter electromyography in clinical urodynamics. J Urol 1981;125:538.

Blaivas JG: Multichannel urodynamic studies. Urology 1984;23:421.

Blaivas JG: Multichannel urodynamic studies in men with benign prostatic hyperplasia: Indications and interpretation. Urol Clin North Am 1990;17:543.

Blaivas JG, Fischer DM: Combined radiographic and urodynamic monitoring: Advances in technique. J Urol 1981;125:693.

Blaivas JG, Salinas JM, Katz GP: The role of urodynamic testing in the evaluation of subtle neurologic lesions. Neurourol Urodynam 1985;4:211.

Cassidenti AP, Ostergard DR: Multichannel urodynamics: Ambulatory versus standard urodynamics. Curr Opin Obstet Gynecol 1999;11:485.

Daneshgari F: Valsalva leak point pressure: Steps toward standardization. Curr Urol Rep 2001;2:388.

Everaert K et al: Urodynamic assessment of voiding dysfunction and dysfunctional voiding in girls and women. Int Urogynecol J Pelvic Floor Dysfunct 2000;11:254.

Gasthuisberg KU, Vereecken RL: A critical view on the value of urodynamics in non-neurogenic incontinence in women. Int Urogynecol J Pelvic Floor Dysfunct 2000;11:188.

Gerber GS: The role of urodynamic study in the evaluation and management of men with lower urinary tract symptoms secondary to benign prostatic hyperplasia. Urology 1996;48: 668.

Kulseng-Hanssen S: Reliability and validity of stationary cystometry, stationary cysto-urethrometry and ambulatory cysto-urethro-vaginometry. Acta Obstet Gynecol Scand Suppl 1997; 166:33.

Lane TM, Shah PJ: Leak-point pressures. BJU Int 2000;86:942.

Lewis P, Abrams P: Urodynamic protocol and central review of data for clinical trials in lower urinary tract dysfunction. BJU Int 2000;85(Suppl 1):20.

Massey A, Abrams P: Urodynamics of the female lower urinary tract. Urol Clin North Am 1985;12:231.

McGuire EJ, Woodside JR: Diagnostic advantages of fluoroscopic monitoring during urodynamic evaluation. J Urol 1981; 125:830.

McLellan A, Cardozo L: Urodynamic techniques. Int Urogynecol J Pelvic Floor Dysfunct 2001;12:266.

O'Donnell PD: Pitfalls of urodynamic testing. Urol Clin North Am 1991;18:257.

Sand PK, Bowen LW, Ostergaard DR: Uninhibited urethral relaxation: An unusual cause of incontinence. Proc Int Continence Soc 1985;15:117.

Schafer W: Urethral resistance? Urodynamic concepts of physiological and pathological bladder outlet function during voiding. Neurourol Urodynam 1985;4:161.

Siroky MB: Urodynamic assessment of detrusor denervation and areflexia. World J Urol 1984;2:181.

Sutherst JR, Brown MC: Comparison of single and multichannel cystometry in diagnosing bladder instability. Br Med J 1984; 288:1720.

Tanagho EA: Membrane and microtransducer catheters: Their effectiveness for profilometry of the lower urinary tract. Urol Clin North Am 1979;6:110.

Thüroff JW: Mechanism of urinary continency: Animal model to study urethral responses to stress conditions. J Urol 1982; 127:1202.

Turner-Warwick R, Brown AD: A urodynamic evaluation of urinary incontinence in the female and its treatment. Urol Clin North Am 1979;6:203.

Turner-Warwick R, Milroy E: A reappraisal of the value of routine urological procedures in the assessment of urodynamic function. Urol Clin North Am 1979;6:63.

van Waalwijk van Doorn ES et al: Ambulatory urodynamics: Extramural testing of the lower and upper urinary tract by Holter monitoring of cystometrogram, uroflowmetry, and renal pelvic pressures. Urol Clin North Am 1996;23:345.

Wein AJ et al: Effects of bethanechol chloride on urodynamic parameters in normal women and in women with significant residual urine volumes. J Urol 1980;124:397.

Urinary Incontinence

Emil A. Tanagho, MD

Urinary incontinence is a major health issue that affects an estimated 10 million patients to some degree. Approximately 50% of all nursing home residents and between 15% and 30% of women over age 65 in retirement communities have urinary incontinence. In excess of $15–20 billion is spent on this problem annually.

PATHOPHYSIOLOGY

Elderly patients frequently accept urinary incontinence as a sign of aging and fail to seek help. In fact, it is a manifestation of an underlying disease; occasionally it is transient and resolves spontaneously, but most often it is chronic and progressive. Transient incontinence may occur after childbirth or may be associated with an acute bladder infection. Chronic urinary incontinence can result from a multitude of causes and can be classified under these main headings:

- Anatomic or genuine urinary stress incontinence
- Urge incontinence
- Neuropathic incontinence
- Congenital incontinence
- False (overflow) incontinence
- Post-traumatic or iatrogenic incontinence
- Fistulous incontinence.

Each entity listed has its own basic mechanism, although a combination of more than one of the varieties of incontinence is not uncommon.

A. ANATOMIC (GENUINE STRESS INCONTINENCE)

Anatomic incontinence is primarily the result of hypermobility of the vesicourethral segment owing to pelvic floor weakness. Its basic features are an essentially intact sphincteric mechanism, a weak pelvic floor support, and an anatomic abnormality. It is easily demonstrable radiologically, and restoration of the anatomy restores function.

B. TRUE URGE INCONTINENCE

The basic features of true urge incontinence are detrusor instability with a normal sphincteric component, normal anatomy, and no neuropathy. Sphincteric instability is less common. Leakage occurs with either detrusor instability and spontaneous contraction or, less commonly, with sphincteric instability and relaxation.

C. NEUROPATHIC INCONTINENCE

Neuropathic incontinence varies, depending on the nerve lesion. The neuropathy is usually identifiable. The incontinence can be active (detrusor hyperreflexia) or passive (sphincteric atony) or, occasionally, a combination of the two.

D. CONGENITAL INCONTINENCE

The causes of congenital incontinence are ectopic ureters, duplicate or single system, with epispadias, exstrophy, or cloacal malformation.

E. FALSE (OVERFLOW) INCONTINENCE

False incontinence is usually the result of an obstructive or neuropathic lesion. It is not true incontinence.

F. TRAUMATIC INCONTINENCE

Traumatic incontinence is associated with a fractured pelvis or with surgical damage to the sphincter during bladder neck resection or extensive internal urethrotomy; it also may result from failure of urethral diverticulectomy or repair of erosion of an artificial sphincter.

G. FISTULOUS COMMUNICATION

The fistula can be ureteral, vesical, or urethral. Most of the time, the cause is iatrogenic, from either pelvic or vaginal surgery.

This chapter discusses the most common and significant disorders: urinary stress incontinence and neuropathic incontinence.

Urinary incontinence is the involuntary loss of urine when the intravesical pressure exceeds maximal urethral pressure. Under resting conditions, continence is effected by an adequate urethral tone, which is the result of smooth and striated muscle activity, tension of the fibroelastic elements in the urethral wall, and the cushioning effect of the soft, compressible, submucosal vascular bed (Figure 28–1).

The major contribution to urethral resistance comes from the smooth and striated muscle components (Figures 28–2 and 28–3). In experimental animals, as well as in humans, the striated external sphincter provides about 50% of static urethral resistance, while smooth muscle is primarily responsible for proximal urethral closure pressure (Figure 28–4). The rise in pressure in the mid urethra results from the combined function of the smooth musculature and the striated muscle fibers

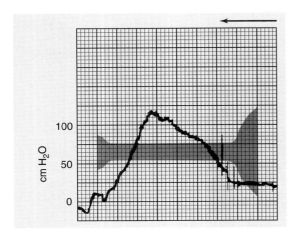

Figure 28–1. Urethral pressure profile in a normal female. Closure pressure at the level of the internal meatus is very low; the pressure rises progressively to reach its maximum at approximately the middle third of the urethra—the site of maximal condensation of striated muscle.

Figure 28–3. Response of the striated component to stimulation of the sacral nerves. Note that the bladder pressure does not change and the proximal urethral pressure (U$_1$) rises only slightly, but that the increase in midurethral pressure (U$_2$) is sharp and sustained.

A

B

Figure 28–2. **A:** Response to stimulation of the pelvic nerve. Note the simultaneous, equal pressure rise in the bladder, proximal urethra (U$_1$), and mid urethra (U$_2$). **B:** Vesical and sphincteric responses to an injection of the parasympathetic drug methacholine chloride. Note again the simultaneous rise in pressure at the bladder, proximal urethra (U$_1$), and mid urethra (U$_2$).

Figure 28–4. **A:** The resistance needed to force the urethra open, overcoming both voluntary and involuntary sphincteric elements. With progressively increasing pressure, the urethra opens at the **critical opening pressure** (in this recording, about 85 mm Hg). Once the urethra is forced open, the resistance to flow drops precipitously and becomes sustained at the level of **sustained urethral resistance** (in this recording, roughly 50 mm Hg). **B:** A similar recording obtained after administration of curare, which completely blocks voluntary sphincteric responses. Note the appreciable drop in both critical opening pressure and sustained resistance. **C:** Recording after administration of both curare and atropine (a combination that eliminates the activity of smooth and voluntary sphincteric elements). The critical opening pressure drops markedly and is now equal to the sustained resistance; both are very low. **D:** An overlap of the 3 recordings shows the contribution of each muscular element: The voluntary component contributes roughly 50% of the total resistance, while the smooth component contributes the other 50%. The minimal residual resistance is a function of the collagen elastic element of the urethral wall; this collagen element has no sphincteric significance.

around it. To maintain continence under stress conditions, the striated urethral sphincter has to resist a raised bladder pressure owing to intra-abdominal pressure increase (Figures 28–5 and 28–6). The activity of the external sphincter helped by the pelvic floor provides for this increased urethral resistance. Involuntary loss of urine with increased intra-abdominal pressure, in the absence of detrusor contraction, is usually labeled stress incontinence. When loss of urine is associated with increased intravesical pressure owing to detrusor contraction, it is commonly referred to as urge incontinence.

Genuine stress incontinence is invariably associated with weakness of the pelvic floor support, permitting hypermobility of the vesicourethral segments, which in turn impairs the efficiency of the sphincteric musculature. The increase in intraurethral pressure observed during coughing results mainly from contraction of the voluntary muscles with sphincteric action. Part of the rise is passive (ie, by direct transmission), but a significant component is active (ie, caused by reflex musculature contraction).

URINARY STRESS INCONTINENCE

Often seen in women after middle age (with repeated pregnancies and vaginal deliveries), urinary stress in-

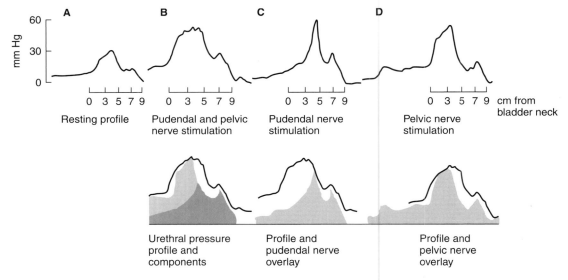

Figure 28–5. Urethral pressure profile. **A:** At rest. **B:** Stimulation of both the pudendal and the pelvic nerves incites the maximal response from both smooth and voluntary sphincteric elements. **C:** Pudendal stimulation alone shows the contribution of the voluntary component. **D:** Pelvic nerve stimulation shows the response of the smooth-muscle component alone. **Bottom tracings:** Total maximal pressure profile obtained by stimulation of pelvic and pudendal nerves shown by overlapping the profile of simultaneous stimulation of both nerves. The contribution and anatomic distribution of each element are clearly seen. Their summation results in the overall total responses recorded in **B** above.

continence is usually a result of weakness of the pelvic floor and poor support of the vesicourethral sphincteric unit. Urethral closure pressure normally responds to bladder filling; a change in position; or stressful events such as coughing, sneezing, and bearing down. The sphincteric mechanism has its own capacity to augment urethral resistance under stress reflexively and thus to prevent leakage.

The urethral pressure profile is a good measure of the activity of the external sphincter. A static profile demonstrates the resting tonus of both components of the sphincteric mechanism (see Figure 28–1); a dynamic profile gives the responses of these sphincteric elements to various activities, such as an increase in bladder volume, assumption of the upright position (Figure 28–7), the prolonged stress of bearing down, or the sudden stress of coughing and sneezing (Figure 28–8). Normally, the urethral closure pressure—the net difference between the intraurethral and intravesical pressures—is maintained or augmented during stress.

Anatomy

In genuine stress incontinence, the assumption is that the intrinsic structure of the sphincter itself is intact and normal. However, it loses efficiency because of excessive mobility and loss of support. Thus, the anatomic feature of genuine stress incontinence is consistently that of hypermobility or a lowering of the position of the vesicourethral segment (or a combination of the two factors) (Figure 28–9).

The relationships among the urethra, the bladder base, and various bony points have been the object of much study. For many years the posterior vesicourethral angle has been considered a key factor indicating the presence of anatomic stress incontinence. Some authors, however, have emphasized the axis of inclination, that is, the angle between the urethral line and the vertical plane. Other investigators stress bony landmarks in the pelvis in their descriptions of the relationship of the bladder base and the vesicourethral junction to the sacrococcygeal inferior pubic point (Figure 28–10).

These descriptions illustrate that abnormal anatomic position and excessive mobility are essential elements in the diagnosis of genuine anatomic stress incontinence. To evaluate this aspect of incontinence, I recommend a simplified cystographic study (a lateral cystogram with a urethral catheter in place) to define the vesicourethral segment clearly. With the patient lying on the flat x-ray

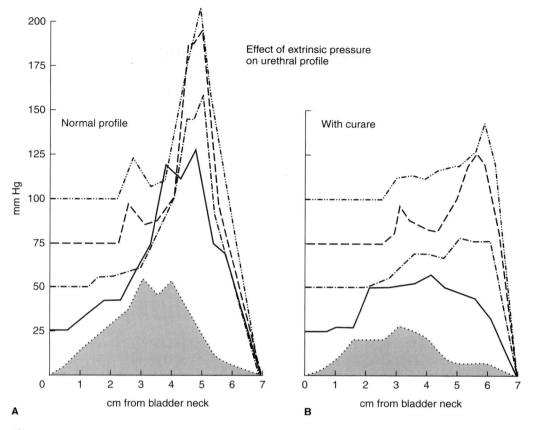

Figure 28–6. Urethral pressure profile at rest and after subjecting an experimental animal to progressively increasing extrinsic pressure applied around the abdomen—not involving any muscular activity. **A:** Extrinsic pressure was increased by 25–mm Hg increments. Note the sharp increase in urethral closure pressure with each increment, marked after 25 and 50 mm Hg, less so after 75 and 100 mm Hg. The increase in urethral closure pressure is far higher than the increase in extrinsic pressure, which denotes not simple transmitted pressure but active muscular function. **B:** Curare administration demonstrates that much of the rise in closure pressure recorded in **A** results from the activity of the voluntary sphincter, which is lost after blockade by curare.

table, a lateral film is obtained, first at rest to determine the position of the vesicourethral segment in relation to the pubic bone and then with straining to ascertain its degree of mobility (Figures 28–11 and 28–12). Normally, the vesicourethral junction is opposite the lower third of the pubic bone and moves 0.5–1.5 cm with straining. It should be emphasized, however, that cystography is not the means of diagnosing stress incontinence. This demonstration of abnormal position or excessive mobility of the vesicourethral segment is helpful in confirming the cause of existing urinary incontinence. Some authors like to classify urinary inconti-

nence in various stages. Stages I and II depend on the degree of hypermobility and usually relate to the amount of urinary leakage. Stage III, which most often is not associated with hypermobility, is usually due to intrinsic sphincteric damage—most often iatrogenic.

Urodynamic Characteristics of Stress Incontinence

A. PRESSURE PROFILE

As would be expected, patients have a low urethral pressure profile with reduced closure pressure. This factor

Figure 28–7. Urethral pressure profile with patient in sitting and upright positions. Approximately a 50% increase in urethral closure pressure occurs when the patient assumes the upright position. Urethral functional length is well sustained.

varies with the severity of the sphincteric impairment as a result of the excessive mobility: The pressure profile might be low-normal when weakness is minimal or it might be quite significant when mobility is severe. Not infrequently, however, this weakness of the pressure profile is not demonstrable when the bladder is partially full. It characteristically becomes more significant when the bladder has been distended (Figure 28–13). Also, the pressure profile may appear normal when the patient is in the resting (sitting) position; when he or she assumes the upright position in the dynamic pressure profile, the weakness becomes more apparent (Figure 28–14).

B. FUNCTIONAL URETHRAL LENGTH

The anatomic length of the urethra is usually maintained, yet the functional length is invariably shorter. The loss is in the proximal urethral segment (Figure 28–15). Although it might not look funneled on the cystogram, this segment has very low closure efficiency, or none at all, and its pressure is almost equal to intravesical pressure. The functional shortening might be minimal or it might involve more than one-half of the length of the urethra. It is important to note that the functional length, like the pressure profile, might appear normal when the bladder is partially full or the patient is in the sitting position.

C. RESPONSE TO STRESS

With the sustained stress of bearing down or the sudden stress of coughing or sneezing, the net urethral closure pressure is reduced, depending on the degree of sphincteric weakness. In severe urinary stress incontinence, any strain or increase in intravesical pressure leads to negative closure pressure and urinary leakage (Figure 28–16).

D. VOLUNTARY INCREASE IN URETHRAL CLOSURE PRESSURE

Patients with mild stress incontinence might be capable of activating their external sphincter maximally and generating a high urethral closure pressure. However, with progression of the anatomic problem and hypermobility, this voluntary increase progressively diminishes; depending on the severity of the weakness and inefficiency of the external sphincter, this weakness becomes more readily apparent.

E. RESPONSE TO BLADDER DISTENTION AND CHANGE IN POSITION

It must be emphasized that, although the features described might be normal in the resting position with minimal bladder filling, all of them can become aggravated with a full bladder or the upright position. In testing these patients urodynamically, one must ascertain the changes that occur with a full bladder and the assumption of the upright position (Figures 28–14 and 28–17).

Diagnosis

A detailed history is important, including the degree of leakage; its relation to activity, position, and state of bladder fullness; the timing of its onset; and the course of its progression. Knowledge of past surgical and obstetric history, medications taken, dietary habits, and systemic diseases (eg, diabetes) can be helpful in the diagnosis. Whether the incontinence is purely stress or purely urge or a combination of the two can be assessed, as can its degree—minimal, moderate, severe, or complete.

Physical examination is essential. The pelvic examination demonstrates laxity of pelvic support, presence

Figure 28–8. **A:** Intravesical and urethral pressure responses to the stresses of coughing, bearing down, and the hold maneuver. Note the sharp increase in intra-abdominal pressure reflected in intravesical pressure with coughing and the simultaneous greater increase in urethral pressure. The response is similar with bearing down. Closure pressure is maintained and even augmented during these periods of stress. The hold maneuver (recording membrane is in the proximal urethra) produces a minimal response in closure pressure of the proximal urethra. **B:** Recording comparable to that in **A,** but the membrane is in the mid urethra. Note again the sustained closure pressure as a result of coughing and bearing down and the marked pressure increase in the midurethral segment with the hold maneuver.

of any degree of prolapse, cystocele, rectocele, and mobility of the anterior vaginal wall. A neurologic examination should be done if neuropathy is suspected. Cystographic study for demonstration of the anatomic abnormality is important, as is urodynamic study to confirm the classic features of urinary incontinence and determine its cause. The goals of cystographic and urodynamic study are, first, to demonstrate the anatomic abnormality and its extent and, second, to assess the activity of the sphincteric mechanism and hence the potential for improvement by correcting the anatomic ab-

normality. In recurrent cases, repeated previous surgeries may have caused so much intrinsic damage to the sphincteric musculature that simple suspension cannot provide satisfactory results. Indirect evidence of the degree of sphincteric weakness can be obtained by measurement of what is called the **leak pressure** (ie, by measuring the intra-abdominal pressure through a rectal transducer during the Valsalva maneuver and noting at what pressure the first leakage of urine occurs). A low reading indicates a severe degree of sphincteric weakness.

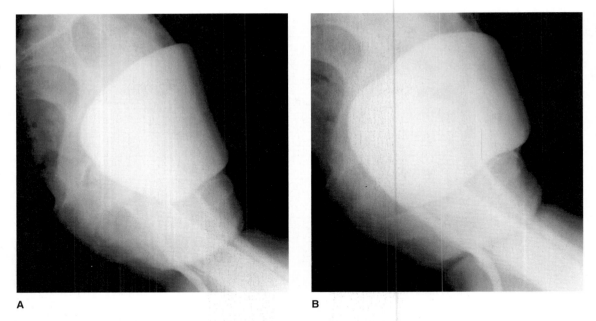

A **B**

Figure 28–9. Lateral cystograms in a 53-year-old woman with stress incontinence. **A:** Preoperative, relaxed. Note slightly low-lying vesicourethral junction. The posterior vesicourethral angle is near normal. **B:** With straining, excessive downward and posterior mobility of the vesicourethral segment is shown. Posterior angle almost disappears.

Figure 28–10. Diagrammatic representation of (**A**) the angles considered when assessing adequacy of bladder support (posterior vesicourethral angle; angle of inclination) and (**B**) the "SCIPP line" (sacrococcygeal inferior pubic point) and its relationship to the bladder base and the vesicourethral segment as a reference to adequate pelvic support.

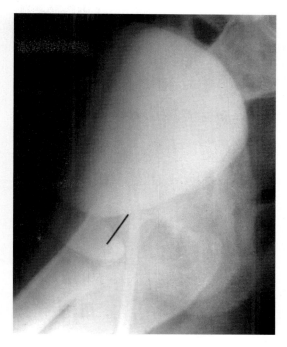

Figure 28–11. Lateral cystograms in 2 continent women in the relaxed state. A perpendicular line from the anterior vesicourethral angle over the long axis of the pubic bone crosses the bone near the junction of the middle and lower thirds.

Treatment

The principal treatment of urinary stress incontinence is proper suspension and support of the vesicourethral segment in a normal position. The rationalization is that, in genuine stress incontinence, the intrinsic sphincteric mechanism is intact but its efficiency is impaired because of excessive mobility in the abnormal position. Once the position is restored, the sphincteric mechanism usually regains its function.

There are numerous approaches to restoring the normal position and providing adequate support—some vaginal, others suprapubic. The suprapubic approach was popularized by the classic Marshall-Marchetti-Krantz (MMK) retropubic suspension described in 1949, in which periurethral tissue is attached to the back of the pubic symphysis. A modification was introduced by Burch in 1961, in which the anterior vaginal wall is fixed to Cooper's ligament. Many urologic surgeons today have found that the latter technique, with modifications, provides the most lasting results (Figures 28–18 and 28–19).

The vaginal suspension has various forms; in some, the tissue is gathered behind the bladder neck (eg, the Kelly procedure), while others rely on sutures in the paravaginal tissues that are passed bluntly to the suprapubic area by a needle to be tied over the rectus sheath. This technique was originally described by Pereyra in 1959 and subsequently was modified—in 1973 by Stamey, who added endoscopic confirmation of suture placement and the degree of compression, and in 1981 by Raz. Most of these techniques have a high initial success rate; however, there is some concern about the long-term results. Hence, the retropubic approach remains the recommended procedure.

With excessive sphincteric damage and intrinsic weakness, suspension alone might not be adequate and sling procedures are advised. Of the various techniques and materials, the most popular uses a strip of the anterior rectus sheath, first reported by McGuire. Raz advocates the vaginal wall sling, in which an island of the anterior vaginal wall is mobilized and used to support the vesicourethral segment. Numerous other sling materials are being used: for example, cadaveric fascia lata and various synthetic materials. Most recently, tension-free vaginal tape has been gaining popularity (Ulmsten, Johnson, and Rezapour, 1999). More recently, in instances of significant intrinsic sphincteric damage, local injection of bulking material such as polytetrafluoroethylene (Teflon), or preferably collagen, is used to

Figure 28–12. Lateral cystograms in two young continent women. **A:** Relaxed state, 28-year-old woman. **B:** With straining, the vesicourethral segment is displaced 0.5 cm downward and posteriorly. **C:** Relaxed state, 34-year-old woman. **D:** With straining, the vesicourethral segment is displaced 0.8 cm downward and 1 cm posteriorly.

increase the bladder outlet resistance to help in patients in whom mobility is not excessive and whose primary problem is intrinsic sphincteric weakness.

NEUROPATHIC INCONTINENCE

Neuropathic incontinence can be broken down into 2 broad classifications: active and passive. **Active neuro-**pathic incontinence is found in patients who have a spastic lesion but in whom the sphincteric mechanism, although not under voluntary control, still exerts adequate closure pressure. The presence of a hyperreflexive detrusor with uninhibited contractions increases the intravesical pressure. When intravesical pressure exceeds sphincteric pressure, there is a leakage of urine (Figure 28–20). Active incontinence is most often as-

Figure 28–13. Urethral pressure profile with minimally filled bladder. Bladder pressure remains constant, but urethral pressure drops progressively. Closure pressure becomes minimal at the end of bladder filling.

sociated with suprasegmental, or upper motor neuron, lesions.

Passive neuropathic incontinence occurs when the sphincteric mechanism is weakened or completely lacking. Even without abnormally high intravesical pressure, any increase in intra-abdominal pressure results in urinary leakage. Passive incontinence is most often associated with lesions involving the micturition center or more distal lesions.

The more common classification of neurogenic incontinence is based on an evaluation of the functions of the lower urinary tract: incontinence owing to failure of the reservoir or to failure of retention.

A. FAILURE OF RESERVOIR FUNCTION

Loss of reservoir function in the contractile or contracted bladder can be caused by poor compliance in the detrusor muscle. Intravesical pressure rises with minimal bladder filling, exceeding the outlet resistance and causing urinary leakage. In contrast to the classification of active incontinence associated with suprasegmental lesions, failure of reservoir function may be found in patients who have meningomyelocele who exhibit other lower motor neuron lesions. Although these patients may have partial lesions with significant striated sphincteric activity, offering some degree of resistance, early loss of bladder compliance increases intra-

Figure 28–14. Urethral pressure profile in moderately severe stress incontinence: closure pressure with patient in the sitting position with half-distended bladder, then after the upright position is assumed. Note that closure pressure is close to 75 cm H_2O with the patient in the sitting position but decreases to approximately 35 cm H_2O with the upright position. Note also the marked shortening of functional urethral length once the upright position is assumed.

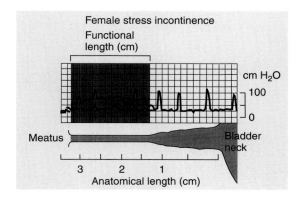

Figure 28–15. Urethral pressure profile in a female patient with moderate urinary stress incontinence. Note the relatively low closure pressure, the short functional urethral length, and the loss of closure pressure of the proximal 1.5 cm of urethra.

Figure 28–16. Urethral pressure profile in moderate stress incontinence. Note that, with the bladder relatively empty, closure pressure is close to the normal range. At the start of bladder filling, resting pressure is again normal; as filling progresses, bladder pressure remains stable and urethral closure pressure decreases progressively to a minimum with full bladder distention.

Figure 28–17. Effect of bladder filling and emptying on urethral pressure. **Top:** Effect of progressive filling, which leads to a gradual drop in urethral pressure. At the end of filling, urethral closure pressure is only a fraction of the relatively normal initial closure pressure. **Bottom:** At the start, the bladder is full. With gradual emptying, note the progressive buildup in urethral resistance and closure pressure.

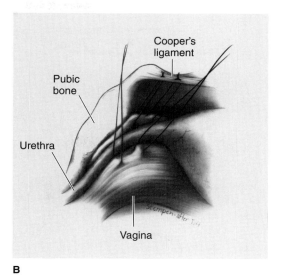

A   B

Figure 28–18. **A:** Diagrammatic depiction of the retropubic space after mobilization of the anterior vaginal wall and placement of sutures, 2 on either side and far from the midline laterally. Distal sutures are opposite the mid urethra, while proximal sutures are at the end of the vesicourethral junction. Sutures are attached to Cooper's ligament. **B:** Side view of suture placement with one side tied. The anterior vaginal wall acts as a broad sling, supporting and lifting the vesicourethral segment. The urethra is free in the retropubic space.

Figure 28–19. **Top:** Cross section shows the urethra free in the retropubic space with the anterior vaginal wall lifting and supporting it. **Bottom:** The urethra is compressed and strangulated against the pubic bone when vaginal sutures are applied close to the urethra and fixed to the symphysis pubis.

vesical pressure with minimal bladder filling, overcoming what outlet resistance there is. These patients, once recognized, must be managed aggressively because they often have a significant back-pressure effect in the upper urinary tract, which can lead to early deterioration and possible vesicoureteral reflux or lower ureteral obstruction.

B. FAILURE OF RETENTION FUNCTION

Complete lesions of the sacral segment or the cauda equina result in a total loss of smooth and striated sphincteric activity. The external sphincter offers minimal resistance. Most patients experiencing such failure can retain some volume, because the bladder musculature becomes atonic and lax and intravesical pressure remains low, but any increase in intravesical pressure can cause leakage, and the bladder never reaches full capacity. Consequently, the integrity of the upper urinary tract is not endangered, as in cases of reservoir failure. It must be stressed, however, that most cases involve the loss of some components, with the patient retaining some activity. For example, if a patient were to retain some activity in the internal sphincter but experience a complete loss of the striated sphincter, the entire pelvic floor would become flaccid and atonic.

Figure 28–20. Urodynamic recording in a patient with evidence of detrusor/sphincter dyssynergia, showing spontaneous activity in the bladder associated with a burst of activity in the external sphincter interrupting voiding. This represents a classic demonstration of upper motor neuron dysfunction leading to urinary incontinence as a result of detrusor hyperactivity or hyperreflexia.

Diagnosis

Diagnostic evaluation of neuropathic urinary incontinence determines whether the condition arises from detrusor or sphincteric dysfunction, or from a combination of the two. In exceptional cases, such as patients with multiple sclerosis with spinal stenosis or those with disk problems in addition to partial traumatic damage to the spinal cord, the neuropathy is less clear.

A complete urologic and neurologic history should be taken, followed by radiographic evaluation to determine the integrity of the upper urinary tract, the status of the reservoir, and the state of the sphincteric mechanism. Intravenous pyelography, cystourethrography, and cinefluoroscopy are also recommended. The following are valuable in determining the underlying cause of incontinence:

1. Bladder responses to progressive filling
2. Sphincteric pressure profile and its response to progressive filling and the initiation of voiding
3. The presence of detrusor hyperreflexia and uninhibited activity (in patients with hyperreflexia)
4. Electromyographic studies of the striated urinary sphincter
5. In selected patients, response to neurostimulation of the sacral roots and pudendal nerve, with or without blocking and measurement of latencies.

Differentiation among incontinence caused by uninhibited detrusor contractions, detrusor hyperreflexia, and poor bladder compliance is a straightforward process. Significant findings include sphincteric weakness, precipitous sphincteric relaxation, and decrease in pressure, as well as a lack of electromyographic activity of the pelvic floor musculature and external sphincter. The proper diagnosis can be achieved by establishing the integrity of the sacral root reflex arc by neurostimulation of the sacral roots, with simultaneous recording of intravesical and intraurethral pressures at the levels of the internal and the external sphincter. One must be alert to the possibility of overlapping causes, and the responses of the external sphincter and pelvic floor musculature to active contraction, progressive bladder filling, and sacral root stimulation can be informative. The extent of one cause relative to another (for example, sphincteric weakness versus detrusor hyperreflexia) should be taken into account, and management should be directed toward the predominating cause of incontinence.

Treatment

Although diagnosis of the causes of incontinence is relatively easy, management is generally difficult. The rehabilitation of the neuropathic condition and the alleviation of the potentially damaging sequelae must be the guiding principles of management. Choices must be made according to the severity and potential progression of the lesion and the integrity of the system. Especially in the previously mentioned cases of patients with spinal cord injury and meningomyelocele, early treatment provides the best chance of preserving the integrity of the entire urinary system.

A. CONSERVATIVE MANAGEMENT

1. Failure of reservoir function—Adequate reservoir function can be restored, allowing patients to maintain dryness for 2–4 h, with successful pharmacologic manipulation to suppress the detrusor hyperreflexia. The response to pharmacologic agents depends on the initial functional bladder capacity, extent of spasticity and hyperreflexia, lack of compliance owing to collagen deposition, and mural changes in the bladder wall. For this reason, an understanding of the function and capacity of the bladder and the role of detrusor hyperreflexia is essential to the conservative management of reservoir dysfunction.

There are 3 categories of pharmacologic agents for the treatment of reservoir dysfunction: Anticholinergic drugs are used primarily to treat detrusor hyperreflexia and uninhibited contractions. Oxybutynin (Ditropan), a tertiary amine anticholinergic drug with antispasmodic action, is the most commonly used, with a dosage of 5 mg 2–4 times a day, depending on the patient's tolerance and responses. Possible side effects include dry mouth, drowsiness, palpitations, and occasional nausea, and patients must be careful to stay below their threshold of tolerance. Oxybutynin is contraindicated in patients with high intraocular pressure. Tolterodine tartrate (Detrol), a new antimuscarinic agent, is effective in reducing detrusor hyperactivity with fewer side effects than oxybutynin. Long-acting formulations are available for both (Ditropan XL, Detrol LA).

Propantheline bromide (Pro-Banthine), although often less effective than oxybutynin, can be a useful supplement to oxybutynin and is better tolerated by some patients. The usual dosage is 15 mg 2–3 times a day, with perhaps a larger dose at bedtime. Side effects include dry mouth, visual disturbances, and increased intraocular pressure.

Imipramine hydrochloride (Tofranil), a tricyclic antidepressant with a strong anticholinergic, antimuscarinic action, has a significant effect on detrusor hyperreflexia. The usual dosage is 25 mg 2–4 times daily. Side effects include dry mouth, constipation, blurred vision, and drowsiness.

Antihistaminic drugs antagonize the histamine-mediated release of acetylcholine to produce an anticholinergic effect. Chlorpheniramine maleate can be taken alone in the long-acting 8-mg capsules or tablets orally twice a day or in combination with 75 mg of phenylpropanolamine hydrochloride (Ornade Spansules). The latter produces an anticholinergic effect on the detrusor as well as alpha-receptor stimulation to improve outlet resistance.

Musculotropic relaxants depress smooth-muscle activity directly. Flavoxate hydrochloride (Urispas, 200 mg), the most common, is taken 3–4 times daily by mouth.

2. Failure of retention mechanism—Intermittent catheterization is the first line of conservative management in these patients. Although such patients have very low outlet resistance, their bladder atonia permits some retention. Most of the time, catheterization every 4–6 h enables them to avoid leakage. When catheterization is not possible and the increase in intravesical pressure becomes excessive, the patient can wear minimal protection.

Pharmacologic manipulation is less successful. Ephedrine sulfate and phentermine (Ionamin) have a stimulating effect on both alpha and beta receptors, which increases urethral sphincteric smooth-muscle activity and partially relaxes the detrusor muscle. The former is usually given in 30- to 60-mg doses 3–4 times daily orally; the latter is usually given in a 15-mg dose 2–3 times daily orally.

B. SURGICAL MANAGEMENT

1. Sphincterotomy—In spastic hyperreflexive situations in male patients, this operation is performed to eliminate outlet resistance so that, with an external appliance or condom catheter, the bladder will remain empty. Although many consider this procedure the easiest way to preserve the upper urinary tract, it is clearly not rehabilitative and might interfere with other treatments.

2. Bladder augmentation—In patients with poor compliance owing to mural changes and chronic hypertrophy, this procedure improves reservoir function. If the sphincteric mechanism is adequate, detubularized bowel segments can be used in patients in whom the bladder will not expand even under anesthesia. Usually patients have to rely on intermittent catheterization postoperatively, but they regain continence and the upper urinary tract is preserved.

3. Artificial sphincter—In patients with severe sphincteric damage and a low-pressure, large-capacity bladder, this device can be useful. In males it is applied around the bulbous urethra. When the device is deflated, the patient can void either by detrusor contraction (if some capability is preserved) or by straining and the Valsalva maneuver. A complete sphincterotomy can

be done first. Intermittent catheterization is hazardous in patients with a urethral cuff and is rarely necessary.

4. Continent urinary diversion—This method should be considered only with progressively deteriorating upper urinary tract function, and even then a simple conduit is preferable. Approaches to be condemned are denervation of the bladder through cystolysis or transvesical transection and resuturing and denervation of the bladder base through phenol or alcohol injection. In the long term, these methods have been complete failures.

5. Neurostimulation—In selected patients with detrusor hyperreflexia, stimulation of the sacral roots has effectively suppressed the hyperactivity, relying on the known reflex response of the detrusor muscle to stimulate the somatic component of the sacral plexus (which aborts and inhibits detrusor contractility). If such patients with spinal cord injury, meningomyelocele, multiple sclerosis, and other neuropathies show significant improvement after temporary testing, a permanent electrode can be placed over the most responsive root, usually S_3.

6. Dorsal rhizotomy—Complete dorsal rhizotomy of S_2–S_4 extra- or intradurally effectively eliminates detrusor hyperreflexia and increases bladder capacity. Increases have been seen from a capacity of 150 or 200 mL to one of 600–800 mL. In patients with suprasegmental lesions and spastic upper motor neuron lesions, sacral root electrode implantation promotes detrusor contraction and bladder evacuation (the so-called bladder pacemaker).

REFERENCES

Abrams P et al: The standardisation of terminology of lower urinary tract function. The International Continence Society Committee on Standardisation of Terminology. Scand J Urol Nephrol 1988;114:5.

Appell RA: Electrical stimulation for the treatment of urinary incontinence. Urology 1998;51(2A Suppl):24.

Ashton-Miller JA, Howard D, DeLancey JO: The functional anatomy of the female pelvic floor and stress continence control system. Scand J Urol Nephrol Suppl 2001;(207):1.

Barnes NM et al: Pubovaginal sling and pelvic prolapse repair in women with occult stress urinary incontinence: Effect on postoperative emptying and voiding symptoms. Urology 2002;59:856.

Bernstein IT: The pelvic floor muscles: Muscle thickness in healthy and urinary-incontinent women measured by perineal ultrasonography with reference to the effect of pelvic floor training. Estrogen receptor studies. Neurourol Urodyn 1997; 16:237.

Bidmead J, Cardozo L: Genuine stress incontinence: Colpocystourethropexy versus sling procedures. Curr Opin Obstet Gynecol 2000;12:421.

Bidmead J, Cardozo L: Retropubic urethropexy (Burch colposuspension). Int Urogynecol J Pelvic Floor Dysfunct 2001; 12:262.

Bosch JLR, Groen J: Sacral nerve neuromodulation in the treatment of refractory motor urge incontinence. Curr Opin Urol 2001;11:399.

Brubaker L: Electrical stimulation in overactive bladder. Urology 2000;55(Suppl 5A):17.

Burch JC: Cooper's ligament urethrovesical suspension for stress incontinence: Nine years' experience—results, complications, technique. Am J Obstet Gynecol 1968;100:764.

Burch JC: Urethrovaginal fixation to Cooper's ligament for correction of stress incontinence, cystocele, and prolapse. Am J Obstet Gynecol 1961;81:281.

Cardozo LD, Stanton SL: Genuine stress incontinence and detrusor instability: A review of 200 patients. Br J Obstet Gynaecol 1980;87:184.

Carey MP, Dwyer PL: Position and mobility of the urethrovesical junction in continent and in stress incontinent women before and after successful surgery. Aust N Z J Obstet Gynaecol 1991;31:279.

Cervigni M, Natale F: Surgical treatment of stress urinary incontinence. Eur J Obstet Gynecol Reprod Biol 1999;85:63.

Chai TC, Steers WD: Neurophysiology of micturition and continence in women. Int Urogynecol J Pelvic Floor Dysfunct 1997;8:85.

Chaliha C, Stanton SL: Complications of surgery for genuine stress incontinence. Br J Obstet Gynaecol 1999;106:1238.

Chapple CR: Muscarinic receptor antagonists in the treatment of overactive bladder. Urology 2000;55(Suppl 5A):33.

Coates KW: Physiologic evaluation of the pelvic floor. Obstet Gynecol Clin North Am 1998;25:805.

Dainer M et al: The Burch procedure: A comprehensive review. Obstet Gynecol Surv 1999;54:49.

DeGroat WC: A neurologic basis for the overactive bladder. Urology 1997;50(6A Suppl):36.

DeLancey JO: The pathophysiology of stress urinary incontinence in women and its implications for surgical treatment. World J Urol 1997;15:268.

DeLancey JO: Structural aspects of the extrinsic continence mechanism. Obstet Gynecol 1988;72:296.

Demirci F, Petri E: Perioperative complications of Burch colposuspension. Int Urogynecol J Pelvic Floor Dysfunct 2000; 11:170.

Denny-Brown D, Robertson GE: On the physiology of micturition. Brain 1933;56:149.

Diokno AC et al: Prevalence of urinary incontinence and other urological symptoms in the noninstitutionalized elderly. J Urol 1986;136:1022.

Dmochowski RR, Appell RA: Advancements in pharmacologic management of the overactive bladder. Urology 2000;56 (Suppl 1):41.

Drouin J et al: Burch colposuspension: Long-term results and review of published reports. Urology 1999;54:808.

Dwyer R, Rosamilia A: Evaluation and diagnosis of the overactive bladder. Clin Obstet Gynecol 2002;45:193.

Eastham JA et al: Risk factors for urinary incontinence after radical prostatectomy. J Urol 1996;156:1707.

Elbadawi A: Functional anatomy of the organs of micturition. Urol Clin North Am 1996;23:177.

Elbadawi A, Diokno AC, Millard RJ: The aging bladder: Morphology and urodynamics. World J Urol 1998;16(Suppl 1):S10.

Elliott DS, Barrett DM: The artificial urinary sphincter in the female: Indications for use, surgical approach and results. Int Urogynecol J Pelvic Floor Dysfunct 1998;9:409.

Enhorning G: Simultaneous recording of intravesical and intraurethral pressure. Acta Chir Scand 1967;30:309.

Everaert K et al: Urodynamic assessment of voiding dysfunction and dysfunctional voiding in girls and women. Int Urogynecol J Pelvic Floor Dysfunct 2000;11:254.

Fantl JA et al: Urinary incontinence in community-dwelling women: Clinical, urodynamic and severity characteristics. Am J Obstet Gynecol 1990;162:946.

Fowler CJ: Bladder afferents and their role in the overactive bladder. Urology 2002;59(Suppl 1):37.

Fry CH et al: The cellular basis of contraction in human detrusor smooth muscle from patients with stable and unstable bladders. Urology 2002;59(Suppl 1):3.

Ghoniem GM, Hassouna M: Alternatives for the pharmacologic management of urge and stress urinary incontinence in the elderly. J Wound Ostomy Continence Nurs 1997;24:311.

Goldman HB, Rackley RR, Appell RA: The in situ anterior vaginal wall sling: Predictors of success. J Urol 2001;166:2259.

Gosling J: Structure of the lower urinary tract and pelvic floor. Clin Obstet Gynaecol 1985;2:285.

Griffiths DJ et al: Urge incontinence and impaired detrusor contractility in the elderly. Neurourol Urodyn 2002;21:126.

Harvey MA, Versi E: Predictive value of clinical evaluation of stress urinary incontinence: A summary of the published literature. Int Urogynecol J Pelvic Floor Dysfunct 2001;12:31.

Hodgkinson CP, Stanton SL: Retropubic urethropexy or colposuspension. In: Stanton SL, Tanagho EA (editors): *Surgery of Female Incontinence.* Springer-Verlag, 1980.

Hu TW: Impact of urinary incontinence on health-care costs. J Am Geriatr Soc 1990;38:292.

Hutch JA: A new theory of the anatomy of the internal urinary sphincter and the physiology of micturition. 5. The base plate and stress incontinence. Obstet Gynecol 1967;30:309.

Jabs CF, Stanton SL: Urge incontinence and detrusor instability. Int Urogynecol J Pelvic Floor Dysfunct 2001;12:58.

Jones JA, Mitchell ME, Rink RC: Improved results using a modification of the Young-Dees-Leadbetter bladder neck repair. Br J Urol 1993;71:555.

Junemann KP: The management of female urinary stress incontinence: II. The use of devices. BJU Int 2001;87:449.

Kjerulff KH et al: Urinary incontinence and hysterectomy in a large prospective cohort study in American women. J Urol 2002; 167:2088.

Kobashi KC, Leach GE: Pelvic prolapse. J Urol 2000;164:1879.

Kohli N, Rosenblatt PL: Neuromodulation techniques for the treatment of the overactive bladder. Clin Obstet Gynecol 2002;45:218.

Kulseng-Hanssen S, Berild GH: Subjective and objective incontinence 5 to 10 years after Burch colposuspension. Neurourol Urodyn 2002;21:100.

Lemack GE, Baseman AG, Zimmern PE: Voiding dynamics in women: A comparison of pressure-flow studies between asymptomatic and incontinent women. Urology 2002;59:42.

Litwiller SE et al: Post-prostatectomy incontinence and the artificial urinary sphincter: A long-term study of patient satisfaction and criteria for success. J Urol 1996;156:1975.

Lockhart JL et al: Periurethral polytetrafluoroethylene injection following urethral reconstruction in female patients with urinary incontinence. J Urol 1988;140:51.

Madersbacher H et al: Urge incontinence in the elderly: Supraspinal reflex incontinence. World J Urol 1998;16(Suppl 1):S35.

Marshall VV, Marchetti AA, Krantz KE: The correction of stress incontinence by simple vesicourethral suspension. J Urol 2002;167(Pt 2):1109.

McGrother C et al: Epidemiology and etiology of urinary incontinence in the elderly. World J Urol 1998;16(Suppl 1):S3.

McGuire EJ: Mixed symptomatology. BJU Int 2000;85(Suppl 3):47.

McGuire EJ, Cespedes RD: Proper diagnosis: A must before surgery for stress incontinence. J Endourol 1996;10:201.

McGuire EJ, English SF: Periurethral collagen injection for male and female sphincteric incontinence: Indications, techniques, and result. World J Urol 1997;15:306.

McGuire EJ, Lytton B: Pubovaginal sling procedure for stress incontinence. J Urol 2002;167(Pt 2):1120.

McGuire EJ, Savastano JA: Stress incontinence and detrusor instability/urge incontinence. Neurourol Urodynam 1985;4:313.

McGuire EJ et al: Clinical assessment of urethral sphincter function. J Urol 1993;150:1452.

McGuire EJ et al: Experience with pubovaginal slings for urinary incontinence at the University of Michigan. J Urol 1987; 138:525.

Miklos JR, Kohli N: Laparoscopic paravaginal repair plus Burch colposuspension: Review and descriptive technique. Urology 2000;56(Suppl 1):64.

Mostwin JL: Current concepts of female pelvic anatomy and physiology. Urol Clin North Am 1991;18:175.

Mostwin JL et al: Anatomic goals in the correction of female stress urinary incontinence. J Endourol 1996;10:207.

Mouritsen L, Lose G, Glavind K: Assessment of women with urinary incontinence. Acta Obstet Gynecol Scand 1998;77:361.

Ouslander JG: Intractable incontinence in the elderly. BJU Int 2000;85(Suppl 3):72.

The Overactive Bladder: From Basic Science to Clinical Management Consensus Conference. Proceedings. London, England, June 29, 1997. Urology 1997;50 (6A Suppl):1.

Payne CK: Epidemiology, pathophysiology, and evaluation of urinary incontinence and overactive bladder. Urology 1998;51 (2A Suppl):3.

Pereyra AJ: A simplified surgical procedure for the correction of stress incontinence in women. J Urol 2002;167(Pt 2):1116.

Pereyra AJ, Lebherz TB: The modified Pereyra procedure. In: Buschbaum HJ, Schmidt JD (editors): *Gynecologic and Obstetric Urology,* 2nd ed. Saunders, 1982.

Petros PE, Ulmsten U: Bladder instability in women: A premature activation of the micturition reflex. Neurourol Urodynam 1993;12:235.

Petros PE, Ulmsten U: An integral theory and its method for the diagnosis and management of female urinary incontinence. Scand J Urol Nephrol 1993;[Suppl]:153:1.

Petros PE, Ulmsten U: Urge incontinence history is an accurate predictor of urge incontinence. Acta Obstet Gynecol Scand 1992;71:537.

Peyrat L et al: Prevalence and risk factors of urinary incontinence in young and middle-aged women. BJU Int 2002;89:61.

Raz S: Modified bladder neck suspension for female stress incontinence. Urology 1981;17:82.

Raz S: Vaginal surgery for stress incontinence. J Am Geriatr Soc 1990;38:348.

Raz S et al: Vaginal wall sling. J Urol 1989;141:43.

Rijkhoff NJ et al: Urinary bladder control by electrical stimulation: Review of electrical stimulation techniques in spinal cord injury. Neurourol Urodyn 1997;16:39.

Robinson D: Urinary incontinence in the elderly: A growing problem that needs attention. Curr Opin Obstet Gynecol 1997; 9:285.

Robinson D, Khullar V, Cardozo L: Pharmacological management of detrusor instability. Int Urogynecol J Pelvic Floor Dysfunct 2001;12:271.

Sampselle CM, DeLancey JO: Anatomy of female incontinence. J Wound Ostomy Continence Nurs 1998;25:63.

Sarver R, Govier FE: Pubovaginal slings: Past, present and future. Int Urogynecol J Pelvic Floor Dysfunct 1997;8:358.

Scott FB, Bradley WE, Timm GW: Treatment of urinary incontinence by an implantable prosthetic urinary sphincter. J Urol 2002;167(Pt 2):1125.

Smith ARB, Hosker GL, Warrell DW: The role of partial denervation of the pelvic floor in the aetiology of genitourinary prolapse and stress incontinence of urine: A neurophysiological study. Br J Obstet Gynaecol 1989;96:24.

Stage P, Fischer-Rasmussen W, Iversen HR: The value of colpocysto-urethrography in female stress and urge incontinence and following operation. Acta Obstet Gynecol Scand 1986; 65:401.

Stamey TA: Endoscopic suspension of the vesical neck for urinary incontinence. Surg Gynecol Obstet 1973;136:547.

Stamey TA: Endoscopic suspension of the vesical neck for urinary incontinence in females: Report on 203 consecutive patients. Ann Surg 1980;192:465.

Stanton SL: Consensus report on pelvic floor weakness of the elderly female. World J Urol 1998;16(Suppl 1):S44.

Stanton SL: Surgical treatment of sphincteric incontinence in women. World J Urol 1997;15:272.

Stanton SL, Zimmern PE: *Female Pelvic Reconstructive Surgery.* Springer-Verlag, 2002.

Stanton SL et al: Clinical and urodynamic factors of failed incontinence surgery in the female. Obstet Gynecol 1978;51:515.

Stoker J, Halligan S, Bartram CI: Pelvic floor imaging. Radiology 2001;218:621.

Su TH et al: Prospective comparison of laparoscopic and traditional colposuspensions in the treatment of genuine stress incontinence. Acta Obstet Gynecol Scand 1997;76:576.

Summitt RL Jr, Bent AE, Ostergard DR: The pathophysiology of genuine stress incontinence. Int Urogynecol J 1990;1:12.

Tanagho EA: The anatomy and physiology of micturition. Clin Obstet Gynaecol 1978;5:3.

Tanagho EA: Colpocystourethropexy, the way we do it. J Urol 1976;116:751.

Tanagho EA: Simplified cystography in stress incontinence. Br J Urol 1974;74:295.

Tanagho EA: Urodynamics of female urinary incontinence with emphasis on stress incontinence. J Urol 1979;122:200.

Tanagho EA, Smith DR: Clinical evaluation of a surgical technique for the correction of complete urinary incontinence. J Urol 1972;107:402.

Tanagho EA, Stoller ML: Urodynamics: Uroflowmetry and female voiding patterns. In: Ostergard D, Bent AE (editors): *Urogynecology and Urodynamics: Theory and Practice,* 3rd ed. Williams & Wilkins, 1991.

Thakar R, Stanton SL: Weakness of the pelvic floor: Urological consequences. Hosp Med 2000;61:259.

Thunedborg P, Fischer-Rasmussen W, Jensen SB: Stress urinary incontinence and posterior bladder suspension defects: Results of vaginal repair versus Burch colposuspension. Acta Obstet Gynecol Scand 1990;69:55.

Thüroff JW et al: Medical treatment and medical side effects in urinary incontinence in the elderly. World J Urol 1998;16 (Suppl 1):S48.

Turner-Warwick R: Observations of the function and dysfunction of the sphincter and detrusor mechanisms. Urol Clin North Am 1979;6:13.

Ulmsten U: Some reflections and hypotheses on the pathophysiology of female urinary incontinence. Acta Obstet Gynecol Scand Suppl 1997;166:3.

Ulmsten U, Asmussen M, Lindstrom KA: A new technique for simultaneous urethrocystometry and measurements of the urethral pressure profile. Urol Int 1977;32:88.

Ulmsten U, Johnson P, Rezapour M: A three-year follow up of tension free vaginal tape for surgical treatment of female stress urinary incontinence. Br J Obstet Gynaecol 1999; 106:345.

Ulmsten U et al: An ambulatory surgical procedure under local anesthesia for treatment of female urinary incontinence. Int Urogynecol J 1996;7:81.

Vancaillie TG: Laparoscopic colposuspension and pelvic floor repair. Curr Opin Obstet Gynecol 1997;9: 244.

Van der Vaart CH et al: The contribution of hysterectomy to the occurrence of urge and stress urinary incontinence symptoms. BJOG 2002;109:149.

Van Kerrebroeck PE: The role of electrical stimulation in voiding dysfunction. Eur Urol 1998;34(Suppl 1):27.

Weber AM: Is urethral pressure profilometry a useful diagnostic test for stress urinary incontinence? Obstet Gynecol Surv 2001;56:720.

Weber AM, Walters MD: Anterior vaginal prolapse: Review of anatomy and techniques of surgical repair. Obstet Gynecol 1997;89:311.

Wein AJ: Pharmacologic treatment of incontinence. J Am Geriatr Soc 1990;38:317.

Weiss BD: Diagnostic evaluation of urinary incontinence in geriatric patients. Am Fam Physician 1998;57:2688.

Zacharin RF: *Pelvic Floor Anatomy and the Surgery of Pulsion Enterocele.* Springer-Verlag, 1985.

Disorders of the Adrenal Glands   29

Christopher J. Kane, MD, FACS

Disorders of the adrenal glands result in classic endocrine syndromes such as Cushing syndrome, hyperaldosteronism, and catechol excess from pheochromocytoma (Figure 29–1). The diagnosis of these disorders requires careful endocrine evaluation and imaging with computed tomography (CT) or magnetic resonance imaging (MRI).

In addition, many adrenal lesions are discovered on cross-sectional imaging performed for other reasons. These "incidentalomas" require metabolic evaluation and assessment to determine their need for treatment.

■ DISEASES OF THE ADRENAL CORTEX

CUSHING SYNDROME

Cushing syndrome is the clinical disorder caused by overproduction of cortisol. Most cases (80%) are due to bilateral adrenocortical hyperplasia stimulated by overproduction of pituitary adrenocorticotropic hormone (corticotropin, ACTH), known as Cushing disease. About 10% of cases are due to the ectopic production of ACTH from nonpituitary tumors. Ectopic ACTH production occurs most frequently in small-cell lung carcinoma; other tumors producing ACTH include carcinoids (lung, thymic, gastrointestinal tract), islet cell tumors of the pancreas, medullary thyroid carcinoma, pheochromocytoma, and small-cell carcinoma of the prostate. Adrenal adenoma is the cause in 5% of cases and carcinoma in 5%. In children, adrenocortical carcinoma is the most common cause of Cushing syndrome.

Pathophysiology

Overproduction of cortisol by adrenocortical tissue leads to a catabolic state. This causes liberation from muscle tissue of amino acids, which are transformed into glucose and glycogen in the liver by gluconeogenesis. The resulting weakened protein structures (muscle and elastic tissue) cause a protuberant abdomen and poor wound healing, generalized muscle weakness, and marked osteoporosis, which is made worse by excessive loss of calcium in the urine.

In addition, glucose is transformed largely into fat and appears in characteristic sites such as the abdomen, supraclavicular fat pads, and cheeks. There is a tendency to diabetes, with an elevated fasting plasma glucose level in 20% of cases and diabetic glucose tolerance curve in 80%.

The cortisol excess also suppresses the immune mechanisms, which makes these patients susceptible to repeated infection. Inhibition of fibroblast function by excess cortisol further interferes with wound healing and host defenses against infection.

Hypertension is present in 90% of cases. Although the aldosterone level is not usually elevated, cortisol itself exerts a hypertensive effect when present in excessive amounts, as does 11-deoxycorticosterone. The hypertension may be accompanied by manifestation of mineralocorticoid excess (hypokalemia and alkalosis), especially in patients with the ectopic ACTH syndrome or adrenocortical carcinoma.

Pathology

The cells in adrenal hyperplasia resemble those of the zona fasciculata of the normal adrenal cortex. Frank adenocarcinoma reveals pleomorphism and invasion of the capsule, the vascular system, or both (Figure 29–2). Local invasion may occur, and metastases are common to the liver, lungs, bone, or brain. Histologic differentiation between adenoma and adenocarcinoma is frequently difficult.

In the presence of adenoma or malignant tumor, atrophy of the cortices of both adrenals occurs because the main secretory product of the tumor is cortisol, which inhibits the pituitary secretion of ACTH. Thus, although the tumor continues to grow, the contralateral adrenal cortex undergoes atrophy.

Clinical Findings

A. SYMPTOMS AND SIGNS (FIGURES 29–3 AND 29–4.)

The presence of at least 3 of the following strongly suggests Cushing syndrome:

1. Obesity (with sparing of the extremities), moon face, and fat pads of the supraclavicular and dorsocervical areas (buffalo hump).

2. Striae (red and depressed) over the abdomen and thighs.

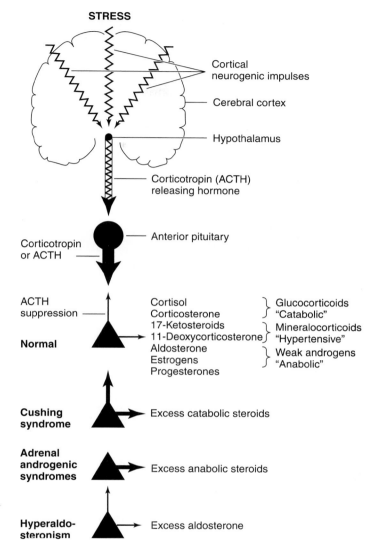

Figure 29–1. The hypothalamic-pituitary-adrenocortical relationships in various adrenocortical syndromes.

3. Hypertension (almost always present).
4. Proximal myopathy with marked weakness, especially in the quadriceps femoris, making unaided rising from a chair difficult.
5. Emotional lability, irritability, difficulty in sleeping, and sometimes psychotic personality.
6. Osteoporosis (common), with back pain from compression fractures of the lumbar vertebrae as well as rib fractures.
7. In 80% of cases, post-prandial hyperglycemia is present, and in 20% there is an elevated fasting plasma glucose level.
8. To a variable extent, there are features of adrenal androgen excess in women with Cushing syndrome; these are absent in the case of adenoma, most severe with carcinoma, and present to an intermediate degree with Cushing disease. They consist of recession of the hairline, hirsutism, small breasts, and generalized muscular overdevelopment, with deepening of the voice.

It is not possible to differentiate the cause from the clinical presentation alone.

The most rapid onset is noted in cases caused by ectopic ACTH-producing tumor with high glucocor-

Figure 29–2. **Left:** Histologic appearance of a typical benign adenoma of the adrenal cortex made up of a large number of identical cells from the zona fasciculata removed from a 39-year-old woman with Cushing syndrome. **Right:** Section of an adenocarcinoma removed from a 36-year-old woman with metastatic adenocarcinoma showing significant pleomorphism of the cells. Invasion of a large vein is not shown in this micrograph. Note that benign adenomas will occasionally have this appearance but without invasion of the bloodstream. (Reproduced, with permission, from Forsham PH: The adrenal cortex. In: Williams RH [editor]: *Textbook of Endocrinology,* 4th ed. Saunders, 1968.)

ticoid output or those due to adrenocortical carcinoma.

B. Laboratory Findings

The leukocyte count may be elevated to the range of 12,000–20,000/μL, usually with fewer than 20% lymphocytes. Eosinophils are few in number or absent. Polycythemia is present in over half the cases, with the hemoglobin ranging from 14 to 16 g/dL. Anemia, however, may occur in patients with malignant tumors ectopically secreting ACTH.

Blood chemical analyses may show an increase in serum Na^+ and CO_2 levels and a decrease in serum K^+ levels. Hyperglycemia may occur.

1. Specific tests for Cushing syndrome—The following tests are performed to determine whether the patient has Cushing syndrome or is an anxious individual with elevated plasma levels of cortisol.

a. 24-h urinary cortisol level—Urine cortisol is measured in a 24-h urine collection by high-performance liquid chromatography (normal range, 10–50 μg/24 h), and urine creatinine is also measured to en-

sure completeness of the collection. A urine cortisol value more than 2-fold elevated is typical of Cushing syndrome. False-positive elevations can occur in acute illness, depression, and alcoholism. However, obesity does not raise the level of urinary free cortisol above normal.

b. Late night salivary cortisol determinations—These are simple and specific and may evolve into a convenient screening test.

c. Suppression of ACTH and plasma cortisol by dexamethasone—Dexamethasone in low doses is used to assess the feedback suppression of ACTH and cortisol production by glucocorticoids. If dexamethasone is given at 11 PM, ACTH is suppressed in normal persons but not in those with Cushing syndrome. Dexamethasone is useful because it has 30 times the potency of cortisol as an ACTH suppressant and it is not measured in current plasma or urine cortisol methods.

The procedure is to give 1 mg of dexamethasone by mouth at 11 PM and to draw blood at 8–9:00 AM for measurement of plasma cortisol. If the level is below 5

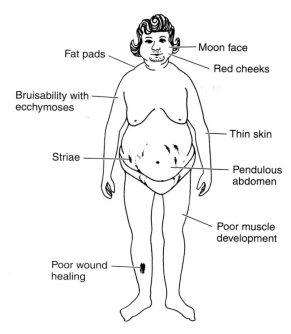

Figure 29–3. Drawing of a typical case of Cushing syndrome showing the principal clinical features. (Reproduced, with permission, from Forsham PH: The adrenal cortex. In: Williams RH [editor]: *Textbook of Endocrinology*, 4th ed. Saunders, 1968.)

Figure 29–4. A patient with Cushing disease. Note the red moon face, receding hairline, buffalo hump over the seventh vertebra, protuberant abdomen, and inappropriately thin arms and legs.

μg/dL (normal is 5–20 μg/dL), Cushing syndrome can be ruled out. If the value is above 10 μg/dL, Cushing syndrome is present (Figure 29–5). A level in the range of 5–10 μg/dL is equivocal, and the test should be repeated or the urine cortisol may be measured.

Women taking birth control pills have high plasma cortisol levels because, as in pregnancy, the estrogen stimulates production of the cortisol-binding globulin. The pills must be withheld for at least 3 weeks before the dexamethasone suppression test. Other conditions causing false-positive responses are acute illness, depression, and alcoholism. Also, about 15% of obese patients do not suppress cortisol with this test.

2. Specific tests for differentiation of causes of Cushing syndrome—The various causes of Cushing syndrome can be determined with great accuracy (95% of cases).

a. Plasma ACTH level—If the diagnosis of Cushing syndrome has been established, this test will differentiate ACTH-dependent causes (Cushing disease and the ectopic ACTH syndrome) from adrenal tumors, which are ACTH-independent. ACTH is currently measured by a sensitive immunoradiometric assay (IRMA) (normal range, 10–50 pg/mL). Patients with Cushing disease have ACTH levels that range from 10 to 200 pg/mL; in the ectopic ACTH syndrome, levels are usually greater than 200 pg/mL; and patients with adrenal tumors have suppressed ACTH levels (< 5 pg/mL with the IRMA ACTH assay) and thus are easily differentiated.

b. Plasma androgen levels—In patients with adrenal adenomas, androgen levels are normal or low, and in adrenocortical carcinoma these levels are often markedly elevated.

C. X-Ray Findings and Special Examinations

1. Localization of source of ACTH excess—When tests suggest Cushing disease or the ectopic ACTH syndrome and an elevated plasma level of ACTH is present, the source of ACTH must be identified. Because the great majority of these patients have Cushing dis-

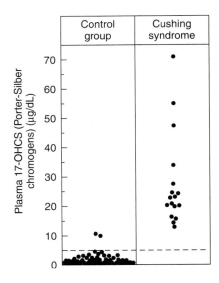

Figure 29–5. Results of the dexamethasone suppression test in obese individuals and patients with Cushing syndrome. See text for procedure. 17-OHCS, 17-hydroxycorticosteroids. (Reproduced, with permission, from Pavlatos FC, Smilo RP, Forsham PH: A rapid screening test for Cushing's syndrome. JAMA 1975;193:720.)

ease and because most of the patients with ectopic ACTH secretion have an obvious malignancy, the first step is to perform pituitary magnetic resonance imaging (MRI). These are positive in 50–60% of patients with Cushing disease; in the remainder, the diagnosis should be established by the sampling of ACTH levels in the venous drainage of the anterior pituitary, that is, the cavernous sinuses and inferior petrosal sinuses. If the MRI and venous sampling do not reveal a pituitary source of ACTH, computed tomography (CT) scans of the chest and abdomen are used to localize an ectopic tumor.

2. Localization of adrenal lesions—Patients with Cushing syndrome with suspected adrenal tumors and suppressed ACTH levels should undergo a CT scan of the abdomen with 3-mm sections through the adrenals. Adrenal tumors causing Cushing syndrome are usually greater than 3 cm in diameter (Figure 29–6) and are therefore easily visualized. Adenomas are usually 3–6 cm in diameter; carcinomas are usually greater than 5 cm in diameter and are frequently locally invasive or metastatic to the liver and lungs at the time of diagnosis. In patients with adrenal tumors, the contralateral adrenal is suppressed and therefore appears atrophic or normal on CT scan. The finding of bilateral adrenal enlargement is typical of Cushing disease or the ectopic

ACTH syndrome. Ultrasound or MRI may also be used for adrenal localization, although these techniques do not appear to offer significant advantage over CT scans.

Complications

Hypertension may lead to cardiac failure or stroke. Diabetes may be a problem but is usually mild. Intractable skin or systemic infections are common. Compression fractures of osteoporotic vertebrae and rib fractures may develop. Renal stones are not uncommon as a result of bone resorption. Psychosis is not uncommon; it usually subsides after successful surgery.

Treatment

A. CUSHING DISEASE

A pituitary microadenoma, which is the most common cause of bilateral adrenocortical hyperplasia, must be located and removed surgically. **Transsphenoidal resection** performed by an experienced neurosurgeon is the method of choice. Success is reported in over 80% of cases, and in most instances the endocrine functions of the pituitary gland are preserved.

B. ECTOPIC ACTH SYNDROME

The treatment of these patients is difficult because most have an advanced malignancy and severe hypercortisolism. Removal of the primary tumor is clearly the therapy of choice; however, curative resection is limited to the few patients with benign tumors such as bronchial carcinoids. Patients with residual or metastatic tumors should be managed first with adrenal inhibitors, and if that is not successful, bilateral adrenalectomy should be considered.

C. TOTAL BILATERAL ADRENALECTOMY

Total bilateral adrenalectomy is indicated in patients with Cushing disease in whom the pituitary tumor is not resectable and in whom radiotherapy and medical therapy fail to control the cortisol excess. At present, it is best to perform bilateral adrenalectomy via a laparoscopic approach. The procedure significantly decreases morbidity and length of hospital stay. Bilateral adrenalectomy is also indicated in patients with ectopic ACTH syndrome who have life-threatening hypercortisolism that cannot be controlled by inhibitors of adrenal secretion.

1. Preoperative preparation—Because removal of the source of excessive cortisol will inevitably lead to temporary or permanent adrenal insufficiency, it is of the utmost importance to administer cortisol preoperatively and to continue substitution therapy after surgery to

Figure 29–6. Noncontrast CT image of a right benign adrenal adenoma. Hounsfield units under 10.

control Addison disease. In the postoperative period, the dose is tapered downward until oral medication provides sufficient control.

2. Postoperative status—The patient feels moderately well following removal of the source of excess ACTH or adrenalectomy or while receiving a high dose of hydrocortisone in excess of the usual daily output of approximately 20 mg. It is important to reduce the steroid substitution gradually over a period of several days. On the day of operation, 200 mg of cortisol is given; the dosage is then reduced gradually on successive days (150, 100, 80, 60, and 40 mg) until a maintenance dosage of 20–30 mg cortisol combined with 0.1 mg fludrocortisone is reached.

D. Adrenal Adenoma and Adenocarcinoma

Virtually all adrenal adenomas and smaller adrenal carcinomas are now removed laparoscopically, again allowing decreased hospital stay and more rapid recovery from surgery. Adrenal carcinomas that are large (greater than 8–10 cm) are likely to be metastatic or locally invasive. Thus, if there is evidence of invasion of adjacent structures or invasion of the adrenal or renal veins or the vena cava, these tumors are best approached by a traditional abdominal incision.

1. Preoperative preparation—Preoperative preparation is the same as that for bilateral hyperplasia, since, in this case, the remaining adrenal gland will be atrophic and thus the patient will be hypoadrenal.

2. Postoperative treatment and follow-up—Cortisol is administered perioperatively in the doses described above and then tapered to a replacement dose of 20–30 mg per day. Hydrocortisone is given orally in a dosage of 10 mg 3 times daily initially and reduced within 2–3 weeks to 10 mg daily given at 7 or 8 AM. Substitution therapy may be necessary for 6 months to 2 years depending on the rate of recovery of the residual gland. Mineralocorticoid therapy is rarely necessary, since the atrophic adrenal usually produces sufficient aldosterone. Patients with adrenocortical carcinoma are usually not cured by surgery and require additional therapy.

E. Medical Therapy

There is no effective method of inhibiting ACTH secretion; however, adrenal hypersecretion can be controlled in many patients by inhibitors of adrenal cortisol secretion. Medical therapy is indicated in patients who either cannot undergo surgery (eg, because of debility, recent myocardial infarction) or in those who have had unsuccessful resection of their pituitary, ectopic, or adrenal tumor.

Ketoconazole is the current drug of choice; it blocks cortisol secretion by inhibiting P450c11 and P450scc. The total dose required is 800–1600 mg/d given in 2 divided doses. Side effects are adrenal insufficiency, abnormal liver function tests, and hepatotoxicity in a few patients.

Metyrapone may be used alone or may be added if ketoconazole alone is unsuccessful in normalizing cortisol levels. The usual dosage is 1–4 g daily given in 4 divided doses.

Aminoglutethimide and trilostane also inhibit adrenal secretion, but they are uncommonly used at present.

Mitotane (*o,p'*-DDD) is both an inhibitor of adrenal secretion and a cytotoxic agent that damages adrenocortical cells. It is used almost exclusively in patients with residual adrenocortical carcinoma, in whom it helps to reduce cortisol hypersecretion. The usual dosage is 6–12 g daily in 3–4 divided doses. About 70% of patients achieve a reduction in steroid secretion and 35% achieve a reduction in tumor size; however, there is no convincing evidence that the drug prolongs survival. Side effects occur in 80% of patients and include nausea, vomiting, diarrhea, depression, and somnolence.

Prognosis

Treatment of hypercortisolism usually leads to disappearance of symptoms and many signs within days to weeks, but osteoporosis usually persists in adults, whereas hypertension and diabetes often improve. Cushing disease treated by pituitary adenomectomy has an excellent early prognosis, and long-term follow-up shows a recurrence rate of about 10%. Patients with the ectopic ACTH syndrome and malignant tumors in general have a poor prognosis; these patients usually die within several months of diagnosis. Patients with benign lesions may be cured by resection of the tumor. Removal of an adrenal adenoma offers an excellent prognosis; and these patients are cured by unilateral adrenalectomy.

The outlook for patients with adrenocortical carcinoma is poor. The antineoplastic drug mitotane (*o,p'*-DDD; Lysodren) given in doses of up to 6–12 g orally daily reduces the symptoms and signs of Cushing syndrome but does little to prolong survival. Radiotherapy and chemotherapy are not successful in these patients.

ADRENAL ANDROGENIC SYNDROMES

Adrenal androgenic syndromes are more common in females. Congenital bilateral adrenal hyperplasia and tumors, both benign and malignant, may be observed. In contrast to Cushing syndrome, which is protein catabolic, the androgenic syndromes are anabolic. In untreated cases, there is a marked recession of the hairline, increased beard growth, and excessive growth of pubic and sexual hair in general in both sexes. In males, there is enlargement of the penis, usually with atrophic testes; in females, enlargement of the clitoris occurs, with atrophy of the breasts and amenorrhea. Muscle mass increases and fat content decreases, leading to a powerful but trim figure. The voice becomes deeper, particularly in females; this condition is irreversible, because it is due to enlargement of the larynx. In both sexes there may be increased physical sexual aggressiveness and libido.

1. Congenital Bilateral Adrenal Androgenic Hyperplasia

Pathophysiology

A congenital defect in certain adrenal enzymes results in the production of abnormal steroids, causing **pseudohermaphroditism** in females and **macrogenitosomia** in males. The enzyme defect is associated with excess androgen production in utero. In females, the müllerian duct structures (eg, ovaries, uterus, and vagina) develop normally, but the excess androgen exerts a masculinizing effect on the urogenital sinus and genital tubercle, so that the vagina is connected to the urethra, which, in turn, opens at the base of the enlarged clitoris. The labia are often hypertrophied. Externally, the appearance is that of severe hypospadias with cryptorchidism.

The adrenal cortex secretes mostly anabolic and androgenic steroids, leading to various degrees of cortisol deficiency depending on the nature of the enzyme block. This increases the secretion of ACTH, which causes hyperplasia of both adrenal cortices. The cortices continue to secrete large amounts of inappropriate anabolic, androgenic, or hypertensive steroids. Absence or reduction of the usual tissue concentration of various enzymes accounts for blocks in the adrenocortical synthetic pathways.

A block at P450scc leads to the rare congenital lipoid adrenal hyperplasia with complete absence of any steroidal hormone production; the infant will die at an early age unless full substitution therapy is given for life.

A block at 3β-hydroxydehydrogenase/isomerase enzyme prevents formation of progesterone, aldosterone, and cortisol. Dehydroepiandrosterone (DHEA) is produced in excess. This uncommon syndrome is characterized by adrenal insufficiency and male pseudohermaphroditism, with females showing unusual sexual development with hirsutism.

A block at P450c21, which is the most common cause of congenital adrenal hyperplasia, does not allow for the transformation of 17α-hydroxyprogesterone to cortisol. This common deficiency occurs in 2 forms: the salt-losing variety, with low to absent aldosterone, and the more frequent non-salt-losing type. Infants present with adrenal insufficiency and ambiguous genitalia; older children develop pseudoprecocious puberty and accelerated growth and skeletal maturation.

A block at P450c17 with lack of 17α-hydroxylase occurs mostly in females and may not be discovered until puberty. Findings include low cortisol levels with high ACTH levels, primary amenorrhea, and sexual infantilism, as neither the glucocorticoids nor the sex steroids are produced in adequate amounts. Rarely, there is male pseudohermaphroditism. Hypertension due to excess mineralocorticoids, notably 11-deoxycorticosterone, is characteristically present.

A block at P450c11 with lack of 11β-hydroxylase prevents formation of cortisol and corticosterone and thus leads to overproduction of adrenal androgens and 11-deoxycorticosterone. Patients usually have clinical features of mild androgen excess with hypertension and hypokalemia.

A block at P450aldo results in the inability to produce aldosterone in the zona glomerulosa; these patients present with isolated mineralocorticoid deficiency with hypotension and hyperkalemia.

Clinical Findings

A. SYMPTOMS AND SIGNS

In newborn girls, the appearance of the external genitalia resembles severe hypospadias with cryptorchidism. Infant boys may appear normal at birth. The earlier in intrauterine life the fetus has been exposed to excess androgen, the more marked the anomalies.

In untreated cases, hirsutism, excess muscle mass, and, eventually, amenorrhea are the rule. Breast development is poor. In males, growth of the phallus is excessive. The testes are often atrophic because of inhibition of gonadotropin secretion by the elevated androgens. On rare occasions, hyperplastic adrenocortical rests in the testes make them large and firm. In most instances, there is azoospermia after puberty.

In both males and females with androgenic hyperplasia, the growth rate is initially increased, so that they are taller than their classmates. At about age 9–10 years, premature fusion of the epiphyses caused by excess androgen causes termination of growth, so that these patients are short as adults.

B. LABORATORY FINDINGS

Urinary 17-ketosteroid levels are higher than normal for sex and age, and plasma anchostenedione, DHEA, DHEA-S, and testosterone are elevated. Plasma ACTH is also elevated, and in patients with the most common defect (ie, 21-hydroxylase deficiency), plasma 17α-hydroxyprogesterone is markedly elevated. Chromosome studies are normal.

C. X-RAY FINDINGS

X-rays show acceleration of bone age.

D. CT SCANS

Scans usually show the hypertrophied adrenals.

E. UROLOGIC EVALUATION

This is indicated to define the anatomic abnormalities.

Differential Diagnosis

Several congenital anomalies that affect the development of the external genitalia resemble adrenal androgenic syndrome. These include (1) severe hypospadias with cryptorchidism, (2) female pseudohermaphroditism of the nonadrenal type (caused by administration of androgens or progestational compounds during the pregnancy), (3) male pseudohermaphroditism, and (4) true hermaphroditism. These children show no hormonal abnormalities, and bone age and maturation are not accelerated.

Treatment

It is imperative to make the diagnosis early. Treatment of the underlying cause is medical, with the goal of suppressing excessive ACTH secretion, thus minimizing excess androgenicity. This is accomplished by adrenal replacement with cortisol or prednisone in doses sufficient to suppress adrenal androgen production and therefore prevent virilization and rapid skeletal growth. In patients with mineralocorticoid deficiency, fludrocortisone (0.05–0.3 mg, depending on severity and age) together with good salt intake is necessary to stabilize blood pressure and body weight.

After puberty, the vagina can be surgically separated from the urethra and opened in the normal position on the perineum. Judicious administration of estrogens or birth control pills feminizes the figure in pseudohermaphrodites and improves their psyche considerably.

Prognosis

If the condition is recognized early and ACTH suppression is begun even before surgical repair of the genital anomaly, the outlook for normal linear growth and development is excellent. Delay in treatment inevitably results in stunted growth. In some female pseudohermaphrodites, menses begin after treatment, and conception and childbirth can occur when the anatomic abnormalities are minimal or have been surgically repaired.

2. Adrenocortical Tumors

Adrenocortical tumors producing androgens are most frequently carcinomas; however, a few benign adenomas have been reported. Most of the carcinomas also hypersecrete other hormones (ie, cortisol or 11-deoxycorticosterone), and thus the clinical presentation is variable. Female patients present with androgen excess, which may be severe enough to cause virilization; many of these patients also have Cushing syndrome and mineralocorticoid excess (hypertension and hypokalemia). In adult males excess androgens may cause no clinical manifestations, and diagnosis in these patients may be delayed until there is abdominal pain or an abdominal mass. These patients may also present with Cushing syndrome and mineralocorticoid excess.

The tumor can be located by CT scan, which is also used to define the extent of tumor spread. Local invasion and distant spread to the liver and lungs are common at the time of diagnosis. The primary therapy is surgical resection of the adrenal tumor, as discussed above; however, surgical cure is rare. These patients are subsequently treated with mitotane and other adrenal inhibitors, as discussed in the section on Cushing syndrome.

THE HYPERTENSIVE, HYPOKALEMIC SYNDROME (PRIMARY ALDOSTERONISM)

Excessive production of aldosterone, due mostly to aldosteronoma or to spontaneous bilateral hyperplasia of the zona glomerulosa of the adrenal cortex, leads to the combination of hypertension, hypokalemia, nocturia, and polyuria. A syndrome resembling nephrogenic diabetes insipidus may occur as a result of reversible damage to the renal collecting tubules. The alkalosis may produce tetany.

Pathophysiology

Excessive aldosterone, acting on most cell membranes in the body, produces typical changes in the distal renal tubule and the small bowel that lead to urinary potassium loss together with increased renal sodium reabsorption and hydrogen ion secretion. This results in potassium depletion, metabolic alkalosis, increased plasma sodium concentration, and hypervolemia. With low serum levels of potassium, the concentrating ability of the kidney is lowered and the tubules no longer respond to the administration of vasopressin by increased reabsorption of water. Finally, impairment of insulin release secondary to potassium depletion increases carbohydrate intolerance in about 50% of cases.

Plasma renin and, secondarily, plasma angiotensin are depressed by excess aldosterone as a result of blood volume expansion. Early in the course of excess aldosterone production, there may be hypertension with a normal serum potassium level. Later, the potassium level will be low as well, and this suggests the diagnosis.

Clinical Findings

A. SYMPTOMS AND SIGNS

Hypertension is usually the presenting manifestation, and the accompanying hypokalemia suggests mineralocorticoid excess. Headaches are common, nocturia is invariably present, and rare episodes of paralysis occur with very low serum potassium levels. Numbness and tingling of the extremities are related to alkalosis that may lead to tetany.

B. LABORATORY FINDINGS

Before the tests outlined below are done, one must ascertain that the patient is not taking oral contraceptives or other estrogen preparations, since these may increase renin and angiotensin levels and therefore aldosterone levels, thus raising the blood pressure artificially. Withdrawal of these medications for 1 week is mandatory. Diuretics must also be discontinued, since they lower blood volume and induce secondary aldosteronism and hypokalemia. Also, if the patient is following a salt-restricted diet, aldosterone is normally elevated.

Before serum electrolytes are measured, the patient receives a loading dose of 6 g of salt for at least 2 days. This will furnish exchangeable sodium in the distal tubule and allow potassium to exchange with sodium, thus clearly revealing the low serum potassium level and electrolyte imbalance. Later, serum potassium must also be replenished, because a very low level of this ion may artificially decrease the secretory rate of aldosterone.

In true aldosterone excess, serum sodium is slightly elevated and CO_2 increased, whereas serum potassium is very low, for example, 3 mEq/L or less. Urine and serum potassium determinations while the patient is receiving good sodium replacement provide a screening test. Potassium wasting is considered to be established if the urinary potassium level is greater than 30 mEq/L/24 h but the serum potassium level is low (3 mEq/L or less).

Definitive diagnosis rests on demonstration of an elevated urine or plasma aldosterone level. The initial step is to obtain simultaneous plasma aldosterone and plasma renin levels. If the aldosterone is elevated and the renin is suppressed with a ratio of greater than 20:1, the diagnosis is established. Further confirmation can be obtained by demonstrating an elevated aldosterone level in a 24-h urine sample.

C. LOCALIZATION

A thin-section CT scan is the initial procedure and will localize an adenoma in approximately 90% of patients (Figure 29–7). If no adenoma is visualized, adrenal vein sampling of aldosterone and cortisol will correctly dif-

Figure 29–7. A typical canary-yellow aldosteronoma associated with the syndrome of hypertension, hypokalemia, and alkalosis. Note the relatively small size of this tumor compared with other types of adrenocortical tumors.

ferentiate adenoma from hyperplasia in virtually all cases.

Differential Diagnosis

Secondary hyperaldosteronism may accompany renovascular hypertension. This too is associated with hypokalemic alkalosis; however, the renin level is elevated rather than suppressed.

Essential hypertension does not cause changes in the electrolyte pattern. Definitive tests for hyperaldosteronism show negative results.

Treatment

A. ALDOSTERONOMA

If the site of the tumor has been established, only the affected adrenal need be removed. Again, the procedure of choice is laparoscopic unilateral adrenalectomy, which is highly successful at resolving the metabolic defect.

B. BILATERAL NODULAR HYPERPLASIA

Most authorities do not recommend resection of both adrenals, since the fall in blood pressure is only temporary and electrolyte imbalance may continue. Medical treatment is recommended.

C. MEDICAL TREATMENT

If surgery must be postponed, if the hypertension is mild in an older person, or if bilateral hyperplasia is the cause, one may treat medically with spironolactone (Aldactone), 25–50 mg orally 4 times daily. Amiloride, a potassium-sparing diuretic, may be given in doses of up to 20–40 mg per day. Other antihypertensive agents may also be necessary.

Prognosis

Following removal of an adrenal adenoma, the hypokalemia resolves. Seventy percent of patients become normotensive and 50% show some lowering of hypertension. Bilateral nodular hyperplasia is not amenable to surgical treatment, and the results of medical treatment are only fair.

■ DISEASES OF THE ADRENAL MEDULLA

PHEOCHROMOCYTOMA

Pheochromocytoma, derived from the neural crest, is one of the surgically curable hypertensive syndromes. There is no sex predilection. Pheochromocytoma accounts for fewer than 1% of cases of hypertension, but it is readily diagnosed if the possibility is kept in mind. It usually occurs spontaneously, but 10% of cases occur in patients with other disorders such as neurofibromatosis or familial syndromes such as multiple endocrine neoplasia type II or von Hippel-Lindau disease. The tumor is bilateral or extra-adrenal in 10% of cases in adults and in an even greater percentage in children and is then most often familial.

Clinical Findings

A. SYMPTOMS AND SIGNS

Hypertension is both systolic and diastolic. Hypertension may be either sustained and indistinguishable from ordinary blood pressure elevation, or paroxysmal, coming on for variable lengths of time and then subsiding to normal levels. Such attacks are usually precipitated by trigger mechanisms of various sorts, for example, emotional upsets or straining at stool.

Headache is a frequent complaint and is commensurate in severity with the degree of hypertension. Increased sweating without appropriate causes such as exertion or environmental heat resembles the phenomenon seen during menopause and may be accompanied by flushing or blanching. Tachycardia with palpitations occurs mainly as a consequence of epinephrine rather than norepinephrine excess. Postural hypotension is a frequent finding, as a result of diminished plasma volume.

Profound weakness may occur after an attack of hypertension. Weight loss is common.

Decreased gastrointestinal motility occurs, leading to nausea and vomiting and constipation. This effect is a direct pharmacologic consequence of excessive circulating catecholamines. Episodes of psychic instability verging on hysteria are frequent and are probably due to increased concentrations of catecholamines and other neurotransmitters in the brain, although circulating catecholamines, unlike some of their precursors, penetrate the blood-brain barrier to only a limited extent.

B. BIOCHEMICAL DIAGNOSIS

The choice of biochemical test and whether to measure plasma or urine values remain controversial, but certain principles are clear: (1) Screening the hypertensive population is not recommended because of the low incidence of pheochromocytoma (about 0.1%). (2) Regardless of the test chosen, specific methodology is essential, and thus methods using high-performance liquid chromatography, radioimmunoassay, or radioenzymatic assays should be selected. (3) Patients with pheochromocytoma who have sustained hypertension usually have clearly elevated catecholamines or metabolites in both urine and plasma. More than 80% of these patients have urine values 2 times greater than normal and total plasma catecholamine (Epi + Norepi) above 2000 ng/L. Levels of this magnitude are unusual in patients without pheochromocytoma except in acute major illness. (4) Patients with only episodic hypertension may have normal random plasma catecholamine levels and normal 24-h urine values. Evaluation of these patients must be directed to obtaining plasma catecholamine during an episode or having the patient collect timed urine values (eg, 2–4 h) from the onset of an episode. (5) Suppression or stimulation tests are not recommended except in the rare instances when the diagnosis cannot be established by routine procedures.

1. Urinary measurements—Urine measurements are the traditional diagnostic procedure. Normal values are shown in Table 29–1, and recent series in patients with

Table 29–1. Catecholamines in urine and plasma.[a]

Urine
Norepinephrine: 10–100 µg/24 h
Epinephrine: Up to 20 µg/24 h
Normetanephrine and metanephrine: < 1.5 mg/24 h
Vanillylmandelic acid (VMA): 2–9 mg/24 h
Plasma
Norepinephrine: 100–200 pg/mL
Epinephrine: 30–50 pg/mL

[a]The values listed represent the means of the normal ranges, which vary for each laboratory.

pheochromocytoma are summarized in Table 29–2. These data suggest that measurements of metanephrines or catecholamine are more useful than measurement of vanillylmandelic acid, since more than 80% of patients have values that were elevated more than 2 times. Spot urinary metanephrines (MN) and normetanephrines (NMN) measured by radioimmunoassay are very simple and highly accurate. At a cutpoint of 500 ng/mL creatinine for either MN or NMN, Ito et al (1998) reported 100% sensitivity and specificity. Patients with only episodic symptoms or episodic hypertension should be studied with shorter urine collections if 24-h studies are normal.

2. Plasma catecholamines—These values, when measured by specific methods, are elevated in most patients with pheochromocytoma; however, the frequency of false-positive values limits diagnostic utility. Thus, in patients with pheochromocytoma and sustained hypertension, 85% have plasma catecholamine values above 2000 ng/L. When patients with only paroxysmal hypertension are included, however, only 75% have values above 2000 ng/L. Values between 600 and 2000 ng/mL are commonly obtained in stressed or anxious patients without pheochromocytoma. This is especially

Table 29–2. 24-h urine measurements in patients with pheochromocytoma.[a]

	Normal No. (%)	1–2X Elevated No. (%)	> 2X Elevated No. (%)
VMA (n = 384)	41 (11)	86 (22)	257 (67)
MN (n = 271)	12 (5)	33 (12)	226 (83)
UFC (n = 319)	14 (4)	30 (10)	275 (86)

[a]Reprinted with permission from Stein PP, Black HR: A simplified diagnostic approach to pheochromocytoma. Medicine 1991; 70:46.

true if samples are obtained by venipuncture without prior placement of an intravenous line with the patient supine for 30 min. Plasma catecholamine measurements do have a role, though, because markedly elevated levels during an episode may be diagnostic; conversely, the finding of normal values during episodes of severe hypertension essentially excludes the diagnosis.

Tumor Localization

Pheochromocytomas are intra-abdominal in 98% of cases, and 90% are intra-adrenal (10% are bilateral, especially in familial syndromes). Extra-adrenal pheochromocytomas are usually within the abdomen and are located along the sympathetic chain, the periaortic areas, and at the bifurcation of the aorta. The tumors may also arise from the bladder. Extra-abdominal pheochromocytomas occur in posterior mediastinum, rarely in the heart or pericardium and rarely in the neck. Tumors less than 2 cm in diameter are rare, and most are greater than 3 cm (Figure 29–8). Thus, the vast majority of pheochromocytomas are larger than the lower limits of resolution of current imaging techniques.

A. CT Scans

CT is currently the initial imaging procedure of choice; with current technology, it demonstrates virtually all intra-abdominal tumors and most of those that are extra-adrenal. Small tumors in the abdomen, pelvis, and chest may be obscured by surrounding structures. CT is not useful in determining whether an adrenal mass is in fact a pheochromocytoma (ie, if the adrenal mass is found coincidentally or the catechol determinations are equivocal, the adrenal mass could be a nonfunctioning adenoma). In this case, MRI or metaiodobenzylguanidine (MIBG) techniques may be useful.

B. MRI

The accuracy of detecting pheochromocytoma with MRI is as good as that obtained with CT, but the cost is greater at most institutions. MRI has the advantage of greater diagnostic specificity in that T2-weighted images or those obtained with gadolinium enhancement show greater signal intensity of the pheochromocytoma (compared with liver) than that obtained with adrenal adenomas. Limited data suggest that MRI may be superior to CT in localizing extra-adrenal tumors.

C. MIBG Scanning

Radionuclide scanning with MIBG has assumed a prominent role in the localization of pheochromocytomas. The compound is taken up by pheochromocytomas, ganglioneuromas, neuroblastomas, and other neural crest tumors as well as some carcinoids. MIBG

Figure 29–8. A typical large pheochromocytoma. Removal was followed by complete remission of hypertension.

scans are positive in 85–90% of patients with pheochromocytomas, which limits their usefulness as a screening procedure. The procedure is extremely useful, however, since false-positive results are rare and a positive scan in the presence of elevated catechols is diagnostic. In addition, MIBG scans have great utility in the localization of (1) small lesions, (2) extra-adrenal lesions, (3) bilateral lesions, and (4) metastatic deposits in patients with malignant tumors.

Diagnostic Strategy

Patients in whom there is a high index of clinical suspicion and those who have greater than a 2-fold elevation of urine catechols should undergo an adrenal CT scan. If the CT scan reveals a unilateral tumor and the contralateral adrenal is normal, the diagnosis is established. Patients with familial syndromes and those in whom cancer is suspected should undergo MIBG scanning to determine the extent of disease. If the adrenal CT is negative, MIBG scanning or MRI of the chest and abdomen is indicated to localize the tumor. This approach localizes virtually all tumors.

If the clinical suspicion is low and urine catechols are normal, imaging procedures are not indicated. However, it is not infrequent that patients at low risk on the basis of clinical manifestations have persisting mild elevations of catecholamines. In this situation, a single negative adrenal imaging procedure should suffice to terminate the evaluation, and the patient may be followed clinically and reevaluated if appropriate.

Therapy

A. Preoperative Management

Once the diagnosis of pheochromocytoma is established, the patient should be prepared for surgery to reduce the incidence of intraoperative complications and postoperative hypotension. The greatest experience is with the long-acting alpha-adrenergic blocker phenoxybenzamine, and its use has minimized surgical mortality and morbidity. The initial dosage is 10 mg twice daily, and patients may require hospitalization for bed rest and intravenous fluids to overcome the initially increased orthostatic hypotension that occurs in most patients. The dose may then be titrated upward every 2–3 days over several weeks until the blood pressure is less than 160/90 mm Hg and symptoms are abolished. Doses in the range of 100–200 mg/d are routinely used; however, no data are available that establish the superiority of these dosage levels. Higher doses of phenoxybenzamine are not associated with a higher risk of postoperative hypotension. Beta blockers are generally unnecessary unless tachycardia and arrhythmias are present, and these occur most frequently in the minority of patients with epinephrine hypersecretion.

Metyrosine (alpha-methylparatyrosine), an inhibitor of catecholamine synthesis, is also useful for preoperative management although current experience is limited. Initial dosage is 250 mg every 6 h, and total daily dosages of 2–4 g are required. Preoperative treatment for 1–2 weeks appears to be sufficient to prevent operative complications. Metyrosine can be used in conjunction with alpha blockers.

Successful preoperative management with prazosin, calcium channel blockers, and labetolol has been reported in a few cases.

B. Surgery

Surgery is the mainstay of therapy for pheochromocytoma; it requires adequate preoperative control of symptoms and hypertension with alpha blockers or metyrosine. Intraoperatively, hypertension is controlled with nitroprusside, and antiarrhythmics are used as needed. Adequate volume replacement is essential and in conjunction with preoperative medical therapy prevents postoperative hypotension.

If CT and MIBG show only a solitary adrenal lesion in patients with sporadic disease, a unilateral laparoscopic approach may be used. Bilateral or malignant disease may require a transabdominal approach, and even if total resection is not feasible, debulking of tumor mass facilitates subsequent medical management of catecholamine excess.

Malignant Pheochromocytoma

The incidence of cancer in pheochromocytoma has been traditionally estimated to be in the range of 10%, although recent series describe a higher incidence. Thus, all patients should undergo serial follow-up to detect early recurrences. Patients with known metastatic disease should undergo surgical debulking of accessible disease. Catecholamine excess can be controlled in most patients with alpha blockade, metyrosine, or both. Despite encouraging reports of chemotherapy or ^{131}I-MIBG therapy, it appears that only a minority of patients have sustained remissions.

Prognosis

In general, the prognosis is good. With better understanding of the disease, surgical deaths are now rare. Blood pressure falls to normal levels in most patients with benign tumors. Patients with cancer have persisting hypertension and require the multiple therapies described above.

INCIDENTALOMA

The most common presentation of adrenal masses is incidental observation on cross-sectional imaging performed for other reasons. The differential diagnosis is quite broad (see Table 29-3) and includes benign adenoma, functional adrenal tumors as previously discussed, metastasis and benign adrenal lesions such as myelolipoma, and neurofibroma. A systematic approach is required to differentiate functional adrenal masses that deserve removal and those lesions with a significant risk of carcinoma from the more common benign nonfunctional adenoma.

Metabolic Evaluation

A careful history and physical examination with focus on obesity pattern, virilization, glucose intolerance, and hypertension is warranted. Laboratory examination with serum electrolytes including glucose and potassium should be done. If hypokalemia exists, then fur-

Table 29–3. Differential diagnosis of adrenal incidentaloma.

Adenoma
Metastasis
Lymphoma
Pheochromocytoma
Neuroblastoma
Adrenocortical carcinoma
Hematoma
Myelolipoma
Adrenal hyperplasia
Adrenal cyst
Granulomatous disease
Hemangioma
Ganglioneuroma

ther tests for aldosteronoma are indicated. A 24-h urinary free cortisol to rule out Cushing syndrome and urinary metanephrines and normetanephrines to rule out pheochromocytoma are recommended. Additional metabolic tests are performed when there are suspicious signs or symptoms or when screening tests are abnormal.

If the test that identified the adrenal mass was an ultrasound or CT, an MRI may be helpful to differentiate the various causes of adrenal masses. Because adrenal adenomas have abundant intracytoplasmic lipid, they can often be confirmed on CT and MRI.

Imaging

Lesions that are primarily cystic on CT or MRI are typically benign and can be followed with serial imaging. Benign adrenal cysts are characterized by thin nonenhancing walls; fluid attenuation on CT and thin calcifications may be present peripherally in about 50%.

Characteristics suspicious for malignancy include solid masses that are large, hemorrhagic, or necrotic. MRI is usually heterogeneous on T1- and T2-weighted images due to internal bleeding.

Masses with gross fat on CT (Hounsfield unit < 30) are myelolipomas, benign nonfunctional adrenal lesions with lipid and myeloid components. Myelolipomas are usually asymptomatic or present with pain if they bleed.

Noncontrast CT sensitivity for benign adenomas ranges from 50–80% depending on the Hounsfield unit (HU) attenuation value threshold chosen (Figure 29–6). If a threshold of under 10 HU is chosen, the specificity is 84–100%. Chemical-shift imaging is an MR technique to identify intracellular lipid. In-phase and out-of-phase T1-weighted images can distinguish water and fat protons from water photons only. Sensitivities of 81–87% with specificities of 92–100% have been reported for chemical-shift MRI (Figure 29–9).

Diagnostic Algorithm

Percutaneous CT-guided biopsy may be appropriate for adrenal masses with imaging characteristics suspicious for metastasis or in patients with known malignancy.

A

B

Figure 29–9. In-phase (**A**) and out-of-phase (**B**) coronal MRI of a patient with bilateral benign nonfunctional adrenal adenomas.

All functional adrenal masses and those over 5 cm should be removed. Laparoscopic adrenalectomy is the preferred technique and is used in most cases except very large masses suspicious for malignancy or with evidence of local extension. Nonfunctional adrenal masses under 5 cm should be assessed for radiographic features concerning for malignancy and removed if they are irregular or hemorrhagic or have demonstrated growth. An individualized approach for nonsuspicious nonfunctional masses under 5 cm can be taken. It may be appropriate to remove lesions in the 3–5 cm range in well-informed younger patients in order to avoid the burden of radiographic follow-up. Those under 3 cm can generally be followed up with serial CTs every 6 months initially, then yearly if stable. There is growing evidence that some incidentalomas that have initial negative screening tests may be causing "subclinical" Cushing disease. Therefore, if a patient with an incidentaloma has symptoms or signs of Cushing disease, additional or repeat screening tests may be appropriate.

NEUROBLASTOMA

Neuroblastomas (Figure 29–10) are of neural crest origin and may therefore develop from any portion of the sympathetic chain. Most arise in the retroperitoneum, and 45% involve the adrenal gland. The latter offer the poorest prognosis. In childhood, neuroblastoma is the third most common neoplastic disease after leukemia and brain tumors. Most are encountered in the first 2½ years of life, but a few are seen as late as the sixth decade, when they seem to be less aggressive. Abnormalities of muscle and heart and hemihypertrophy have been observed in association with neuroblastoma.

Metastases spread through both the bloodstream and lymphatics. Common sites in children include the skull and long bones, regional lymph nodes, liver, and lungs. Local invasion is common. In infants, who enjoy the best prognosis, metastases are usually limited to the liver and subcutaneous fat.

The following staging of neuroblastoma is generally accepted:

Stage I: Tumors confined to the structure of origin.

Stage II: Tumors extending in continuity beyond the organ but not crossing the midline. Ipsilateral lymph nodes may be involved.

Stage III: Tumors extending in continuity beyond the midline. Regional lymph nodes may be involved.

Stage IV: Remote disease involving skeletal organs, soft tissues, and distant lymph node groups.

Stage IV-S: Stage I or II patients with remote spread of tumor confined to one or more of the following sites: liver, skin, or bone marrow.

Figure 29–10. Neuroblastoma of adrenal gland. Plain film, child age 7 years, showing large mass occupying left flank. Punctate calcification in upper portion is typical of neuroblastoma.

Clinical Findings

A. SYMPTOMS

An abdominal mass is usually noted by parents, the physician, or the patient. About 70% of patients have metastases when first seen. Symptoms relating to metastases include fever, malaise, bone pain, failure to thrive, and constipation or diarrhea.

B. SIGNS

A flank mass is usually palpable and may even be visible; it often extends across the midline. The tumor is usually nodular and fixed, since it tends to be locally invasive. Evidence of metastases may be noted: ocular proptosis from metastases to the skull, enlarged nodular liver, or a mass in bone. Hypertension is often found.

C. LABORATORY FINDINGS

Anemia is common. Urinalysis and renal function are normal. Because 70% of neuroblastomas elaborate increased levels of norepinephrine and epinephrine, urinary vanillylmandelic acid and homovanillic acid levels should be measured. Serial estimations of these substances during definitive treatment can be used as tumor markers. A return to normal levels is encouraging, while rising levels imply residual or progressive tumor. Bone marrow aspiration may reveal tumor cells.

D. X-Ray Findings

Plain radiographs may show a mass and displacement of the kidneys or other organs. CT scans are used to define tumor size, vascular invasion (eg, of the vena cava), local tumor spread, and distant metastases. Further evaluation includes CT of the chest to determine whether lung metastases are present and a bone scan to define skeletal metastases. Many of these tumors take up ^{131}I-MIBG; thus this test can be used for staging.

Differential Diagnosis

Wilms tumor is also a disease of childhood. Intravenous urograms show the caliceal distortion characteristic of an intrinsic renal tumor; no such distortion is shown in neuroblastoma, which merely displaces the kidney. Hydronephrosis, polycystic renal disease, and neonatal adrenal hemorrhage may be confused with neuroblastoma. CT is very useful in differentiating the various lesions. Neuroblastomas cause the excretion of large amounts of catecholamines (eg, vanillylmandelic acid), which is not present with the other disorders.

Treatment

Surgical excision of a tumor is standard care of stage I and stage II patients. Although neuroblastoma is radiosensitive, radiation therapy is typically used as part of multimodality therapy of high-risk disease. In stage IV and high-risk stage III disease, chemotherapy is typically given followed by surgery and radiation therapy for residual disease. Useful drugs include cisplatin, cyclophosphamide, doxorubicin, and etoposide. There is evidence that after chemotherapy and surgery/radiation for residual disease, bone marrow transplant followed by 13-*cis*-retinoic acid prolongs disease-specific survival in high-risk patients and is now standard care.

Prognosis

Patients with stage I and II disease have an 80% survival rate. Including all patients, however, long-term survival occurs in only 15% of patients. Infants have the best prognosis; their 2-year survival rate approaches 60%, and if the tumor is confined to the primary site with or without adjacent regional spread, the cure rate is about 80%. Factors that define high-risk neuroblastoma include age over 1 year, metastasis, amplification of the MYCN oncogene, and particular histologic findings.

In a few infants, spontaneous maturation of neuroblastoma to ganglioneuroma has been observed. It is thought by some that x-ray treatment and chemotherapy can also accomplish this.

Serial estimation of urinary catecholamines following therapy usually indicates the presence of residual tumor.

REFERENCES

General

Brunt LM et al: Outcomes analysis in patients undergoing laparoscopic adrenalectomy for hormonally active adrenal tumors. Surgery 2001;130:629.

Hsu TH, Gill IS: Bilateral laparoscopic adrenalectomy: Retroperitoneal and transperitoneal approaches. Urology 2002;59:184.

Lockhart ME et al: Imaging of adrenal masses. Eur J Radiol 2002; 41:95.

MacGillivray DC et al: Laparoscopic resection of large adrenal tumors. Ann Surg Oncol 2002;9:480.

Ross NS, Aron DC: Hormonal evaluation of the patient with an incidentally discovered adrenal mass. N Engl J Med 1990; 323:1401.

Smith CD, Weber CJ, Amerson JR: Laparoscopic adrenalectomy: New gold standard. World J Surg 1999;23:389.

Winfield HN et al: Laparoscopic adrenalectomy: The preferred choice? A comparison to open adrenalectomy. J Urol 1998; 160:325.

Cushing Syndrome & Adrenocortical Tumors

Atkinson AB: The treatment of Cushing's syndrome. Clin Endocrinol 1991;34:507.

Benecke R et al: Plasma level monitoring of mitotane (*o,p′*-DDD) and its metabolite (*o,p′*-DDE) during long-term treatment of Cushing's disease with low doses. Eur J Clin Pharmacol 1991;41:259.

Boushey RP, Dackiw AP: Adrenal cortical carcinoma. Curr Treat Options Oncol 2001;2:355.

Brennan MF: Adrenocortical carcinoma. CA Cancer J Clin 1987; 37:348.

Decker RA et al: Eastern Cooperative Oncology Group Study 1879: Mitotane and Adriamycin in patients with advanced adrenocortical carcinoma. Surgery 1991;110:1006.

Doherty GM et al: Time to recovery of the hypothalamic-pituitary-adrenal axis after curative resection of adrenal tumors in patients with Cushing's syndrome. Surgery 1990;108:1085.

Dwyer AJ et al: Pituitary adenomas in patients with Cushing's disease: Initial experience with Gd-DTPA-enhanced MR imaging. Radiology 1987;163:421.

Findling JW, Tyrrell JB: Occult ectopic secretion of corticotropin. Arch Intern Med 1986;146:929.

Findling JW, Raff H: Diagnosis and differential diagnosis of Cushing's syndrome. Endocrinol Metab Clin North Am 2001; 30:729.

Flack MR et al: Urine free cortisol in the high-dose dexamethasone suppression test for the differential diagnosis of the Cushing syndrome. Ann Intern Med 1992;116:211.

Grus JR, Nelson DH: ACTH-producing pituitary tumors. Endocrinol Metab Clin North Am 1991;20:319.

Jones KL: The Cushing syndromes. Pediatr Clin North Am 1990; 37:1313.

Kaye TB, Crapo L: The Cushing's syndrome: An update on diagnostic tests. Ann Intern Med 1990;112:434.

Luton J-P et al: Clinical features of adrenocortical carcinoma, prognostic factors, and the effect of mitotane therapy. N Engl J Med 1990;322:1195.

Mampalam TJ, Tyrrell JB, Wilson CB: Transsphenoidal microsurgery for Cushing's disease. Ann Intern Med 1988; 109:487.

Oldfield EH et al: Petrosal sinus sampling with and without corticotropin-releasing hormone for the differential diagnosis of Cushing's syndrome. N Engl J Med 1991;325:897.

Orth DN: Cushing's syndrome. N Engl J Med 1995;32:791.

Sheeler LR: Cushing's syndrome. Urol Clin North Am 1989; 16:447.

Styne DM et al: Treatment of Cushing's disease in childhood and adolescence by transsphenoidal microadenomectomy. N Engl J Med 1984;B310:889.

Tabarin A et al: Use of ketoconazole in the treatment of Cushing's disease and ectopic ACTH syndrome. Clin Endocrinol 1991; 34:63.

Trainer PJ, Grossman A: The diagnosis and differential diagnosis of Cushing's syndrome. Clin Endocrinol 1991;34:317.

Tyrrell JB et al: An overnight high-dose dexamethasone suppression test: Rapid differential diagnosis of Cushing's syndrome. Ann Intern Med 1986;104:180.

Watson RGK et al: Results of adrenal surgery for Cushing's syndrome: 10 years' experience. World J Surg 1986;10:531.

Adrenal Androgenic Syndromes

Cumming DC et al: Treatment of hirsutism with spironolactone. JAMA 1982;247:1295.

Ehrmann DA, Rosenfield RL: Hirsutism: Beyond the steroidogenic block. N Engl J Med 1990;323:909.

Killeen AA et al: Prevalence of nonclassical congenital adrenal hyperplasia among women self-referred for electrolytic treatment of hirsutism. Am J Med Genet 1992;42:197.

Marshburn PB, Carr BR: Hirsutism and virilization: A systematic approach to benign and potentially serious causes. Postgrad Med 1995;97:99.

Masiakos PT, Flynn CE, Donahoe PK: Masculinizing and feminizing syndromes caused by functioning tumors. Semin Pediatr Surg 1997;6:147.

Mendonca BB et al: Clinical, hormonal and pathological findings in a comparative study of adrenocortical neoplasms in childhood and adulthood. J Urol 1995;154:2004.

Miller WL: Congenital adrenal hyperplasias. Endocrinol Metab Clin North Am 1991;20:721.

Miller WL: Genetics, diagnosis, and management of 21-hydroxylase deficiency. J Clin Endocrinol Metab 1994;78:241.

Moltz L, Schwartz U: Gonadal and adrenal androgen secretion in hirsute females. Clin Endocrinol Metab 1986;15:229.

Sciarra F, Tosti-Croce C, Toscano V: Androgen-secreting adrenal tumors. Minerva Endocrinologica 1995;20:63.

Siegel SF et al: ACTH stimulation tests and plasma dehydroepiandrosterone sulfate levels in women with hirsutism. N Engl J Med 1990;323:849.

Hyperaldosteronism

Biglieri EG: The spectrum of mineralocorticoid hypertension. Hypertension 1991;18:251.

Ganguly A: Primary aldosteronism. N Engl J Med 1998; 339:1828.

Gomez-Sanchez CE: Primary aldosteronism and its variants. Cardiovasc Res 1998;37:8.

Gordon RD: Primary aldosteronism. J Endocrinol Invest 1995; 18:495.

Gordon RD et al: High incidence of primary aldosteronism in 199 patients referred with hypertension. Clin Exp Pharmacol Physiol 1994;21:315.

Ikeda DM et al: The detection of adrenal tumors and hyperplasia in patients with primary aldosteronism: Comparison of scintigraphy, CT, and MR imaging. Am J Roentgenol 1989; 153:301.

Irony I et al: Correctable subsets of primary aldosteronism: Primary adrenal hyperplasia and renin responsive adenoma. Am J Hypertens 1990;3:576.

Kater CE et al: Stimulation and suppression of the mineralocorticoid hormones in normal subjects and adrenocortical disorders. Endocr Rev 1989;11:149.

Schalekamp MA, Wenting GJ, Man in't Veld AJ: Pathogenesis of mineralocorticoid hypertension. Clin Endocrinol Metab 1981;10:397.

Shen WT et al: Laparoscopic vs open adrenalectomy for the treatment of primary hyperaldosteronism. Arch Surg 1999; 134:628.

Siren J et al: Laparoscopic adrenalectomy for primary aldosteronism. Surg Laparosc Endosc 1999;9:9.

Vallotton MB: Primary aldosteronism. Part I. Diagnosis of primary hyperaldosteronism. Clin Endocrinol 1996;45:47.

Vallotton MB: Primary aldosteronism. Part II. Differential diagnosis of primary hyperaldosteronism and pseudoaldosteronism. Clin Endocrinol 1996;45:53.

Young WF Jr, Hogana MJ: Renin-independent hypermineralocorticoidism. Trends Endocrinol Metab 1994;5:97.

Young WF Jr et al: Primary aldosteronism: Adrenal venous sampling. Surgery 1996;120:913.

Pheochromocytomas & Related Tumors

Averbuch SD et al: Malignant pheochromocytoma: Effective treatment with a combination of cyclophosphamide, vincristine, and dacarbazine. Ann Intern Med 1988;109:267.

Bouloux PMG, Fakeeh M: Investigation of phaeochromocytoma. Clin Endocrinol 1995;43:657.

Bravo EL: Plasma or urinary metanephrines for the diagnosis of pheochromocytoma? That is the question. Ann Intern Med 1996;125:331.

Caty MG et al: Current diagnosis and treatment of pheochromocytoma in children: Experience with 22 consecutive tumors in 14 patients. Arch Surg 1990;125:978.

Chevinsky AH, Minton JP, Falko JM: Metastatic pheochromocytoma associated with multiple endocrine neoplasia syndrome type II. Arch Surg 1990;125:935.

Eigelberger MS, Duh QY: Pheochromocytoma. Curr Treat Options Oncol 2001;2:321.

Francis IR, Korobkin M: Pheochromocytoma. Radiol Clin North Am 1996;34:1101.

Golub MS, Tuck ML: Diagnostic and therapeutic strategies in pheochromocytoma. The Endocrinologist 1992;2:101.

Heron et al: The urinary metanephrine-to-creatinine ratio for the diagnosis of pheochromocytoma. Ann Intern Med 1996; 125:300.

Ito Y et al: Efficacy of single voided urine metanephrine and normetanephrine assay for diagnosing pheochromocytoma. World J Surg 1998;22:684.

Joris JL et al: Hemodynamic changes and catecholamine release during laparoscopic adrenalectomy for pheochromocytoma. Anesth Analg 1999;88:16.

Kebebew E, Duk Q-Y: Benign and malignant pheochromocytoma: Diagnosis, treatment and follow-up. Surg Oncol Clin North Am 1998;7:765.

Lenders JWM et al: Plasma metanephrines in the diagnosis of pheochromocytoma. Ann Intern Med 1995;123:101.

Loh K-C et al: The treatment of malignant pheochromocytoma with iodine-131 metaiodobenzylguanidine ([131]1-MIBG): A comprehensive review of 116 reported patients. J Endocrinol Invest 1997;20:648.

Peaston RT, Lennard TWJ, Lai LC: Overnight excretion of urinary catecholamines and metabolites in the detection of pheochromocytoma. J Clin Endocrinol Metab 1996;81:1379.

Proye C et al: High incidence of malignant pheochromocytoma in a surgical unit: 26 cases out of 100 patients operated from 1971 to 1991. J Endocrinol Invest 1992;15:651.

Sheps SG et al: Recent developments in the diagnosis and treatment of pheochromocytoma. Mayo Clin Proc 1990;65:88.

Stein PP, Black HR: A simplified diagnostic approach to pheochromocytoma: A review of the literature and report of one institution's experience. Medicine 1991;70:46.

Whalen RK, Althausen AF, Daniels GH: Extra-adrenal pheochromocytoma. J Urol 1992;147:1.

Young WF: Pheochromocytoma: 1926–1993. Trends Endocrinol Metab 1993;4:122.

Incidentaloma

Boland GW et al: Characterization of adrenal masses using unenhanced CT: An analysis of the CT literature. AJR 1998; 171:201.

Herts BR, Remer EM: The role of percutaneous biopsy in the evaluation of renal and adrenal mass. AUA Update Series; 2000; Vol. 19, Lesson 36.

Kievit J, Haak HR: Diagnosis and treatment of adrenal incidentaloma: A cost-effectiveness analysis. Endocrinol Metab Clin North Am 2000;29:69.

Korobkin M et al: Characterization of adrenal masses with chemical shift and gadolinium-enhanced MR imaging. Radiol 1995;197:411.

Ross NS, Aron DC: Hormonal evaluation of the patient with an incidentally discovered adrenal mass. N Engl J Med 1990; 323:1401.

Terzolo M et al: Adrenal incidentaloma: A new cause of the metabolic syndrome? J Clin Endocrinol Metab 2002;87:998.

Vaughan ED: Diagnosis of surgical adrenal disorders. AUA Update Series, 1997; Vol. 16, Lesson 39.

Neuroblastoma

Evans AE, D'Angio GJ, Randolph J: A proposed staging for children with neuroblastoma. Cancer 1979;27:374.

Evans AE et al: Prognostic factors in neuroblastoma. Cancer 1987; 59:1853.

Evans AE et al: A review of 17 IV-S neuroblastoma patients at the Children's Hospital of Philadelphia. Cancer 1980;45:833.

Forman HP et al: Congenital neuroblastoma: Evaluation with multimodality imaging. Radiology 1990;175:365.

Hann H-WL et al: Biologic differences between neuroblastoma stages IV-S and IV: Measurement of serum ferritin and E-rosette inhibition in 30 children. N Engl J Med 1981; 305:425.

Matthay KK: Neuroblastoma: Biology and therapy. Oncology (Huntingt) 1997;11:1857.

Matthay KK et al: Treatment of high risk neuroblastoma with intensive chemotherapy, radiotherapy, autologous bone marrow transplantation, and 13-*cis*-retinoic acid. N Engl J Med 1999; 341:1165.

Smith EI, Castleberry RP: Neuroblastoma. Curr Probl Surg 1990; 27:573.

Snyder HM et al: Pediatric oncology. In: Walsh et al (editors): *Campbell's Urology*, 7th ed, pp. 2210–2256. Saunders, 1997.

Disorders of the Kidneys

Jack W. McAninch, MD

■ CONGENITAL ANOMALIES OF THE KIDNEYS

Congenital anomalies occur more frequently in the kidney than in any other organ. Some cause no difficulty, but many (eg, hypoplasia, polycystic kidneys) cause impairment of renal function. It has been noted that children with a gross deformity of an external ear associated with ipsilateral maldevelopment of the facial bones are apt to have a congenital abnormality of the kidney (eg, ectopy, hypoplasia) on the same side as the visible deformity. Lateral displacement of the nipples has been observed in association with bilateral renal hypoplasia.

A significant incidence of renal agenesis, ectopy, malrotation, and duplication has been observed in association with congenital scoliosis and kyphosis. Unilateral agenesis, hypoplasia, and dysplasia are often seen in association with supralevator imperforate anus.

For a better understanding of these congenital abnormalities, see the discussion of the embryology and development of the kidney in Chapter 2.

AGENESIS

Bilateral renal agenesis is extremely rare; no more than 400 cases have been reported. The children do not survive. The condition does not appear to have any predisposing factors. Prenatal suspicion of the anomaly exists when oligohydramnios is present on fetal ultrasound examination. Pulmonary hypoplasia and facial deformities (Potter facies) are usually present. Abdominal ultrasound examination usually establishes the diagnosis.

One kidney may be absent (estimated incidence: 1 in 450–1000 births). In some cases, this may be because the ureteral bud (from the wolffian duct) failed to develop or, if it did develop, did not reach the metanephros (adult kidney). Without a drainage system, the metanephric mass undergoes atrophy. The ureter is absent on the side of the unformed kidney in 50% of cases, although a blind ureteral duct may be found. (See Chapter 2.)

Renal agenesis causes no symptoms; it is usually found by accident on abdominal or renal imaging. It is not an easy diagnosis to establish even though on inspection of the bladder the ureteral ridge is absent and no orifice is visualized, for the kidney could be present but be drained by a ureter whose opening is ectopic (into the urethra, seminal vesicle, or vagina). If definitive diagnosis seems essential, isotope studies, ultrasonography, and computed tomography (CT) should establish the diagnosis.

There appears to be an increased incidence of infection, hydronephrosis, and stones in the contralateral organ. Other congenital anomalies associated with this defect include cardiac, vertebral column, and anal anomalies as well as anomalies of the long bones, hands, and genitalia.

HYPOPLASIA

Hypoplasia implies a small kidney. The total renal mass may be divided in an unequal manner, in which case one kidney is small and the other correspondingly larger than normal. Some of these congenitally small kidneys prove, on pathologic examination, to be dysplastic. Unilateral or bilateral hypoplasia has been observed in infants with fetal alcohol syndrome, and renal anomalies have been reported in infants with in utero cocaine exposure (Rosenstein, Wheeler, and Heid, 1990).

Differentiation from acquired atrophy is difficult. Atrophic pyelonephritis usually reveals typical distortion of the calyces. Vesicoureteral reflux in infants may cause a dwarfed kidney even in the absence of infection. Stenosis of the renal artery leads to shrinkage of the kidney.

Such kidneys have small renal arteries and branches and are associated with hypertension, which is relieved by nephrectomy. Selective renal venography is helpful in differentiating between a congenitally absent kidney and one that is small and nonvisualized.

SUPERNUMERARY KIDNEYS

The presence of a third kidney is very rare; the presence of 4 separate kidneys in one individual has been reported only once. The anomaly must not be confused with duplication (or triplication) of the renal pelvis in one kidney, which is not uncommon.

DYSPLASIA & MULTICYSTIC KIDNEY

Renal dysplasia has protean manifestations. Multicystic kidney of the newborn is usually unilateral, nonhereditary, and characterized by an irregularly lobulated mass of cysts; the ureter is usually absent or atretic. It may develop because of faulty union of the nephron and the collecting system. At most, only a few embryonic glomeruli and tubules are observed. The only finding is the discovery of an irregular mass in the flank. Nothing is shown on urography, but in an occasional case, some radiopaque fluid may be noted. If the cystic kidney is large, its mate is usually normal. However, when the cystic organ is small, the contralateral kidney is apt to be abnormal. The cystic nature of the lesion may be revealed by sonography, and the diagnosis can be established in utero. If the physician feels that the proper diagnosis has been made, no treatment is necessary. If there is doubt about the diagnosis, nephrectomy is considered the procedure of choice. Dimmick et al (1989) noted neoplastic changes in multicystic renal dysplasia.

Multicystic kidney is often associated with contralateral renal and ureteral abnormalities. Contralateral ureteropelvic junction obstruction is one of the common problems noted. Diagnostic evaluation of both kidneys is required to establish the overall status of anomalous development.

Dysplasia of the renal parenchyma is also seen in association with ureteral obstruction or reflux that was probably present early in pregnancy. It is relatively common as a segmental renal lesion involving the upper pole of a duplicated kidney whose ureter is obstructed by a congenital ureterocele. It may also be found in urinary tracts severely obstructed by posterior urethral valves; in this instance, the lesion may be bilateral.

Microscopically, the renal parenchyma is "disorganized." Tubular and glomerular cysts may be noted; these elements are fetal in type. Islands of metaplastic cartilage are often seen. The common denominator seems to be fetal obstruction.

ADULT POLYCYSTIC KIDNEY DISEASE

Adult polycystic kidney disease is an autosomal dominant hereditary condition and almost always bilateral (95% of cases). The disease encountered in infants is different from that seen in adults, although the literature reports a small number of infants with the adult type. The former is an autosomal recessive disease in which life expectancy is short, whereas that diagnosed in adulthood is autosomal dominant; symptoms ordinarily do not appear until after age 40. Cysts of the liver, spleen, and pancreas may be noted in association with both forms. The kidneys are larger than normal and are studded with cysts of various sizes.

Etiology & Pathogenesis

The evidence suggests that the cysts occur because of defects in the development of the collecting and uriniferous tubules and in the mechanism of their joining. Blind secretory tubules that are connected to functioning glomeruli become cystic. As the cysts enlarge, they compress adjacent parenchyma, destroy it by ischemia, and occlude normal tubules. The result is progressive functional impairment.

Pathology

Grossly, the kidneys are usually much enlarged. Their surfaces are studded with cysts of various sizes (Figure 30–1). On section, the cysts are found to be scattered throughout the parenchyma. Calcification is rare. The fluid in the cyst is usually amber-colored but may be hemorrhagic.

Microscopically, the lining of the cysts consists of a single layer of cells. The renal parenchyma may show

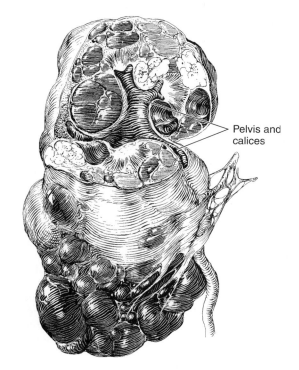

Pelvis and calices

Figure 30–1. Polycystic kidney. Multiple cysts deep in the parenchyma and on the surface. Note distortion of the calyces by the cysts.

peritubular fibrosis and evidence of secondary infection. There appears to be a reduction in the number of glomeruli, some of which may be hyalinized. Renal arteriolar thickening is a prominent finding in adults.

Clinical Findings

A. Symptoms

Pain over one or both kidneys may occur because of the drag on the vascular pedicles by the heavy kidneys, from obstruction or infection, or from hemorrhage into a cyst. Gross or microscopic total hematuria is not uncommon and may be severe; the cause for this is not clear. Colic may occur if blood clots or stones are passed. The patient may notice an abdominal mass.

Infection (chills, fever, renal pain) commonly complicates polycystic disease. Symptoms of vesical irritability may be the first complaint. When renal insufficiency ensues, headache, nausea and vomiting, weakness, and loss of weight occur.

B. Signs

One or both kidneys are usually palpable. They may feel nodular. If infected, they may be tender. Hypertension is found in 60–70% of these patients. Evidence of cardiac enlargement is then noted.

Fever may be present if pyelonephritis exists or if cysts have become infected. In the stage of uremia, anemia and loss of weight may be evident. Ophthalmoscopic examination may show changes typical of moderate or severe hypertension.

C. Laboratory Findings

Anemia may be noted, caused either by chronic loss of blood or, more commonly, by the hematopoietic depression accompanying uremia. Proteinuria and microscopic (if not gross) hematuria are the rule. Pyuria and bacteriuria are common.

Progressive loss of concentrating power occurs. Renal clearance tests show varying degrees of renal impairment. About one-third of patients with polycystic kidney disease are uremic when first seen.

D. X-Ray Findings

Both renal shadows are usually enlarged on a plain film of the abdomen, even as much as 5 times normal size. Kidneys more than 16 cm in length are suspect.

The renal masses are usually enlarged and the caliceal pattern is quite bizarre (spider deformity). The calyces are broadened and flattened, enlarged, and often curved, as they tend to hug the periphery of adjacent cysts. Often the changes are only slight or may even be absent on one side, leading to the erroneous diagnosis of tumor of the other kidney.

If cysts are infected, perinephritis may obscure the renal and even the psoas shadows.

E. CT Scanning

CT is an excellent noninvasive technique used to establish the diagnosis of polycystic disease. The multiple thin-walled cysts filled with fluid and the large renal size make this imaging method extremely accurate (95%) for diagnosis.

F. Isotope Studies

Photoscans reveal multiple "cold" avascular spots in large renal shadows.

G. Ultrasonography

Sonography appears to be superior to both excretory urography and isotope scanning in diagnosis of polycystic disorders.

H. Instrumental Examination

Cystoscopy may show evidence of cystitis, in which case the urine will contain abnormal elements. Bleeding from a ureteral orifice may be noted. Ureteral catheterization and retrograde urograms are rarely indicated.

Differential Diagnosis

Bilateral hydronephrosis (on the basis of congenital or acquired ureteral obstruction) may present bilateral flank masses and signs of impairment of renal function, but ultrasonography shows changes quite different from those of the polycystic kidney.

Bilateral renal tumor is rare but may mimic polycystic kidney disease perfectly on urography. Tumors are usually localized to one portion of the kidney, whereas cysts are quite diffusely distributed. The total renal function should be normal with unilateral tumor but is usually depressed in patients with polycystic kidney disease. CT may be needed at times to differentiate between the 2 conditions.

In **von Hippel-Lindau disease** (angiomatous cerebellar cyst, angiomatosis of the retina, and tumors or cysts of the pancreas), multiple bilateral cysts or adenocarcinomas of both kidneys may develop. The presence of other stigmas should make the diagnosis. CT, angiography, sonography, or scintiphotography should be definitive.

Tuberous sclerosis (convulsive seizures, mental retardation, and adenoma sebaceum) is typified by hamartomatous tumors often involving the skin, brain, retinas, bones, liver, heart, and kidneys (see Chapter 21). The renal lesions are usually multiple and bilateral and microscopically are angiomyolipomas. The presence of other stigmas and use of CT or sonography should make the differentiation.

A **simple cyst** (see section following) is usually unilateral and single; total renal function should be normal. Urograms usually show a single lesion (Figure

30–2), whereas polycystic kidney disease is bilateral and has multiple filling defects.

Complications

For reasons that are not clear, pyelonephritis is a common complication of polycystic kidney disease. It may be asymptomatic; pus cells in the urine may be few or absent. Stained smears or quantitative cultures make the diagnosis. A gallium-67 citrate scan will definitely reveal the sites of infection, including abscess.

Infection of cysts is associated with pain and tenderness over the kidney and a febrile response. The differential diagnosis between infection of cysts and pyelonephritis may be difficult, but here again a gallium scan will prove helpful.

In rare instances, gross hematuria may be so brisk and persistent as to endanger life.

Treatment

Except for unusual complications, the treatment is conservative and supportive.

A. GENERAL MEASURES

The patient should be placed on a low-protein diet (0.5–0.75 g/kg/d of protein) and fluids forced to 3000 mL or more per day. Physical activity may be permitted within reason, but strenuous exercise is contraindicated. When the patient is in the state of absolute renal insufficiency, one should treat as for uremia from any cause. Hypertension should be controlled. Hemodialysis may be indicated.

B. SURGERY

There is no evidence that excision or decompression of cysts improves renal function. If a large cyst is found to be compressing the upper ureter, causing obstruction and further embarrassing renal function, it should be resected or aspirated. When the degree of renal insufficiency becomes life-threatening, chronic dialysis or renal transplantation should be considered.

C. TREATMENT OF COMPLICATIONS

Pyelonephritis must be rigorously treated to prevent further renal damage. Infection of cysts requires surgical drainage. If bleeding from one kidney is so severe that exsanguination is possible, nephrectomy or embolization of the renal or, preferably, the segmental artery must be considered as a lifesaving measure.

Concomitant diseases (eg, tumor, obstructing stone) may require definitive surgical treatment.

Prognosis

When the disease affects children, it has a very poor prognosis. The large group presenting clinical signs and symptoms after age 35–40 has a somewhat more favorable prognosis. Although there is wide variation, these patients usually do not live longer than 5 or 10 years after the diagnosis is made unless dialysis is made available or renal transplantation is done.

SIMPLE (SOLITARY) CYST

Simple cyst (Figures 30–2 and 30–3) of the kidney is usually unilateral and single but may be multiple and multilocular and, more rarely, bilateral. It differs from polycystic kidneys both clinically and pathologically.

Etiology & Pathogenesis

Whether simple cyst is congenital or acquired is not clear. Its origin may be similar to that of polycystic kidneys, that is, the difference may be merely one of degree. On the other hand, simple cysts have been produced in animals by causing tubular obstruction and local ischemia; this suggests that the lesion can be acquired.

As a simple cyst grows, it compresses and thereby may destroy renal parenchyma, but rarely does it destroy so much renal tissue that renal function is impaired. A solitary cyst may be placed in such a position as to compress the ureter, causing progressive hydronephrosis. Infection may complicate the picture.

Feiner, Katz, and Gallo (1981) have noticed that acquired cystic disease of the kidney is commonly observed as an effect of chronic dialysis. The spontaneous regression of cysts has occasionally been noted.

Pathology

Simple cysts usually involve the lower pole of the kidney. Those that produce symptoms average about 10 cm in diameter, but a few are large enough to fill the entire flank. They usually contain a clear amber fluid. Their walls are quite thin, and the cysts are "blue-domed" in appearance. Calcification of the sac is occasionally seen. About 5% contain hemorrhagic fluid, and possibly one-half of these have papillary cancers on their walls.

Simple cysts are usually superficial but may be deeply situated. When a cyst is situated deep in the kidney, the cyst wall is adjacent to the epithelial lining of the pelvis or calyces, from which it may be separated only with great difficulty. Cysts do not communicate with the renal pelvis (Figure 30–2). Microscopic examination of the cyst wall shows heavy fibrosis and hyalinization; areas of calcification may be seen. The adjacent renal tissue is compressed and fibrosed. A number of cases of simple cysts have been reported in children.

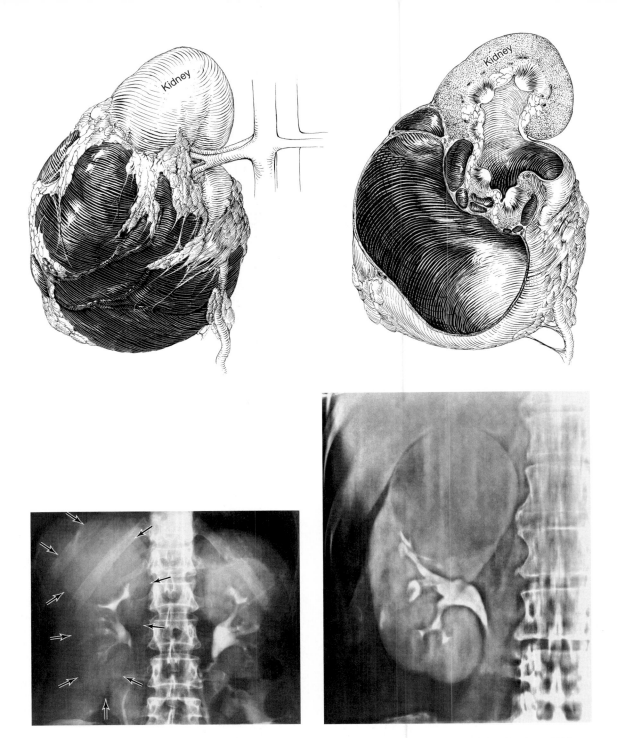

Figure 30–2. Simple cyst. **Upper left:** Large cyst displacing lower pole laterally. **Upper right:** Section of kidney showing one large and a few small cysts. **Lower left:** Excretory urogram showing soft-tissue mass in upper pole of right kidney. Elongation and distortion of upper calyces by cyst. **Lower right:** Infusion nephrotomogram showing large cyst in upper renal pole distorting upper calyces and dislocating upper portion of kidney laterally.

Figure 30–3. Left renal cyst. **Left:** Computed tomography (CT) scan shows a homogeneous low-density mass (C) arising from anterior border of left kidney just posterior to tail of the pancreas. The CT attenuation value was similar to that of water, indicating a simple renal cyst. **Right:** After intravenous injection of contrast material, the mass did not increase in attenuation value, adding further confirmatory evidence of its benign cystic nature.

However, large cysts are rare in children; the presence of cancer must therefore be ruled out.

Multilocular renal cysts may be confused with tumor on urography. Sonography usually makes the diagnosis. Occasionally, CT and magnetic resonance imaging (MRI) may be necessary.

Clinical Findings

A. SYMPTOMS

Pain in the flank or back, usually intermittent and dull, is not uncommon. If bleeding suddenly distends the cyst wall, pain may come on abruptly and be severe. Gastrointestinal symptoms are occasionally noted and may suggest peptic ulcer or gallbladder disease. The patient may discover a mass in the abdomen, although cysts of this size are unusual. If the cyst becomes infected, the patient usually complains of pain in the flank, malaise, and fever.

B. SIGNS

Physical examination is usually normal, although occasionally a mass in the region of the kidney may be palpated or percussed. Tenderness in the flank may be noted if the cyst becomes infected.

C. LABORATORY FINDINGS

Urinalysis is usually normal. Microscopic hematuria is rare. Renal function tests are normal unless the cysts are multiple and bilateral (rare). Even in the face of extensive destruction of one kidney, compensatory hypertrophy of the other kidney will maintain normal total function.

D. CT SCANNING

CT appears to be the most accurate means of differentiating renal cyst and tumor (Figure 30–3). Cysts have an attenuation approximating that of water, whereas the density of tumors is similar to that of normal parenchyma. Parenchyma is made more dense with the intravenous injection of radiopaque fluid, but a cyst remains unaffected. The wall of a cyst is sharply demarcated from the renal parenchyma; a tumor is not. The wall of a cyst is thin; that of a tumor is not. CT may well supplant cyst puncture in the differentiation of cyst and tumor in many cases.

E. RENAL ULTRASONOGRAPHY

Renal ultrasonography is a noninvasive diagnostic technique that in a high percentage of cases differentiates between a cyst and a solid mass. If findings on ultrasonography are also compatible with a cyst, a needle can be introduced into the cyst under ultrasonographic control and the cyst can be aspirated.

F. ISOTOPE SCANNING

A rectilinear scan clearly delineates the mass but does not differentiate cyst from tumor. The technetium scan, made with the camera, reveals that the mass is indeed avascular.

G. PERCUTANEOUS CYST ASPIRATION WITH CYSTOGRAPHY

If the studies listed leave some doubt about the differentiation between cyst and tumor, aspiration may be done. (See Treatment, following, and p. 516.)

Differential Diagnosis

Carcinoma of the kidney also occupies space but tends to lie more deeply in the organ and therefore causes more distortion of the calyces. Hematuria is common with tumor, rare with cyst. If a solid tumor overlies the psoas muscle, the edge of the muscle is obliterated on the plain film; it can be seen through a cyst, however. Evidence of metastases (ie, loss of weight and strength, palpable supraclavicular nodes, chest film showing metastatic nodules), erythrocytosis, hypercalcemia, and increased sedimentation rate suggest cancer. It must be remembered, however, that the walls of a simple cyst may undergo cancerous degeneration. Sonography, CT scan, or MRI should be almost definitive in differential diagnosis. It is wise to assume that all space-occupying lesions of the kidneys are cancers until proved otherwise.

Polycystic kidney disease is almost always bilateral. Diffuse caliceal and pelvic distortion is the rule. Simple cyst is usually solitary and unilateral. Polycystic kidney disease is usually accompanied by impaired renal function and hypertension; simple cyst is not.

Renal carbuncle is a rare disease. A history of skin infection a few weeks before the onset of fever and local pain may be obtained. CT scan of the kidney usually defines a carbuncle. The kidney may be fixed; this can be demonstrated by comparing the position of the kidney when the patient is supine and upright. Angiography demonstrates an avascular lesion. A gallium-67 scan demonstrates the inflammatory nature of the lesion, but an infected simple cyst might have a similar appearance.

Hydronephrosis may present the same symptoms and signs as simple cyst, but the urograms are quite different. Cyst causes calyceal distortion; with hydronephrosis, dilatation of the calyces and pelvis due to an obstruction is present. Acute or subacute hydronephrosis usually produces more local pain because of increased intrapelvic pressure and is more apt to be complicated by infection.

Extrarenal tumor (eg, adrenal, mixed retroperitoneal sarcoma) may displace a kidney, but rarely does it invade it and distort its calyces.

If an echinococcal cyst of the kidney does not communicate with the renal pelvis, it may be difficult to differentiate from solitary cyst, for no scoleces or hooklets will be present in the urine. The wall of a hydatid cyst often reveals calcification on x-ray examination (Figure 14–5). A skin sensitivity test (Casoni) for hydatid disease may prove helpful.

Complications (Rare)

Spontaneous infection in a simple cyst is rare, but when it occurs, it is difficult to differentiate from carbuncle. Hemorrhage into the cyst sometimes occurs. If sudden, it causes severe pain. The bleeding may come from a complicating carcinoma arising on the wall of the cyst.

Hydronephrosis may develop if a cyst of the lower pole impinges on the ureter. This in itself may cause pain from back pressure of urine in the renal pelvis. This obstruction may lead to renal infection.

Treatment

A. Specific Measures

1. If renal sonography, CT, or MRI does not lead to a definitive diagnosis, renal angiography or needle aspiration of the cyst may be necessary. Should aspiration be necessary, it can be done under sonographic guidance. The recovery of clear fluid is characteristic of a benign cyst, which should be confirmed by cytologic evaluation. In some centers, contrast radiopaque fluid is injected into the cyst after aspiration for a more thorough evaluation of the cyst wall. A smooth cyst wall, free of irregularities, supports the presence of a benign cyst.

   If the aspirate contains blood, surgical exploration should be considered, because the chances are great that the growth is cancerous.

2. If the diagnosis can be clearly established, one should consider leaving the cyst alone, since it is rare for a cyst to harm the kidney. Sonography is useful in follow-up of patients with cysts.

B. Treatment of Complications

If the cyst becomes infected, intensive antimicrobial therapy should be instituted, although Muther and Bennett (1980) found that antimicrobial drugs attained very low concentrations in the cyst fluid. Therefore, percutaneous drainage is often required. Surgical excision of the extrarenal portion of the cyst wall and drainage are curative when percutaneous drainage fails.

If hydronephrosis is present, excision of the obstructing cyst will relieve the ureteral obstruction.

Pyelonephritis in the involved kidney should suggest urinary stasis secondary to impaired ureteral drainage. Removal of the cyst and consequent relief of urinary back pressure make antimicrobial therapy more effective.

Prognosis

Simple cysts can be diagnosed with great accuracy using sonography and CT. Yearly sonography is recommended as a method of following the cyst for changes in size, configuration, and internal consistency. CT may be done if changes suggest carcinoma, and aspiration may then be performed if necessary to establish a diagnosis. Most cysts cause little difficulty.

RENAL FUSION

About 1 in 1000 individuals has some type of renal fusion, the most common being the horseshoe kidney. The fused renal mass almost always contains 2 excretory systems and therefore 2 ureters. The renal tissue may be divided equally between the 2 flanks, or the entire mass may be on one side. Even in the latter case, the 2 ureters open at their proper places in the bladder.

Etiology & Pathogenesis

It appears that this fusion of the 2 metanephroi occurs early in embryologic life, when the kidneys lie low in the pelvis. For this reason, they seldom ascend to the high position that normal kidneys assume. They may even remain in the true pelvis. Under these circumstances, such a kidney may derive its blood supply from many vessels in the area (eg, aorta, iliacs).

In patients with both ectopia and fusion, 78% have extraurologic anomalies and 65% exhibit other genitourinary defects.

Pathology (Figure 30–4)

Because the renal masses fuse early, normal rotation cannot occur; therefore, each pelvis lies on the anterior surface of its organ. Thus, the ureter must ride over the isthmus of a horseshoe kidney or traverse the anterior surface of the fused kidney. Some degree of ureteral compression may arise from this or from obstruction by one or more aberrant blood vessels. The incidence of hydronephrosis and, therefore, infection is high. Vesicoureteral reflux has frequently been noted in association with fusion.

In horseshoe kidney, the isthmus usually joins the lower poles of each kidney; each renal mass lies lower than normal. The axes of these masses are vertical, whereas the axes of normal kidneys are oblique to the spine, because they lie along the edges of the psoas muscles.

On rare occasions, the 2 nephric masses are fused into one mass containing 2 pelves and 2 ureters. The mass may lie in the midline in order to open into the bladder at the proper point (crossed renal ectopy with fusion).

Clinical Findings

A. SYMPTOMS

Most patients with fused kidneys have no symptoms. Some, however, develop ureteral obstruction. Gastrointestinal symptoms (renodigestive reflex) mimicking peptic ulcer, cholelithiasis, or appendicitis may be noted. Infection is apt to occur if ureteral obstruction and hydronephrosis or calculus develops.

B. SIGNS

Physical examination results are usually negative unless the abnormally placed renal mass can be felt. With horseshoe kidney, it may be possible to palpate a mass over the lower lumbar spine (the isthmus). In the case of crossed ectopy, a mass may be felt in the flank or lower abdomen.

C. LABORATORY FINDINGS

Urinalysis is normal unless there is infection. Renal function is normal unless disease coexists in each of the fused renal masses.

D. X-RAY FINDINGS

In the case of horseshoe kidney, the axes of the 2 kidneys, if visible on a plain film, are parallel to the spine. At times the isthmus can be identified. The plain film may also reveal a large soft-tissue mass in one flank yet not show a renal shadow on the other side.

Excretory urograms establish the diagnosis if the renal parenchyma has been maintained. The increased density of the renal tissue may make the position or configuration of the kidney more distinct. Urograms also visualize the pelvis and ureters.

1. With horseshoe kidney, the renal pelves lie on the anterior surfaces of their kidney masses, whereas the normal kidney has its pelvis lying mesial to it. The most valuable clue to the diagnosis of horseshoe kidney is the presence of calyces in the region of the lower pole that point medially and lie medial to the ureter (Figure 30–4).

2. Crossed renal ectopy with fusion shows 2 pelves and 2 ureters. One ureter must cross the midline in order to empty into the bladder at the proper point (Figure 30–4).

3. A cake or lump kidney may lie in the pelvis (fused pelvis kidney), but again its ureters and pelves will be shown (Figure 30–4). It may compress the dome of the bladder.

CT clearly outlines the renal mass but is seldom necessary for diagnosis. With pelvic fused kidney or one lying in the flank, the plain film taken with ureteral catheters in place gives the first hint of the diagnosis. Retrograde urograms show the position of the pelves and demonstrate changes compatible with infection or obstruction. Renal scanning delineates the renal mass and its contour, as does sonography.

Differential Diagnosis

Separate kidneys that fail to undergo normal rotation may be confused with horseshoe kidney. They lie along the edges of the psoas muscles, whereas the poles of a horseshoe kidney lie parallel to the spine and the lower

Figure 30–4. Renal fusion. **Upper left:** Crossed renal ectopy with fusion. The renal mass lies in the left flank. The right ureter must cross over the midline. **Upper right:** Example of "sigmoid" kidney. **Lower left:** Horseshoe kidney. Pelves are anterior. Note aberrant artery obstructing left ureter and the low position of renal mass. **Lower right:** Pelvic kidney. Pelves are placed anteriorly. Note aberrant blood supply.

poles are placed on the psoas muscles. The calyces in the region of the isthmus of a horseshoe kidney point medially and lie close to the spine.

The diagnosis of fused or lump kidney may be missed on excretory urograms if one of the ureters is markedly obstructed, so that a portion of the kidney, pelvis, and ureter fails to visualize. Infusion urograms or retrograde urograms demonstrate both excretory tracts in the renal mass.

Complications

Fused kidneys are prone to ureteral obstruction because of a high incidence of aberrant renal vessels and the necessity for one or both ureters to arch around or over the renal tissue. Hydronephrosis, stone, and infection, therefore, are common.

A large fused kidney occupying the concavity of the sacrum may cause dystocia.

Treatment

No treatment is necessary unless obstruction or infection is present. Drainage of a horseshoe kidney may be improved by dividing its isthmus. If one pole of a horseshoe is badly damaged, it may require surgical resection.

Prognosis

In most cases, the outlook is excellent. If ureteral obstruction and infection occur, renal drainage must be improved by surgical means so that antimicrobial therapy will be effective.

ECTOPIC KIDNEY

Congenital ectopic kidney usually causes no symptoms unless complications such as ureteral obstruction or infection develop.

Simple Ectopy

Simple congenital ectopy usually refers to a low kidney on the proper side that failed to ascend normally. It may lie over the pelvic brim or in the pelvis. Rarely, it may be found in the chest. It takes its blood supply from adjacent vessels, and its ureter is short. It is prone to ureteral obstruction and infection, which may lead to pain or fever. At times such a kidney may be palpable, leading to an erroneous presumptive diagnosis (eg, cancer of the bowel, appendiceal abscess).

Excretory urograms reveal the true position of the kidney. Hydronephrosis, if present, is evident. There is no redundancy of the ureter, as is the case with neph-

roptosis or acquired ectopy (eg, displacement by large suprarenal tumor).

Obstruction and infection may complicate simple ectopy and should be treated by appropriate means.

Crossed Ectopy Without Fusion

In crossed ectopy without fusion, the kidney lies on the opposite side of the body but is not attached to its normally placed mate. Unless 2 distinct renal shadows can be seen, it may be difficult to differentiate this condition from crossed ectopy with fusion (Figure 30–4). Sonography, angiography, or CT should make the distinction.

ABNORMAL ROTATION

Normally, when the kidney ascends to the lumbar region, the pelvis lies on its anterior surface. Later, the pelvis comes to lie mesially. Such rotation may fail to occur, although this seldom leads to renal disease. Urography demonstrates the abnormal position.

MEDULLARY SPONGE KIDNEY (CYSTIC DILATATION OF THE RENAL COLLECTING TUBULES)

Medullary sponge kidney is a congenital autosomal recessive defect characterized by widening of the distal collecting tubules. It is usually bilateral, affecting all of the papillae, but it may be unilateral. At times, only one papilla is involved. Cystic dilatation of the tubules is often present also. Infection and calculi are occasionally seen as a result of urinary stasis in the tubules. It is believed that medullary sponge kidney is related to polycystic kidney disease. Its occasional association with hemihypertrophy of the body has been noted.

The only symptoms are those arising from infection and stone formation. The diagnosis is made on the basis of excretory urograms or contrast-enhanced CT scan (Figure 30–5). The pelvis and calyces are normal, but dilated (streaked) tubules are seen just lateral to them; many of the dilated tubules contain round masses of radiopaque material (the cystic dilatation). If stones are present, a plain film will reveal small, round calculi in the pyramidal regions just beyond the calyces.

The differential diagnosis includes tuberculosis, healed papillary necrosis, and nephrocalcinosis. Tuberculosis is usually unilateral, and urography shows ulceration of calyces; tubercle bacilli are found on bacteriologic study. Papillary necrosis may be complicated by calcification in the healed stage but may be distinguished by its typical calyceal deformity, the presence of

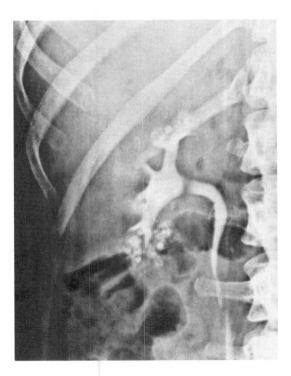

Figure 30–5. Medullary sponge kidneys. **Left:** Plain film of right kidney showing multiple small stones in its mid portion. **Right:** Excretory urogram showing relationship of calculi to calyces. Typically, the calyces are large; the stones are located in the dilated collecting tubules.

infection, and, usually, impaired renal function. The tubular and parenchymal calcification seen in nephrocalcinosis is more diffuse than that seen with sponge kidney (Figure 16–3); the symptoms and signs of primary hyperparathyroidism or renal tubular acidosis may be found.

There is no treatment for medullary sponge kidney. Therapy is directed toward the complications (eg, pyelonephritis and renal calculi). Only a small percentage of people with sponge kidney develop complications. The overall prognosis is good. A few patients may pass small stones occasionally.

ABNORMALITIES OF RENAL VESSELS

A single renal artery is noted in 75–85% of individuals and a single renal vein in an even higher percentage. Aberrant veins and, especially, arteries occur. An aberrant artery passing to the lower pole of the kidney or crossing an infundibulum can cause obstruction and hydronephrosis. These causes of obstruction can be diagnosed on angiography or spiral CT.

■ ACQUIRED LESIONS OF THE KIDNEYS

ANEURYSM OF THE RENAL ARTERY

Aneurysm of the renal artery usually results from degenerative arterial disease that weakens the wall of the artery so that intravascular pressure may balloon it out. It is most commonly caused by arteriosclerosis or polyarteritis nodosa, but it may develop secondary to trauma or syphilis. Well over 300 cases have been reported. Congenital aneurysm has been recorded. Most cases represent an incidental finding on angiography.

Aneurysmal dilatation has no deleterious effect on the kidney unless the mass compresses the renal artery, in which case some renal ischemia and, therefore, atrophy are to be expected. A true aneurysm may rupture, producing a false aneurysm. This is especially likely to occur during pregnancy. The extravasated blood in the retroperitoneal space finally becomes encapsulated by a fibrous covering as organization occurs. An aneurysm may involve a small artery within the renal parenchyma. It may rupture into the renal pelvis or a calyx.

Most aneurysms cause no symptoms unless they rupture, in which case there may be severe flank pain and even shock. If an aneurysm ruptures into the renal pelvis, marked hematuria occurs. The common cause of death is severe hemorrhage from rupture of the aneurysm. Hypertension is not usually present. A bruit should be sought over the costovertebral angle or over the renal artery anteriorly. If spontaneous or traumatic rupture has occurred, a mass may be palpated in the flank.

A plain film of the abdomen may show an intrarenal or extrarenal ringlike calcification (Figure 30–6). Urograms may be normal or reveal renal atrophy. Some impairment of renal function may be noted if compression or partial obstruction of the renal artery has developed. Aortography delineates the aneurysm. Sonography and CT scanning may prove helpful.

The differential diagnosis of rupture of an aneurysm and injury to the kidney is difficult unless a history or evidence of trauma is obtained. A hydronephrotic kidney may present a mass, but renal imaging clarifies the issue.

Because a significant number of noncalcified and large calcified aneurysms rupture spontaneously, the presence of such a lesion is an indication for operation, particularly during pregnancy. The repair of extrarenal aneurysms may be considered, but complications (eg, thrombosis) are not uncommon. If an intrarenal aneurysm is situated in one pole, heminephrectomy may be feasible. If it is in the center of the organ, however, nephrectomy is required. Therapeutic occlusion of an aneurysm by intra-arterial injection of autologous muscle tissue has been reported. Those few patients with hypertension may become normotensive following definitive surgery.

RENAL INFARCTS

Renal infarcts are caused by arterial occlusion. The major causes are subacute infective endocarditis, atrial or ventricular thrombi, arteriosclerosis, polyarteritis nodosa, and trauma. A thrombotic process in the abdominal aorta may gradually extend upward to occlude the renal artery. Renal infarcts may be unilateral or bilateral.

If smaller arteries or arterioles become obstructed, the tissue receiving blood from such a vessel will first become swollen and then undergo necrosis and fibrosis.

Figure 30–6. Intrarenal aneurysm of renal artery. **Left:** Plain film showing calcified structure over right renal shadow. **Right:** Excretory urogram relating calcific mass to pelvis and upper calyx. (Courtesy of CD King.)

Multiple infarcts are the rule. If the main renal artery becomes occluded, the entire kidney will react in kind. The kidney may become functionless and atrophic, therefore, as it undergoes necrosis and fibrosis.

Partial renal infarction is a silent disease, but it can result in flank pain and microscopic or gross hematuria. Sudden and complete infarction may cause renal or chest pain and at times gross or microscopic hematuria. Proteinuria and leukocytosis are found. "Epitheluria," representing sloughing of renal tubular cells, has been noted. Tenderness over the flank may be elicited. The kidney is not significantly enlarged by arterial occlusion.

CT may fail to have contrast enhancement in a portion of the kidney with partial infarction; with complete infarction, none of the radiopaque fluid is excreted. If complete renal infarction is suspected, a radioisotope renogram should be performed. A completely infarcted kidney shows little or no radioactivity. A similar picture is seen on CT scans performed after injection of radiopaque contrast medium. Even though complete loss of measurable function has occurred, renal circulation may be restored spontaneously in rare instances.

Renal angiography or CT makes the definitive diagnosis. A dynamic technetium scan will reveal no perfusion of the affected renal vasculature.

During the acute phase, infarction may mimic ureteral stone. With stone, the excretory urogram may also show lack of renal function, but even so there is usually enough medium in the tubules for a "nephrogram" to be obtained (Figure 16–3). This will not occur with complete infarction. Evidence of a cardiac or vascular lesion is helpful in arriving at a proper diagnosis.

The complications are related to those arising from the primary cardiovascular disease, including emboli to other organs. In a few cases, hypertension may develop a few days or weeks after the infarction. It may later subside.

Although emergency surgical intervention has been done, it has become clear that anticoagulation therapy is the treatment of choice. It has been shown that an infusion of streptokinase may dissolve the embolus. Renal function returns in most cases.

THROMBOSIS OF THE RENAL VEIN

Thrombosis of the renal vein is rare in adults. It is frequently unilateral and usually associated with membranous glomerulonephritis and nephrotic syndrome. Invasion of the renal vein by tumor or retroperitoneal disease can be the cause. Thrombosis of the renal vein may occur as a complication of severe dehydration and hemoconcentration in children with severe diarrhea

from ileocolitis. The thrombosis may extend from the vena cava into the peripheral venules or may originate in the peripheral veins and propagate to the main renal vein. The severe passive congestion that develops causes the kidney to swell and become engorged. Degeneration of the nephrons ensues. There is usually flank pain, and hematuria may be noted. A large, tender mass is often felt in the flank. Thrombocytopenia may be noted. The urine contains albumin and red cells. In the acute stage, urograms show poor or absent secretion of the radiopaque material in a large kidney. Stretching and thinning of the calyceal infundibula may be noted. Clots in the pelvis may cause filling defects. Later, the kidney may undergo atrophy.

Ultrasonography shows the thrombus in the vena cava in 50% of cases. The involved organ is enlarged. CT scan is also a valuable diagnostic tool; visualization of the thrombus can be noted in a high percentage of cases. Recently, MRI has proved to be a very sensitive diagnostic tool. Renal angiography reveals stretching and bowing of small arterioles. In the nephrographic phase, the pyramids may become quite dense. Late films may show venous collaterals. Venacavography or, preferably, selective renal venography demonstrates the thrombus in the renal vein (Figure 30–7) and, at times, in the vena cava.

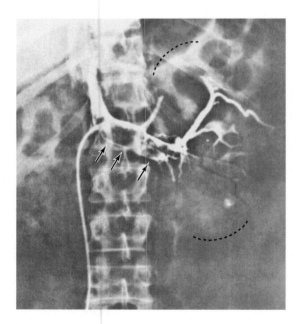

Figure 30–7. Thrombosis of renal vein. Selective left renal venogram showing almost complete occlusion of vein. Veins to lower pole failed to fill. Note large size of kidney.

The symptoms and signs resemble obstruction from a ureteral calculus. The presence of a stone in the ureter should be obvious; some degree of dilatation of the ureter and pelvis also should be expected. Clot obstruction in the ureter must be differentiated from an obstructing calculus.

While thrombectomy and even nephrectomy have been recommended in the past, it has become increasingly clear that medical treatment is usually efficacious. The use of heparin anticoagulation in the acute phase and warfarin chronically offers satisfactory resolution of the problems in most patients. In infants and children, it is essential to correct fluid and electrolyte problems and administer anticoagulants. Fibrinolytic therapy has also been successful. Renal function is usually fully recovered.

ARTERIOVENOUS FISTULA

Arteriovenous fistula may be congenital (25%) or acquired. A number of these fistulas have been reported following needle biopsy of the kidney or trauma to the kidney. A few have occurred following nephrectomy secondary to suture or ligature occlusion of the pedicle. These require surgical repair. A few have been recognized in association with adenocarcinoma of the kidney.

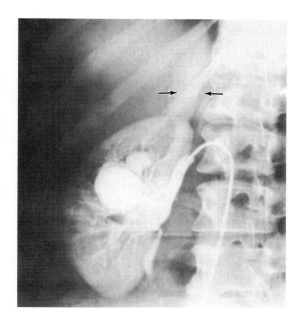

Figure 30–8. Arteriovenous aneurysm. Selective renal angiogram. Note aneurysm in center of kidney, with prompt filling of the vena cava (shown by arrows).

Figure 30–9. Nephroduodenal fistula and small-bowel obstruction from renal staghorn calculus. **Left:** Excretory urogram showing nonfunction of right kidney; staghorn stone. **Right:** Patient presented with symptoms and signs of bowel obstruction 4 years later. Plain film showing dilated loops of small bowel down to a point just proximal to ileocecal valve. Obstruction due to stone extruded into duodenum. (Courtesy of CD King.)

A thrill can often be palpated and a murmur heard both anteriorly and posteriorly. In cases with a wide communication, the systolic blood pressure is elevated and a widened pulse pressure is noted. Renal angiography or isotopic scan establishes the diagnosis. CT scan, sonography, and, recently, duplex ultrasound with color flow are particularly helpful. Arteriovenous fistula involving the renal artery and vein requires surgical repair or nephrectomy. Most, however, can be occluded by embolization, balloon, or steel coil. Those that develop secondary to renal biopsy tend to heal spontaneously.

ARTERIOVENOUS ANEURYSM

About 100 instances of this lesion have been reported (Figure 30–8). Most follow trauma. Hypertension is to be expected and is associated with high-output cardiac failure. A bruit is usually present. Nephrectomy is usually indicated.

RENOALIMENTARY FISTULA

Over 100 instances of renoalimentary fistula have been reported. They usually involve the stomach, duodenum, or adjacent colon, although fistula formation with the esophagus, small bowel, appendix, and rectum has been reported.

The underlying cause is usually a pyonephrotic kidney or renal cell carcinoma that becomes adherent to a portion of the alimentary tract and then ruptures spontaneously, thus creating a fistula (Figure 30–9). A few cases following trauma have been reported. The patient is apt to have symptoms and signs of acute pyelonephritis. Urography may show radiopaque material escaping into the gastrointestinal tract. Gastrointestinal series may also reveal the connection with the kidney. The treatment is nephrectomy with closure of the opening into the gut.

RENOBRONCHIAL FISTULA

Renobronchial fistulas are rare. They are caused by rupture of an infected, calculous kidney through the diaphragm.

REFERENCES

Congenital Anomalies

General

Bruno D et al: Genitourinary complications of sickle cell disease. J Urol 2001;166:803.

Donohue RE, Fauver HE: Unilateral absence of the vas deferens: A useful clinical sign. JAMA 1989;261:1180.

Elder JS et al: Evaluation of fetal renal function: Unreliability of fetal urinary electrolytes. J Urol 1990;144:574.

Johnson CE et al: The accuracy of antenatal ultrasonography in identifying renal abnormalities. Am J Dis Child 1992;146:1181.

Mandell J et al: Human fetal compensatory renal growth. J Urol 1993;150:790.

Mandell J et al: Structural genitourinary defects detected in utero. Radiology 1991;178:193.

Patten RM et al: The fetal genitourinary tract. Radiol Clin North Am 1990;28:115.

Pope JC IV et al: Congenital anomalies of the kidney and urinary tract: Role of the loss of function mutation in the pluripotent angiotensin type 2 receptor gene. J Urol 2001;165:196.

Sanders RC: Prenatal ultrasonic detection of anomalies with a lethal or disastrous outcome. Radiol Clin North Am 1990;28:163.

Scott JE, Renwick M: Urological anomalies in the Northern Region Fetal Abnormality Survey. Arch Dis Child 1993;68 (1 Spec No):22.

Sheih CP et al: Renal abnormalities in schoolchildren. Pediatrics 1989;84:1086.

Takebayashi S et al: Transarterial embolization and ablation of renal arteriovenous malformations: Efficacy and damages in 30 patients with long-term followup. J Urol 1998;159:696.

Warne SA et al: Renal outcome in patients with cloaca. J Urol 2002;167:2548.

Agenesis

Acien P et al: Renal agenesis in association with malformation of the female genital tract. Am J Obstet Gynecol 1991;165:1368.

Hill LM, Rivello D: Role of transvaginal sonography in the diagnosis of bilateral renal agenesis. Am J Perinatol 1991;8:395.

Ouden van den D et al: Diagnosis and management of seminal vesicle cysts associated with ipsilateral renal agenesis: A pooled analysis of 52 cases. Eur Urol 1998;33:433.

Robson WL, Leung AK, Rogers RC: Unilateral renal agenesis. Adv Pediatr 1995;42:575.

Sanders RC: Prenatal ultrasonic detection of anomalies with a lethal or disastrous outcome. Radiol Clin North Am 1990;28:163.

Sheih CP et al: Cystic dilatations within the pelvis in patients with ipsilateral renal agenesis or dysplasia. J Urol 1990;144:324.

Hypoplasia

Rosenstein BJ, Wheeler JS, Heid PL: Congenital renal abnormalities in infants with in utero cocaine exposure. J Urol 1990;144:110.

Saborio P, Scheinman J: Genetic renal disease. Curr Opin Pediatr 1998;10:174.

Sheih CP et al: Cystic dilatations within the pelvis in patients with ipsilateral renal agenesis or dysplasia. J Urol 1990;144:324.

Dysplasia & Multicystic Kidney

Atiyeh B, Husmann D, Baum M: Contralateral renal abnormalities in patients with renal agenesis and noncystic renal dysplasia. Pediatrics 1993;91:812.

Carey PO, Howards SS: Multicystic dysplastic kidneys and diagnostic confusion on renal scan. J Urol 1988;139:83.

Corica FA et al: Cystic renal cell carcinoma is cured by resection: A study of 24 cases with long-term followup. J Urol 1999; 161:408.

Corrales JG, Elder JS: Segmental multicystic kidney and ipsilateral duplication anomalies. J Urol 1996;155:1398.

Dimmick JE et al: Wilms tumorlet, nodular renal blastema and multicystic renal dysplasia. J Urol 1989;142:484.

Pinto E, Guignard JP: Renal masses in the neonate. Biol Neonate 1995;68:175.

Sanders RC, Nussbaum AR, Solez K: Renal dysplasia: Sonographic findings. Radiology 1988;167:623.

Strife JL et al: Multicystic dysplastic kidney in children: US followup. Radiology 1993;186:785.

Wolf JS Jr: Evaluation and management of solid and cystic renal masses. J Urol 1998;159:1120.

Polycystic Kidneys

Dunn MD et al: Laparoscopic cyst marsupialization in patients with autosomal dominant polycystic kidney disease. J Urol 2001;165:1888.

Fick GM et al: Causes of death in autosomal dominant polycystic kidney disease. J Am Soc Nephrol 1995;5:2048.

Fleming TW, Barry JM: Bilateral open transperitoneal cyst reduction surgery for autosomal dominant polycystic kidney. J Urol 1998;159:44.

Levine E et al: Current concepts and controversies in imaging of renal cystic diseases. Urol Clin North Am 1997;24:523.

MacDermot KD et al: Prenatal diagnosis of autosomal dominant polycystic kidney disease PKD1 presenting in utero and prognosis for very early onset disease. J Med Genet 1998;35:13.

Maher ER, Kaelin WG Jr: von Hippel-Lindau disease. Medicine (Baltimore) 1997;76:381.

Martinez JR, Grantham JJ: Polycystic kidney disease: Etiology, pathogenesis, and treatment. Dis Mon 1995;41:693.

Reichard EAP, Roubidoux MA, Dunnick NR: Renal neoplasms in patients with renal cystic diseases. Abdom Imaging 1998; 23:237.

Romanowski CA, Cavallin LI: Tuberous sclerosis, von Hippel-Lindau disease, Sturge-Weber syndrome. Hosp Med 1998;59: 226.

Thomsen HS et al: Renal cystic diseases. Eur Radiol 1997;7:1267.

Vinocur L et al: Follow-up studies of multicystic dysplastic kidneys. Radiology 1988;167:311.

Watson ML, Macnicol AM, Wright AF: Adult polycystic kidney disease. Br Med J 1990;300:62.

Simple Cyst

Blazer S et al: Natural history of fetal simple renal cysts detected in early pregnancy. J Urol 1999;162:812.

Eilenberg SS et al: Renal masses: Evaluation with gradient-echo Gd-DTPA-enhanced dynamic MR imaging. Radiology 1990; 176:333.

Feiner HD, Katz LA, Gallo GR: Acquired cystic disease of kidney in chronic dialysis patients. Urology 1981;17:260.

Muther RS, Bennett WM: Concentration of antibiotics in simple renal cysts. J Urol 1980;124:596.

Renal Fusion

Dalla Palma L et al: Radiological anatomy of the kidney revisited. Br J Radiol 1990;63:680.

Decter RM: Renal duplication and fusion anomalies. Pediatr Clin North Am 1997;44:1323.

Pitts WR Jr, Muecke EC: Horseshoe kidneys: A 40-year experience. J Urol 1975;113:743.

Ectopic Kidney

Bolton DM, Stoller ML: Pseudo-crossed renal ectopia secondary to ureteropelvic junction obstruction. J Urol 1995;153:397.

Hertz M et al: Crossed renal ectopia: Clinical and radiological findings in 22 cases. Clin Radiol 1977;28:339.

Medullary Sponge Kidney

Ginalski JM, Portmann L, Jaeger P: Does medullary sponge kidney cause nephrolithiasis? AJR 1990;155:299.

Indridason OS, Thomas L, Berkoben M: Medullary sponge kidney associated with congenital hemihypertrophy. J Am Soc Nephrol 1996;7:1123.

Nunley JR, Sica DA, Smith V: Medullary sponge kidney and staghorn calculi. Urol Int 1990;45:118.

Acquired Lesions

General

Matin SF, Novick AC: Renal dysfunction associated with staged bilateral partial nephrectomy: The importance of operative positioning. J Urol 2001;165:880.

Rawashdeh YF et al: The intrarenal resistive index as a pathophysiological marker of obstructive uropathy. J Urol 2001;165: 1397.

Tsushima Y et al: Determination of glomerular filtration rate per unit renal volume using computerized tomography: Correlation with conventional measures of total and divided renal function. J Urol 2001;165:382.

Zhang JQ, Fielding JR, Zou KH: Etiology of spontaneous perirenal hemorrhage: A meta-analysis. J Urol 2002;167:1593.

Infection-related Renal Disorders

Best CD et al: Clinical and radiological findings in patients with gas-forming renal abscess treated conservatively. J Urol 1999; 162:1273.

Foresman WH, Hulbert WC Jr, Rabinowitz R: Does urinary tract ultrasonography at hospitalization for acute pyelonephritis predict vesicoureteral reflux? J Urol 2001;165(6 Pt 2):2232.

Meng MV, Mario LA, McAninch JW: Current treatment and outcomes of perinephric abscesses. J Urol 2002;168:1337.

Shekarriz B et al: Laparoscopic nephrectomy for inflammatory renal conditions. J Urol 2001;166:2091.

Wan Y-L et al: Predictors of outcome in emphysematous pyelonephritis. J Urol 1998;159:369.

Aneurysm of the Renal Artery

Cinat M, Yoon P, Wilson SE: Management of renal artery aneurysms. Semin Vasc Surg 1996;9:236.

Cooper GG, Atkinson AB, Barros D'Sa AA: Simultaneous aortic and renal artery reconstruction. Br J Surg 1990;77:194.

Helenon O et al: Renovascular disease: Doppler ultrasound. Semin Ultrasound CT MR 1997;18:136.

Jebara VA et al: Renal artery pseudoaneurysm after blunt abdominal trauma. J Vasc Surg 1998;27:362.

Renal Infarcts

Bartolozzi C, Neri E, Caramella D: CT in vascular pathologies. Eur Radiol 1998;8:679.

Gasparini M, Hofmann R, Stoller M: Renal artery embolism: Clinical features and therapeutic options. J Urol 1992;147:567.

Thrombosis of the Renal Vein

Hibbert J et al: The ultrasound appearances of neonatal renal vein thrombosis. Br J Radiol 1997;70:1191.

Laplante S et al: Renal vein thrombosis in children: Evidence of early flow recovery with Doppler US. Radiology 1993; 189:37.

Witz M et al: Renal vein occlusion: A review. J Urol 1996;155: 1173.

Arteriovenous Fistula

Crotty KL, Orihuela E, Warren MM: Recent advances in the diagnosis and treatment of renal arteriovenous malformations and fistulas. J Urol 1993;150:1355.

Fogazzi GB, Moriggi M, Fontanella U: Spontaneous renal arteriovenous fistula as a cause of haematuria. Nephrol Dial Transplant 1997;12:350.

Morton MJ, Charboneau JW: Arteriovenous fistula after biopsy of renal transplant: Detection and monitoring with color flow and duplex ultrasonography. Mayo Clin Proc 1989;64:531.

Renoalimentary Fistula

Tan SM, The CH, Tan PK: Duodeno-ureteric fistula secondary to chronic duodenal ulceration. Ann Acad Med Singapore 1997; 26:850.

Diagnosis of Medical Renal Diseases

31

Flavio G. Vincenti, MD, & William J.C. Amend, Jr., MD

Medical renal diseases are those that involve principally the parenchyma of the kidneys. Many of the symptoms and signs of urinary tract disease are common to both medical and surgical diseases of the kidneys. Hematuria, proteinuria, pyuria, oliguria, polyuria, pain, renal insufficiency with azotemia, acidosis, anemia, electrolyte abnormalities, hypertension, and auditory and ocular involvement may occur in a wide variety of disorders affecting any portion of the parenchyma of the kidney, the blood vessels, or the excretory tract.

A complete medical history and physical examination, a thorough examination of the urine, and blood chemistry examinations as indicated are essential initial steps in the workup of any patient.

History

A. FAMILY HISTORY

The family history may reveal disease of genetic origin, for example, tubular metabolic anomalies, polycystic kidneys, unusual types of nephritis, or vascular or coagulation defects that may be essential clues to the diagnosis.

B. PAST HISTORY

The past history should cover infections, injuries, and exposure to toxic agents, anticoagulants, or drugs that may produce toxic or sensitivity reactions. A history of diabetes, hypertensive disease, and autoimmune disease may be obtained. The inquiry must also elicit symptoms of uremia, debilitation, and the vascular complications of chronic renal disease.

Physical Examination

One must look for such physical signs as pallor, edema, hypertension, retinopathy, and stigmas of congenital and hereditary disease.

Urinalysis

Examination of the urine is the essential part of the investigation.

A. PROTEINURIA

Proteinuria of any significant degree (2–4+) is suggestive of medical renal disease (parenchymal involvement). Formed elements present in the urine additionally establish the diagnosis. Significant proteinuria occurs in immune-mediated glomerular diseases or disorders with glomerular involvement such as diabetes mellitus, myeloma, or amyloidosis. Interstitial nephritis, polycystic kidneys, and other tubular disorders are not associated with significant proteinuria.

B. ERYTHROCYTE CASTS

When red blood cell (erythrocyte) casts are not present, microscopic hematuria may or may not be of glomerular origin. Phase contrast microscope study may reveal dysmorphic changes in the erythrocytes present in the urine in patients with parenchymal renal disorders.

C. FATTY CASTS AND OVAL FAT BODIES

Tubular cells showing fatty changes occur in degenerative diseases of the kidney (nephrosis, glomerulonephritis, autoimmune disease, amyloidosis, and damage due to toxins such as mercury).

D. OTHER FINDINGS

Abnormal urinary chemical constituents may be the only indication of a metabolic disorder involving the kidneys. These disorders include diabetes mellitus, renal glycosuria, aminoacidurias (including cystinuria), oxaluria, gout, hyperparathyroidism, hemoglobinuria, and myoglobinuria.

Examination of the Kidneys & Urinary Tract

Roentgenographic, sonographic, and radioisotopic studies provide information about the size, structure, blood supply, and function of the kidneys.

Renal Biopsy

Renal biopsy is a valuable diagnostic procedure. The technique has become well established, providing sufficient tissue for light and electron microscopy and for immunofluorescence examination. Contraindications for percutaneous kidney biopsy may include the anatomic presence of only one kidney; severe malfunction of one kidney even though function is adequate in the other; bleeding diathesis; and an uncooperative patient.

Clinical indications for renal biopsy, in addition to the necessity for establishing a diagnosis, include the need to determine prognosis, to follow progression of a lesion and response to treatment, to confirm the presence of a generalized disease (autoimmune disorder, amyloidosis, sarcoidosis), and to diagnose renal dysfunction in a transplanted kidney.

GLOMERULONEPHRITIS

The clinical manifestations of renal disease are apt to consist only of varying degrees of hematuria, excretion of characteristic formed elements in the urine, proteinuria, and renal insufficiency and its complications. Excluding diabetes, purported immunologic renal diseases are the most common cause of proteinuria and the nephrotic syndrome.

Alterations in glomerular architecture as observed in tissue examined by light microscopy are also apt to be minimal, nonspecific, and difficult to interpret. For these reasons, specific diagnoses of renal disease require targeted immune fluorescent techniques for demonstrating a variety of antigens, antibodies, and complement fractions. Electron microscopy has complemented these immunologic methods. Tissue analysis can be complemented by serologic studies of immunoglobulins, complement, and other mediators of inflammation.

The two important humoral mechanisms leading to deposition of antibodies within the glomerulus are based on the location of the antigen, whether fixed within the kidney or present in soluble form in circulation. The fixed antigens are either a natural structural element of the glomerulus or foreign materials that have been trapped within the glomerulus for a variety of immunologic or physiochemical reasons. The best examples of the fixed natural antigens are those associated with the glomerular basement membrane. These antigens are evenly distributed in the glomerular basement membrane and cause characteristic linear immunoglobulin (IgG) deposition, as determined in immunofluorescence studies. This process represents 5% of cases of immune-mediated glomerular disease and is referred to as anti-GBM (glomerular basement membrane) disease. However, most patients with glomerular immune deposits have discontinuous immune aggregates caused by antibody binding to native renal cell antigens or to antigens trapped within the glomerulus. In addition, immune complexes formed in the circulation can deposit and accumulate in the glomerular basement membrane and the mesangium.

A group of immune-mediated nephrities characterized by necrotizing and crescentic architecture and rapid progression are referred to as pauci-immune glomerular nephrities because, while antibodies may contribute to the pathogenesis of the disease, they are rarely demonstrated within the glomeruli. These are known as antineutrophil cytoplasmic antibody (ANCA) diseases. Circulating antibodies against myeloperoxidase, MPO (P-ANCA) and proteinase 3, PR3 (C-ANCA) have been noted in microscopic angiitis and Wegener granulomatosis, respectively.

Cellular immune processes are likely to be stimulated and contribute in different ways in various forms of glomerulonephrities.

The current classification of glomerulonephritis is based on the mechanism, the presence, and the localization of immune aggregates in the glomeruli.

I. Immunologic Mechanisms Likely

    A. Subepithelial Immune Deposits:
Glomerulonephritis associated with post-infectious glomerulonephritis such as post-streptococcal glomerulonephritis
Membranous nephropathy idiopathic or secondary to other causes such as systemic lupus erythematosus, cancer, gold penicillamine

    B. Subendothelial Immune Deposits:
Glomerulonephritis associated with systemic lupus erythematosus, type I membranoproliferative glomerulonephritis, glomerulonephritis associated with hepatitis C infection, bacterial endocarditis, and shunt nephritis

    C. Mesangial Immune Deposits
IgA nephropathy, Schönlein-Henoch purpura

    D. Anti-GBM Disease
Diffuse linear deposition of immunoglobulin

II. Immunologic Mechanisms Not Clearly Established

    Minimal change nephropathy
    Focal glomerulosclerosis
    Hemolytic-uremic syndrome and thrombotic thrombocytopenic purpura
    ANCA-associated disease: Wegener granulomatosis and small-vessel vasculitis
    Type II membranoproliferative glomerulonephritis (dense deposit disease)

1. Post-Streptococcal Glomerulonephritis

Essentials of Diagnosis

- History of streptococcal infection.
- Mild generalized edema, mild hypertension, retinal hemorrhages.
- Gross hematuria; protein, erythrocyte casts, granular and hyaline casts, white blood cells (leukocytes), and renal epithelial cells in urine.
- Elevated antistreptolysin O titer, hypocomplementemia.

General Considerations

Glomerulonephritis is a disease affecting both kidneys. In most cases recovery from the acute stage is complete, but progressive involvement may destroy renal tissue, leading to renal insufficiency. Acute glomerulonephritis is most common in children aged 3–10 years. By far the most common cause is an antecedent infection of the pharynx and tonsils or of the skin with group A β-hemolytic streptococci, certain strains of which are nephritogenic. Nephritis occurs in 10–15% of children and young adults who have clinically evident infection with a nephritogenic strain. In children under age 6, pyoderma (impetigo) is the most common antecedent; in older children and young adults, pharyngitis is a common antecedent. Rarely, nephritis may follow infection due to other agents.

The pathogenesis of the glomerular lesion has been further elucidated by the use of new immunologic techniques (immunofluorescence) and electron microscopy. A likely sequel to infection is injury to the mesangial cells in the intercapillary space. The glomerulus may then become more easily damaged by antigen-antibody complexes developing from the immune response to the streptococcal infection. Complement is deposited in association with IgG or alone in a granular pattern on the epithelial side of the basement membrane.

Gross examination of the involved kidney shows only punctate hemorrhages throughout the cortex. Microscopically, the primary alteration is in the glomeruli, which show proliferation and swelling of the mesangial and endothelial cells of the capillary tuft. The proliferation of capsular epithelium occurs in and around the tuft there are collections of leukocytes, erythrocytes, and exudate. Edema of the interstitial tissue and cloudy swelling of the tubular epithelium are common. When severe, typical histologic findings in glomerulitis are enlarging crescents that become hyalinized and converted into scar tissue and obstruct the circulation through the glomerulus. Degenerative changes occur in the tubules, with fatty degeneration, necrosis, and ultimately scarring of the nephron.

Clinical Findings

A. SYMPTOMS AND SIGNS

Often the disease is mild, and there may be no reason to suspect renal involvement unless the urine is examined. In severe cases, about 2 weeks after the acute streptococcal infection, the patient has headache, malaise, mild fever, puffiness around the eyes and face, flank pain, and oliguria. Hematuria is usually noted as "bloody" or, if the urine is acid, as "brown" or "coffee-colored." There may be moderate tachycardia, dyspnea, and moderate to marked elevation of blood pressure. Tenderness in the costovertebral angle is common.

B. LABORATORY FINDINGS

The diagnosis is confirmed by examination of the urine, which may be grossly bloody or coffee-colored (acid hematin) or may show only microscopic hematuria. In addition, the urine contains protein (1–3+) and casts. Hyaline and granular casts are commonly found in large numbers, but the classic sign of glomerulitis, occasionally noted, is the erythrocyte cast. The erythrocyte cast is usually of small caliber, is intensely orange or red, and may show the mosaic pattern of the packed erythrocytes held together by the clot of fibrin and plasma protein.

With the impairment of renal function (decrease in glomerular filtration rate and blood flow) and with oliguria, plasma or serum urea nitrogen and creatinine become elevated, the levels varying with the severity of the renal lesion. A mild normochromic anemia may result from fluid retention and dilution. Infection of the throat with nephritogenic streptococci is frequently followed by increasing antistreptolysin O titers in the serum, whereas high titers are usually not demonstrable following skin infections. Serum complement levels are usually low.

Confirmation of diagnosis is made by examination of the urine, although the history and clinical findings in typical cases leave little doubt. The finding of erythrocytes in a cast is proof that erythrocytes were present in the renal tubules and did not arise from elsewhere in the genitourinary tract.

Treatment

There is no specific treatment. Eradication of infection, prevention of overhydration and hypertension, and prompt treatment of complications such as hypertensive encephalopathy and heart failure require careful management.

Prognosis

Most patients with the acute disease recover completely; 5–20% show progressive renal damage. If oliguria, heart failure, or hypertensive encephalopathy is severe, death may occur during the acute attack. Even with severe acute disease, however, recovery is the rule, particularly in children.

2. Iga Nephropathy

Primary hematuria (idiopathic benign and recurrent hematuria, Berger disease) is now known to be an immune complex glomerulopathy in which deposition of IgA occurs in a granular pattern in the mesangium of the glomerulus. The associated light microscope findings are variable and range from normal to extensive crescentic glomerulonephritis.

Recurrent macroscopic and microscopic hematuria and mild proteinuria are usually the only manifestations of renal disease. Most patients with IgA nephropathy are between the ages of 16 and 35 years at the time of diagnosis. The disease occurs much more frequently in males than females and is the most common cause of glomerulonephritis in Asians. While most patients continue to have episodes of gross hematuria or microscopic hematuria, the renal function is likely to remain stable. However, approximately 30% of patients will have progressive renal dysfunction and develop end-stage renal disease. Clinical features that indicate a poor prognosis include male sex, older age at onset of disease, the presence of nephrotic-range proteinuria, and hypertension.

There is no satisfactory therapy for IgA nephropathy. The role of immunosuppressive drugs such as steroids and cytotoxic agents is not clear, and there have been few rigorously performed controlled trials. A more intriguing approach is the use of omega-3 fatty acids (fish oils) to delay progression of the renal disease. A large prospective randomized placebo-controlled trial in patients with IgA nephropathy using 12 g of omega-3 fatty acids has shown that fish oils probably can reduce the deterioration of renal function and the number of patients in whom end-stage renal disease develops.

3. Rapidly Progressive Glomerulonephritis (RPGN)

The patient usually gives a history of recent hemoptysis and often of malaise, anorexia, and headache. A severe acute glomerulonephritis may be accompanied by diffuse hemorrhagic inflammation of the lungs. The urine shows gross or microscopic hematuria, and laboratory findings of severely suppressed renal function are usually evident. Biopsy shows glomerular crescents, glomerular adhesions, and inflammatory infiltration interstitially. Electron microscope examination shows an increase in basement membrane material and deposition of fibrin beneath the capillary endothelium. In cases of antiglomerular basement membrane disease, circulating antibody against glomerular basement membrane can be identified. IgG, C3, and, often, other components of the classic complement pathway can be demonstrated as linear deposits on the basement membranes of the glomeruli and the lung.

Large doses of corticosteroids in combination with immunosuppressive therapy may be useful. Plasmapheresis to remove circulating antibody has been reported to be effective in some patients. Transplantation should be delayed until circulating antiglomerular basement antibodies have disappeared.

In contrast, some patients have crescenteric glomerulonephritis but do not show any immune deposits or antibody deposition by immunofluorescence studies. They have pauci-immune idiopathic rapidly progressive glomerulonephritis. Many of these patients are serologically ANCA-positive. High-dose prednisone pulse therapy and cytotoxic agents may result in prolonged remission.

NEPHROTIC SYNDROME

Essentials of Diagnosis

- Edema.
- Proteinuria > 3.5 g/d.
- Hypoalbuminemia < 3 g/dL.
- Hyperlipidemia: Cholesterol > 300 mg/100 mL.
- Lipiduria: Free fat, oval fat bodies, fatty casts.

General Considerations

Because treatment and prognosis vary with the cause of nephrotic syndrome, renal biopsy is important. Light microscopy, electron microscopy, and immunofluorescence identification of immune mechanisms diagnose most causes of nephrosis.

Glomerular diseases associated with nephrosis include the following:

A. Minimal Glomerular Lesions

Minimal-change nephropathy (Nil disease) accounts for about 20% of cases of nephrosis in adults. No abnormality is visible by examination of biopsy material with the light microscope. With the electron microscope, alterations of the glomerular basement membrane, with effacement of foot processes of the epithelial cells, are evident. There is no evidence of immune disease by immunofluorescence studies. The response to treatment with corticosteroids is good, but for patients who have frequent relapses with steroids or are steroid-resistant, a course of cyclophosphamide or chlorambucil may induce a prolonged remission. Patients who do not respond to these agents may show a favorable response with cyclosporine. Renal function usually remains stable.

B. Focal Glomerulosclerosis

Focal glomerulosclerosis is the second most common cause of nephrotic syndrome in children and an increasing cause of the nephrotic syndrome in adults. The diagnosis is based on light microscope findings of segmental hyalinosis and sclerosis associated with effacement of the foot processes on electron microscopy. Focal glomerulosclerosis is frequently idiopathic but can be associated with human immunodeficiency virus infection and heroin use. A secondary form of focal glomerulosclerosis without the diffuse changes in foot processes may occur in patients with a solitary kidney, hyperfiltration syndromes, and reflux nephropathy. There are reports of familial variants. The response of the idiopathic form of focal glomerulosclerosis to therapy is suboptimal. Prolonged corticosteroid therapy produces remission in approximately 40% of patients. Over a 10-year period, approximately 50% of patients will have chronic renal failure. Focal glomerulosclerosis has a recurrence rate of 25% after transplantation.

C. Membranous Nephropathy

Examination of biopsy material with the light microscope shows thickening of the glomerular cells but no cellular proliferation. With the electron microscope, irregular lumpy deposits appear between the basement membrane and the epithelial cells, and new basement membrane material protrudes from the glomerular basement membrane as spikes or domes. Immunofluorescence studies show diffuse granular deposits of immunoglobulins (especially IgG) and complement (C3 component). As the membrane thickens, glomeruli become sclerosed and hyalinized.

The pathogenesis of most cases of membranous nephropathy in humans is unclear. Several mechanisms have been suggested. They include trapping of circulating immune complexes or binding of an antibody to scattered glomerular antigens (either present already or "planted" after a nonrenal-source antigen lodges in the glomerulus).

There is considerable controversy regarding the effectiveness of therapy with steroids or immunosuppressive agents. Therapy should be reserved for patients at high risk of progressive renal failure with the following criteria: proteinuria > 10, hypertension, and elevated serum creatinine.

D. Membranoproliferative Glomerulonephritis—Type I

Light microscopy shows thickening of glomerular capillaries, accompanied by mesangial proliferation and obliteration of glomeruli. With the electron microscope, subendothelial deposits and growth of mesangium into capillary walls are demonstrable. Immunofluorescence studies show the presence of the C3 component of complement and, rarely, the presence of immunoglobulins. The most common cause of membranoproliferative glomerulonephritis type I is chronic hepatitis C virus infection. This condition is usually associated with high levels of IgG/IgM cryoimmunoglobulins with normal or slightly reduced levels of complement. There is no known effective treatment.

E. Membranoproliferative Glomerulonephritis—Type II

Type II is characterized by dense deposits visible by electron microscopy and lack of findings by immunofluorescence studies. Treatment is unsatisfactory, and there is a high rate of recurrence after kidney transplantation.

F. Miscellaneous Diseases

Many metabolic, autoimmune, infectious, and neoplastic diseases and reactions to drugs and other toxic substances can produce glomerular disease. These include diabetic glomerulopathy, systemic lupus erythematosus, ANCA-positive renal disease (including Wegener granulomatosis), amyloid disease, multiple myeloma, lymphomas, carcinomas, syphilis, reaction to toxins, reaction to drugs (eg, trimethadione), and exposure to heavy metals.

Two recent glomerular lesions have been described with nephrotic syndrome: fibrillary and immunotactoid glomerular nephritis. The lesions of fibrillary glomerulonephritis are characterized by randomly oriented fibril deposits 10–30 nm in diameter located within the mesangium and capillary wall. Immunotactoid glomerulopathy is characterized by deposits of microtubular structures of 18–19 nm and has been associated with lymphoproliferative disorders. In contrast to amyloid, the deposits in both diseases are Congo red–negative. Treatment is generally unsatisfactory.

Clinical Findings

A. Symptoms and Signs

Edema may appear insidiously and increase slowly; often it appears suddenly and accumulates rapidly. Symptoms other than those related to the mechanical effects of edema and serous sac fluid accumulation are not remarkable.

On physical examination, massive peripheral edema is apparent. Signs of hydrothorax and ascites are common. Pallor is often accentuated by the edema, and striae commonly appear in the stretched skin of the extremities.

B. LABORATORY FINDINGS

The urine contains large amounts of protein, 4–10 g or more per 24 h. The sediment contains casts, including the characteristic fatty and waxy varieties; renal tubular cells, some of which contain fatty droplets (oval fat bodies); and variable numbers of erythrocytes. A mild normochromic anemia is common, but anemia may be more severe if renal damage is great. Nitrogen retention varies with the severity of impairment of renal function. The plasma is often lipemic, and the blood cholesterol is usually greatly elevated. Plasma protein is greatly reduced. The albumin fraction may fall to less than 2 g/dL or even below 1 g/dL. Serum complement is usually low in active disease. The serum electrolyte concentrations are often normal, although the serum sodium may be slightly low; total serum calcium may be low, in keeping with the degree of hypoalbuminemia and decrease in the protein-bound calcium moiety. During edema-forming periods, urinary sodium excretion is very low and urinary aldosterone excretion is elevated. If renal insufficiency (see preceding discussion) is present, the blood and urine findings are usually altered accordingly.

Renal biopsy is essential to confirm the diagnosis and to indicate prognosis.

Differential Diagnosis

The nephrotic syndrome (nephrosis) may be associated with a variety of renal diseases, including primary glomerular disease, collagen-vascular diseases (eg, disseminated lupus erythematosus, polyarteritis), diabetic nephropathy, amyloid disease, thrombosis of the renal vein, myxedema, multiple myeloma, malaria, syphilis, reaction to toxins or heavy metals, reactions to drugs, and constrictive pericarditis.

Treatment

An adequate diet with restricted sodium intake (0.5–1 g/d) and prompt treatment of intercurrent infection are the basis of therapy. Diuretics may be given but are often only partially effective. Salt-free albumin and other oncotic agents are of little help, and their effects are transient. The corticosteroids have been shown to be of value in treating nephrotic syndrome when the underlying disease is minimal glomerular lesion, focal segmental glomerulosclerosis, systemic lupus erythematosus, or proliferative and crescentic glomerulonephritis. These drugs are less often effective in the treatment of membranous disease and membranoproliferative lesions of the glomerulus.

Alkylating agents, azathioprine, mycophenolate mofetil, and cyclosporine have been used in the treatment of nephrotic syndrome. Encouraging early results have been reported in children and adults with proliferative or membranous lesions and with systemic lupus erythematosus. Improvement was noted in the glomerular changes and renal function in many patients. It is not known what percentage of patients can be expected to benefit from these drugs.

Both corticosteroids and cytotoxic agents are commonly associated with serious side effects. At present, this form of therapy should be employed only in patients in whom the disease has proved refractory to well-established treatment regimens.

Reduction in proteinuria and improvement in nephrotic edema have been reported using low-protein diets and angiotensin-converting enzyme inhibitors. Most recently, studies have shown some improvements with lipid-lowering drugs.

Prognosis

The course and prognosis depend on the basic disease responsible for nephrotic syndrome. In most children with nephrosis (probably secondary to minimal change nephropathy), the disease appears to run a rather benign course when properly treated and to leave insignificant sequelae. Of the remaining children, most go inexorably into renal insufficiency. Adults with nephrosis fare less well. Hypertension, heavy proteinuria, and renal dysfunction are poor prognosticators.

RENAL INVOLVEMENT IN COLLAGEN DISEASES

Although it may not be accurate to classify all of these disorders as collagen diseases, disseminated lupus erythematosus, polyarteritis nodosa, scleroderma, Wegener granulomatosis, and thrombotic thrombocytopenic purpura have been implicated in cases of glomerulonephritis. The urine sediment is often diagnostic, containing erythrocytes and erythrocyte casts; renal tubular cells, including some filled with fat droplets; and waxy and granular broad casts. The presence of these formed elements is indicative of active glomerular and tubular disease. The symptoms and signs of the primary disease, involving extrarenal findings (eg, pulmonary or ear, nose, or throat changes with Wegener granulomatosis; dermatologic abnormalities or carditis with systemic lupus erythematosus; dysphagia with scleroderma), as well as the presence of ANCA, help to differentiate the form of collagen disease present. Complete renal recovery from the disease is not likely to occur, although steroid and immunosuppressive drugs (alone or in combination) may be effective for long-term amelioration.

DISEASES OF THE RENAL TUBULES & INTERSTITIUM

1. Interstitial Nephritis

Acute interstitial diseases are usually due to sensitivity to drugs, including antibiotics (penicillin, sulfonamides), nonsteroidal anti-inflammatory drugs, and phenytoin. The hallmark of acute interstitial nephritis is the infiltration of inflammatory cells in the interstitium. A typical presentation is a rapid deterioration in renal function associated with a recent introduction of a new drug. The finding of eosinophiluria is very suggestive of allergic interstitial nephritis. Recovery may be complete, especially if the offending drug is withdrawn. A short course with corticosteroids may hasten the recovery.

Chronic interstitial nephritis is characterized by focal or diffuse interstitial fibrosis accompanied by infiltration, with inflammatory cells ultimately associated with extensive tubular atrophy. It represents a nonspecific reaction to a variety of causes: analgesic abuse, lead and cadmium toxicity, nephrocalcinosis, urate nephropathy, radiation nephritis, sarcoidosis, Balkan nephritis, and some instances of obstructive uropathy.

2. Analgesic Nephropathy

Analgesic nephropathy typically occurs in patients with chronic and recurrent headaches or with chronic arthritis who habitually consume large amounts of the drugs. Phenacetin was implicated initially, but with elimination of phenacetin from the mixtures, the incidence of analgesic nephropathy has not decreased. Chronic use of nonsteroidal anti-inflammatories is a frequent cause of this condition. The ensuing damage to the kidneys usually is detected late, after renal insufficiency has developed. Careful history taking or the detection of analgesic metabolites in the urine can lead to this diagnosis. The history of excessive use of analgesics may be concealed by the patient.

The kidney lesion is pathologically nonspecific, consisting of peritubular and perivascular inflammation with degenerative changes of the tubular cells (chronic interstitial nephritis). There are often no glomerular changes. Renal papillary necrosis extending into the medulla may involve many papillae.

Hematuria is a common presenting complaint. Renal colic occurs when necrotic renal papillae slough away. Polyuria may be prominent. Signs of acidosis (hyperpnea), dehydration, and pallor of anemia are common. Infection is a frequent complication. The urine usually is remarkable only for the presence of blood and small amounts of protein. Elevated blood urea nitrogen and creatinine and the electrolyte changes characteristic of renal failure are typically present. Urinary concentrating impairments are usually present. Urograms show cavities and ring shadows typical of areas of destruction of papillae.

3. Uric Acid Nephropathy

Crystals of urate produce an interstitial inflammatory reaction. Urate may precipitate out in acid urine in the calyces to form uric acid stones. Patients with myeloproliferative disease under treatment are subject to occlusion of the upper urinary tract by uric acid crystals. Alkalinization of the urine and a liberal fluid intake help prevent crystal formation. Allopurinol is a useful drug to prevent hyperuricemia and hyperuricosuria. Recently, it has been suggested that many instances considered to be chronic "gouty nephropathy" are instead related to chronic lead renal injury and not due to primary uric acid depositions.

4. Obstructive Uropathy

Interstitial nephritis due to obstruction may not be associated with infection. Tubular conservation of salt and water is impaired. Partial-to-full renal recovery follows relief of the obstruction.

5. Myelomatosis

Features of myelomatosis that contribute to renal disease include proteinuria (including filtrable Bence Jones protein and κ and λ chains) with precipitation in the tubules leading to accumulation of abnormal proteins in the tubular lumen. A Fanconi-like syndrome may develop.

Plugging of tubules, tubular atrophy, and, occasionally, the accumulation of amyloid may also be present. Renal failure may occur acutely or develop slowly. Hemodialysis may rescue the patient during efforts to control the myeloma with chemical agents.

HEREDITARY RENAL DISEASES

The importance of inheritance and the familial incidence of disease warrants the inclusion of a classification of hereditary renal diseases. Although relatively uncommon in the population at large, hereditary renal disease must be recognized to permit early diagnosis for detection and genetic counseling.

1. Chronic Hereditary Nephritis

Evidence of the disease usually appears in childhood, with episodes of hematuria. Renal insufficiency commonly develops in males but only rarely in females. Survival beyond age 40 is rare.

In many families, deafness and abnormalities of the eyes accompany the renal disease (so-called Alport disease). Another form of the disease is accompanied by polyneuropathy. Infection of the urinary tract is a common complication.

There is splitting and thickening of the glomerular basement membrane or podocyte proliferation and thickening of Bowman's capsule. Recently, kindreds have been described that have "thin-membrane disease." This condition is characterized by microscopic hematuria and, often, later progression to chronic renal failure. This, like Alport disease, may represent inherited abnormalities or deficiencies in type 4 collagen in the glomerular basement membrane. This affects both genders.

Laboratory findings with these conditions are commensurate with existing renal function. Treatment is symptomatic.

2. Cystic Diseases Of The Kidney

Congenital structural anomalies of the kidney must be considered in any patient with hypertension, pyelonephritis, or renal insufficiency. Many of these patients are at increased risk of urinary tract infection.

Polycystic Kidneys

Polycystic kidney disease is familial and often involves not only the kidney but the liver and pancreas as well. It is clear that at least 2 genetic loci can lead to autosomal dominant polycystic kidney disease.

The formation of cysts on the cortex of the kidney is thought to result from failure of union of the collecting tubules and convoluted tubules of some nephrons. Intrarenal cysts may be of a proximal or a distal luminal type, differing on analysis by their cyst electrolyte content. This is important if one or more of these cysts become infected, and an antibiotic (with varying cyst-type penetrance) is chosen. New cysts do not form, but those present enlarge and, by exerting pressure, cause destruction of adjacent tissue. The incidence of cerebral vessel aneurysms and cardiac valve prolapse is higher than normal.

Cases of polycystic disease are discovered during the investigation of hypertension, by diagnostic study in patients presenting with pyelonephritis or hematuria, or by investigation of families of patients with polycystic disease. At times, flank pain due to hemorrhage into a cyst occurs. Otherwise the symptoms and signs are those commonly seen in hypertension or renal insufficiency. On physical examination, the enlarged, irregular kidneys are often easily palpable.

The urine may contain leukocytes and erythrocytes. With bleeding into the cysts, there may also be bleeding into the urinary tract. The blood chemistry findings reflect the degree of renal insufficiency. Examination by sonography, CT scan, or x-ray shows the enlarged kidneys, and urography demonstrates the classic elongated calyces and renal pelves stretched over the surface of the cysts.

No specific therapy is available, and surgical interference is only indicated to decompress very large cysts in patients with severe pain.

Patients with polycystic kidney disease live in reasonable comfort with slowly advancing uremia; both hemodialysis and renal transplantation extend the life of these patients. Nephrectomy is indicated only in patients with recurrent infections, severe recurrent bleeding, or markedly enlarged kidneys.

Cystic Disease of the Renal Medulla

Medullary cystic disease is a familial disease that may become symptomatic during adolescence. Anemia is usually the initial manifestation, but azotemia, acidosis, and hyperphosphatemia soon become evident. The urine is not remarkable, although there is often an inability to concentrate and renal salt wasting often occurs. Many small cysts are scattered through the renal medulla. Renal transplantation is indicated by the usual criteria.

Medullary sponge kidney is asymptomatic and is discovered by the characteristic appearance of tubular ectasia in the urogram. Enlargement of the papillae and calyces and small cavities within the pyramids is demonstrated by the contrast media in the excretory urogram. Many small calculi often occupy the cysts, and infection may be troublesome. Life expectancy is not affected, and only therapy for ureteral stone or for infection is required.

3. Anomalies Of the Proximal Tubule

Defects of Amino Acid Reabsorption

A. CONGENITAL CYSTINURIA

Increased excretion of cystine results in the formation of cystine calculi in the urinary tract. Ornithine, arginine, and lysine are also excreted in abnormally large quantities. There is also a defect in absorption of these amino acids in the jejunum. Nonopaque stones should be examined chemically to provide a specific diagnosis.

Treatment goals include a large fluid intake and keeping the urine pH above 7.0 by giving sodium bicarbonate and sodium citrate plus acetazolamide at bedtime to ensure an alkaline night urine. In refractory cases, a low-methionine (cystine precursor) diet may be necessary. Penicillamine has proved useful in some cases.

B. AMINOACIDURIA

Many amino acids may be poorly absorbed, resulting in unusual losses. Failure to thrive and the presence of other tubular deficits suggest the diagnosis. There is no treatment.

C. HEPATOLENTICULAR DEGENERATION (WILSON DISEASE)

In this congenital familial disease, aminoaciduria and renal tubular acidosis are associated with cirrhosis of the liver and neurologic manifestations. Hepatomegaly, evidence of impaired liver function, spasticity, athetosis, emotional disturbances, and Kayser-Fleischer rings around the cornea constitute a unique syndrome. There is a decrease in synthesis of ceruloplasmin, with a deficit of plasma ceruloplasmin and an increase in free copper that may be etiologically specific.

Penicillamine is given to chelate and remove excess copper. Edathamil (EDTA) may also be used to remove copper.

Multiple Defects of Tubular Function (De Toni-Fanconi-Debre Syndrome)

Aminoaciduria, phosphaturia, glycosuria, and a variable degree of renal tubular acidosis characterize this syndrome. Osteomalacia is a prominent clinical feature; other clinical and laboratory manifestations are associated with specific tubular defects described previously.

Treatment consists of replacing cation deficits (especially potassium), correcting acidosis with bicarbonate or citrate, replacing phosphate loss with isoionic neutral phosphate (mono- and disodium salts) solution, and ensuring a liberal calcium intake. Vitamin D is useful, but the dose must be controlled by monitoring levels of serum calcium and phosphate.

Defects of Phosphorus & Calcium Reabsorption

Several sporadic, genetically transmitted, and acquired disorders are grouped under this category and are characterized by persisting hypophosphatemia because of excessive phosphaturia and an associated metabolic bone disorder, rickets in childhood, and osteomalacia in adulthood. Response to vitamin D therapy (1,25,-dihydroxycholecalciferol, the active analog of vitamin D) is variable.

Defects of Glucose Absorption (Renal Glycosuria)

Renal glycosuria results from an abnormally poor ability to reabsorb glucose and is present when blood glucose levels are normal. Ketosis is not present. The glucose tolerance response is normal. There is no treatment for renal glycosuria, just reassurance.

Defects of Bicarbonate Reabsorption

Proximal renal tubular acidosis (RTA, type II) is due to a reduced bicarbonate reclamation in the proximal tubule, with resultant loss of bicarbonate in the urine and decreased bicarbonate concentration in extracellular fluid. There are increased K^+ losses into the urine and retrieval of CL^- instead of HCO_3^-. The acidosis is therefore associated with hypokalemia and hyperchloremia. Transport of glucose, amino acids, phosphate, and urate may be deficient as well (Fanconi syndrome).

4. Anomalies Of the Distal Tubule

Defects of Hydrogen Ion Secretion & Bicarbonate Reabsorption (Classic Renal Tubular Acidosis, Type I)

Failure to secrete hydrogen ion and to form ammonium ion results in loss of "fixed base" sodium, potassium, and calcium. There is also a high rate of excretion of phosphate. Vomiting, poor growth, and symptoms and signs of chronic metabolic acidosis are accompanied by weakness due to potassium deficit and bone discomfort due to osteomalacia. Nephrocalcinosis, with calcification in the medullary portions of the kidney, occurs in about one-half of cases. The urine is alkaline and contains larger than normal quantities of sodium, potassium, calcium, and phosphate. An abnormality in urinary anion gap (U.Na$^+$ + U.K.$^+$ − U.C$^-$) is noted (low), which is associated with the reduced NH_4^+ production. This abnormality differentiates this condition from type II RTA and from the metabolic acidosis seen with diarrhea. The blood chemistry findings are those of metabolic acidosis with low serum potassium.

Treatment consists of replacing deficits and increasing the intake of sodium, potassium, calcium, and phosphorus. Sodium and potassium should be given as bicarbonate or citrate. Additional vitamin D may be required.

Excess Potassium Secretion (Potassium "Wastage" Syndrome)

Excessive renal secretion or loss of potassium may occur in 4 situations: (1) moderate renal insufficiency with diminished H$^+$ secretion; (2) renal tubular acidosis (proximal and distal RTA)(3) hyperaldosteronism and hyperadrenocorticism; and (4) tubular secretion of potassium, the cause of which is unknown. Hypokalemia indicates that the deficit is severe. Muscle weakness and polyuria and dilute urine are signs attributable to hypokalemia. Treatment consists of correcting the primary disease and giving supplementary potassium.

Reduced Potassium Secretion

Reduced potassium secretion is noted in conditions in which extrarenal aldosterone is reduced or when intrarenal production of renin (and secondary hypoaldosteronism) occurs. The latter condition is termed RTA, type IV, and is associated with impaired H^+ and K^+ secretion in the distal tubule. Drug-induced interstitial nephritis, gout, and diabetes mellitus are clinical circumstances that may produce type IV RTA and resulting hyperkalemia and mild metabolic acidosis. Treatment is to promote kaliuresis (with loop diuretics) to prescribe potassium-binding gastrointestinal resins (Kayexalate), or to provide the patient with a mineralocorticoid, fludrocortisone acetate.

Defects of Water Absorption (Renal Diabetes Insipidus)

Nephrogenic diabetes insipidus occurs more frequently in males than females. Unresponsiveness to antidiuretic hormone is the key to differentiation from pituitary diabetes insipidus.

In addition to congenital refractoriness to antidiuretic hormone, obstructive uropathy, lithium, methoxyflurane, and demeclocycline also may render the tubule refractory to vasopressin.

Symptoms are related to an inability to reabsorb water, with resultant polyuria and polydipsia. The urine volume approaches 12 L/d, and osmolality and specific gravity are low.

Treatment consists primarily of an adequate water intake. Chlorothiazide may ameliorate the diabetes; the mechanism of action is unknown, but the drug may act by increasing isosmotic reabsorption in the proximal segment of the tubule.

5. Unspecified Renal Tubular Abnormalities

In idiopathic hypercalciuria, decreased reabsorption of calcium predisposes to the formation of renal calculi. Serum calcium and phosphorus are normal. Urine calcium excretion is high; urine phosphorus excretion is low. Microscopic hematuria may be present. See treatment of urinary stones containing calcium (Chapter 16).

REFERENCES

General

Kaplan BS et al: The pathogenesis and treatment of hemolytic uremic syndrome. J Am Soc Nephrol 1998;9:1126.

Klotman PE: HIV-associated nephropathy. Kidney Int 1999;59: 1161.

Pham PT et al: Renal abnormalities in sickle cell disease. Kidney Int 2000;57:1.

Pirson Y: Making the diagnosis of Alport's Syndrome. Kidney Int 1999;56:760.

Ronco PM: Paraneoplastic glomerulopathies: New insights into an old entity. Kidney Int 1999;56:355.

Qian Q et al: Treatment prospects for autosomal-dominant polycystic kidney disease. Kidney Int 2001;59:2005.

Glomerulonephritis

Bartosik LP et al: Predicting remission in IgA nephropathy. Am J Kidney Dis 2001;38:728.

Cameron JS: Lupus nephritis. J Am Soc Nephrol 1999;10:413.

Cattran DC (editor) : Management of glomerulonephritis. Kidney Int 1999(Suppl 70)55:S1.

Cunningham MA et al: Prominence of cell-mediated immunity effectors in "pauci-immune" glomerulonephritis. J Am Soc Nephrol 1999;10:499.

D'Amico G: Natural history of idiopathic IgA nephropathy: Role of clinical and histologic prognostic factors. Am J Kidney Dis 2000;36:227.

Daugas E et al: Antiphospholipid syndrome nephropathy in systemic lupus erythematosus. J Am Soc Nephrol 2002;13:42.

Donadio JV et al: A randomized trial of high-dose compared with low-dose omega-3 fatty acids in severe IgA nephropathy. J Am Soc Nephrol 2001;12:791.

Floege J, Feehally J: IgA nephropathy: Recent developments. J Am Soc Nephrol 2000;11:2395.

Hrick D et al: Glomerulonephritis. N Engl J Med 1998;339:888.

Kluth D, Rees AJ: Anti-glomerular basement membrane disease. J Am Soc Nephrol 1999;10:2446.

Rai A et al: Henoch-Schönlein purpura nephritis. J Am Soc Nephrol 1999;10:2637.

Savage COS: ANCA-associated renal vasculitis. Kidney Int 2001; 60:1614.

Savige J et al: Antineutrophil cytoplasmic antibodies and associated diseases: A review of the clinical and laboratory features. Kidney Int 2000;57:846.

Nephrotic Syndrome

Cattran D: Idiopathic membranous glomerulonephritis. Kidney Int 2001;59:1983.

Cattran D et al: Cyclosporine in patients with steroid-resistant membranous nephropathy: A randomized trial. Kidney Int 2001;59:1484.

Durkan AM et al: Immunosuppressive agents in childhood nephrotic syndrome: A meta-analysis of randomized controlled trials. Kidney Int 2001;59:1919.

Fogo AG: Progression and potential regression of glomerulosclerosis. Kidney Int 2001;59:804.

Orth SR, Ritz E: The nephrotic syndrome. N Engl J Med 1998;33:1202.

Interstitial Nephritis

Gambaro G et al: Risks for renal failure in nephrolithiasis. Am J Kidney Dis 2001;37:233.

Hruska KA: Treatment of chronic tubulointerstitial disease: A new concept. Kidney Int 2002;61:1911.

Rossert J: Drug-induced acute interstitial nephritis. Kidney Int 2001;60:804.

Yagisawa T et al: Contributory metabolic factors in the development of nephrolithiasis in patients with medullary sponge kidney. Am J Kidney Dis 2001;37:1140.

Tubular Disorders

Caravaca F et al: Metabolic acidosis in advanced renal failure: Differences between diabetic and nondiabetic patients. Am J Kidney Dis 1999;33:892.

Cochat P: Primary hyperoxaluria type 1. Kidney Int 1999;58:2533.

Leumann E, Hoppe B: The primary hyperoxalurias. J Am Soc Nephrol 2001;12:1986.

Soleimani M, Burnham CE: Physiologic and molecular aspects of the $Na^+:HCO_3$-cotransporter in health and disease. Kidney Int 2000;57:371.

Oliguria; Acute Renal Failure

William J.C. Amend, Jr., MD, & Flavio G. Vincenti, MD

Oliguria literally means "reduced" urine volume—less than that necessary to remove endogenous solute loads that are the end products of metabolism. If the patient concentrates urine in a normal fashion, oliguria (for that person) is present at urine volumes under 400 mL/d, or approximately 6 mL/kg body weight. If the kidney concentration is impaired and the patient can achieve a specific gravity of only 1.010, oliguria is present at urine volumes under 1000–1500 mL/d.

Acute renal failure is a condition in which the glomerular filtration rate is abruptly reduced, causing a sudden retention of endogenous and exogenous metabolites (urea, potassium, phosphate, sulfate, creatinine, administered drugs) that are normally cleared by the kidneys. The urine volume is usually low (under 400 mL/d). If renal concentrating mechanisms are impaired, the daily urine volume may be normal or even high (**high-output or nonoliguric renal failure**). Rarely, there is no urine output at all (anuria) in acute renal failure.

The causes of acute renal failure are listed in Table 32–1. Prerenal renal failure is reversible if treated promptly, but a delay in therapy may allow it to progress to a fixed intrinsic renal failure (eg, acute tubular necrosis). The other causes of acute renal failure are classified on the basis of their involvement with vascular lesions, intrarenal disorders, or postrenal disorders.

PRERENAL RENAL FAILURE

The term **prerenal** denotes inadequate renal perfusion or lowered effective arterial circulation. The most common cause of this form of acute renal failure is dehydration due to renal or extrarenal fluid losses from diarrhea, vomiting, excessive use of diuretics, and so on. Less common causes are septic shock, "third spacing" with extravascular fluid pooling (eg, pancreatitis), and excessive use of antihypertensive drugs. Heart failure with reduced cardiac output also can reduce effective renal blood flow. Careful clinical assessment may identify the primary condition responsible for prerenal renal failure, but many times several conditions can coexist. In the hospital setting, these circulatory abnormalities often lead to more fixed, acute renal failure (acute tubular necrosis).

Acute reductions in glomerular filtration rate may also be noted in patients with cirrhosis (hepatorenal failure) or in patients taking cyclosporine, tacrolimus, nonsteroidal anti-inflammatory drugs, or angiotensin-converting enzyme inhibitors. It is felt that these conditions represent significant intrarenal hemodynamic functional derangements. In these clinical circumstances, the urinary findings may mimic prerenal renal failure, but the patient's clinical assessment does not demonstrate the extrarenal findings seen in common prerenal conditions, as noted in the following section. Improvements in glomerular filtration rate are usually noted after drug discontinuance or, in cases of hepatorenal renal failure, with management of the liver disease or liver transplantation.

Clinical Findings

A. SYMPTOMS AND SIGNS

Except for rare cases with associated cardiac or "pump" failure, patients usually complain of thirst or of dizziness in the upright posture (orthostatic dizziness). There may be a history of overt fluid loss. Weight losses reflect the degree of dehydration.

Physical examination frequently reveals decreased skin turgor, collapsed neck veins, dry mucous membranes, and, most important, orthostatic or postural changes in blood pressure and pulse.

B. LABORATORY FINDINGS

1. Urine—The urine volume is usually low. Accurate assessment may require bladder catheterization followed by hourly output measurements (which will also rule out lower urinary tract obstruction; see discussion following). High urine specific gravity (> 1.025) and urine osmolality > 600 mOsm/kg) also are noted in this form of acute apparent renal failure. Routine urinalysis usually shows no abnormalities.

2. Urine and blood chemistries—The blood urea nitrogen-creatinine ratio, normally 10:1, is usually increased with prerenal renal failure. Other findings are set forth in Table 32–2. Because mannitol, radiocontrast dyes, and diuretics affect the delivery and tubular handling of urea, sodium, and creatinine, urine and blood chemistry tests performed after these agents have been given produce misleading results.

3. Central venous pressure—A low central venous pressure indicates hypovolemia. If severe cardiac failure

Table 32–1. Causes of acute renal failure.

I. **Prenatal renal failure:**
   1. Dehydration
   2. Vascular collapse due to sepsis, antihypertensive drug therapy, "third spacing"
   3. Reduced cardiac output
II. **Functional–hemodynamic:**
   1. Angiotensin-converting enzyme inhibitor drugs
   2. Nonsteroidal anti-inflammatory drugs
   3. Cyclosporine; tacrolimus
   4. Hepatorenal syndrome
III. **Vascular:**
   1. Atheroembolism
   2. Dissecting arterial aneurysms
   3. Malignant hypertension
IV. **Parenchymal (intrarenal):**
   1. Specific:
      a. Glomerulonephritis
      b. Interstitial nephritis
      c. Toxin, dye-induced
      d. Hemolytic uremic syndrome
   2. Nonspecific:
      a. Acute tubular necrosis
      b. Acute cortical necrosis
V. **Postrenal:**
   1. Calculus in patients with solitary kidney
   2. Bilateral ureteral obstruction
   3. Outlet obstruction
   4. Leak, post-traumatic

Table 32–2. Acute renal failure versus prerenal azotemia.

	Acute Renal Failure	Prerenal Azotemia
Urine osmolarity (mOsm/L)	< 350	> 500
Urine/plasma urea	< 10	> 20
Urine/plasma creatinine	< 20	> 40
Urine Na (mEq/L)	> 40	< 20
Renal failure index[a] = $\dfrac{U_{Na}}{U/P_{cr}}$	> 1	< 1
$FE_{Na} = \dfrac{U/P_{Na}}{U/P_{Cr}} \times 100$	> 1	< 1

[a]Excreted fraction of filtered sodium. See Espinel CH: JAMA 1976;236:579; and Miller TR et al: Ann Intern Med 1978; 89:47.

is the principal cause of prerenal renal failure (it is rarely the sole cause), reduced cardiac output and high central venous pressure are apparent.

4. Fluid challenge—An increase in urine output in response to a carefully administered fluid challenge is both diagnostic and therapeutic in cases of prerenal renal failure. Rapid intravenous administration of 300–500 mL of physiologic saline is the usual initial treatment. Urine output is measured over the subsequent 1–3 h. A urine volume increase of more than 50 mL/h is considered a favorable response that warrants continued intravenous infusion. If the urine volume does not increase, the physician should carefully review the results of blood and urine chemistry tests, reassess the patient's fluid status, and repeat the physical examination to determine whether an additional fluid challenge (with or without furosemide) might be worthwhile.

Treatment

In states of dehydration, fluid losses must be rapidly corrected to treat oliguria. Inadequate fluid management may cause further renal hemodynamic deterioration and eventual renal tubular ischemia (with fixed acute tubular necrosis; see discussion following). If oliguria and hypotension persist in a well-hydrated patient, vasopressor drugs are indicated in an effort to correct the hypotension associated with sepsis or cardiogenic shock. Pressor agents that restore systemic blood pressure while maintaining renal blood flow and renal function are most useful. Dopamine, 1–5 µg/kg/min, may increase renal blood flow without systemic pressor responses. Higher doses of 5–20 µg/kg may be necessary if systemic hypotension persists after volume correction. Discontinuance of antihypertensive medications or diuretics can, by itself, cure the apparent acute renal failure resulting from prerenal conditions.

VASCULAR RENAL FAILURE

Common causes of acute renal failure due to vascular disease include atheroembolic disease, dissecting arterial aneurysms, and malignant hypertension. Atheroembolic disease is rare before age 60 and in patients who have not undergone vascular procedures or angiographic studies. Dissecting arterial aneurysms and malignant hypertension are usually clinically evident.

Rapid assessment of the arterial blood supply to the kidney requires arteriography or other noncontrast blood flow studies (eg, magnetic resonance imaging or Doppler ultrasound). The cause of malignant hypertension may be identified on physical examination (eg, scleroderma). Primary management of the vascular process is necessary to affect the course of these forms of acute renal failure.

INTRARENAL DISEASE STATES; INTRARENAL ACUTE RENAL FAILURE

Diseases in this category can be divided into specific and nonspecific parenchymal processes.

1. Specific Intrarenal Disease States

The most common causes of intrarenal acute renal failure are acute or rapidly progressive glomerulonephritis, acute interstitial nephritis, toxic nephropathies, and hemolytic uremic syndrome.

Clinical Findings

A. SYMPTOMS AND SIGNS

Usually the history shows some salient data such as sore throat or upper respiratory infection, diarrheal illness, use of antibiotics, or intravenous use of drugs (often illicit types). Bilateral back pain, at times severe, is occasionally noted. Gross hematuria may be present. It is unusual for pyelonephritis to present as acute renal failure unless there is associated sepsis, obstruction, or involvement of a solitary kidney. Systemic diseases in which acute renal failure occurs include Henoch-Schönlein purpura, systemic lupus erythematosus, and scleroderma. Human immunodeficiency virus (HIV) infection may present with acute renal failure from HIV nephropathy.

B. LABORATORY FINDINGS

1. Urine—Urinalysis discloses variably active sediments: many red or white cells and multiple types of cellular and granular casts. Phase contrast microscopy usually reveals dysmorphic red cells in the urine. In allergic interstitial nephritis, eosinophils may be noted. The urine sodium concentration may range from 10 to 40 mEq/L.

2. Blood test—Components of serum complement are often diminished. In a few conditions, circulating immune complexes can be identified. Other tests may disclose systemic diseases such as lupus erythematosus. Thrombocytopenia and altered red cell morphologic structure are noted in peripheral blood smears in the hemolytic uremic syndrome. Rapidly progressive glomerulonephritis can be evaluated with tests for ANCA (antineutrophil cytoplasmic antibodies) and anti-GBM titres (anti-glomerular basement membrane antibodies).

3. Renal biopsy—Biopsy examination shows characteristic changes of glomerulonephritis, acute interstitial nephritis, or glomerular capillary thrombi (in hemolytic

uremic syndrome). There may be extensive crescents involving Bowman's space.

C. X-RAY FINDINGS

Dye studies should be avoided because of the risk of dye-induced renal injury. For this reason, sonography is preferable to rule out obstruction.

Treatment

Therapy is directed toward eradication of infection, removal of antigen, elimination of toxic materials and drugs, suppression of autoimmune mechanisms, removal of autoimmune antibodies, or a reduction in effector-inflammatory responses. Immunotherapy may involve drugs or the temporary use of plasmapheresis. Initiation of supportive dialysis may be required (see discussion below).

2. Nonspecific Intrarenal States

Nonspecific intrarenal causes of acute renal failure include acute tubular necrosis and acute cortical necrosis. The latter is associated with intrarenal intravascular coagulation and has a poorer prognosis than the former. These forms of acute renal failure usually occur in hospital settings. Various morbid conditions leading to septic syndrome–like physiologic disturbances are often present.

Degenerative changes of the distal tubules (lower nephron nephrosis) are believed to be due to ischemia. With dialysis, most of these patients recover—usually completely—provided intrarenal intravascular coagulation and cortical necrosis does not occur.

Elderly patients are more prone to have this form of oliguric acute renal failure develop following hypotensive episodes. It appears that exposure to some drugs such as nonsteroidal anti-inflammatory agents may increase the risk of acute tubular necrosis. Although the classic picture of lower nephron nephrosis may not develop, a similar nonspecific acute renal failure is noted in some cases of mercury (especially mercuric chloride) poisoning and following exposure to radiocontrast agents, especially in patients with diabetes mellitus or myeloma.

Clinical Findings

A. SYMPTOMS AND SIGNS

Usually the clinical picture is that of the associated clinical state. Dehydration and shock may be present concurrently, but the urine output and acute renal failure fail to improve following administration of intravenous fluids, in contrast to patients who have prerenal renal failure (see preceding discussion). On the other hand, there may be signs of excessive fluid retention in patients with acute renal failure following radiocontrast exposure. Symptoms of uremia per se (eg, altered mentation or gastrointestinal symptoms) are unusual in acute renal failure (in contrast to chronic renal failure).

B. LABORATORY FINDINGS

(See also Table 32–2.)

1. Urine—The specific gravity is usually low or fixed in the 1.005–1.015 range. Urine osmolality is also low (< 450 mOsm/kg and U/P osmolal ratio < 1.5:1). Urinalysis often discloses tubular cells and granular casts; the urine may be muddy brown. If the test for occult blood is positive, one must be concerned about the presence of myoglobin or hemoglobin. Tests for differentiating myoglobin pigment are available.

2. Central venous pressure—This is usually normal to slightly elevated.

3. Fluid challenges—There is no increase in urine volume following intravenous administration of mannitol or physiologic saline. Occasionally following the use of furosemide or "renal doses" of dopamine (1–5 μg/kg/min), a low urine output is converted to a high fixed urine output (low-output renal failure to high-output renal failure).

Treatment

If there is no response to the initial fluid or mannitol challenge, the volume of administered fluid must be sharply curtailed to noted losses. An assessment of serum creatinine and blood urea nitrogen and of the concentrations of electrolytes is necessary to predict the possible use of dialysis. With appropriate regulation of the volume of fluid administered, solutions of glucose and essential amino acids to provide 30–35 kcal/kg are used to correct or reduce the severity of the catabolic state accompanying acute tubular necrosis.

Serum potassium must be closely monitored to ensure early recognition of hyperkalemia. This condition can be treated with (1) intravenous sodium bicarbonate administration, (2) Kayexalate, 25–50 g (with sorbitol) orally or by enema, (3) intravenous glucose and insulin, and (4) intravenous calcium preparations to prevent cardiac irritability.

Peritoneal dialysis or hemodialysis should be used as necessary to avoid or correct uremia, hypokalemia, or fluid overload. Hemodialysis in patients with acute renal failure can be either intermittent or continuous (with arteriovenous or venovenous hemofiltration techniques). Vascular access is obtained with percutaneous catheters. The continuous dialysis techniques allow for easier management in many hemodynamically unstable patients in intensive care units.

Prognosis

Most cases are reversible within 7–14 days. Residual renal damage may be noted, particularly in elderly patients.

POSTRENAL ACUTE RENAL FAILURE

The conditions listed in Table 32–1 involve primarily the need for urologic diagnostic and therapeutic interventions. Following lower abdominal surgery, urethral or ureteral obstruction should be considered as a cause of acute renal failure. The causes of bilateral ureteral obstruction are (1) peritoneal or retroperitoneal neoplastic involvement, with masses or nodes; (2) retroperitoneal fibrosis; (3) calculous disease; and (4) postsurgical or traumatic interruption. With a solitary kidney, ureteral stones can produce total urinary tract obstruction and acute renal failure. Urethral or bladder neck obstruction is a frequent cause of renal failure, especially in elderly men. Post-traumatic urethral tears are discussed in Chapter 17.

Clinical Findings

A. SYMPTOMS AND SIGNS

Renal pain and renal tenderness often are present. If there has been an operative ureteral injury with associated urine extravasation, urine may leak through a wound. Edema from overhydration may be noted. Ileus is often present along with associated abdominal distention and vomiting.

B. LABORATORY FINDINGS

Urinalysis is usually not helpful. A large volume of urine obtained by catheterization may be both diagnostic and therapeutic for lower tract obstruction.

C. X-RAY FINDINGS

Radionuclide renal scans may show a urine leak or, in cases of obstruction, retention of the isotope in the renal pelvis. Ultrasound examination often reveals a dilated upper collecting system with deformities characteristic of hydronephrosis.

D. INSTRUMENTAL EXAMINATION

Cystoscopy and retrograde ureteral catheterization demonstrate ureteral obstruction.

Treatment

For further discussion of ureteral injuries, see Chapter 17.

REFERENCES

Forni LG, Hilton PJ: Continuous hemofiltration in the treatment of acute renal failure. N Engl J Med 1997;336:1303.

Gines P, Arroyo V: Hepatorenal syndrome. J Am Soc Nephrol 1999;10:1833.

Intensive care nephrology. J Am Soc Nephrol 2001;12(Suppl 17):S1.

Marik PE et al: Low-dose dopamine does not prevent acute renal failure in patients with septic shock and oliguria. Am J Med 1999;107:387.

Murphy SW et al: Contrast nephropathy. J Am Soc Nephrol 2000; 11:177.

Nolan CR, Anderson RJ: Hospital-acquired acute renal failure. J Am Soc Nephrol 1998;9:710.

Schiffl H et al: Daily hemodialysis and the outcome of acute renal failure. N Engl J Med 2002;346:305.

Schor N: Acute renal failure and the sepsis syndrome. Kidney Int 2002;61:764.

Star RA: Treatment of acute renal failure. Kidney Int 1998;54: 1817.

Tepel M et al: Prevention of radiographic-contrast-agent-induced reductions in renal function by acetylcysteine. N Engl J Med 2000; 343:180.

Chronic Renal Failure & Dialysis

33

William J.C. Amend, Jr., MD, & Flavio G. Vincenti, MD

In chronic renal failure, reduced clearance of certain solutes principally excreted by the kidney results in their retention in the body fluids. The solutes are end products of the metabolism of substances of exogenous origin (eg, food) or endogenous origin (eg, catabolism of tissue). The most commonly used indicators of renal failure are blood urea nitrogen and serum creatinine. The clearance of creatinine can be used as a reasonable measure of glomerular filtration rate (GFR).

Renal failure may be classified as acute or chronic depending on the rapidity of onset and the subsequent course of azotemia. An analysis of the acute or chronic development of renal failure is important in understanding physiologic adaptations, disease mechanisms, and ultimate therapy. In individual cases, it is often difficult to establish the duration of renal failure. Historical clues such as preceding hypertension or radiologic findings such as small, shrunken kidneys tend to indicate a more chronic process. Acute renal failure may progress to irreversible chronic renal failure. For a discussion of acute renal failure, see Chapter 32.

The incidence of severe chronic renal failure leading to end-stage renal disease is 280 cases per million population per year. These patients require chronic dialysis or renal transplantation. All age groups are affected. The severity and the rapidity of development of uremia are hard to predict. The use of dialysis and transplantation is expanding rapidly worldwide. Over 233,000 such patients in the United States are currently treated with dialysis. A trend toward increasingly older patients has been noted. At the present time, 94,000 patients have functioning kidney transplants.

Historical Background

There are various causes of progressive renal dysfunction leading to end-stage or terminal renal failure. In the 1800s, Bright described several patients who presented with edema, hematuria, and proteinuria and ended in death. Chemical analyses of sera drew attention to retained nonprotein nitrogen (NPN) compounds, and an association was made between this and the clinical findings of uremia. Although the pathologic state of uremia was well described, long-term survival was not achieved until chronic renal dialysis and renal transplantation became available after 1960–1970. Significant improvements in patient survival have been made in the past 40 years.

Etiology

A variety of disorders are associated with end-stage renal disease. Either a primary renal process (eg, glomerulonephritis, pyelonephritis, congenital hypoplasia) or a secondary one (owing to a systemic process such as diabetes mellitus or lupus erythematosus) may be responsible. Superimposed physiologic alterations secondary to dehydration, infection, or hypertension often "tip the scale" and put a borderline patient into uncompensated chronic uremia.

Clinical Findings

A. SYMPTOMS AND SIGNS

Symptoms such as pruritus, generalized malaise, lassitude, forgetfulness, loss of libido, nausea, and easy fatigability are frequent and nonfocal complaints in this chronic disorder. There is often a strong family history of renal disease. Growth failure is a primary complaint in preadolescent patients. Symptoms of a multisystem disorder (eg, systemic lupus erythematosus) may be present coincidentally. Most patients with renal failure have elevated blood pressure secondary to volume overload or from hyperreninemia. However, the blood pressure may be normal or low if patients have marked renal salt-losing tendencies (eg, medullary cystic disease). The pulse and respiratory rates are rapid as manifestations of anemia and metabolic acidosis. Clinical findings of uremic fetor, pericarditis, neurologic findings of asterixis, altered mentation, and peripheral neuropathy are often present. Palpable kidneys suggest polycystic disease. Ophthalmoscopic examination may show hypertensive or diabetic retinopathy. Alterations involving the cornea have been associated with metabolic disease (eg, Fabry disease, cystinosis, and Alport hereditary nephritis).

B. LABORATORY FINDINGS

1. Urine composition—The urine volume varies depending on the type of renal disease. Quantitatively normal amounts of water and salt losses in urine can be associated with polycystic and interstitial forms of disease. Usually, however, urine volumes are quite low when the GFR falls below 5% of normal. Daily salt losses become more fixed, and, if they are low, a state of sodium retention occurs soon after. Proteinuria can be variable. Urinalysis examinations may reveal mononuclear white blood cells (leukocytes) and occasionally broad waxy casts, but usually the urinalysis is nonspecific and inactive.

2. Blood studies—Anemia is the rule with normal platelet counts. Platelet dysfunction or thrombasthenia is characterized by abnormal bleeding times. Several abnormalities in serum electrolytes and mineral metabolism become manifest when the GFR drops below 30 mL/min. Progressive reduction of body buffer stores and an inability to excrete titrable acids result in progressive acidosis characterized by reduced serum bicarbonate and compensatory respiratory hyperventilation. The metabolic acidosis of uremia is associated with a normal anion gap, hyperchloremia, and normokalemia. Hyperkalemia is not usually seen unless the GFR is below 5 mL/min. In patients with interstitial renal diseases, gouty nephropathy, or diabetic nephropathy, hyperchloremic metabolic acidosis with hyperkalemia (renal tubular acidosis, type IV) may develop. In these cases the acidosis and hyperkalemia are out of proportion to the degree of renal failure and are related to a decrease in renin and aldosterone secretion. Multiple factors lead to an increase in serum phosphate and a decrease in serum calcium. The hyperphosphatemia develops as a consequence of reduced phosphate clearance by the kidney. In addition, vitamin D activity is diminished because of reduced conversion of vitamin D2 to the active form of vitamin D3 in the kidney. These alterations lead to secondary hyperparathyroidism with skeletal changes of both osteomalacia and osteitis fibrosa cystica. Uric acid levels are frequently elevated but rarely lead to calculi or gout during chronic uremia.

C. X-Ray Findings

Patients with reduced renal function should not be routinely subjected to contrast studies. Renal sonograms are helpful in determining renal size and cortical thickness and in localizing tissue for percutaneous renal biopsy. Bone x-rays may show retarded growth, osteomalacia (renal rickets), or osteitis fibrosa. Soft-tissue or vascular calcification may be present.

D. Renal Biopsy

Renal biopsies may not reveal much except nonspecific interstitial fibrosis and glomerulosclerosis. There may be pronounced vascular changes consisting of thickening of the media, fragmentation of elastic fibers, and intimal proliferation, which may be secondary to uremic hypertension or due to primary arteriolar nephrosclerosis. Percutaneous or open biopsies of end-stage shrunken kidneys are associated with a high morbidity rate, particularly bleeding.

Treatment

Management should be conservative until it becomes impossible for patients to continue their customary lifestyles. Conservative management includes restriction of dietary protein (0.5 g/kg/d), potassium, and phosphorus, as well as maintenance of close sodium balance in the diet so that patients become neither sodium-expanded nor -depleted. This is best done by the accurate and frequent monitoring of the patient's weight. Use of bicarbonate can be helpful when moderate acidemia occurs. Anemia can be treated with recombinant erythropoietin. Prevention of possible uremic osteodystrophy and secondary hyperparathyroidism requires close attention to calcium and phosphorus balance. Phosphate-retaining antacids and calcium or vitamin D supplements may be needed to maintain the balance.

A. Chronic Peritoneal Dialysis

Chronic peritoneal dialysis is used electively or when circumstances (ie, no available vascular access) prohibit chronic hemodialysis. Improved soft catheters can be used for repetitive peritoneal lavages. In comparison to hemodialysis, small molecules (such as creatinine and urea) are cleared less effectively than larger molecules, but excellent treatment can be accomplished. Intermittent thrice-weekly treatment (IPPD), continuous cycler-assisted peritoneal dialysis (CCPD), or chronic ambulatory peritoneal dialysis (CAPD) is possible. With the latter, the patient performs 3–5 daily exchanges using 1–2 L of dialysate at each exchange. Bacterial contamination and peritonitis are becoming less common with improvements in technology.

B. Chronic Hemodialysis

Chronic hemodialysis using semipermeable dialysis membranes is now widely performed. Access to the vascular system is provided by an arteriovenous fistula, vascular grafts (with saphenous vein or synthetic material), or by a subclavian permcatheter (placed either surgically or with interventional radiology). The actual dialyzers are of various geometries. Body solutes and excessive body fluids can be easily cleared by using dialysate fluids of known chemical composition. Newer, high-efficiency membranes (high/flux) are serving to reduce dialysis treatment time.

Treatment is intermittent—usually 3–5 h 3 times weekly. Computer modeling, using measurements of urea kinetics, has provided more precise hemodialysis prescriptions. Treatments may be given in a kidney center, a satellite unit, or the home. Home dialysis is optimal because it provides greater scheduling flexibility and is generally more comfortable and convenient for the patient, but only 30% of dialysis patients meet the requirements for this type of therapy.

More widespread use of dialytic techniques has permitted greater patient mobility. Treatment on vacations and business trips can be provided by prior arrangement.

Common problems with either type of chronic dialysis include infection, bone symptoms, technical accidents, persistent anemia, and psychological disorders. The morbidity associated with atherosclerosis often occurs with long-term treatment. It is now recognized that chronically uremic patients, despite dialysis, can develop wasting syndrome, cardiomyopathy, polyneuropathy, and secondary dialysis-amyloidosis so that kidney transplant must be urgently done. Routine bilateral nephrectomy should be avoided because it increases the transfusion requirements of dialysis patients. Nephrectomy in dialysis patients should be performed in cases of refractory hypertension, reflux with infection, and polycystic disease with recurrent bleeding and pain. The dialysis patient can occasionally have acquired renal-cystic disease. Such patients need close monitoring for the development of in situ renal cell carcinoma.

Yearly costs range from an average of $35,000 for patients who receive dialysis at home to as much as $35,000–60,000 for patients treated at dialysis centers, but much of this is absorbed under HR-1 (Medicare) legislation. If the patient has no other systemic problems (eg, diabetes), the mortality rates are 8–10%/year once maintenance dialysis therapy is instituted. Despite these medical, psychological, social, and financial difficulties, most patients lead productive lives while receiving dialysis treatment.

C. RENAL TRANSPLANTATION

After immunosuppression techniques and genetic matching were developed, renal homotransplantation became an acceptable alternative to maintenance hemodialysis. Improved transplantation results are now noted owing to the development of newer immunosuppressant drugs. Currently employed post-transplant drugs include prednisone, azathioprine, mycophenolate mofetil, cyclosporine, and tacrolimus. The great advantage of transplantation is reestablishment of nearly normal constant body physiology and chemistry. Diet can be less restrictive. The disadvantages include bone marrow suppression, susceptibility to infection, cushingoid body habitus, and the psychological uncertainty of the homograft's future. Most of the disadvantages of transplantation are related to the medicines given to counteract the rejection. Later problems with transplantation include recurrent disease in the transplanted kidney and an increased incidence of cancer. Genitourinary infection appears to be of minor importance if structural urologic complications (eg, leaks) do not occur.

Nephrology centers, with close cooperation between medical and surgical staff, attempt to use these treatment alternatives of dialysis and transplantation in an integrated fashion.

For a more detailed review, see Chapter 34.

REFERENCES

Aljama P et al: New insights in ESRD. Kidney Int 2002; (Suppl 80)61:S1.

Ifudu O: Care of patients undergoing hemodialysis. N Engl J Med 1998;339:1054.

Kliger AS, Haley WE: Clinical practice guidelines in end-stage renal disease: A strategy for implementation. J Am Soc Nephrol 1999;10:872.

Levey AS et al: Dietary protein restriction and the progression of chronic renal disease: What have all the results of the MDRD study shown? J Am Soc Nephrol 1999;10:2426.

Lewis EJ et al: Renoprotective effect of the angiotensin receptor antagonist Irbesartan in patients with nephropathy due to Type 2 diabetes. N Engl J Med 2001;345:851.

Nassar GM, Ajus JC: Infectious complications of the hemodialysis access. Kidney Int 2001;60:1.

Remuzzi G et al: Chronic renal diseases: Renoprotective benefits of renin-angiotensin system inhibition. Ann Intern Med 2002; 136:304.

U.S. Renal Data System 2000 Annual Data Report [Excerpts]. Am J Kidney Dis 2000;36(Suppl 6):1.

Vanholder R, DeSmet R: Pathophysiologic effects of uremic retention solutes. J Am Soc Nephrol 1999;10:1815.

Wolfe RA et al: Comparison of mortality in all patients on dialysis, patients on dialysis awaiting transplantation and recipients of a first cadaveric transplant. N Engl J Med 1999;341:1725.

Renal Transplantation

34

Peter N. Bretan, Jr, MD

Renal transplantation is the procedure of choice and the most cost-effective strategy for the management of patients with end-stage renal disease. Although major advances have been made in both dialysis and renal transplantation in the last 15 years, current knowledge firmly supports the notion that successful renal transplant is associated with a substantial improvement in quality of life and significant reduction in morbidity and mortality from end-stage renal disease (Mathur, Bretan, and Tomlanovich, 1994). Today more than 13,000 renal transplants are performed annually in the United States. This number is likely to increase, but more important it is hoped that the current high rate of success will continue to improve through advances in preservation, the use of laparoscopic nephrectomy for live donors, and development of more specific forms of immunosuppression. Much of our philosophy regarding the surgical and medical management of renal transplant candidates and patients has evolved from recent experience, and is summarized here.

Selection & Preparation of Recipients

The causes of renal failure in the United States include diabetes, 36%; hypertension nephrosclerosis, 30%; chronic glomerulonephritis, 24%; and autosomal dominant polycystic kidney disease, 12% (Urban Institute, 1986). Renal failure patients in the pediatric age group (< 18 years of age) have congenital urologic conditions (hydronephrosis with obstruction or congenital atrophy) as the major causes (45%) of renal failure (McEnery et al, 1992). Although there are no categories of patients that are deemed untransplantable, these patients will have increased morbidity and mortality posttransplantation. Today, there are few absolute contraindications to renal transplantation, other than active infection and active malignant disease. Improved graft and patient survival has led to less restrictive policies regarding the determination of candidacy for renal transplant. Usually the upper age limit for consideration of transplantation is 70 years; however, all decisions must be individualized, and patients with a life expectancy of less than 5 years probably should be maintained on dialysis. Determination of transplant candidacy depends on identification of risk factors that are associated with increased mortality and graft loss. The following risk factors define high-risk patients who

require specific studies or therapies to help assess candidacy.

A. Cardiac Status

Potential transplant candidates who are at high risk for coronary artery disease, such as patients with a history of coronary artery disease, older men, or diabetics, should undergo coronary arteriography (Steinmuller, 1983). Noninvasive studies such as Doppler ultrasonography are helpful, although these tests are not reliable enough to differentiate patients with surgical correctable disease from those with high mortality risk or noncorrectable lesions (Philipson et al, 1986). In the former group, mortality risks can be reduced substantially if a bypass procedure is successfully accomplished (Braun et al, 1983).

B. Malignant Disease

Active malignant disease is an absolute contraindication to renal transplantation. Concurrent use of immunosuppressive drugs can enhance growth of microscopic metastases. The safe waiting period for transplantation after surgical removal of solid tumors varies and depends on the grade and stage of tumor on presentation and the associated risk of subsequent metastasis. These waiting times range from 1–2 years for tumors with low metastatic potential to 5–6 years for patients at high risk. Specific risks have been determined using data from the 1993 Transplant Tumor Registry (Tables 34–1, 34–2, 34–3) (Penn, 1993). Most recurrences after transplantation reported by Penn occur within 2 years (Figure 34–1). Transplantation can be performed safely after removal of tumor if there has been adequate follow-up to determine whether the risk of subsequent metastasis or recurrence of disease is acceptable.

Patients with renal failure who have a prostatic nodule, elevated prostate-specific antigen (PSA > 4.0 ng/mL), should have a systematic prostate biopsy prior to renal transplantation. Patients with a PSA greater than 10.0 ng/mL or a positive biopsy result are at high risk for transplant.

C. Infection

Active infection is an absolute contraindication to transplantation. For urinary tract infections, it is important to distinguish between bacterial colonization

Table 34–1. Pretransplant tumors: Low recurrence rates.

Type	N	Recurrence Rate (%)	Deaths
Incidental			
Renal	59	0(0)	0
Testicular	34	1(3)	0
Cervix	59	3(5)	2
Thyroid	39	3(8)	1
Lymphoma	29	3(10)	2

Table 34–3. Pretransplant tumors: High recurrence rates.

Type	N	Recurrence Rate (%)	Deaths
Bladder	42	11(26)	4
Sarcomas	14	4(28)	2
Melanoma	20	6(30)	6
Symptomatic renal	169	51(30)	39
Nonmelanoma skin	79	49(62)	1
Myeloma	8	7(88)	7

and true tissue penetration of bacteria as noted in cystitis, pyelonephritis, or prostatitis. In the former, bacteria can be adequately treated with a 3-way Foley catheter and antibiotic bladder irrigations along with systemic antibiotics before the bladder is opened during renal transplantation. When any questions arise as to the cause of recurrent urinary tract infections in a potential transplant candidate, a full urologic evaluation should be carried out prior to renal transplantation.

Patients who have the human immunodeficiency virus (HIV) are considered to have active infection, which precludes transplantation in all cases because of the subsequent development of the acquired immunodeficiency syndrome (AIDS).

D. Systemic and Metabolic Disease

Viral hepatitis (C antibody–positive and hepatitis B antigenicity) is associated with a 2- to 3-fold increase in morbidity and mortality from progressive cirrhosis. Despite these relative contraindications, transplantation may be justified if there is no histologic evidence of active hepatic dysfunction; informed consent is obtained because of the possibility of future problems. Similarly, the activity and extent of systemic diseases such as Fabry disease, cystinosis, vasculitis, systemic lupus erythematosus, amyloidosis, and oxalosis necessitate individualized and careful assessment before a final decision on transplantation is made. The basic rationale to perform a transplant is based on an overall judgment that the benefits exceed the relative risks of subsequent complications.

E. Gastrointestinal Disease

Patients with active peptic ulcer disease should be treated appropriately; complete resolution of this process should be obtained prior to transplantation. Endoscopy can be performed just before transplantation if there is suspicion of peptic ulcer disease, and if necessary, the transplant should be postponed. Lower tract abnormality, suggested by symptoms or stools

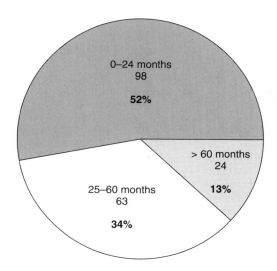

Figure 34–1. Tumor recurrences related to pretransplant treatment time. Three different waiting time periods prior to transplantation are shown, with the relative proportion of patients in whom cancer recurrence developed after renal transplantation. Note that the longer the wait, the less likely the tumors are to recur. (Modified with permission from Penn I: The effect of immunosuppression in pre-existing cancers. Transplantation 1993;55:742.)

Table 34–2. Pretransplant tumors: Intermediate recurrence rates.

Type	N	Recurrence Rate (%)	Deaths
Uterus	19	2(11)	2
Wilms	61	10(16)	8
Colon	38	8(21)	5
Prostate	21	5(21)	1
Breast	64	16(25)	13

positive for occult blood, may require a sodium diatri-zoate (Hypaque) enema or colonoscopy to screen for inflammatory bowel disease or occult malignant disease. Close observation is maintained after transplantation if a history of diverticulitis exists.

F. Genitourinary Tract Abnormalities

Patients with a history of urologic dysfunction or recurrent urinary tract infections should have a voiding cystourethrogram to rule out vesicoureteral reflux and to assess lower urinary tract function. If a significant postvoid residual exists, cystourethrometry (urodynamic profile) may be required to rule out spastic bladder or bladder neck, sphincteric, and urethral obstruction. Vesicoureteral reflux greater than grade 3 (hydronephrosis) may require bilateral nephrectomy. When high-grade > 3 reflux exists with a small non-compliant bladder, augmentation may be required to create a low-pressure urinary reservoir. Ileal conduits have been performed for urinary drainage of a renal transplant when the bladder is not repairable or usable, with acceptable results (MacGregor et al, 1986; Hatch et al, 1993); nevertheless, bladder augmentation may provide a better quality of life. For example, an internal reservoir is often preferred to an external appliance. In addition, supravesical urinary diversion in males is associated with a 20% incidence of subsequent pyocystitis. Internal continent urinary reservoirs made up of portions of stomach, ileum, and colon have been used to augment the bladder. Each method has an inherent and specific complication profile (Gold et al, 1992), and routine use has been questioned (Churchill et al, 1993). The native dilated ureter has been used to augment the bladder. The procedure of augmentation native ureterocystoplasty has been used to augment neurogenic bladders in preparation for transplantation (Koyle et al, 1994). Since nephrectomy is often required for recurrent pyelonephritis from high-grade reflux associated with neurogenic bladder, this procedure can be done instead and seems ideal for these pathologic processes, avoiding the complications that occur when the gastrointestinal tract is used.

G. Distal Urinary Obstruction

Incomplete urethral strictures or prostatic hypertrophy can be surgically corrected post-transplantation. The production of urine post-transplantation in these patients, who often have had anuric renal failure in the past, diminishes the incidence of bladder neck contracture and subsequent stenosis. In addition, although the full recovery of detrusor function after transplantation may require some time, it is expected in most cases. During this interim period of adaptation, the patient can be maintained on intermittent clean straight catheterization, or with a suprapubic tube.

H. Acquired Renal Cystic Disease (ARCD) and Risk of Renal Cell Carcinoma (RCCa)

Chronic renal failure has been shown to be a significant risk factor in the development of ARCD and RCCa (Sasagawa, Terasawa, and Sekino, 1992; Bretan et al, 1986). ARCD is a bilateral and premalignant state with up to 45% of cases developing in patients who have had renal failure for longer than 3 years. Of the patients who have ARCD, in 20% renal tumors will develop, with an overall metastatic rate of 1–2%. Baseline ultrasonography is used to screen for RCCa pretransplantation in patients with end-stage renal disease. This screening should be carried out in those with single high-risk factors (flank pain, history of renal mass, or gross hematuria) or those with double (any 2) moderate-risk factors (ARCD with increasing size, more than 4 years of dialysis, male sex, or questionable renal mass) (Levine, 1992). Questionable renal masses should be followed up periodically with radiologic screening (computed tomography is preferred), and established renal masses should be removed via radical nephrectomy.

I. Peritoneal Dialysis (PD)

PD catheters can be removed in most living related transplant recipients just after completion of the transplant, during the same anesthesia. Removal of PD catheters in many recipients of cadaveric renal transplants can be delayed in those with delayed graft function or with high immunologic risk factors. If PD is required, it can be performed immediately postoperatively. After renal function has returned, the PD catheter can be removed without difficulty (1–8 weeks postoperatively, and often under local anesthesia).

J. Pretransplant Bilateral Native Kidney Nephrectomy

Native kidney nephrectomies are seldom required pretransplantation. Common indications include pyelonephritis, medically uncontrolled renin-mediated hypertension, malignant disease, and nephrotic syndrome. Other, less common indications are extremely large polycystic kidneys. Bilateral laparoscopic nephrectomy has obvious advantages over the open approach. For patients with bilateral high-grade vesicoureteral reflux, a thorough examination of the bladder should be conducted to assess the need for augmentation. If this is required, the procedure of choice is use of both native dilated ureters as augmentation vascularized patch grafts.

The availability of synthetic erythropoietin diminishes the validity of old arguments to leave problematic and symptomatic native kidneys in situ.

K. Transplant Allograft Nephrectomy

It often is not necessary, for patients undergoing retransplantation, to remove a failed, chronically rejected but asymptomatic allograft if the contralateral side can be used as an implant site. Prognosis in the retransplant patient is strongly associated with the time period in which the primary graft was lost. If loss is secondary to rejection within 6 months of the first transplant, the success rate is greatly diminished compared with the rate in those who have lost kidneys more than 6 months after the initial transplant. Indications for allograft nephrectomy include acute rejection while on dialysis, fevers, gross hematuria, myalgias consistent with systemic inflammation and reaction, malaise, graft tenderness, infection, and uncontrolled hypertension. The subcapsular allograft nephrectomy is the safest approach to prevent iliac vessel injury.

SELECTION OF DONORS

Types of Donors

A. Living Related Donors (LRDs)

The potential donor must be free of any condition that could increase the risk of any complication from the operation, diminish the function of the remaining kidney, or change their baseline quality of life. First-order LRDs continue to provide significantly higher success rates in renal transplantation than cadaveric donors. When strict policies are enforced to ensure that only medically suitable donors are selected, long-term studies of these patients (up to 45 years of follow-up) have consistently demonstrated that donation can be performed with acceptable perioperative morbidity, no renal compromise, and negligible perioperative mortality (Dunn et al, 1986; Torres, Offord, and Anderson, 1987; Bohannon, Norman, and Barry, 1987; Williams, Oler, and Jorkasky, 1986; Narkun-Burgess et al, 1993).

Current allograft half-life is more than 10 years greater for LRD transplants than for cadaveric donor transplants (13.4 versus 8.2 years) (Yuge and Burgos, 1992). Cyclosporine-treated human leukocyte antigen (HLA)-mismatched (1-haplotype) recipients of transplants from LRDs enjoy similar graft and patient survival to that of recipients of HLA-identical (2-haplotype, or haploididentical) LRD transplants (Leivestad et al, 1986). Thus LRD continues to be a valuable and important resource for transplantation not only because of the superior results but also because of the growing shortage of cadaver organs.

B. Living-Unrelated Donors (LURDs)

Recent advances in laparoscopic live donor nephrectomy has catapulted live donors to the fastest-growing organ source for transplant recipients (Meng et al, 2001; Buell et al, 2002). In addition, there has been increasing use of LURDs as an important method to circumvent the worldwide shortage of organs; published reports of 1-year graft survival in recipients of these kidneys range from 83% to 93%. However, donor selection standards are often not stated. Physicians in underdeveloped countries have used kidneys from total strangers who were paid for their donation; poor donor patient survival times (71–85% at 1 year) and graft survival times (63–82% at 1 year) are reported. In addition, there were 5 cases of HIV transmission to recipient patients in this study population (Daar and Sells, 1990). Thus overt commercialism of human organ tissues and transplantation is unacceptable. LURD should be considered only when medically and ethically appropriate. It is medically acceptable if better results can be expected compared with cadaveric renal transplantation. It is ethically appropriate if an enduring relationship between the donor and recipient exists, such as in spousal donation. Any compromise of these minimum standards regarding LURD would hurt the spirit of altruism of organ donation and would be detrimental to all aspects of renal transplantation. When these criteria are used, the results of LURD transplants continue to be superior regarding graft and patient survival to those of transplants from cadaveric donors, and are equivalent to the results in LRD transplants. The excellent physiologic quality (no preservation or ischemic injury) of these kidneys is one of the major factors responsible for these outstanding results (Wyner et al, 1993; Park et al, 1990; Pirsch, 1990).

C. Cadaver Donors

Cadaver donors should not have any generalized disease that could adversely affect renal vascular integrity or perfusion, such as chronic hypertension, diabetes, malignant disease (with significant metastatic potential), or infections (Khauli, 1986). In older donors (> 60 years of age) or in those with questionable or minimal systemic disease (eg, hypertension), a renal biopsy should be considered. A biopsy finding of significant glomerulosclerosis (> 10–20%), intimal hyperplasia, interstitial fibrosis, tubular atrophy, or evidence of disseminated intravascular coagulopathy renders the donor suboptimal to unacceptable. Any member of a group at high risk for HIV is not an acceptable donor. Hemodynamically stable, heart-beating donors are preferred to prevent hypotension-induced oliguria and subsequent acute tubular necrosis (ATN). Young adult donors are much more resistant to ATN, and every attempt to use organs from that age group should be made. Donors between 2 and 60 years of age are associated with the highest success rates. Donors younger than 2 years of age can be successfully used if induction antibody immunotherapy is instituted in conjunction with a policy to minimize donor-recipient size differences. Pediatric donor kidneys (< 2 years of age or (< 14 kg) either en bloc (Bretan et al, 1992), or as single kidneys (Bretan, Banafsche, and Garovoy, 1994) have been used with excellent results when adhering to specific immunosuppressive protocols.

Procedures for Donors

A. DONOR PRETREATMENT

Cadaveric donor pretreatment principles are simple yet often are difficult to institute properly. The difficulty often arises in the interim period in which a ventilator-dependent "brain-dead" patient is going through the final process of aggressive neurologic management prior to being established as an irreversible, global, brain-dead patient. At this time, fluid often is restricted in order to prevent cerebral edema. In addition, most (74%) patients with isolated central nervous system pathology have diabetes insipidus (Keogh et al, 1988), causing a relative diuresis that can lead to systemic hypotension and subsequent renal shutdown. The importance of adequate hydration and volume status of donors preharvest is underscored by the great variability of recipient ATN rates worldwide (5–50%), which may reflect that donor situations and pretreatment managements are not as standardized as are harvest and transplant techniques.

B. BLOOD TRANSFUSION

Historically, recipient blood transfusions produced a positive effect on subsequent graft survival; however, in the postcyclosporine and synthetic erythropoietin era it is evident that the degree of benefit from donor-specific or third-party transfusions depends on the efficacy of the post-transplant immunosuppressive regimen (Kerman, 1987; Flechner et al, 1986; Kahan, 1987).

In addition to transmitting viral hepatitis and cytomegalovirus, a blood transfusion may lead to sensitization and render less likely the chance of achieving a negative cross-match for potential transplant recipients. For this reason, blood transfusions will continue to play a minor role in future immunosuppressive protocols for living donor and cadaveric renal recipients.

C. HLA TISSUE MATCHING

The strong positive correlation between histocompatibility matching for A, B, and DR locus antigens and allograft survival has been widely accepted for LRD renal transplants. With first-degree relatives (sibling, parent, and offspring), there is a consistent inherited homogeneity to these antigen histocompatibility complexes found on the sixth chromosome, and thus matching these loci in closely related individuals implies matching for most of the whole chromosome (haplotype).

HLA matching is less useful in cadavers and unrelated donor populations because of the greater heterogeneity in these groups compared with living related donors. Results of matching these loci in cadaver renal transplants have been less impressive, and the clinical effects on allograft survival continue to be controversial. Single centers report both favorable (Takiff et al, 1988; Leivestad, Berger, and Thorsby, 1992; Gjertson and Terasaki, 1991; Opelz, 1992) and nonsignificant (Matas et al, 1990; Hayes et al, 1993) influences on HLA (ABDR) matching. Nevertheless, it is generally accepted based on overwhelming experience that 6-antigen (6-AG)-matched kidneys have superior results compared with other, less well-matched kidneys (Takemoto, Carnahan, and Terasaki, 1990). The United Network of Organ Sharing (UNOS) 6-AG-matched or zero-mismatched program reports an 87% 1-year graft survival and 13-year half-life compared with 79% graft survival and 7-year half-life in controls. In addition, there are fewer rejection episodes noted per patient with these matched recipients.

We analyzed our results with shared 6-AG and other ABDR-matched cadaveric renal recipients to determine the clinical influences of HLA matching. The outcome was determined in all cadaveric renal transplants performed (N = 1420) between January 1984 and September 1992 at UCSF in the cyclosporine era. The HLA-matched groups studied were 6-AG (57), 2-DR (133), 1-DR (418), and 0-DR (734). HLA matching had a significant inverse impact on *rejection episodes*. The mean number of rejection episodes per patient (Figure 34–2) was significantly different for the 6-AG ($P < .008$) and 2-DR ($P < .03$) groups when each was compared with the 1- and 0-DR matched groups. Overall, HLA matching had a positive and significant ($P < .05$) impact on graft survival (Figure 34–3). Thus in our experience, 6-AG-matched kidney recipients had superior graft survival (92% 1-year graft survival) and significantly fewer rejection episodes. This result supports previous reports recommending continuation of the mandatory UNOS national sharing program. DR matching had a positive graded effect on graft survival and was associated with diminution of rejection episodes; this finding also was significant but to a lesser extent. Nevertheless, DR matching should be strongly considered in the allocation of organs within a local region. On the national level, the beneficial effect of less than perfect (6-AG) matching would be offset by the increase in preservation time incurred in attempting to match these recipients with donor organs that are a long distance away.

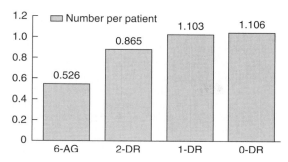

Figure 34–2. Impact of human leukocyte antigen (HLA) matching on rejection episodes. HLA matching had a significant inverse impact on subsequent rejection episodes. The mean number of rejection episodes per patient is significantly less for 6-AG ($P < .008$) and 2-DR ($P < .03$) matched groups than for the 1 + 0-DR matched groups. UCSF Renal Transplant Registry data. (N = 1420 cadaver kidneys.) Time period 1984–1992.

Extracorporeal Renal Preservation

A. Simple Hypothermic Storage and Flush Solutions

Kidneys for transplantation can be stored using preservation methods of simple cold storage or continuous hypothermic pulsatile perfusion. These methods and indications have been previously described in detail (Bretan, 1989). The most commonly used method is simple cold (hypothermic) storage. In this method, the kidneys are removed from the donor and flushed out immediately with cold preservation solution. For most living donor kidneys, an extracellular (lactated Ringer's)

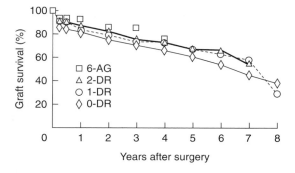

Figure 34–3. Impact of human leukocyte antigen (HLA) matching on graft survival. HLA matching had a positive and significant impact on graft survival, ($P < .04$). UCSF Renal Transplant Registry data. (N = 1420 cadaver kidneys.) Time period 1984–1992.

solution can be used, since the total cold ischemia time (CIT) is minimal (1–3 h). Longer CITs require an intracellular solution to prevent cell swelling, which is caused by free water moving into the cells. To counteract this effect, high-osmotic solutions are used. Currently, the most popular cold storage flush solution is University of Wisconsin solution (UW-1). Since the advent of UW-1 solution, liver preservation has improved significantly. Because most organ donors are combined multiple organ donors (eg, liver, kidney, and pancreas), UW-1 is now the preferred flush and storage preservation solution for abdominal organs and thus is preferred for most cadaveric kidneys.

B. Pulsatile Perfusion

Pulsatile perfusion is most commonly used for kidneys of questionable viability; however, its use is limited because of the distribution and transportation disadvantages associated with sharing kidneys stored and the required bulky machinery needed for this technique (Barry et al, 1980; Gregg et al, 1986; Halloran and Aprile, 1987).

C. Results

Viability is consistently good with either method if the transplantation is performed prior to 24 h of CIT. With total preservation times of greater than 48 h, concerns arise because of a significant increase in the incidence of ATN and delayed renal function. Kidneys with prolonged delayed function are susceptible to undiagnosed rejection episodes, because the functional clinical renal parameters that are usually monitored in immediately functioning kidneys to assess and treat allograft rejection properly are not present. In our experience, cadaver kidneys transplanted within total preservation times of less than 24 h have significantly better graft survival ($P < .04$) than kidneys with CITs greater than 24 h (Figure 34–4). This experience is from the cyclosporine era of 1984–1992 and represents clinical experience with 1420 cadaver kidneys. Other major registries have validated our experience with reports that diminished graft survival is strongly associated with prolonged preservation time (Opelz, 1986). Much research progress has been made in developing and understanding new renal preservation maneuvers during simple cold storage (Bretan et al, 1991; Bretan, 1994; Bretan, Paul, and Sharma, 1993). It is hoped that continued progress not only will decrease the incidence of delayed function in suboptimally preserved kidneys but also will translate to increased graft survival.

Donor Nephrectomy

As previously discussed, the best results in renal transplantations are obtained by using highly screened, healthy living donors. Nevertheless, there exists a

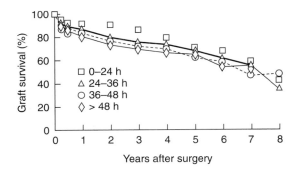

Figure 34–4. Impact of cold ischemia time (CIT) on graft survival. There was a significant ($P < .04$) increase in graft survival in kidney transplants with a total CIT of less than 24 h, compared with those with a CIT greater than 24 h. UCSF Renal Transplant Registry data. (N = 1420 cadaver kidneys.) Time period 1984–1992.

chronic shortage of organs, and transplantation using cadaveric donors not only is a suitable alternative but also is a significant (> 50% of all renal transplants) method for renal transplantation in the world today.

A. LIVING DONORS

1. Evaluation—In addition to the rationales previously delineated, potential living donors are primarily identified on the basis of the ABO blood group compatibility, optimum HLA typing, and preliminary serologic cross-matching. The general health of the living donor is assessed, and if it is acceptable, renal function is quantified. Subsequently, excretory urography and renal arteriography are performed to assess the urologic and vascular status of the donor's kidneys. The donor is always left with the better kidney.

2. Surgical technique—While multiple approaches for living donor nephrectomy have been described, the most commonly used approach is the **intraperitoneal laparoscopic** (Bartlett 2002), which has recently replaced the previous standard extraperitoneal flank approach via a superior 11th or 12th rib incision (Streem and Bretan, 1992). Based on preoperative arteriography, multiple vessels are usually avoided, as most people (> 60%) have a single renal artery at least on one side. Nevertheless, bilateral multiple renal arteries are encountered, and reconstruction can be performed during hypothermic conditions (cold bench surgery) by the recipient transplant surgeon to simplify the final in situ donor-to-recipient arterial anastomosis. Reconstruction of double or triple vessels can be revascularized end-to-side to the largest artery. Smaller upper pole arteries (< 2 mm) often can be sacrificed, while the lower pole vessels cannot because of a risk to the ureteral blood supply.

B. CADAVER DONORS

The donor patient is declared brain dead, usually by 2 independent physicians designated by the referring hospital. Family consent is obtained for organ donation. Because most donors are multiple-organ donors, they require removal of the liver, and often the heart and pancreas, in addition to the kidneys. The retrieval is often performed by a combination of a liver and a heart procurement team.

Technique of Transplantation

Either iliac fossa is acceptable for the transplant. However, the right external iliac vessels are more nearly horizontal with respect to each other, and this facilitates the anastomoses, making the right side the preferred choice. A lower quadrant curvilinear incision is made, and the iliac vessels are exposed through a retroperitoneal approach.

The renal-to-iliac-vein anastomosis is usually performed first, in an end-to-side fashion with 5-0 permanent monofilament. No heparin is needed. For the end-to-end arterial anastomosis, the internal iliac artery is isolated and transected. In men with a compromised bilateral internal iliac artery, such as in diabetes, the development of impotence postoperatively is common, because vascular insufficiency to the corpus cavernosum is exacerbated. Thus, patients with these risk factors should not undergo internal iliac anastomoses. Because of these factors, we prefer an end-to-side anastomosis of the renal artery to the external iliac artery.

An extravesical ureteroneocystostomy (often the Gregoir-Lich technique) is the preferred method to reimplant the transplant ureter. This technique does not require a large vesicotomy as does the traditional Politano-Leadbetter ureteral reimplant procedure. In addition to being faster, the Lich implant procedure is associated with less obstruction.

Immediate Pretransplant & Post-Transplant Care

Preoperative and postoperative care can be divided into surgical and immunosuppressive issues. Immunosuppressive regimens are discussed in the following section.

Preoperative surgical assessment is obtained prior to the patient's pretransplant admission to the hospital for a potential cadaveric renal transplant as an extensive outpatient evaluation to determine transplant candidacy. Central venous pressures should be kept at the high end of normal to maintain adequate preload (normal range 1–11 cm water), and urine output is replaced milliliter for milliliter. Urine outputs greater than 1 mL/kg/h are desirable, and low-dose dopamine (2–3 μg/kg/min) is used routinely. If these parameters are met and urine output is poor, other factors must be taken into consideration. Extended cold preservation or warm ischemia times predispose to ATN in the immediately postoperative period and should be anticipated. Nevertheless, technical problems also must be considered. A Doppler ultrasound study is the most convenient test; it can confirm anastomotic patency indirectly via graft blood flow and determine whether ureteral dilation is present. Fluid overload can cause pulmonary edema; this situation can be prevented if fluid is limited and furosemide (Lasix) is given in the immediate postoperative period when central venous pressures are excessively high (> 14 cm water).

Many transplant patients have baseline ultrasound and renal scintiphotography performed in the first few days postoperatively. Information from these 2 studies is overlapping and confirmatory. Information ascertained on ultrasound includes vascular patency, presence of ureteral obstruction or hydronephrosis, lymphocele formation, and indirect evidence of rejection. Common ultrasound findings with acute rejection include graft swelling, increased vascular resistivity (resistive index > 70%), pelvi-infundibular thickening, reduced sinus fat, and prominent medullary pyramids. Renal scintiphotography using Tc-99m mercaptoacetyltriglycerine (^{99m}Tc-MAG-3) has largely supplanted the ^{131}I-orthoiodohippurate scan (O'Malley, Ziessman, and Chantarapitak, 1993). This scan gives important information on blood flow and renal function. Allograft uptake, accumulation, clearance, and excretion of isotope can be used to assess renal function and help differentiate pathologic states such as rejection, ATN, and hydronephrosis. The **Bretan scale** evaluates overall renal allograft function based on these specific renal isotope criteria (Zaki et al, 1990). This simple and accurate method for grading post-transplant renal function by renal isotope scan is as follows:

- Grade 0—no uptake
- Grade 1—can define kidney outline, no excretion, and no peak accumulation
- Grade 2—excretion with no peak accumulation
- Grade 3—excretion, delayed peak accumulation, and delayed clearance
- Grade 4—excretion, normal peak accumulation, and delayed clearance
- Grade 5—excretion, normal peak accumulation, and normal clearance

Increase in grade by renal scan correlated well with the subsequent clinical function of the graft. For example, a grade between 0 and 1 predicted dialysis requirements for the first week post-transplant in more than 77% of the patients (grade 2, 50%; grade 3, 19%).

Grades 4 and 5 predicted no dialysis requirement for delayed function (Figure 34–5).

Transplant Immunobiology & Rejection

Transplantation antigens are glycoproteins expressed on the surface of an individual's cells. Every individual has a unique set of inherited transplant antigens—the **human leukocyte antigens (HLA)**—which are genetically encoded on chromosome 6. Each parent contributes one HLA-containing chromosome to the offspring, and each is coexpressed in the offspring. The purpose of these antigens is to help the body recognize what is self and what is not. In this manner, bacteria and other pathogens harmful to the individual can be sensed as nonself and destroyed by the immune system. When an organ is transplanted between unrelated people (allotransplantation), that organ is recognized as nonself because of unrecognized HLA, and can be destroyed; thus, the phenomenon of rejection. In the same fashion, organs transplanted between identical twins are recognized as self and not rejected. The first successful human transplant took advantage of this premise—the kidney was transplanted between identical twins.

Three types of rejection may take place in renal transplant patients: **hyperacute, acute, and chronic. Hyperacute** rejection is analogous to a blood transfu-

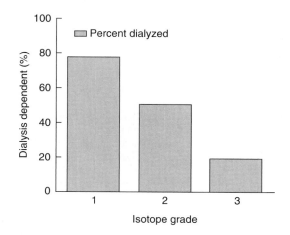

Figure 34–5. Relation between isotope grade and dialysis dependence. Bretan Scale of Renal Isotope grades on first postoperative day. The higher the grade, the less likely dialysis will be required after transplantation. (N = 138.) (Reproduced, with permission, from Zaki SK et al: A simple and accurate grading system for orthoiodohippurate renal scans in the assessment of post-transplant renal function. J Urol 1990;143:1099.)

sion reaction, as it is a humoral response mediated by preformed recipient antibodies against the HLA expressed on the donor renal vascular endothelium. To have these preformed antibodies, the recipient must be sensitized by a previous blood transfusion, a previous pregnancy, or a previous transplant. All potential recipients are screened for these antibodies preoperatively by placement of donor lymphocytes with recipient serum. If this cross-match is positive, that is, antibodies are present in the recipient serum against the donor HLA, transplant surgery is contraindicated. Clinically, hyperacute rejection is seen as soon as blood flow to the donor kidney is established. The graft turns from white to a mottled bluish black and should be removed immediately. Hyperacute rejection is rarely (1:1000) observed because of current sensitive cross-match screening.

Acute rejection occurs in the first weeks to months after transplant. The most common differential diagnosis includes ATN and ureteral obstruction. Interleukin-2 inhibitor (cyclosporine or tacrolimus) toxicity can occur, but it remains a diagnosis of exclusion. Approximately 25–55% of patients have an episode of acute rejection after renal transplantation, with 5–12% having 2 or more (Sutherland et al, 1993; Pirsch et al, 1992; Cecka, Cho, and Terasaki, 1992; Frey et al, 1992; Hayes, 1993). Most episodes of acute rejection can be treated successfully with immunosuppressive drugs, although in a minority of cases the graft is lost secondary to unrelenting and severe acute rejection (< 10%) (Basadonna et al, 1993; Tesi et al, 1993; Bertolatus, 1992).

The T lymphocyte is the main cell involved in this process. Receptors found on the T lymphocyte cell surface (T-cell receptor–CD3 complex) are stimulated by foreign transplantation antigens (HLA) found on allotransplants. Other cell surface antigens found on T cells are CD2, CD4, CD8, and CD25 receptors. With T-cell stimulation, a cascade of events is initiated. Intimately involved with this cascade is interleukin-1 production by donor and recipient antigen-presenting cells and interleukin-2 production by recipient T-helper-lymphocyte CD4+ cells. In this milieu, class II–stimulated CD4+ cells undergo clonal expansion. Recipient CD8+ cytotoxic cells, stimulated by foreign class I antigens, cause graft destruction in the presence of interleukin-2. Clinically, patients with acute rejection may be febrile and have tenderness over the graft; however, these signs and symptoms are often absent, and suspicion arises only because of worsening renal function. Although rejection can be diagnosed clinically in many patients, the gold standard is renal biopsy, which is performed in most patients prior to treatment of steroid-resistant acute rejection (Pozniak, Dodd, and Kelcz, 1992; Delaney et al, 1993; Olsen et al, 1989). With the advent of cyclosporine, more than 80% of cadaveric and 90% of living related allografts are functioning after 1 year

(Sutherland et al, 1993; Pirsch et al, 1992; Cecka, Cho, and Terasaki, 1992; Frey et al, 1992; Hayes, 1993).

Chronic rejection is defined as a process of gradual, progressive decrease in renal function that cannot be attributed to another cause. Other causes of graft dysfunction such as acute rejection, infection, or obstruction uropathy must be excluded before this diagnosis is made. Unlike the cases of hyperacute and acute rejection, the underlying immune mechanism of chronic rejection is not well understood. Chronic rejection is the single most important cause of late graft failure, with an attrition rate of approximately 5–7% per year after the first year in cadaveric kidney recipients. Thus, although 1-year cadaveric graft survival is greater than 80%, at 5 years graft survival has dropped to 60% (Hayes, 1993; Pirsch et al, 1992; Gray and Kasiske, 1992). Factors implicated in chronic rejection include donor source, incidence and timing of acute rejection, post-transplant infections, ischemic renal injury, suboptimal immunosuppression, and noncompliance with drug therapies. There is no known treatment for chronic rejection, and many patients in the late transplant period return to dialysis treatment. Investigation of the cause, pathogenesis, and treatment of chronic rejection remains a high priority in transplant research.

Immunosuppression

As discussed, hyperacute rejection is mediated by antibodies and is rarely encountered with the use of current screening techniques (cross-matching). The exact mechanisms responsible for chronic rejection have not been elucidated, although research is increasing in this area. Immunosuppressive therapy has focused, therefore, on preventing or reversing acute rejection. Although a significant proportion of renal transplant patients have at least one episode of acute rejection despite maintenance immunosuppression, these episodes are usually reversible.

Immunosuppressive agents can be used in one of three ways: (1) as an induction agent used immediately after transplantation, (2) for maintenance immunosuppressive therapy initiated once serum creatinine has normalized, or (3) for treatment of acute rejection.

Azathioprine, a purine analog, was discovered to have immunosuppressive effects in the early 1960s and, along with steroids, has been the mainstay of most past immunosuppressive regimens, but has recently been replaced by mycophenolate mofetil. Azathioprine and its metabolites are incorporated into DNA and inhibit cell mitosis and proliferation. The major complication associated with this drug is bone marrow suppression exemplified by leukopenia. Azathioprine is useful for induction and maintenance immunotherapy, but is not useful as therapy for an acute rejection episode.

Corticosteroids also have been used since the early 1960s. They have a diverse array of immunosuppressive and anti-inflammatory effects, inducing inhibition of interleukin-1 release for antigen-presenting cells. Because of this, the overall effect of corticosteroids is nonspecific, and secondary complications are common, especially with prolonged high-dose therapy. Steroids are used for induction, maintenance immunosuppression, and acute rejection episodes.

Cyclosporine A was introduced into clinical use approximately in the year 1978. Cyclosporine revolutionized the field of solid organ transplants; 1-year cadaveric renal allograft survival increased from 50% to nearly 90% after its introduction.

Antilymphocyte/antithymocyte globulins (ALG/ATG) are xenoantibodies produced by immunizing laboratory animals with human lymphocytes. Antilymphocyte/antithymocyte globulin is used both for induction and for reversing acute rejection episodes. Because of significant side effects, it is not useful for maintenance therapy.

OKT3 is a murine monoclonal antibody specific for the CD3 portion of the T-lymphocyte-receptor complex. It was developed as a specific immunosuppressive agent against T lymphocytes.

New Antibody Immunotherapy

New DNA technology has been used to help alleviate some of the clinical problems associated with the use of both monoclonal (OKT3) and polyclonal (ALG/ATG) antilymphocyte antibodies as previously described. For example, both chimeric (basiliximab; Simulect [Novartis]) and humanized (daclizumab; Xenapac [Roche]) monoclonal antibodies have been generated against specific T-cell surface proteins (CD3 receptors). By reducing xenogenic epitomes, a decrease in development of antixenogenic antibodies and thus serum sickness is achieved. These new monoclonal antibodies appear to decrease acute rejection without toxicity; thus they have replaced most polyclonal antibodies currently used for sequential immunotherapy.

FK506 (tacrolimus; ProGraft [Fujisawa Healthcare, Inc]) is an immunosuppressive agent discovered recently. It has similar properties and modes of action to cyclosporine. It also suppresses interleukin-2 production from the CD4+ cells. The experience with FK506 in kidney transplant patients indicates similar efficacy to cyclosporine A. Like cyclosporine, FK506 is used for maintenance immunosuppression therapy. FK506 can rescue grafts undergoing rejection when substituted for cyclosporine.

Rapamycin (sirolimus, rapamune) is another immunosuppressive agent that blocks the effect of interleukin-2. Unlike FK506 and cyclosporine, rapamycin does not seem to be nephrotoxic. Rapamycin can be combined with cyclosporine as there is some synergy between them.

Mycophenolate mofetil (MMF) (Cellcept [Roche]) is an antimetabolite drug that inhibits the synthesis of purines. Its effect is different from and more lymphocyte-specific than that of azathioprine, thus has replaced azathioprine in most current immunosuppressive regimens. Results favor its use in induction and maintenance immunotherapy with an associated decrease in acute rejection rate (first year post-transplantation) of almost 50%.

Current immunosuppressive regimens vary according to center preference and requirements of ongoing clinical trials. Most institutions in the United States use a combination of prednisone, an antimetabolite, with or without anti-CD3 or -CD25 antibodies for induction immunosuppression. This regimen avoids the deleterious effect of induction cyclosporine or FK506 on early graft function. Typically methylprednisolone (7 mg/kg) is given intraoperatively for primary first-time living related renal transplant recipients. Oral cyclosporine (5 mg/kg/12 h) or tacrolimus (0.1 mg/kg/12 h) is started the next day and titrated to therapeutic levels of 200–250 µg/L or 10–15 µg/L, respectively (HPLC assay), in addition to MMF. Cadaveric recipients with expected ATN or delayed function or with high immunogenic risk (previous transplant or Panel Reactive Antibodies [PRA] > 15%) are given either OKT3 (5 mg) intraoperatively or daclizumab (1 mg/kg) preoperatively. Patients are given these drugs until serum creatinine levels have normalized (< 2.5 mg/dL), which usually takes 5–14 days. Cyclosporine (5 mg/kg/12 h) or tacrolimus (0.1 mg/kg/12 h) is then started, and the antibody preparations are discontinued when adequate serum cyclosporine levels are achieved. Individual drug doses are gradually adjusted, and the patients are sent home on this maintenance drug combination. This protocol is called **quadruple therapy with sequential interleukin-2 inhibitor institution.** For patients undergoing acute rejection episodes, high-dose steroids, 7 mg/kg, are usually given for 3 days. If patients are unresponsive to steroids, biopsies are taken and therapy is determined based on findings. Often OKT3 (5 mg) is used for 7–14 days for moderate to severe rejection episodes. CD3 cell levels are monitored, and the dose is increased if the absolute count is greater than 50 cells/mm^3.

Results

Great improvements in 1-year patient and graft survival have been made in the last 3 decades. One-year patient survival has increased from approximately 50% to about 92% (Gray and Kasiske, 1992). Similarly, graft survival has paralleled this trend, with 1-year graft survival currently at 80–85% for cadaveric and greater than 90% for living related renal transplants (Sutherland et al, 1993; Pirsch et al, 1992; Cecka, Cho, and Terasaki, 1992; Frey et al, 1992; Hayes, 1993; Gray and Kasiske, 1992). However, graft attrition over a 10-year period remains high, as discussed previously, secondary to chronic rejection as well as patient death. Death with a functioning graft is the second major cause of graft loss. Most deaths after the first year are cardiovascular in origin in patients with functioning grafts (Pirsch et al, 1992; Gray and Kasiske, 1992). After 10 years, therefore, not more than 40–50% of cadaveric grafts can be expected to be functioning. The cause of long-term graft failure is uncertain. Graft loss secondary to patient noncompliance with medications has been estimated at 10%. Although late acute rejection episodes can account for some late graft failures, most grafts undergo a slow, chronic, progressive deterioration, ending in graft failure. Only recently has chronic rejection become a major focus, since it is apparent that cyclosporine has not really affected long-term graft attrition (Pirsch et al, 1992; Hayes, 1993; Gray and Kasiske, 1992; Paul, 1993; Kuo and Monaco, 1993; Paul et al, 1993). Elucidating the mechanisms of late graft failure/chronic rejection is a current focus in transplantation clinical research.

Complications

A. TECHNICAL

Various technical complications can occur post-transplantation, including renal artery or vein occlusion, renal artery stenosis, ureteral leak or occlusion, and lymphocele.

Immediate renal artery occlusion is unusual (< 1% incidence) but may be the cause of a sudden decrease or cessation of urine output post-transplantation. In a diuresing kidney, acute cessation of urine output in the immediately postoperative period should prompt emergent reexploration once Foley catheter occlusion has been eliminated as a cause. Prompt recognition and treatment offer the only chance for graft salvage.

Delayed transplant renal artery stenosis is a well-recognized complication. The true incidence of this complication has been estimated in recent retrospective studies to range from 1.5 to 8% (Sutherland et al, 1993; Roberts et al, 1989; Macia et al, 1991). Both technical and immunologic causes have been postulated (Sutherland et al, 1993; Macia et al, 1991). Patients may present with poorly controlled hypertension, a bruit over the transplant, or gradually worsening renal function (Sutherland et al, 1993; Roberts et al, 1989). Stenosis must be considered in this scenario, although rejection or cyclosporine toxicity is more common. Diagnosis is made by renal angiogram, although duplex and color Doppler ultrasonography are useful noninvasive screening techniques with excellent reported accuracy (Pozniak, Dodd, and Kelcz, 1992). Treatment options include surgical correction and percutaneous transluminal angioplasty. Although somewhat controversial, percutaneous transluminal angioplasty is favored for small segmental or intraparenchymal stenoses and in patients who are at high risk for further surgery (Farrugia and Schwab, 1992).

Urologic complications are unusual, with a range of 2–5% in most series (Loughlin, Tilney, and Richie, 1984; Brayman et al, 1992). Specific technical complications include anastomotic leaks, ureteral or anastomotic stricture formation, ureteral obstruction, and ureterovesical disruption. Clinical signs include decreased output and graft dysfunction. Diagnosis of most complications can be made by ultrasound or renal scan. Lymphocele formation is another complication seen postoperatively. This is thought to arise from lymphatic disruption during iliac artery dissection. The reported incidence is variable, ranging from 6% to 18% in several large series. Most are asymptomatic, and most resolve spontaneously over several months (Khauli et al, 1993). Clinical presentation may include wound swelling, ipsilateral leg edema, or graft dysfunction, depending upon which pelvic structures are being compressed. Diagnosis is made by ultrasound (Pozniak, Dodd, and Kelcz, 1992). In a recent multivariate analysis, acute rejection was implicated as the main factor in the development of symptomatic lymphoceles. The treatment of choice is laparoscopic marsupialization and drainage into the peritoneal cavity. Percutaneous drainage should be performed only for diagnostic purposes and is not therapeutic.

Primary acute renal failure, or ATN in the transplanted kidney, is seen in 5–40% of kidneys from cadaver donors (Cecka, Cho, and Terasaki, 1992; Delaney et al, 1993; Olsen et al, 1989). This injury is usually attributed to cold preservation ischemia or prolonged anastomotic times. Older and unstable donors are more susceptible. The diagnosis of ATN is confirmed by renal scan demonstrating good blood flow and poor tubular function and by duplex scanning to exclude other possible causes such as urinary obstruction. Treatment is expectant and supportive; ATN may take several weeks to resolve (Pozniak, Dodd, and Kelcz, 1992). Morphologically, transplant ATN differs from native kidney ATN; the former has increased interstitial infiltrates and necrotic tubular cells (Olsen et al, 1989). It is controversial whether ATN is associated with a worse long-term prognosis or predisposes to acute chronic rejection. Immunosuppressive strategies during ATN include sequential use of ALG/ATG or antitac (anti-CD25) monoclonal antibodies, followed by careful monitoring of interleukin-2 inhibitor (cyclosporine or tacrolimus) levels and biopsy to detect presence of unsuspected rejection.

B. NONTECHNICAL

Important nontechnical complications include infection and cancer. A recent study confirmed that post-transplant infections are the second most frequent cause of death following renal transplantation (Brayman et al, 1992; Dlugosz et al, 1989). Prophylactic antibiotics are used perioperatively and have been shown to reduce significantly the incidence of wound infections in renal transplant patients to approximately 1% (Brayman et al, 1992; Paul et al, 1993). Trimethoprim-sulfamethoxazole (TMP-SMX) given daily has been shown to decrease the incidence of urinary tract infections and *Pneumocystis carinii* 4-fold and is used routinely. For patients with allergies to sulfa drugs, inhaled pentamidine is an effective alternative (Brayman et al, 1992). Although bladder irrigation with an antibiotic/antifungal solution has not been studied in a randomized fashion, many centers routinely use this procedure (Goodman and Hargreave, 1989).

Opportunistic infections predominate throughout the next 2–6 months. Transplant patients are most susceptible to viruses and intracellular infectious agents because immunosuppressive agents inhibit the cellular component of the immune response. The major viral pathogen during this period is the cytomegalovirus (CMV), causing symptomatic disease in 35% and death in 2% of renal transplant recipients (Farrugia and Schwab, 1992). Seronegative recipients of positive donor kidneys are at the highest risk (50–60%) of having symptomatic CMV disease (Farrugia and Schwab, 1992). The initial clinical manifestations are those of a flulike illness including fever, fatigue, malaise, myalgias, and arthralgias. If it is untreated, manifestations of site-specific disease occur; usually the respiratory, urinary, or gastrointestinal tract is affected. Common initial laboratory findings include elevated serum transaminases and an atypical lymphocytosis. Leukopenia and thrombocytopenia are also commonly seen. Cell culture currently is the most widely used method of detecting active infection. Treatment of established CMV infection involves decreasing immunosuppressive therapy, providing supportive treatment such as hydration and antipyretics, and administering the antiviral agent ganciclovir. In infected renal transplant patients, ganciclovir decreases rates of viral shedding, alleviates symptoms, and arrests progression of CMV disease (Farrugia and Schwab, 1992). The prophylactic administration of oral acyclovir for the first 6 months post-transplantation has been shown to suppress virus infection. Prophylaxis with ganciclovir has substantially decreased the incidence of CMV when given to patients taking OKT3.

Another effect of immunosuppression is the increased incidence of cancer (Penn, 1987; Cockfield et al, 1993). Analysis of malignant disease occurrences since the advent of cyclosporine therapy reveals an increase in lymphoma and Kaposi sarcoma (Penn, 1987). Post-transplant lymphoproliferative disorders (PTLD) have an incidence of 2.5% in cadaveric renal allografts (Cockfield et al, 1993). Mean time of onset of PTLD with cyclosporine use was about 15 months, with 32% occurring within 4 months of allografting. Primary infection with Epstein-Barr virus at the time of transplantation seems to be a major risk factor. Patients may present with or without renal allograft involvement. By immunohistochemistry, lesions can be identified as polyclonal or monoclonal populations of B lymphocytes. A reduction or cessation of immunotherapy may allow the host immune system to bring the disease under control. Monoclonal lesions tend to have a worse prognosis, although if immunosuppression is stopped early enough, these also have been reported to regress (Cockfield et al, 1993).

REFERENCES

Barry JM et al: Comparison of intracellular flushing and cold storage to machine perfusion for human kidney preservation. J Urol 1980;123:14.

Bartlett ST: Laparoscopic donor nephrectomy after seven years. Am J Transplantation 2002;2:896.

Basadonna G et al: Early versus late acute renal allograft rejection: Impact on chronic rejection. Transplantation 1993;55:993.

Bertolatus J: Clinical immunosuppressive regimens and clinical results in renal transplantation. Semin Nephrol 1992;12:332.

Bohannon LL, Norman DJ, Barry JM: Renal functional consequences of kidney donation: A long term follow-up study. Clin Transplant 1987;I:225.

Braun WE et al: The course of coronary artery disease in diabetics with and without renal allografts. Transplantation Proc 1983; 15:1114.

Brayman KL et al: Analysis of infectious complications occurring after solid organ transplant. Arch Surg 1992;127:38.

Bretan PN: Characterization of improved renal transplant preservation mechanisms using PB-2 flush solution by HPLC assay. Transplant Int (Suppl 1) 1994;5465.

Bretan PN: Extracorporeal renal preservation. In: Novick AC (editor): *Stewart Textbook of Operative Urology*. Williams & Wilkins, 1989.

Bretan PN, Banafsche R, Garovoy M: Minimizing recipient/donor size differences improves long-term graft survival using single pediatric cadaver kidneys. Transplantation 1994;26:28.

Bretan PN, Paul G, Sharma J: Improved renal preservation with PB-3 flush solution during 72 hours cold storage: Demonstration of a salutary effect on isolated mitochondrial respiration. Transplantation Proc 1993;25:3215.

Bretan PN et al: Chronic renal failure: A significant risk factor in the development of acquired renal cyst and renal cell carcinoma. Case reports and reviews of the literature. Cancer 1986;57:1871.

Bretan PN et al: Improved allograft survival using en bloc renal transplants from pediatric donors less than 14 kg: Technical and immunologic considerations. J Urol 1992;147:342A.

Bretan PN et al: Improved renal transplant preservation using PB-2 flush solution: Characterization of intracellular mechanisms by renal clearance, HPLC, 31P-MRS and EM studies. Urol Res 1991;19:73.

Buell JF et al: Hand-assisted laparoscopic living-donor nephrectomy as an alternative to traditional laparoscopic living-donor nephrectomy. Am J Transplantation 2002;2:983.

Cecka J, Cho Y, Terasaki P: Analysis of the UNOS scientific renal transplant registry at three years: Early events affecting transplant success. Transplantation 1992;53:59.

Churchill BM et al: Ureteral bladder augmentation. J Urol 1993; 150:716.

Cockfield SM et al: Post-transplant lymphoproliferative disorder in renal allograft recipients. Transplantation 1993;56:88.

Daar AJ, Sells RA: Living nonrelated donor renal transplantation: A reappraisal. Transplant Rev 1990;4:128.

Delaney V et al: Comparison of fine-needle aspiration biopsy, Doppler ultrasound, and radionuclide scintigraphy in the diagnosis of acute allograft dysfunction in renal transplant recipients: Sensitivity, specificity, and cost analysis. Nephron 1993;63:263.

Dlugosz BA et al: Causes of death in kidney transplant recipients. Transplantation Proc 1989;21:2168.

Dunn JF et al: Living related kidney donors: A 14 year experience. Ann Surg 1986;203:637.

Farrugia E, Schwab T: Subspecialty clinics: Nephrology. Mayo Clin Proc 1992;67:879.

Flechner SM et al: Long-term results of cyclosporine therapy in recipients of mismatched living related kidneys. Transplantation Proc (Suppl 1) 1986;18:47.

Frey D et al: Sequential therapy: A prospective randomized trial of MALG versus OKT3 for prophylactic immunosuppression in cadaver renal allograft recipients. Transplantation 1992; 54:50.

Gjertson DW, Terasaki PL: National allocation of cadaveric kidneys by HLA matching: Projected effect on outcome and cost. N Engl J Med 1991;324:1032.

Gold BD et al: Gastrointestinal complications of gastrocystoplasty. Arch Dis Child 1992;67:1272.

Goodman CM, Hargreave TB: Survey of antibiotic prophylaxis in European renal transplantation practice. Int J Urol Nephrol 1989;22:173.

Gray J, Kasiske B: Patient and renal allograft survival in the late posttransplant period. Semin Nephrol 1992;12:343.

Gregg CM et al: Recovery of glomerular and tubular function in autotransplanted dog kidneys preserved by hypothermic storage or machine perfusion. Transplantation 1986;42:453.

Halloran P, Aprile M: A randomized prospective trial of cold storage versus pulsatile perfusion for cadaver kidney preservation. Transplantation 1987;43:827.

Hatch DA et al: Fate of renal allograft transplanted in patients with urinary diversion. Transplantation 1993;56:838.

Hayes JM: The immunobiology and clinical use of current immunosuppressive therapy for renal transplantation. J Urol 1993;149:437.

Hayes JM et al: A single center experience with shared 6 Ag matched cadaver renal transplants. Transplantation 1993; 55:669.

Kahan BD: Blood transfusion. (Editorial) Transpl Immunol Lett 1987;4:1.

Keogh AM et al: Pituitary function in brain stem dead organ donors: A prospective survey. Transplantation Proc 1988; 20:729.

Kerman RH: To be or not to be transfused? That is the question in the cyclosporine era! Transpl Immunol Lett 1987;4:2.

Khauli RB: Current policies in renal procurement and transplantation. In: Stamey T (editor): *Monographs in Urology.* Medical Directions Publishing Co., Inc, Monterde, FL, 1986.

Khauli RB et al: Post-transplant lymphoceles: A critical look into the risk factors, pathophysiology and management. J Urol 1993;150:22.

Koyle MA et al: Bladder reconstruction with the dilated ureter for renal transplantation. Transplantation Proc 1994;26:35.

Kuo P, Monaco AP: Chronic rejection and suboptimal immunosuppression. Transplantation Proc 1993;25:2082.

Leivestad T, Berger L, Thorsby E: Beneficial effect of DR matching on cadaveric renal graft survival in Scandian transplant. Transplantation Proc 1992;24:2447.

Leivestad T et al: Renal transplants from HLA-haploid identical living-related donors: The influence of donor-specific transfusions and different immunosuppressive regimens. Transplantation 1986;42:35.

Levine E: Chronic renal failure and renal cell carcinoma in uremic acquired renal cystic disease: Incidence, detection and management. Urol Radiol 1992;13:203.

Loughlin KR, Tilney NL, Richie JP: Urologic complications in 718 renal transplant patients. Surgery 1984;95:297.

MacGregor P et al: Renal transplantation in end stage renal disease patients with existing urinary diversion. J Urol 1986; 135:686.

Macia M et al: Posttransplant renal artery stenosis: A possible immunological phenomenon. J Urol 1991;145:251.

Matas AJ et al: The impact of HLA matching on graft survival and on sensitization after a failed transplant. Transplantation 1990;50:599.

Mathur VS, Bretan PN, Tomlanovich SJ: Management of ESRD-transplantation versus dialysis. In: Novick AC (editor): *Current Opinion in Urology.* Current Science, 1994.

McEnery PT et al: Renal transplantation in children: A report from the North American Pediatric Cooperative Study. N Engl J Med 1992;326:1727.

Meng M et al: Laparoscopic live donor nephrectomy at the University of California San Francisco. In: Cecka J and Terasaki P (editors): *Clinical Transplants 2001.* UCLA Immunogenetics Center, Los Angeles, Calif.

Narkun-Burgess DM et al: Forty-five-year follow-up after uninephrectomy. Kidney Int 1993;43:1110.

Olsen S et al: Primary acute renal failure (acute tubular necrosis) in the transplanted kidney: Morphology and pathogenesis. Medicine 1989;68:173.

O'Malley JP, Ziessman HA, Chantarapitak N: Tc-99m MAG3 as an alternative to Tc-99m DTPA and I-131 Hippuran for renal transplant evaluation. Clin Nucl Med 1993;18:22.

Opelz G: How unusual are the University of Minnesota HLA matching results? Transplantation 1992;53:694.

Opelz G: Multicenter impact of cyclosporine on cadaver kidney graft survival. Prog Allergy 1986;38:329.

Park K et al: Single-center experience of unrelated living-donor renal transplantation in the cyclosporine era. In: Terasaki P (editor): *Clinical Transplants*. UCLA Tissue Typing Laboratory, 1990.

Parlevliet K, Schellekens P: Monoclonal antibodies in renal transplantation: A review. Transplant Int 1992;5:234.

Paul LC: Chronic rejection of organ allografts: Magnitude of the problem. Transplantation Proc 1993;25:2024.

Paul LC et al: Diagnostic criteria for chronic rejection/accelerated graft atherosclerosis in heart and kidney transplants: Joint proposal from the fourth Alexis Carrel Conference on chronic rejection and accelerated arteriosclerosis in transplanted organs. Transplantation Proc 1993;25:2022.

Penn I: Cancers following cyclosporine therapy. Transplantation 1987;43:32.

Penn I: The effect of immunosuppression in pre-existing cancers. Transplantation 1993;55:742.

Philipson JB et al: Evaluation of cardiovascular risk for renal transplantation in diabetic patients. Am J Med 1986;81:630.

Pirsch J et al: The effect of donor age, recipient age, and HLA match on immunologic graft survival in cadaver renal transplant recipients. Transplantation 1992;53:55.

Pirsch JD: Living-unrelated renal transplantation at the University of Wisconsin. In: Terasaki P (editor): *Clinical Transplants*. UCLA Tissue Typing Laboratory, 1990.

Pozniak M, Dodd G, Kelcz F: Ultrasonographic evaluation of renal transplantation. Radiol Clin North Am 1992;30:1053.

Roberts PP et al: Transplant renal artery stenosis. Transplantation 1989;48:580.

Sasagawa I, Terasawa KI, Sekino H: Acquired cystic disease of kidney and renal cell carcinoma in hemodialysis patients. Br J Urol 1992;70:236.

Steinmuller DR: Evaluation and selection of candidates for renal transplantation. Urol Clin North Am 1983;10:217.

Streem SB, Bretan PN: Considerations in donor nephrectomy. In: Droller MJ (editor): *Surgical Management of Urologic Disease: An Anatomic Approach*. Mosby Year Book, 1992.

Sutherland R et al: Renal artery stenosis after renal transplantation: The impact of the hypogastric artery anastomosis. J Urol 1993;149:980.

Takemoto S, Carnahan E, Terasaki PL: Report on 604 6-Ag matched transplants. In: Terasaki P (editor): *Clinical Transplants*. UCLA Tissue Typing Laboratory, 1990.

Takiff H et al: Dominant effect of histocompatibility on ten-year kidney transplant survival. Transplantation 1988;45:410.

Tesi R et al: OKT3 for primary therapy of the first rejection episode in kidney transplants. Transplantation 1993;55:1023.

Tilney NL et al: Factors contributing to the declining mortality rate in renal transplantation. N Engl J Med 1978;299:1321.

Torres VE, Offord KP, Anderson CF: Blood pressure determinants in living-related renal allograft donors and their recipients. Kidney Int 1987;31:1383.

Urban Institute: Medicare ESRD incidence per million by primary diagnosis. The Urban Institute 1980–1986. Based on HCFA data. 1986.

Williams SL, Oler J, Jorkasky DK: Long-term renal function in kidney donors: A comparison of donors and their siblings. Ann Intern Med 1986;105:1.

Wyner LM et al: Improved success of living unrelated renal transplantation with cyclosporine immunosuppression. J Urol 1993;149:706.

Yuge J, Burgos D: Long term kidney graft survival. In: Terasaki PI, Cecka JM (editors): *Clinical Transplants*. UCLA Tissue Typing Laboratory, 1992.

Zaki SK et al: A simple and accurate grading system for orthoiodohippurate renal scans in the assessment of post-transplant renal function. J Urol 1990;143:1099.

Disorders of the Ureter & Ureteropelvic Junction

35

Barry A. Kogan, MD

The ureter is a complex functional conduit carrying urine from the kidneys to the bladder. Any pathologic process that interferes with this activity can cause renal abnormalities, the most common sequels being hydronephrosis (see Chapter 11) and infection. Disorders of the ureter can be classified as congenital or acquired.

■ CONGENITAL ANOMALIES OF THE URETER

Congenital ureteral malformations are common and range from complete absence to duplication of the ureter. They may cause severe obstruction requiring urgent attention, or they may be asymptomatic and of no clinical significance. The nomenclature can be confusing and has been standardized to prevent ambiguity (Glassberg et al, 1984).

URETERAL ATRESIA

The ureter may be absent entirely, or it may end blindly after extending only part of the way to the flank. The anomaly is caused during embryologic development, either by failure of the ureteral bud to form from the mesonephric duct or by an arrest in its development before it comes in contact with the metanephric blastema. The genetic determinants of ureteral bud development and the causes of bud abnormalities are being elucidated and so far the PAX-2 and RET genes have been shown to play an important role (Brophy et al, 2001; Tang et al, 2002). In any event, the end result of an atretic ureteral bud is an absent or multicystic, dysplastic kidney. The multicystic kidney is usually unilateral and asymptomatic and of no clinical significance. In rare cases it can be associated with hypertension (Javadpour et al, 1970), infection (Yoshida and Sakamoto, 1986), or tumor. Contralateral vesicoureteral reflux is common, and many clinicians recommend a voiding cystourethrogram as part of the initial workup (Selzman and Elder, 1995). There is a natural tendency of these kidneys to involute (Rotten-

berg, Gordon, and DeBruyn, 1997); hence, most clinicians feel observation is the best treatment. A few recommend nephrectomy owing to the small risk of neoplasia and the relatively small morbidity (Homsy et al, 1997).

DUPLICATION OF THE URETER

Complete or incomplete duplication of the ureter is one of the most common congenital malformations of the urinary tract. Nation (1944) found some form of duplication of the ureter in 0.9% of a series of autopsies. The condition occurs more frequently in females than in males and is often bilateral. The mode of inheritance is autosomal dominant, although the gene is of incomplete penetrance (Atwell et al, 1974).

Incomplete (Y) type of duplication is caused by branching of the ureteral bud before it reaches the metanephric blastema. In most cases, this anomaly is associated with no clinical abnormality. However, disorders of peristalsis may occur near the point of union (Figure 35–1) (O'Reilly et al, 1984).

In complete duplication of the ureter, the presence of 2 ureteral buds leads to the formation of 2 totally separate ureters and 2 separate renal pelves. Because the ureter to the upper segment arises from a cephalad position on the mesonephric duct, it remains attached to the mesonephric duct longer and consequently migrates farther, ending medial and inferior to the ureter draining the lower segment (Weigert-Meyer law). Thus, the ureter draining the upper segment may migrate too far caudally and become ectopic and obstructed, whereas the ureter draining the lower segment may end laterally and have a short intravesical tunnel that leads to vesicoureteral reflux (Figure 35–2) (Tanagho, 1976).

Although many patients with duplication of the ureter are asymptomatic, a common presentation is persistent or recurrent infections. In females, the ureter to the upper pole may be ectopic, with an opening distal to the external sphincter or even outside the urinary tract. Such patients have classic symptoms: incontinence characterized by constant dribbling, and at the same time, a normal pattern of voiding. In males, because the mesonephric duct becomes the vas and

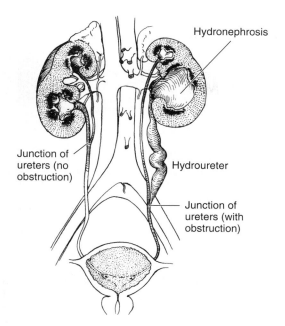

Figure 35–1. Duplication of the ureter. Incomplete (Y) type with hydronephrosis of lower pole of left kidney. Ureteroureteral (yo-yo) reflux can also occur and account for the radiographic appearance.

Figure 35–2. Duplication of the ureter. Complete duplication with reflux to lower pole of right kidney and chronic pyelonephritic scarring. Upper-pole ureter of left kidney is ectopic, and its associated renal parenchyma is often dysplastic.

seminal vesicles, the ectopic ureter is always proximal to the external sphincter, and associated incontinence does not occur. In recent years, prenatal ureteral ultrasonography has led to the diagnosis in many asymptomatic neonates.

Excretory urography and voiding cystourethrography have been the classic studies for detecting duplication of the ureter. The excretory urogram shows the duplication in most cases. Occasionally, one segment of the kidney functions so poorly that it is not visualized. In such cases, the diagnosis can be inferred from the displacement of the visualized calyces or ureter or from the discrepancy between the amount of renal parenchyma and the relatively small number of visualized calyces. The voiding cystourethrogram discloses vesicoureteral reflux and may demonstrate the presence of a ureterocele. At the present time, the excretory urogram has been supplanted by sonography, which usually can visualize a hydronephrotic upper pole and a dilated distal ureter and can readily evaluate parenchymal thickness and the presence of bladder anomalies. Renal scanning (especially with ^{99m}Tc-dimercaptosuccinic acid) is helpful for estimating the degree of renal function in each renal segment (Carter, Malone, and Lewington, 1998) (Figure 35–3).

The treatment of reflux alone should not be influenced by the presence of ureteral duplication (Lee et al, 1991). Lower grades of reflux are generally treated medically and higher grades of reflux surgically. Because of anatomic variations, many surgical options are available (Decter, 1997). If upper-pole obstruction or ectopy is present, surgery is almost always required. Numerous operative approaches have been recommended (Belman, Filmer, and King, 1974). If renal function in one segment is very poor, heminephrectomy is the most appropriate procedure (Barrett, Malek, and Kelalis, 1975). In an effort to preserve renal parenchyma, treatment by pyeloureterostomy, ureteroureterostomy, or ureteral reimplantation are all appropriate (Amar, 1970; Amar, 1978; Bieri et al, 1998).

URETEROCELE

A ureterocele is a sacculation of the terminal portion of the ureter (Figure 35–4). It may be either intravesical or ectopic; in the latter case, some portion is located at the bladder neck or in the urethra. Intravesical ureteroceles are associated most often with single ureters, whereas

Figure 35–3. Duplication of the ureter and the ureterocele. **Upper left:** Excretory urogram shows duplication of the right kidney (arrowheads on upper pole) and visualization of only the lower pole (arrows on lower pole) of the left kidney (white arrow). There is a filling defect on the left side of the bladder. **Upper right:** Cystogram confirms the filling defect. There is no reflux. **Lower left:** Renal scan with ^{99m}Tc-dimercaptosuccinic acid shows some functioning parenchyma in upper pole to left kidney. **Lower right:** After excision of ureterocele and reimplantation of both ureters on left, repeat excretory urogram shows improved excretion of contrast medium from upper pole of left kidney.

Figure 35–4. Ureterocele. **Left:** Orthotopic ureterocele associated with a single ureter. **Right:** Ureterocele associated with ureteral duplication and poor function of upper pole of kidney.

ectopic ureteroceles nearly always involve the upper pole of duplicated ureters. Ectopic ureteroceles are 4 times more common than those that are intravesical (Snyder and Johnston, 1978). Ureterocele occurs 7 times more often in girls than in boys, and about 10% of cases are bilateral. Mild forms of ureterocele are found occasionally in adults examined for unrelated reasons.

Ureterocele has been attributed to delayed or incomplete canalization of the ureteral bud leading to an early prenatal obstruction and expansion of the ureteral bud prior to its absorption into the urogenital sinus (Tanagho, 1976). The cystic dilation forms between the superficial and deep muscle layers of the trigone. Large ureteroceles may displace the other orifices, interfere with the muscular backing of the bladder, or even obstruct the bladder outlet. There is nearly always significant hydroureteronephrosis, and a dysplastic segment of the upper pole of the kidney may be found in association with a ureterocele.

Clinical findings vary considerably. Patients commonly present with infection, but bladder outlet obstruction or incontinence may be the initial complaint. Occasionally, a ureterocele may prolapse through the female urethra (Ahmed, 1984). Calculi can develop secondary to urinary stasis and are often seen in the distal

ureter. Currently, many cases are diagnosed by antenatal maternal ultrasound (Gloor, Ogburn, and Matsumoto, 1996). Although excretory urography (Figures 35–3 and 35–5) is usually diagnostic, sonography has replaced the excretory urogram in most centers. Voiding cystourethrography should always be part of the workup (Bauer and Retik, 1978). It may demonstrate reflux into the lower pole or contralateral ureter and occasionally shows eversion of the ureterocele during urination, in which case the ureterocele has the appearance of a diverticulum. Renal scanning is helpful for estimating renal function (Geringer et al, 1983).

Treatment must be individualized. Transurethral incision was used previously only in very ill children with pyohydronephrosis; however, it has been recognized as the definitive procedure in many instances, particularly in patients with intravesical ureteroceles (Blyth et al, 1993; Pfister et al, 1998) and especially in neonates (Coplen, 2001; Upadhyay et al, 2002). When an open operation is needed, the procedure must be chosen on the basis of the anatomic location of the ureteral meatus, the position of the ureterocele, and the degree of hydroureteronephrosis and impairment of renal function. In general, choices range from heminephrectomy and ureterectomy (Husmann et al, 1995) to excision of the ureterocele, vesical reconstruction, and ureteral

Figure 35–5. Ureterocele. **Left:** Excretory urogram in a woman shows "cobra head" deformity of distal ends of both ureters, bilateral ureteroceles causing minimal obstruction, and pressure on the bladder from the uterus. No treatment is indicated. **Right:** Excretory urogram in an 8-year-old girl shows a space-occupying lesion (left side of bladder) caused by ureterocele. Absence of calyceal system in upper portion of left kidney (arrows) implies duplication of ureters and renal pelves and a nonfunctioning upper pole (advanced hydronephrosis); the dilated ureter from that pole drains into an obstructing ureterocele and displaces the visualized ureter laterally just below the kidney.

reimplantation. Often, a second procedure is necessary (Caldamone, Snyder, and Duckett, 1984).

ECTOPIC URETERAL ORIFICE

Although an ectopic ureteral orifice most commonly occurs in association with duplication of the ureter (see preceding sections), single ectopic ureters do occur (Gotoh et al, 1983). They are caused by a delay or failure of separation of the ureteral bud from the mesonephric duct during embryologic development. Again, the genetic determinants of these ureteral bud abnormalities are currently being determined, but at least the PAX-2 and RET genes are involved (Brophy et al, 2001; Tang et al, 2002). In anatomic terms, the primary anomaly may be an abnormally located ureteral bud; that explains the high incidence of dysplastic kidneys associated with single ectopic ureters.

The clinical picture varies according to the sex of the patient and the position of the ureteral opening. Boys are seen because of urinary tract infection or epididymi-tis. In these cases, the ureter may drain directly into the vas deferens or seminal vesicle (Umeyama et al, 1985). In girls, the ureteral orifice may be in the urethra, vagina, or perineum. Although infection may be present, incontinence is the rule. Continual dribbling despite normal voiding is pathognomonic. Urgency and urge incontinence may confound the diagnosis (Johnson and Perlmutter, 1980).

Sonography and voiding cystourethrography help delineate the problem. However, because an ectopic kidney may be both tiny and in an abnormal location, it may be difficult to find by ultrasound; and magnetic resonance imaging, cystoscopy, or laparoscopy may be necessary to confirm the diagnosis (Borer et al, 1998). During cystoscopy, a hemitrigone may be seen and the ectopic orifice may be visualized directly or demonstrated by retrograde catheterization (Figures 35–6 and 35–7). Renal scanning is also helpful in estimating relative renal function. As in ureteroceles and duplication of the ureter, the clinical picture and the degree of renal function dictate the therapeutic approach.

Figure 35–6. Ectopic ureter. **Top:** Excretory urogram demonstrates no right renal outline and no excretion of contrast medium on right. **Lower left:** Endoscopic injection of contrast medium into ejaculatory duct demonstrates seminal vesicle and stump of ectopic ureter (arrows). **Lower right:** Same anatomy visualized on a vasogram. (Courtesy of DW Ferguson.)

Figure 35–7. Ectopic ureter. **Left:** Cystoscopy in a 6-year-old girl with a lifelong history of urinary incontinence revealed 2 ureteral orifices on the right and one on the left; these were catheterized and urograms obtained. **Right:** Same patient. An ectopic ureteral orifice near the urethral meatus was catheterized. Retrograde urogram demonstrates second hydronephrotic renal pelvis on left. Resection of upper pole and ureter cured incontinence.

ABNORMALITIES OF URETERAL POSITION

Retrocaval ureter (also called circumcaval ureter and postcaval ureter) is a rare condition in which an embryologically normal ureter becomes entrapped behind the vena cava because of abnormal persistence of the right subcardinal (as opposed to the supracardinal) vein. This forces the right ureter to encircle the vena cava from behind. The ureter descends normally to approximately the level of L3, where it curves back upward in the shape of a reverse J to pass behind and around the vena cava. Obstruction generally results.

Traditionally, the diagnosis of retrocaval ureter was made by excretory urography. However, since sonography is now usually the first test performed, the radiologist must be suspicious of the anomaly based on a dilated proximal (but not distal) ureter. Currently, magnetic resonance imaging is the best single study to delineate the anatomy clearly and noninvasively. Surgical repair for retrocaval ureter, when indicated, consists of dividing the ureter (preferably across the dilated portion), bringing the distal ureter from behind the vena cava, and reanastomosing it to the proximal end. The procedure has been performed laparoscopically to reduce morbidity (Polascik and Chen, 1998).

OBSTRUCTION OF THE URETEROPELVIC JUNCTION

In children, primary obstruction of the ureter usually occurs at the ureteropelvic junction or the ureterovesical junction (Figure 35–8). Obstruction of the ureteropelvic junction is probably the most common congenital abnormality of the ureter. It is seen more often in boys than in girls (5:2 ratio) and, in unilateral cases, more often on the left than on the right side (5:2 ratio). Bilateral obstruction occurs in 10–15% of cases and is especially common in infants (Johnston et al, 1977). The abnormality may occur in several members of the same family, but it shows no clear genetic pattern.

The exact cause of obstruction of the ureteropelvic junction often is not clear. Ureteral polyps and valves have been reported but are very rare (Punjani, 1983; Sant, Barbalias, and Klauber, 1985). There is almost always an angulation and kink at the junction of the dilated renal pelvis and ureter. This by itself can cause obstruction, but it is unclear whether this is primary or merely secondary to another obstructive lesion. True stenosis is found rarely; however, a thin-walled, hypoplastic proximal ureter is observed frequently. Characteristic histologic and ultrastructural changes are ob-

Figure 35–8. Congenital ureteral obstruction. **Left:** Right ureteropelvic junction obstruction with hydronephrosis. **Right:** Left ureterovesical junction obstruction (obstructed megaureter) with hydroureteronephrosis.

served in this area and could account for abnormal peristalsis through the ureteropelvic junction and consequent interference with pelvic emptying (Hanna et al, 1976). Two other findings sometimes seen at operation are a high origin of the ureter from the renal pelvis and an abnormal relationship of the proximal ureter to a lower-pole renal artery. It is debatable whether these findings are the result or the cause of pelvic dilatation, but Stephens (1982) has suggested that abnormal rotation of the renal pelvis allows the ureter to become entrapped in the blood vessels of the lower pole of the kidney, ultimately leading to obstruction. Using careful studies at the time of operation, it is possible to define whether the principal lesion is intrinsic or extrinsic (Koff et al, 1986; Johnston, 1969).

Clinical findings vary depending on the patient's age at diagnosis. Recent improvements in prenatal ultrasonography now allow most cases to be diagnosed in utero (Mandell et al, 1991). Later, pain and vomiting are the most common symptoms; however, hematuria and urinary infection also may be seen. A few patients

have complications such as calculi (Figure 35–9), trauma to the enlarged kidney, or (rarely) hypertension.

The diagnosis is made most often by sonography. In equivocal cases, diuretic renography or (rarely) antegrade urography with pressure-flow studies is helpful (Thrall, Koff, and Keyes, 1981; Whitaker, 1973). Many surgeons consider a voiding cystourethrogram a routine part of the preoperative workup, since radiographic findings in vesicoureteral reflux may be similar to those in ureteropelvic junction obstruction. This fact is especially relevant when the ureter is well seen or dilated (or both) below the ureteropelvic junction (Maizels, Smith, and Firlit, 1984).

Symptomatic obstruction of the ureteropelvic junction should be treated surgically. Because most cases are now detected by hydronephrosis on prenatal ultrasonography and the infants are asymptomatic, it becomes important to assess the significance of the hydronephrosis. On the one hand, early surgery may prevent future urinary tract infections, stones, or other complications; on the other hand, many of the patients could live their

Figure 35–9. Ureteropelvic junction obstruction with calculi. **Upper left:** Plain film of abdomen shows radiopacities in region of right kidney. **Bottom left:** Early film from excretory urogram demonstrates dilation of calyces on right and layering of calculi in large right renal pelvis. **Bottom Right:** Delayed film from excretory urogram shows a typical right ureteropelvic junction obstruction.

whole lives without experiencing a consequence of the hydronephrosis. This remains an area of considerable controversy. Early surgery is recommended for patients who have kidneys with diminished function, massive hydronephrosis, infection, or stones. Nonoperative surveillance with good follow-up is thought to be safe (Onen et al, 2002), although about 25% of patients will ultimately require an operative repair for pain, urinary infection, or reduced renal function on repeat nuclear scan (Palmer et al, 1998). This subject remains particularly controversial (Peters, 2002).

Because of anatomic variations, no single procedure is sufficient for all situations (Smart, 1979). Regardless of the technique used, all successful repairs have in common the creation of a dependent and funnel-shaped ureteropelvic junction of adequate caliber. Although preservation of the intact ureteropelvic junction is feasible in some circumstances (Perlberg and Pfau, 1984), when the obstruction appears to be caused by a dyskinetic segment of proximal ureter, the most popular operation is a dismembered pyeloureteroplasty (Anderson, 1963). Dismembered pyeloureteroplasty is also favored when the proximal ureter is hooked over a lower-pole blood vessel. When there is a dilated extrarenal renal pelvis, dismembered pyeloureteroplasty can be combined with a Foley Y-V plasty to create a more funnel-shaped ureteropelvic junction (Foley, 1937). Pelvic flap procedures (Culp and DeWeerd, 1951; Scardino and Prince, 1953) are suited ideally to cases in which the ureteropelvic junction has remained in a dependent position despite significant pelvic dilation. They also have the advantage of interfering less with the ureteral blood supply; this is particularly relevant when distal ureteral surgery (eg, ureteral reimplantation) is contemplated in the future. In most centers, the dismembered pyeloureteroplasty is the mainstay of repairs.

Both the Y-V plasty and the flap techniques are useful in managing ureteropelvic junction obstructions in horseshoe or pelvic kidneys, in which the anatomy may prevent creation of a dependent ureteropelvic junction if a dismembered technique is attempted. The use of stenting catheters and proximal diversion at the time of pyeloplasty has been the subject of debate, and the issue has not been resolved. Excellent results have been reported both with and without stents and diversions (Smith et al, 2002).

The prognosis is generally good. In several large series, the reported reoperation rate has been only 2–4%, but the postoperative radiographic appearance of the area may be disappointing. There can be marked improvement when a large extrarenal renal pelvis has prevented massive calyceal distortion; however, in most cases considerable deformity persists despite adequate drainage of the kidney. Furthermore, it is usually many years before the radiographic appearance improves (Amling et al, 1996).

The recent explosion in the field of endourology as a subspecialty of urology has encouraged use of percutaneous techniques for the repair of ureteropelvic junction obstruction in selected patients (Ramsay et al, 1984; Badlani, Eshghi, and Smith, 1986; Van Cangh et al, 1989). The technique is similar to that reported by Davis (1943) but is done entirely endoscopically. The technique may be applied antegrade, via a nephrostomy tract, or retrograde, using either a ureteroscope (for direct vision) or an Acusize (Applied Urology, Laguna Beach, Calif.) balloon catheter with fluoroscopic visualization. In adults the procedure is clearly an option, with an anticipated success rate of 80–85% and a marked reduction in morbidity (Aslan and Preminger, 1998). In children, retrograde endopyelotomy also has an 85% success rate, but this is still considerably less than 98% and the benefit in terms of reduced morbidity is less significant (Bogaert et al, 1996). An intriguing new option that is becoming commonplace in some centers is laparoscopic pyeloplasty (Moore et al, 1997; Yeung et al, 2001).

OBSTRUCTED MEGAURETER

Obstruction at the ureterovesical junction is 4 times more common in boys than in girls. It may be bilateral and is usually asymmetric. The left ureter is slightly more often involved than the right.

The embryogenesis of the lesion is uncertain. It is clear that in most cases there is no stricture at the ureterovesical junction. At operation, a retrograde catheter or probe can usually be passed through the area of obstruction. Close observation either at operation or by fluoroscopy reveals a failure of the distal ureter to transmit the normal peristaltic wave, resulting in a functional obstruction. Moreover, on fluoroscopy, retrograde peristalsis is seen. This transmits abnormal pressures up to the kidney, resulting in calyceal dilation out of proportion with the renal pelvic dilation. Histologic findings include an excess of circular muscle fibers and collagen in the distal ureter that may account for the problem (Tanagho, Smith, and Guthrie, 1970). Ultrastructural studies show that this obstruction is similar in appearance to obstruction of the ureteropelvic junction.

Currently, most cases are discovered on prenatal sonography; however, a few come to light because of hematuria or infection. Sonography usually shows the pathognomonic configuration of a dilated distal ureter, a less dilated proximal ureter, a relatively normal-appearing renal pelvis, and calyces blunted out of proportion to the renal pelvis (Figure 35–10).

It was assumed previously that surgery was indicated in most cases. Ureteral reimplantation with excision of the distal ureter is curative. Because of the excessive

Figure 35–10. Obstructed megaureter. Follow-up study in a 9-month-old boy with unilateral hydronephrosis detected by ultrasonography in utero. Excretory urogram shows the classic configuration of a dilated distal ureter, a less dilated proximal ureter, and blunted calyces.

dilation of the ureter, ureteral tapering or folding may be necessary (Hendren, 1969; Hanna, 1982; Ehrlich, 1985). Because the ureteral muscle is generally healthy, these cases have an excellent prognosis (Peters et al, 1989). However, in recent years it has become obvious that at least 50% of cases will have spontaneous resolution. A period of observation is nearly always appropriate when the diagnosis is made in an asymptomatic patient (Baskin et al, 1994). Because of the high risk of infection, 1–2 years of prophylactic antibiotics are recommended in neonates.

UPPER URINARY TRACT DILATATION WITHOUT OBSTRUCTION

It should not be assumed that every dilated upper urinary tract is obstructed. A voiding cystourethrogram is an essential part of the evaluation, not only to rule out reflux but also to ensure that no abnormality of the lower urinary tract is responsible for the upper urinary

tract dilatation. Other cases in which diagnosis may be difficult include residual dilatation in a previously obstructed system, dilatation associated with bacterial infection (presumably related to a direct effect of endotoxin on the ureteral musculature), neonatal hydronephrosis (Homsy, Williot, and Danais, 1986), and prolonged polyuria in patients with diabetes insipidus.

In such cases, the usual investigations may not provide sufficient information. A radionuclide diuretic renogram is especially helpful in distinguishing nonobstructive from obstructive dilation and in determining whether renal functional injury has occurred (Figure 35–11) (Thrall, Koff, and Keyes, 1981). However, the procedure must be performed carefully, as technical problems may confuse the results (Nguyen et al, 1997; Gungor et al, 2002). Use of percutaneous renal puncture is occasionally beneficial; in the dilated system, it carries minimal risk, making antegrade urography and pressure-flow studies feasible in selected cases. Measurement of the renal pelvic pressure during infusion of saline into the renal pelvis at high rates (10 mL/min) (**the Whitaker test**) may help differentiate nonobstructive from obstructive dilation (Wolk and Whitaker, 1982). Unfortunately, there is no true "gold standard," and these studies do not always agree; clinical judgment is the final arbiter (Lupton et al, 1985).

ACQUIRED DISEASES OF THE URETER

Nearly all acquired diseases of the ureter are obstructive in nature. Although they are seen frequently, their actual incidence is unknown. Their clinical manifestations, effects on the kidney, complications, and treatment are similar to those described previously. The lesions can be broadly categorized as either intrinsic or extrinsic.

Intrinsic Ureteral Obstruction

The most common causes of intrinsic ureteral obstruction are as follows:

(1) Ureteral stones (see Chapter 16).
(2) Transitional cell tumors of the ureter (see Chapter 20).
(3) Chronic inflammatory changes of the ureteral wall (usually due to tuberculosis or schistosomiasis) leading to contracture or insufficient peristalsis (see Chapter 14 and Figures 14–2 and 14–4).

Extrinsic Ureteral Obstruction

The most frequent causes of extrinsic ureteral obstruction are:

(1) Severe constipation, sometimes with bladder obstruction, seen primarily in children but in adult women as well.

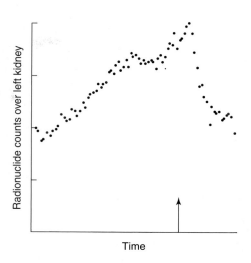

Figure 35–11. Upper urinary tract dilatation. **Left:** Three months after resection of posterior urethral valves, hydronephrosis in the right kidney has completely resolved. The left collecting system remains dilated. (Dashed lines outline kidneys.) **Right:** Radionuclide diuretic renography was performed to determine if there was secondary ureteropelvic or ureterovesical obstruction. Renogram demonstrates clear-cut "washout" of radionuclide following injection of furosemide (arrow). There is no significant obstruction.

(2) Secondary obstruction due to kinks or fibrosis around redundant ureters. The primary process is either distal obstruction or massive reflux.

(3) Benign gynecologic disorders such as endometriosis or right ovarian vein syndrome (Gourdie and Rogers, 1986).

(4) Local neoplastic infiltration associated with carcinoma of the cervix, bladder, or prostate (Richie, Withers, and Ehrlich, 1979).

(5) Pelvic lymphadenopathy associated with metastatic tumors.

(6) Iatrogenic ureteral injuries, primarily after extensive pelvic surgery (Figure 35–12) and also after extensive radiotherapy.

(7) Retroperitoneal fibrosis.

RETROPERITONEAL FIBROSIS (Retroperitoneal Fasciitis, Chronic Retroperitoneal Fibroplasia, Ormond Disease)

One or both ureters may be compressed by a chronic inflammatory process that involves the retroperitoneal tissues over the lower lumbar vertebrae. There are numerous causes of retroperitoneal fibrosis. Malignant diseases (most commonly Hodgkin's disease, carcinoma of the breast, and carcinoma of the colon) should always be suspected and ruled out. Some medications have been implicated, most notably methysergide (Sansert), an ergot derivative used to treat migraine headaches. Rarely, membranous glomerulonephritis (Shirota et al, 2002), inflammatory bowel disease (Siminovitch and Fazio, 1980) or an aortic aneurysm (Brock and Soloway, 1980; Peters and Cowie, 1978) is responsible. The remainder of cases are idiopathic, a condition sometimes referred to as Ormond disease.

The symptoms are nonspecific and include low back pain, malaise, anorexia, weight loss, and, in severe cases, uremia. Infection is uncommon. The diagnosis is usually made by excretory urography (Figure 35–13). There is medial deviation of the ureters with proximal dilation. A long segment of ureter is usually involved, and in some cases there is a pipestem appearance caused by aperistalsis related to the fibrosis. A retrograde ureterogram is necessary when renal function is poor and, in any case, helps to delineate the length of the affected segment of ureter. Ultrasonography is useful, not only for diagnosis but also for monitoring the response

Figure 35–12. Ureteral obstruction. Excretory urogram obtained 2 weeks after Wertheim operation shows bilateral ureteral obstruction and marked hydronephrosis on right.

Figure 35–13. Retroperitoneal fibrosis. Right and left kidneys of same patient as shown by excretory urography. Note medial deviation of upper portions of ureters (arrows) with marked obstruction. (Courtesy of JA Hutch.)

to therapy. Computed tomography scanning or magnetic resonance imaging is essential for evaluating the retroperitoneum itself, as well as for imaging the ureters (Hricak, Higgins, and Williams, 1983). Recently, positron emission tomography scanning has been advocated (Cheung et al, 2002).

Spontaneous regression has been reported (Kume and Kitamura, 2001); however, treatment is usually surgical. A course of corticosteroids may be tried first and in an occasional series, remarkable success has been reported (Kardar et al, 2002). When the response to corticosteroids is poor or the obstruction is severe, the ureter must be dissected surgically from the fibrous plaque. After it is freed, it should either be placed intraperitoneally or wrapped in omentum in an attempt to prevent recurrence (Lepor and Walsh, 1979). Rarely, autotransplantation is necessary (Deane, Gingell, and Pentlow, 1983). Numerous biopsies of the fibrous tissue should be obtained at the time of operation to determine whether there is a malignant tumor.

URETERAL OBSTRUCTION SECONDARY TO MALIGNANT DISEASE

Ureteral obstruction associated with widespread malignant disease was at one time a terminal event. Because therapy for malignant diseases has improved, however, urinary diversion is indicated more frequently in such cases. Diversion usually is necessary for relatively short periods of time; either the tumor is progressive, or if therapy is effective, the obstruction resolves. Thus, the goal of treatment is to leave the urinary tract intact and effect as little morbidity as possible. This can be accomplished with indwelling stents passed either retrogradely during cystoscopy (Hepperlen, Mardis, and Kammandel, 1979) or antegradely using percutaneous techniques (Elyaderani et al, 1982).

REFERENCES

Congenital Anomalies

General

Glassberg KI et al: Suggested terminology for duplex systems, ectopic ureters and ureteroceles. J Urol 1984;132:1153.

Ureteral Atresia

Brophy PD et al: Regulation of ureteric bud outgrowth by Pax2-dependent activation of the glial derived neurotrophic factor gene. Development 2001;128:4747.

Homsy Y et al: Wilms tumor and multicystic kidney disease. J Urol 1997;158:2256.

Javadpour N et al: Hypertension in a child caused by a multicystic kidney. J Urol 1970;104:918.

Rottenberg G, Gordon I, DeBruyn R: The natural history of the multicystic dysplastic kidney in children. Br J Radiol 1997; 70:347.

Selzman A, Elder J: Contralateral vesicoureteral reflux in children with a multicystic kidney. J Urol 1995;113:1252.

Tang MJ et al: Ureteric bud outgrowth in response to RET activation is mediated by phosphatidylinositol 3-kinase. Dev Biol 2002;243:128.

Yoshida T, Sakamoto K: Bilateral blind-ending duplex ureters. Br J Urol 1986;58:459.

Duplication of the Ureter

Amar AD: Ipsilateral ureteroureterostomy for single ureteral disease in patients with ureteral duplication: A review of 8 years of experience with 16 patients. J Urol 1978;119:472.

Amar AD: Ureteropyelostomy for relief of single ureteral obstruction in cases of ureteral duplication. Arch Surg 1970;101: 379.

Atwell JD et al: Familial incidence of bifid and double ureters. Arch Dis Child 1974;49:390.

Barrett DM, Malek RS, Kelalis PP: Problems and solutions in surgical treatment of 100 consecutive ureteral duplications in children. J Urol 1975;114:126.

Belman AB, Filmer RB, King LR: Surgical management of duplication of the collecting system. J Urol 1974;112:316.

Bieri M et al: Ipsilateral ureteroureterostomy for single ureteral reflux or obstruction in a duplicate system. J Urol 1998;159: 1016.

Carter C, Malone P, Lewington V: Lower moiety heminephroureterectomy in the duplex refluxing kidney: The accuracy of isotopic scintigraphy in functional assessment. Br J Urol 1998;81:356.

Decter RM: Renal duplication and fusion anomalies. Pediatr Clin North Am 1997;44:1323.

Lee PH et al: Duplex reflux: A study of 105 children. J Urol 1991; 146:657.

Nation EF: Duplication of the kidney and ureter: A statistical study of 230 new cases. J Urol 1944;51:456.

O'Reilly PH et al: Ureteroureteric reflux: Pathologic entity or physiological phenomenon? Br J Urol 1984;56:159.

Sole GM, Randall J, Arkell DG: Ureteropyelostomy: A simple and effective treatment for symptomatic ureteroureteric reflux. Br J Urol 1987;60:325.

Tanagho EA: Embryologic basis for lower ureteral anomalies: A hypothesis. Urology 1976;7:451.

Ureterocele

Ahmed S: Prolapsed single system ureterocele in a girl. J Urol 1984; 132:1180.

Bauer SB, Retik AB: The non-obstructive ectopic ureterocele. J Urol 1978;119:804.

Blyth B et al: Endoscopic incision of ureteroceles: Intravesical versus ectopic. J Urol 1993;149:556.

Caldamone AA, Snyder HM III, Duckett JW: Ureteroceles in children: Follow-up of management with upper tract approach. J Urol 1984;131:1130.

Coplen DE: Management of the neonatal ureterocele. Curr Urol Rep 2001;2:102.

Geringer AM et al: The diagnostic approach to ectopic ureterocele and the renal duplication complex. J Urol 1983;129:539.

Gloor JM, Ogburn P, Matsumoto J: Prenatally diagnosed ureterocele presenting as fetal bladder outlet obstruction. J Perinatol 1996;16:285.

Husmann DA et al: Ureterocele associated with ureteral duplication and a nonfunctioning upper pole segment: Management by partial nephroureterectomy alone. J Urol 1995;154:723.

Pfister C et al: The value of endoscopic treatment for ureteroceles during the neonatal period. J Urol 1998;159:1006.

Snyder HM, Johnston JH: Orthotopic ureteroceles in children. J Urol 1978;119:543.

Tanagho EA: Embryologic basis for lower ureteral anomalies: A hypothesis. Urology 1976;7:451.

Upadhyay J et al: Impact of prenatal diagnosis on the morbidity associated with ureterocele management. J Urol 2002;167: 2560.

Ectopic Ureteral Orifice

Borer JG et al: A single-system ectopic ureter draining an ectopic dysplastic kidney: Delayed diagnosis in the young female with continuous urinary incontinence. Br J Urol 1998;81: 474.

Brophy PD et al: Regulation of ureteric bud outgrowth by Pax2-dependent activation of the glial derived neurotrophic factor gene. Development 2001;128:4747.

Gotoh T et al: Single ectopic ureter. J Urol 1983;129:271.

Johnson DK, Perlmutter S: Single system ectopic ureteroceles. J Urol 1980;123:81.

Tang M et al: Ureteric bud outgrowth in response to RET activation is mediated by phosphatidylinositol 3-kinase. Dev Biol 2002;243:128.

Umeyama T et al: Ectopic ureter presenting with epididymitis in childhood: Report of 5 cases. J Urol 1985;134:131.

Abnormalities of Ureteral Position

Polascik TJ, Chen RN: Laparoscopic ureteroureterostomy for retrocaval ureter. J Urol 1998;160:121.

Obstruction of the Ureteropelvic Junction

Amling CL et al: Renal ultrasound changes after pyeloplasty in children with ureteropelvic junction obstruction: Long-term outcome in 47 renal units. J Urol 1996;156:2020.

Anderson JC: *Hydronephrosis.* Heinemann, 1963.

Aslan P, Preminger GM: Retrograde balloon cautery incision of ureteropelvic junction obstruction. Urol Clin North Am 1998;25:295.

Badlani G, Eshghi M, Smith AD: Percutaneous surgery for uretero-pelvic junction obstruction (endopyelotomy): Technique and early results. J Urol 1986;135:26.

Bogaert GA et al: Efficacy of retrograde endopyelotomy in children. J Urol 1996;156:734.

Culp OS, DeWeerd JH: A pelvic flap operation for certain types of ureteropelvic obstruction. Mayo Clin Proc 1951;26:483.

Davis DM: Intubated ureterotomy: A new operation for ureteral and ureteropelvic strictures. Surg Gynecol Obstet 1943;76: 513.

Foley FEB: A new plastic operation for stricture at the ureteropelvic junction. J Urol 1937;38:643.

Hanna MK et al: Ureteral structure and ultrastructure. 1. The normal human ureter. 2. Congenital ureteropelvic junction obstruction and primary obstructive megaureter. J Urol 1976; 116:718, 725.

Johnston JH: The pathogenesis of hydronephrosis in children. Br J Urol 1969;41:724.

Johnston JH et al: Pelvic hydronephrosis in children: A review of 219 personal cases. J Urol 1977;117:97.

Koff SA, Campbell K: Nonoperative management of unilateral neonatal hydronephrosis. J Urol 1992;148:525.

Koff SA et al: Pathophysiology of ureteropelvic junction obstruction: Experimental and clinical observations. J Urol 1986; 136:336.

Maizels M, Smith CK, Firlit CF: The management of children with vesicoureteral reflux and ureteropelvic junction obstruction. J Urol 1984;131:722.

Mandell J et al: Structural genitourinary defects detected in utero. Radiology 1991;178:193.

Moore RG et al: Laparoscopic pyeloplasty: Experience with the initial 30 cases. J Urol 1997;157:459.

Onen A et al: Long-term followup of prenatally detected severe bilateral newborn hydronephrosis initially managed nonoperatively. J Urol 2002;168:1118.

Palmer LS et al: Surgery versus observation for managing obstructive grade 3 to 4 unilateral hydronephrosis: A report from the Society for Fetal Urology. J Urol 1998;159:222.

Perlberg S, Pfau A: Management of ureteropelvic junction obstruction associated with lower polar vessels. Urology 1984;23:13.

Peters CA: Editorial: The long-term followup of prenatally detected severe bilateral newborn hydronephrosis initially managed nonoperatively. J Urol 2002;168:1121.

Punjani HM: Transitional cell papilloma of the ureter causing hydronephrosis in a child. Br J Urol 1983;55:572.

Ramsay JWA et al: Percutaneous pyelolysis: Indications, complications and results. Br J Urol 1984;56:586.

Sant GR, Barbalias GA, Klauber GT: Congenital ureteral valves: An abnormality of ureteral embryogenesis? J Urol 1985;133: 427.

Scardino PL, Prince CL: Vertical flap ureteropelvioplasty. South Med J 1953;46:325.

Smart WR: Surgical correction of hydronephrosis. In: Harrison JH et al (editors): *Campbell's Urology*, vol. 3. Saunders, 1979.

Smith KE et al: Stented versus nonstented pediatric pyeloplasty: A modern series and review of the literature. J Urol 2002;168: 1127.

Stephens FD: Ureterovascular hydronephrosis and the "aberrant" renal vessels. J Urol 1982;128:984.

Thrall JH, Koff SA, Keyes JW Jr: Diuretic radionuclide renography and scintigraphy in the differential diagnosis of hydro-ureteronephrosis. Semin Nucl Med 1981;11:89.

Van Cangh PJ et al: Endoureteropyelotomy: Percutaneous treatment of ureteropelvic junction obstruction. J Urol 1989;141: 1317.

Whitaker RH: Methods of assessing obstruction in dilated ureters. Br J Urol 1973;45:15.

Yeung CK et al: Retroperitoneoscopic dismembered pyeloplasty for pelvi-ureteric junction obstruction in infants and children. BJU Int 2001;87:509.

Obstructed Megaureter

Baskin LS et al: Primary dilated megaureter: Long-term followup. J Urol 1994;152:618.

Ehrlich RM: The ureteral folding technique for megaureter surgery. J Urol 1985;134:668.

Hanna MK: Recent advances and further experience with surgical techniques for one-stage total remodeling of massively dilated ureters. Urology 1982;19:495.

Hendren WH: Operative repair of megaureter in children. J Urol 1969;101:491.

Peters CA et al: Congenital obstructed megaureter in early infancy: Diagnosis and treatment. J Urol 1989;142:641.

Tanagho EA, Smith DR, Guthrie TH: Pathophysiology of functional ureteral obstruction. J Urol 1970;104:73.

Upper Urinary Tract Dilatation Without Obstruction

Gungor F et al: Effect of the size of regions of interest on the estimation of differential renal function in children with congenital hydronephrosis. Nucl Med Commun 2002;23:147.

Homsy YL, Williot P, Danais S: Transitional neonatal hydronephrosis: Fact or fantasy? J Urol 1986;136:339.

Lupton EW et al: A comparison of diuresis renography, the Whitaker test and renal pelvic morphology in idiopathic hydronephrosis. Br J Urol 1985;57:119.

Nguyen HT et al: Changing the technique of background subtraction alters calculated renal function on pediatric mercaptoacetyltriglycine renography. J Urol 1997;158:1252.

Thrall JH, Koff SA, Keyes JW Jr: Diuretic radionuclide renography and scintigraphy in the differential diagnosis of hydroureteronephrosis. Semin Nucl Med 1981;11:89.

Wolk FN, Whitaker RH: Late follow-up of dynamic evaluation of upper urinary tract obstruction. J Urol 1982;128:346.

Acquired Diseases

General

Gourdie RW, Rogers ACN: Bilateral ureteric obstruction due to endometriosis presenting with hypertension and cyclical oliguria. Br J Urol 1986;58:244.

Richie JP, Withers G, Ehrlich RM: Ureteral obstruction secondary to metastatic tumors. Surg Gynecol Obstet 1979;148:355.

Retroperitoneal Fibrosis

Brock J, Soloway MS: Retroperitoneal fibrosis and aortic aneurysm. Urology 1980;15:14.

Cheung WS et al: Ormond's disease: Appearance in [F-18]FDG PET imaging. Nuklearmedizin 2002;41:N44.

Deane AM, Gingell JC, Pentlow BD: Idiopathic retroperitoneal fibrosis: The role of autotransplantation. Br J Urol 1983; 55:254.

Hricak H, Higgins CB, Williams RD: Nuclear magnetic resonance imaging in retroperitoneal fibrosis. AJR 1983;141:35.

Kardar AH et al: Steroid therapy for idiopathic retroperitoneal fibrosis: Dose and duration. J Urol 2002;168:550.

Kume H, Kitamura T: Spontaneous regression of bilateral hydronephrosis due to retroperitoneal fibrosis. Scand J Urol Nephrol 2001;35:255.

Lepor H, Walsh PC: Idiopathic retroperitoneal fibrosis. J Urol 1979;122:1.

Peters JL, Cowie AG: Ureteric involvement with abdominal aortic aneurysm. Br J Urol 1978;50:313.

Shirota S et al: Retroperitoneal fibrosis associated with membranous nephropathy effectively treated with steroids. Intern Med 2002;41:20.

Siminovitch JM, Fazio VW: Ureteral obstruction secondary to Crohn's disease: A need for ureterolysis? Am J Surg 1980; 139:95.

Ureteral Obstruction Secondary to Malignant Disease

Andriole GL et al: Indwelling double-J ureteral stents for temporary and permanent urinary drainage: Experience with 87 patients. J Urol 1984;131:239.

Ball AJ et al: The indwelling ureteric stent: The Bristol experience. Br J Urol 1983;55:622.

Elyaderani MK et al: Facilitation of difficult percutaneous ureteral stent insertion. J Urol 1982;128:1173.

Hepperlen TW, Mardis HK, Kammandel H: The pigtail ureteral stent in the cancer patient. J Urol 1979;121:17.

Disorders of the Bladder, Prostate, & Seminal Vesicles

36

Emil A. Tanagho, MD

■ CONGENITAL ANOMALIES OF THE BLADDER

EXSTROPHY

Exstrophy of the bladder is a complete ventral defect of the urogenital sinus and the overlying skeletal system (see Chapter 2). Other congenital anomalies are frequently associated with it. The lower central abdomen is occupied by the inner surface of the posterior wall of the bladder, whose mucosal edges are fused with the skin. Urine spurts onto the abdominal wall from the ureteral orifices.

The rami of the pubic bones are widely separated. The pelvic ring thus lacks rigidity, the femurs are rotated externally, and the child "waddles like a duck." Since the rectus muscles insert on the rami, they are widely separated from each other inferiorly. A hernia, made up of the exstrophic bladder and surrounding skin, is therefore present. Epispadias almost always accompanies it.

Many untreated exstrophic bladders reveal fibrosis, derangement of the muscularis mucosae, and chronic infection. These changes tend to defeat efforts to form a bladder of proper capacity. About 60 instances of adenocarcinoma developing in such bladders have been reported.

Renal infection is common, and hydronephrosis caused by ureterovesical obstruction may be found on urography. These films also reveal separation of the pubic bones.

During the last few years, there have been encouraging reports of complete reconstruction of this defect. Earlier, urinary diversion and resection of the bladder, with later repair of the epispadiac penis, was usually accomplished. With improved techniques and early surgery before the bladder deteriorates, however, good results are being obtained with complete reconstruction. Lattimer et al (1978), pioneers in this field, followed up their 17 patients with reconstructed bladders for as long as 20 years. They reported that the quality of life of these patients was good.

Ansel (1979) performed reconstruction in 28 patients in the neonatal period in an attempt to protect the bladder from later serious changes. Half of these patients did well, and most were continent. DeMaria et al (1980) found the renal function and urine cultures of their patients to be normal. Eight of their patients had complete continence, while 12 had enuresis. Toguri et al (1978) reported that all of their 23 patients were continent.

Lima et al (1981) reconstructed the bladder with human dura mater to increase vesical capacity; they were successful in 8 cases. They perform osteotomy as part of the first stage and recommend that the surgery be performed when patients are 3–18 months old. Enterocystoplasty is currently the method of choice to augment bladder capacity and aid reservoir function. Mollard (1980) recommends the following steps for satisfactory repair of bladder exstrophy: (1) bladder closure with sacral osteotomy in order to close the pelvic ring at the pubic symphysis, plus lengthening of the penis; (2) antiureteral reflux procedure and bladder neck reconstruction; and (3) repair of the epispadiac penis. He completed 16 such 3-step procedures, with satisfactory results in 11. In 1983 and 1989, respectively, Jeffs and Gearhart reported results of staged reconstruction: 86% of patients who underwent primary repair were continent, and renal function was preserved in approximately 90%. Urethral and genital reconstruction have been equally successful. These are the best reported results. In small-capacity bladders, augmentation cystoplasty might be needed (Oesterling and Jeffs, 1987; Gearhart and Jeffs, 1988; Gearhart, 1999).

When the bladder is small, fibrotic, and inelastic, functional closure becomes inadvisable, and urinary diversion with cystectomy is the treatment of choice. Some physicians perform ureteroileocutaneous anastomosis, while others prefer to use the colon for the diversion. A continent reservoir is a current consideration and is preferable. Spence, Hoffman, and Pate (1975) employ ureterosigmoidostomy. Turner, Ransley, and Williams (1980) noted that, although untreated newborns have normal upper urinary tracts, urinary diversion often causes hydronephrosis or pyelonephritis in these patients.

The common complication of total reconstruction is urinary incontinence, but Light and Scott (1983) reported on the implantation of an artificial sphincter in 11 patients who were still incontinent after total reconstruction. They claimed 10 perfect results. Ikeme (1981) reported on 2 patients who became pregnant after repair of bladder exstrophy; one woman had 3 successful pregnancies, and the other had one. Complete primary closure appears to be the best choice for improved continence with reduced morbidity (Grady, Carr, and Mitchell, 1999).

PERSISTENT URACHUS

Embryologically, the allantois connects the urogenital sinus with the umbilicus. Normally, the allantois is obliterated and is represented by a fibrous cord (urachus) extending from the dome of the bladder to the navel (see Chapter 2). Urachal formation is directly related to bladder descent. Lack of descent is more commonly associated with patent urachus than with bladder outlet obstruction.

Incomplete obliteration sometimes occurs. If obliteration is complete except at the superior end, a draining umbilical sinus may be noted. If it becomes infected, the drainage will be purulent. If the inferior end remains open, it will communicate with the bladder, but this does not usually produce symptoms. Rarely, the entire tract remains patent, in which case urine drains constantly from the umbilicus. This is apt to become obvious within a few days of birth. If only the ends of the urachus seal off, a cyst of that body may form and may become quite large, presenting a low midline mass (Figure 36–1). If the cyst becomes infected, signs of general and local sepsis will develop.

Adenocarcinoma may occur in a urachal cyst, particularly at its vesical extremity, and tends to invade the tissues beneath the anterior abdominal wall. It may be seen cystoscopically. Stones may develop in a cyst of the urachus. These can be identified on a plain x-ray film.

Treatment consists of excision of the urachus, which lies on the peritoneal surface. If adenocarcinoma is present, radical resection is required.

Unless other serious congenital anomalies are present, the prognosis is good. The complication of adenocarcinoma offers a poor prognosis.

CONTRACTURE OF THE BLADDER NECK

There is considerable debate about the incidence of congenital narrowing of the bladder neck. Some feel that its presence is a common cause of vesicoureteral reflux, vesical diverticula, a bladder of large capacity, and the syndrome of irritable bladder associated with enuresis. A few observers consider this contracture a rare phenomenon and believe that the diagnosis is purely presumptive. The diagnosis is based on endoscopic observation, which is an unreliable method. Voiding cystourethrography has been used to depict such narrowing, but interpretation of the films varies from urologist to urologist and radiologist to radiologist.

Nunn (1965) studied the intravesical and urethral pressures during voiding in patients with the signs mentioned previously and found no evidence of bladder neck obstruction. The 2 recorded pressures were essentially equal. It appears that the bladder neck would have to be extremely stenotic to truly obstruct urine flow. It is becoming increasingly clear that in young girls, the obstructive lesion is spasm of the periurethral striated muscle, which develops secondary to distal urethral stenosis (see Chapter 39).

Empirical treatment is often employed; this consists of suprapubic bladder neck revision or transurethral resection. Making the bladder neck incompetent in

Figure 36–1. Types of persistent urachus. **Left:** Communicating urachus continuous with the bladder. This is a "pseudodiverticulum" and usually causes no symptoms. **Center:** Urachal cyst; usually causes no symptoms or signs unless it becomes larger or infected. **Right:** Patent urachus. There is constant drainage of urine from the umbilicus.

young boys may cause later retrograde ejaculation and, therefore, infertility. Revision of the bladder neck in females may cause urinary incontinence and is never advised. The diagnosis must therefore be made with caution.

Genuine functional bladder neck obstruction can be detected only in the presence of already high voiding pressures combined with lower resistance in the external sphincteric segment associated with a low flow rate. This condition is highly suggestive of functional bladder neck obstruction, although not 100% diagnostic.

■ ACQUIRED DISEASES OF THE BLADDER

INTERSTITIAL CYSTITIS (HUNNER'S ULCER, SUBMUCOUS FIBROSIS)

Interstitial cystitis is primarily a disease of middle-aged women. It is characterized by fibrosis of the vesical wall, with consequent loss of bladder capacity. Frequency, urgency, and pelvic pain with bladder distention are the principal symptoms.

Pathogenesis & Pathology

Infection does not appear to be the cause of fibrosis of the bladder wall, because the urine is usually normal. It has been postulated that the fibrosis is due to obstruction of the vesical lymphatics secondary to pelvic surgery or infection, but many of these patients fail to give such a history. Fibrosis may be secondary to thrombophlebitis complicating acute infections of the bladder or pelvic organs; may be the result of prolonged intrinsic arteriolar spasm secondary to vasculitis or psychogenic impulses; or could be of neuropathic origin. Endocrinologic factors are also suggested. Investigators are currently studying the role of mast cells and bladder surface glycosaminoglycans (GAGs) in the pathogenesis of interstitial cystitis. Currently, it is believed that interstitial cystitis is a neuroimmunoendocrine disorder. It might be primarily a neurogenic inflammation that leads to the release of neuropeptides that activate the differential secretion of potent mast cell mediators. It is thought that mast cells, through their vasoactive and nociceptive secretions, have a major role in the etiology of interstitial cystitis.

The primary change is fibrosis in the deeper layers of the bladder. The capacity of the organ is decreased, sometimes markedly. The mucosa is thinned, especially where mobility is greatest as the bladder fills and emp-

ties (ie, over the dome), and small ulcers or cracks in the mucous membrane may be seen in this area. In the most severe cases, the normal mechanism of the ureterovesical junctions is destroyed, leading to vesicoureteral reflux. Hydroureteronephrosis and pyelonephritis may ensue.

Microscopically, the mucosa may be thinned or even denuded. The capillaries of the tunica propria are often engorged, and signs of inflammation are apparent. The muscle is replaced by varying amounts of fibrous tissue, which is often quite avascular. The lymphatics may be engorged. Increased mast cells and lymphocytic infiltration are seen.

There has been a tendency recently to overdiagnose interstitial cystitis, particularly in patients with excessive frequency, urgency, and suprapubic or pelvic pain, even though they lack the pathologic manifestations and usually have normal or large bladder capacity. These patients have voiding dysfunction. Although we may not know the exact cause of their symptoms, these patients should not be labeled as having interstitial cystitis and should not be treated as such.

Clinical Findings

Interstitial cystitis should be considered when a middle-aged woman with clear urine complains of severe frequency and nocturia and suprapubic pain on vesical distention.

A. Symptoms

There is a long history of slowly progressive frequency and nocturia, both of which may be severe. The history does not suggest infection (burning on urination, cloudy urine). Suprapubic pain is usually marked when the bladder is full. Pain may also be experienced in the urethra or perineum; it is relieved on voiding. Gross hematuria is occasionally noted, usually when urination has had to be postponed (ie, following vesical overdistention). The patient is tense and anxious. Whether the anxiety is secondary to the prolonged and severe symptoms or is the primary cause of the vesical changes is not clear. A history of allergy may be obtained.

B. Signs

Physical examination is usually normal. Some tenderness in the suprapubic area may be noted. There may be some tenderness in the region of the bladder when it is palpated through the vagina.

C. Laboratory Findings

If the patient has had no previous treatment (eg, instrumentation), the urine is almost always free of infection. Microscopic hematuria may be noted. Results of renal function tests are normal except in the occasional patient in whom vesical fibrosis has led to vesicoureteral reflux or obstruction.

D. X-Ray Findings

Excretory urograms are usually normal unless reflux has occurred, in which case hydronephrosis is found. The accompanying cystogram reveals a bladder of small capacity; reflux into a dilated upper tract may be noted on cystography.

E. Instrumental Examination

Cystoscopy is usually diagnostic. As the bladder fills, increasing suprapubic pain is experienced. The vesical capacity may be as low as 60 mL. In a patient not previously treated (by fulguration or hydraulic overdistention), the bladder lining may look fairly normal. However, if a second distention is done (Messing and Stamey, 1978), punctate hemorrhagic areas may appear over the most distensible portion of the wall. With further distention, an arcuate split in the mucosa will occur and may bleed profusely. Mucosal changes are usually diffuse. Congestion, edematous reaction, and petechial hemorrhages (glomerulation) are common findings.

Differential Diagnosis

Tuberculosis of the bladder may cause true ulceration but is most apt to involve the region of the ureteral orifice that drains the tuberculous kidney. Typical tubercles may be identified, pyuria is present, and tubercle bacilli usually can be found. Furthermore, urograms often show the typical lesion of renal tuberculosis.

Vesical ulcers due to schistosomiasis cause symptoms similar to those of interstitial cystitis. The diagnosis is suggested if the patient lives in an area in which schistosomiasis is endemic. Most patients are males. The typical ova found in the urine and the pathognomonic appearance of the bladder confirm the diagnosis.

Nonspecific vesical infection seldom causes ulceration. Pus and bacteria are found in the urine. Antimicrobial treatment is effective.

Complications

Gradual ureteral stenosis or reflux and its sequelae (eg, hydronephrosis) may develop.

Treatment

A. Specific Measures

There appears to be no definitive treatment for interstitial cystitis. The therapy usually employed frequently affords partial relief, but it may be completely ineffective.

Hydraulic overdistention, with or without anesthesia, sometimes gradually improves the bladder capacity. Vesical lavage with increasing strengths of silver nitrate (1:5000–1:100) may have the same effect. Superficial (transcystoscopic) electrocoagulation of the split mucosa is commonly performed and may afford temporary relief of pain.

Occasionally, symptomatic relief follows the instillation of 50 mL of 50% dimethyl sulfoxide (DMSO) into the bladder every 2 weeks. It is left in for 15 min.

Messing and Stamey (1978) claim their best results were obtained with vesical irrigations of 0.4% oxychlorosene sodium (Clorpactin WCS-90). At 10 cm of water pressure, the bladder is repeatedly filled to capacity until 1 L has been used. This must be done under anesthesia. Cystography should be done before instituting this therapy. The presence of vesicoureteral reflux has caused ureteral fibrosis.

Parsons, Schmidt, and Pollen (1983) observed the results obtained in patients who failed to respond to hydraulic distention or the instillation of DMSO. They found that the bladder mucosa needs a layer of sulfonated GAGs on its surface to protect the transitional cells from the effect of urine, and this substance was absent from the mucosa of these patients. They administered sodium pentosanpolysulfate (Elmiron) orally, in doses of either 50 mg 4 times a day or 150 mg twice daily, for 4–8 weeks. Of 24 patients, 20 noted at least 80% relief of urgency, frequency, and nocturia, and 2 noted 50–80% relief. These 22 patients continue to improve. Two patients experienced no apparent relief.

Cortisone acetate, 100 mg, or prednisone (Meticorten), 10–20 mg/d, in divided doses orally for 21 days, followed by decreasing amounts for an additional 21 days, has also been found effective. Transcystoscopic injection of the lesions with prednisone has its proponents.

Antihistamines (eg, tripelennamine [Pyribenzamine], 50 mg 4 times a day) may also afford some relief. Heparin sodium (long-acting), 20,000 units intravenously daily, also blocks the action of histamine, and its use in the treatment of interstitial cystitis is encouraging.

If the bladder becomes fibrotic and the capacity small, ceco- or ileocystoplasty can be done to augment vesical capacity. Most patients are cured or greatly improved; those who are not may require urinary diversion.

Denervation by presacral and sacral neurectomy and perivesical procedures (cystolysis, cystoplasty, transvaginal neurotomy) is to be condemned, as it is rarely of lasting benefit. In severe contracture, augmentation cystoplasty is indicated.

B. General Measures

General or vesical sedatives may be prescribed but seldom afford relief. If urinary infection is found (usually following instrumentation), it should be treated with appropriate antibiotics. If senile urethritis is discovered, diethylstilbestrol vaginal suppositories may prove helpful.

Prognosis

Most patients respond to one of the conservative measures mentioned previously. Those who do not may require surgery.

INTERNAL VESICAL HERNIATION

One side of the bladder may become involved in an inguinal hernia (in men) or a femoral hernia (in women) (Figure 36–2). Such a mass may recede on urination. It is most often found as a previously unsuspected complication during surgical correction of a hernia (Bell and Witherington, 1980). Weitzenfeld et al (1980) reported

a case in which the right kidney and ureter as well as the left ureter were in scrotal inguinal hernias.

URINARY INCONTINENCE

Partial or complete urinary incontinence may develop after prostatectomy, particularly radical or transurethral prostatectomy. Intrinsic damage to the smooth muscle urethral sphincter is implied. Although it is common to incriminate damage to or resection of the external voluntary sphincter, this is very rare. Such a patient can stop the voiding stream by contraction of the latter sphincter, but prolonged control is impossible because of fatigue of striated muscle. Only the smooth muscle with its constant tone can afford continence.

Scott, Bradley, and Timm (1974) and Light and Scott (1983) have described an ingenious method for affording urinary control by means of an artificial

Figure 36–2. Internal vesical hernia: Female, 6 months old. Cystogram of excretory urogram showing tongue of bladder in right femoral hernia (see arrows). (Courtesy of John A. Hutch.)

sphincter. It consists of a reservoir of fluid in a Silastic bag placed deep to the abdominal wall near the bladder and a collar of Silastic material that can encircle either the bladder neck or the bulbar urethra. The former is used in females, the latter in males. One Silastic bulb is implanted in one scrotal (or labial) sac. This bulb has a special pressurized valve that inflates or deflates the cuff around the urethra; compressed fluid passes from the cuff to the reservoir, permitting free voiding. The cuff refills spontaneously after a delay of 2 min. This device has been successful in affording control in most instances. Results are perfect in 75% or more of cases. Most failures follow technical difficulties with the prosthesis, for example, leakage, which requires reoperation.

Tanagho and Smith (1972) have designed a procedure based on sound anatomic principles that has been quite successful in restoring urinary continence. A rectangular flap of the heavy layer of the middle circular layer of the detrusor muscle, anteriorly, is formed into a tube, thus affording sphincteric action. This is anastomosed to the prostatic urethra. With this procedure, 44 of 50 patients who had post-prostatectomy incontinence were cured. Williams and Snyder (1976) have used this procedure successfully in children.

ENURESIS

Enuresis originally meant incontinence of urine, but usage has caused the term to be restricted to bedwetting after age 3 years. Most children have achieved normal bladder control by that time, girls earlier than boys. At age 6 years, 10% have enuresis. Even at age 14 years, 5% still wet the bed. It is difficult to be sure, but it seems that more than 50% of cases are caused by delayed maturation of the nervous system or an intrinsic myoneurogenic bladder dysfunction; 30% are of psychological origin; and 20% are secondary to more obvious organic disease. Most children with functional enuresis spontaneously gain nocturnal control by age 10 years. The current thinking is that children with enuresis have high nocturnal urine production; some have normal bladder capacity, others reduced capacity.

Psychodynamics

Training in bladder control should begin after age 1½ years; attempts made before this time are usually fruitless and may be harmful. If the parents fail in this teaching, the child may not develop cerebral inhibitory control over the infantile uninhibited bladder until much later in childhood. If the parents are emotionally unstable, their anxieties may be transmitted to the child, who may express tension through enuresis.

The birth of a sibling may cause loss of the child's paramount position in the family. The child may then regress to an infancy pattern in an attempt to recapture the parents' affection. An acute illness may be accompanied or followed by recurrence of incomplete nocturnal control. Physiologic or psychological stress (fear and anxiety) may reestablish an uninhibited bladder.

Possibly 40% of enuretic children have electroencephalograms that are borderline or compatible with epilepsy or delayed maturation of the central nervous system.

Clinical Findings

A. SYMPTOMS

A child may wet the bed occasionally or regularly. Careful questioning of the parents or observation by the physician reveals that the patient voids a free stream of normal caliber. This tends to rule out obstruction of the lower tract as a cause of the enuresis. Children with daytime incontinence are apt to have more than psychogenic enuresis. Many void frequently and are found to have a diminished vesical capacity, although capacity is normal under anesthesia. This is probably a reflection of delayed maturation. There is no burning, although frequency and urgency are common. The urine is clear.

Observation of the parents often reveals that they are anxious and tense, traits that can only be aggravated by the child's bedwetting.

B. SIGNS

General physical and urologic examinations are normal.

C. LABORATORY FINDINGS

In the emotional and delayed maturation groups, all tests, including urinalysis, are normal. An electroencephalogram may be abnormal, however.

D. X-RAY FINDINGS

Excretory urograms show no abnormality. The accompanying cystogram reveals no trabeculation; a film of the bladder taken immediately after voiding shows no residual urine.

E. INSTRUMENTAL EXAMINATION

A catheter of suitable size passes readily to the bladder, thereby ruling out stricture. If the catheter is passed after urination, no residual urine is found. Urethrocystoscopy is normal. Cystometric studies are usually abnormal, and a curve typical of the "uninhibited" (hyperirritable) neuropathic bladder is often obtained. Unless infection or some more obvious organic disease is discovered, instrumentation, x-ray, and urodynamic studies are not necessary. Genetic factors are currently considered the primary cause of enuresis.

Differential Diagnosis

A. OBSTRUCTION

Lower tract obstruction (eg, posterior urethral valves, meatal stenosis) causes a urinary stream of decreased caliber. Painful, frequent urination during the day and night, pyuria, and fever (eg, pyelonephritis) are often present, and the bladder may be distended. Urinalysis usually reveals evidence of infection. Anemia and impairment of renal function may be demonstrated.

Excretory urograms may show dilatation of the bladder and the upper urinary tract. Incomplete vesical emptying may be seen on the postvoiding film. Cystography may demonstrate distal urethral stenosis or reflux. Urethrocystoscopy reveals the organic cause.

Severe obstruction from severe spasm of the entire pelvic floor musculature on a psychosomatic basis can cause damage to the bladder and kidneys; infection is the rule.

B. INFECTION

Chronic urinary tract infection not due to obstruction usually produces frequency both day and night and pain on urination, although such infections may occur without symptoms of vesical irritability. Recurrent fever with exacerbations is common.

General examination may be normal. Anemia may be noted. Urinalysis shows pus cells or bacteria, or both. Renal function may be deficient. Excretory urograms may be essentially normal, although changes compatible with healed pyelonephritis are often seen. Cystoscopy shows the changes caused by infection. Urine specimens obtained by ureteral catheter may reveal renal infection. Cystography may show vesicoureteral reflux.

C. NEUROGENIC DISEASE

Children who have sacral cord or root abnormality (eg, myelodysplasia) may have incomplete urinary control both day and night. Since they ordinarily have significant amounts of residual urine, infection is usually found on urinalysis. The passage of a catheter or the postvoiding film taken in conjunction with excretory urograms demonstrates the presence of residual urine. A plain film of the abdomen may reveal spina bifida.

The cystometrogram is usually typical of a flaccid neurogenic bladder. Cystoscopy demonstrates an atonic bladder with moderate trabeculation and evidence of infection.

D. DISTAL URETHRAL STENOSIS

Distal urethral stenosis, a congenital anomaly, is the cause of enuresis in many young girls, even in the absence of cystitis. Urethral calibration establishes this diagnosis.

Complications

The complications of functional enuresis are psychological, not organic. These children are particularly disturbed when they begin to attend school; even more pressure is brought to bear by their parents. These children find it impossible to stay overnight at the homes of their playmates. Unhealthy introversion may be their lot. Enuresis may be prolonged because of undue emphasis on dryness or as a result of punitive or shaming measures.

Late Sequels

Occasionally an adult is seen who, under stress, develops nocturnal frequency without comparable diurnal frequency. Thorough urologic investigation proves to be negative. Many of these people give histories of enuresis of long duration in childhood. It is suggested that their cerebrovesical pathways again break down with excessive emotional tension; nocturnal frequency may be the adult expression of enuresis.

Treatment

Treatment should be considered if enuresis persists after age 3 years.

A. GENERAL MEASURES

Fluids should be limited after supper. The bladder should be completely emptied at bedtime, and the child should be completely awakened a little before the usual time of bedwetting and allowed to void.

Drug therapy has its proponents.

1. Imipramine has been reported to cure 50–70% of patients and is probably the drug of choice. The starting dose is 25 mg before dinner, which is increased as needed to 50 mg. Usually, 25 mg is sufficient.

2. Parasympatholytic drugs such as atropine or belladonna, by decreasing the tone of the detrusor, may at times be of value. Methantheline bromide, 25–75 mg at bedtime, is more potent.

3. Sympathomimetic drugs, for example, dextroamphetamine sulfate, 5–10 mg at bedtime, may cause enough wakefulness so that the child perceives the urge to void.

4. Desmopressin is an antidiuretic that increases renal reabsorption of water, reducing urine out-

put in patients with a decreased nocturnal peak in antidiuretic hormone. Given as a nasal spray by night, it has been successful in 70% of patients with increased nocturnal urine output.

5. Phenytoin has been found to control symptoms in some children whose electroencephalograms are abnormal.

The use of mechanical devices such as metal-covered pads that when wet cause an alarm to ring may be of benefit in cases of delayed maturation by setting up a conditioned reflex.

Urologic treatments (eg, urethral dilation, urethral instillations of silver nitrate), though often recommended, should be condemned in the absence of demonstrable local disease. They are physically and psychologically traumatic and can only cause further apprehension and fear in an already disturbed child.

B. Psychotherapy

Analytic evaluation and treatment may be indicated for some enuretic children and their parents. Responsibility for correction of the patient's feelings of insecurity rests with the parents, who must be cautioned not to punish the child or in any way increase existing feelings of guilt and insecurity. The handling of the parents may prove difficult, in which case psychiatric referral may be necessary.

Prognosis

Retraining the enuretic child and, above all, reeducating the parents are difficult and time-consuming tasks. Psychiatric referral for the parents and, at times, for the child may be necessary. Most patients conquer their enuresis by age 10 years. A few, however, do not, and they may later develop vesical irritability of the psychogenic type in response to acute or chronic tension or anxiety.

FOREIGN BODIES INTRODUCED INTO THE BLADDER & URETHRA

Numerous objects have been found in the urethra and bladder of both men and women. Some of them find their way into the urethra in the course of inquisitive self-exploration. Others are introduced (in the male) as contraceptive devices in the hope that plugging the urethra will block emission of the ejaculate.

The presence of a foreign body causes cystitis. Hematuria is not uncommon. Embarrassment may cause the victim to delay medical consultation. A plain x-ray of the bladder area discloses metal objects. Nonopaque objects sometimes become coated with calcium. Cystoscopy visualizes them all.

Cystoscopic or suprapubic removal of the foreign body is indicated. If not removed, the foreign body will lead to infection of the bladder. If the infecting organisms are urea-splitting, the alkaline urine (which causes increased insolubility of calcium salts) contributes to rapid formation of stone on the foreign object (Figure 16–13).

VESICAL MANIFESTATIONS OF ALLERGY

So many mucous membranes are affected by allergens that the possibility of allergic manifestations involving the bladder must be considered. Hypersensitivity is occasionally suggested in cases of recurrent symptoms of acute "cystitis" in the absence of urinary infection or other demonstrable abnormality. During the attack, general erythema of the vesical mucosa may be seen and some edema of the ureteral orifices noted.

A careful history may reveal that these attacks follow the ingestion of a food not ordinarily eaten (eg, fresh lobster). Sensitivity to spermicidal creams is occasionally observed. If vesical allergy is suspected, it may be aborted by the subcutaneous injection of 0.5–1 mL of 1:1000 epinephrine. Control may also be afforded by the use of one of the antihistamines. Skin testing has not generally proved helpful in determining the source of allergy.

DIVERTICULA

Most vesical diverticula are acquired and are secondary to either obstruction distal to the vesical neck or the upper motor neuron type of neurogenic bladder. Increased intravesical pressure causes vesical mucosa to insinuate itself between hypertrophied muscle bundles, so that a mucosal extravesical sac develops. Often this sac lies just superior to the ureter and causes vesicoureteral reflux (Hutch saccule; Figure 12–6). The diverticulum is devoid of muscle and therefore has no expulsive power; residual urine is the rule, and infection is perpetuated. If the diverticulum has a narrow opening that interferes with its emptying, transurethral resection of its neck will improve drainage. Carcinoma occasionally develops on its wall. Mićić and Ilić (1983) discovered 13 diverticula harboring malignant tumors: 9 transitional cell tumors, 2 squamous cell tumors, and 2 adenocarcinomas. Gerridzen and Futter (1982) saw 48 cases of vesical diverticula. Transitional cell tumors were found in 5 of these patients, but almost all the rest had abnormal histopathology: chronic inflammation and metaplasia. These authors stress the need for visualizing the interior of diverticula during endoscopy. At the time of open prostatectomy, resection of a diverticulum should be considered.

VESICAL FISTULAS

Vesical fistulas are common. The bladder may communicate with the skin, intestinal tract, or female reproductive organs. The primary disease is usually not urologic. The causes are as follows: (1) primary intestinal disease—diverticulitis, 50–60%; cancer of the colon, 20–25%; and Crohn disease, 10% (Badlani et al, 1980); (2) primary gynecologic disease—pressure necrosis during difficult labor; advanced cancer of the cervix; (3) treatment for gynecologic disease following hysterectomy, low cesarean section, or radiotherapy for tumor; and (4) trauma.

Malignant tumors of the small or large bowel, uterus, or cervix may invade and perforate the bladder. Inflammations of adjacent organs may also erode through the vesical wall. Severe injuries involving the bladder may lead to perivesical abscess formation, and these abscesses may rupture through the skin of the perineum or abdomen. The bladder may be inadvertently injured during gynecologic or intestinal surgery; cystotomy for stone or prostatectomy may lead to a persistent cutaneous fistula.

Clinical Findings

A. VESICOINTESTINAL FISTULA

Symptoms arising from a vesicointestinal fistula include vesical irritability, the passage of feces and gas through the urethra, and usually a change in bowel habits (eg, constipation, abdominal distention, diarrhea) caused by the primary intestinal disease. Signs of bowel obstruction may be elicited; abdominal tenderness may be found if the cause is inflammatory. The urine is always infected.

A barium enema, upper gastrointestinal series, or sigmoidoscopic examination may demonstrate the communication. Following a barium enema, centrifuged urine should be placed on an x-ray cassette and an exposure made. The presence of radiopaque barium establishes the diagnosis of vesicocolonic fistula. Cystograms may reveal gas in the bladder or reflux of the opaque material into the bowel (Figure 36–3). Cystoscopic examination, the most useful diagnostic procedure, shows a severe localized inflammatory reaction from which bowel contents may exude. Catheterization of the fistulous tract may be feasible; the instillation of radiopaque fluid often establishes the diagnosis.

B. VESICOVAGINAL FISTULA

This relatively common fistula is secondary to obstetric, surgical, or radiation injury or to invasive cancer of the cervix. The constant leakage of urine is most distressing to the patient. Pelvic examination usually reveals the fistulous opening, which also can be visualized with the cystoscope. It may be possible to pass a ureteral catheter through the fistula into the vagina. Vaginography often successfully shows ureterovaginal, vesicovaginal, and rectovaginal fistulas. A 30-mL Foley catheter is inserted into the vagina, and the balloon is distended. A radiopaque solution is then instilled, and appropriate x-rays are taken. Biopsy of the edges of the fistula may show carcinoma.

Differential Diagnosis

It is necessary to differentiate ureterovaginal from vesicovaginal fistula. Phenazopyridine (Pyridium) is given by mouth to color the urine orange. One hour later, 3 cotton pledgets are inserted into the vagina, and methylene blue solution is instilled into the bladder. The patient should then walk around, after which the pledgets are examined. If the proximal cotton ball is wet or stained orange, the fistula is ureterovaginal. If the deep cotton pledget contains blue fluid, the diagnosis is vesicovaginal fistula. If only the distal pledget is blue, the patient probably has urinary incontinence (Raghavaiah, 1974).

Treatment

A. VESICOINTESTINAL FISTULA

If the lesion is in the rectosigmoid, treatment consists of proximal colostomy. When the inflammatory reaction has subsided, the involved bowel may be resected, with closure of the opening in the bladder. The colostomy can be closed later. Some authors recommend that the entire procedure be performed in one stage, thus avoiding the need for preliminary colostomy. Small bowel or appendiceal vesical fistulas require bowel or appendiceal resection and closure of the vesical defect.

B. VESICOVAGINAL FISTULA

Tiny fistulous openings may become sealed following the introduction of an electrode into the fistula. As the electrode is withdrawn, the fistula is coagulated with the electrosurgical unit to destroy the epithelium of the tract. An indwelling catheter should be left in place for 2 weeks or more. Occasionally, good results are noted in cases of small vesicovaginal fistulas treated by inserting a metal screw through the vaginal end of the fistula. It is moved up and down to act as a curet. The vaginal mucosa is then closed and an indwelling catheter placed for 3 weeks.

Larger fistulas secondary to obstetric or surgical injuries respond readily to surgical repair, which may be

Figure 36–3. Vesical fistulas. **Above left:** Primary carcinoma of the sigmoid, with perforation through bladder wall. **Above right:** Injury to base of bladder following delivery by forceps. **Below:** Cystogram showing radiopaque fluid entering sigmoid containing multiple diverticula; right ureteral reflux, gallbladder calculi.

done either through the vagina or transvesically. Persky, Herman, and Guerrier (1979) advise repairing such fistulas immediately rather than waiting for 3–6 months as counseled by most surgeons. Fistulas that develop following radiation therapy for cancer of the cervix are much more difficult to close because of the avascularity of the tissues. Surgical closure of fistulas that arise from direct invasion of the bladder by cervical carcinoma is impossible; diversion of the urinary stream above the level of the bladder (eg, ureterosigmoidostomy) is therefore necessary.

C. Vesicoadnexal Fistula

These fistulas are cured by removal of the involved female reproductive organs, with closure of the opening in the bladder.

Prognosis

The surgical repair of fistulas caused by benign disease or operative trauma is highly successful. Postirradiation necrosis offers a more guarded prognosis. Fistulas secondary to invading cancers present difficult problems.

PERIVESICAL LIPOMATOSIS

The cause of perivesical lipomatosis is not known. The disorder seems to affect principally black men in the 20- to 40-year age group. There are no pathognomonic symptoms. There may be some dysuria or mild urinary obstructive symptoms. Examination may demonstrate a distended or enlarged pear-shaped bladder. Excretory urograms and cystography may show dilatation of both upper tracts and an upward displacement and lateral compression of the bladder. In the perivesical area, x-ray reveals areas of radiolucency compatible with fatty tissue. A barium x-ray may show extrinsic pressure on the rectosigmoid. Angiography shows no evidence of neoplastic vessels.

Computed tomography scan in association with the preceding findings establishes the diagnosis by clearly demonstrating the fatty nature of the perivesical tissue. Church and Kazam (1979) found sonography equally helpful.

On surgical exploration, lipomatous tissue is found surrounding the bladder and rectosigmoid. Though it is tempting to proceed with its resection, there are no cleavage planes. Such dissections usually fail to relieve the ureteral obstruction.

Ballesteros (1977) believes that surgical excision is feasible and reported excellent results in one such case. Crane and Smith (1977) found, after a 5-year follow-up, that hydronephrosis progressed in most. Many patients finally required urinary diversion.

RADIATION CYSTITIS

Many women receiving radiation treatment for carcinoma of the cervix develop some degree of vesical irritability. These symptoms may develop months after cessation of treatment. The urine may or may not be sterile. Vesical capacity is usually appreciably reduced. Cystoscopy reveals a pale mucous membrane with multiple areas of telangiectatic blood vessels. Vesical ulceration may be noted, and vesicovaginal fistulas may develop. If symptoms are severe and prolonged, diversion of urine from the bladder may be necessary.

NONINFECTIOUS HEMORRHAGIC CYSTITIS

Some patients, following radiotherapy for carcinoma of the cervix or bladder, are prone to intermittent, often serious vesical hemorrhage. The same is true of those given cyclophosphamide.

In the case of the latter, the drug must be stopped. To control bleeding, cystoscopic fulguration can be tried, though it usually fails. The instillation of 3.9% formalin (prepared by diluting the standard 39% solution 10 times) is more efficacious. The catheter is clamped for 30 min and the bladder lavaged with 10% alcohol. A second or third instillation may be necessary on subsequent days. Holstein et al (1973) recommend the transurethral placement of a large balloon in the bladder. The balloon is filled to a pressure level equal to the systolic blood pressure and left in place for 6 h.

Giulani et al (1979) have reported success by selective transcatheter embolization of the internal iliac arteries. Ostroff and Chenault (1982) believe that the best and least harmful method of treatment is continuous irrigation with 1% alum solution (the ammonium or potassium salt) through a 3-way Foley catheter.

Despite these measures, the mortality rate is significant. Droller, Saral, and Santos (1982) have evolved a plan for reducing the incidence of cyclophosphamide-induced hemorrhagic cystitis: they produce diuresis and have the patient void frequently (or use open catheter drainage). This reduces the concentration of cyclophosphamide metabolites and the duration of their contact with bladder mucosa. Before the institution of this regimen, 8 of 97 such patients died; afterward, 1 of 198 patients died.

EMPYEMA OF THE BLADDER

If supravesical diversion of the urine is performed without cystectomy, severe infection of the bladder may develop because of lack of washout. In males, cystostomy or cutaneous vesicostomy may be necessary. In females, the formation of a vesicovaginal fistula permits drainage

(Spence and Allen, 1971). Occasionally, cystectomy may be necessary.

CONGENITAL ANOMALIES OF THE PROSTATE & SEMINAL VESICLES

Congenital anomalies of the prostate are rare. Cysts of the prostate and the seminal vesicles have been reported. Enlargements of the prostatic utricle are often found in association with penoscrotal or perineal hypospadias. The cysts are usually small, lying in the midline posterior to the prostate and emptying through the verumontanum. These cysts represent embryologic remnants of the distal end of the müllerian ducts (see Chapter 2). Rarely, they become large enough to be easily palpable rectally or even abdominally. Through local pressure, they may cause symptoms of obstruction of the bladder neck.

BLOODY EJACULATION

Hemospermia is not an uncommon complaint of middle-aged men. It is the wife who usually recognizes the symptom. It is thought by some to be caused by hyperplasia of the mucosa of the seminal vesicles. For this reason, the use of diethylstilbestrol, 5 mg/d for 1 week, has been suggested. In my hands, it has worked well. Thorough urologic investigation of men without other symptoms rarely reveals a pathologic lesion. The cause is therefore not clear.

REFERENCES

Exstrophy

Ansel JS: Surgical treatment of exstrophy of the bladder with emphasis on neonatal primary closure. Personal experience with 28 consecutive cases treated at the University of Washington hospitals from 1962 to 1977: Techniques and results. J Urol 1979;121:650.

Ben-Chaim J, Gearhart JP: Current management of bladder exstrophy. Tech Urol 1996;2:22.

Ben-Chaim J et al: Bladder exstrophy from childhood into adult life. J R Soc Med 1996;89:39P.

Connor JP et al: Long-term followup of 207 patients with bladder exstrophy: An evolution in treatment. J Urol 1989;142:793, 795.

DeMaria JE et al: Renal function in continent patients after surgical closure of bladder extrophy. J Urol 1980;124:85.

Gearhart JP: Bladder exstrophy: Staged reconstruction. Curr Opin Urol 1999;9:499.

Gearhart JP, Jeffs RD: Augmentation cystoplasty in the failed exstrophy reconstruction. J Urol 1988;139:790.

Gearhart JP, Jeffs RD: Bladder exstrophy: Increase in capacity following epispadias repair. J Urol 1989;142:525.

Gearhart JP, Jeffs RD: Management of the failed exstrophy closure. J Urol 1991;146:610.

Gearhart JP et al: Techniques to create continence in the failed bladder exstrophy closure patient. J Urol 1993;150:441.

Grady RW, Carr MC, Mitchell ME: Complete primary closure of bladder exstrophy: Epispadias and bladder exstrophy repair. Urol Clin North Am 1999;26:95.

Hollowell JG et al: Bladder function and dysfunction in exstrophy and epispadias. Lancet 1991;338:926.

Ikeme AC: Pregnancy in women after repair of bladder exstrophy: Two case reports. Br J Obstet Gynaecol 1981;88:327.

Jeffs RD: Complications of exstrophy surgery. Urol Clin North Am 1983;10:509.

Johnson P et al: Inferior vesical fissure. J Urol 1995;154:1478.

Lattimer JK et al: Long-term follow-up after exstrophy closure: Late improvement and good quality of life. J Urol 1978; 119:664.

Light JK, Scott FB: Treatment of the epispadias-exstrophy complex with the AS792 artificial urinary sphincter. J Urol 1983; 129:738.

Lima SVC et al: Bladder exstrophy: Primary reconstruction with human dura mater. Br J Urol 1981;53:119.

Merguerian PA et al: Continence in bladder exstrophy: Determinants of success. J Urol 1991;145:350.

Mitchell ME, Brito CG, Rink RC: Cloacal exstrophy reconstruction for urinary continence. J Urol 1990;144:554, 562.

Mollard P: Bladder reconstruction in exstrophy. J Urol 1980; 124:525.

Oesterling JE, Jeffs RD: The importance of a successful initial bladder closure in the surgical management of classical bladder exstrophy: Analysis of 414 patients at the Johns Hopkins Hospital from 1975 to 1985. J Urol 1987;139:790.

Perlmutter AD, Weinstein MD, Reitelman C: Vesical neck reconstruction in patients with epispadias-exstrophy complex. J Urol 1991;146:613.

Spence HM, Hoffman WW, Pate VA: Exstrophy of the bladder. 1. Long-term results in a series of 37 cases treated by ureterosigmoidostomy. J Urol 1975;114:133.

Stein R, Thüroff JW: Hypospadias and bladder exstrophy. Curr Opin Urol 2002;12:195.

Toguri AG et al: Continence in cases of bladder exstrophy. J Urol 1978;119:538.

Turner WR, Ransley PG, Williams DI: Patterns of renal damage in the management of vesical exstrophy. J Urol 1980;124:412.

Woodhouse CR: The fate of the abnormal bladder in adolescence. J Urol 2001;166:2396.

Persistent Urachus

al-Hindawi MK, Aman S: Benign non-infected urachal cyst in an adult: Review of the literature and a case report. Br J Radiol 1992;65:313.

Bauer SB, Retik AB: Urachal anomalies and related umbilical disorders. Urol Clin North Am 1978;5:195.

Cilento BG Jr et al: Urachal anomalies: Defining the best diagnostic modality. Urology 1998;52:120.

Holten I et al: The ultrasonic diagnosis of urachal anomalies. Australas Radiol 1996;40:2.

Mesrobian HG et al: Ten years of experience with isolated urachal anomalies in children. J Urol 1997;158(3 Pt 2):1316.

Scheye T et al: Anatomic basis of pathology of the urachus. Surg Radiol Anat 1994;16:135.

Stone NN, Garden RJ, Weber H: Laparoscopic excision of a urachal cyst. Urology 1995;45:161.

Suita S, Nagasaki A: Urachal remnants. Semin Pediatr Surg 1996; 5:107.

Yu JS et al: Urachal remnant diseases: Spectrum of CT and US findings. Radiographics 2001;21:451.

Contracture of the Bladder Neck

Elliott JP Jr et al: Post prostatectomy bladder neck contractures. J Miss State Med Assoc 1991;32:41.

Kulb TB et al: Prevention of postprostatectomy vesical neck contracture by prophylactic vesical neck incision. J Urol 1987; 137:230.

Nunn IN: Bladder neck obstruction in children. J Urol 1965; 93:693.

Smith DR: Critique on the concept of vesical neck obstruction in children. JAMA 1969;207:1686.

Interstitial Cystitis

Andersson KE: Neurotransmission and drug effects in urethral smooth muscle. Scand J Urol Nephrol Suppl 2001;(207):26.

Andersson KE: Neurotransmitters and neuroreceptors in the lower urinary tract. Curr Opin Obstet Gynecol 1996;8:361.

Awad SA et al: Idiopathic reduced bladder storage versus interstitial cystitis. J Urol 1992;148:409.

Baskin LS, Tanagho EA: Pelvic pain without pelvic organs. J Urol 1992;147:683.

Chaiken DC, Blaivas JG, Blaivas ST: Behavioral therapy for the treatment of refractory interstitial cystitis. J Urol 1993; 149:1445.

Duncan JL, Schaeffer AJ: Do infectious agents cause interstitial cystitis? Urology 1997;49(5A Suppl):48.

Elbadawi A: Interstitial cystitis: A critique of current concepts with a new proposal for pathologic diagnosis and pathogenesis. Urology 1997;49(5A Suppl):14.

Hohenfellner M et al: Interstitial cystitis: Increased sympathetic innervation and related neuropeptide synthesis. J Urol 1992;147:587.

Hurst RE et al: Urinary glycosaminoglycan excretion as a laboratory marker in the diagnosis of interstitial cystitis. J Urol 1993;149:31.

Irwin P, Galloway NT: Impaired bladder perfusion in interstitial cystitis: A study of blood supply using laser Doppler flowmetry. J Urol 1993;149:890.

Johansson SL, Fall M: Clinical features and spectrum of light microscopic changes in interstitial cystitis. J Urol 1990; 143:1118.

Jones CA, Nyberg LE: Epidemiology of interstitial cystitis. Urology 1997 (May);49(5A Suppl):2.

Kusek JW, Nyberg LM: The epidemiology of interstitial cystitis: Is it time to expand our definition? Urology 2001;57(Suppl 1):95.

Liebert M: Basic science research on the urinary bladder and interstitial cystitis: New genetic approaches. Urology 2001; 57(Suppl 1):7.

Messing EM, Stamey TA: Interstitial cystitis: Early diagnosis, pathology and treatment. Urology 1978;12:381.

Nickel JC, Emerson L, Cornish J: The bladder mucus (glycosaminoglycan) layer in interstitial cystitis. J Urol 1993; 149:716.

Oberpenning F, van Ophoven A, Hertle L: Interstitial cystitis: An update. Curr Opin Urol 2002;12:321.

Parsons CL: Interstitial cystitis: Epidemiology and clinical presentation. Clin Obstet Gynecol 2002;45:242.

Parsons CL, Mulholland SG: Successful therapy of interstitial cystitis with pentosanpolysulfate. J Urol 1987;138:513.

Parsons CL, Schmidt JD, Pollen JJ: Successful treatment of interstitial cystitis with sodium pentosanpolysulfate. J Urol 1983; 130:51.

Pontari MA, Hanno PM, Wein AJ: Logical and systematic approach to the evaluation and management of patients suspected of having interstitial cystitis. Urology 1997;49(5A Suppl):114.

Ratner V: Interstitial cystitis: A chronic inflammatory bladder condition. World J Urol 2001;19:157.

Sant GR, Theoharides TC: The role of the mast cell in interstitial cystitis. Urol Clin North Am 1994;21:41.

Simon LJ et al: The Interstitial Cystitis Data Base Study: Concepts and preliminary baseline descriptive statistics. Urology 1997;49(5A Suppl):64.

Slade D, Ratner V, Chalker R: A collaborative approach to managing interstitial cystitis. Urology 1997;49(5A Suppl):10.

Theoharides TC et al: Interstitial cystitis: A neuroimmunoendocrine disorder. Ann N Y Acad Sci 1998;840:619.

Wesselmann U: Neurogenic inflammation and chronic pelvic pain. World J Urol 2001;19:180.

Internal Vesical Herniation

Austin RC, Kaisary A, Winslet MC: Obturator herniation following radical cystoprostatectomy. Br J Urol 1995;76:800.

Bell ED, Witherington R: Bladder hernias. Urology 1980;15:127.

Catalano O: Incisional herniation of the bladder: CT findings. Rofo Fortschr Geb Rontgenstr Neuen Bildgeb Verfahr 1996; 165:508.

Catalano O: US evaluation of inguinoscrotal bladder hernias: Report of three cases. Clin Imaging 1997;21:126.

Weitzenfeld MB et al: Scrotal kidney and ureter: An unusual hernia. J Urol 1980;123:437.

Urinary Incontinence

Furlow WL: Postprostatectomy urinary incontinence: Etiology, prevention, and selection of surgical treatment. Urol Clin North Am 1978;5:347.

Hetzenauer A, Bazzanella A, Reider W: Unstable female urethra: Incidence and significance. Proc Int Continence Soc 1985; 15:111.

Langer R et al: Detrusor instability following colposuspension for urinary stress incontinence. Br J Obstet Gynaecol 1988; 95:607.

Ouslander JG: Geriatric urinary incontinence. Dis Mon 1992; 38(2):65.

Rousseau P, Fuentevilla-Clifton A: Urinary incontinence in the aged. Part 1: Patient evaluation. Geriatrics 1992;47(6):22, 33.

Rousseau P, Fuentevilla-Clifton A: Urinary incontinence in the aged. Part 2: Management strategies. [Published erratum appears in Geriatrics 1992;47(9):87.] Geriatrics 1992;47(6):37, 45, 48.

Scott FB, Bradley WE, Timm GW: Treatment of urinary incontinence by implantable prosthetic urinary sphincter. J Urol 1974;112:75.

Tanagho EA: Bladder neck reconstruction for total urinary incontinence: 10 years of experience. J Urol 1981;125:321.

Tanagho EA, Smith DR: Clinical evaluation of a surgical technique for the correction of complete urinary incontinence. J Urol 1972;107:402.

Westby M, Asmussen M: Anatomical and functional changes in the lower urinary tract after radical hysterectomy with lymph node dissection as studied by dynamic urethrocystography and simultaneous urethrocystometry. Gynecol Oncol 1985; 21:261.

Williams DI, Snyder H: Anterior detrusor tube repair for urinary incontinence in children. Br J Urol 1976;48:671.

Enuresis

Butler R, Stenberg A: Treatment of childhood nocturnal enuresis: An examination of clinically relevant principles. BJU Int 2001;88:563.

Butler RJ: Combination therapy for nocturnal enuresis. Scand J Urol Nephrol 2001;35:364.

Butler RJ, Holland P: The three systems: A conceptual way of understanding nocturnal enuresis. Scand J Urol Nephrol 2000; 34:270.

Desmopressin for nocturnal enuresis. Med Lett Drugs Ther (April) 1990;32:38.

Djurhuus JC, Matthiesen TB, Rittig S: Similarities and dissimilarities between nocturnal enuresis in childhood and nocturia in adults. BJU Int 1999;84(Suppl 1):9.

Djurhuus JC, Rittig S: Current trends, diagnosis, and treatment of enuresis. Eur Urol 1998;33(Suppl 3):30.

Djurhuus JC, Rittig S: Nocturnal enuresis. Curr Opin Urol 2002; 12:317.

Hjalmas K: Nocturnal enuresis: Basic facts and new horizons. Eur Urol 1998;33(Suppl 3):53.

Howe AC, Walker CE: Behavioral management of toilet training, enuresis, and encopresis. Pediatr Clin North Am 1992; 39:413.

Klauber GT: Clinical efficacy and safety of desmopressin in the treatment of nocturnal enuresis. J Pediatr 1989;114:719.

Lettgen B: Differential diagnoses for nocturnal enuresis. Scand J Urol Nephrol Suppl 1997;183:47.

Mark SD, Frank JD: Nocturnal enuresis. Br J Urol 1995;75:427.

Moffatt ME: Nocturnal enuresis: Psychologic implications of treatment and nontreatment. J Pediatr 1989;114:697.

Moffatt ME et al: Desmopressin acetate and nocturnal enuresis: How much do we know? [See comments.] Pediatrics 1993; 92:420.

Neveus T et al: Enuresis—background and treatment. Scand J Urol Nephrol Suppl 2000;(206)1.

Nørgaard JP, Rittig S, Djurhuus JC: Nocturnal enuresis: An approach to treatment based on pathogenesis. J Pediatr 1989; 114:705.

Nørgaard JP et al: Experience and current status of research into the pathophysiology of nocturnal enuresis. Br J Urol 1997; 79:825.

Rushton HG: Nocturnal enuresis: Epidemiology, evaluation, and currently available treatment options. J Pediatr 1989; 114:691.

Ullom-Minnich MR: Diagnosis and management of nocturnal enuresis. Am Fam Physician 1996;54:2259.

Van Gontard A et al: The genetics of enuresis: A review. J Urol 2001;166:2438.

Van Kerrebroeck PE: Experience with the long-term use of desmopressin for nocturnal enuresis in children and adolescents. BJU Int 2002;89:420.

Wolfish NM: Sleep/arousal and enuresis subtypes. J Urol 2001; 166:2444.

Foreign Bodies Introduced Into the Bladder & Urethra

Bjornerem A, Tollan A: Intrauterine device—primary and secondary perforation of the urinary bladder. Acta Obstet Gynecol Scand 1997;76:383.

Cardozo L: Recurrent intra-vesical foreign bodies. Br J Urol 1997;80:687.

Chitale SV, Burgess NA: Endoscopic removal of a complex foreign body from the bladder. Br J Urol 1998;81:756.

Maskey CP et al: Vesical calculus around an intra-uterine contraceptive device. Br J Urol 1997;79:654.

Prasad S et al: Foreign bodies in urinary bladder. Urology 1973; 2:258.

Van Ophoven A, deKernion JB: Clinical management of foreign bodies of the genitourinary tract. J Urol 2000;164:274.

Vesical Manifestations of Allergy

Pastinszky I: The allergic diseases of the male genitourinary tract with special reference to allergic urethritis and cystitis. Urol Int 1960;9:288.

Rubin L, Pincus MD: Eosinophilic cystitis: The relationship of allergy in the urinary tract to eosinophilic cystitis and the pathophysiology of eosinophilia. J Urol 1974;112:457.

Diverticula

Barrett DM, Malek RS, Kelalis PP: Observations on vesical diverticulum in childhood. J Urol 1976;116:234.

Das S, Amar AD: Vesical diverticulum associated with bladder carcinoma: Therapeutic implications. J Urol 1986;136:1013.

Gerridzen R, Futter NG: Ten-year review of vesical diverticula. Urology 1982;10:33.

Keeler LL, Sant GR: Spontaneous rupture of a bladder diverticulum. J Urol 1990;143:349.

Mićić S, Ilić V: Incidence of neoplasm in vesical diverticula. J Urol 1983;129:734.

Shah B et al: Tumour in a giant bladder diverticulum: A case report and review of literature. Int Urol Nephrol 1997;29:173.

Yu CC et al: Intradiverticular tumors of the bladder: Surgical implications—an eleven-year review. Eur Urol 1993;24:190.

Vesical Fistulas

Anderson GA, Goldman IL, Mulligan GW: 3-dimensional computerized tomographic reconstruction of colovesical fistulas. J Urol 1997;158(3 Pt 1):795.

Ayhan A et al: Results of treatment in 182 consecutive patients with genital fistulas. Int J Gynaecol Obstet 1995;48:43.

Badlani G et al: Enterovesical fistulas in Crohn disease. Urology 1980;16:599.

Bazeed M et al: Urovaginal fistulae: 20 years' experience. Eur Urol 1995;27:34.

Birkhoff JD, Wechsler M, Romas NA: Urinary fistulas: Vaginal repair using labial fat pad. J Urol 1977;177:595.

Blaivas JG, Heritz DM, Romanzi LJ: Early versus late repair of vesicovaginal fistulas: Vaginal and abdominal approaches. J Urol 1995;153:1110.

Carr LK, Webster GD: Abdominal repair of vesicovaginal fistula. (Editorial). Urology 1996;48:10.

Cruikshank SH: Early closure of posthysterectomy vesicovaginal fistulas. South Med J 1988;81:1525.

Driver CP et al: Vesico-colic fistulae in the Grampian region: Presentation, assessment, management and outcome. J R Coll Surg Edinb 1997;42:182.

Dupont MC, Raz S: Vaginal approach to vesicovaginal fistula repair. (Editorial.) Urology 1996(Jul);48:7.

Elkins TE: Surgery for the obstetric vesicovaginal fistula: A review of 100 operations in 82 patients. Am J Obstet Gynecol 1994;170:1108.

Gilmour DT, Dwyer PL, Carey MP: Lower urinary tract injury during gynecologic surgery and its detection by intraoperative cystoscopy. Obstet Gynecol 1999;94(5 Pt 2):883.

Hsieh JH et al: Enterovesical fistula: 10 years experience. Chung Hua I Hsueh Tsa Chih (Taipei) 1997;59:283.

Iselin CE, Aslan P, Webster GD: Transvaginal repair of vesicovaginal fistulas after hysterectomy by vaginal cuff excision. J Urol 1998;160(3 Pt 1):728.

Margolis T, Mercer LJ: Vesicovaginal fistula. Obstet Gynecol Surv 1994;49:840.

Moss RL, Ryan JA Jr: Management of enterovesical fistulas. Am J Surg 1990;159:514.

Nesrallah LJ, Srougi M, Gittes RF: The O'Conor technique: The gold standard for supratrigonal vesicovaginal fistula repair. J Urol 1999;161:566.

Persky L, Herman G, Guerrier K: Nondelay in vesico-vaginal fistula repair. Urology 1979;13:273.

Raghavaiah NV: Double-dye test to diagnose various types of vaginal fistulas. J Urol 1974;112:811.

Semelka RC et al: Pelvic fistulas: Appearances on MR images. Abdom Imaging 1997;22:91.

Simoneaux SF, Patrick LE: Genitourinary complications of Crohn's disease in pediatric patients. AJR 1997;169:197.

Waaldijk K: Surgical classification of obstetric fistulas. Int J Gynaecol Obstet 1995;49:161.

Woo HH, Rosario DJ, Chapple CR: The treatment of vesicovaginal fistulae. Eur Urol 1996;29:1.

Perivesical Lipomatosis

Ambos MA et al: The pear-shaped bladder. Radiology 1977;122:85.

Ballesteros JJ: Surgical treatment of perivesical lipomatosis. J Urol 1977;118:329.

Church PA, Kazam E: Computed tomography and ultrasound in diagnosis of pelvic lipomatosis. Urology 1979;14:631.

Crane DB, Smith MJV: Pelvic lipomatosis: Five-year follow-up. J Urol 1977;118:547.

Halachmi S et al: The use of an ultrasonic assisted lipectomy device for the treatment of obstructive pelvic lipomatosis. Urology 1996;48:128.

Heyns CF et al: Pelvic lipomatosis associated with cystitis glandularis and adenocarcinoma of the bladder. J Urol 1991;145:364.

Masumori N, Tsukamoto T: Pelvic lipomatosis associated with proliferative cystitis: Case report and review of the Japanese literature. Int J Urol 1999;6:44.

Mordkin RM et al: The radiographic diagnosis of pelvic lipomatosis. Tech Urol 1997;3:228.

Radiation Cystitis

Capelli-Schellpfeffer M, Gerber GS: The use of hyperbaric oxygen in urology. J Urol 1999;162:(3 Pt 1):647.

Crew JP, Jephcott CR, Reynard JM: Radiation-induced haemorrhagic cystitis. Eur Urol 2001;40:111.

Del Pizzo JJ et al: Treatment of radiation induced hemorrhagic cystitis with hyperbaric oxygen: Long-term followup. J Urol 1998;160(3 Pt 1):731.

Lowe BA, Stamey TA: Endoscopic topical placement of formalin soaked pledgets to control localized hemorrhage due to radiation cystitis. J Urol 1997;158:528.

Russo P: Urologic emergencies in the cancer patient. Semin Oncol 2000;27:284.

Sanchiz F et al: Prevention of radioinduced cystitis by orgotein: A randomized study. Anticancer Res 1996;16:2025.

Suzuki K et al: Successful treatment of radiation cystitis with hyperbaric oxygen therapy: Resolution of bleeding event and changes of histopathological findings of the bladder mucosa. Int Urol Nephrol 1998;30:267.

Weiss JP, Neville EC: Hyperbaric oxygen: Primary treatment of radiation-induced hemorrhagic cystitis. J Urol 1989;142:43.

Noninfectious Hemorrhagic Cystitis

Bennett AH: Cyclophosphamide and hemorrhagic cystitis. J Urol 1974;111:603.

deVries CR, Freiha FS: Hemorrhagic cystitis: A review. J Urol 1990;143:1.

Donahue LA, Frank IN: Intravesical formalin for hemorrhagic cystitis: Analysis of therapy. J Urol 1989;141:809.

Droller MJ, Saral K, Santos G: Prevention of cyclophosphamide-induced hemorrhagic cystitis. Urology 1982;20:256.

Giulani L et al: Gelatin foam and isobutyl-2-cyanoacrylate in the treatment of life-threatening bladder haemorrhage by selective transcatheter embolisation of the internal iliac arteries. Br J Urol 1979;51:125.

Holstein P et al: Intravesical hydrostatic pressure treatment: New method for control of bleeding from bladder mucosa. J Urol 1973;109:234.

Ilhan O et al: Hemorrhagic cystitis as a complication of bone marrow transplantation. J Chemother 1997;9:56.

Miller J, Burfield GD, Moretti KL: Oral conjugated estrogen therapy for treatment of hemorrhagic cystitis. J Urol 1994; 151:1348.

Ostroff EB, Chenault OW Jr: Alum irrigation for the control of massive bladder hemorrhage. J Urol 1982;128:929.

Ratliff TR, Williams RD: Hemorrhagic cystitis, chemotherapy, and bladder toxicity. (Editorial.) J Urol 1998;159:1044.

Stillwell TJ, Benson RC Jr: Cyclophosphamide-induced hemorrhagic cystitis. A review of 100 patients. Cancer 1988;61:451.

West NJ: Prevention and treatment of hemorrhagic cystitis. Pharmacotherapy 1997;17:696.

Empyema of the Bladder

Adeyoju AB, Lynch TH, Thornhill JA: The defunctionalized bladder. Int Urogynecol J Pelvic Floor Dysfunct 1998;9:48.

Dretler SP: The occurrence of empyema cystitis: Management of the bladder to be defunctionalized. J Urol 1972;108:82.

Spence HM, Allen TD: Vaginal vesicostomy for empyema of the defunctionalized bladder. J Urol 1971;106:862.

Congenital Anomalies of the Prostate & Seminal Vesicles

Barzilai M, Ginesin Y: A müllerian prostatic cyst protruding into the base of the urinary bladder. Urol Int 1998;60:194.

Feldman RA, Weiss RM: Urinary retention secondary to Müllerian duct cyst in a child. J Urol 1972;108:647.

McDermott VG et al: Prostatic and periprostatic cysts: Findings on MR imaging. AJR 1995;164:123.

Ng KJ, Milroy EJ, Rickards D: Intraprostatic cyst—a cause of bladder outflow obstruction. J R Soc Med 1996;89:708.

Sanchez-Chapado M, Angulo JC: Giant Müllerian duct cyst mimicking prostatic malignancy. Scand J Urol Nephrol 1995; 29:229.

Terris MK: Transrectal ultrasound guided drainage of prostatic cysts. J Urol 1997;158:179.

Yasumoto R et al: Is a cystic lesion located at the midline of the prostate a müllerian duct cyst? Analysis of aspirated fluid and histopathological study of the cyst wall. Eur Urol 1997; 31:187.

Bloody Ejaculation

Munkel Witz R et al: Current perspectives on hematospermia: A review. J Androl 1997;18:6.

Male Sexual Dysfunction

37

Tom F. Lue, MD

A better understanding of male sexual dysfunction has been made possible by innovative laboratory and clinical research in the mechanism, neurophysiology, and pharmacology of penile erection. Erectile function can now be evaluated in the office setting by intracavernous injection of vasoactive agents or the response to oral phosphodiesterase inhibitor at home. Improved diagnostic tests can differentiate among types of impotence. More oral and transurethral drugs are being developed, and the latest generation of penile prostheses is more sophisticated and durable than earlier ones. Continuing research may offer a more physiologic and disease-specific solution to various types of erectile dysfunction (ED).

PHYSIOLOGY OF PENILE ERECTION

Innervation of the Penis

The autonomic spinal erection center is located in the intermediolateral nuclei of the spinal cord at levels $S_2–S_4$ and $T_{12}–L_2$. Nerve fibers from the thoracolumbar (sympathetic) and sacral (parasympathetic) spinal segments join to form inferior hypogastric and pelvic plexuses, which sends branches to the pelvic organs. The fibers innervating the penis (the cavernous nerves) travel along the posterolateral aspect of the seminal vesicles and prostate and then accompany the membranous urethra through the genitourinary diaphragm (Walsh and Donker, 1982; Figure 37-1). Some of these fibers enter the corpora cavernosa and corpus spongiosum with the cavernous and bulbourethral arteries. Others travel further distally with the dorsal nerve and enter the corpus cavernosum and corpus spongiosum in various locations to supply the mid- and distal portions of the penis. The terminal branches of the cavernous nerves innervate the helicine arteries and the trabecular smooth muscle and are responsible for the vascular events during tumescence and detumescence (Paick, Donatucci, and Lue, 1993).

The center for somatic motor nerves is located at the ventral horn of the $S_2–S_4$ segment. The motor fibers join the pudendal nerve to innervate the bulbocavernosus and ischiocavernosus muscles. The somatic sensory nerves originate at the receptors in the penis to transmit pain, temperature, touch, and vibratory sensations. The pathway and center for erotic feeling from genital stimulation has not been elucidated. The brain has a modulatory effect on the spinal pathways of erection. Various supraspinal areas that have a role in erectile function include the hypothalamus and limbic system, ventral thalamus, tegmentum of mid brain and lateral substantia nigra, and ventrolateral pons and medulla. Specifically, the medial preoptic area (MPOA) and the paraventricular nucleus of the hypothalamus, the periaqueductal gray of the mid brain, and the nucleus paragigantocellularis of the medulla are the centers intimately involved in the control of penile erection (McKenna, 1998).

Three types of erections are noted in humans: genital-stimulated (contact or reflexogenic), central-stimulated (noncontact or psychogenic), and central-originated (nocturnal). Genital-stimulated erection is induced by tactile stimulation of the genital area. This kind of erection can be preserved in upper spinal cord lesions, although erections are usually short in duration and poorly controlled by the individual. Central-stimulated erection is more complex, resulting from memory, fantasy, or visual or auditory stimuli. The central-originated erection can occur spontaneously without stimulation or during sleep. Most of the sleep erections occur during rapid eye movement (REM) sleep. The mechanism that triggers REM sleep is located in the pontine reticular formation. During REM sleep, the cholinergic neurons in the lateral pontine tegmentum are activated while the adrenergic neurons in the locus ceruleus and the serotonergic neurons in the mid brain raphe are silent. This differential activation may be responsible for the nocturnal erections during REM sleep. The number and duration of erections are markedly reduced in hypogonadism and in men receiving antiandrogen therapy.

Anatomy & Hemodynamics of Penile Erection

The tunica of the corpora cavernosa is a bilayered structure with multiple sublayers. The inner circular bundles support and contain the cavernous tissue. From this inner layer radiate intracavernosal pillars that act as struts to augment the septum; both of these structures provide essential support to the erectile tissue (Hsu et al 1992). The outer-layer bundles are oriented longitudinally and extend from the glans penis to the proximal

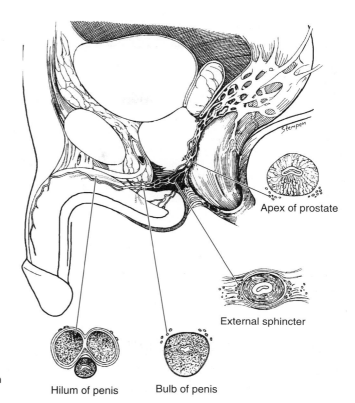

Apex of prostate

External sphincter

Hilum of penis   Bulb of penis

Figure 37–1. Location of cavernous nerves in relation to urethra.

crura. These fibers insert into the inferior pubic ramus but are absent between the 5 and 7 o'clock positions. In contrast, the corpus spongiosum lacks an outer layer or intracorporeal struts, ensuring a lower-pressure structure during erection. The tunica is composed of elastic fibers forming a network on which the collagen fibers rest. Emissary veins run between the inner and outer layers for a short distance, often piercing the outer bundles obliquely. Branches of the dorsal artery take a more direct perpendicular route, however, and are surrounded by a periarterial fibrous sheath.

The paired internal pudendal artery is the major carrier of the blood supply to the penis. The terminal portion of this artery divides into 3 branches: the bulbourethral artery, the dorsal artery, and the cavernous artery (deep artery). The cavernous artery supplies the corpora cavernosa; the dorsal artery, the skin, subcutaneous tissue, and the glans penis; and the bulbourethral artery, the corpus spongiosum. Accessory pudendal arteries from external iliac or obturator arteries may supply a major portion of the penis in some cases. Collaterals among the 3 branches are often observed (Breza et al, 1989). The venous drainage of the glans is mainly through the deep dorsal vein. The corpus spongiosum

is drained via the circumflex, urethral, and bulbar veins, but the drainage of the corpora cavernosa is more complex: The mid and distal shafts are drained by the deep dorsal vein to the preprostatic plexus; the proximal portion is drained by the cavernous and the crural veins to the preprostatic plexus and internal pudendal vein. The drainage of all 3 corpora originates in the subtunical venules, which unite to form emissary veins that pierce the tunica albuginea. The glans penis possesses numerous large and small veins that communicate freely with the dorsal veins. The penile skin and subcutaneous tissue are drained by superficial dorsal veins, which then empty into the saphenous veins.

Activation of the autonomic nerve produces a full erection, that is, filling and trapping of blood in the cavernous bodies. After full erection is achieved, contraction of the ischiocavernosus muscle (from activation of the somatic nerves) compresses the proximal corpora and raises the pressure in the entire corpora well above the systolic blood pressure, resulting in rigid erection (Table 37–1) This rigid phase occurs naturally during masturbation or sexual intercourse but can also occur from slight bending of the penis, without muscular action. The erection process can be divided into phases,

Table 37–1. Phases of the erection process.[a]

Flaccid phase (1)

Minimal arterial and venous flow; blood gas values equal those of venous blood. Flow rate: 2.5–8 mL/100 g/min (Wagner and Uhrenholdt, 1980); 0.5–6.5 mL/100 g/min (Shirai et al, 1978).[b]

Latent (filling) phase (2)

Increased flow in the internal pudendal artery during both systolic and diastolic phases. Decreased pressure in the internal pudendal artery; unchanged intracavernous pressure. Some elongation of the penis.

Tumescent phase (3)

Rising intracavernous pressure until full erection is achieved. Penis shows more expansion and elongation with pulsation. The arterial flow rate decreases as the pressure rises. When intracavernous pressure rises above diastolic pressure, flow occurs only in the systolic phases.

Full erection phase (4)

Intracavernous pressure can rise to as much as 80–90% of the systolic pressure. Pressure in the internal pudendal artery increases but remains slightly below systemic pressure. Arterial flow is much less than in the initial filling phase but is still higher than in the flaccid phase. Although the venous channels are mostly compressed, the venous flow rate is slightly higher than during the flaccid phase. Blood gas values approach those of arterial blood.

Skeletal or rigid erection phase (5)

As a result of contraction of the ischiocavernous muscle, the intracavernous pressure rises well above the systolic pressure, resulting in rigid erection. During this phase, almost no blood flows through the cavernous artery; however, the short duration prevents the development of ischemia or tissue damage.

Detumescent phase (6)

After ejaculation or cessation of erotic stimuli, sympathetic tonic discharge resumes, resulting in contraction of the smooth muscles around the sinusoids and arterioles. This effectively diminishes the arterial flow to flaccid levels, expels a large portion of blood from the sinusoidal spaces, and reopens the venous channels. The penis returns to its flaccid length and girth.

[a]Numbers 1–6 correspond to phases shown in Fig 37–2.
[b]Wagner G, Uhrenhold A: Blood flow measurement by the clearance method in the human corpus cavernosum in the flaccid and erect states. In: Zogniotti AW, Rossi G (editors): *Vasculogenic Impotence.* (Proceedings of the First International Conference on Corpus Cavernosum Revascularization.) Thomas, 1980. Shirai M et al: Hemodynamic mechanism of erection in the human penis. Arch Androl 1978;1:345.

as shown in Table 37–1 and Figure 37–2. The hemodynamic of the glans penis is somewhat different. Arterial flow increases in the glans in a manner similar to that in the shaft. Because it lacks the tunica albuginea, however, the glans functions as an arteriovenous fistula during the full erection phase. Nevertheless, during rigid erection, most of the venous channels are temporarily compressed, and further engorgement of the glans can be observed (Lue, 2000).

Mechanism of Penile Erection

The anatomic mechanism of penile erection was discovered in the 1980s by electron microscopy of corrosion penile casts made in the flaccid state and during erection (Fournier et al, 1987; Banya et al, 1989). In these models, the flaccid corpus cavernosum shows contracted sinusoids with constricted arteries and arterioles, and the draining venules form a plexus under the tunica albuginea. During erection, dilation of the arterial tree, expansion of the sinusoids, and compression of the subtunical and emissary veins are clearly seen. From these studies and observation of vasodilator-induced erections, it appears that the smooth muscles in the arterial tree and the trabeculae are the key to the erectile process.

The intrinsic smooth-muscle tone and, possibly, the adrenergic tonic discharge maintain contraction of the smooth muscles and the arterioles in the flaccid state. When the smooth muscles relax owing to release of neurotransmitters, the resistance to incoming flow

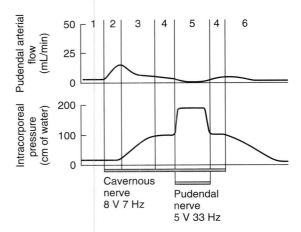

Figure 37–2. Phases of penile erection (induced in monkeys via neurostimulation). Numbers correspond to phases outlined in Table 37–1. (Lower tracing = intracavernous pressure; upper tracing = flow within the internal pudendal artery.)

drops to a minimum. This allows arterial and arteriolar vasodilatation and expansion of the sinusoids to receive a large increase of flow. Trapping of blood causes the penis to lengthen and widen rapidly until the capacity of the tunica albuginea is reached. Meanwhile, expansion of the sinusoidal walls against one another and against the tunica albuginea results in compression of the subtunical venular plexus. Meanwhile, uneven stretching of the layers of the tunica albuginea also compresses the emissary veins and effectively reduces the venous flow to a minimum (Lue, 2000; Figure 37–3A and B).

Hormones & Sexual Function

Androgens are essential for male sexual maturity. Testosterone regulates gonadotropin secretion and muscle development; dihydrotestosterone mediates all other aspects of male sexual maturation, including hair growth, acne, male pattern baldness, and spermatogenesis. In adults, androgen deficiency results in loss of sexual interest and impaired seminal emission. The frequency, magnitude, and latency of nocturnal penile erections are reduced. However, studies have shown that erection in response to visual sexual stimulation is preserved in hypogonadal men, suggesting that andro-

gen enhances but is not essential for erection (Bancroft and Wu, 1983).

In a longitudinal study of middle-aged men for 7–10 years, it was noted that total testosterone level declined at 0.8% per year of age, whereas both free and albumin-bound testosterone declined at about 2% per year. Sex hormone–binding globulin increased at 1.6% per year. Dehydroepiandrosterone, dehydroepiandrosterone sulfate, cortisol, and estrone showed significant longitudinal declines, whereas dihydrotestosterone, pituitary gonadotropins, and prolactin rose longitudinally. The significance of these hormone changes in the pathogenesis of ED is not clear (Feldman et al, 2002).

Neurotransmitters & Pharmacology of Erection

Neural control of penile erection involves the adrenergic, cholinergic, and nonadrenergic-noncholinergic (NANC) neuroeffector systems. Adrenergic nerves mediate intracavernous smooth-muscle contraction, which maintains the penis in a flaccid state. Cholinergic nerves may contribute to smooth-muscle relaxation and penile erection through (1) inhibition of adrenergic nerves via inhibitory interneurons and (2) release of nitric oxide (NO) from the endothelium by acetylcholine

Figure 37–3. The mechanism of penile erection. In the flaccid state (**A**), the arteries, arterioles, and sinusoids are contracted. The intersinusoidal and subtunical venular plexuses are wide open, with free flow to the emissary veins. In the erect state (**B**), the muscles of the sinusoidal wall and the arterioles relax, allowing maximal flow to the compliant sinusoidal spaces. Most of the venules are compressed between the expanding sinusoids. Even the larger intermediary venules are sandwiched and flattened by distended sinusoids and the noncompliant tunica albuginea. This effectively reduces the venous capacity to a minimum.

(Saenz de Tejada et al, 1988a). The principal neuro-transmitter for penile erection is NO from parasympathetic, NANC nerve terminals. Once blood rushes into the sinusoids, the shear stress can also release NO from endothelium to augment smooth-muscle relaxation and erection (Ignarro et al, 1990; Hurt et al, 2002). In addition, oxygen tension (Kim et al, 1993) and substances secreted by endothelium lining the sinusoidal spaces may also be involved in penile erection and detumescence. These include prostaglandins (Saenz de Tejada et al, 1988b), endothelins (Holmquist, Andersson, and Hedlund, 1990), and angiotensin (Becker et al, 2001). The agents capable of inducing erection and causing detumescence are summarized in Table 37–2. Although the actions of different agents vary, when given in large doses, all erection-inducing agents cause the smooth muscles to relax, and all detumescence-inducing agents cause them to contract.

Molecular Mechanism of Smooth-Muscle Contraction & Relaxation

Smooth-muscle contraction is regulated by Ca^{2+}. When the cytosolic free Ca^{2+} increases from a resting level of 120–270 to 500–700 nM, calmodulin-4 Ca^{2+} complex binds to the myosin light-chain kinase (Murray, 1996). The activated kinase then phosphorylates the light chain, which ceases to inhibit the myosin-actin interaction and initiates a contraction cycle.

When cytosolic free Ca^{2+} falls to the resting level, the Ca^{2+} dissociates from calmodulin, which in turn dissociates from the myosin light-chain kinase, thus inactivating it. Dephosphorylated myosin light chain resumes its action of inhibiting the binding of the myosin

head to actin and relaxes the smooth muscle (Murray, 1996).

Signal Transduction in Penile Erection

During sexual stimulation, NO released from nerve ending and endothelium diffuses into the trabecular and arterial smooth-muscle cells to activate guanylyl cyclase, which catalyzes the formation of second messenger cyclic guanosine monophosphate (cGMP) (Trigo-Rocha et al, 1993). cGMP in turn activates protein kinase G, which phosphorylates potassium and calcium channels, resulting in hyperpolarization and reduced intracytosolic calcium. The end result is dissociation of myosin head from actin and smooth-muscle relaxation. In addition to the NO-cGMP pathway, several neurotransmitters (eg, vasoactive intestinal polypeptide [VIP] and calcitonin gene related peptide [CGRP]) and drugs (eg, alprostadil) combine with membrane receptor and activate the cyclic adenosine monophosphate (cAMP) pathway, which also phosphorylates ion channels and causes smooth-muscle relaxation. On the other hand, norepinephrine, phenylephrine, and endothelin appear to activate phospholipase C, which leads to the formation of inositol triphosphate and diacylglycerol, which in turn increases cytoplasmic calcium and induces smooth-muscle contraction.

Detumescence occurs following degradation of cGMP and cAMP to GMP and AMP, respectively, by specific phosphodiesterases. Eleven classes of phosphodiesterases have been identified. The penis is rich in phosphodiesterase type V (GMP specific), and therefore specific type V phosphodiesterase inhibitors (sildenafil, vardenafil, and tadalafil) are able to improve penile erections in patients with ED.

Intercellular Communication

Gap junctions are aqueous intercellular channels that have been demonstrated to interconnect the cytoplasm of adjacent cells in many tissues. In the penis, smooth-muscle cells are sparsely innervated by the terminal branches of the cavernous nerves. Therefore, gap junctions play a vital role in the intercellular communication within the corpus cavernosum, which enables the penis to function as a unit (Melman and Christ, 2001).

■ MALE SEXUAL DYSFUNCTION

Male sexual dysfunction, denoting the inability to achieve a satisfactory sexual relationship, may involve inadequacy of erection or problems with emission, ejaculation, or orgasm.

Table 37–2. Agents that have been reported to induce or inhibit penile erection.

Inducers	Inhibitors
Papaverine	Phenylephrine
Phentolamine	Epinephrine
Phenoxybenzamine	Norepinephrine
Thymoxamine	Metaraminol
Alprostadil (prostaglandin E$_1$)	Ephedrine
Vasoactive intestinal polypeptide (VIP)	
Calcitonin gene related peptide (CGRP)	
Nitric oxide donor	
Guanylate cyclase activator	
Dopamine receptor agonist	
Phosphodiesterase inhibitors	
Rho kinase inhibitors	
Melanocortin receptors agonist	

Erectile dysfunction (impotence) is the inability to obtain or maintain penile erection (or both) sufficient for satisfactory sexual performance (NIH Consensus Panel on Impotence, 1993).

Premature (rapid) ejaculation refers to persistent or recurrent occurrence of ejaculation with minimal sexual stimulation before, on, or shortly after penetration and before the person wishes it.

Retarded ejaculation is undue delay in reaching a climax during sexual activity.

Retrograde ejaculation denotes backflow of semen into the bladder during ejaculation owing to an incompetent bladder neck mechanism.

Anorgasmia is the inability to achieve an orgasm during conscious sexual activity, although nocturnal emission may occur.

EPIDEMIOLOGY

In the Massachusetts Male Aging Study, a community-based survey of men between 40 and 70 years of age, 52% of respondents reported some degree of ED: 17% mild, 25% moderate, and 10% complete. Although the prevalence of mild ED remained constant (17%) between the ages of 40 and 70, there was a doubling in the number of men reporting moderate ED (from 17% to 34%) and a tripling in the number of men reporting complete ED (from 5% to 15%). Among the major predictors of ED are diabetes mellitus, heart disease, hypertension, and decreased high-density lipoprotein level. There is a higher prevalence of ED in men who have undergone radiation or surgery for prostate cancer. The psychological correlates of ED include depression and anger (Feldman et al, 1994). In the National Health and Social Life Survey in men aged 18–59, other male sexual dysfunctions were also found to be highly prevalent: premature ejaculation (28.5%), lack of sexual interest (15.8%), anxiety about sexual performance (17%), and lack of pleasure in sex (8.1%) (Laumann et al, 1994).

Classification & Pathogenesis

A new classification of ED has been recommended by the International Society of Impotence Research (Lizza and Rosen, 1999, Table 37–3). In the 1950s, 90% of cases of ED were believed to be psychogenic. Most authors now believe that mixed organic and psychogenic ED is the most common.

Psychological Disorders

Many psychologic conditions (performance anxiety, strained relationship, lack of sexual arousal, depression, and schizophrenia) can either cause or aggravate ED.

Table 37–3. New classification of ED recommended by the International Society of Impotence Research

I. Psychogenic
1. Generalized Type
   A. Generalized unresponsiveness
      a. Primary lack of sexual arousability
      b. Aging-related decline in sexual arousability
   B. Generalized inhibition
      a. Chronic disorder of sexual intimacy
2. Situational Type
   A. Partner related
      a. Lack of arousability in specific relationship
      b. Lack of arousability due to sexual object preference
      c. High central inhibition due to partner conflict or threat
   B. Performance related
      a. Associated with other sexual dysfunction/s (eg, rapid ejaculation)
      b. Situational performance anxiety (eg, fear of failure)
   C. Psychological distress or adjustment related
      a. Associated with negative mood state (eg, depression) or major life stress (eg, death of partner)

II. Organic
1. Neurogenic
2. Hormonal
3. Arterial
4. Cavernosal (venogenic)
5. Drug-induced

III. Mixed organic/psychogenic (Most common type)

The pathogenesis of psychogenic ED is still speculative. The most cited include imbalance of central neurotransmitters, over-inhibition of spinal erection center by the brain, inadequate NO release, and sympathetic overactivity.

Neurogenic Disorders

ED can be caused by disease or dysfunction of the brain, spinal cord, or cavernous and pudendal nerves. In men with spinal cord injury, the degree of erectile function depends on the nature, location, and the extent of the lesion. Peripheral neuropathy as seen in diabetes mellitus, chronic alcohol abuse, or vitamin deficiency may affect the nerve endings and result in a deficiency of neurotransmitters. Direct injury to the cavernous or pudendal nerves from trauma or radical prostatic or rectal surgery also can cause disruption of the neural pathway and result in ED.

Hormonal Disorders

Hypogonadism due to hypothalamic or pituitary tumors, estrogen or antiandrogen therapy, or orchiectomy can suppress sexual interest and nocturnal erections. However, these patients may achieve varying degree of erections during visual sexual stimulation (Bancroft and Wu, 1983), and thus, the erectile ability is preserved. Similarly, ED resulting from hyperprolactinemia is probably caused by suppressed sexual interest. Hyperthyroidism, hypothyroidism, Cushing syndrome, and Addison disease are all reported to cause decreased libido and ED. Whether the hormonal disturbance or other factors are responsible for the ED needs further investigation.

Arterial Disorders

Although arteriogenic ED may be due to trauma or may be congenital, most often it is part of a generalized systemic arterial disease. The distribution and severity of the disease, however, differ from person to person. Some patients with severe arterial disease may still be potent as long as the arterial flow exceeds the venous flow; conversely, some patients with minimal arterial disease may be partially or completely impotent because of relatively large venous outflow, cavernous smooth-muscle dysfunction, or inadequate neurotransmitter release.

Arterial disease can be classified as extra- or intrapenile arterial insufficiency. Extrapenile arterial disease is amenable to surgical repair and comprises diseases of the internal pudendal artery, internal and common iliac arteries and aorta, the pelvic steal syndrome, and pelvic trauma. Intrapenile arterial disease such as that resulting from aging, arteriosclerosis, or diabetes mellitus does not respond well to currently available surgical techniques.

Cavernosal Disorders

Cavernous (venous) impotence can be divided into 5 types according to cause: In type 1, large veins exit the corpus cavernosum (this type is probably congenital); in type 2, venous channels are enlarged as a result of distortion of the tunica albuginea (as in Peyronie disease or the weakening associated with aging); in type 3, the cavernous smooth muscle is unable to relax because of fibrosis, degeneration, or dysfunction of gap junctions; in type 4, there is inadequate neurotransmitter release (in neurologic or psychological impotence or endothelial dysfunction); and in type 5, there is abnormal communication between the corpus cavernosum and the spongiosum or glans (congenital, traumatic, or consequent to shunt procedure for priapism) (Lue, 2000).

Electron microscope studies of cavernous erectile tissue obtained during implantation of penile prostheses reveal a high incidence of smooth-muscle atrophy, fibrous replacement, and endothelial disruption in patients with diabetes mellitus and atherosclerosis (Mersdorf et al, 1991). Studies of penile tissue obtained by needle biopsy have also revealed changes in the smooth muscle–collagen ratio, decreased endothelium, and diminished elastic fibers in impotent patients and impaired smooth–muscle relaxation in diabetic patients (Saenz de Tejada et al, 1989; Sattar et al, 1995).

Other Causes

Other causes may affect one or more of the factors controlling the erectile mechanism. Because of the lack of scientific studies, however, their precise pathogenetic relationship remains speculative.

A. Drugs

Many drugs have been reported to cause ED, although the mechanism of action is largely unknown and there are few controlled studies on the sexual effects of a particular drug. In general, drugs that interfere with central neuroendocrine or local neurovascular control of penile smooth muscle have the potential to cause ED. Central neurotransmitter pathways, including serotonergic, noradrenergic, and dopaminergic pathways involved in sexual function, may be disturbed by antipsychotics, antidepressants, and centrally acting antihypertensive drugs.

Alpha-adrenergic blocking drugs, such as prazosin, terazosin, and doxazosin, may cause retrograde ejaculation owing to relaxation of the bladder neck. Beta-adrenergic blocking drugs may cause ED by potentiating α_{-1} adrenergic activity in the penis. Thiazide diuretics have been reported to cause ED, but the cause is unknown. Spironolactone can cause erectile failure as well as decrease in libido and gynecomastia.

Cigarette smoking may induce vasoconstriction and penile venous leakage because of its contractile effect on the cavernous smooth muscle. Alcohol in small amounts improves erection and increases libido because of its vasodilatory effect and the suppression of anxiety; however, large amounts can cause central sedation, decreased libido, and transient ED. Chronic alcoholism may cause hypogonadism and polyneuropathy, which may affect penile nerve function. Cimetidine, a histamine-H_2 receptor antagonist, has been reported to decrease libido and cause erectile failure; it acts as an antiandrogen and can cause hyperprolactinemia. Other drugs known to cause ED are estrogens and drugs with antiandrogenic action, such as ketoconazole and cyproterone acetate.

B. Systemic Disease, Aging, and Other Disorders

About 50% of men with chronic diabetes mellitus reportedly have ED. In addition to the disease's effect on small vessels, it may also affect the cavernous nerve terminals, cavernous smooth muscle, and endothelial cells. The harmful effect of long-term diabetes on both neural and vascular components makes diabetic ED one of the least responsive to oral sildenafil therapy.

Sexual function progressively declines in "healthy" aging men. For example, the latent period between sexual stimulation and erection increases, erections are less turgid, ejaculation is less forceful, ejaculatory volume decreases, and the refractory period between erections lengthens. There is also a decrease in penile sensitivity to tactile stimulation.

Men with severe pulmonary disease may have ED because of fear of aggravating dyspnea during sexual intercourse. Men with angina, myocardial infarction, or heart failure may have ED from anxiety, depression, or concomitant penile arterial insufficiency, which is quite common in these patients. Chronic renal failure has frequently been associated with diminished erectile function, impaired libido, and infertility. In men with chronic renal failure and ED, many were found to have cavernous artery occlusive disease and veno-occlusive dysfunction. The mechanism is probably multifactorial: low serum testosterone concentrations, diabetes mellitus, vascular insufficiency, multiple medications, autonomic and somatic neuropathy, and psychological stress. Other systemic disorders such as cirrhosis, chronic debilitation, and cachexia can cause ED due to loss of libido or neurovascular dysfunction.

DIAGNOSIS & TREATMENT

A detailed medical and psychosexual history and a thorough physical examination are the most important steps in the differential diagnosis of sexual dysfunction. Interviewing the partner, if available, is very helpful in eliciting a reliable history, planning treatment, and obtaining a successful outcome. ED is often associated with a variety of diseases such as diabetes mellitus, coronary artery disease, hyperlipidemia, hypertension, spinal cord compression, and pituitary tumor. Therefore, a routine workup aimed at determining the cause should be performed in all patients. This should include basic laboratory tests such as a complete blood count, urinalysis, fasting blood glucose, serum creatinine, lipid profile, morning serum testosterone, and prolactin levels. The physician should then assess the findings, inquire about the goals and preferences of the man (and his partner), and discuss further diagnostic and therapeutic options so that his (or their) participation in the decision-making process will be well informed (Lue, 1989). Some men may benefit from a referral for further testing and treatment. The indications for referral include complex gonadal or other endocrine disorders; neurologic deficit suggestive of brain or spinal cord disease; deep-seated psychologic or psychiatric problems; and active cardiovascular disease, especially if the patient wishes to take sildenafil. If the man is taking a drug known to cause ED or recreational drugs, or has vascular risk factors, a change in medication or lifestyle may be helpful.

A variety of self-report measures for assessing the levels of male sexual function are now available. The most commonly used is International Index of Erectile Function (IIEF) (Rosen et al, 1997). It has 15 items and addresses and quantifies 5 domains: erectile function, orgasmic function, sexual desire, intercourse satisfaction, and overall satisfaction (Rosen et al, 1997). An abridged 5-item version of the IIEF has also been developed for office use (Rosen et al, 1999). ED severity is classified into 5 categories based on the IIEF 5: severe (5–7), moderate (8–11), mild to moderate (12–16), mild (17–21), no ED (22–25).

In patients with complicated problems, a variety of vascular and neurologic tests are available to further identify the cause of ED (Table 37–4). These are discussed below.

Table 37–4. Tests suggested for various treatment options (Lue, 1989).[a]

---

1. Oral medication, transurethral therapy, or vacuum constriction device
   No further testing
2. Intracavernous injection therapy
   CIS test
3. Penile prosthesis
   CIS test or NPT test or duplex scanning
4. Venous surgery
   CIS test
   Duplex scanning or cavernous arterial occlusion pressure test
   Cavernosometry and cavernosography
5. Arterial surgery (or combined arterial and venous surgery)
   CIS test
   Duplex scanning or cavernous arterial occlusion pressure
   Cavernosometry and cavernosography
   Pharmacologic arteriography

CIS, combined injection and stimulation; NPT, nocturnal penile tumescence.
[a]Regardless of desired treatment, all patients must undergo history, physical examination, and basic laboratory testing.

Advanced Testing for ED

A. Nocturnal Penile Tumescence (NPT) Test

Nocturnal erections occur in healthy males of all ages. Of the nocturnal erections, about 80% occur during REM sleep. The average man has 3–5 episodes of NPT each night, with each episode yielding 30–60 min of erection time. Total NPT time declines with increasing age. NPT has been measured by several methods: stamp test, Snap Gauges, strain gauges, NPTR (Rigiscan, Timm Medical Technologies, [Levine and Lenting, 1995]) sleep lab NPTR and NPT electrobioimpedance (NEVA, American Medical Systems, [Knoll and Abrams, 1999]).

In its classic form, NPT monitoring devices measure the number of erectile episodes, maximal penile rigidity, tumescence (circumference), and duration of the nocturnal erections. These data are recorded in conjunction with electroencephalographic, electro-oculographic, and electromyographic, nasal air flow, and oxygen saturation data, to document REM sleep, the presence or absence of hypoxia, and abnormal limb movement (Karacan, 1988). Because of its expense, sleep lab NPT has been replaced by simpler outpatient devices such as Rigiscan and NEVA. These newer devices have the advantage of electronically recording the number, duration, rigidity, and circumference of penile erections. NPT was originally designed to differentiate psychogenic from organic ED. In the United States, it is now mostly used in medicolegal or complicated cases.

B. Psychological Evaluation

The contemporary definition of psychogenic ED is, "persistent inability to achieve or maintain erection satisfactory for sexual performance which is due to predominantly or exclusively to psychological or interpersonal factors" (Lizza and Rosen, 1999). Therefore, a skillful diagnostic interview is the mainstay of a good psychological evaluation. The diagnostic interview should focus more on the current sexual problem and its immediate causation, partner relationship, and any psychiatric symptoms. Because psychogenic impotence is the result of changes in affect and mood, it usually occurs in a specific pattern. A suggestive history includes sudden onset, selective dysfunction (eg, rigid erection with one partner and poor erection with others, or normal erection during masturbation or fantasy but not during intercourse), and normal pattern of nocturnal erections but abnormal pattern during waking hours. This is often associated with anxiety, guilt, fear, emotional stress, and religious or parental inhibition.

Although psychological consultation is not indicated for most patients, it is very useful in evaluating and treating men with deep-seated psychological problems.

Three groups of psychometric instruments are available: (1) personality questionnaires; (2) the depression inventory; and (3) questionnaires for sexual dysfunction and relationship factors. The Minnesota Multiphasic Personality Inventory (MMPI)-2 is a valuable tool for evaluating the patient's personality and its relevance to sexual dysfunction. The Beck Depression Inventory is a self-reported test for which a score exceeding 18 is considered indicative of significant clinical depression. For relationship assessment, the Short Marital Adjustment Test (for married couples) and the Dyadic Adjustment Inventory (for unmarried people) can be used to determine overall relationship quality.

C. Neurologic Tests

There are 3 types of erections: nocturnal, psychogenic, and reflexogenic. In a broader sense, neurologic testing should assess peripheral, spinal, and supraspinal centers as well as both somatic and autonomic pathways associated with all 3 types of erection and sexual arousal. However, the effect of neurologic deficit on penile erection is a complicated phenomenon and, with a few exceptions, neurologic testing will rarely change management. Therefore the aim of neuro-urologic testing is to (1) uncover reversible neurologic disease such as dorsal nerve neuropathy secondary to long-distance bicycling; (2) assess the extent of neurologic deficit from a known neurologic disease such as diabetes mellitus or pelvic injury; and (3) determine whether a referral to a neurologist is necessary (eg, workup for possible spinal cord tumor).

1. Biothesiometry—This test is designed to measure the sensory perception threshold to various amplitudes of vibratory stimulation produced by a hand-held electromagnetic device (biothesiometer) placed on the pulp of the index fingers, both sides of the penile shaft, and the glans penis (Bemelmans et al, 1995).

2. Bulbocavernosus reflex latency—This test is performed by placing 2 stimulating ring electrodes around the penis, one near the corona and the other 3 cm proximal. Concentric needle electrodes are placed in the right and left bulbocavernous muscles to record the response. Square-wave impulses are delivered via a direct current stimulator. The latency period for each stimulus response is measured from the beginning of the stimulus to the beginning of the response. An abnormal bulbocavernosus reflex (BCR) latency time, defined as a value greater than 3 standard deviations above the mean (30–40 msec), carries a high probability of neuropathology.

3. Genitocerebral evoked potential—This test involves electrical stimulation of the dorsal nerve of the penis as described for the BCR latency test. Instead of recording EMG responses, this study records the evoked potential waveforms overlying the sacral spinal cord and cerebral cortex.

4. Smooth muscle EMG—This involves direct recording of cavernous electrical activity with a needle electrode. The normal resting flaccid electrical activity from the corpora cavernosa was a rhythmic slow wave with an intermittent burst of activity. These bursts virtually ceased during visual sexual stimulation or after intracavernous injection of a smooth-muscle relaxant. Patients with suspected autonomic neuropathy demonstrated a discoordination pattern with continuing electrical activity during visual sexual stimulation or after intracavernous injection of a smooth-muscle relaxant (Jünemann, Buhrle, and Stief, 1993).

5. Tests for penile vascular function—

    a. CIS (Combined Intracavernous Injection and Stimulation) test—Office pharmacotesting consists of an intracavernous injections, visual or manual sexual stimulation, and a rating of the subsequent erection. This test is the most commonly performed diagnostic procedure for ED. This screening test allows the clinician to bypass neurogenic and hormonal influences and to evaluate the vascular status of the penis directly and objectively. The most commonly used vasodilator is 10 μg of alprostadil or 0.3 mL of a mixture of papaverine and phentolamine. A rigid erection lasting for more than 20 min is indicative of normal venous function (Virag et al, 1984; Donatucci & Lue, 1992). However, the same conclusion cannot be made for arterial function because some men with mild arterial insufficiency can also have the same response.

    b. Duplex ultrasonography (gray-scale and color-coded)—When further vascular diagnostic testing is indicated, the color duplex ultrasound study—which consists of an intracavernous pharmacotest and measurement of blood flow by duplex Doppler ultrasound—is the most reliable and least invasive evidence-based assessment of ED (Lue et al, 1985; Figure 37–4). Normal arterial response is a peak flow velocity measured at the base of penis of more than 30 cm/s, a sharp upstroke of the waveform, and absence of diastolic flow after sexual stimulation. Ultrasound can also be used to detect penile abnormalities such as Peyronie's plaque, calcification, thickened vessel wall, and intracavernous fibrosis. The parameters useful in diagnosing venous leakage include a diastolic venous flow velocity of > 5 cm/s, a resistive index (RI) of < 0.75, or both (Naroda et al, 1994). RI = peak flow velocity (PSV) − end diastolic flow velocity (EDV)/PSV.

    The **Pulsed Doppler study** test is performed with a portable Midus pulsed Doppler unit. It records the

Figure 37–4. Duplex ultrasonography and Doppler analysis of the arterial response to intracavernous papaverine injection. In the flaccid state (**A**), the luminal diameter of the cavernous artery is 0.06 cm; after papaverine injection (**B**), this increases to 0.13 cm. Wave analysis (**C**) shows normal flow in the cavernous artery (peak velocity, 39 cm/s).

Doppler waveform of the cavernous arteries without providing a real-time image. Cavernous artery blood flow is studied in a similar fashion to duplex Doppler.

c. Cavernous arterial occlusion pressure—This test involves infusing saline solution into the corpora after intracavernous injection of vasodilators to raise the intracavernous pressure above the systolic blood pressure. A pencil Doppler transducer is then applied to the side of the penile base. The saline infusion is stopped, and the intracavernous pressure is allowed to fall. The pressure at which the cavernous arterial flow becomes detectable is defined as the cavernous artery systolic occlusion pressure (CASOP). A gradient between the cavernous and brachial artery pressures of less than 35 mm Hg and equal pressure between the right and left cavernous arteries have been defined as normal.

d. Cavernosometry and cavernosography—Pharmacologic cavernosometry involves intracavernous injection of a vasodilator combination (papaverine + phentolamine + alprostadil) followed by saline infusion and simultaneous monitoring of intracavernous pressure. In men with normal venous function, the maintenance flow should be less than 10 mL/min at 100 mm Hg intracavernous pressure, and the intracavernous pressure drop rate after the infusion is stopped should be less than 50 mm Hg in 30 seconds (Padma-Nathan, 1989).

Cavernosography involves the infusion of diluted radiocontrast solution into the corpora cavernosa during an artificial erection to visualize the site of venous leakage. It should always be performed after activation of the veno-occlusive mechanism by intracavernous injection of vasodilators. Minimal or no contrast is seen outside the corpora cavernosa in men with normal veno-occlusive function. In patients with venous leakage of congenital or traumatic origin, the leakage is seen most often in the crura or at the site of injury, respectively (Figure 37–5). The typical finding in men with intrinsic disease of the corpus cavernosum or the tunica albuginea is a diffuse leakage through all penile venous channels.

e. Arteriography—Arteriography is reserved for the evaluation of the complex patient when revascularization surgery is contemplated. The study is performed by intracavernous injection of a vasodilating agent (papaverine, papaverine + phentolamine, or alprostadil) followed by selective cannulation of the internal pudendal artery and injection of a diluted contrast solution of low osmolarity. The anatomy and radiographic appearance of the cavernous arteries are then evaluated (Figure 37–6). The evaluation should include the size and length of the inferior epigastric arteries as well as the cavernous and dorsal arteries of the penis.

A

B

C

Figure 37–5. Cavernosography after intracavernous injection of papaverine. In a normal man (**A**), the cavernosogram shows opacification of the erect corpora cavernosa and nonvisualization of penile veins. In (**B**), the patient has a large leak through both superficial dorsal veins (arrows) to the saphenous veins (arrowheads). Film (**C**) shows abnormal venous drainage via the cavernous veins (solid arrow) into the preprostatic plexus (open arrow) and the internal pudendal veins (arrowhead). (Reproduced, with permission, from Lue TF, Tanagho EA: Physiology of erection and pharmacological management of impotence. J Urol 1987;137:829. © by Williams & Wilkins, 1987.)

A

B

Figure 37–6. Internal iliac arteriogram in the flaccid penis (**A**) shows poor visualization of penile arteries, simulating occlusion (arrow). After intracavernous injection of 60 mg of papaverine (**B**), all the branches of the penile artery are well visualized.

NONSURGICAL TREATMENT OF ERECTILE DYSFUNCTION

Although the penile prosthesis remains one of the most effective treatments for all types of ED, nonsurgical management has replaced prosthetic surgery as the preferred choice in the last decade. Both specific and nonspecific treatments are available. The former include psychotherapy, change of offending medications, and hormonal therapy; the latter include sildenafil, vacuum constriction device, transurethral therapy and intracavernous injection. Although nonspecific therapies appear to be more effective for most cases of ED, the patient should also be made aware of specific therapies.

Lifestyle Changes

It is well known that ED is intimately related to the atherosclerotic coronary and peripheral vascular dis-eases. Although it is difficult to prove its beneficial effect, a change of lifestyle should be encouraged (regular exercise, a healthy diet, smoking cessation, alcohol in moderation only). Long-distance bicycling is another risk factor that should be discussed. The detrimental effects of perineal compression on penile arteries may be lessened by changes in seat design and riding practices.

Changing Medications

When a patient complains of sexual dysfunction after taking a particular medication, it is important to determine whether the problem is related to loss of sexual drive, impaired erection, or rapid/delayed ejaculation. In many situations, changing the medication to a different class of agents is a feasible first step. Antihypertension agents therapeutically lower blood pressure; this primary effect has long been thought the mechanism of their adverse actions on erection. Switching patients to newer agents such as alpha-adrenoceptor antagonists, calcium channel blockers, and angiotensin-converting enzyme inhibitors may reverse ED in some patients. Patients complaining of sexual dysfunction while taking antidepressants may benefit from changing to trazodone or bupropion.

Psychosexual Therapy

Therapies such as a sildenafil, vacuum constriction device, or intracavernous injection may provide a faster relief for patients than a prolonged course of psychosexual therapy. However, in patients with obvious psychologic problems, a referral to a psychologist or sex therapist is highly recommended because elimination of the specific underlying cause may result in a cure. Moreover, in some patients with mixed psychogenic and organic ED, psychosexual therapy may help relieve the anxiety and remove unrealistic expectations associated with medical or surgical therapy.

Hormonal Therapy

Referral to endocrinology is recommended for patients with thyroid, adrenal, pituitary or hypothalamic dysfunction. The urologist should be aware that aging men with ED may show a variety of symptoms when hypogonadism coexists: low libido, depression, decreased intellectual abilities, decreased lean body mass, decreased bone mineral density, decreased skin turgor, changes in body hair distribution, changes in sleep patterns, and increased visceral fat. This discussion is limited to treatment of hypogonadism and hyperprolactinemia as they relate to ED.

In the patient with documented hypogonadism and ED, it is reasonable to initiate androgen therapy. Parenteral depo-preparations of testosterone such as testosterone cypionate and enanthate are the cheapest form of androgen supplementation and are effective in restoring serum levels of testosterone to normal. They are administered through deep intramuscular injection; resulting in supraphysiologic levels of testosterone for 72 h with gradual steady decline over 2–3 weeks. Enanthate and cypionate are generally administered every 2–4 weeks at dosages of 200–400 mg. Testosterone propionate has a shorter half-life requiring dosing every other day. Transcutaneous dosing more closely simulates normal circadian levels of testosterone if patients apply the patch in the morning.

There are currently 3 FDA-approved preparations available in the United States: Testoderm/Testoderm TTS (Alza Pharmaceuticals), Androderm (Glaxo-SmithKline), and AndroGel (Unimed Pharmaceuticals, Inc). Testoderm comes in 2 sizes, delivering 4 mg/d or 6 mg/d. Physiologic blood levels can be achieved in 65% of patients who apply the system to the scrotum. Testoderm TTS may be applied daily as a 5-mg patch to the arm, back, or upper buttocks, avoiding the inconveniences of scrotal therapy. Androderm comes as a patch that delivers 2.5 mg or 5 mg. The most common adverse reactions to both Testoderm TTS and Androderm are itching, chronic skin irritation, and allergic contact dermatitis. Patients should alternate sites of application and avoid sun-exposed sites, and they may be helped by local application of cortisone cream to irritated skin. Androgel 1% is a cream designed to deliver 50 mg of testosterone, applied once daily in the morning to clean, dry skin over the shoulders, upper arms, or abdomen. It is supplied in packets of 25 mg and 50 mg. The most common adverse reaction is also skin-site irritation. The oral forms available in the United States are 17α-methyl testosterone preparations. When taken orally, these preparations are largely rendered metabolically inactive during the "first pass" circulation through the liver. These preparations are toxic to the liver and can lead to hepatitis, cholestatic jaundice, hepatomas, hemorrhagic liver cysts, and hepatocarcinoma (Bagatell and Bremner, 1996). Testosterone undecenoate is an oral testosterone ester relatively free of liver toxicity but is not available in the United States.

A discussion of **potential adverse effects** is in order. In a young hypogonadal man, testosterone replacement is clearly the treatment of choice. However, the risks may outweigh the benefits in some patients. Supraphysiologic levels of testosterone will suppress luteinizing hormone and follicle-stimulating hormone production and can result in infertility, breast tenderness, and gynecomastia. Erythrocytosis is the most common laboratory alteration noted with long-term therapy. Androgens may also induce or worsen sleep apnea. Cardiovascular risks are increased in some patients by increases in red cell mass and thromboxane A_2 as well as platelet aggregation (Ajayi, Mathur, and Halushka, 1995). Many practitioners have raised concerns about the potential risks of androgen therapy in elderly patient with prostate symptoms or occult prostate cancer. Several studies in the literature suggest that androgen replacement does not induce prostate cancer in men with normal prostates, and placebo-controlled studies show little difference in prostate volume, prostate-specific antigen levels, and obstructive symptoms (Cooper et al, 1998; Nomura et al, 1998). The fear of exacerbating an occult cancer of the prostate remains a major concern. Nevertheless, there are some older hypogonadal patients whose libido and erectile function can be restored by testosterone therapy and who should not be denied the option. When a patient desires this, we routinely perform a digital rectal examination and obtain a serum prostate-specific antigen level. When one is in doubt, ultrasound-guided biopsy is also done before androgen therapy is given. The presence of prostate or breast cancer is an absolute contraindication to androgen supplementation. Patients are followed up every 6 months with a rectal examination and serum prostate-specific antigen test as long as they are receiving therapy. Laboratory surveillance should also include hemoglobin/hematocrit levels, liver function tests, and a cholesterol and lipid profile. The efficacy of testosterone supplementation is reasonably determined by clinical response rather than blood level of testosterone.

In patients with hyperprolactinemia with or without hypogonadism, testosterone therapy does not improve sexual function. Treatment should first be aimed at eliminating the offending drugs, such as estrogens, morphine, sedatives, or neuroleptics. Bromocriptine is a dopamine agonist that lowers the prolactin level and restores testosterone to normal. It is used to reduce tumor size of a prolactin-secreting adenoma. Neurosurgery may occasionally be needed if the response is not satisfactory or if there are changes in the visual field secondary to optic nerve compression.

Phosphodiesterase (PDE) Inhibitors

Sildenafil citrate (Viagra, Pfizer Pharmaceuticals) is a selective inhibitor of phosphodiesterase-5 (PDE5), the enzyme that breaks down the intracellular second messenger of erection cGMP and thus enhances penile erection. The clinical efficacy and safety of sildenafil was evaluated in many placebo-controlled, double-blind trials and open-label studies (Goldstein et al, 1998, Morales et al, 1998). Improvement in erections was reported in 56–84% of subjects taking 25–100 mg of sildenafil and 25% in the placebo group. Treatment effect was principally assessed by items 3 and 4 of the IIEF-15 questionnaires (ability to initiate and maintain erection). Overall responses to sildenafil appear to be dosage related over the range 25–100 mg, with little ED benefit and considerably more side effects above 100 mg. Sildenafil is effective in patients with organic, psychogenic, and mixed-etiology ED. An overall beneficial treatment effect was seen in 70% of patients. As fas as specific etiologies of ED, sildenafil was effective in 70% of hypertensive patients, 57% of diabetic patients, 43% of radical prostatectomy patients, and 80% of spinal cord injury patients. Since PDE5 inhibitor proerectile effects are only seen with sexual stimulation and depend on intact cavernous nerve function (release of NO), a positive treatment effect would not be expected in patients with cavernous nerve injury due to non-nerve sparing pelvic surgery.

The peak blood level is achieved about 1 h following oral administration. A high-fat meal slows the rate of absorption and may delay peak plasma concentrations by 2 h and in some cases reduce peak plasma concentrations by 25%. Older age (> 65 years), hepatic impairment, drugs that inhibit the cytochrome P450 isoenzyme (cimetidine, ketoconazole, erythromycin), and severe renal insufficiency are associated with increased plasma levels of sildenafil; therefore, the dosage should be reduced in these patients.

Principal adverse events with a dose of 25–100 mg are headache (15.8%), flushing (10.5%), dyspepsia (6.5%), nasal congestion (4.2%), altered vision (2.7%), diarrhea (2.6%), dizziness (2.2%), and arthralgia (2.0%). Sildenafil is absolutely contraindicated for men using nitrates (oral, sublingual, or topical) because sildenafil potentiates the hypotensive effects of all nitrates. ED is common among men who have atherosclerotic coronary artery disease. Data from the Framingham Heart Study suggest that the risk of myocardial infarction in a healthy 50-year-old US male is 1% per year or 1 per million men per hour. The risk of myocardial infarction is 2 in a million during and within 2 h after sexual activity (Moller et al, 2001). The American College of Cardiology and American Heart Association guidelines caution that sildenafil dosing is potentially hazardous in men with coronary ischemia (positive exercise test), men with congestive heart failure and borderline low blood pressure and low blood volume, and men taking complicated multidrug antihypertensives (Cheitlin et al, 1999). In these patients a referral to cardiology is strongly recommended if the patient desires sildenafil therapy.

Yohimbine

Yohimbine is a centrally acting alpha-2-adrenergic antagonist obtained from the bark of the yohim tree. Although it has been highly effective in castrated rats, several clinical studies have shown only moderate success in men. In clinical studies, yohimbine seems to be effective in patients with psychogenic but not organic ED. As an initial treatment 5.4 mg 3 times daily has been recommended; others have reported efficacy by doubling that dosage or using on an as-needed basis (2 tablets 1–2 h prior to anticipated sexual activity). Side effects of yohimbine include palpitations, headache, agitation, anxiety, and increase in blood pressure (precautions are advised in men with cardiovascular disease).

Trazodone

Trazodone is a commonly prescribed mild antidepressant with a rare incidence of priapism. Several small clinical trials have shown a positive effect on nocturnal penile erection (Saenz de Tejada et al, 1991) and a modest effect on sexually stimulated erection. A dual mechanism of (peripheral) alpha-adrenergic blocking and (central) inhibition of serotonin reuptake (increasing 5HT-1c) is the proposed mechanism of action. Dosages ranging from 25 mg to 200 mg nightly have been used. A combination of trazodone and yohimbine has also been reported to improve erectile function in some patients (Montorsi et al, 1994). Side effects include drowsiness, nausea, emesis, blood pressure changes (both hypotension and hypertension are reported), urinary retention, and priapism (especially at therapeutic antidepressant levels).

Apomorphine

Apomorphine is a D1/D2 dopamine receptor agonist, activating D1 and D2 receptors. Dopaminergic stimulation is proerectile; early reports of patients treated for Parkinson disease showed increased spontaneous erections, without increased libido. A sublingual form of apomorphine (Uprima) has been approved for ED in Europe but has not been approved by the FDA in the United States.

In a double-blind, placebo-controlled study, at dosages of 2 and 4 mg, subjects reporting erections firm enough for intercourse were 45% and 55%, respectively, with placebo responses of 35% and 36%. Sexual attempts resulting in intercourse were 40% and 49%, respectively, on 2 and 4 mg; placebo dosing resulted in intercourse in 30% of attempts. Self-assessment of success was 47% at 2-mg dosing and 59.9% at 4-mg dosing (Heaton, 2001).

The drug has a rapid onset of action, with a window of sexual opportunity of approximately 2 h from ingestion. Maximal plasma concentrations are reached in 50 min. Adverse events described in clinical trials were nausea, 16.9%; dizziness, 8.3%; sweating, 5%; somnolence, 5.8%; yawning, 7.9%; and emesis, 3.7%. At the highest recommended dosage syncope occurred in 0.6% of patients and was accompanied by a clear prodrome suggestive of a vasovagal event: nausea, vomiting, sweating, dizziness, and lightheadedness (Heaton, 2001). There were no documented food/drug interactions in clinical trials (with the exception of ethanol) and specifically no documented pharmacologic interactions for subjects using nitrate drugs.

Transurethral Therapy

Alprostadil, the synthetic formulation of PGE_1, is the only pharmacologic agent approved by the FDA for the management of ED via intracavernous and transurethral routes. Alprostadil stimulates adenyl cyclase to increase intracellular levels of cAMP, lowering intracellular concentrations of calcium, thus relaxing arterial and trabecular smooth muscle. Drug is transferred from urethra to corpus spongiosum to corpus cavernosum. MUSE (medicated urethral system for erection) consists of a very small semisolid pellet (3 × 1 mm) administered into the distal urethra (3 cm) by a proprietary applicator (MUSE VIVUS Inc, Menlo Park, CA).

Clinical trials showed that 66% of men responded to an in-office trial; of these, 65% had successful intercourse at least once at home with MUSE, for a rate of 43% (Padma-Nathan, 1997). With MUSE therapy, the rigidity can be enhanced by an elastic ring placed at the base of the penis (ACTIS, Vivus Inc), to mechanically assist veno-occlusion (Lewis, 1998).

Penile pain is a ubiquitous side effect of alprostadil-based therapies and is clearly dosage-related; in MUSE patients the discomfort can include a dull ache in the penis and the scrotum. The reported penile pain rate was 33% in MUSE trials. Hypotension and syncope have been noted in 1–5.8% of patients, thus mandating that initial administration be in the office setting.

Intracavernous Injection

One of the most dramatic changes in urology has been the introduction of intracavernous injection of vasoactive drugs for the diagnosis and treatment of ED. A list of drugs that have been used clinically is presented in Table 37–5.

A. PAPAVERINE

Papaverine is an alkaloid isolated from the opium poppy. Its molecular mechanism of action is through its inhibitory effect on phosphodiesterase, leading to increased cAMP and cGMP in penile erectile tissue and thus relaxing cavernous smooth muscle and penile vessels. Papaverine is metabolized in the liver, and the plasma half-life is about 1–2 h.

The average dose for papaverine injection ranges from 15 to 60 mg. Papaverine has been shown to be ef-

Table 37–5. Intracavernous vasodilator injection therapy.[a]

Drug	Test Dose	Therapeutic Dose
Papaverine	15–30 mg	15–60 mg
Alprostadil	5–10 µg	5–60 µg
Papaverine (30 mg) + Phentolamine (1 mg)	0.1–0.3 mL	0.2–1 mL
Papaverine (30 mg) + Phentolamine (1 mg) + Alprostadil (10 µg)	0.1–0.3 mL	0.2 –1 mL

[a]Lower doses for management of neurogenic and psychogenic impotence.

fective in psychogenic and neurogenic ED (Virag, 1982). The advantages are its low cost and stability at room temperature. The major disadvantages are the higher incidence of corporal fibrosis (1–33%), thought to be a result of low acidity (pH 3–4), and occasional elevation of liver enzymes.

B. PHENTOLAMINE METHYLATE (REGITINE)

Phentolamine methylate is a competitive alpha-adrenoceptor antagonist with equal affinity for alpha-1 and alpha-2 receptors. Systemic hypotension, reflex tachycardia, nasal congestion, and gastrointestinal upset are the most common systemic side effects. It has a short plasma half-life (30 min). When injected intracorporally alone, it increases corporal blood flow but does not result in a significant rise in intracorporal pressure.

C. ALPROSTADIL (PROSTAGLANDIN E₁)

Alprostadil is the synthetic form of a naturally occurring unsaturated 20-carbon fatty acid (ie, alprostadil refers to the exogenous form; prostaglandin E_1 to the endogenous compound). It causes smooth-muscle relaxation, vasodilation, and inhibition of platelet aggregation through elevation of intracellular cAMP. Alprostadil is metabolized by the enzyme prostaglandin 15-hydroxydehydrogenase, which has been shown to be active in human corpus cavernosum (Roy et al, 1989). After intracavernous injection, 96% of alprostadil is locally metabolized within 60 min and no change in peripheral blood levels has been observed (van Ahlen et al, 1994).

In the United States, 2 formulations of alprostadil have been approved by the FDA for intracavernous therapy: Caverject (Pharmacia & Upjohn, Peapack, NJ) and Edex (Schwarz Pharma, Milwaukee, WI). Caverject is a lyophilized alprostadil powder developed for intracavernous injection. Edex is lyophilized alprostadil contained in an alpha cyclodextrin inclusion complex.

At a dosage of 10–20 µg, alprostadil produced full erections in 70–80% of patients with ED (Stackl, Hasun, and Marberger, 1988). The most frequent side effects were pain at the injection site or during erection (occurring in 16.8% of patients), hematoma/ecchymosis (1.5%), and prolonged erection/priapism (1.3%). Systemic side effects occurred rarely (Linet and Ogrinc, 1996).

D. Drug Combinations

Various drug combinations have been used for intracavernous injection therapy. The most commonly used are bimix (papaverine/phentolamine) and trimix (papaverine/phentolamine/alprostadil) in various concentrations. A study comparing papaverine or phentolamine alone with a papaverine/phentolamine combination in men with organic ED found that full erection occurred in 40% with papaverine alone, in 7% with phentolamine alone, and in 87% with papaverine/phentolamine (Zorgniotti and Lefleur, 1985; Stief and Wetterauer, 1988). Prolonged erection has been reported in 1–23% and fibrosis in 1.4–16% of patients receiving bimix therapy. The most commonly used formula contains 30 mg of papaverine and 1 mg of phentolamine per milliliter.

Regarding papaverine/phentolamine/alprostadil combinations, theoretically, because each of the 3 drugs has a different mechanism of action, the combination should take advantage of the synergism among them and permit a much lower dose of each to be used, avoiding the side effects of high dosages. In the study by Bennett, Carpenter, and Barada (1991), 89% of the patients tested had adequate erection and went on to home injection therapy. Overall, 74% of the 78 patients were maintained at a dose of < 0.25 mL per injection with a frequency averaging 3.1 uses per month. Two patients had a prolonged erection that required treatment. In another report from the same group of patients with 12–28 months of follow-up, 65% were continuing injection therapy and, of these, 89% were satisfied with the drug combination. Seven (5.6%) had prolonged erections > 3 h. No patient had fibrosis or nodules.

In a randomized crossover study of 228 patients, McMahon (1991) compared the triple-drug combination with papaverine/phentolamine and alprostadil alone. Statistically, the triple-drug combination was more effective in patients with severe arteriogenic or mild veno-occlusive dysfunction. The incidence of prolonged erection was lower when compared with papaverine/phentolamine but not significantly different from that in alprostadil alone. The triple-drug combination has been shown to be very effective in patients with organic ED (up to 89% response rate), but has a much lower incidence of painful erection.

E. Patient Acceptance and Dropout Rate

In several studies, the percentage of patients accepting injection therapy when offered in the office ranges from 49% to 84% (Gerber and Levine, 1991). The reasons for declining include penile pain, inadequate response, fear of the needle, unnaturalness, and loss of sex drive. In long-term studies, 13–60% of patients drop out for a number of reasons. These include loss of interest, loss of the partner, poor erectile response, penile pain, concomitant illness, recovery of spontaneous erection, and ultimate choice of other therapy.

F. Serious Adverse Effects

Priapism and fibrosis are the 2 more serious side effects associated with intracavernous injection therapy. Linet and Ogrinc (1996) calculated that priapism occurred in 1.3% of 8090 patients in 48 studies with alprostadil. The incidence was found to be about 5 times lower with alprostadil than with papaverine or the combination of papaverine and phentolamine (1.5% vs 10% vs 7%). Fibrosis can occur as a nodule, diffuse scarring, plaque, or curvature. The incidence is about 10 times lower with alprostadil than with papaverine or papaverine/phentolamine (1% vs 12% vs 9% of patients), although one study reported a 12% incidence with alprostadil.

G. Dosage and Administration

Patients must have the first injection performed by medical personnel and receive appropriate training and education before home injection. For alprostadil, an initial dose of 2.5 µg is recommended. If the response is inadequate, increases in 2.5-µg increments can be given until a full erection is achieved or a maximum of 60 µg is reached.

For drug combinations, one should start with a small dose (eg, 0.1 mL) and titrate the amount according to erectile response. The goal is to achieve a full erection of less than 1-h duration to avoid priapism. Compression of the needle puncture site for at least 5 minutes is recommended to prevent bleeding and fibrosis.

H. Treatment of Prolonged Erection or Priapism

The best treatment is prevention; patient should be warned not to increase the dose or repeat the injection without consulting the physician. If the erection lasted more than 4 h, the patient should either call the physician or go to the emergency room for treatment. The best regimen for averting priapism is intracavernous injection of diluted phenylephrine 250 to 500 µg every 3–5 min until detumescence. In patients with cardiovascular disease, monitoring blood pressure and pulse is recommended.

I. CONTRAINDICATIONS

The use of intracavernous injection therapy is contraindicated in patients with sickle cell anemia, schizophrenia or a severe psychiatric disorder, or severe venous incompetence. In patients taking an anticoagulant or aspirin, compressing the injection site for 7–10 min after injection is recommended. In patients with poor manual dexterity, the sexual partner can be instructed to perform the injection.

Vacuum Constriction Device

The vacuum constriction device consists of a plastic cylinder connected directly or by tubing to a vacuum-generating source (manual or battery-operated pump). After the penis is engorged by the negative pressure, a constricting ring is applied to the base to maintain the erection. To avoid injury, the ring should not be left in place for longer than 30 min.

The erection produced by a vacuum device is different from a physiologic erection or one produced by intracavernous injection. The portion of the penis proximal to the ring is not rigid, which may produce a pivoting effect. The penile skin may be cold and dusky, and ejaculation may be trapped by the constricting ring. The ring can be uncomfortable or even painful. However, in many patients the device can produce an erection that is close to normal and with rigidity sufficient for coitus. The device also engorges the glans and is useful for patients with glanular insufficiency. In patients with severe vascular insufficiency, the device may not produce adequate erection. In these cases, combining intracavernous injection with the vacuum constriction device may enhance the erection.

Complications include penile pain and numbness, difficult ejaculation, ecchymosis, and petechiae. Patients taking aspirin or warfarin sodium (Coumadin) should exercise caution when using these devices.

The patient's satisfaction rate has been reported to range from 68% to 83% (Cookson and Nadig, 1993). The device is more acceptable to older men in a steady relationship than to young single men in search of a partner. It is safe when used properly and is one of the least costly treatment options available.

PENILE VASCULAR SURGERY

Isolated stenosis or occlusion of the extrapenile arteries is amenable to surgical repair. Restoration of potency has been reported after surgery of the internal iliac and internal pudendal arteries. Currently, the most commonly used technique for penile revascularization is a bypass from the inferior epigastric artery to the dorsal artery or deep dorsal vein of the penis. This procedure is indicated only in young men with congenital or trau-

matic arterial insufficiency (Hakim et al, 1995). In men with generalized vascular disease secondary to hyperlipidemia, diabetes mellitus, chronic hypertension, and similar conditions, this procedure does not produce durable results and therefore is not recommended.

Penile venous surgery is also indicated only in young men with congenital or traumatic venous leakage. In congenital venous leakage, the venous insufficiency is typically through abnormal crural veins or superficial dorsal veins and is amenable to surgical cure (Lue, 1999). Traumatic venous leak is usually due to localized damage to the tunica albuginea or formation of a "fistula" between the corpus cavernosum and corpus spongiosum. Repair of the tunica or closure of the fistula can result in significant improvement of erectile function. In older men with chronic systemic diseases, the cause of leakage is atrophy of the cavernous smooth muscle and intracavernous fibrosis; ligation of the penile vein will only produce transient improvement and is not recommended.

PENILE PROSTHESIS

Penile prostheses are divided into 3 general types: malleable (semirigid), mechanical, and inflatable devices. The malleable devices are made of silicone rubber and several models contain a central intertwined metallic core. The mechanical device is also made of silicone rubber but contains polytetrafluoroethylene-coated interlocking polysulfone rings in a rod column, which provides rigidity when the rings are lined up in a straight line and flaccidity when the penis is bent.

Inflatable (hydraulic) devices are further divided into 2-piece and 3-piece devices. Two-piece inflatable prostheses consist of a pair of cylinders attached to a scrotal pump-reservoir. Three-piece inflatable penile prostheses consist of paired the penile cylinders, a scrotal pump, and a suprapubic fluid reservoir (Table 37–6).

Table 37–6. Types of penile protheses.

Semirigid
AMS 600 and 650 (malleable)
Mentor malleable
Acu-Form
Hinged
DuraPhase
One-piece inflatable
DynaFlex
Two-piece inflatable
Mark II (Mentor)
Ambicor (AMS)
Three-piece inflatable
Alpha-1, Alpha-1 narrow base (Mentor)
CX, CXM, Ultrex (AMS)

In general, the malleable devices last longer than the inflatable ones. Patients should be informed that a 5–15% failure rate is expected in the first 5 years and most of the devices will fail in 10–15 years and will need a replacement. Potential complications include mechanical failures, cylinder leaks, tubing leaks, infection, perforation, persistent pain, and autoinflation (Mulcahy, 2000; Montague et al, 2001; Anastasiadis et al, 2001).

MALE SEXUAL DYSFUNCTION INVOLVING EMISSION, EJACULATION, & ORGASM

Physiology of Emission, Ejaculation, & Orgasm

Different mechanisms are involved in erection, emission, ejaculation, and orgasm, and these events can be dissociated from one another (eg, a frequent complaint of impotent patients is ejaculating through a "limp penis"). Except for nocturnal emissions, or "wet dreams," emission and ejaculation require stimulation of the external genitalia. Impulses traveling from the pudendal nerves reach the upper lumbar spinal sympathetic nuclei. Efferent signals traveling in the hypogastric nerve activate secretions and transport sperm from the distal epididymis, vasa deferentia, seminal vesicles, and prostate to the prostatic urethra. Coordinated closing of the internal urethral sphincter and relaxation of the external sphincter direct the semen into the bulbous urethra (emission). Subsequent rhythmic contractions of the bulbocavernous muscles force the semen through a pressurized conduit—the much narrowed urethral lumen compressed by the engorged corpora cavernosa—to produce the 2- to 5-mL ejaculate. The external ejaculation process involves the somatomotor efferent of the pudendal nerve to contract the bulbocavernous muscle. Since this action is involuntary, however, integrated autonomic and somatic action is required.

The mechanism of orgasm is the least understood of the sexual processes. It probably involves cerebral interpretation and response to sexual stimulation. Along with emission and ejaculation, several nongenital responses also occur. These include involuntary rhythmic contractions of the anal sphincter, hyperventilation, tachycardia, and elevation of blood pressure.

Disorders Affecting Emission, Ejaculation, & Orgasm

Bilateral sympathectomy at the L2 level has resulted in ejaculatory dysfunction in about 40% of patients. High bilateral retroperitoneal lymphadenectomy causes an even higher percentage of emission failures. Retrograde ejaculation is usually the result of dysfunction of the internal sphincter or the bladder neck, as seen after prostatectomy, with alpha-blocker therapy, and in autonomic neuropathy due to diabetes.

Successful emission and ejaculation without orgasm occur in some patients with spinal cord injury. Phantom orgasm in a paraplegic man also has been described. A history of disease or surgery is helpful in differentiating emission failure from retrograde ejaculation. If microscopic examination confirms the presence of sperm in bladder urine after a dry ejaculation, retrograde ejaculation can be diagnosed. If no sperm is found, emission failure is the cause.

Treatment

Elimination of alpha-adrenergic blockers results in cure for some patients with emission failure or retrograde ejaculation. Alpha sympathomimetics such as ephedrine or a combination of chlorpheniramine maleate and phenylpropanolamine hydrochloride (Ornade) have been used successfully in patients with retrograde ejaculation. Electroejaculation via a rectal probe has been applied in patients with spinal cord injury with some success (Perkash et al, 1985; Ohl et al, 1991). Patients who have normal wet dreams but cannot achieve orgasm and ejaculation may benefit from psychosexual counseling. Premature ejaculation can be treated by desensitization, the squeezing technique (Masters and Johnson, 1976), or application of a local anesthetic (Berkovitch, Keresteci, and Koren, 1995; Xin et al, 1997) or a condom to reduce the sensitivity of the glans and frenulum. Selective serotonin reuptake inhibitors (fluoxetine, sertraline, and clomipramine) are also reported to be useful in prolonging the intravaginal ejaculation latency time in patients with premature ejaculation (Kim and Seo, 1998).

REFERENCES

Ajayi AAL, Mathur R, Halushka PV: Testosterone increases human platelet thromboxane A2 receptor density and aggregation responses. Circulation 1995;91:2742.

Anastasiadis AG et al: Long-term outcomes of inflatable penile implants: Reliability, patient satisfaction, and complication management. Curr Opin Urol 2001;11(6):619.

Bagatell CJ, Bremner WJ: Androgens in men: Uses and abuses. N Engl J Med 1996;334(11):707.

Bancroft J, Wu FCW: Changes in erectile responsiveness during androgen replacement therapy. Arch Sex Behav 1983;12:59.

Banya Y et al: Two circulatory routes within the human corpus cavernosum penis: A scanning electron microscopic study of corrosion casts. J Urol 1989;142:879.

Becker AJ et al: Possible role of bradykinin and angiotensin II in the regulation of penile erection and detumescence. Urology 2001;57(1):193.

Bemelmans BL et al: Comparison of biothesiometry and neuro-urophysiological investigations for the clinical evaluation of patients with erectile dysfunction. J Urol 1995;153(5):1483.

Bennett AH, Carpenter AJ, Barada JH: An improved vasoactive drug combination for a pharmacological erection program. J Urol 1991;146:1564.

Berkovitch M, Keresteci AG, Koren G: Efficacy of prilocaine-lidocaine cream in the treatment of premature ejaculation. J Urol 1995;154:1360.

Breza J et al: Detailed anatomy of penile neurovascular structures: Surgical significance. J Urol 1989;141:437.

Cheitlin MD et al: Use of sildenafil (Viagra) in patient with cardiovascular disease. J Am Coll Cardiol 1999;33:273.

Cookson MS, Nadig PW: Long-term results with vacuum constriction device. J Urol 1993;149(2):290.

Cooper CS et al: Effects of exogenous testosterone on prostate volume, serum and semen prostate specific antigen levels in healthy young men. J Urol 1998;159:441.

Donatucci CF, Lue TF: The combined intracavernous injection and stimulation test: Diagnostic accuracy. J Urol 1992; 148:61.

Feldman HA et al: Age trends in the level of serum testosterone and other hormones in middle-aged men: Longitudinal results from the Massachusetts male aging study. J Clin Endocrinol Metab 2002;87(2):589.

Feldman HA et al: Impotence and its medical and psychosocial correlates: Results of the Massachusetts Male Aging Study. J Urol 1994;151:54.

Fournier GR Jr et al: Mechanism of venous occlusion during canine penile erection: Anatomic demonstration. J Urol 1987; 137:163.

Gerber GS, Levine LA: Pharmacological erection program using prostaglandin E_1. J Urol 1991;146(3):789.

Goldstein I et al: Oral sildenafil in the treatment of erectile dysfunction. Sildenafil Study Group. N Engl J Med 1998;338: 1397.

Hakim LS et al: Penile microvascular arterial bypass surgery: Microsurgery 1995;16(5):296.

Heaton JP: Characterising the benefit of apomorphine SL (Uprima) as an optimised treatment for representative populations with erectile dysfunction. Int J Impot Res 2001;13 (Suppl 3):S35.

Holmquist F, Andersson K-E, Hedlund H: Actions of endothelin on isolated corpus cavernosum from rabbit and man. Acta Physiol Scand 1990;139:113.

Hsu G-L et al: The three dimensional structure of the human tunica albuginea: Anatomical and ultrastructure levels. Int J Impotence Res 1992;4:117.

Hurt KJ et al: Akt-dependent phosphorylation of endothelial nitric-oxide synthase mediates penile erection. Proc Natl Acad Sci U S A 2002;99(6):4061.

Ignarro LJ et al: Nitric oxide and cyclic GMP formation upon electrical stimulation cause relaxation of corpus cavernosum smooth muscle. Biochem Biophys Res Commun 1990; 170:843.

Jünemann KP, Buhrle CP, Stief CG: Current trends in corpus cavernosum EMG. Int J Impotence Res 1993;5:105.

Karacan I: Sleep environment important in assessing NPT. Urology 1988;32:180.

Kim N et al: Oxygen tension regulates the nitric oxide pathway: Physiological role in penile erection. J Clin Invest 1993;91 (2):437.

Kim SC, Seo KK: Efficacy and safety of fluoxetine, sertraline and clomipramine in patients with premature ejaculation: A double-blind, placebo controlled study. J Urology 1998;159:425.

Knoll LD, Abrams JH: Nocturnal electrobioimpedance volumetric assessment of patients with erectile dysfunction. Urology 1999;53(6):1200.

Laumann EO et al: *The Social Organization of Sexuality: Sexual Practice in the United States.* University of Chicago Press, 1994.

Levine LA, Lenting EL: Use of nocturnal penile tumescence and rigidity in the evaluation of male erectile dysfunction. Urol Clin North Am 1995;22(4):775.

Lewis R: Combined use of transurethral alprostadil and an adjustable penile constriction band in men with erectile dysfunction: Results from a multicenter trial. Int J Impotence Res 1998;10:S49.

Linet OI, Ogrinc FG: Efficacy and safety of intracavernosal alprostadil in men with erectile dysfunction: The Alprostadil Study Group. N Engl J Med 1996;334(14):873.

Lizza EF, Rosen RC: Definition and classification of erectile dysfunction: Report of the Nomenclature Committee of the International Society of Impotence Research. Int J Impot Res 1999;11(3):141.

Lue TF: Erectile dysfunction. N Engl J Med 2000;342:1802.

Lue TF: Patient's goal-directed impotence management. Urol Grand Rounds 1989;29:1.

Lue TF: Surgery for crural venous leakage. Urology 1999;54 (4):739.

Lue TF et al: Vasculogenic impotence evaluated by high-resolution ultrasonography and pulsed Doppler spectrum analysis. Radiology 1985;155:777.

Masters WH, Johnson VE: Principles of the new sex therapy. Am J Psychol 1976;133:548.

McKenna KE: Central control of penile erection. Int J Impotence Res 1998;(Suppl 1):S25.

McMahon CG: A comparison of the response to the intracavernous injection of a combination of papaverine and phentolamine, prostaglandin E_1, and a combination of all three agents in the management of impotence. Int J Impotence Res 1991;3:113.

Melman A, Christ GJ: Integrative erectile biology: The effects of age and disease on gap junctions and ion channels and their potential value to the treatment of erectile dysfunction. Urol Clin North Am 2001;28(2):217.

Mersdorf A et al: Ultrastructural changes in impotent penile tissue: Comparison of 65 patients. J Urol 1991;145:749.

Moller J et al: Sexual activity as a trigger of myocardial infarction: A case-crossover analysis in the Stockholm Heart Epidemiology Programme (SHEEP). Heart 2001;86(4):387.

Montague DK, Angermeier KW, Lakin MM: Penile prosthesis infections. Int J Impot Res 2001;13(6):326.

Montorsi F et al: Effect of yohimbine-trazodone on psychogenic impotence: A randomized, double-blind, placebo-controlled study. Urology 1994;44(5):732.

Morales A et al: Clinical safety of oral sildenafil citrate (VIAGRA) in the treatment of erectile dysfunction. Int J Impotence Res 1998;10:69.

Mulcahy JJ: Surgical management of penile prosthesis complications. Int J Impot Res 2000;12 Suppl 4:S108.

Murray RK: Muscle. In: Murray RK et al (editors): *Harper's Biochemistry,* 24th ed. Appleton & Lange, 1996.

Naroda T et al: Evaluation of resistance index of the cavernous artery with color Doppler ultrasonography for venogenic impotence. Int J Impotence Res 1994;6(1):D62.

NIH Consensus Panel on Impotence: Impotence. JAMA 1993;270:83.

Nomura A et al: Prediagnositic serum hormones and the risk of prostate cancer. Cancer Res 1998;48:3515.

Ohl DA et al: Electroejaculation following retroperitoneal lymphadenectomy. J Urol 1991;145:980.

Padma-Nathan H: Evaluation of the corporal veno-occlusive mechanism: Dynamic infusion cavernosometry and cavernosonography. Semin Interventional Radiol 1989;6:205.

Padma-Nathan H et al: Treatment of men with erectile dysfunction with transurethral alprostadil: Medicated Urethral System for Erection (MUSE) Study Group. N Engl J Med 1997;336:1.

Paick J-S, Donatucci CF, Lue TF: Anatomy of cavernous nerves distal to prostate: Microdissection study in adult male cadavers. Urology 1993;42:145.

Perkash I et al: Reproductive biology of paraplegics: Results of semen collection, testicular biopsy and serum hormone evaluation. J Urol 1985;134:284.

Rosen RC et al: Development and evaluation of an abridged, 5-item version of the International Index of Erectile Function (IIEF-5) as a diagnostic tool for erectile dysfunction. Int J Impot Res 1999;11(6):319.

Rosen RC et al: The international index of erectile function (IIEF): A multidimensional scale for assessment of erectile dysfunction. Urology 1997;49(6):822.

Roy AC et al: Prostaglandin 15-hydroxydehydrogenase activity in human penile corpora cavernosa and its significance in prostaglandin-mediated penile erection. Br J Urol 1989;64(2):180.

Saenz de Tejada I et al: Cholinergic neurotransmission in human corpus cavernosum. I. Response of isolated tissue. Am J Physiol 1988a;254:H459.

Saenz de Tejada I et al: Impaired neurogenic and endothelium-mediated relaxation of penile smooth muscle from diabetic men with impotence. N Engl J Med 1989;320:1025.

Saenz de Tejada I et al: Pathophysiology of prolonged penile erection associated with trazodone use. J Urol 1991;145(1):60.

Saenz de Tejada I et al: Prostaglandin production by human corpus cavernosum endothelial cells (HCC EC) in culture. J Urol 1988b;139:252A.

Sattar AA, Schulman CC, Wespes E: Objective quantification of cavernous endothelium in potent and impotent men. J Urol 1995;153:1136.

Stackl W, Hasun R, Marberger M: Intracavernous injection of prostaglandin E_1 in impotent men. J Urol 1988;140:66.

Stief CG, Wetterauer U: Responses to intracavernous papaverine and phentolamine: Comparison of single and combined delivery. J Urol 1988;140(6):1415.

Trigo-Rocha F et al: Nitric oxide and cyclic guanosine monophosphate: Mediators of pelvic nerve-stimulated erection in dogs. Am J Physiol 1993;264 (Heart Circ Physiol 33):H419.

van Ahlen H et al: Pharmacokinetics of vasoactive substances administered into the human corpus cavernosum. J Urol 1994;151(5):1227.

Virag R: Intracavernous injection of papaverine for erectile failure. Lancet 1982;2:938.

Virag R et al: Intracavernous injection of papaverine as a diagnostic and therapeutic method in erectile failure. Angiology 1984;35:79.

Walsh PC, Donker PJ: Impotence following radical prostatectomy: Insight into etiology and preservation. J Urol 1982;128:492.

Xin ZC et al: Efficacy of a topical agent SS-cream in the treatment of premature ejaculation: Preliminary clinical studies. Yonsei Med J 1997;38:91.

Zorgniotti AW, Lefleur RS: Auto-injection of the corpus cavernosum with a vasoactive drug combination for vasculogenic impotence. J Urol 1985;133:39.

Disorders of the Penis & Male Urethra

38

Jack W. McAninch, MD

■ CONGENITAL ANOMALIES OF THE PENIS

APENIA

Congenital absence of the penis (apenia) is extremely rare. In this condition, the urethra generally opens on the perineum or inside the rectum.

Patients with apenia should be considered for assignment to the female gender. Castration and vaginoplasty should be considered in combination with estrogen treatment as the child develops.

MEGALOPENIS

The penis enlarges rapidly in childhood (megalopenis) in boys with abnormalities that have increased the production of testosterone, for example, interstitial cell tumors of the testicle, hyperplasia, or tumors of the adrenal cortex. Management is by correction of the underlying endocrine problem.

MICROPENIS

Micropenis is a more common anomaly and has been attributed to a testosterone deficiency that results in poor growth of organs that are targets of this hormone. A penis smaller than 2 standard deviations from the norm is considered a micropenis (see Table 38–1). The testicles are small and frequently undescended. Other organs, including the scrotum, may be involved. Early evidence suggests that the ability of the hypothalamus to secrete luteinizing hormone-releasing hormone (LHRH) is decreased. The pituitary-gonadal axis appears to be intact, since the organs respond to testosterone, although this response may be sluggish at times. Studies have shown that topical application of 5% testosterone cream causes increased penile growth, but its effect is due to absorption of the hormone, which systemically stimulates genital growth. Patients with micropenis must be carefully evaluated for other endocrine and central nervous system anomalies. Retarded bone growth, anosmia, learning disabilities, and deficiencies of adrenocorticotropic hormone and thyrotropin have been associated with micropenis. In addition, the possibility of intersex problems must be carefully investigated before therapy is begun.

The approach to management of micropenis has undergone gradual change in recent years, but androgen replacement is the basic requirement. The objective is to provide sufficient testosterone to stimulate penile growth without altering growth and closure of the epiphyses. Allen (1980) recommends giving testosterone in doses of 25 mg orally every 3 weeks for no more than 4 doses. Penile growth is assessed by measuring the length of the stretched penis (pubis to glans) before and after treatment. Therapy should be started by age 1 year and aimed at maintaining genital growth commensurate with general body growth. Repeat courses of therapy may be required if the size of the penis falls behind as the child grows. For undescended testicles, orchiopexy should be done before the child is 2 years old. In the future, treatment with LHRH may correct micropenis as well as cause descent of the testicles, but at present, LHRH is not approved for such use.

ADULT PENILE SIZE

In recent years, penile augmentation and enhancement procedures have been done with increasing frequency, although no validation of success has been documented. Suspensory ligament release with pubic fat pad advancement, fat injections, and dermal fat grafts have been used in attempts to enhance penile size. Many consider that these procedures have not been proved safe or efficacious in normal men. Recently, Wessells, Lue, and McAninch (1996) evaluated penile size in the flaccid and erect state in otherwise normal adult men and found very good correlation between stretched and erect length ($R^2 = 0.793$; Table 38–2). This information can provide a guideline for physicians whose patients are concerned with their penile dimensions.

Table 38–1. Size of unstretched penis and testis from infancy to adulthood.

Age (Years)	Length of Penis (cm ± SD)	Diameter of Testis (cm ± SD)
0.2–2	2.7 ± 0.5	1.4 ± 0.4
2.1–4	3.3 ± 0.4	1.2 ± 0.4
4.1–6	3.9 ± 0.9	1.5 ± 0.6
6.1–8	4.2 ± 0.8	1.8 ± 0.3
8.1–10	4.9 ± 1	2 ± 0.5
10.1–12	5.2 ± 1.3	2.7 ± 0.7
12.1–14	6.2 ± 2	3.4 ± 0.8
14.1–16	8.6 ± 2.4	4.1 ± 1
16.1–18	9.9 ± 1.7	5 ± 0.5
18.1–20	11 ± 1.1	5 ± 0.3
20.1–25	12.4 ± 1.6	5.2 ± 0.6

Source: Reproduced, with permission, from Winter JSD, Faiman C: Pituitary-gonadal relations in male children and adolescents. Pediatr Res 1972;6:126.

CONGENITAL ANOMALIES OF THE URETHRA

DUPLICATION OF THE URETHRA

Duplication of the urethra is rare. The structures may be complete or incomplete. Resection of all but one complete urethra is recommended.

URETHRAL STRICTURE

Congenital urethral stricture is uncommon in infant boys. The fossa navicularis and membranous urethra are the 2 most common sites. Severe strictures may cause bladder damage and hydronephrosis (see Chapter 11), with symptoms of obstruction (urinary frequency

Table 38–2. Adult penile size: Relationships among flaccid, stretched, and erect measurements.[a]

Penile State	Length (cm)	Circumference (cm)
Flaccid	8.8	9.7
Stretched	12.4	—
Erect	12.9	12.3

[a]Data represent the mean of measurements in 80 men and are drawn from Wessells H, Lue TF, McAninch JW: Penile length in the flaccid and erect states: Guidelines for penile augmentation. J Urol 1996;156:995.

and urgency) or urinary infection. A careful history and physical examination are indicated in patients with these complaints. Excretory urography and excretory voiding urethrography often define the lesion and the extent of obstruction. Retrograde urethrography (Figure 38–1) may also be helpful. Cystoscopy and urethroscopy should be performed in all patients in whom urethral stricture is suspected.

Strictures can be treated at the time of endoscopy. Diaphragmatic strictures may respond to dilation or visual urethrotomy. Other strictures should be treated under direct vision by internal urethrotomy with the currently available pediatric urethrotome. It may be necessary to repeat these procedures in order to stabilize the stricture. Single-stage open surgical repair by anastomotic urethroplasty, buccal mucosa graft, or penile flap is desirable if the obstruction recurs.

POSTERIOR URETHRAL VALVES

Posterior urethral valves, the most common obstructive urethral lesions in infants and newborns, occur only in males and are found at the distal prostatic urethra. The valves are mucosal folds that look like thin membranes; they may cause varying degrees of obstruction when the child attempts to void (Figure 38–2).

Clinical Findings

A. SYMPTOMS AND SIGNS

Children with posterior urethral valves may present with mild, moderate, or severe symptoms of obstruction. They often have a poor, intermittent, dribbling urinary stream. Urinary infection and sepsis occur frequently. Severe obstruction may cause hydronephrosis (see Chapter 11), which is apparent as a palpable abdominal mass. A palpable midline mass in the lower abdomen is typical of a distended bladder. Occasionally, palpable flank masses indicate hydronephrotic kidneys. In many patients, failure to thrive may be the only significant symptom, and examination may reveal nothing more than evidence of chronic illness.

B. LABORATORY FINDINGS

Azotemia and poor concentrating ability of the kidney are common findings. The urine is often infected, and anemia may be found if infection is chronic. Serum creatinine and blood urea nitrogen levels and creatinine clearance are the best indicators of the extent of renal failure.

C. X-RAY FINDINGS

Voiding cystourethrography is the best radiographic study available to establish the diagnosis of posterior

Figure 38–1. **Upper left:** Retrograde urethrogram showing congenital diaphragmatic stricture. **Upper right:** Posterior urethral valves revealed on voiding cystourethrography. Arrow points to area of severe stenosis at distal end of prostatic urethra. **Lower left:** Posterior urethral valves. Patient would not void with cystography. Retrograde urethrogram showing valves (arrow). **Lower right:** Cystogram, same patient. Free vesicoureteral reflux and vesical trabeculation with diverticula.

Figure 38–2. Posterior urethral valves. **Left:** Dilatation of the prostatic urethra, hypertrophy of vesical wall and trigone in stage of compensation; bilateral hydroureters secondary to trigonal hypertrophy. **Right:** Attenuation of bladder musculature in stage of decompensation; advanced ureteral dilatation and tortuosity, usually secondary to vesicoureteral reflux.

urethral valves. The presence of large amounts of residual urine is apparent on initial catheterization done in conjunction with radiographic studies, and an uncontaminated urine specimen should be obtained via the catheter and sent for culture. The cystogram may show vesicoureteral reflux and the severe trabeculations of long-standing obstruction, and the voiding cystourethrogram often demonstrates elongation and dilatation of the posterior urethra, with a prominent bladder neck (Figure 38–1). Excretory urograms may reveal hydroureter and hydronephrosis when obstruction is severe and long-standing.

D. ULTRASONOGRAPHY

Ultrasonography can be used to detect hydronephrosis, hydroureter, and bladder distention in children with severe azotemia. It can also detect fetal hydronephrosis, which is typical of urethral valves, as early as 28 weeks of gestation; when the obstruction is from valves, an enlarged bladder with bilateral hydroureteronephrosis is usually present.

E. INSTRUMENTAL EXAMINATION

Urethroscopy and cystoscopy, performed with the patient under general anesthesia, show vesical trabeculation and cellules and, occasionally, vesical diverticula. The bladder neck and trigone may be hypertrophied. The diagnosis is confirmed by visual identification of the valves at the distal prostatic urethra. Supravesical compression shows that the valves cause obstruction.

Treatment

Treatment consists of destruction of the valves, but the approach depends on the degree of obstruction and the general health of the child. In children with mild to moderate obstruction and minimal azotemia, transurethral fulguration of the valves is usually successful. Occasionally, catheterization, cystoscopy, or urethral dilation by perineal urethrostomy destroys the valves.

The more severe degrees of obstruction create varying grades of hydronephrosis requiring individualized management. Treatment of children with urosepsis and azotemia associated with hydronephrosis includes use of antibiotics, catheter drainage of the bladder, and correction of the fluid and electrolyte imbalance. Vesicostomy may be of benefit in patients with reflux and renal dysplasia.

In the most severe cases of hydronephrosis, vesicostomy or removal of the valves may not be sufficient, because of ureteral atony, obstruction of the ureterovesical junction from trigonal hypertrophy, or both. In such cases, percutaneous loop ureterostomies may be done to preserve renal function and allow resolution of the hydronephrosis. After renal function is stabilized, valve ablation and reconstruction of the urinary tract can be done.

The period of proximal diversion should be as short as possible, since vesical contracture can be permanent after prolonged supravesical diversion.

Johnston (1979) found that approximately 50% of children with urethral valves had vesicoureteral reflux and that the prognosis is worse if the reflux is bilateral. After removal of the obstruction, reflux ceases spontaneously in about one-third of patients. In the remaining two-thirds of patients, the reflux should be corrected surgically.

Long-term use of antimicrobial drugs is often required to prevent recurrent urosepsis and urinary tract infection even though the obstruction has been relieved.

Prognosis

Early detection is the best way to preserve kidney and bladder function. This can be accomplished by ultrasonography in utero, by careful physical examination and observation of voiding in the newborn, and by thorough evaluation of children who have urinary tract infections. Children in whom azotemia and infection persist after relief of obstruction have a poor prognosis.

ANTERIOR URETHRAL VALVES

Signs of anterior urethral valves, a rare congenital anomaly, are urethral dilatation or diverticula proximal to the valve, bladder outlet obstruction, postvoiding incontinence, and infection. Enuresis may be present. Urethroscopy and voiding cystourethrography will demonstrate the lesion, and endoscopic electrofulguration will effectively correct the obstruction.

URETHRORECTAL & VESICORECTAL FISTULAS

Urethrorectal and vesicorectal fistulas are rare and are almost always associated with imperforate anus. Failure

of the urorectal septum to develop completely and separate the rectum from the urogenital tract permits communication between the 2 systems (see Chapter 2). The child with such a fistula passes fecal material and gas through the urethra. If the anus has developed normally (ie, if it opens externally), urine may pass through the rectum.

Cystoscopy and panendoscopy usually show the fistulous opening. Radiographic contrast material given by mouth will reach the blind rectal pouch, and the distance between the end of the rectum and the perineum can be seen on appropriate radiograms.

Imperforate anus must be opened immediately and the fistula closed, or if the rectum lies quite high, temporary sigmoid colostomy should be performed. Definitive surgery, with repair of the urethral fistula, can be done later.

HYPOSPADIAS

In hypospadias, the urethral meatus opens on the ventral side of the penis proximal to the tip of the glans penis (Figure 38–3).

Sexual differentiation and urethral development begin in utero at approximately 8 weeks and are complete by 15 weeks. The urethra is formed by the fusion of the urethral folds along the ventral surface of the penis, which extends to the corona on the distal shaft. The glandular urethra is formed by canalization of an ectodermal cord that has grown through the glans to communicate with the fused urethral folds (see Chapter 2). Hypospadias results when fusion of the urethral folds is incomplete.

Hypospadias occurs in one in every 300 male children. Estrogens and progestins given during pregnancy are known to increase the incidence. Although a familial pattern of hypospadias has been recognized, no specific genetic traits have been established.

Classification

There are several forms of hypospadias, classified according to location: (1) glandular, that is, opening on the proximal glans penis; (2) coronal, that is, opening at the coronal sulcus; (3) penile shaft; (4) penoscrotal; and (5) perineal. About 70% of all cases of hypospadias are distal penile or coronal.

Hypospadias in the male is evidence of feminization. Patients with penoscrotal and perineal openings should be considered to have potential intersex problems requiring appropriate evaluation. Hypospadiac newborns should not be circumcised, because the preputial skin may be useful for future reconstruction.

Figure 38–3. Hypospadias and epispadias. **Upper left:** Hypospadias, penoscrotal type. Redundant dorsal foreskin that is deficient ventrally; ventral chordee. **Upper right:** Hypospadias, midscrotal type. Chordee more marked. Penis often small. **Lower left:** Epispadias. Redundant ventral foreskin that is absent dorsally; severe dorsal chordee. **Lower right:** Traction on foreskin reveals dorsal defect.

Clinical Findings

A. SYMPTOMS AND SIGNS

Although newborns and young children seldom have symptoms related to hypospadias, older children and adults may complain of difficulty directing the urinary stream and stream spraying. Chordee (curvature of the penis) causes ventral bending and bowing of the penile shaft, which can prevent sexual intercourse. Perineal or penoscrotal hypospadias necessitates voiding in the sitting position, and these proximal forms of hypospadias in adults can be the cause of infertility. An additional complaint of almost all patients is the abnormal (hooded) appearance of the penis, caused by deficient or absent ventral foreskin. The hypospadiac meatus may be stenotic and should be carefully examined and calibrated. (A meatotomy should be done when stenosis exists.) There is an increased incidence of undescended testicles in children with hypospadias; scrotal examination is necessary to establish the position of the testicles.

B. LABORATORY, X-RAY, AND ENDOSCOPIC FINDINGS

Since children with penoscrotal and perineal hypospadias often have a bifid scrotum and ambiguous genitalia, a buccal smear and karyotyping are indicated to help establish the genetic sex. Urethroscopy and cystoscopy are of value to determine whether internal male sexual organs are normally developed. Excretory urography is also indicated in these patients to detect additional congenital anomalies of the kidneys and ureters.

Some authors recommend routine use of excretory urography for all patients with hypospadias; however, this seems to be of little value in the more distal types of the disorder, because there appears to be no increased incidence of upper urinary tract anomalies.

Differential Diagnosis

Any degree of hypospadias is an expression of feminization. Perineal and scrotal urethral openings should be carefully evaluated to ascertain that the patient is not a female with androgenized adrenogenital syndrome. Urethroscopy and cystoscopy will aid in evaluating the development of internal reproductive organs.

Treatment

For psychological reasons, hypospadias should be repaired before the patient reaches school age; in most cases, this can be done before age 2. More than 150 methods of corrective surgery for hypospadias have been described. Currently, one-stage repairs using island flap grafts are performed by more and more urologists. Bladder epithelium has also been used successfully (Keating, Cartwright, and Duckett, 1990). It now appears that buccal mucosa grafts are

more advantageous than others and should be considered the primary grafting technique (Baskin and Duckett, 1995). Fistulas occur in 15–30% of patients, but the fistula repair is considered a small, second-stage reconstruction.

All types of repair involve straightening the penis by removal of the chordee. The chordee removal can be confirmed by producing an artificial erection in the operating room following urethral reconstruction and advancement. Most successful techniques for repair of hypospadias use local skin and foreskin in developing the neourethra. In recent years, advancement of the urethra to the glans penis has become technically feasible and cosmetically acceptable.

Prognosis

After corrective surgery, most patients are able to void in the standing position as well as to deposit semen into the vagina. The overall cosmetic appearance and the prevention of fistula formation remain the greatest challenges in these repairs.

CHORDEE WITHOUT HYPOSPADIAS

Congenital ventral chordee without hypospadias is seen occasionally and is caused by a short urethra, fibrous tissues surrounding the corpus spongiosum, or both. The urethral opening is in the normal position on the glans penis; only with erection does the penis bow, thus preventing satisfactory vaginal penetration. During examination, if the patient cannot achieve an erection naturally, erection can be induced by injecting saline solution into the corpus cavernosum after placing a tourniquet at the base of the penis. This technique should also be used during corrective surgery to be certain that the penis will be straight after the operation.

If the penis is adequate in length, the dorsal surface can be shortened (1) by excising elliptic portions of the tunica albuginea on the dorsum of the penis on either side of the midline or (2) by making transverse cuts in a similar position and then closing them longitudinally, thus shortening the dorsum. Fibrous tissue found in association with the urethra and corpus spongiosum should be totally excised.

EPISPADIAS

The incidence of complete epispadias is approximately 1 in 120,000 males and 1 in 450,000 females. The urethra is displaced dorsally, and classification is based on its position in males. In glandular epispadias, the urethra opens on the dorsal aspect of the glans, which is broad and flattened. In the penile type, the urethral meatus, which is often broad and gaping, is located between the pubic symphysis and the coronal sulcus. A distal groove usually extends from the meatus through the splayed glans. The penopubic type has the urethral opening at the penopubic junction, and the entire penis has a distal dorsal groove extending through the glans.

Patients with glandular epispadias seldom have urinary incontinence. However, with penopubic and penile epispadias, incontinence is present in 95% and 75% of cases, respectively.

Females with epispadias have a bifid clitoris and separation of the labia. Most are incontinent.

Urinary incontinence is a common problem because of maldevelopment of the urinary sphincters. Dorsal curvature of the penis (dorsal chordee) is also present (Figure 38–3). The pubic bones are separated as in exstrophy of the bladder. Epispadias is a mild form of bladder exstrophy, and in severe cases, exstrophy and epispadias coexist.

Surgery is required to correct the incontinence, remove the chordee to straighten the penis, and extend the urethra out onto the glans penis. Repair of the urinary sphincter has not been very successful, but Tanagho and Smith (1972) obtained complete continence by interposing a tube graft of anterior bladder wall between the bladder and prostatic urethra. Chordee excision and urethroplasty with advancement of the meatus have been successful in achieving acceptable cosmetic and functional results. Bladder augmentation combined with the artificial sphincter may be required in patients in whom incontinence cannot be corrected.

■ ACQUIRED DISEASES & DISORDERS OF THE PENIS & MALE URETHRA

PRIAPISM

Priapism is an uncommon condition of prolonged erection. It is usually painful for the patient, and no sexual excitement or desire is present. The disorder is idiopathic in 60% of cases, while the remaining 40% of cases are associated with diseases (eg, leukemia, sickle cell disease, pelvic tumors, pelvic infections), penile trauma, spinal cord trauma, or use of medications. Currently, intracavernous injection therapy for impotence may be the most common cause. Although the idiopathic type often is initially associated with prolonged sexual stimulation, cases of priapism due to the other causes are unrelated to psychic sexual excitement.

Priapism may be classified into high- and low-flow types. High-flow priapism (nonischemic) usually occurs secondary to perineal trauma, which injures the central penile arteries and results in loss of penile blood-flow regulation. Aneurysms of one or both central arteries have been observed. Aspiration of penile blood for blood-gas determination demonstrates high oxygen and normal carbon dioxide levels. Arteriography is useful to demonstrate aneurysms that will respond to embolization; erectile function is usually preserved.

The patient with low-flow priapism (ischemic) usually presents with a history of several hours of painful erection. The glans penis and corpus spongiosum are soft and uninvolved in the process. The corpora cavernosa are tense with congested blood and tender to palpation. The current theories regarding the mechanism of priapism remain in debate, but most authorities believe the major abnormality to be physiologic obstruction of the venous drainage. This obstruction causes buildup of highly viscous, poorly oxygenated blood (low O_2, high CO_2) within the corpora cavernosa. If the process continues for several days, interstitial edema and fibrosis of the corpora cavernosa will develop, causing impotence.

Priapism must be considered a urologic emergency. Epidural or spinal anesthesia can be used. The sludged blood can then be evacuated from the corpora cavernosa through a large needle placed through the glans. The addition of adrenergic agents administered via intracavernous irrigation has proved helpful. Monitoring intracavernous pressure ensures that recurrence is not imminent (Lue et al, 1986). Multiple wedges of tissue can be removed via a Travenol biopsy needle to create a shunting fistula between the glans penis and corpora cavernosa (Winter and McDowell, 1988). This technique, which has been very successful, provides an internal fistula to keep the corpora cavernosa decompressed. To maintain continuous fistula drainage, pressure should be exerted intermittently (every 15 min) on the body of the penis. The patient can do this manually after he has recovered from anesthesia.

If the shunt described fails, another shunting technique may be used. Barry (1976) described an easy method of accomplishing shunting by anastomosing the superficial dorsal vein to the corpora cavernosa. Other effective shunting methods are corpora cavernosa to corpus spongiosum shunt by perineal anastomosis; saphenous vein to corpora cavernosa shunt; and pump decompression.

Patients with sickle cell disease have benefited from massive blood transfusions, exchange transfusions, or both. Hyperbaric oxygen also has been suggested for these patients. Patients with leukemia should receive prompt chemotherapy. Appropriate management of any underlying cause should be instituted without delay. Such treatment should not prevent aggressive management of the priapism if the erection persists for several hours.

Impotence is the worst sequel of priapism. It is more common after prolonged priapism (several days). Early recognition (within hours) and prompt treatment of priapism offer the best opportunity to avoid this major problem.

PEYRONIE DISEASE

Peyronie disease (plastic induration of the penis) was first described in 1742 and is a well-recognized clinical problem affecting middle-aged and older men. Patients present with complaints of painful erection, curvature of the penis, and poor erection distal to the involved area. The penile deformity may be so severe that it prevents satisfactory vaginal penetration. The patient has no pain when the penis is in the nonerect state.

Examination of the penile shaft reveals a palpable dense, fibrous plaque of varying size involving the tunica albuginea. The plaque is usually near the dorsal midline of the shaft. Multiple plaques are sometimes seen. In severe cases, calcification and ossification are noted and confirmed by radiography. Although the cause of Peyronie disease remains obscure, the dense fibrous plaque is microscopically consistent with findings in severe vasculitis. The condition has been noted in association with Dupuytren's contracture of the tendons of the hand, in which the fibrosis resembles that of Peyronie disease when examined microscopically.

Spontaneous remission occurs in about 50% of cases. Initially, observation and emotional support are advised. If remission does not occur, *p*-aminobenzoic acid powder or tablets or vitamin E tablets may be tried for several months. However, these medications have limited success. In recent years, a number of operative procedures have been used in refractory cases. Excision of the plaque with replacement with a dermal or vein graft has been successful, as has the use of tunica vaginalis grafts after plaque incision. Other authors have incised the plaque and inserted penile prostheses in the corpora cavernosa. Additional methods include radiation therapy and injection of steroids, dimethyl sulfoxide, or parathyroid hormone into the plaque. The success of such treatments is poorly documented.

PHIMOSIS

Phimosis is a condition in which the contracted foreskin cannot be retracted over the glans. Chronic infection from poor local hygiene is its most common cause. Most cases occur in uncircumcised males, although excessive skin left after circumcision can become stenotic and cause phimosis. Calculi and squamous cell carcinoma may develop under the foreskin. Phimosis can

occur at any age. In diabetic older men, chronic balanoposthitis may lead to phimosis and may be the initial presenting complaint. Children under 2 years of age seldom have true phimosis; their relatively narrow preputial opening gradually widens and allows for normal retraction of foreskin over the glans. Circumcision for phimosis should be avoided in children requiring general anesthesia; except in cases with recurrent infections, the procedure should be postponed until the child reaches an age when local anesthesia can be used.

Edema, erythema, and tenderness of the prepuce and the presence of purulent discharge usually cause the patient to seek medical attention. Inability to retract the foreskin is a less common complaint.

The initial infection should be treated with broad-spectrum antimicrobial drugs. The dorsal foreskin can be slit if improved drainage is necessary. Circumcision, if indicated, should be done after the infection is controlled.

PARAPHIMOSIS

Paraphimosis is the condition in which the foreskin, once retracted over the glans, cannot be replaced in its normal position. This is due to chronic inflammation under the redundant foreskin, which leads to contracture of the preputial opening (phimosis) and formation of a tight ring of skin when the foreskin is retracted behind the glans. The skin ring causes venous congestion leading to edema and enlargement of the glans, which make the condition worse. As the condition progresses, arterial occlusion and necrosis of the glans may occur.

Paraphimosis usually can be treated by firmly squeezing the glans for 5 min to reduce the tissue edema and decrease the size of the glans. The skin can then be drawn forward over the glans. Occasionally, the constricting ring requires incision under local anesthesia. Antibiotics should be administered and circumcision should be done after inflammation has subsided.

CIRCUMCISION

Although circumcision is routinely performed in some countries for religious or cultural reasons, it is usually not necessary if adequate penile cleanliness and good hygiene can be maintained. There is a higher incidence of penile carcinoma in uncircumcised males, but chronic infection and poor hygiene are usually underlying factors in such instances. Circumcision is indicated in patients with infection, phimosis, or paraphimosis (see preceding sections).

URETHRAL STRICTURE

Acquired urethral stricture is common in men but rare in women. (Congenital urethral stricture is discussed earlier in the chapter.) Most acquired strictures are due to infection or trauma. Although gonococcal urethritis is seldom a cause of stricture today, infection remains a major cause—particularly infection from long-term use of indwelling urethral catheters. Large catheters and instruments are more likely than small ones to cause ischemia and internal trauma. External trauma, for example, pelvic fractures (see Chapter 17), can partially or completely sever the membranous urethra and cause severe and complex strictures. Straddle injuries can produce bulbar strictures.

Urethral strictures are fibrotic narrowings composed of dense collagen and fibroblasts. Fibrosis usually extends into the surrounding corpus spongiosum, causing spongiofibrosis. These narrowings restrict urine flow and cause dilation of the proximal urethra and prostatic ducts. Prostatitis is a common complication of urethral stricture. The bladder muscle may become hypertrophic, and increased residual urine may be noted. Severe, prolonged obstruction can result in decompensation of the ureterovesical junction, reflux, hydronephrosis, and renal failure. Chronic urinary stasis makes infection likely. Urethral fistulas and periurethral abscesses commonly develop in association with chronic, severe strictures.

Clinical Findings

A. Symptoms and Signs

A decrease in urinary stream is the most common complaint. Spraying or double stream is often noted, as is postvoiding dribbling. Chronic urethral discharge, occasionally a major complaint, is likely to be associated with chronic prostatitis. Acute cystitis or symptoms of infection are seen at times. Acute urinary retention seldom occurs unless infection or prostatic obstruction develops. Urinary frequency and mild dysuria may also be initial complaints.

Induration in the area of the stricture may be palpable. Tender enlarged masses along the urethra usually represent periurethral abscesses. Urethrocutaneous fistulas may be present. The bladder may be palpable if there is chronic retention of urine.

B. Laboratory Findings

If urethral stricture is suspected, urinary flow rates should be determined. The patient is instructed to accumulate urine until the bladder is full and then begin voiding; a 5-s collection of urine should be obtained during midstream maximal flow and its volume recorded. After the patient repeats this procedure 8–10 times over several days in a relaxed atmosphere, the mean peak flow can be calculated. With strictures creating significant problems, the flow rate will be less than 10 mL/s (normal, 20 mL/s).

Urine culture may be indicated. The midstream specimen is usually bacteria-free, with some pyuria [8–10 white blood cells (leukocytes) per high-power field] in a carefully obtained first aliquot of urine. If the prostate is infected, bacteria will be present in a specimen obtained after prostatic massage. In the presence of cystitis, the urine will be grossly infected.

C. X-Ray Findings

A urethrogram or voiding cystourethrogram (or both) will demonstrate the location and extent of the stricture. Sonography has also been a useful method of evaluating the urethral stricture (McAninch, Laing, and Jeffrey, 1988). Urethral fistulas and diverticula are sometimes noted. Vesical stones, trabeculations, or diverticula may also be seen.

D. Instrumental Examination

Urethroscopy allows visualization of the stricture. Small-caliber strictures prevent passage of the instrument through the area. Direct visualization and sonourethrography aid in determining the extent, location, and degree of scarring. Additional areas of scar formation adjacent to the stricture may be detected by urethroscopy.

The stricture can be calibrated by passage of bougies à boule.

Differential Diagnosis

Benign or malignant prostatic obstruction can cause symptoms similar to those of stricture. After prostatic surgery, bladder neck contracture can develop and induce stricturelike symptoms. Rectal examination and panendoscopy adequately define such abnormalities of the prostate. Urethral carcinoma is often associated with stricture; urethroscopy demonstrates a definite irregular lesion, and biopsy establishes the diagnosis of carcinoma.

Complications

Complications include chronic prostatitis, cystitis, chronic urinary infection, diverticula, urethrocutaneous fistulas, periurethral abscesses, and urethral carcinoma. Vesical calculi may develop from chronic urinary stasis and infection.

Treatment

A. Specific Measures

1. Dilation—Dilation of urethral strictures is not usually curative, but it fractures the scar tissue of the stricture and temporarily enlarges the lumen. As healing occurs, the scar tissue re-forms.

Dilation may initially be required because of severe symptoms of chronic retention of urine. The urethra should be liberally lubricated with a water-soluble medium before instrumentation. A filiform is passed down the urethra and gently manipulated through the narrow area into the bladder. A follower can then be attached (see Chapter 10) and the area gradually dilated (with successively larger sizes) to approximately 22F. A 16F silicone catheter can then be inserted. If difficulty arises in passing the filiform through the stricture, urethroscopy should be used to guide the filiform under direct vision.

An alternative method of urethral dilation employs Van Buren sounds. These instruments are best used by an experienced urologist familiar with the size and extent of the stricture involved. First, a 22F sound should be passed down to the stricture site and gentle pressure applied. If this fails, a 20F sound should be used. Smaller sounds should be used with care, because they can easily perforate the urethral wall and produce false passages. Bleeding and pain are major problems caused by dilation.

2. Urethrotomy under endoscopic direct vision—
Lysis of urethral strictures can be accomplished using a sharp knife attached to an endoscope. The endoscope provides direct vision of the stricture during cutting. A filiform should be passed through the stricture and used as a guide during lysis. The stricture is usually incised dorsally, but multiple incisions in other areas may be required to open a narrow segment. A 22F instrument

should pass with ease. A catheter is left in place for a short time to prevent bleeding and pain. Results of this procedure have been satisfactory in short-term follow-up in 70–80% of patients, but long-term success rates are much lower. The procedure has several advantages: (1) Minimal anesthesia is required—in some cases, only topical anesthesia combined with sedation; (2) it is easily repeated if the stricture recurs; and (3) it is very safe, with few complications.

3. Surgical reconstruction—If urethrotomy under direct vision fails, open surgical repair should be performed. Short strictures (≤ 2.0 cm) of the anterior urethra should be completely excised and primary anastomosis done. If possible, the segment to be excised should extend 1 cm beyond each end of the stricture to allow for removal of any existing spongiofibrosis and improve postoperative healing.

Strictures more than 2 cm in length can be managed by patch graft urethroplasty. The urethra is incised in the midline for the full length of the stricture plus an additional 0.5 cm proximal and distal to its ends. A full-thickness skin graft is obtained—preferably from the penile skin or buccal mucosa—and all subcutaneous tissue is carefully removed. The graft is then tailored to cover the defect and meticulously sutured into place (Figure 38–4).

In very long, densely fibrotic strictures, the distal penile fasciocutaneous flap technique has been successful in more than 80% (McAninch and Morey, 1998). This single-stage procedure can be combined with buccal

Figure 38–4. **Left:** Urethrogram demonstrating multiple anterior urethral strictures. **Right:** Voiding cystourethrogram following a patch skin graft of 14 cm in the same patient. There are no residual strictures.

mucosa grafting in panurethral strictures (Wessells, Morey, and McAninch, 1997). In adults, grafts from buccal mucosa or penile skin should be applied with an onlay technique in the bulbar region of the urethra to maximize graft vascularization from the corpus spongiosum (Morey and McAninch, 1996b).

Strictures involving the membranous urethra ordinarily result from external trauma (see Chapter 17) and present problems in reconstruction. Most can be corrected by a perineal approach with excision of the urethral rupture defect and direct anastomosis of the bulbar urethra to the prostatic urethra (Figure 38–5). At times, partial pubectomy from the perineal approach can be done to improve urethral approximation without tension on the anastomosis. Rarely, total pubectomy combined with the perineal approach is required to accomplish the direct end-to-end anastomosis.

These single-stage procedures have a high success rate and create a urethra free of hair—a major problem seen with 2-stage procedures. Although seldom required, 2-stage procedures are important reconstructive techniques to be considered in complex urethral strictures.

B. TREATMENT OF COMPLICATIONS

Urinary tract infection in patients with strictures requires specific antimicrobial therapy, followed by long-term prophylactic therapy until the stricture has been corrected. Periurethral abscesses require drainage and use of antimicrobial drugs. Urethral fistulas usually require surgical repair.

Prognosis

A stricture should not be considered "cured" until it has been observed for at least 1 year after therapy, since it may recur at any time during that period. Urinary flow rate measurements and urethrograms are helpful to determine the extent of residual obstruction.

URETHRAL CONDYLOMATA ACUMINATA (URETHRAL WARTS)

Condylomata acuminata are uncommon in the urethra and are almost always preceded by lesions on the skin. They are wartlike papillomas caused by a papilloma virus and are usually transmitted by direct sexual contact but may be transmitted nonsexually.

Patients commonly complain of bloody spotting from the urethra and occasionally have dysuria and urethral discharge. Examination of the urethral meatus often reveals a small, protruding papilloma. If a lesion is not found in this location, the meatus should be separated with the examining fingers so that the distal urethra can be inspected. About 90% of such lesions are situated in the distal urethra. Complete urethroscopy must be done to be certain other lesions do not exist.

Lesions of the meatus can be treated by local excision. A local anesthetic is applied to the area at the base of the lesions, and the pedunculated lesions are sharply incised with small scissors. The area is then fulgurated by electrocautery. Meatotomy may be indicated for excision of lesions in the fossa navicularis and glandular urethra.

Deeper lesions may be fulgurated transurethrally with a resectoscope or Bugby electrode. Recently, lesions have been successfully destroyed using a carbon dioxide laser. Laser therapy does minimal damage to the urethral mucosa, and stricture formation seems less likely with its use.

Multiple lesions have also been treated with fluorouracil, 5% solution or cream. The drug is instilled in the urethra for 20 min twice a week for 5 weeks. Care must be taken to protect the penile skin and scrotum from coming in contact with the medication, since it may produce severe irritation.

Lesions may become infected and ulcerated. This suggests carcinoma, and histopathologic confirmation of the diagnosis should be obtained. Rarely, giant condylomata (Buschke-Löwenstein tumors) involving the glans penis and often the urethra may be seen. Such lesions suggest carcinoma and a biopsy must be done. Surgical excision is the treatment of choice.

Figure 38–5. Voiding urethrogram following repair of traumatic posterior urethral stricture. Arrow indicates that area of repair is stricture-free.

To prevent recurrence of condylomata acuminata, the sexual partner must also be examined and treated if necessary.

STENOSIS OF THE URETHRAL MEATUS

Newborns are often suspected of having meatal stenosis of some degree. This condition is thought to be secondary to ammonia dermatitis following circumcision and resulting in prolonged irritative meatitis.

Calibration is important, since the visual appearance of the meatus does not correlate well with its actual size. The urethra should easily accept the tip of an 8F pediatric feeding tube. The significance of meatal stenosis is debated, but a meatal caliber less than 5F in children under 10 years of age is an indication for meatotomy.

PENILE PHLEBOTHROMBOSIS & LYMPHATIC OCCLUSION

Superficial veins and lymphatic vessels of the dorsal penile shaft just proximal to the corona may become irritated and inflamed. A careful history usually indicates that minor trauma to the area (eg, from prolonged sexual intercourse) has occurred. Examination reveals a tender, indurated, cordlike structure on the distal penile shaft. Slight erythema may be present.

For clinical purposes, there is no need to distinguish lymphatic and venous causes, since both penile phlebothrombosis and lymphatic occlusion will resolve spontaneously. The patient must be reassured.

REFERENCES

Congenital Anomalies

Penis & Urethra

Akman Y et al: Penile anatomy under the pubic arch: Reconstructive implications. J Urol 2001;166:225.

Allen TD: Congenital microphallus. In: Kaufman JJ (editor): *Current Urologic Therapy.* Saunders, 1980.

Churchill BM et al: The dartos flap as an adjunct in preventing urethrocutaneous fistulas in repeat hypospadias surgery. J Urol 1996;156:2047.

Darewicz B et al: Ultrastructure of the tunica albuginea in congenital penile curvature. J Urol 2001;166:1766.

Gad YZ et al: 5 alpha-reductase deficiency in patients with micropenis. J Inherit Metab Dis 1997;20:95.

Hinman F Jr: Microphallus: Distinction between anomalous and endocrine types. J Urol 1980;123:412.

Ishii T, Higashionna T, Hiratsuka Y: Transrectal ultrasound findings of pelvic arteriovenous malformation. J Urol 2001; 166:999.

Karnak I et al: Rare congenital abnormalities of the anterior urethra. Pediatr Surg Int 1997;12:407.

Wessells H, Lue TF, McAninch JW: Penile length in the flaccid and erect states: Guidelines for penile augmentation. J Urol 1996;156:995.

Wilson SA, Walker RD: Megalourethra and hypospadias. J Urol 1983;129:556.

Wittkopf JE, Cooper CS, Hawtrey CE: Penile agenesis with a separated scrotum and normal renal function in an identical twin. J Urol 2002;167(2 Pt 1):687.

Urethral Stricture

Aragona F et al: Familial occurrence of congenital stricture of bulbar urethra. Urol Int 1991;46:112.

Hoebeke PB et al: Membrano-bulbo-urethral junction stenosis: Posterior urethra obstruction due to extreme caliber disproportion in the male urethra. Eur Urol 1997;32:480.

Narborough GC, Elliott S, Minford JE: Congenital stricture of the urethra. Clin Radiol 1990;42:402.

Scherz HC, Kaplan GW: Etiology, diagnosis, and management of urethral strictures in children. Urol Clin North Am 1990; 17:389.

Posterior Urethral Valves

Hulbert WC et al: The predictive value of ultrasonography in evaluation of infants with posterior urethral valves. J Urol 1992; 148:122.

Johnston JH: Vesicoureteric reflux with urethral valves. Br J Urol 1979;51:100.

Parkhouse HF, Woodhouse CR: Long-term status of patients with posterior urethral valves. Urol Clin North Am 1990;17:373.

Peters CA et al: The urodynamic consequences of posterior urethral valves. J Urol 1990;144:122.

Reinberg Y, de Castano I, Gonzalez R: Influence of initial therapy on progression of renal failure and body growth in children with posterior urethral valves. J Urol 1992;148:532.

Reinberg Y, de Castano I, Gonzalez R: Prognosis for patients with prenatally diagnosed posterior urethral valves. J Urol 1992; 148:125.

Anterior Urethral Valves

Takeda M et al: Application of flexible renoureteroscope for antegrade urethroscopy in the treatment of congenital anterior urethral valve. Eur Urol 1992;22:190.

Urethrorectal, Vesicorectal, & Urethroperineal Fistulas

Bates DG, Lebowitz RL: Congenital urethroperineal fistula. Radiology 1995;194:501.

Hypospadias

Asopa HS: Newer concepts in the management of hypospadias and its complications. Ann R Coll Surg Engl 1998;80:161.

Baskin LS: Hypospadias and urethral development. J Urol 2000; 163:951.

Baskin LS, Duckett JW: Buccal mucosa grafts in hypospadias surgery. Br J Urol 1995;76(Suppl 3):23.

Baskin LS, Duckett JW, Lue TF: Penile curvature. Urology 1996; 48:347.

Bleustein CB et al: Mechanism of healing following the Snodgrass repair. J Urol 2001;165:277.

Duckett JW: Island flap technique for hypospadias repair. Urol Clin North Am 1981;8:503.

Duckett JW, Snyder HM III: Meatal advancement and glanuloplasty hypospadias repair after 1,000 cases: Avoidance of meatal stenosis and regression. J Urol 1992;147:665.

Hensle TW et al: Hypospadias repair in adults: Adventures and misadventures. J Urol 2001;165:77.

Hinman F JR: The blood supply to preputial island flaps. J Urol 1991;145:1232.

Kass EJ, Bolong D: Single stage hypospadias reconstruction without fistula. J Urol 1990;144:520, 530.

Keating MA, Cartwright PC, Duckett JW: Bladder mucosa in urethral reconstructions. J Urol 1990;144:827.

Powell CR et al: Comparison of flaps versus grafts in proximal hypospadias surgery. J Urol 2000;163:1286.

Rober PE, Perlmutter AD, Reitelman C: Experience with 81, 1-stage hypospadias/chordee repairs with free graft urethroplasties. J Urol 1990;144:526.

Smith EP, Wacksman J: Evaluation of severe hypospadias. J Pediatr 1997;131:344.

Chordee without Hypospadias

Devine CJ Jr et al: The surgical treatment of chordee without hypospadias in men. J Urol 1991;146:325.

Kaplan GW, Lamm DL: Embryogenesis of chordee. J Urol 1975; 114:769.

Epispadias

Arap S et al: Incontinent epispadias: Surgical treatment of 38 cases. J Urol 1988;140:577.

Ben-Chaim J, Gearhart JP: Current management of bladder exstrophy. Scand J Urol Nephrol 1997;31:103.

Diamond DA, Ransley PG: Male epispadias. J Urol 1995; 154:2150.

Kaefer M et al: Continent urinary diversion: The Children's Hospital experience. J Urol 1997;157:1394.

Perlmutter AD, Weinstein MD, Reitelman C: Vesical neck reconstruction in patients with epispadias-exstrophy complex. J Urol 1991;146:613.

Peters CA, Gearhart JP, Jeffs RD: Epispadias and incontinence: The challenge of the small bladder. J Urol 1988;140:1199.

Tanagho EA, Smith DR: Clinical evaluation of a surgical technique for the correction of complete urinary incontinence. J Urol 1972;107:402.

Acquired Diseases & Disorders

DeCastro BJ, Morey AF: Fibrin sealant for the reconstruction of Fournier's gangrene sequelae. J Urol 2002;167:1774.

Park S et al: Extramammary Paget's disease of the penis and scrotum: Excision, reconstruction and evaluation of occult malignancy. J Urol 2001;166:2112.

Priapism

Barry JM: Priapism: Treatment with corpus cavernosum to dorsal vein of penis shunts. J Urol 1976;116:754.

Brock G et al: High flow priapism: A spectrum of disease. J Urol 1993;150:968.

Hamre MR et al: Priapism as a complication of sickle-cell disease. J Urol 1991;145:1.

Ilkay AK, Levine LA: Conservative management of high-flow priapism. Urology 1995;46:419.

Levine JF et al: Recurrent prolonged erections and priapism as a sequela of priapism: Pathophysiology and management. J Urol 1991;145:764.

Lue TF et al: Priapism: Refined approach to diagnosis and treatment. J Urol 1986;136:104.

Mabjeesh NJ, Shemesh D, Abramowitz HB: Posttraumatic high flow priapism: Successful management using duplex guided compression. J Urol 1999;161:215.

Mulhall JP, Honig SC: Priapism: Etiology and management. Acad Emerg Med 1996;3:810.

Patel AG, Mukherji K, Lee A: Priapism associated with psychotropic drugs. Br J Hosp Med 1996;55:315.

Ricciardi R Jr et al: Delayed high flow priapism: Pathophysiology and management. J Urol 1993;149:119.

Secil M et al: The prediction of papaverine induced priapism by color Doppler sonography. J Urol 2001;165:416.

Shapiro RH, Berger RE: Post-traumatic priapism treated with selective cavernosal artery ligation. Urology 1997;49:638.

Volkmer BG et al: Prepubertal high flow priapism: Incidence, diagnosis and treatment. J Urol 2001;166:1018.

Winter CC, McDowell G: Experience with 105 patients with priapism: Update review of all aspects. J Urol 1988;140:980.

Peyronie Disease

Carson CC: Penile prosthesis implantation in the treatment of Peyronie's disease. Int J Impotence Res 1998;10:125.

Gelbard MK, Dorey F, James K: The natural history of Peyronie's disease. J Urol 1990;144:1376.

Jordan GH, Angermeier KW: Preoperative evaluation of erectile function with dynamic infusion cavernosometry/cavernosography in patients undergoing surgery for Peyronie's disease: Correlation with postoperative results. J Urol 1993;150: 1138.

Lue TF, El-Sakka AI: Lengthening shortened penis caused by Peyronie's disease using circular venous grafting and daily stretching with a vacuum erection device. J Urol 1999;161: 1141.

Lue TF, El-Sakka AI: Venous patch graft for Peyronie's disease. Part I: Technique. J Urol 1998;160:2047.

Mufti GR et al: Corporeal plication for surgical correction of Peyronie's disease. J Urol 1990;144:281.

Mulhall JP et al: Basic fibroblast growth factor expression in Peyronie's disease. J Urol 2001;165:419.

O'Donnell PD: Results of surgical management of Peyronie's disease. J Urol 1992;148:1184.

Pryor JP: Correction of penile curvature and Peyronie's disease: Why I prefer the Nesbit technique. Int J Impotence Res 1998;10:129.

Wilson SK, Cleves MA, Delk JR II: Long-term followup of treatment for Peyronie's disease: Modeling the penis over an inflatable penile prosthesis. J Urol 2001;165:825.

Phimosis

Langer JC, Coplen DE: Circumcision and pediatric disorders of the penis. Pediatr Clin North Am 1998;45:801.

Simpson ET, Barraclough P: The management of the paediatric foreskin. Aust Fam Physician 1998;27:381.

Paraphimosis

Olson C: Emergency treatment of paraphimosis. Can Fam Physician 1998;44:1253.

Raveenthiran V: Reduction of paraphimosis: A technique based on pathophysiology. Br J Surg 1996;83:1247.

Circumcision

Baskin LS et al: Treating complications of circumcision. Pediatr Emerg Care 1996;12:62.

Collins S et al: Effects of circumcision on male sexual function: Debunking a myth? J Urol 2002;167:2111.

Fink KS, Carson CC, DeVellis RF: Adult circumcision outcomes study: Effect on erectile function, penile sensitivity, sexual activity and satisfaction. J Urol 2002;167:2113.

Langer JC, Coplen DE: Circumcision and pediatric disorders of the penis. Pediatr Clin North Am 1998;45:801.

Niku SD, Stock JA, Kaplan GW: Neonatal circumcision. Urol Clin North Am 1995;22:57.

Urethral Stricture

Angermeier KW, Jordan GH, Schlossberg SM: Complex urethral reconstruction. Urol Clin North Am 1994;21:567.

Armenakas NA, Morey AF, McAninch JW: Reconstruction of resistant strictures of the fossa navicularis and meatus. J Urol 1998;160:359.

Barbagli G, Palminteri E, Rizzo M: Dorsal onlay graft urethroplasty using penile skin or buccal mucosa in adult bulbourethral strictures. J Urol 1998;160:1307.

Barbagli G et al: Long-term outcome of urethroplasty after failed urethrotomy versus primary repair. J Urol 2001;165:1918.

Barry JM: Visual urethrotomy in the management of the obliterated membranous urethra. Urol Clin North Am 1989;16:319.

Carney KJ, McAninch JW: Penile circular fasciocutaneous flaps to reconstruct complex anterior urethral strictures. Urol Clin North Am 2002;29:397.

Coursey JW et al: Erectile function after anterior urethroplasty. J Urol 2001;166:2273.

el-Kasaby AW et al: The use of buccal mucosa patch graft in the management of anterior urethral strictures. J Urol 1993;149:276.

Gary R, Cass AS, Koos G: Vascular complications of transurethral incision of post-traumatic urethral strictures. J Urol 1988;140:1539.

McAninch JW: Pubectomy in repair of membranous urethral stricture. Urol Clin North Am 1989;16:297.

McAninch JW, Laing FC, Jeffrey RB Jr: Sonourethrography in the evaluation of urethral strictures: A preliminary report. J Urol 1988;139:294.

McAninch JW, Morey AF: Penile circular fasciocutaneous skin flap in one-stage reconstruction of complex anterior urethral strictures. J Urol 1998;159:1209.

Morey AF: Urethral plate salvage with dorsal graft promotes successful penile flap onlay reconstruction of severe pendulous strictures. J Urol 2001;166:1376.

Morey AF, McAninch JW: Reconstruction of posterior urethral disruption injuries: Outcome analysis in 82 patients. J Urol 1997;157:506.

Morey AF, McAninch JW: Sonographic staging of anterior urethral strictures. J Urol 2000;163:1070.

Morey AF, McAninch JW: Ultrasound evaluation of the male urethra for assessment of urethral stricture. J Clin Ultrasound 1996a;24:473.

Morey AF, McAninch JW: When and how to use buccal mucosal grafts in adult bulbar urethroplasty. Urology 1996b;48:194.

Morey AF et al: American Urological Association symptom index in the assessment of urethroplasty outcomes. J Urol 1998;159:1192.

Mundy AR: Urethroplasty for posterior urethral strictures. Br J Urol 1996;78:243.

Santucci RA, Mario LA, McAninch JW: Anastomotic urethroplasty for bulbar urethral stricture: Analysis of 168 patients. J Urol 2002;167:1715.

Wessells H, Morey AF, McAninch JW: Single-stage reconstruction of complex anterior urethral strictures: Combined tissue-transfer techniques. J Urol 1997;157:1271.

Urethral Condylomata Acuminata

Fralick RA et al: Urethroscopy and urethral cytology in men with external genital condyloma. Urology 1994;43:361.

Volz LR, Carpiniello VL, Malloy TR: Laser treatment of urethral condyloma: A five-year experience. Urology 1994;43:81.

Penile Thrombophlebitis & Lymphatic Occlusion

Bird V et al: Traumatic thrombophlebitis of the superficial dorsal vein of the penis: An occupational hazard. Am J Emerg Med 1997;15:67.

Shapiro RS: Superficial dorsal penile vein thrombosis (penile Mondor's phlebitis): Ultrasound diagnosis. J Clin Ultrasound 1996;24:272.

Disorders of the Female Urethra

39

Emil A. Tanagho, MD

■ CONGENITAL ANOMALIES OF THE FEMALE URETHRA

DISTAL URETHRAL STENOSIS IN INFANCY & CHILDHOOD (Spasm of the External Urinary Sphincter)

There has been considerable confusion about the site of lower tract obstruction in young girls who have enuresis, a slow and interrupted urinary stream, recurrent cystitis, and pyelonephritis, and who, on thorough examination, often exhibit vesicoureteral reflux. Treatment has been directed largely to the bladder neck on rather empiric grounds. Most of these children, however, have congenital distal urethral stenosis with secondary spasm of the striated external sphincter rather than bladder neck obstruction due to functional or organic causes.

At birth, calibration of the urethra with bougies à boule reveals no evidence of a distal ring of urethral stenosis (Fisher et al, 1969). Within a few months, however, such a ring develops as a normal anatomic structure. After puberty, the ring disappears. The inference is that the absence of estrogens leads to the development of this lesion. Lyon and Tanagho (1965) found that the ring calibrates at 14F at age 2 and at 16F between the ages of 4 and 10. Even though from the hydrodynamic standpoint such a stenotic area should not be obstructive, almost all observers agree that dilatation of the ring does relieve symptoms in these children and that it results in cure or amelioration of persistent infection or vesical dysfunction in 80% of cases. Lyon and Tanagho thought it possible that the basic cause of these urinary difficulties might be reflex spasm of periurethral striated sphincter and noted that voiding cystourethrograms supported that view (Figure 39–1).

Tanagho et al (1971) measured pressures in the bladder and in the proximal and mid urethra simultaneously in symptomatic girls and found high resting pressures, some as high as 200 cm of water (normal, 100 cm of water) in the midurethral segment. Attempts at voiding caused intravesical pressures as high as 225 cm of water (normal, 30–40 cm of water) to develop. Under curare, the urethral closing pressures dropped to normal (40–50 cm of water), proving that these obstructing pressures were caused by spasm of the striated sphincter muscle. If the distal urethral ring was treated and symptoms abated, repeat pressure studies showed normal midurethral and intravesical voiding pressures. If, on the other hand, symptoms persisted, pressures were found to remain at extremely high levels. It seems clear, therefore, that the major cause of urinary problems in young girls is spasm of the external sphincter and not vesical neck stenosis (Smith, 1969).

In addition to recurrent urinary tract infections, these patients have hesitancy in initiating micturition and a slow, hesitant, or interrupted urinary stream. Enuresis and involuntary loss of urine during the day are common complaints. Abdominal straining may be required in order to void. Small amounts of residual urine are found, which impair the vesical defense mechanism. A voiding cystourethrogram may reveal an open bladder neck and ballooning of the proximal urethra secondary to spasm of the external sphincter (Figure 39–1).

The voiding cystourethrogram may reveal evidence of the distal ring, but typical findings are not always seen, particularly if the flow rate is slow. Definitive diagnosis is made by bougienage.

The simplest and least harmful treatment is overdilatation with sounds up to 32–36F or with the Kollmann dilator (Lyon and Tanagho, 1965; Lyon and Marshall, 1971; Hendry, Stanton, and Williams, 1973). With either method, the ring "cracks" anteriorly, with some bleeding. Recurrence of the ring is rare. Internal urethrotomy has its proponents (Immergut and Gilbert, 1973; Hradec et al, 1973), but Kaplan, Sammons, and King (1973) found that results with urethrotomy were poor, since incising the urethra along its entire length does not cut the external sphincter, whose abnormal tone is the cause of the obstruction, whereas "cracking" the ring by overdilatation accomplishes this purpose.

In 80% of affected children, destruction of the ring of distal urethral stenosis helps to overcome enuresis and achieve a normal free voiding pattern and to cure recurrent cystitis or persistent bacteriuria (Lyon and Marshall, 1971). Spontaneous resolution of reflux is possible only in the case of "borderline" values that tend to give way in the presence of increased voiding pressure and infection.

627

Figure 39–1. Distal urethral stenosis with reflux spasm of voluntary urethral sphincter. **Left:** Voiding cystourethrogram showing bilateral vesicoureteral reflux, a wide-open vesical neck, and severe spasm of the striated urethral sphincter in the mid portion of the urethra (arrow) secondary to distal urethral stenosis. **Right:** Postvoiding film. The bladder is empty and the vesical neck open, but the dilated urethra contains radiopaque fluid proximal to the stenotic zone. Bacteria in the urethra thus can flow back into the bladder. (Courtesy of AD Amar.)

Since the ring normally disappears at puberty, it is possible to await spontaneous cure; however, the ring should be broken if symptoms have been severe enough to bring the child to the attention of a urologist.

LABIAL FUSION (SYNECHIA VULVAE)

Some children with recurring urinary infection are found to have fused labia minora, which are apt to obstruct the flow of urine, causing it to pool in the vagina. Local application of estrogen cream twice daily for 2–4 weeks usually causes spontaneous separation. Forceful separation or dissection has its advocates (Christensen and Oster, 1971).

■ ACQUIRED DISEASES OF THE FEMALE URETHRA

ACUTE URETHRITIS

Acute urethritis frequently occurs with gonorrheal infection in women. Urinary symptoms are often present at the onset of the disease. Cultures and smears establish the diagnosis. Prompt cure can be achieved with antimicrobial drugs.

The detergents in bubble bath and some spermicidal jellies may cause vaginitis and urethritis. Symptoms of vesical irritability may occur.

CHRONIC URETHRITIS

Chronic urethritis is one of the most common urologic problems of females. The distal urethra normally harbors pathogens, and the risk of infection may be increased by wearing contaminated diapers, by insertion of an indwelling catheter, by spread from cervical or vaginal infections, or by intercourse with an infected partner. Urethral inflammation may also occur from the trauma of intercourse or childbirth, particularly if urethral stenosis, either congenital or following childbirth, is present.

Clinical Findings

The urethral mucosa is reddened, quite sensitive, and often stenotic. Granular areas are often seen, and polypoid masses may be noted just distal to the bladder neck.

A. SYMPTOMS

The symptoms resemble those of cystitis, although the urine may be clear. Complaints include burning on urination, frequency, and nocturia. Discomfort in the urethra may be felt, particularly when walking.

B. SIGNS

Examination may disclose redness of the meatus, hypersensitivity of the meatus and of the urethra on vaginal palpation, and evidence of cervicitis or vaginitis. There is no urethral discharge.

C. LABORATORY FINDINGS

When the initial and midstream urine are collected in separate containers, the first glass contains pus and the second does not (Marshall, Lyon, and Schieble, 1970). *Ureaplasma urealyticum* (formerly called T strains of mycoplasmas) is often identifiable in the first glass. These findings are similar to those of nongonococcal (chlamydial) urethritis in males. Clinically, the presence of white blood cells (leukocytes) in the absence of bacteria on a routine stain or culture suggests nongonococcal urethritis. In other cases, various bacteria (eg, *Streptococcus faecalis, Escherichia coli*) may be cultured from both the urethral washings and a specimen taken from the introitus.

D. INSTRUMENTAL EXAMINATION

A catheter, bougie à boule, or sound may meet resistance because of urethral stenosis. Panendoscopy reveals redness and a granular appearance of the mucosa. Inflammatory polyps may be seen in the proximal portion of the urethra. Cystoscopy may show increased injection of the trigone (trigonitis), which often accompanies urethritis.

Differential Diagnosis

Differentiation of urethritis from cystitis depends on bacteriologic study of the urine; panendoscopy demonstrates the urethral lesion. Both urethritis and cystitis may be present.

Psychological disorders may cause symptoms identical to those of chronic urethritis. A history of short bouts of frequency without nocturia is suggestive of functional illness. The neurotic makeup of the patient is usually obvious.

Treatment & Prognosis

Gradual urethral dilatations (up to 36F in adults) are indicated for urethral stenosis; this allows for some inevitable contracture. Immergut and Gilbert (1973) prefer internal urethrotomy. *U urealyticum* is fairly sensitive to tetracycline or erythromycin. Chlamydial urethritis usually responds to sulfonamides or tetracyclines. For ascending bacterial infections, Bruce et al (1973) recommend the regular, local application of an antiseptic (eg, hexachlorophene, chlorhexidine cream) to the introitus in order to prevent bacteria from the area of the perineum, vagina, and vulva from reinfecting the urethra.

SENILE URETHRITIS

After physiologic (or surgical) menopause, hypoestrogenism occurs and retrogressive (senile) changes take place in the vaginal epithelium, so that it becomes rather dry and pale. Similar changes develop in the lower urinary tract, which arises from the same embryologic tissues as the female reproductive organs. Some eversion of the mucosa about the urethral orifice, from foreshortening of the vaginal canal, is usually seen. This is commonly misdiagnosed as caruncle.

Clinical Findings

A. SYMPTOMS

Many postmenopausal women have symptoms of vesical irritability (burning, frequency, urgency) and stress incontinence. They may complain of vaginal and vulval itching and some discharge.

B. SIGNS

The vaginal epithelium is dry and pale. The mucosa at the urethral orifice is often reddened and hypersensitive; eversion of its posterior lip from foreshortening of the urethrovaginal wall is common.

C. LABORATORY FINDINGS

The urine is usually free of microorganisms. The diagnosis can be made by the following procedure: A dry smear of vaginal epithelial cells is stained with Lugol's solution. The slide is then washed with water and immediately examined microscopically while wet. In hypoestrogenism, the cells take up the iodine poorly and are therefore yellow. When the mucosa is normal, these cells stain a deep brown because of their glycogen content. The diagnosis may also be confirmed by a Papanicolaou smear.

D. INSTRUMENTAL EXAMINATION

Panendoscopy usually demonstrates a reddened and granular urethral mucosa. Some urethral stenosis may be noted.

Differential Diagnosis

Senile urethritis is often mistaken for urethral caruncle. Eversion of the posterior lip of the urinary meatus is evident in both conditions; however, a hypersensitive vascular tumor is not present in senile urethritis.

Before operations to relieve stress incontinence are performed, estrogen (or androgen) therapy should be tried.

Treatment

Senile urethritis responds well to diethylstilbestrol vaginal suppositories, 0.1 mg nightly for 3 weeks. Estrogen creams applied locally are also effective. Estrogen urethral suppositories have been recommended, but they offer no advantages and are difficult to insert. After 3 weeks of treatment, the drug is withheld for 1 week and the course is repeated. Three or more courses are occasionally indicated, depending on the symptoms and the appearance of the vaginal smear stained as outlined previously.

If vaginal irritation or bleeding on discontinuation of estrogen suppositories is a problem, methyltestosterone buccal tablets can be used as vaginal suppositories. One 5-mg tablet is inserted vaginally daily for 5–8 weeks. Diethylstilbestrol, 0.1 mg/d orally, is also effective.

Prognosis

Senile urethritis usually responds promptly to estrogen or androgen therapy.

URETHRAL CARUNCLE

Urethral caruncle is a benign, red, raspberrylike, friable vascular tumor involving the posterior lip of the external urinary meatus. It is rare before the menopause. Microscopically, it consists of connective tissue containing many inflammatory cells and blood vessels and is covered by an epithelial layer.

Clinical Findings

Symptoms include pain on urination, pain with intercourse, and bloody spotting from even mild trauma. A sessile or pedunculated red, friable, tender mass is seen at the posterior lip of the meatus.

Differential Diagnosis

Carcinoma of the urethra may involve the urethral meatus. Palpation reveals definite induration. Biopsy establishes the true diagnosis.

Senile urethritis is often associated with a polypoid reaction of the urinary meatus and in fact is the most common cause of masses in this region. The diagnosis can be made by verifying the patient's hypoestrogenic status and by demonstrating a favorable response to estrogen replacement therapy. Biopsy should be done if doubt exists.

Thrombosis of the urethral vein presents as a bluish, swollen, tender lesion involving the posterior lip of the urinary meatus. It has the appearance of the thrombosed hemorrhoid. It subsides without treatment.

Treatment

Local excision is indicated only if symptoms are troublesome.

Prognosis

True caruncle is usually cured by excision, but in a few instances it does recur.

PROLAPSE OF THE URETHRA

Prolapse of the female urethra is not common. It usually occurs only in children or in paraplegics suffering from a lower motor neuron lesion. The protruding urethral mucosa presents as an angry red mass that may become gangrenous if it is not reduced promptly. When a young girl has a protruding mass, urethral prolapse must be differentiated from prolapse of a ureterocele.

After reduction, cystoscopy should be done to rule out ureterocele. Recurrences are rare following reduction; the accompanying inflammation probably "fixes" the tissue in place as healing progresses. If the prolapsed urethra cannot be reduced or if it recurs, an indwelling catheter should be inserted, traction placed on it, and a heavy piece of suture material tightly tied over the tissue and catheter just proximal to the mass. The tissue later sloughs off. Using this same technique, the tissue can be resected, preferably with an electrosurgical cautery.

URETHROVAGINAL FISTULA

Urethrovaginal fistulas may follow local injury secondary to fracture of the pelvis or obstetric or surgical injury (see Chapter 16). A common cause is accidental trauma to the urethra or its blood supply in the course of surgical repair of a cystocele or excision of urethral diverticula. Vaginal urethroplasty is indicated.

URETHRAL DIVERTICULUM

Diverticulation of the urethral wall is not common. Diverticula are at times multiple. Most cases are probably secondary to obstetric urethral trauma or severe urethral infection. A few cases of carcinoma in such diverticula have been reported. Urethral diverticula are usually associated with recurrent attacks of cystitis. Purulent urethral discharge is sometimes noted as the infected diverticulum empties. Dyspareunia sometimes results. On occasion, the diverticulum may be large enough to be discovered by the patient.

The diagnosis is usually made on feeling a rounded cystic mass in the anterior wall of the vagina that leaks pus from the urethral orifice when pressure is applied. Endoscopy may reveal the urethral opening. The postvoiding film of an excretory urographic series may demonstrate the lesion. It may be possible to introduce a small catheter through which radiopaque fluid can be instilled. Appropriate x-ray films are then exposed (Figure 39–2). The plain film may show a stone in the diverticulum. If these methods fail, the following procedures can be used:

(1) Empty the diverticulum manually. Via a catheter, instill 5 mL of indigo carmine and 60 mL of contrast medium into the bladder. Remove the catheter and have the patient begin to void. Occlude the meatus with a finger. This maneuver usually causes the diverticulum to fill with the test solution. Take appropriate x-rays, and perform panendoscopy to look for leakage of blue dye from the mouth of the diverticulum.

(2) Insert a Davis-TeLinde catheter. This looks like a Foley catheter but is surrounded by a second movable balloon. Pass the catheter to the bladder and inflate the proximal balloon. While exerting tension on the catheter, slide the second balloon against the urinary meatus and inflate it. Then inject contrast medium into the catheter. The radiopaque fluid will escape from the catheter through a hole between the balloons and will fill the urethra and diverticulum, after which x-rays can be exposed. Occasionally, urethral diverticulum is elusive and difficult to visualize. Transvaginal ultrasonography or pelvic magnetic resonance imaging can be helpful in diagnosis.

Treatment consists of removal of the sac through an incision in the anterior vaginal wall, care being taken not to injure the urethral sphincteric musculature. Incision is carried down to the diverticular mucosa, and the plane of cleavage is followed all around to the neck of

Figure 39–2. Urethral diverticulum containing stone. **Left:** Plain film showing stone. Arrows outline bladder. **Right:** Diverticulum filled with radiopaque fluid instilled through ureteral catheter. Bladder outlined by arrows.

the diverticulum. The diverticular sac is completely excised and the defect in the urethra repaired. Elik (1957) recommends that the diverticulum be opened, stuffed with absorbable cellulose (Oxycel), and then closed; the resulting inflammatory reaction destroys the cyst. A suprapubic cystostomy should be left in place for 15 days following surgical excision of the diverticulum.

The outcome is usually good unless the diverticulum is so situated that its excision injures the external urinary sphincter mechanism. In a few cases, urethrovaginal fistula may develop. If the fistula does not close with adequate suprapubic drainage, surgical repair will be necessary 2–3 months later.

URETHRAL STRICTURE

True organic stricture of the adult female urethra is not common. (Functional urethral obstruction is more common.) It may be congenital or acquired. The trauma of intercourse and especially of childbirth may lead to periurethral fibrosis with contracture, or the stricture may be caused by the surgeon during vaginal repair. It may develop secondary to acute or chronic urethritis.

Persistent hesitancy in initiating urination and a slow urinary stream are the principal symptoms of stricture. Burning, frequency, nocturia, and urethral pain may occur from secondary urethritis or cystitis. If secondary infection of the bladder is present, pus and bacteria will be found in the urine. A fairly large catheter (22F) may pass to the bladder only with difficulty. Panendoscopy may demonstrate the point of narrowness and disclose evidence of urethritis. Cystoscopy often reveals trabeculation (hypertrophy) of the bladder wall.

Chronic cystitis may cause similar symptoms, but urinalysis reveals evidence of infection. Cancer of the urethra causes progressive narrowing of the urethra, but induration and infiltration of the urethra are found on vaginal examination. Panendoscopy with biopsy establishes the diagnosis. Vesical tumor involving the bladder neck causes hesitancy and impairment of the urinary stream. Cystoscopy is definitive. Chronic urethritis commonly accompanies urethral stenosis; either may be primary. Recurrent or chronic cystitis is often secondary to stenosis.

Treatment consists of gradual urethral dilatation (up to 36F) at weekly intervals. Slight overstretching is necessary, since some contracture will occur after therapy is discontinued. Measures to combat urethritis and cystitis also must be employed. Internal urethrotomy has its proponents.

With proper overdilatation of the urethra and specific therapy of the urethritis that is usually present, the prognosis is good.

REFERENCES

Distal Urethral Stenosis

Archimbaud JP, Leriche A, Mottet N: Urethral stenosis and urinary incontinence in the female: 149 cases. Ann Urol 1989; 23:340.

Farrar DJ, Green NA, Ashken MH: An evaluation of the Otis urethrotomy in female patients with recurrent urinary tract infections: A review after 6 years. Br J Urol 1980;52:68.

Fisher RE et al: Urethral calibration in newborn girls. J Urol 1969; 102:67.

Hendry WF, Stanton SL, Williams DI: Recurrent urinary infections in girls: Effects of urethral dilatation. Br J Urol 1973; 45:72.

Hojsgaard A: The urethral pressure profile in female patients with meatal stenosis. Scand J Urol Nephrol 1976;10:97.

Hradec E et al: Significance of urethral obstruction in girls. Urol Int 1973;28:440.

Immergut MA, Gilbert EC: Internal urethrotomy in recurring urinary infections in girls. J Urol 1973;109:126.

Kaplan GW, Sammons TA, King LR: A blind comparison of dilatation, urethrotomy and medication alone in the treatment of urinary tract infection in girls. J Urol 1973;109:917.

Leadbetter GW: Re: Internal urethrotomy in girls and its impact on the urethral intrinsic and extrinsic continence mechanisms. (Letter.) J Urol 1988;139:142.

Lyon RP, Marshall S: Urinary tract infections and difficult urination in girls: Long-term follow-up. J Urol 1971;105:314.

Lyon RP, Tanagho EA: Distal urethral stenosis in little girls. J Urol 1965;93:379.

Smith DR: Critique on the concept of vesical neck obstruction in children. JAMA 1969;207:1686.

Tanagho EA, Lyon RP: Urethral dilatation versus internal urethrotomy. J Urol 1971;105:242.

Tanagho EA et al: Spastic external sphincter and urinary tract infection in girls. Br J Urol 1971;43:69.

Uehling DT: The normal caliber of the adult female urethra. J Urol 1978;120:176.

Van Gool J, Tanagho EA: External sphincter activity and recurrent urinary tract infection in girls. Urology 1977;10:348.

Vermillion CD, Halverstadt DB, Leadbetter GW Jr: Internal urethrotomy and recurrent urinary tract infection in female children. 2. Long-term results in the management of infection. J Urol 1971;106:154.

Walker D, Richard GA: A critical evaluation of urethral obstruction in female children. Pediatrics 1973;51: 272.

Labial Fusion

Aribarg A: Topical oestrogen therapy for labial adhesions in children. Br J Obstet Gynaecol 1975;82:424.

Christensen EH, Oster J: Adhesions of labia minora (synechia vulvae) in childhood: A review and report of fourteen cases. Acta Paediatr Scand 1971;60:709.

Evruke C et al: Labial fusion in a pubertal girl: A case report. J Pediatr Adolesc Gynecol 1996;9:81.

Gibbon KL, Bewley AP, Salisbury JA: Labial fusion in children: A presenting feature of genital lichen sclerosus? Pediatr Dermatol 1999:16;388.

McCann J, Voris J, Simon M: Labial adhesions and posterior fourchette injuries in childhood sexual abuse. Am J Dis Child 1988;142:659.

Norbeck JC, Ritchey MR, Bloom DA: Labial fusion causing upper urinary tract obstruction. Urology 1993;42:209.

Runsza ME: Gonorrheal vulvovaginitis, labial fusion and imperforate hymen. Am J Dis Child 1989;143:381.

Wheeler RA, Burge DM: Urinary obstruction due to labial fusion. Br J Urol 1991;67:102.

Acute Urethritis

Bass HN: "Bubble bath" as an irritant to the urinary tract of children. Clin Pediatr 1968;7:174.

Fihn SD, Johnson C, Stamm WE: *Escherichia coli* urethritis in women with symptoms of acute urinary tract infection. J Infect Dis 1988;157:196.

Horner PJ et al: Association of *Mycoplasma genitalium* with acute non-gonococcal urethritis. Lancet 1993; 342:582.

Marshall S: The effect of bubble bath on the urinary tract. J Urol 1965;93:112.

Taylor-Robinson D, Furr PM: Genital mycoplasma infections. Wien Klin Wochenschr 1997;109(14–15):5785.

Taylor-Robinson D, Gilroy CB, Hay PE: Occurrence of *Mycoplasma genitalium* in different populations and its clinical significance. Clin Infect Dis 1993;17(Suppl 1):S66.

Waugh MA: Azithromycin in gonorrhoea. Int J STD AIDS 1996;7(Suppl 1):2.

Chronic Urethritis

Baldwin HE: STD update: Screening and therapeutic options. Int J Fertil Women's Med 2001;46:79.

Batra SC, Iosif CS: Female urethra: Target for estrogen action. J Urol 1983;129:418.

Bodner DR: The urethral syndrome. Urol Clin North Am 1988; 15:699.

Bruce AW et al: Recurrent urethritis in women. Can Med Assoc J 1973;108:973.

Farrar DJ, Green NA, Ashken MH: An evaluation of Otis urethrotomy in female patients with recurrent urinary tract infections: A review after 6 years. Br J Urol 1980;52:68.

Gittes RF, Nakamura RM: Female urethral syndrome. A female prostatitis? West J Med 1996;164:435.

Karafin LJ, Coll ME: Lower urinary tract disorders in the postmenopausal woman. Med Clin North Am 1987;71:111.

Krieger JN et al: Evaluation of chronic urethritis: Defining the role for endoscopic procedures. Arch Intern Med 1988;148:703.

Marshall S, Lyon RP, Schieble J: Nonspecific urethritis in females. Calif Med (June) 1970;112:9.

O'Neil AGB: The bacterial content of the female urethra: A new method of study. Br J Urol 1981;53:368.

Uuskula A, Kohl PK: Genital mycoplasmas, including *Mycoplasma genitalium,* as sexually transmitted agents. Int J STD AIDS 2002;13:79.

Senile Urethritis

Murphy JT: Urological problems in aged patients. Aust Fam Physician 1977;6:17, 21, 25.

Quinlivan LG: The treatment of senile vaginitis with low doses of synthetic estrogens. Am J Obstet Gynecol 1965;92:172.

Smith P: Age changes in the female urethra. Br J Urol 1972; 44:667.

Zweig S: Urinary tract infections in the elderly. Am Fam Physician 1987;35:123.

Urethral Caruncle

Lee WH, Tan KH, Lee YW: The aetiology of postmenopausal bleeding—A study of 163 consecutive cases in Singapore. Singapore Med J 1995;36:164.

Neilson D, Grant JB, Smith CE: Squamous intra-epithelial neoplasia presenting as a urethral caruncle. Br J Urol 1989;64:200.

Young RH et al: Urethral caruncle with atypical stromal cells simulating lymphoma or sarcoma—A distinctive pseudoneoplastic lesion of females. A report of six cases. Am J Surg Pathol 1996;20:1190.

Prolapse of the Urethra

Anveden-Hertzberg L, Gauderer MW, Elder JS: Urethral prolapse: An often misdiagnosed cause of urogenital bleeding in girls. Pediatr Emerg Care 1995;11:212.

Devine PC, Kessel HC: Surgical correction of urethral prolapse. J Urol 1980;123:856.

Fernandes ET et al: Urethral prolapse in children. Urology 1993; 41:240.

Johnson CF: Prolapse of the urethra: Confusion of clinical and anatomic characteristics with sexual abuse. Pediatrics 1991; 87:722.

Klaus H, Stein RT: Urethral prolapse in young girls. Pediatrics 1973;52:645.

Kleinjan JH, Vos P: Strangulated urethral prolapse. Urology 1996; 47:599.

Mitre A et al: Urethral prolapse in girls: Familial case. J Urol 1987; 137:115.

Rudin JE, Geldt VG, Alecseev EB: Prolapse of urethral mucosa in white female children: Experience with 58 cases. J Pediatr Surg 1997;32:423.

Valerie E et al: Diagnosis and treatment of urethral prolapse in children. Urology 1999;54:1082.

Urethrovaginal Fistula

Creatsas G et al: Reconstruction of urethrovaginal fistula and vaginal atresia in an adolescent girl after an abdominoperineal-vaginal pull-through procedure. Fertil Steril 1997;68:556.

Fall M: Vaginal wall bipedicled flap and other techniques in complicated urethral diverticulum and urethrovaginal fistula. J Am Coll Surg 1995;180:150.

Gil-Vernet JM, Gil-Vernet A, Campos JA: New surgical approach for treatment of complex vesicovaginal fistula. J Urol 1989; 141:513.

Gray L: Urethrovaginal fistulas. Am J Obstet Gynecol 1968; 101:28.

Hedlund H, Lindstedt E: Urovaginal fistulas: 20 years of experience with 45 cases. J Urol 1987;137:926.

Hilton P: Urodynamic findings in patients with urogenital fistulae. Br J Urol 1998;81:539.

Kliment J, Berats T: Urovaginal fistulas: Experience with the management of 41 cases. Int Urol Nephrol 1992;24:119.

Krogh J, Kay L, Hjortrup A: Treatment of urethrovaginal fistula. Br J Urol 1989;63:555.

Leach GE: Urethrovaginal fistula repair with Martius labial fat pad graft. Urol Clin North Am 1991;18:409.

Tancer ML: A report of thirty-four instances of urethrovaginal and bladder neck fistulas. Surg Gynecol Obstet 1993;177:77.

Tehan TJ, Nardi JA, Baker R: Complications associated with surgical repair of urethrovaginal fistula. Urology 1980;15:31.

Urethral Diverticulum

Baert L, Willemen P, Oyen R: Endovaginal sonography: New diagnostic approach for urethral diverticula. J Urol 1992; 147:464.

Debaere C et al: MR imaging of a diverticulum in a female urethra. J Belge Radiol 1995;78:345.

Dretler SP, Vermillion CD, McCullough DL: The roentgenographic diagnosis of female urethral diverticula. J Urol 1972; 107:72.

Elik M: Diverticulum of the female urethra: A new method of ablation. J Urol 1957;77:243.

Fall M: Vaginal wall bipedicled flap and other techniques in complicated urethral diverticulum and urethrovaginal fistula. J Am Coll Surg 1995;180:150.

Fortunato P, Schettini M, Gallucci M: Diagnosis and therapy of the female urethral diverticula. Int J Urogynecol Pelvic Floor Dysfunct 2001;12:51.

Fortunato P, Schettini M, Gallucci M: Diverticula of the female urethra. Br J Urol 1997;80:628.

Ganabathi K et al: Experience with the management of urethral diverticulum in 63 women. J Urol 1994;152(5 Pt 1):1445.

Golimbu M, al-Askari S: High pressure voiding urethrography. Urology 1974;3:717.

Jensen LM et al: Female urethral diverticulum: Clinical aspects and a presentation of 15 cases. Act Obstet Gynecol Scand 1996; 75:748.

Kato H et al: Carcinoembryonic antigen positive adenocarcinoma of a female urethral diverticulum: Case report and review of the literature. Int J Urol 1998;5:291.

Keefe B et al: Diverticula of the female urethra: Diagnosis by endovaginal and transperineal sonography. AJR 1991; 156:1195.

Kim B, Hricak H, Tanagho EA: Diagnosis of urethral diverticula in women: Value of MR imaging. AJR 1993;161:809.

Marshall S, Hirsch K: Carcinoma within urethral diverticula. Urology 1977;10:161.

Moran PA, Carey MP, Dwyer PL: Urethral diverticula in pregnancy. Aust N Z J Obstet Gynaecol 1998;38:102.

Mouritsen L, Bernstein I: Vaginal ultrasonography: A diagnostic tool for urethral diverticulum. Acta Obstet Gynecol Scand 1996;75:188.

Mueller EJ, Drake GL: A new surgical procedure for the removal of the wide-mouthed urethral diverticulum in females. Surg Gynecol Obstet 1989;168:269.

Nakamura Y et al: A case of adenocarcinoma arising within a urethral diverticulum diagnosed only by the surgical specimen. Gynecol Obstet Invest 1995;40:69.

Neitlich JD et al: Detection of urethral diverticula in women: Comparison of a high resolution fast spin echo technique with double balloon urethrography. J Urol 1998;159:408.

Nezu FM, Vasavada SP: Evaluation and management of female urethral diverticulum. Tech Urol 2001;7:169.

Pauwels M, Wyndaele JJ: Female urethral diverticula: A report of 5 cases. Acta Urol Belg 1996;64:27.

Presman D, Rolnick D, Zumerchek J: Calculus formation within a diverticulum of the female urethra. J Urol 1964;91:376.

Siegel CL et al: Sonography of the female urethra. AJR 1998; 170:1269.

Spence HM, Duckett JW Jr: Diverticulum of the female urethra: Clinical aspects and presentation of a simple operative technique for cure. J Urol 1970;104:432.

Spencer WF, Streem SB: Diverticulum of the female urethral roof managed endoscopically. J Urol 1987;138:147.

Summit RL Jr, Stovall TG: Urethral diverticula: Evaluation by urethral pressure profilometry, cystourethroscopy, and the voiding cystourethrogram. Obstet Gynecol 1992;80:695.

Vargas-Serrano B et al: Transrectal ultrasonography in the diagnosis of urethral diverticula in women. J Clin Ultrasound 1997;25:21.

Urethral Stricture

Essenhigh DM, Ardran GM, Cope V: A study of the bladder outlet in lower urinary tract infections in women. Br J Urol 1968;40:268.

Immergut MA, Gilbert EC: The clinical response of women to internal urethrotomy. J Urol 1973;109:90.

Surgical Repair

Bass JS, Leach GE: Surgical treatment of concomitant urethral diverticulum and stress incontinence. Urol Clin North Am 1991;18:365.

Hricak H et al: Female urethra: MR imaging. Radiology 1991; 178:527.

Steward M, Bretland PM, Stidolph NE: Urethral diverticula in the adult female. Br J Urol 1981;53:353.

Symmonds RE, Hill LM: Loss of the urethra: A report on 50 patients. Am J Obstet Gynecol 1978;53:130.

van Geelen JM et al: The clinical and urodynamic effects of anterior vaginal repair and Burch colposuspension. Am J Obstet Gynecol 1988;159:137.

Woodhouse CRJ et al: Urethral diverticulum in females. Br J Urol 1980;52:305.

Timothy G. Berger, MD

■ INFLAMMATORY DERMATOSES

The patient with skin disease of the external genitalia should be questioned about and examined for other possible areas of involvement. Scabies must always be considered in cases of genital pruritus. Patients, fearing genital infection, frequently overtreat genital lesions. Repeated scratching and rubbing tend to prolong and complicate genital conditions.

CONTACT DERMATITIS

Contact dermatitis includes both irritant dermatitis and allergic contact dermatitis. True allergic contact dermatitis is pruritic, erythematous, edematous, and weepy. Possible causes are feminine hygiene products, condoms, and plants (poison oak and ivy). Twice-daily cool water compresses followed immediately by the application of a mild, nonfluorinated topical steroid (1% hydrocortisone ointment or 1% Pramasone [hydrocortisone 1% plus pramoxine] ointment) is usually effective.

CIRCUMSCRIBED NEURODERMATITIS (Lichen Simplex Chronicus)

The labia majora and scrotum are predisposed to this chronic skin condition, caused by an itch-scratch cycle. Stress exacerbates the condition. The skin becomes thickened. The scratching may be subconscious and occur during sleep. The treatment is the same as that for contact dermatitis (described previously) plus stopping the scratching. The addition of pramoxine hydrochloride 1%, topical doxepin cream 5% (Zonalon) or EMLA (eutectic mixture local anesthetic—lidocaine 2.5% and prilocaine 2.5%) to topical steroid treatment may be of benefit. Intralesional injections of triamcinolone acetonide 5 mg/cc control refractory cases.

INTERTRIGO

Intertrigo describes the moist plaques that occur in areas of persistent maceration. It is often complicated by bacterial and yeast overgrowth. It occurs in the groin, abdominal skin folds, inframammary areas, and axillae, usually in obese individuals. It is more common in hot, humid weather. Simply allowing the occluded areas to be exposed to air may result in healing. Further treatment consists of twice-daily cool soaks with Burrow's solution 1:20, followed by application of nystatin ointment plus 1% hydrocortisone ointment (see Candidiasis, following).

DRUG ERUPTIONS

Most drug eruptions are widespread, but they may first appear in the groin. Fixed drug eruption, due usually to laxatives (phenolphthalein), sulfonamides, or nonsteroidal anti-inflammatory drugs (NSAIDs), commonly presents on the genitalia. These medications are available over-the-counter and are often taken only intermittently, so the association with the offending medication is often missed. Two percent of all genital ulcers are fixed drug eruptions. Lesions often begin within a day of drug exposure and present as bright red to violaceous macules that quickly blister and erode. The erosion is superficial and broad (usually > 1 cm). Fixed drug eruption occurs in the same site with each exposure to the drug. Treatment is to stop the offending medication.

PSORIASIS

Psoriasis may involve flexural surfaces (inverse psoriasis), such as the groin and the cleft of the buttocks. In moist surfaces the lesions of psoriasis are bright red and usually free of scale. Itching may be intense or nonexistent. A solitary plaque may present on the glans penis, leading to confusion with high-grade dysplasia (erythroplasia of Queyrat). The diagnosis usually can be made by inspection and by noting other areas of involvement such as the scalp, elbows, knees, and nails. Hydrocortisone cream, 1%, plus an imidazole cream (clotrimazole, 1%; miconazole, 2%; or ketoconazole, 2%) is usually efficacious. The condition is chronic and relapsing and often flares after intercourse due to the exposure of the psoriatic lesion to *Candida*. Washing the glans after intercourse is critical in controlling penile psoriasis. The skin lesions of Reiter's syndrome in the genitalia are identical to that of psoriasis and favor the glans penis (circinate balanitis). HIV infection–associated psoriasis and Reiter's syndrome frequently affect the genitalia.

SEBORRHEIC DERMATITIS

Seborrheic dermatitis of the groin and penis appears similar to psoriasis in these areas. Seborrhea favors hairy areas and usually involves the base of the penis, inner thighs, and pubic area. The treatment is identical to that of psoriasis in the groin.

LICHEN PLANUS

Lichen planus may affect the glans penis or the labia majora and minora and vaginal mucosa. The genitalia may be the only site of involvement. The lesions are polygonal, violet-hued, flat-topped papules about 0.5–1 cm in diameter, with milky striations over their shiny surfaces. Vaginal lesions are often erosive. Lesions may be asymptomatic, pruritic, or painful if eroded. Vulvar erosive disease often coexists with oral erosive disease (vulvovaginal-gingival syndrome). The condition may mimic lichen sclerosus completely, making clinical distinction impossible. A biopsy may be required. Superpotent topical corticosteroids and topical tacrolimus 0.1% ointment may be helpful in relieving symptoms and healing erosions. The disease may disappear after months to years.

LICHEN SCLEROSUS

Lichen sclerosus (LS) on the skin surface is characterized by flat-topped white papules that coalesce to form white patches without infiltration. Lesions evolve to marked atrophy, leaving the epithelium resembling very thin parchment paper. LS almost inevitably involves the anogenital regions, where severe pruritus or painful erosions may develop. LS of the glans penis (balanitis xerotica obliterans) may lead to phimosis and urethral stenosis. Squamous cell carcinoma of the genitalia may complicate LS, but prophylactic surgery of these genital lesions is not called for.

Superpotent topical steroids are the treatment of choice for all forms of genital LS, in children and adults. Initially treatment is twice daily, with gradual tapering to once daily, then several times weekly. An initial trial should be 6 weeks of treatment. Atrophy reverses despite the use of potent steroids on thin genital skin. Once the patient is in remission, milder steroids or bland emollients may be used for maintenance. Topical testosterone is not beneficial. Childhood LS may not improve during puberty or adulthood.

■ COMMON SUPERFICIAL INFECTIONS

ARTHROPODS

Pediculosis Pubis (Pubic Lice, Crabs)

Pediculosis pubis may be sexually or nonsexually transmitted. Itching may be intense, leading to scratching and pyoderma. The nits are found on the hair shafts in the pubic area and the eyelids. Treatment consists of application of lindane (gamma benzene hexachloride), 1% shampoo for 4 minutes. All hairy areas contiguous with the genital area, which may be a significant portion of the male body (chest, abdomen, legs, and axilla), should be treated. Permethrin crème rinse 1% for 10 minutes or 5% permethrin cream for 8 h are acceptable alternatives. The sexual partner(s) should also be examined and treated. All clothing, bedding, and towels should be washed and heat dried or dry cleaned. If lice are found 1 week later, the treatment should be repeated.

Scabies

Infestation with the human mite *Sarcoptes scabiei* usually causes a severely pruritic, widespread eruption. In males, very itchy papules or nodules with a central crust are common on the penile shaft or glans and on the scrotum and are virtually pathognomonic of scabies. These nodules may persist for weeks to months after treatment. In adults, scabies is a sexually transmitted disease. Treatment consists of overnight (8–12 h) application of 5% permethrin cream to the whole body from the neck down. The treatment may be repeated in 1 week. All members of the household and all sexual partners of the index case should be treated simultaneously. Lindane, 1% lotion, may be used similarly. All clothing, bedding, and towels should be washed and heat dried or dry cleaned. Potent topical steroids may be used to treat persistent genital nodules.

FUNGAL INFECTIONS (Tinea Cruris)

Tinea cruris is characterized by marginated, slightly elevated, peripherally scaling patches on the inner thighs and in the groin. Tinea cruris does not affect the scrotum and is less intense deep in the inguinal. This is in contrast to candidiasis, which characteristically affects the scrotum and is accentuated deep in the inguinal folds (the moistest area). Pruritus may be intense. Direct microscopic examination of skin scrapings in potassium hydroxide solution reveals hyphae.

Miconazole, clotrimazole, ketoconazole, econazole, ciclopirox olamine, terbinafine, or butenafine creams are all effective. All are applied twice daily except the last two, which are applied once daily. 1% hydrocortisone cream may be used concomitantly. In severe or refractory cases, oral antifungal treatment may be required. Griseofulvin ultramicronized (Grispeg), 250 mg twice daily for 4–6 weeks; itraconazole, 200 mg twice daily with food and an acid beverage for 7 days; or terbinafine, 250 mg once daily for 2–4 weeks, is usually adequate, even in the most severe cases.

CANDIDIASIS

Erythematous, weeping lesions with peripheral satellite vesiculopustules characterize infection with *Candida albicans.* Lesions occur most commonly on the inner thighs and buttocks, with a predilection for the depths of the creases. Scrotal involvement is common in candidiasis. Pregnancy, diabetes mellitus, obesity, broad-spectrum antibiotics, and immunosuppression are predisposing factors. The skin involvement may be secondary to vaginal infection. Lesions occur under the prepuce (candidal balanitis). High-power microscopic examination of skin scrapings in potassium hydroxide solution shows clusters of tiny spores and fine mycelial filaments. Nystatin ointment or cream is effective in most instances. Miconazole, clotrimazole, ketoconazole, and econazole applied twice daily are alternatives to nystatin but may cause burning on application. Nystatin can be applied to eroded areas. In severe cases in women, fluconazole tablets (100–200 mg) once daily for 1 week, followed by 150 mg once weekly, is often dramatically effective.

BACTERIAL INFECTIONS (Pyoderma)

Staphylococcus aureus is the most common cause of primary bacterial infections in the genital area. Culture may confirm the diagnosis. *S aureus* produces 2 types of primary lesions, a follicular pustule (folliculitis) and a superficial blister (impetigo).

Staphylococcal folliculitis begins as a superficial infection of the follicle but may extend deeply (furunculosis). It is usually acute but may be chronic or recurrent. Chronic folliculitis is usually due to nasal carriage of *Staphylococcus.* Deep, draining abscesses are rarely due to bacteria alone and suggest the presence of a chronic suppurative disorder, for example, inflammatory bowel disease, lymphogranuloma venereum, or hidradenitis suppurativa. Recurrent folliculitis in the groin is common in AIDS.

Topical treatment alone is often inadequate for bacterial folliculitis. A penicillinase-resistant penicillin (dicloxacillin) or first-generation cephalosporin is the treatment of choice. Penicillin-allergic individuals may be treated with doxycycline. Treatment is continued until all lesions are healed. Adding rifampin to the described treatment is recommended for frequent recurrences.

Staphylococcal impetigo starts as a very superficial blister that quickly breaks, leaving a crusted, weeping erosion. Treatment is the same as for staphylococcal folliculitis but usually of shorter duration.

VIRAL INFECTIONS
Genital Warts

External genital warts, caused by human papilloma viruses, are the most common sexually transmitted disease. One percent of all sexually active adults have genital warts, and up to 10% can be documented to have active human papilloma virus infection by sensitive techniques such as polymerase chain reaction. Elevated genital warts, condyloma acuminata, are due to low-risk human papilloma virus types (usually 6 and 11). They are most common on the vulva, under the prepuce, and on the penile shaft. The vaginal, anal, and oral mucosa may also be affected.

Since current treatments can eradicate only the clinical lesions (the warts) and not the infectious agent (the virus), recurrence is very common (> 25%). In addition, treating the sexual partners of infected persons has no effect on the outcome of the treatment in the index case. Warts may spontaneously resolve. It is no longer recommended to search for and treat "subclinical warts"—those seen with acetic acid soaking or identified by special immunologic techniques. The goal of treatment is to provide wart-free intervals with the least discomfort and long-term sequelae to the patient. In monogamous couples the option of no treatment should be discussed. Certain "high-risk" genital human papilloma virus types, usually 16 and 18, cause bowenoid papulosis, flat hyperpigmented papules on the genital skin. Bowenoid papulosis is a high-grade intraepithelial lesion and is associated with penile, vaginal, and cervical dysplasia. Regular gynecologic examination with Pap smears is mandatory. Bowenoid papulosis may be treated like external genital warts.

There are two basic forms of therapy: patient applied and health care worker applied. Patient-applied treatment is either podophyllotoxin or imiquimod. Podophyllotoxin is applied twice daily for 3 days per week for 6–10 weeks. About half of patients clear their warts with one course of therapy. It is less irritating and more effective than health care worker–applied podophyllum resin. It is contraindicated in pregnancy. Imiquimod is an immune modulator that results in the local production of interferon. It is applied once daily for 3 times per week (usually Monday, Wednesday, and Friday). The response rate is about 40% for men and over 75% for women. Treatment duration is prolonged, with average time to final response being over 2 months. Physician-applied treatments include liquid nitrogen cryotherapy (75% response, 50% durable remission) and electrocautery (100% response, 75% durable remission). Laser therapy and intralesional or systemic interferon are second-line treatments and are rarely indicated for external genital warts.

Molluscum Contagiosum

Molluscum contagiosum is a common cutaneous infection that is sexually transmitted in adults. The characteristic lesion is a smooth-surfaced, firm, pearly papule 2–5 mm in diameter with a central umbilication. Most infected persons have 5–15 lesions located on the lower abdomen, upper thighs, or skin of the genitalia. Extensive molluscum contagiosum outside the genital area in adults is rare except in immunosuppressed patients, especially those infected with HIV. Treatment involves local destruction of the lesions by cryotherapy or electrodesiccation.

Herpes Simplex

Genital herpes simplex virus (HSV) is usually caused by HSV 2, but, increasingly, HSV 1 genital herpes due to orogenital sex has been reported. Most infections cause no symptoms initially. Viral culture or Tzanck smear will confirm the diagnosis. First-episode genital HSV is treated with acyclovir (200 mg) 5 times daily, valacyclovir (500 mg) twice daily, or famciclovir (250 mg) twice daily, for 7–10 days.

Recurrent disease is frequent, often preceded by tingling at the soon-to-be-affected site (the prodrome). It is virtually always caused by HSV 2. It presents as grouped blisters localized to 1 site and lasting about 1 week. Most patients do not require treatment if the outbreaks are mild. For individual outbreaks, acyclovir (200 mg) 5 times daily, valacyclovir (500 mg) twice daily, or famciclovir (125 mg) twice daily for 3 days only may be used to shorten the duration and severity of the eruption. For frequent recurrences (> 6–12 per year), suppression may be better than intermittent treatment. Acyclovir (400 mg) twice daily (or 800 mg once daily), valacyclovir (500 mg–1 g) once daily, or famciclovir (250 mg) twice daily may be used. Suppressive treatment will reduce outbreaks by 85% and reduce the amount of virus shed by 95%. It is not clear if this reduces transmission.

Herpes simplex is the most common cause of persistent genital ulceration in immunosuppressed patients. In severe cases, intravenous acyclovir may be required. Acyclovir resistance can occur in the setting of immunosuppression and is treated with foscarnet.

REFERENCES

General

Odom RB et al: *Andrew's Diseases of the Skin,* 9th ed. Saunders, 2000.

Inflammatory Dermatoses

Meffert JJ et al: Lichen sclerosus. J Am Acad Dermatol 1995;32:393.

Common Superficial Infections

Bertner KR et al: Genital warts and their treatment. Clin Inf Dis 1999;28:537.

Lesher JL Jr: Oral therapy of common superficial fungal infections. J Am Acad Dermatol 1999;40:531.

Sacks SL: Improving the management of genital herpes. Hospital Practice 1999;34:41.

Abnormalities of Sexual Determination & Differentiation

41

Laurence S. Baskin, MD

Sexuality is defined as the constitution of an individual in relation to sexual attitudes or activity. What defines our sexuality is a complex interaction between our genetic makeup, environmental stimulus, and cultural influences. The origins of our sexuality occur at the time of conception when the genetic material from 2 sources of the opposite sex coalesces into a new individual. From that moment, sexual differentiation occurs by a highly organized process. Sex chromosomes and autosomes dictate the development of gonads; the gonads in turn produce hormones, which then direct the development of the internal and external genitalia. Disorders of sexual differentiation arise from abnormalities in chromosomes, gonadal development, or hormonal production/activity.

Patients with disorders of sexual differentiation may present (1) during the newborn period as having ambiguous genitalia, (2) as having inappropriate pubertal development, (3) as having delayed pubertal development, or (4) later in life as having infertility.

NORMAL SEXUAL DIFFERENTIATION

Chromosomal Sex

The genetic material necessary for the development of the male phenotype is normally located on the short arm of the Y chromosome. The critical gene or sex-determining region on the Y chromosome is known as the SRY region. The gene products of the SRY genetic cascade will subsequently direct the development of the testis by interacting with multiple other genes such as SOX-9. Genetic information that is necessary for male and female development beyond gonadal differentiation is located on the X chromosome and on the autosomes.

Gonadal Differentiation

The gonads develop from the urogenital ridges (Figure 41–1), which are formed during the fourth week of gestation by the proliferation of the coelomic epithelium and condensation of the underlying mesenchyme along the mesonephros. The germ cells, located in the endoderm of the yolk sac, migrate to the genital ridges. At the early stage of development the gonad is bipotential, capable of forming into either a testis or an ovary. During the sixth to seventh week of gestation, at least 4 different genes (Wilms tumor suppressor gene (WT-1), Fushi-Tarza Factor-1 (FTZ-F1), steroidogenic factor-1 (SF-1), and LIM-1) induce the development of the testis. The primordial germ cells differentiate into the Sertoli cells and associated Leydig cells, which aggregate into spermatogenic cords. Loose mesenchymal tissue condenses into a thick layer, the tunica albuginea, which surrounds the testis and separates its connection with the coelomic epithelium, thereby preventing further migration of mesonephric cells into the testis.

Classic teaching is that the female phenotype is the default developmental pathway in the absence of the SRY cascade. It is now known that at least one gene, dosage-sensitive sex reversal (DAX-1), is essential for ovarian development. DAX-1 is located on the short arm of the X chromosome. The gene products of SRY and DAX-1 competitively compete to stimulate the steroidogenic acute regulatory protein (StAR). The StAR protein is the first step in steroidogenesis, facilitating the conversion of cholesterol to pregnenolone. In the normal XY male, SRY overwhelms the one functional DAX-1 gene, stimulating testicular development and subsequent testosterone production. In the normal XX female, 2 DAX-1 genes are present without the competitive SRY, downregulating StAR, hence inhibiting testicular development, which results in ovarian development. In the fetal ovaries, the germ cells differentiate and are arrested in the last phase of meiotic prophase, forming the oocytes. The cells in the genital ridges develop into granulosa cells, which surround the oocytes and complete the formation of the ovaries.

Hormones

At 3.5 weeks' gestation, the wolffian system appears as 2 longitudinal ducts connecting cranially to the mesonephros and caudally draining into the urogenital sinus (Figure 41–2). At approximately the sixth week of gestation, the müllerian duct develops as an evagination in the coelomic epithelium just lateral to the wolffian duct.

Figure 41–1. Sex-determining genes involved in testes and ovarian development.

During the eighth to ninth week of gestation, Sertoli cells of the fetal testis secrete a glycoprotein, müllerian inhibiting substance (MIS), or anti-müllerian hormone. This protein induces the regression of the müllerian ducts through the dissolution of the basement membrane and condensation of mesenchymal cells around the müllerian duct. Because MIS acts locally, müllerian duct regression occurs only on the ipsilateral side of the fetal testis producing this hormone. MIS also induces the formation of seminiferous tubules and further differentiation of the testis. At the ninth or 10th week of gestation, the Leydig cells appear in the testis and begin to synthesize testosterone. This hormone transforms the wolffian duct into the male genital tract, which is completed by the end of the 11th week of gestation.

Beginning in the ninth week of gestation, testosterone also induces the development of the external genitalia (Figure 41–3) from the genital tubercle, urogenital sinus, and genital swellings. At the molecular level testosterone is converted to 5α-dihydrotestosterone (DHT) by the microsomal enzyme, type 2 5α-reductase, for complete differentiation of the penis with a male-type urethra and glans. Testosterone dissociates from its carrier proteins in the plasma and enters cells via passive diffusion. Once in the cell, testosterone binds to the androgen receptor (AR) and induces changes in conformation, protecting it from degradation by proteolytic enzymes. This conformational change is also required for AR dimerization, DNA binding, and transcriptional activation, all necessary for testosterone to be expressed.

Androgen binding also displaces heat shock proteins, possibly relieving constraints on receptor dimerization or DNA binding. After entering the nucleus, the AR complex then binds androgen response element DNA regulatory sequences within the androgen responsive genes and activates them. DHT also binds the AR, with enhanced androgenic activity, in part because of its slow dissociation rate from the AR.

DHT then binds to nuclear receptors, forming a complex that regulates the transformation of these tissues into the glans penis, penile and cavernous urethra, Cowper's glands, prostate, and scrotum. Between the 28th and 37th week of gestation, testicular descent into the scrotum begins. While the mechanism of this process is not completely understood, it is clearly androgen-dependent.

Development of the Female Genitalia

The female internal genitalia develop from the müllerian ducts. Without the hormones produced by the testis, the wolffian ducts regress at the ninth week of gestation. At the same time, the müllerian ducts begin to differentiate; the cranial portions form the fallopian tubes, while the caudal portions fuse to form the uterus, cervix, and the upper portion of the vagina. Concurrently, the external genitalia defined as the lower portion of the vagina, the vestibule, Bartholin and Skene glans, the clitoris, and labia minora and majora develop from the urogenital sinus and genital tubercles. Like the testis, the ovary undergoes a partial transabdominal descent. However, transinguinal descent of the ovary does not occur, leaving the ovaries just below the rim of the true pelvis. The role of estrogen in the differentiation of the female phenotype is unclear.

Development of the Male External Genitalia

Formation of the external male genitalia is a complex developmental process involving the SRY genetic programming, cell differentiation, hormonal signaling, enzyme activity, and tissue remodeling. By the end of the first month of gestation, the hindgut and future urogenital system reach the ventral surface of the embryo at the cloacal membrane. The urorectal septum divides the cloacal membrane into a posterior, or anal, half and an anterior half, the urogenital membrane. Three protuberances appear around the latter. The most cephalad is the genital tubercle. The other two, the genital swellings, flank the urogenital membrane on each side. Up to this point, the male and female genitalia are essentially indistinguishable. Under the influence of testosterone in response to a surge of luteinizing hor-

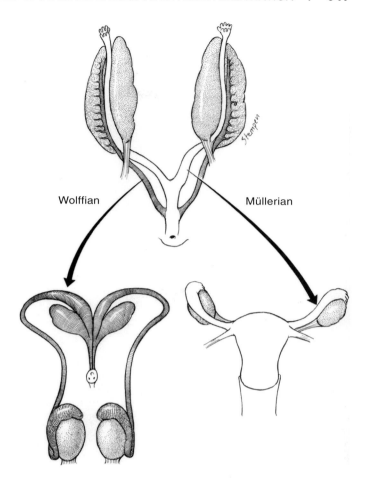

Figure 41–2. Schematic of male (wolffian) and female (müllerian) internal and external genital development from a common origin.

mone from the pituitary, masculinization of the external genitalia takes place. One of the first signs of masculinization is an increase in the distance between the anus and the genital structures, followed by elongation of the phallus, formation of the penile urethra from the urethral groove, and development of the prepuce.

At 8 weeks' gestation, the external genitalia remain in the indifferent stage. The urethral groove on the ventral surface of the phallus is between the paired urethral folds. The penile urethra forms as a result of fusion of the medial edges of the endodermal urethral folds. As development progresses, the ectodermal edges of the urethral groove begin to fuse to form the median raphe (Figure 41–4A). By 11–12 weeks the coronal sulcus separates the glans from the shaft of the penis. By 16 weeks' gestation the urethral folds have completely fused in the midline on the ventrum of the penile shaft (Figure 41–4B). Note the normal ventral penile curva-

ture, or chordee, that occurs during development and resolves by the 20th week (Figure 41–4C).

The glandular urethra, which consists of a squamous epithelial-lined tube different from the urothelial-lined anterior urethra, also completes formation during this period. The mechanism of the glandular urethral formation remains controversial. Evidence suggests 2 possible explanations (Figure 41–5): (1) endodermal cellular differentiation where the glandular urethra forms by an extension of urogenital sinus epithelium that undergoes transdifferentiation versus (2) primary intrusion of the ectodermal tissue from the skin of the glans penis. Cross-sectional histologic analysis at 24 weeks' gestation reveals complete penile development (Figure 41–6A–H). Note the extensive neuronal innervation just above the tunica of the corporeal bodies. Three-dimensional reconstruction of the fetal male penis illustrates the extensive neuronal distribution (Figure

MALE DEVELOPMENT

FEMALE DEVELOPMENT

Figure 41–3. Differentiation of the male and female external genitalia from the indifferent stage to full differentiation (8–16 weeks). Illustrations by Dr Hiep Nguyen.

41–7). Note the nerve density in the glans (Figure 41–7E and F).

Anatomical and immunohistochemical studies advocate the new theory of endodermal differentiation, which shows that epithelium of the entire urethra is of urogenital sinus origin. The entire male urethra, including the glandular urethra, is formed by dorsal growth of the urethral plate into the genital tubercle and ventral growth and fusion of the urethral folds. Under proper mesenchymal induction, urothelium has the ability to differentiate into a stratified squamous phenotype with characteristic keratin staining, thereby explaining the cell type of the glans penis. There is no

evidence of an ectodermal ingrowth or a solid ectodermal cord filling the glans, as was historically proposed (old theory).

The future prepuce is forming at the same time as the urethra and is dependent on normal urethral development. At about 8 weeks' gestation, low preputial folds appear on both sides of the penile shaft, which join dorsally to form a flat ridge at the proximal edge of the corona. The ridge does not entirely encircle the glans because it is blocked on the ventrum by incomplete development of the glandular urethra. Thus, the preputial fold is transported distally by active growth of the mesenchyme between it and the glandular lamella.

Figure 41–4. Male human fetal external genitalia during gestation. **A:** 11 weeks. Note the urethra is open and urethral fold (uf) and groove are prominent in the transillumination view of the phallus. **B:** At 16.5 weeks. Note the normal ventral curvature (vc) is shown as well as the foreskin, which is almost completely formed. **C:** At 20 weeks' gestation, penile and urethral development looks complete, with the prepuce covering the glans and the penile curvature resolving. **D:** At 24 weeks the prepuce covers the whole glans. Note the midline seam (ms). Note the progression of natural curvature to a straight phallus during development.

The process continues until the preputial fold (foreskin) covers all of the glans, forming a midline seam (Figure 41–4D). The fusion is usually present at birth, but subsequent desquamation of the epithelial fusion allows the prepuce to retract. If the genital folds fail to fuse, the preputial tissues do not form ventrally; consequently, in hypospadias, preputial tissue is absent on the ventrum, and excessive dorsally.

DISORDERS OF SEXUAL DIFFERENTIATION

Disorders of abnormal sexual differentiation may be divided into the three categories.

Disorders of Chromosomal Sex

These result from abnormalities in the number or structure of the sex chromosomes. These abnormalities may arise from nondisjunction, deletion, breakage, rearrangement, and translocation of genetic material on these chromosomes. These disorders are summarized in Table 41–1.

Disorders of Gonadal Sex

These result from abnormalities in gonadal development. In these disorders, the karyotype is normal (ie, 46XX or 46XY). However, mutations in the sex chromosomes or autosomes, teratogens, or trauma to the gonads interferes with their normal development. These disorders are summarized in Table 41–2.

Disorders of Phenotypic Sex

These result from abnormalities in hormonal production or activity. The etiologies include defective synthesis by the gonads, abnormal production by the adrenal glands, presence of exogenous sources, or abnormalities in receptor activity. These disorders are summarized in Table 41–3.

CLINICAL EVALUATION OF PATIENTS WITH AMBIGUOUS GENITALIA

The accurate diagnosis of a patient with ambiguous genitalia is a challenging process. Based on the diagnosis, decisions will be made for gender assignment, which will have a great impact not only on the patient but also on the patient's family. In most societies the accepted norm is 2 sexes, either male or female. When a new baby arrives and the proclamation as to whether it's a boy or a girl cannot be made immediately, an anticipated celebration turns into a stressful family dilemma. With prenatal amniocentesis and routine ultrasound, sex determination is often known well before

Ectodermal ingrowth theory

Ectodermal differentiation theory

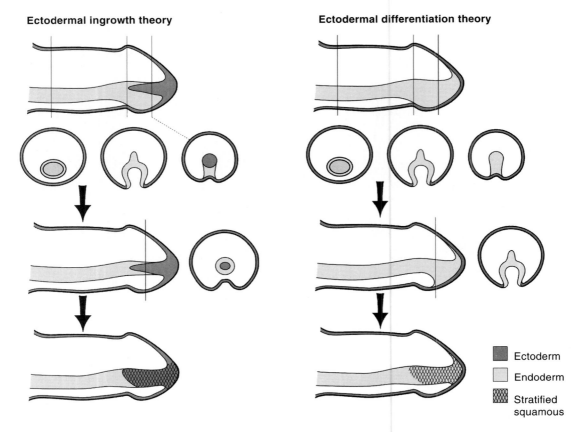

Ectoderm

Endoderm

Stratified squamous

Figure 41–5. Theories of human penile urethral development. The ectodermal ingrowth theory as described in most textbooks of embryology postulates that the glandular urethra is formed by ingrowth of epidermis. More recent data support the formation of the entire urethra via endodermal differentiation alone.

birth. This can compound the emotional trauma when the known and anticipated genotype does not match the newborn's phenotype. Furthermore, in cases such as severe salt-wasting congenital adrenal hyperplasia, accurate diagnosis is lifesaving.

History

A detailed history is of great importance. Since many of the disorders such as XX male syndrome and true hermaphrodites are hereditary, a family history should carefully be examined for similarly affected individuals, unexplained death during infancy, infertility, amenorrhea, and hirsutism. Furthermore, drugs ingested during pregnancy (such as progesterone) and virilizing signs in the mother during pregnancy should be ascertained.

Physical Examination

The abdomen and rectum should be carefully palpated for midline structures such as a uterus. These examinations will provide information regarding the presence of müllerian duct derivatives. Other helpful physical findings include dehydration, failure to thrive, pigmentation (in patients with salt-wasting congenital adrenal hyperplasia), and the presence of other associated anomalies such as cardiac murmurs or web neck (in patients with Turner or Klinefelter syndrome).

It is important to palpate for gonads in the labioscrotal fold or the scrotum. Since ovaries do not descend, it is likely to be a testis and hence unlikely to represent a case of female pseudohermaphroditism. Based on the presence or absence of gonads, an algorithm can be followed to determine the differential di-

Figure 41–6. Normal human fetal penis, 24 weeks. Transverse histologic sections show immunohistochemical localization with the neuronal marker S-100 (25×). Note localization of S-100 nerve marker (dark staining) completely surrounding the cavernous bodies up to the junction with the urethral spongiosum along the penile shaft except at the 12 o'clock position (**A–D**). On the proximal penis at the point where the corporeal bodies split into two (**E**) and continue in a lateral fashion inferior and adjacent to the pubic rami, the nerves localize to an imaginary triangular area at the 11 o'clock and 1 o'clock positions. At this point (**E**) the nerves reach their furthest vertical distance from the corporeal body (~ one-half the diameter of the corporeal body) and continue (**F–H**) in a tighter formation at the 11 o'clock and 1 o'clock positions well away from the urethra.

agnosis of patients with ambiguous genitalia (Figure 41–8). It is important to look at the size of phallus (Table 41–4) and the location of the urethral meatus. Any patients with bilateral cryptorchidism or with unilateral cryptorchidism with hypospadias should be suspected of having abnormalities in sexual differentiation. As noted, other helpful physical findings include hyperpigmentation of the areola and labioscrotal fold, common in patients with congenital adrenal hyperplasia.

Chromosomal Evaluation

Examination of buccal mucosal cells for Barr body (inactivated second X chromosome) provides a rapid

method of determining chromosomal sex. In normal females, the Barr body is found in greater than 20% of the cells while in males it is found in less than 2% of cells. However, this test has high false-positive and false-negative rates and cannot be relied on to make an accurate diagnosis in patients with ambiguous genitalia.

A more accurate but more time-consuming method (2–3 days) is the direct assessment of chromosomes from cultured peripheral blood leukocytes. This method provides the exact chromosomal complements, presence of mosaicism, and structural features of the chromosomes. In the case of mosaicism, several different tissue samples may be required to accurately determine the presence of mosaicism.

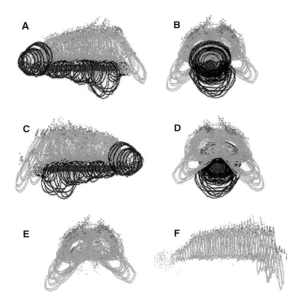

Figure 41–7. Normal human fetal penis, 45 weeks' gestation. Four views of a computer-generated three-dimensional reconstruction (**A**, side; **B**, front; **C**, side; **D**, back; **E**, front (without urethra); **F**, side (without urethra). Note the nerves along the outside of the tunica of the corporeal bodies and their absence at the 12 o'clock position. Note the impressive glandular innervation in **E** and **F**.

Biochemical Evaluation

In the case of congenital adrenal hyperplasia, the specific enzyme defect can be determined based on the presence or absence and the type of steroid excreted in the urine. Figure 41–9 depicts the steroid synthesis pathway from cholesterol to aldosterone, steroids, or dihydrotestosterone. Note the enzymes necessary for conversion from precursors to products (also see Table 41–3).

In other disorders caused by hormonal abnormalities (such as 5α-reductase deficiency and androgen resistance), direct measurement of plasma testosterone is often not helpful, since abnormalities in testosterone levels in these pathologic states have not been consistently characterized. A more useful test is the testosterone response following stimulation by hCG (2000 IU per day for 4 days). If plasma testosterone levels rise more than 2 ng/mL from baseline, the abnormality is consistent with androgen resistance rather than a defect in testosterone synthesis. In addition, this test is also used to diagnose 5α-reductase type 2 deficiency. A post-hCG stimulation ratio of testosterone to DHT greater than 30 establishes this diagnosis.

Radiographic Evaluation

In patients with intersex disorders, ultrasonography provides the least invasive and safest means of imaging the abdomen and pelvis. Identification of müllerian-derived structures such as the uterus and fallopian tubes will be important in determining the diagnosis (Figure 41–10A). The adrenal glands can also be examined for enlargement. While this finding is not diagnostic for CAH, it is suggestive and can direct further evaluation. Magnetic resonance imaging can provide a more detailed examination of the abdomen for internal genital structures. However, in most cases, anesthesia is needed for a good-quality magnetic resonance imaging examination. Injecting radiographic contrast material through the opening in the urogenital sinus is helpful in delineating the internal duct structures. It is most useful in assessing the presence of vagina, cervix, fallopian tube, utricle, and the connection with the urethra (Figure 41–10B and C). Genitography will also provide needed anatomical information for future reconstructive surgery.

Diagnostic Laparotomy or Laparoscopy

Occasionally, surgery is needed to delineate the internal genitalia and obtain a biopsy specimen of the gonads. It is indicated in patients in whom the biopsy result will influence sex assignment. In addition, surgery may be needed to remove streak or dysgenetic gonads in patients who are at risk for cancer (incomplete testicular feminization, Turner Y variant, and mixed gonadal dysgenesis). Laparoscopic surgery has provided an alternative to open surgery in patients with intersex disorders. It can be performed safely in newborns and only requires 1–3 3-mm incisions for placement of the laparoscopic ports. Simple surgical procedures such as hernia repair, orchidopexy, and resection of discordant organs can readily be performed laparoscopically. More complex procedures may require 5-mm ports and instruments.

Sex Assignment

In the past the baby born with ambiguous genitalia was considered incomplete until either a male or female sex was assigned. Unfortunately, a prompt but inappropriate assignment, although timely and comforting for family, physicians, nurses and staff, can lead to more complex problems in the future. The issue of sexual determination remains complex. We reaffirm the teaching of our mentors by advocating an immediate attempt to make a definitive and accurate diagnosis. Fortunately, for most patients with ambiguous genitalia (ie, congenital adrenal hyperplasia) this can be accomplished. In patients where ambiguity remains after initial testing

Table 41–1. Disorders of Chromosomal Sex.

Disorder	Pathology	Chromosomes	Incidence	Gonads	Internal Genitalia	External Genitalia	Other Features	Risk of Cancer	Treatment
Klinefelter syndrome	Extra X chromosome	47 XXY 46 XY/47XXY	1 in 500	Hyalinized testis No spermato-genesis	Wolffian	Male	Gynecomastia Tall stature Mild mental retardation Elevated FSH/LH Low testosterone Elevated estradiol Infertility	Breast Extragonadal germ cell	Supplemental androgens Surgery to severe gynecomastia
XX male	No Y chromo-some Usually TDF (+)	46 XX	1 in 20,000 to 24,000	Hyalinized testis No spermato-genesis	Wolffian	Male	Gynecomastia Short stature Inc. incidence of hypospadias Normal mental status May be familial	Rare germ cell	Same as Klinefelter
Turner syndrome	Absence of X chromosome	45 X 46 XX/45 X Some contain Y chrom. elements	1 in 2700	Streak gonads No germ cells	Müllerian	Immature female	Short stature Little breast development Web neck and other somatic abn. Cardiovascular abn. (ie, coarctation) Renal abn. (Horseshoe or malrotation) Autoimmune dz. (hypothyroid, diabetes) Infertility Amenorrhea	Germ cell in Y-chrom mosaic	Supplemental estrogen Removal of streak gonads in Y-chrom. mosaic

(continued)

Table 41–1. Disorders of Chromosomal Sex. (continued)

Disorder	Pathology	Chromosomes	Incidence	Gonads	Internal Genitalia	External Genitalia	Other Features	Risk of Cancer	Treatment
Mixed gonadal dysgenesis	Incompl. virilization & müllerian regression	45 X/46 XY (70%) Undetected mosaic		One testis (usually undescended) and streak gonad	Wolffian and Müllerian	Usually ambiguous 60% reared as female	Somatic features like 45 X	Germ cell	Female —Prophylatic gonadectomy Male —Streak gonads removed —intra-abd. testis excised unless can be relocated and no ipsilateral müllerian structure present
True hermaphrodite	Unknown	46 XX (70%) 46 XY (10%) Mosaic	Unknown	Bilateral ovitestis (20%) Ovitestis & ovary or testis (40%) One overy & testis (40%)	Wolffian and müllerian	Usually ambiguous 70% reared as male	Gynecomastia at puberty Menstruation at puberty May be familial	Rare germ cell	Reconstructuve surgery Poss. remove gonads

Table 41–2. Disorders of Gonadal Sex.

Disorder	Pathology	Chromosomes	Incidence	Gonads	Internal Genitalia	External Genitalia	Other Features	Risk of Cancer	Treatment
Pure gonadal dysgenesis	Unknown mutation prevents nl. differentiation of gonads	46 XX 46 XY	1 in 8000	Bilateral streak gonads	Müllerian	Immature female	Normal to tall stature Minimal somatic abn. Female: estrogen def. Male: testosterone def. May be familial	Germ cell in 46 XY	Estrogen supplement Remove gonads in 46 XY
Absent testes syndrome	Mutation, teratogen or trauma to testis	46 XY	Unknown	Absent/rudiment testis No streak gonads	Wolffian	Var. virilization	Normal	Usually none	Female: —Estrogen supplement —Reconstructive surgery Male: —Androgen supplement

649

Table 41–3. Disorders of Phenotypic Sex.

Disorder	Pathology	Chromosomes	Incidence	Gonads	Internal Genitalia
3 β-Hydroxysteroid dehydrogenase def.	Excess androgens	46 XX	Second most common of CAH	Ovary	Müllerian
11 β-hydroxylase def.	Excess androgens	46 XX	Rare	Ovary	Müllerian
21 α-hydroxylase def. —Partial	Excess androgens	46 XX	1 in 5000 to 15,000	Ovary	Müllerian
—Severe	Excess androgens	46 XX		Ovary	Müllerian
Excess maternal androgens	Excess androgens	46 XX		Ovary	Müllerian
20,22 Desmolase def.	Defect in testosterone synthesis	46 XY		Testis	Wolffian
3 β-hydroxysteroid dehydrogenase def.	Defect in testosterone synthesis	46 XY	Second most common in CAH	Testis	Wolffian
17 α-hydroxylase def.	Defect in testosterone synthesis	46 XY		Testis	Wolffian
17,20 Desmolase def.	Defect in testosterone synthesis	46 XY	Rare	Testis	Wolffian
17 β-hydroxysteroid dehydrogenase def.	Defect in testosterone synthesis	46 XY	Most common	Testis	Wolffian
5 α-reductase def.	Defect in androgen action	46 XY —Autosomal rec.		Testis with spermato- genesis	Wolffian
Complete testicular feminization	Androgen receptor defect	46 XY —X linked	1 in 20,000 to 64,000	Testis not fertile	Absent
Incomplete testicular feminization	Androgen receptor defect	46 XY —X linked rec.	1/10th of complete	Testis not fertile	Wolffian
Relfenstein syndrome	Androgen receptor defect	46 XY —X linked rec.		Testis not fertile	Wolffian
Infertile male syndrome	Androgen receptor defect	46 XY —X linked rec.		Testis not fertile	Wolffian
				Testis not fertile	Wolffian
Receptor + resistance	Androgen receptor defect	Unknown		Testis not fertile	Wolffian
Persistant müllerian duct	Persistent müllerian duct syndrome	Unknown		Testis	Wolffian with rudimentary uterus and tubes

External Genitalia	Other Features	Urinary Steroids	Risk of Cancer	Treatment
Mild ambiguous	Severe salt wasting No cortisol No aldosterone	DEAS	None	Replacement mineralocorticoids and glucocorticoids Reconstruction as needed
Ambiguous	Hypertension Dec. cortisol Dec. aldosterone	11 DCS 11 DOC	None	Replacement glucocorticoids
Ambiguous	Normal cortisol Inc. aldosterone	17 OH-P	None	Reconstruction as needed
Ambiguous	Severe salt wasting Dec. cortisol Dec. aldosterone	17 OH-P	None	Replacement mineralocorticoids and glucocorticoids Reconstruction as needed
Ambiguous	Drugs such as progestational agents Virilizing ovarian Adrenal tumors	None	None	None
Ambiguous	Severe salt wasting No cortisol No aldosterone	None	None	Replacement mineralcocorticoids and glucocorticoids
Ambiguous	Severe salt wasting No cortisol No aldosterone	DEAS	None	Replacement mineralcocorticoids and glucocorticoids Reconstruction as needed
Ambiguous	Hypokalemic alkalosis Hypertension Dec. cortisol Dec. aldosterone Gynecomastia	CS 11 DCS	None	Replacement glucocorticoids
Ambiguous	Normal cortisol and aldosterone		None	Supplemental testosterone
Ambiguous	Virilization at puberty	ASD	None	Decision reared as female or male
Female	No gynecomastia nl testosterone nl. virilization	None	None	None
Female reared as female	Inc. testosterone Inc. estrogen	None	Germ cells	Remove gonads after puberty Estrogen replacement
Female	Inc. testosterone Inc. estrogen	None	Germ cells	Remove gonads prior to puberty Estrogen replacement
Hypospadias male	Gynecomastia Inc. testosterone Inc. estrogen	None	None	Reconstruction as needed
Male	Infertility	None	None	None
Ambiguous	Nl. or inc. testosterone Nl. or inc. estrogen	None	None	None
Male usually cryptorchid	Nl. or inc. testosterone Nl. or inc. estrogen Nl. testosterone Nl. estrogen	None	None	Orchipexy Leave uterus and tubes

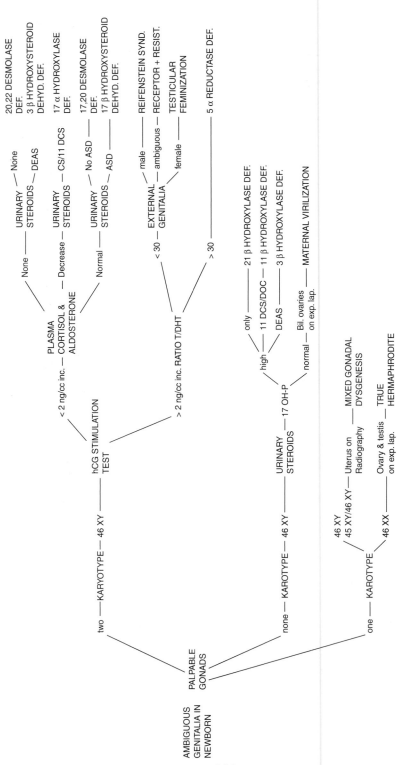

Figure 41–8. Clinical approach to intersex. Algorithm based on palpating gonads. bil., bilateral; def., deficiency; dehyd., dehydration; exp. lap., experimental laparoscopy; resist, resistance; synd., syndrome; T/DHT, testosterone/dihydrotestosterone.

Table 41–4. Normal values for stretched penile length.

Age	Length (cm) (Mean ± SD)
Premature 30 wk	2.5 ± 0.4
Full-term newborn	3.5 ± 0.4
0–5 months	3.9 ± 0.8
6–12 months	4.3 ± 0.8
1–2 y	4.7 ± 0.8
2–3 y	5.1 ± 0.9
3–4 y	5.5 ± 0.9
5–6 y	6.0 ± 0.9
10–11 y	6.4 ± 1.1
Adult	12.4 ± 2.7

and the diagnosis cannot be made, or when the diagnosis is clear but sex assignment remains difficult, we would now advocate for a more cautious approach. Foremost, this would include a reversible or nonbinding sex assignment. Experience has shown that the patients themselves will reassign their sex. For example, in cases of cloacal exstrophy or iatrogenic penile injuries, past treatment was based on the absence of an "adequate" phallic structure. These patients were converted

from genetic males to females with surgical orchiectomy, removal of any excess male genitalia, vaginoplasty, and future hormonal treatment for breast development. Although surgical results can be anatomically successful, these women will not menstruate or have fertility potential, and their sexual function is not known. As many of these patients went through adolescence, they identified with their genetic sex and demanded or reassigned their sex from female to male. In cases where the genotype does not match the phenotype, it is clear that surgical reconstruction from male to female does not guarantee a successful sexual identity.

The clinical experience exemplifies the complexity of sexual determination. It is clear that social factors, or the "nurturing" hypothesis, and biologic factors, or the "genetic" hypothesis, both play a role in determining our sexual identity. The nurturing hypothesis is based on the parent's perception of their child's genitalia. This perception will influence interactions such as naming, clothes, play orientation, and social organization. Clearly, how a parent perceives his or her child and the type of environment used to raise the baby is critical to the child's identity.

In contrast, the genetic hypothesis states that sexual identity is predetermined by the genetic makeup. Increasing laboratory evidence is accumulating to support

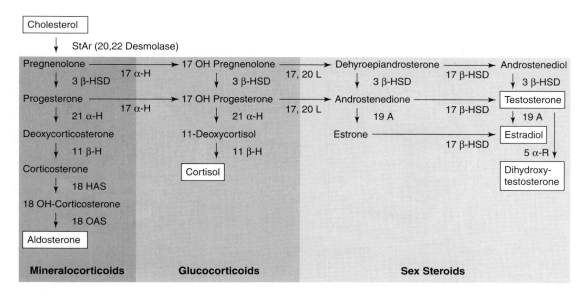

Figure 41–9. Pathway of steroid hormone biosynthesis and possible enzyme deficiencies. 3β-HSD, 3β-hydroxysteroid dehydrogenase; 21α-H, 21α-hydroxylase; 11β-H, 11β hydroxylase; 17β-HSD, 17β-hydroxysteroid dehydrogenase; 18 HAS, 18 hydroxy-aldosterone synthetase; 18 OAS, 18 oxidase-aldosterone synthetase; 5α-R, 5α reductase; 19A, 19 aromatase; StAR, steroidogenic acute regulatory protein.

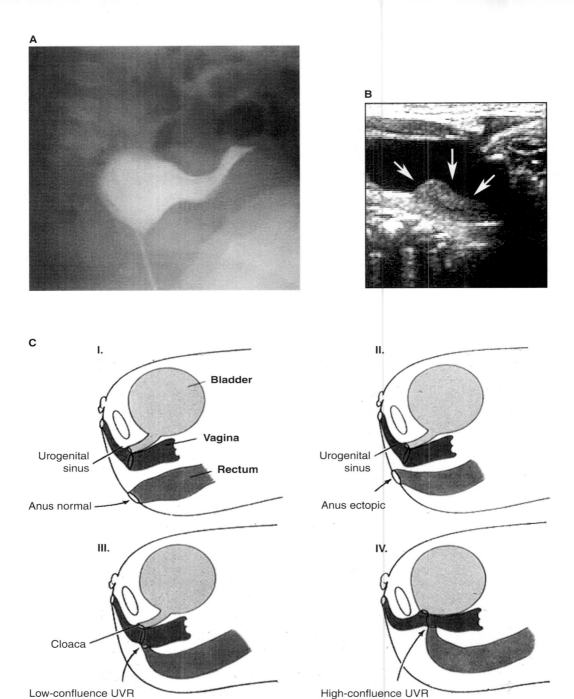

Figure 41–10. **A:** Newborn sonogram revealing a uterus behind the bladder in a patient with congenital adrenal hyperplasia. Note the endometrial streak within the uterus. **B:** Genitogram showing the uterus and left fallopian tube (arrows). **C:** Schematic of possible genitogram findings: I. and II. Urogenital sinus anomalies note 2 openings on the perineum (common urogenital sinus and rectum). III. and IV. Cloacal anomalies with 1 perineal opening. Note the low and high confluence of the urethra, vagina, and rectum (UVR). (Modified with permission from Dr Hardy Hendron.) Genitogram showing the common urogenital sinus.

the genetic hypothesis. For example, animal experimentation supports the concept of steroid or androgen imprinting of the brain. The human evidence supporting masculinization of the brain is supported by (1) iatrogenic penile ablation in males raised as females, and (2) males with 5α-reductase deficiency who were raised as females. The common theme in these patients is the high level of in utero exposure to androgens theoretically masculinizing the brain and inferring a male identity. Another example of hormonal influence on sexual orientation can be found in women exposed to diethylstilbestrol. Human retrospective studies looking at these women reveal an increase in bisexual and homosexual orientation.

The process of sexual identity in both humans and experimental animals is not an all-or-none process, meaning that male and female characteristics exist as a continuum. For example, although the garbage removal, plumbing, and TV-channel-flipping gene seems to exist almost exclusively on the Y chromosome, these traits may also be found in the female sex.

Two issues must be separated when evaluating patients with intersex or ambiguous genitalia: (1) gender identity (Is the person's sense of identity male or a female?) and (2) sexual orientation. The incidence of discordant gender identity is approximately 1 in 30,000 males and 1 in 100,000 females. The incidence of same-sex orientation in both males and females is estimated to be approximately 5% of the population.

Practical Approach to the Diagnosis of Intersex

In the newborn period, patients with ambiguous genitalia can be approached in a logical fashion (Figure 41–11). As noted above, history, physical examination, laboratory evaluation, and radiographic and in some cases surgical exploration are necessary to make an accurate diagnosis. Once the karyotype is known, along with the gonadal status, an appropriate test can lead to a diagnosis (Figure 41–11 and Table 41–5). Patients may also present at puberty (inappropriate or delayed development) with sexual differentiation abnormalities or later in life with infertility. The differential diagnosis for these disorders is diagrammed in Figure 41–12.

TREATMENT OF SPECIFIC DISORDERS

Female Pseudohermaphrodites

Female pseudohermaphrodites are characterized by a 46 XX genotype, nonpalpable gonads or normal ovaries, and variable degrees of virilization of the external genitalia.

A. Congenital Adrenal Hyperplasia (CAH)

CAH is the most common cause of female ambiguous genitalia or pseudohermaphroditism and accounts for approximately 70% of all patients with ambiguous genitalia. CAH accounts for greater than 95% of the cases of female pseudohermaphroditism, with exposure to maternal androgens accounting for the remaining 5%. Mutations in 1 of 5 genes result in impaired cortisol secretion, which in turn causes excess secretion of adrenocorticotropic hormone (ACTH) and consequently, adrenal hyperplasia. Four of the 5 genes code for enzymes necessary for steroid hormone synthesis, and the fifth encodes for an intracellular cholesterol transport protein (StAR) (Figure 41–9). Deficiencies in 21α-hydroxylase and 11β-hydroxylase result in masculinization of the female fetus, while they have no effects on the genitalia of the male fetuses. In contrast, infants with deficiencies in 3β-hydroxysteroid dehydrogenase, 17α-hydroxylase, and StAR have defects in both the synthesis of cortisol and steroid hormones. Affected

Figure 41–11. Algorithm for initial workup of intersex based on physical examination and karyotype.

Table 41–5. Differential diagnosis for a newborn with ambiguous genitalia.

	Common Karyotype	Gonad Status	Genitalia	Uterus	Urinary/Serum Steroids
Female pseudohermaphrodite (CAH)	XX	Ovary	Hypospadias	Present	Elevated
Male pseudohermaphrodite	XY	Testes	Hypospadias/micropenis	Absent	Normal
Mixed gonadal genesis	XY/XO	Streak dysgenetic	Hypospadias	Variable/rudimentary	Normal
True hermaphrodite	XX/mosaic	Ovotestis or ovary and testes	Hypospadias	Variable/rudimentary	Normal

males have varying degree of ambiguous genitalia due to deficiency in testosterone synthesis, while affected females may or may not be virilized.

21α-hydroxylase deficiency is the most common cause of CAH, accounting for 90% of cases. The metabolites 17-hydroxyprogesterone and 17-hydroxypregnenolone, which build up above the 21α-hydroxylase deficiency, are metabolized to androgens, resulting in virilization of the female external genitalia. Three forms of 21α-hydroxylase deficiency exist: classic, simple virilizing, and nonclassic. Each of these disorders is characterized by the activity level of the gene. Patients with the classic disease have both virilization and salt wasting, those with simple virilizing have masculinization without salt losing, and the nonclassic patients present after puberty with virilization.

Figure 41–12. Differential diagnosis of patients with inappropriate pubertal development, impaired pubertal development, and infertility. Def., deficiency; devel., development; DOC, deoxycorticosterone; exp. lap., experimental laparoscopy; synd., syndrome.

In general the classic form of 21α-hydroxylase deficiency exhibits the more severe forms of virilization (Figure 41–13). Impaired cortisol and aldosterone secretion leads to electrolytes and fluid losses, producing hyponatremia, hyperkalemia, acidosis, increased plasma renin, dehydration, and eventual vascular collapse unless recognized and treated. In affected males, deficiency in 21α-hydroxylase does not result in abnormal genitalia and consequently, salt loss may occur unnoticed. Aggressive fluid resuscitation with normal saline should be instituted immediately and repeat serum electrolyte measurement should be obtained to monitor the progress of the resuscitation. Diagnosis is based on an elevated level of 17-hydroxyprogesterone in the urine and blood. After diagnosis and stabilization, replacement therapy should be instituted with glucocorticoids, mineralocorticoids, and salt. Regular measurement of serum electrolytes, renin, and ACTH helps to monitor the adequacy of hormonal replacement. Untreated patients with 21α-hydroxylase deficiency exhibit excessive growth, virilization, advanced bone age, and early closure of epiphyseal growth plates.

11β-hydroxylase deficiency accounts for most of the remaining cases of CAH (~ 9%). Patients with 11β-hydroxylase accumulate 17-hydroxyprogesterone as well as deoxycorticosterone (DOC) and 11-deoxycortisol, which results in salt accumulation leading to hypertension. Patients with 11β-hydroxylase deficiency are more likely to present with hypertension secondary to the salt-retaining metabolites DOC and 11-deoxycortisol, in contrast to the hypovolemic shock associated with 21α-hydroxylase deficiency. Hypokalemia is also common secondary to an increase in mineralocorticoid activity.

Since CAH is hereditary, it is possible to counsel and offer treatment to families wishing further children. Maternal treatment with dexamethasone prior to the 10th week of gestation can significantly reduce the risk of masculinization of the female fetus. Standard prenatal treatment is 20 μg/kg 2 times daily beginning as soon as the pregnancy is confirmed (fifth week of gestation) in a family with a positive history of CAH. At 9–10 weeks' gestation, chorionic villus sampling can confirm karyotype and test for the presence of the gene *CYP 21,* which is present in 21α-hydroxylase deficiency (90% of CAH cases). If the karyotype is XY or the CAH gene *CYP 21* is not present, the maternal dexamethasone treatment is stopped. Statistically, 50% of the fetuses will be male and of the females, only 25%

Figure 41–13. Patient with severe masculinization from congenital adrenal hyperplasia.

will be affected secondary to the recessive inheritance pattern of 21α-hydroxylase deficiency. Unfortunately, this will result in unnecessary prenatal steroid exposure in 7 of 8 fetuses with unknown long-term health consequences, such as hypertension. Although the short-term success of decreasing female virilization has been documented, long-term follow-up of fetuses exposed to steroids needs to be documented.

B. MATERNAL HORMONAL SOURCES OF VIRILIZATION

Maternal tumors are a rare cause of virilization of the female fetus. The most common type is luteomas of the ovary, which also virilize the mother. Diagnosis can be made by maternal blood samples and imaging studies (sonogram and magnetic resonance imaging). Maternal ingestion of medication is another rare cause of abnormalities in genital development (Table 41–6). Progesterone is a common agent being used early in pregnancy to prevent abortion and during in vitro fertilization treatments. The female fetus that is exposed to high concentrations of progesterone can virilize secondary to direct action of progesterone on the androgen receptor. In the male fetus, hypospadias can develop by progesterone-inhibiting testosterone synthesis and downregulating the androgen receptor. A prenatal history of progesterone exposure should be elicited in the differential diagnosis of patients with abnormalities of the external genitalia.

Male Pseudohermaphrodites

Male pseudohermaphrodites are characterized by a 46 XY genotype, normal testes (usual palpable), and partial or complete masculinization of the external genitalia. The differential diagnosis is outlined in (Figure 41–14).

Two forms of androgen resistance related to male pseudohermaphrodites are complete androgen insensitivity and partial androgen insensitivity.

A. COMPLETE ANDROGEN INSENSITIVITY

Androgen resistance ranges from partial to complete due to a defect in the androgen receptor. Patients with

Table 41–6. Drugs that may induce intersex disorders if taken during pregnancy.

C21-steroid medroxyprogesterone acetate (progesterone)
Finasteride (Proscar)
Leuprolide acetate (Lupron)
Stilbestrol
Danazol
Norethynodrel
Ethisterone
Norethindrone

complete androgen resistance or androgen insensitivity syndrome (AIS) (previously called testicular feminization) have a 46 XY karyotype but have unambiguous female external genitalia, hypoplastic labia majora, a blind vaginal pouch, and an absent uterus. Since a functional androgen receptor is necessary for the development of axillary and pubic hair, complete AIS patients have sparse to nonexistent hair growth in these areas. Complete AIS patients either inherit the disease by an X-linked recessive pattern or develop a spontaneous mutation that renders the androgen receptor nonfunctional. Patients with complete AIS appear to identify as females. Presumably the functional defect in the androgen receptor also exists in the brain, preventing "masculinization." There is not enough long-term follow-up to assess issues with sexual identity in these patients.

Complete androgen resistance should be suspected in phenotypic females who present with an inguinal hernia that contains a testis (approximately 1% of all prepubertal females undergoing hernia repair). The most common presentation for complete AIS is amenorrhea in adolescent females. Breast development occurs in AIS patients secondary to the peripheral conversion of testosterone to estradiol from aromatase enzyme. After puberty, the testes have approximately a 10% risk of developing cancer, the most common tumor being a seminomatous germ cell. Because of the significantly increased cancer risk, removal of the gonads is recommended after postpubertal breast development. Alternatively, the gonads can be removed at the time of diagnosis, with estrogen replacement therapy initiated in the pubertal time period. Since the vagina may be inadequate in length, some patients may need augmentation procedures. Self-vaginal dilation is the most common technique, followed by vaginal augmentation procedures using skin grafts or bowel.

B. PARTIAL ANDROGEN INSENSITIVITY

In contrast to complete AIS, patients with partial androgen resistance may have external genitalia ranging from mild to severe hypospadias (with and without cryptorchidism) to micropenis or clitorimegaly with partial labial fusion (Figure 41–15). The testes may be located in the labia, inguinal canal, or abdomen. The testes are histologically normal before puberty. However, after puberty spermatogenesis is usually absent and there is Leydig cell hyperplasia. The testes are predisposed to malignant transformation in 4–9% of the patients.

The defect in partial androgen resistance is typically due to a single base pair mutation in the androgen receptor. Inheritance may be X-linked or autosomal recessive or from a spontaneous mutation. Interestingly, the same genetic defect within a family may have a dif-

Müllerian duct structure

No   Yes

Abnormalities in testosterone
synthesis or action

**Dysgenetic male
pseudohermaphroditism**
Differential Diagnosis

1. XY gonadal dysgenesis
   (incomplete)
2. XO/XY mosaicism
3. Deny Drash
4. Wilms, aniridia GU anomalies
   Mental retardation (WAGR)
5. Testicular regression syndrome

hCG stimulation

< 2 ng/cc
testosterone

> 2 ng/cc
testosterone

Testosterone precursors

T/DHT

Decreased   **Increased**

**LH receptor mutation
StAR mutation**

**17 α-D deficiency:
progesterone
& pregnenolone
3 β-HSD deficiency: DHEA**

**17 β-HSD deficiency:
androstenediol**

< 30   > 30

Androgen receptor defects
**Testicular feminization
Reifenstein syndrome
Receptor and resistence**

5 α-Reductase deficiency

Figure 41–14. Differential diagnosis of patients with male pseudohermaphroditism. DHEA, dehydroepiandrosterone; GU, genitourinary;_hCG, human chorionic gonadotropin; LH, luteinizing hormone; StAR, steroidogenic acute regulatory protein; T/DHT, testosterone/dihydrotestosterone.

Figure 41–15. Partial androgen receptor defect resulting in severe hypospadias with curvature (**A**) and a small phallus (**B**).

ferent phenotypic expression. The variability of phenotypic expression makes counseling difficult in affected families.

In patients with partial androgen resistance, the sex of rearing depends on the degree of androgen resistance and the degree of genital ambiguity. In patients who respond to high-dose androgen therapy (2 mg/kg initially followed by 4 mg/kg) by phallic growth, the sex of rearing as male has been successful. Genital reconstruction, repairing the hypospadias and undescended testes is performed at an early age. Patients who have a poor response to androgen stimulation fall into a difficult category of intersex. In the past, patients who were raised as females had feminizing genital surgery and gonadectomy typically in the first year of life. At time of puberty, estrogen replacement is instituted. Presumably, in partial androgen insensitivity, sexual identity is influenced by the effects of androgens on central imprinting. A discordance may exist between the external genitalia that partially responds to androgen stimulation versus the effects of androgens on determining sexual identity in the brain. The fact that some patients with severe hypospadias and a small phallus have had difficulty with sexual identity in adulthood makes sex assignment difficult. Presently, it seems reasonable to delay irreversible surgery until after the patient has developed a sexual identity and can drive the decision for reconstructive surgery.

5α-Reductase Type 2 Deficiency

5α-reductase type 2 deficiency is an autosomal recessive transmitted disorder affecting the formation of the male genitalia. 5α-reductase is responsible for the conversion of the less potent testosterone to the 5–10 times more potent dihydrotestosterone. Type 2 5α-reductase predominates in the tissue of the external genitalia and the prostate, whereas type 1 5α-reductase localizes to the skin and nongenital tissues. Numerous mutations have been described in the 5α-reductase type 2 gene consistent with the variation in clinical spectrum seen in patients with this defect. Immunohistochemical localization of 5α-reductase type 2 reveals that the enzyme is located in the midline urethral seam (Figure 41–16). The midline seam localization is consistent with the formation of hypospadias in patients with 5α-reductase type 2 gene defects in that the epithelial edges of the urethral seam would fail to fuse, resulting in hypospadias.

Clinically, patients with 5α-reductase type 2 present with a small phallus, severe hypospadias, bifid scrotum, and a residual prostatic utricle or blind-ending vaginal pouch (Figure 41–17). The testes are often undescended in the inguinal canal. Untreated patients will typically virilize during puberty when elevated levels of the less potent testosterone either overwhelm the functioning androgen gene or the functioning 5 α-reductase type 1 enzyme cross-reacts with the excess testosterone, converting it to dihydrotestosterone.

Sexual identity appears to be intact for karyotype XY males with 5α-reductase type 2 deficiency, presumably from an intact masculinization of the brain. In specific geographic areas such as the Dominican Republic, where the incidence of 5α-reductase type 2 is relatively high, it is generally accepted that these children will change from an initial "in-between" sex to a male sexual identity at the time of puberty.

The diagnosis of 5α-reductase type 2 deficiency should be considered in severe phenotypes of hypospadias, especially with associated scrotal anomalies and

Figure 41–16. Immunohistochemical localization of 5α-reductase type 2 (**A–D**) and the androgen receptor (AR) (**E–H**) in the same human fetal penis at 16.5 weeks of gestation (reduced from 25×). Note strong expression of 5α-reductase type 2 along the urethral seam area (arrows).

Figure 41–17. A patient with 5α-reductase type 2 deficiency. Note severe hypospadias with a small phallus, bifid scrotum, and visible prostatic utricle or blind-ending vaginal pouch.

undescended testes. Diagnosis is based on an increase in ratio of testosterone to dihydrotestosterone. Since these patients have a small phallus, attempts at enlargement with dihydrotestosterone cream are reasonable, although dihydrotestosterone is difficult to obtain in the United States. Reconstructive surgery for the hypospadias and undescended testes is indicated. Fertility has not been reported in patients with 5α-reductase type 2, although sperm production has been documented.

Persistent Müllerian Duct Syndrome

Müllerian inhibiting substance (MIS) or factor (anti-müllerian duct hormone) causes regression of the structures that would have formed the uterus, fallopian tube, and upper part of the vagina. Defects in the MIS gene or MIS receptor result in retained müllerian structures typically inherited as an autosomal recessive defect. Male siblings of affected patients, especially with cryptorchidism, should undergo screening; they have a 25% chance of being affected.

Clinically, patients with persistent müllerian duct syndrome present, unexpectedly, at the time of surgery for cryptorchidism (Figure 41–18). Hence the alternate name for persistent müllerian duct syndrome, hernia uterine inguinale. Within the hernia sac a fallopian tube, uterus, or both are found attached to the testicular cord structures. What makes the treatment difficult is that these structures and hence the diagnosis are found unexpectedly at the time of surgery for cryptorchidism. If persistent müllerian duct structures are found during orchiopexy, it is reasonable to abort the procedure until a correct diagnosis can be determined. At the initial exploration, a clear description of gonad and surrounding müllerian structures should be documented, with a biopsy specimen of the gonad taken and a karyotype obtained.

Once a definitive diagnosis is made, reconstructive surgery can than be performed. Separation of inappropriate müllerian structures from the cord without disturbing the vas deferens, the testicular artery, or both is the goal; however, this may be impossible if the vas runs through the müllerian structures, which is a common outcome. Fertility is usually impaired in patients with persistent müllerian duct syndrome even though testosterone levels may be normal. Whether this is a consequence of primary gonadal dysfunction or secondary to the cryptorchid testes is controversial. Efforts should be made to remove the müllerian structures and deliver the testes into the scrotum or at least a palpable position in the groin for subsequent cancer surveillance. Testes cancer has been reported in 2–10% of patients. In patients where the testes remains in the abdomen or cannot be separated from the müllerian structures, orchiectomy is indicated.

Abnormal Gonadal Function Syndromes

A. TURNER SYNDROME

Turner syndrome is relatively common, occurring in 1 in every 2000 female births. The genotype in patients with Turner syndrome is complete or mosaic X monosomy, (45,X, or 45,X/46,XX). Turner stigmata consist of a web neck, shield chest, aortic valve defects, coarctation of the aorta, horseshoe kidney, short stature, and absent puberty. During fetal development in patients with Turner syndrome the ovaries develop but subsequently degenerate to streak gonads. The streak gonads are not at risk for cancer and therefore do not need to be removed. Therapy is directed toward growth augmentation with growth hormone therapy in childhood. Subsequently estrogen replacement is begun in late adolescence so as not to interfere with maximum growth.

B. PURE GONADAL DYSGENESIS

Patients with 46, XX complete gonadal dysgenesis are typically diagnosed following a workup for delayed puberty or primary amenorrhea. Patients have a normal

Figure 41–18. Hernia uterine inguinale, or persistent müllerian duct syndrome. Note the presence of a fallopian tube and uterus attached to the testicular cord structures.

female phenotype without the stigmata of Turner syndrome, normal external and internal müllerian structures, and bilateral streak gonads. Sexual identity is female. Unlike patients with 46, XY gonadal dysgenesis, risk of tumor formation is rare and treatment is directed at hormonal replacement, with removal of the streaks gonads unnecessary.

C. XY GONADAL DYSGENESIS

Patients with 46, XY gonadal dysgenesis are characterized by absent testicular function in the presence of a Y chromosome. Classically, patients with 46, XY gonadal dysgenesis have a female phenotype. Patients come to medical attention if the prenatal karyotype (XY) is discordant with the child's phenotype (female), delayed puberty, amenorrhea, or precocious puberty from a hormonally functional gonadal tumor. The incidence of gonadal tumors is as high as 60%, with gonadoblastoma being the most common, although dysgerminomas, seminomas, and nonseminomatous germ cell tumors have also been reported.

In pure XY gonadal dysgenesis, müllerian duct structures usually are present secondary to failure of müllerian inhibiting factor secretion, and wolffian duct structures are vestigial or absent secondary to lack of testosterone secretion. Laboratory analysis reveals female levels of baseline testosterone with no increase in response to hCG stimulation. Surgical exploration reveals streak gonads, fallopian tubes, and a uterus. With a 60% chance of tumor, the gonads need to be removed once the diagnosis is confirmed. These patients should

be raised as females with estrogen replacement at the time of puberty.

D. MIXED GONADAL DYSGENESIS

Patients with mixed gonadal dysgenesis usually have a 45,X/46,XY, 46XY, or other mosaic karyotype. They typically have one streak and one dysgenetic testis. Most children with mixed gonadal dysgenesis have incomplete virilization resulting in ambiguous genitalia or hypospadias with cryptorchidism. The other classic presentation is a mosaic genotype diagnosed on prenatal amniocentesis. Interestingly, the subsequent phenotype of patients with a prenatal karyotype of 45,X/46,XY is 90% normal male external genitalia. However, with a prenatal genotype of 45,X/46,XY the patient is at risk for progressive gonadal changes leading to fibrosis and decreased fertility and low testosterone levels. The incidence of gonadal tumors does not seem to be increased. Most notably, 20% of these children have mental retardation or autism.

In patients who present with ambiguous genitalia, one gonad is typically palpable in the scrotum or inguinal canal and the other gonad (streak) nonpalpable. The phallus size is typically small with a proximal or more severe hypospadias (Figure 41–19). Testosterone levels are normal with an appropriate response to hCG. MIF levels are usually normal. At surgery, the dysgenetic gonad (streak) may grossly appear normal but have microscopic abnormalities such as hypoplastic tubules surrounded by ovarian or fibrotic stroma. Variable müllerian duct structures, such as fallopian tubes

Figure 41–19. Presentation of mixed gonadal dysgenesis with ambiguous genitalia and a unilateral palpable gonad on the right side.

and uterus, are present depending on the degree of gonadal dysgenesis. On biopsy, the contralateral gonad in the scrotum or inguinal canal is either a normal or dysgenetic testis. In patients with mixed gonadal dysgenesis, the risk of gonadoblastoma is 15–30%. Gonadoblastoma is a steroid hormone–secreting gonadal tumor composed of large germ cells, Sertoli cells, and stromal derivatives. The incidence of gonadoblastoma appears to be higher in more undervirilized patients and the most common associated karyotype is 46 XY. Sixty percent of gonadoblastomas arise in an indeterminate gonad, 22% in streak gonads, and 18% in dysgenetic cryptorchid testis. Two cases occurring in a testis located in the scrotum have been reported. One-third of the patients have bilateral disease. Sixty percent of gonadoblastomas are associated with subsequent malignant germ cell tumor (germinoma, seminoma, and dysgerminoma but also embryonal teratoma, embryonal carcinoma, endodermal sinus tumor, or choriocarcinoma). Metastases develop in 10% of patients with germinomas arising within the gonadoblastoma.

In children who are undervirilized, female sex assignment is recommended, and the streak and dysge-

netic gonads should be removed at time of diagnosis due to increased risk of malignancy. Hormonal replacement with estrogen will be necessary during adolescence. If male gender is assigned, management of the scrotal testis is controversial, ranging from serial observation to surveillance biopsy. In the virilized patients who are raised as males, the testis will inevitably reveal poor hormonal and fertility potential. These patients will require testosterone supplementation in adulthood.

In 5% of patients, mixed gonadal dysgenesis is associated with Wilms tumor, ambiguous genitalia, and progressive glomerulopathy known as the Denys-Drash syndrome. Wilms tumor occurs in the first 2 years of life and is often bilateral. Classic presentation is an infant with ambiguous genitalia, hypertension, and nephrotic syndrome.

E. 17β-HYDROXYSTEROID DEHYDROGENASE DEFICIENCY

Patients with a defect in the enzyme 17β-hydroxysteroid dehydrogenase do not efficiently convert androstenedione to testosterone. 17β-hydroxysteroid dehydrogenase is predominantly located in the testes. The rare disorder of 17β-hydroxysteroid dehydrogenase deficiency is inherited via an autosomal recessive pattern. This disorder is indigenous to the Arab population of the Gaza strip in the Middle East. Clinical presentation in a patient with XY genotype is mild virilization of the external genitalia, with clitoral hypertrophy and a blind-ending utricle (vagina). The testes are undescended in the abdomen or inguinal canal or descended into the labioscrotal folds. If the virilization is mild, the diagnosis becomes apparent at puberty, with penile growth and male secondary sexual characteristics. At puberty, the increased levels of androstenedione are converted by nongenital, nonmutant 17α-hydroxysteroid dehydrogenase to testosterone. These patients may also present with gynecomastia at puberty by the peripheral conversion of androstenedione to estradiol by aromatase. Diagnosis is based on an increased ratio of androstenedione to testosterone postpubertal or in the prepubertal state in response to an hCG stimulation test.

If the diagnosis is suspected in infancy, treatment with testosterone, reconstruction of the hypospadias, and male sex assignment is indicated. At puberty in the Gaza strip, gender conversion from female to male is common practice. Long-term outcomes of patients raised as females initially and reassigned to males at puberty await documentation.

True Hermaphroditism

True hermaphroditism is defined as the presence of both ovarian and testicular tissue within the same individual (Figure 41–20). The most common karyotype in patients with true hermaphroditism is 46 XX (predominately in African Americans), followed by 46 XY/46 XX mosaicism. The latter karyotype in a patient with ambiguous genitalia strongly suggests the diagnosis of true hermaphroditism. Only 7% of patients with this disorder have a 46 XY karyotype. Interestingly, not all true hermaphrodites express the SRY gene, suggesting that non-SRY genes play a role in the development of the testes in these patients.

In patients with true hermaphroditism, the gonads are a combination of ovotestis, ovaries, or testis. The most common configuration is ovotestis/ovary in 35%, followed by bilateral ovotestis in 25%, separate ovary and testes in 25%, and ovotestis/testes in the remaining 15%. One or both gonads are palpable in at least 60% of the patients. For unexplained reasons the testes is more likely to be found on the right side. The testis and ovaries are located in their respective normal position, and the level of descent of the ovotestis is dependent on the amount of testicular tissue. While ovarian histology and function may be normal, testicular histology and function is usually abnormal. Ovotestis can be bilobar in configuration, with the ovarian and testicular tissue relatively separate, or the ovarian and testicular tissue may be intermingled and difficult to surgically separate. At the time of diagnosis, deep biopsies are necessary to determine the histologic status of the gonad. The internal structures tend to correlate with the type of gonad. Approximately 80% of true hermaphrodites will have a functional or rudimentary uterus. The uterus may be

Figure 41–20. Finding at the time of surgical exploration in a true hermaphrodite. On the patient's right side, note the testes, and on the left, note the fallopian tube, uterus, and biopsy-proven ovary.

found in the abdomen or associated with an inguinal hernia. In patients with normal uterine structures and ovarian histology, fertility and normal pregnancies have been reported.

The external genitalia are usually ambiguous, although 60% of patients are masculinized, with a well-developed hypospadiac phallus. The hypospadias can be severe perineal or penile-scrotal with incomplete fusion of the labioscrotal folds. The degree of masculinization is dependent on the amount of functional testicular tissue present. In childhood, testicular tissue has been documented to have normal spermatogonia. With maturation, however, testicular fibrosis occurs, with fertility in males a rare event. Testicular tumor is uncommon, occurring in 1–2% of the patients.

The diagnosis of true hermaphroditism should be suspected in patients with virilized ambiguous genitalia who have a 46 XX (African American) or mosaic genotype 46 XX/XY associated with the finding of müllerian structures. Diagnosis is confirmed by gonadal biopsy confirming the presence of both ovarian and testicular tissue. After a decision regarding sex gender assignment has been made, gonadal tissue inappropriate for sex gender assignment should be removed. In patients who are raised as females, removal of all functioning testicular tissue is critical to prevent virilization at puberty. Surgical correction of the urogenital sinus to expose the vagina is necessary. In patients raised as males—who account for approximately 30% of all true hermaphrodites—the hypospadias and undescended testes should be reconstructed. In males, since testicular failure is common at puberty, testosterone supplementation may be required.

Unclassified Forms of Abnormal Sexual Differentiation

A. Hypospadias

Hypospadias is not a form of intersex (Figure 41–21). The etiology can be defined in less than 5% of patients. This leaves most cases without a defined etiology. The variable expression of the androgen receptor in the ventral versus the dorsal urethra may play a role in the etiology of hypospadias (Figure 41–22). Recent theories suggest an abnormality in closure of the midline urethral seam. Another possible etiology explaining the increase in incidence of hypospadias in Western countries over the last 25 years is an increase in exposure to environmental endocrine disruptors.

In controlled studies most patients with hypospadias undergo successful surgical reconstruction and have acceptable long-term outcomes. Patients with hypospadias have an unambiguous male sexual identity. In severe forms of hypospadias with perineal or scrotal urethral openings, severe curvature and the phallus buried within the scrotum are the critical issues confirming the correct diagnosis. This is also the case for patients with hypospadias and a nonpalpable or undescended testis. If any doubt exists, patients with severe hypospadias, hypospadias in association with an undescended testis, or both, a karyotype should be checked to document genotype. In severe cases of hypospadias where penile size is difficult to assess secondary to severe chordee, an hCG stimulation will assess the gonadal axis and confirm an intact androgen receptor by eliciting penile growth.

B. Micropenis

A small penis defined as less than 2.5 cm in length without hypospadias in a full-term male is defined as micropenis (Figure 41–23 and Table 41–4). Micropenis can be caused by multiple etiologies, the most common being fetal testosterone deficiency followed by partial defects in the androgen receptor or 5α-reductase enzyme (Table 41–7). Fetal testosterone synthesis can be divided into 2 categories: (1) primary testicular failure (Leydig cell) and (2) central failure. Central failure can be from congenital hypopituitarism or isolated gonadotropin deficiency. Patients with decreased fetal testosterone production either from Leydig cell failure or lack of Leydig cell stimulation from gonadotropin deficiency respond to treatment with supplementary testosterone enanthate intramuscular injections 25–50 mg each month for 3 consecutive months.

Long-term outcomes of patients with micropenis have documented that final adult penile length is normal for greater than 90% of patients treated with multiple short courses of testosterone enanthate. In addition, patients with micropenis identified with the male gender had normal erections, ejaculation, and orgasm. In the rare patient who does not respond to testosterone stimulation, gender conversion to female had been advocated in the past. Presently, gender conversion would not be considered based on solely on the small phallus size.

Reassignment to the female gender with removal of the gonads and feminizing genitoplasty in patients with penile agenesis and iatrogenic penile amputation or circumcision injury has been standard treatment. In complete penile agenesis, the testicles are normal, corporeal bodies are absent, and the urethra opens into the anterior rectum or perineum. These patients have normal prenatal androgen levels and hence the brain has received signals for male sexual identity. The same is true for the rare patient who has a severe penile injury during circumcision. As in micropenis, gender conversion would now not be considered based solely on the absence or small size of the phallus. Penile reconstruction, although not technically ideal, may provide the best overall outcome.

Figure 41–21. The spectrum of hypospadias, which is not an ambiguous or intersex condition. **A:** Anterior, where the meatus is on the inferior surface of the glans penis. **B:** Coronal, where the meatus is in the balanopenile furrow. **C:** Distal, on the distal third of the shaft. **D:** Penoscrotal, at the base of the shaft in front of the scrotum. **E:** Scrotal, on the scrotum or between the genital swellings. **F:** Perineal, where the meatus is behind the scrotum or genital swellings.

C. CLOACAL AND EXSTROPHY ANOMALIES

In the past, patients with the most severe and rare form of lower abdominal congenital malformation, cloacal exstrophy (incidence of 1:200,000 live births), were usually left to die. Significant problems associated with surgical reconstruction of cloacal exstrophy include omphalocele; numerous gastrointestinal anomalies such as short gut, malrotation, duplication, duodenal atresia, and Meckel's diverticulum; and significant genitourinary anomalies such as separate bladder halves, upper tract renal anomalies, and bifid genitalia. Patients with cloacal exstrophy can also have neurologic and orthopedic anomalies such as tethered cord, myelomeningocele, lower extremity paralysis, clubfoot, and hip dislocation.

Historically, newborn males with cloacal exstrophy (Figure 41–24) were often gender-converted to female as a result of inadequate genital development and the poor prognosis for surgically developing a normal male phenotype. In rearing genetic males as females, although the surgical reconstruction can match the assigned female phenotype, a new set of issues was created, such as the need for hormonal replacement with estrogen during adolescence and the issue of a nonmenstruating infertile female. In addition, the fetal and neonatal androgen imprinting on the brain does not seem to be reversible.

Because some of these XY, gender-converted females have self-reassigned their sex during adolescence to coincide with their genetic karyotype, there has been reevaluation of the practice of rearing genetic males as females. With the exact determinates of sexually identity not completely defined, a pragmatic approach is to delay any irreversible surgery such as orchiectomy or phallic removal/reduction in these patients. With modern surgical techniques and a multidisciplinary approach to their care, children with this complex disorder can have a normal sexual identity.

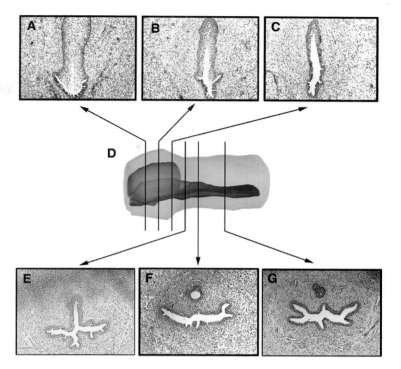

Figure 41–22. Androgen receptor (AR) expression in the human fetal penis at 16.5 weeks. A greater density of AR-positive cells is seen in the ventral portion of the urethral epithelium in the distal glans (**A**), mid glans (**B**), and proximal glans (**C**). In the distal (**E**), mid (**F**), and proximal (**G**) shaft of the penis, all portions of the urethral epithelium show the same density of expression. Three-dimensional reconstruction was performed to demonstrate the urethral AR expression pattern (**D**). Note the weaker density of AR in the dorsal aspect of the glandular urethra.

Figure 41–23. Micropenis. Normal corporeal bodies are palpable within the foreskin. The urethral meatus is at a terminal position within the glans. Stretched penile length is less than 2.5 cm in this full-term infant.

SURGICAL MANAGEMENT OF INTERSEX

The surgical management of patients with intersex is undergoing a reevaluation. The determination of a patient's sexual identity is strongly influenced by the genetic karyotype and steroid/androgen action on the developing brain. The environmental and social impacts are certainly important but presently seem to have a less dominating influence.

We would advocate surgical management of patients with intersex when the diagnosis is clearly established and the long-term outcome for the diagnosis is favorable. Surgery falls into 5 categories: (1) diagnostic/biopsy, (2) gonadectomy and removal of inappropriate müllerian structures, (3) clitoral reduction, (4) vaginoplasty, and (5) phallic reconstruction.

Diagnostic techniques have improved with the widespread use of laparoscopy to assess the morphology of the internal genital structures. Laparoscopic techniques allow the gonads and associated structures to be visualized and in some cases have a biopsy specimen taken without the need for a laparotomy open incision. Once the diagnosis is established, it is possible to remove an inappropriate gonad, müllerian remnant, or both via laparoscopic techniques.

Table 41–7. Etiologies of micropenis.

I. Deficient Testosterone Secretion
  A. Hypogonadotrophic hypogonadism
    1. Kallmann syndrome
    2. Prader-Willi syndrome
    3. Laurence-Moon syndrome
    4. Bardet-Biedl syndrome
    5. Rudd syndrome
  B. Primary hypogonadism ("Bum Gonads")
    1. Anorchia
    2. Klinefelter syndrome
    3. Gonadal dysgenesis (partial)
    4. LH receptor defects (partial)
    5. Noonan syndrome
    6. Trisomy 21
    7. Robinow syndrome
    8. Bardet-Biedl syndrome
    9. Laurence-Moon syndrome
    10. Testosterone synthesis defects (partial)
II. Defects in testosterone action
  A. Androgen receptor defects (partial)
  B. 5α-Reductase deficiency
  C. Growth hormone/insulin growth factor-1 deficiency
  D. Fetal hydantoin syndrome
III. Developmental anomalies
  A. Aphallia
  B. Cloacal exstrophy
  C. Iatrogenic injuries
    1. Circumcision
    2. Trauma

Clitoroplasty

Clitoroplasty is presently a controversial topic. No studies exist to clearly document whether androgen stimulation resulting in a large clitoris requires reduction or can be left intact. Clearly, surgery on the clitoral structures can result in nerve damage and removal of erectile tissue.

Historically, the enlarged clitoris/phallic structure has been dealt with by amputation. Subsequently, more refined techniques such as recession clitoroplasty were developed where the entire clitoral organ is preserved by imbricating and burying the proximal corporeal shaft and excess glans clitoris. The disadvantage of the clitoral recession procedures may not become apparent until puberty, when the recessed corporeal bodies become enlarged and painful during sexual stimulation. This leads to the need for a procedure involving subtotal resection of the shaft of the clitoris with preservation of the glans.

In cases where clitoroplasty is performed, the goal is to re-create the normal female anatomy. Presently, more conservative procedures have been employed to preserve both the sensory and cosmetic aspects of the clitoris. An understanding of normal female anatomy has benefited the design of reconstructive surgery in patients with congenital adrenal hyperplasia (Figures 41–25 and 41–26). A contemporary reduction clitoroplasty is based on anatomical observations from fetal anatomical dissections. Presently, the tunica of the cor-

Figure 41–24. **A:** Male with cloacal exstrophy. **B:** Female with cloacal exstrophy. In the male note the split scrotal appearance and the small hemi-phallus (arrows). In the female the clitoral bodies/genitalia are not visi-

Figure 41–25. Normal human fetal clitoris at 24 weeks' gestation (40×) immunostained with the neuronal marker S-100 (dark stain). **A:** Clitoral hood, labia minora and majora. **B:** Nerves on top of the erectile body and top of glans clitoris. **C–E:** Glans clitoris and erectile bodies. **F–G:** Lower part of glans clitoris with midline cleft. **H:** End of glans clitoris and vaginal introitus.

poral body can be preserved to spare as much of the dorsal nerve as possible. The concept of lifting the dorsal nerve off the tunica at the 11 and 1 o'clock positions seems inconsistent with the fact that the nerves fan out extensively around the dorsal and lateral aspects of the clitoral body.

A second issue is the removal of erectile tissue. In severe cases of masculinization of the genitalia, it seems reasonable to reduce the amount of erectile tissue. Standard treatment was to amputate the erectile body of the clitoris at the pubic arch, leaving each crural body and the neurovascular bundle with a strip of dorsal tunica. The long-term effects of removing this erectile tissue on sexual function are unknown. In contrast, leaving too much erectile tissue has been reported to cause pain in patients at the time of puberty. This, however, may be from fixing the corporeal tissue to the pubic bone, a practice that is no longer advocated. A compromise is to incise the corpora cavernosal body on the ventral surface at the 6 o'clock position and remove erectile tissue within the tunica to reduce the size of the erectile body, thereby preserving some erectile tissue and the nerves of the clitoris (Figure 41–27).

The final issue is the reduction of the glans clitoris, which may be the only surgical procedure required for reconstruction if used in conjunction with recession of the clitoral erectile tissue in less severe cases. Anatomical studies would support reduction on the ventral aspect of the glans, where the innervation is less dense than on the dorsal aspect (Figures 41–25 and 41–26). This should maximize sensation and hence sexual function (Figure 41–28).

Vaginoplasty

The timing of vaginoplasty is also a controversial issue in genital reconstruction. The presence of a vagina is not necessary until puberty and initially only to allow the passage of menstrual fluids. Later the vagina is necessary for vaginal penetration, fertility and, in most females, a healthy female sexual identity. This may not be the case for all females, for example, a women with a small vagina and a female sexual identity with a female sexual preference may not desire a larger vagina. In patients with absent müllerian structures (specifically a functional uterus) who have a female sexual identity, menstruation is not an issue and timing of vaginoplasty can be driven by the patient's wishes and motivation. In patients with a common urogenital sinus and hidden vagina, there are advantages and disadvantages of early

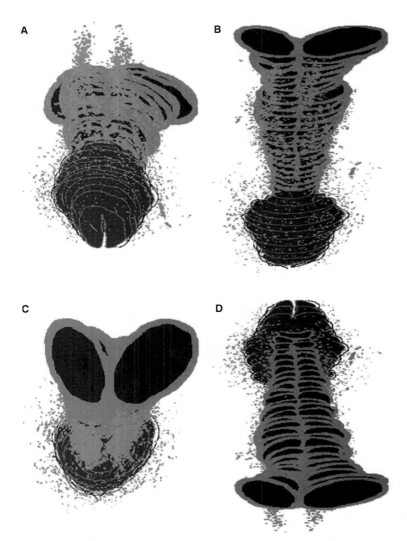

A   B

C   D

Figure 41–26. Normal human fetal clitoris, 24 weeks' gestation. Four views of a computer-generated three-dimensional reconstruction (**A:** top; **B:** bottom; **C:** back/top; **D:** bottom.) Note the pathway of the nerves (light gray) with a paucity of nerves on the bottom of the clitoris as well as in the top midline.

surgery in the first year of life versus late surgery prior to puberty. The advantage of early vaginoplasty is the closeness of the vagina to the perineum and the reported decreased bleeding in the early years of life. The major disadvantages are the smallness of the structures and that secondary surgery at the time of puberty may be necessary to correct vaginal stenosis. In contrast, delaying surgery has the advantages of operating on larger structures and the possibility that the patient can perform postoperative vaginal dilation to prevent stenosis.

The type of vaginoplasty depends on the level of masculinization. For low urogenital sinus anomalies, a flap vaginoplasty will usual allow for an adequate introitus with separation of the urethral and vagina. For high urogenital sinus anomalies, mobilization of the common urogenital sinus may be necessary. In the case of an absent vagina or a very short vagina, substitution vaginoplasty with bowel or skin grafting may be required.

A. FLAP VAGINOPLASTY

For the low-confluence urogenital (UG) sinus (Figure 41–29), a flap vaginoplasty can be used to bring the vaginal opening to the perineum. To perform a flap vaginoplasty, insert a urethral catheter into the bladder and a vascular balloon angiocatheter into the vagina. An inverted U- shaped/omega incision is made from the inferior aspect of the UG sinus opening to each ischial tuberosity. A thick subcutaneous tissue flap is developed after infiltration with lidocaine (1%) with

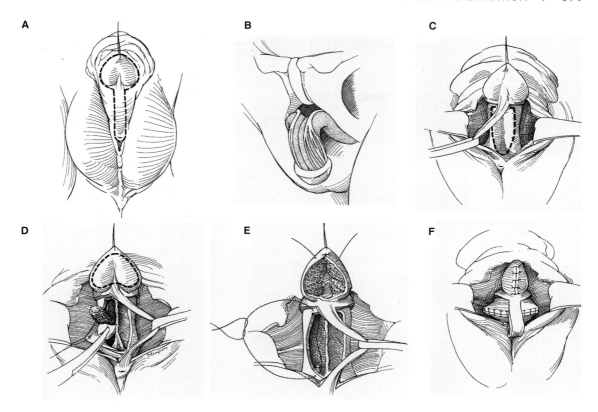

Figure 41–27. Schematic of feminizing genitoplasty based on neuroanatomical studies. **A:** Clitoroplasty incision. **B:** Schematic representation of nerves based on anatomical studies. **C:** Mobilization of urethral plate and outline for ventral incision into corporal bodies. **D:** Reduction of erectile tissue and incision for glans reduction. **E:** Corporal and glans reduction. **F:** Reduced glans clitoris with erectile preservation. (Used with permission from Baskin LS et al: Anatomical studies of the human clitoris. J Urol 1999;162(3 Pt 2):1015.)

Figure 41–28. A patient with congenital adrenal hyperplasia and virilization before (**A**) and after (**B**) feminizing genitoplasty.

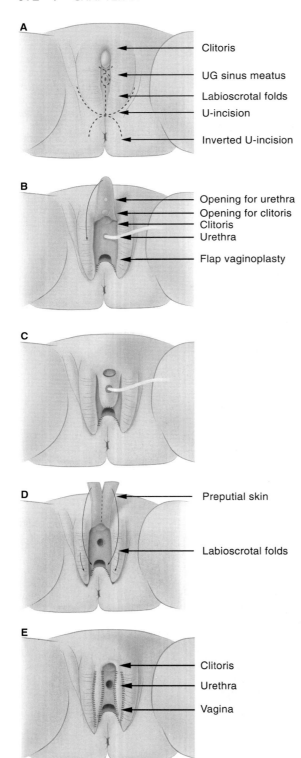

A
Clitoris
UG sinus meatus
Labioscrotal folds
U-incision
Inverted U-incision

B
Opening for urethra
Opening for clitoris
Clitoris
Urethra
Flap vaginoplasty

C

D
Preputial skin
Labioscrotal folds

E
Clitoris
Urethra
Vagina

1:100,000 of epinephrine to minimize bleeding. Since the confluence is distal, the UG sinus can be opened directly over the balloon catheter. Sutures are placed into the vaginal opening for retraction and hemostasis. A posterior incision into the vagina allows for creation of a wide vaginal opening that can accept the posterior flap.

The anterior flap for the vagina can be created using the phallic skin or the distal portion of the UG sinus. If a clitoroplasty is concurrently being performed, 2 openings are created in the midline of the preputial skin flap to accommodate the clitoris and the urethra. The preputial skin flap is then brought down and sutured to the anterior wall of the vagina. Alternatively, in more severe cases, the distal portion of the UG sinus can be used to create the anterior wall of the vagina.

B. TOTAL UG SINUS MOBILIZATION

Total UG sinus mobilization involves the circumferential mobilization of the entire UG sinus, thereby bringing the vagina and separated urethra to the perineum. This technique allows midlevel urogenital confluences to easily reach the perineum and high vaginal confluences to be better visualized, making vaginoplasty less technically demanding (Figure 41–30). Total UG sinus mobilization decreases the risk of fistula and vaginal stenosis. Long-term follow-up results in respect to continence and vaginal stenosis are not yet available. Stress incontinence in ambulatory patients as they mature through puberty is a concern.

Urethral and vascular catheters are placed into the bladder and vagina, respectively. An incision is made

Figure 41–29. Female external genitalia reconstruction in patients with a low confluence using a flap vaginoplasty. **A:** Surgical schematic of the perineum in patients with common urogenital sinus. **B:** The anterior flap for the vagina can be created using the phallic skin or the distal portion of the urogenital sinus. If a clitoroplasty is concurrently being performed, 2 openings are created in the midline of the preputial skin flap to accommodate the clitoris and urethra. The preputial skin flap is then brought down and sutured to the anterior wall of the vagina. **C:** The completed repair. **D:** Alternatively, the preputial skin can be split in the midline and used for reconstruction of the vaginal introitus and the anterior vaginal wall. **E:** The completed repair. (Used with permission from Nguyen HT, Baskin LS: *A Child with Ambiguous Genitalia.* American Urological Association Patient Management Problems, vol. 6, issue 2. Decker Electronic Publishing Inc, 2002.)

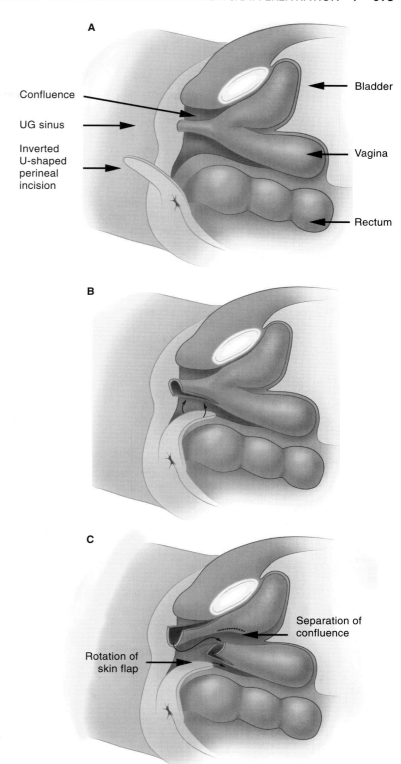

Figure 41–30. Urogenital sinus mobilization. **A:** The urogenital (UG) sinus is separated from the rectum posteriorly and the pubic bone anteriorly. **B:** The posterior skin flap (arrows) is assessed for length to reach the vagina. **C:** The confluence of the vagina and urethra (arrow) is separated. (Used with permission from Nguyen HT, Baskin LS: *A Child with Ambiguous Genitalia.* American Urological Association Patient Management Problems, vol. 6, issue 2. Decker Electronic Publishing Inc, 2002.)

circumferentially around the UG sinus meatus. In addition, an inverted U-shaped/omega incision with its apex at the perineal body and its bases at the ischial tuberosities is made above the anal opening (Figure 41–29A). A second true U-shaped incision is made at the base of the labioscrotal folds. Finally, a midline incision is made, extending from the phallus to the base of the labioscrotal folds. The dissection around the UG sinus is performed in the midline posteriorly, separating the perineal musculature that exists between the UG sinus and rectum. The dissection is carried cranially, exposing the entire posterior wall of the vagina and reflecting the cranial peritoneum superiorly. Next, the dissection is performed anteriorly, separating the UG sinus from the phallus and pubis. Finally, the avascular ligaments from the pubis to the UG sinus are divided, allowing the UG sinus to move downward toward the perineum. If the vagina is near the perineum, the sinus is opened ventrally and the posterior wall of the vagina is opened. The previously created U-shaped flap is then sewn to the spatulated posterior wall of the vagina. The resultant UG sinus tissue flap is then brought anteriorly to form a mucosal lining of the vestibule to the clitoris.

If the vagina is still high after mobilization, the anterior wall of the vagina is separated from the sinus and the posterior wall is opened. The opening in the sinus is then closed to form the urethra. The distal portion of the newly formed urethra is then opened dorsally to create a flap that is then inverted to form the anterior wall of the vagina. The previously created U-shaped flap is then sewn to the spatulated posterior wall of the vagina to complete the vaginoplasty.

The separated labioscrotal folds are brought posteriorly to form anatomical labia majoras. To complete the labioplasty, the preputial skin is divided in the midline and sutured around the clitoris and to the perineal flap, lateral vaginal wall, and opened UG sinus to create labia minora. These maneuvers allow the vagina to be brought into the introitus and the labia to be positioned next to the vagina in the normal anatomical position.

C. REPLACEMENT VAGINOPLASTY

Replacement vaginal reconstruction should be performed when the patient is ready to assume appropriate care of the newly constructed vagina. Typically this is in the later teenage years when tampon use is developmentally appropriate or sexual activity is considered, or both. The patient must be willing to actively take part in the postoperative care, which may involve performing self-dilation or wearing a vaginal mold, depending on the means of vaginal reconstruction that is chosen. In essence, the patient needs to request the procedure and demonstrate both the physical and psychological capacity to manage the vaginal reconstruction.

The surgical strategy for vaginal reconstruction, like all types of surgery, is dependent on the experience and bias of the surgeon. The 2 substantial tissues are skin and bowel. The technique of split-thickness skin graft as described by McIndoe (1950) has been the most popular form of vaginal reconstruction over the last 3 decades and certainly has withstood the test of time. The criticism of this technique is that long-term regular home dilation may be required. There may be complications of inadequate vaginal depth, dyspareunia, and vaginal stenosis.

The McIndoe procedure can be performed from a perineal approach and does not risk the complications of using a segment of bowel. This procedure continues to be favored by the plastic surgeons and gynecologists who are more likely to treat the patients who present in the teenage years, such as those with Mayer-Rokitansky syndrome (vaginal agenesis and unilateral renal dysplasia).

Vaginal reconstruction can also be performed by bowel substitution. Ileum, cecum, transverse colon, sigmoid colon, rectum, and a rudimentary bladder from a cloacal variant can all be adapted for vaginal reconstruction. The classic approach is to use a 10-cm segment of sigmoid colon or cecum. In patients with a rudimentary vagina (androgen insensitivity syndrome and Mayer-Rokitansky syndrome), a direct anastomosis to the short vagina will require less bowel in the introitus. In contrast, in patients with a flat perineum a slightly longer bowel segment to provide adequate length is required. It is also critical that when a direct perineal anastomosis is required, an adequate amount of space is created for a tension-free anastomosis that will comfortably accept the new bowel vagina. This point needs to be emphasized in that an inadequate space will lead to stenosis and the requirement of self-dilation, reoperation, or both. Despite adequate mobilization of retroperitoneal bowel mesentery, the situation may arise where a tension-free anastomosis of the bowel segment to the perineum is tenuous. In this case it is possible to bridge the gap with a short segment of ileum. When ileum is used, the segment must be folded onto itself to provide for adequate caliber. We also recommend fixation of the bowel segment to the retroperitoneum/sacral promontory to prevent wandering or prolapse of the neovagina. Another trick that is useful for patients with a flat perineum is mobilization of a U-shaped skin flap that can then be recessed into the perineum. This allows the mucosal edge of the bowel skin anastomosis to be within the hymenal ring in a less conspicuous place.

When one is performing a bowel substitution vaginoplasty, the direction of peristalsis of the bowel segment does seem to matter. Excess mucus production has not been a major factor in cecal neovaginas or colonic or sigmoid neovaginas (or both). Occasionally, daily vaginal irrigations using daily vaginal douching may be needed to evacuate mucus from the bowel segment.

Theoretically, a small amount of mucus production will allow for natural lubrication, thereby obviating the need for additional lubrication. Dyspareunia has not been a problem in patients with an adequate-sized neovagina. Retrospective analysis also shows that patients who had vaginal reconstruction prior to the onset of puberty uniformly required revisions. This is because patient and family motivation in this age group is suboptimal, yet critical for the success of the repair.

In summary, the critical factor is to use an adequate amount of bowel as well as to create an adequate space for the bowel to reside in. In all cases of vaginal reconstruction, careful preoperative counseling and an assessment of the patient's motivation are essential for a good result. In patients who have complained of dyspareunia, examination has revealed 3 problems: (1) a stenotic perineal anastomosis, (2) kinking of the vagina secondary to inadequate fixation, or (3) inadequate vaginal depth.

D. TECHNIQUES OF SIGMOID VAGINOPLASTY

An 8- to 10-cm segment of distal sigmoid is isolated, preserving the vasculature from the left colic or superior hemorrhoidal vessels (Figure 41–31). The segment size is selected to allow for adequate length of the neovagina. An additional segment of sigmoid distal to the isolated segment is discarded to provide greater length on the vascular pedicle of the neovagina. Similarly, the proximal vascular mesentery of the isolated segmented is also divided to allow greater mobilization of the neovagina into the pelvis.

A

B

Left colic

Superior hemorrhoidal

8—10 cm

Discarded segment

C

Figure 41–31. Sigmoid vaginoplasty: **A:** A U-shaped flap is created on the perineum so the sigmoid bowel segment can be recessed within the vaginal introitus. **B:** An 8- to 10-cm segment of distal sigmoid is isolated, preserving the vasculature from left colic or superior hemorrhoidal vessels. An additional segment of sigmoid distal to the isolated segment is discarded to provide greater length on the vascular pedicle of the neovagina. **C:** The sigmoid segment is rotated 180 degrees on its mesentery and brought into the perineum (**arrow**). (Used with permission from Nguyen HT, Baskin LS: *A Child with Ambiguous Genitalia.* American Urological Association Patient Management Problems, vol. 6, issue 2. Decker Electronic Publishing Inc, 2002.)

The sigmoid segment is rotated 180 degrees on its mesentery and brought into the perineum. The proximal end of the neovagina is then closed in 2 layers. The neovagina should be fixed to the retroperitoneum to prevent prolapse. The sigmoid colon is reanastomosed anterior to the neovagina.

The distal end of the segment is anastomosed to the vaginal remnant or directly onto the perineum. If the latter is performed, an inverted U-shaped flap should be created to allow the neovagina to be recessed inside the introitus.

Phallic Reconstruction

Phallic reconstruction is a formidable task. Nevertheless, it is critical that reconstructive efforts continue in this area, especially for patients with penile agenesis or iatrogenic injuries and a XY genotype and functional androgen receptor. Several techniques have been devised, such as free microanastomosis, innervated radial forearm flaps, tubed abdominal flaps with a penile prosthesis, and rectus abdominus myocutaneous flaps. In the free radial forearm flap, the pudendal nerve is anastomosed to the lateral cutaneous nerve of the forearm. The radial artery and vein are anastomosed to the inferior epigastrics, the internal pudendals, or the femoral vessels. The major complications with these procedures are fistula, prosthesis erosion, and poor sensation. The technical nuances of microvascular anastomosis require that the procedures be performed in adolescents and adulthood. The psychological implications of relatively late reconstruction have not been determined. With newer tissue engineering techniques, better phallic reconstruction procedures may be on the horizon.

REFERENCES

Ahmed SF et al: Phenotypic features, androgen receptor binding, and mutational analysis in 278 clinical cases reported as androgen insensitivity syndrome. J Clin Endocrinol Metab 2000;85(2):658.

Baskin LS: Hypospadias: A critical analysis of cosmetic outcomes using photography. Br J Urol Int 2001;87:534.

Baskin LS et al: Anatomical studies of the human clitoris. J Urol 1999;162(3 Pt 2):1015.

Baskin LS et al: Anatomical studies of hypospadias. J Urol 1998;160(3 Pt 2):1108.

Baskin LS et al: Hypospadias and endocrine disruption: Is there a connection? Environ Health Perspect 2001;109:1175.

Birnbacher R et al: Gender identity reversal in an adolescent with mixed gonadal dysgenesis. J Pediatr Endocrinol Metab 1999; 12(5):687.

Chang HJ et al: The phenotype of 45,X/46,XY mosaicism: An analysis of 92 prenatally diagnosed cases. Am J Hum Genet 1990;46(1):156.

Chase C: Psychological evaluation of intersex children. Arch Sex Behav 1999;28(1):103.

Creighton S, Minto C: Managing intersex. BMJ 2001;323 (7324):1264.

Daaboul J, Frader J: Ethics and the management of the patient with intersex: A middle way. J Pediatr Endocrinol Metab 2001;14(9):1575.

Farkas A et al: 1-Stage feminizing genitoplasty: 8 years of experience with 49 cases. J Urol 2001;165(6 Pt 2):2341.

Glassberg KI: The intersex infant: Early gender assignment and surgical reconstruction. J Pediatr Adolesc Gynecol 1998;11 (3):151.

Griffin J et al: The androgen resistance syndromes: Steroid 5 alpha-reductase deficiency, testicular feminization and related disorders. In: Scriver C: *The Metabolic and Molecular Bases of Inherited Disease,* vol. 3, p. 2967. McGraw-Hill, 1995.

Gross R, Crigler R: Clitorectomy for sexual abnormalities, indications and techniques. J Surg 1966;59:300.

Hendren WH: Surgical approach to intersex problems. Semin Pediatr Surg 1998;7(1):8.

Hensle TW, Dean GE: Vaginal replacement in children. J Urol 1992;148(2 Pt 2):677.

Hrabovszky Z, Hutson JM: Surgical treatment of intersex abnormalities: A review. Surgery 2002;131(1):92.

Jirasek J et al: The relationship between the development of gonads and external genitals in human fetuses. Am J Obstet Gynecol 1968;101:830.

Kim KS et al: Expression of the androgen receptor and 5 alpha-reductase type 2 in the developing human fetal penis and urethra. Cell Tissue Res 2002;307(2):145.

Kolon TF et al: Clinical and molecular analysis of XX sex reversed patients. J Urol 1998;160(3 Pt 2):1169, discussion 1178.

Kurzrock E et al: Ontogeny of the male urethra: Theory of endodermal differentiation. Differentiation 1999;64:115.

Levin HS: Tumors of the testis in intersex syndromes. Urol Clin North Am 2000;27(3):543.

Ludwikowski B et al: Total urogenital sinus mobilization: Expanded applications. BJU Int 1999;83(7):820.

McAleer IM, Kaplan GW: Is routine karyotyping necessary in the evaluation of hypospadias and cryptorchidism? J Urol 2001; 165(6 Pt 1):2029, discussion 2031.

McIndoe A: The treatment of congenital absence and obliterative conditions of the vagina. Br J Plast Surg 1950;2:254.

Melton L: New perspectives on the management of intersex. Lancet 2001;357(9274):2110.

Meyer-Bahlburg HF: Gender and sexuality in classic congenital adrenal hyperplasia. Endocrinol Metab Clin North Am 2001; 30(1):155.

Migeon CJ, Wisniewski AB: Human sex differentiation: From transcription factors to gender. Horm Res 2000;53(3):111.

Migeon CJ et al: Ambiguous genitalia with perineoscrotal hypospadias in 46,XY individuals: Long-term medical, surgical, and psychosexual outcome. Pediatrics 2002;110(3):31.

Migeon CJ et al: 46,XY intersex individuals: Phenotypic and etiologic classification, knowledge of condition, and satisfaction with knowledge in adulthood. Pediatrics 2002;110(3):32.

Miller W: Dexamethasone treatment of congenital hyperplasia in utero: An experimental therapy of unproven safety. J Urol 1999;162:537.

Mittwoch U: Genetics of sex determination: Exceptions that prove the rule. Mol Genet Metab 2000;71(1–2):405.

Morel Y et al: Aetiological diagnosis of male sex ambiguity: A collaborative study. Eur J Pediatr 2002;161(1):49.

Morland I: Management of intersex. Lancet 2001;358(9298):2085.

Mureau MA et al: Satisfaction with penile appearance after hypospadias surgery: The patient and surgeon view. J Urol 1996;155(2):703.

Pachter EM et al: True hermaphrodite. Urology 1998;52(2):318.

Pang SY et al: Prenatal treatment of congenital adrenal hyperplasia due to 21-hydroxylase deficiency. N Engl J Med 1990; 322(2):111.

Rey RA et al: Evaluation of gonadal function in 107 intersex patients by means of serum antimullerian hormone measurement. J Clin Endocrinol Metab 1999;84(2):627.

Schober JM: A surgeon's response to the intersex controversy. J Clin Ethics 1998;9(4):393.

Schober JM: Sexual behaviors, sexual orientation and gender identity in adult intersexuals: A pilot study. J Urol 2001;165(6 Pt 2):2350.

Shapiro E: The sonographic appearance of normal and abnormal fetal genitalia. J Urol 1999;162(2):530.

van der Werff JF et al: Normal development of the male anterior urethra. Teratology 2000;61(3):172.

Warne GL et al: Androgen insensitivity syndrome in the era of molecular genetics and the Internet: A point of view. J Pediatr Endocrinol Metab 1998;11(1):3.

Wilson BE, Reiner WG: Management of intersex: A shifting paradigm. J Clin Ethics 1998;9(4):360.

Wilson JD et al: Steroid 5 alpha-reductase 2 deficiency. Endocr Rev 1993;14(5):577.

Wisniewski AB, Migeon CJ: Gender identity/role differentiation in adolescents affected by syndromes of abnormal sex differentiation. Adolesc Med 2002;13(1):119.

Wisniewski AB et al: Complete androgen insensitivity syndrome: Long-term medical, surgical, and psychosexual outcome. J Clin Endocrinol Metab 2000;85(8):2664.

Woodhouse CR: Prospects for fertility in patients born with genitourinary anomalies. J Urol 2001;165(6 Pt 2):2354.

Male Infertility

42

Paul J. Turek, MD

Infertility is defined as the inability to conceive after 1 year of unprotected sexual intercourse. Infertility affects approximately 15% of couples. Roughly 40% of cases involve a male contribution or factor, 40% involve a female factor, and the remainder involve both sexes. The evaluation of male infertility is undertaken methodically to acquire several kinds of information. Before discussing the diagnosis and treatment of male infertility, a review of basic reproductive tract physiology is in order.

■ MALE REPRODUCTIVE PHYSIOLOGY

THE HYPOTHALAMIC-PITUITARY-GONADAL AXIS

The physiology of the hypothalamic-pituitary-gonadal (HPG) axis plays a critical role in each of the following processes, the last 2 of which are relevant for reproduction:

1. Phenotypic gender development during embryogenesis
2. Sexual maturation during puberty
3. Endocrine function of the testis: testosterone production
4. Exocrine function of the testis: sperm production

Basic Endocrine Concepts

A. HORMONE CLASSES (FIGURE 42–1)

Two kinds of hormones classically mediate communication in the reproductive hormone axis: peptide and steroid. Peptide hormones are small secretory proteins that act via receptors on the cell surface membrane. Hormone signals are transduced by one of 3 second-messenger pathways, as outlined in Figure 42–1. Ultimately, most peptide hormones induce the phosphorylation of various proteins that alter cell function. Examples of peptide hormones are luteinizing hormone (LH) and follicle-stimulating hormone (FSH).

In contrast, steroid hormones are derived from cholesterol and are not stored in secretory granules; consequently, steroid secretion rates directly reflect production rates. In plasma, these hormones are usually bound to carrier proteins. Since they are lipophilic, steroid hormones are generally cell membrane–permeable. After binding to an intracellular receptor, steroids are translocated to DNA recognition sites within the nucleus and regulate the transcription of target genes. Examples of reproductive steroid hormones are testosterone and estradiol.

B. FEEDBACK LOOPS

Normal reproduction depends on the cooperation of numerous hormones, and thus the signals that hormones generate must be well controlled. Feedback control is the principal mechanism through which this occurs. With feedback, a hormone can regulate the synthesis and action of itself or of another hormone. Further coordination is provided by hormone action at multiple sites and eliciting multiple responses. In the HPG axis, negative feedback activity is responsible for minimizing hormonal perturbations and maintaining homeostasis.

Components of the HPG Axis (Figure 42–2)

A. HYPOTHALAMUS

As the integrative center of the HPG axis, the hypothalamus receives neuronal input from many brain centers, including the amygdala, thalamus, pons, retina, and cortex, and is the pulse generator for the cyclical secretion of pituitary and gonadal hormones. It is anatomically linked to the pituitary gland by both a portal vascular system and neuronal pathways. By avoiding the systemic circulation, the portal vascular system provides a direct mechanism for the delivery of hypothalamic hormones to the anterior pituitary. Of the several hypothalamic hormones that act on the pituitary gland, the most important one for reproduction is gonadotropin-releasing or LH-releasing hormone (GnRH or LHRH), a 10–amino acid peptide secreted from the neuronal cell bodies in the preoptic and arcuate nuclei. At present, the only known function of GnRH is to stimulate the secretion of LH and FSH from the anterior pituitary. Once secreted into the pituitary portal circulation, GnRH has a half-life of approximately 5–7 min,

Figure 42–1. Two kinds of hormone classes mediate intercellular communication in the reproductive hormone axis: peptide and steroid.

almost entirely removed on the first pass through the pituitary either by receptor internalization or enzymatic degradation.

GnRH secretion by the hypothalamus results from integrated input from a variety of influences, including the effects of stress, exercise, and diet from higher brain centers, gonadotropins secreted from the pituitary, and circulating gonadal hormones. Known substances that regulate GnRH secretion are listed in Table 42–1.

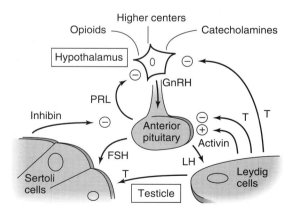

Figure 42–2. Major components of the HPG axis and recognized hormone feedback pathways. GnRH, gonadotropin-releasing hormone; PRL, prolactin; T, testosterone; FSH, follicle-stimulating hormone; LH, luteinizing hormone; +, positive feedback; −, negative feedback.

Table 42–1. Substances that modulate GnRH secretion.

GnRH Modulator	Type of Feedback	Examples
Opioids	Negative/inhibitory	β-Endorphin
Catecholamines	Variable	Dopamine
Peptide hormones	Negative/inhibitory	FSH, LH
Sex steroids	Negative/inhibitory	Testosterone
Prostaglandins	Positive/stimulatory	PGE_2

FSH, follicle-stimulating hormone; LH, luteinizing hormone; PGE_2, prostaglandin E_2.

GnRH secretion is pulsatile in nature. This secretory pattern governs the concomitant cyclic release of the gonadotropins LH and FSH (to a lesser extent) from the pituitary. The pulse frequency appears to vary from once hourly to as seldom as once or twice in 24 h. The importance of the pulsatile GnRH secretory pattern in normal reproductive function is aptly demonstrated by the ability of the exogenously given GnRH agonists Lupron or Zoladex (leuprolide acetate) to halt testosterone production within the testicle by changing the pituitary exposure to GnRH from a cyclic to a constant pattern.

B. ANTERIOR PITUITARY

The anterior pituitary gland, located within the bony sella turcica of the cranium, is the site of action of GnRH. GnRH stimulates the production and release of FSH and LH by a calcium flux-dependent mechanism. These peptide hormones were named after their elucidation in the female, but it is recognized that they are equally important in the male. The sensitivity of the pituitary gonadotrophs for GnRH varies with patient age and hormonal status.

LH and FSH are the primary pituitary hormones that regulate testis function. They are both glycoproteins composed of 2 polypeptide chain subunits, termed α and β, each coded by a separate gene. The α subunit of each hormone is identical and is similar to that of all other pituitary hormones; biologic and immunologic activity are conferred by the unique β subunit. Both subunits are required for endocrine activity. Sugars linked to these peptide subunits, consisting of oligosaccharides with sialic acid residues, differ in content between FSH and LH and may account for differences in signal transduction and plasma clearance of these hormones.

Secretory pulses of LH vary in frequency from 8 to 16 pulses in 24 h and vary in amplitude by 1- to 3-fold. These pulse patterns generally reflect GnRH release. Both androgens and estrogens regulate LH secretion through negative feedback. On average, FSH pulses occur approximately every 1.5 h and vary in amplitude by 25%. The FSH response to GnRH is more difficult to measure than that of LH because of a smaller amplitude response and a longer serum half-life. The recently discovered gonadal proteins inhibin and activin may exert significant effects on FSH secretion and are thought to account for the relative secretory independence of FSH from GnRH secretion. They will be discussed in the Testis section.

The only known effects of FSH and LH are in the gonads. They activate adenylate cyclase, which leads to increases in intracellular cAMP. In the testis, LH stimulates steroidogenesis within Leydig cells by inducing the mitochondrial conversion of cholesterol to pregnenolone and testosterone. FSH binds to Sertoli cells and spermatogonial membranes within the testis and is the major stimulator of seminiferous tubule growth during development. FSH is essential for the initiation of spermatogenesis at puberty. In the adult, the major physiologic role of FSH is to stimulate quantitatively normal levels of spermatogenesis.

A third anterior pituitary hormone, prolactin, can also have effects on the HPG axis and fertility. Prolactin is a large, globular protein of 199 amino acids (23 kDa) that is known to affect milk synthesis during pregnancy and lactation in women. The normal role of prolactin in men is less clear, but it may increase the concentration of LH receptors on the Leydig cell and help sustain normal, high intratesticular testosterone levels. It may also potentiate the effects of androgens on the growth and secretions of the male accessory sex glands. Normal prolactin levels may be important in the maintenance of libido. Although low prolactin levels are not necessarily pathologic, evidence suggests that hyperprolactinemia abolishes gonadotropin pulsatility by interfering with episodic GnRH release.

C. The Testis

Normal male virility and fertility requires the collaboration of both the exocrine and endocrine testis. Both units are under the direct control of the HPG axis. The interstitial compartment, composed mainly of Leydig cells, is responsible for steroidogenesis. The seminiferous tubules have an exocrine function with spermatozoa as the product.

1. Endocrine testis—Normal testosterone production in men is approximately 5 g/d, and secretion occurs in a damped, irregular, pulsatile manner. In normal men, approximately 2% of testosterone is "free" or unbound and considered the biologically active fraction. The remainder is almost equally bound to albumin or sex hormone-binding globulin (SHBG) within the blood. SHBG can also bind estradiol in the peripheral blood, but the binding affinity is lower than that of testosterone. Several pathologic conditions can alter SHBG

levels within the blood and, as a consequence, change the amount of free or bioactive testosterone available for tissues. Elevated estrogens and thyroid hormone decrease plasma SHBG and therefore increase the free testosterone fraction, whereas androgens, growth hormone, and obesity increase SHBG levels and decrease the active androgen fraction. Testosterone is a profound regulator of its own production through negative feedback on the HPG axis.

Testosterone is metabolized into 2 major active metabolites in the target tissue: (1) the major androgen dihydrotestosterone (DHT) from the action of 5 α-reductase and (2) the estrogen estradiol through the action of aromatases. DHT is a much more potent androgen than is testosterone. In most peripheral tissues, testosterone reduction to DHT is required for androgen action, but in the testis and probably skeletal muscle, conversion to DHT is not essential for hormonal activity.

2. Exocrine testis—The primary site of FSH action is on Sertoli cells within the seminiferous tubules. In response to FSH binding, Sertoli cells are stimulated to make a host of secretory products important for germ cell growth, including androgen-binding protein (an effect augmented by testosterone), transferrin, lactate, ceruloplasmin, clusterin, plasminogen activator, prostaglandins, and several growth factors. Through these FSH-mediated actions, seminiferous tubule growth is stimulated during development and sperm production is initiated during puberty. In adults it is thought that FSH is required for normal spermatogenesis.

3. Inhibin and activin—Inhibin is a 32-kDa protein derived from Sertoli cells that specifically inhibits FSH release from the pituitary. Within the testis, inhibin production is stimulated by FSH and acts by negative feedback at the pituitary or hypothalamus. Recently, activin, a protein hormone with close structural homology to transforming growth factor-β, has also been purified and cloned and appears to exert a stimulatory effect on FSH secretion. Activin consists of a combination of 2 of the same β subunits found in inhibin and is also derived from the testis. Activin receptors are found in a host of extragonadal tissues, suggesting that this hormone may have a variety of growth factor or regulatory roles in the body.

SPERMATOGENESIS

Spermatogenesis is a complex process by which primitive, totipotent stem cells divide to either renew themselves or produce daughter cells that become spermatozoa. These processes occur within the seminiferous tubules of the testis. In fact, 90% of testis volume is determined by the seminiferous tubules and germ cells at various developmental stages.

Sertoli Cells

The seminiferous tubules are lined with Sertoli cells that rest on the tubular basement membrane and extend into its lumen with a complex cytoplasm. Sertoli cells are linked by tight junctions, the strongest intercellular barriers in the body. These junctional complexes divide the seminiferous tubule space into basal (basement membrane) and adluminal (lumen) compartments. This anatomic arrangement forms the basis for the blood-testis barrier, allowing spermatogenesis to occur in an immunologically privileged site. The importance of this sanctuary effect becomes clear when we remember that spermatozoa are produced at puberty and are considered foreign to an immune system that develops self-recognition during the first year of life.

Sertoli cells serve as "nurse" cells for spermatogenesis, nourishing germ cells as they develop. These specialized support cells also participate in germ cell phagocytosis. High-affinity FSH receptors exist on Sertoli cells and FSH binding induces the production of androgen-binding protein, which is then secreted into the tubular luminal fluid. By binding testosterone, androgen-binding protein ensures that high levels of androgen ($20-50 \times$ that of serum) exist within the seminiferous tubules. Evidence also suggests that inhibin is Sertoli cell–derived. Ligand-receptor complexes, such as c-*kit* and kit ligand, may also mediate communication between germinal and Sertoli cells.

Germ Cells

Within the tubule, germ cells are arranged in a highly ordered sequence from the basement membrane to the lumen. Spermatogonia lie directly on the basement membrane, followed by primary spermatocytes, secondary spermatocytes, and spermatids toward the tubule lumen. In all, 13 different germ cell stages have been identified in humans. The tight junction barrier supports spermatogonia and early spermatocytes within the basal compartment and all subsequent germ cells within the adluminal compartment. Germ cells are staged by their morphologic appearance; there are dark type A (Ad) and pale type A (Ap) and type B spermatogonia and preleptotene, leptotene, zygotene, and pachytene primary spermatocytes, secondary spermatocytes, and Sa, Sb, Sc, Sd_1, and Sd_2 spermatids.

Cycles & Waves

A cycle of spermatogenesis involves the division of primitive spermatogonial stem cells into subsequent germ cells. Several cycles of spermatogenesis coexist within the germinal epithelium at any one time. The duration of an entire spermatogenic cycle within the human testis is 74 days. During spermatogenesis, cohorts of germ cells at the same point in development are linked by cytoplasmic bridges and pass through the process together. There is also a specific organization of the steps of the spermatogenic cycle within the tubular space, termed spermatogenic waves. In humans, this is likely a spiral cellular arrangement, which probably exists to ensure that sperm production is a continuous and not a pulsatile process.

MEIOSIS & MITOSIS

Basic Processes

Somatic cells replicate by mitosis, in which genetically identical daughter cells are formed. Germ cells replicate by meiosis, in which the genetic material is halved to allow for reproduction. Meiosis and sexual reproduction generate genetic diversity, providing a richer source of material on which natural selection can act. The life of a cell is divided into cycles, each of which is associated with different activities. About 5–10% of the cell cycle is spent in the mitotic phase (M), in which DNA and cellular division occurs. Cell replication by mitosis is a precise, well-orchestrated sequence of events involving duplication of the genetic material (chromosomes), breakdown of the nuclear envelope, and equal division of the chromosomes and cytoplasm into 2 daughter cells (Table 42–2). The essential difference between mitotic and meiotic replication is that a single DNA duplication step is followed by only 1 cell division in mitosis, but 2 cell divisions in meiosis (4 daughter cells). As a consequence, daughter cells contain only half of the chromosome content of the parent cell. Thus, a diploid (2*n*) parent cell becomes a haploid (*n*) gamete. Figure 42–3 illustrates how the DNA content of the dividing cell changes with mitosis and meiosis. Other major differences between mitosis and meiosis are outlined in Table 42–3.

Table 42–2. Phases of the cell cycle and mitosis.

Mitotic Phase	Cell Cycle	Description of Events
Interphase	G_1, S, G_2	DNA doubling occurs.
Prophase	M	Nuclear envelope dissolves; spindle forms.
Metaphase	M	Chromosomes align at cell equator.
Anaphase	M	Duplicated chromosomes separate.
Telophase	M	Chromosomes to poles, cytoplasm divides.

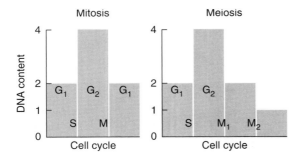

Figure 42–3. Changes in nuclear DNA content with mitosis and meiosis. G, growth phase; S, DNA synthesis phase; M, mitotic phase.

Making Sperm

The mature spermatozoan is an elaborate, specialized cell produced in massive quantity, up to 300 per g of testis per second. Type B spermatogonia divide mitotically to produce diploid primary spermatocytes (2n), which then duplicate their DNA during interphase. After the first meiotic division, each daughter cell contains one partner of the homologous chromosome pair, and they are called secondary spermatocytes (2n). These cells rapidly enter the second meiotic division in which the chromatids then separate at the centromere to yield haploid early round spermatids (n). Thus, each primary spermatocyte theoretically yields 4 spermatids, although fewer actually result, as the complexity of meiosis is associated with germ cell loss.

Table 42–3. Essential differences between mitosis and meiosis.

Mitosis	Meiosis
Occurs in somatic cells	Occurs in sexual cycle cells
1 cell division, 2 daughter cells	2 cell divisions, 4 daughter cells
Chromosome number maintained	Chromosome number halved
No pairing, chromosome homologs	Synapse of homologs, prophase I
No crossovers	> 1 crossover per homolog pair
Centromeres divide, anaphase	Centromeres divide, anaphase II
Identical daughter genotype	Genetic variation in daughter cells

The process by which spermatids become mature spermatozoa within the Sertoli cell can take several weeks and consists of several events:

1. The acrosome is formed from the Golgi apparatus.
2. A flagellum is constructed from the centriole.
3. Mitochondria reorganize around the midpiece.
4. The nucleus is compacted to about 10% of its former size.
5. Residual cell cytoplasm is eliminated.

The nucleus of the round spermatid is spherical but the shape changes from spherical to asymmetric as chromatin condenses. It is theorized that many cellular elements contribute to the reshaping process, including chromosome structure, associated chromosomal proteins, the perinuclear cytoskeletal theca layer, the manchette of microtubules in the nucleus, subacrosomal actin, and Sertoli cell interactions.

With completion of spermatid elongation, the Sertoli cell cytoplasm retracts around the developing sperm, stripping it of all unnecessary cytoplasm and extruding it into the tubule lumen. The mature sperm has remarkably little cytoplasm.

Sperm Maturation: The Epididymis

Spermatozoa within the testis have very poor or no motility and are incapable of fertilizing an egg. They become functional only after traversing the epididymis and the additional maturation process that it entails. Anatomically, the epididymis is classically divided into 3 regions: caput or head, corpus or body, and cauda or tail. Passage through the epididymis induces many changes to the newly formed sperm, including alterations in net surface charge, membrane protein composition, immunoreactivity, phospholipid and fatty acid content, and adenylate cyclase activity. These changes are thought to improve the membrane structural integrity and increase fertilization ability. The transit time of sperm through the fine tubules of the epididymis is thought to be 10–15 days in humans.

FERTILIZATION

Fertilization normally occurs within the ampullary portion of the fallopian tubes. During the middle of the female menstrual cycle the cervical mucus changes, becoming more abundant and watery. These changes facilitate the entry of sperm into the uterus and protect the sperm from the highly acidic vaginal secretions. Within the female reproductive tract, sperm undergo physiologic changes, generally referred to as capacitation. After sperm contact with the egg, a new type of flagellar motion is initiated, termed hyperactive motility, characterized by large, lashing motions of the sperm tail. Sperm release lytic enzymes from the acrosome region to help penetrate the egg investments, termed the acrosome reaction. Direct contact between the sperm and egg appears to be mediated by specific receptors on the surface of each gamete. As a result of the interactions and changes, the sperm is incorporated into the cytoplasm of the egg.

After penetration of the egg, a "zona reaction" occurs in which the zona pellucida becomes impenetrable to more sperm, providing a block to polyspermy. In addition, the egg resumes its meiosis and begins to form a metaphase II spindle. The sperm centriole within the midpiece is crucial for early spindle formation within the fertilized egg.

■ DIAGNOSIS OF MALE INFERTILITY

Given that a male factor can be identified as the cause of infertility in 30–40% of couples and is a contributing factor in 50% of cases, it is important to evaluate the male and female partners in parallel. Although infertility is defined as a failure to conceive after 1 year of unprotected sexual intercourse, couples may be anxious to proceed with an evaluation sooner and this may be appropriate. A complete urologic evaluation is important because male infertility may be the presenting symptom of otherwise occult but significant systemic disease. The evaluation involves collecting 4 types of information, as outlined in Figure 42–4.

HISTORY

The cornerstone of the male partner evaluation is the history. It should note the duration of infertility, earlier pregnancies with present or past partners, and whether there was previous difficulty with conception. A comprehensive list of information relevant to the fertility history is given in Table 42–4.

A sexual history should be addressed. Most men (80%) do not know how to precisely time intercourse to achieve a pregnancy. Since sperm reside within the cervical mucus and crypts for 1–2 days, an appropriate frequency of intercourse is every 2 days for most men. Lubricants can influence sperm motility and should be avoided. Commonly used products such as K-Y Jelly, Surgilube, Lubifax, most skin lotions, and saliva significantly reduce sperm motility in vitro. If needed, acceptable lubricants include vegetable, safflower, and peanut oils.

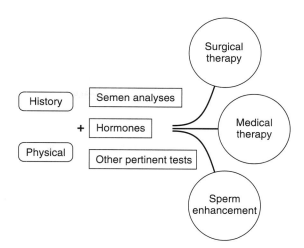

Figure 42–4. The male infertility evaluation consists of 4 kinds of information: the history, physical examination, semen analysis, and hormone assessment. Several therapeutic directions are possible once this information is collected.

A general medical and surgical history is also important. Any generalized insult such as a fever, viremia, or other acute infection can decrease testis function and semen quality. The effects of such insults are not noted in the semen until 2–3 months after the event, because spermatogenesis requires 75 days to complete. Surgical procedures on the bladder, retroperitoneum, or pelvis can also lead to infertility, by causing either retrograde ejaculation of sperm into the bladder or anejaculation (aspermia), in which the muscular function within the entire reproductive tract is inhibited. Hernia surgery can also result in vas deferens obstruction in 1% of cases; this incidence may be rising because of the recent increased use of mesh patches that tend to be inflammatory to tissues.

Childhood diseases may also affect fertility. A history of mumps can be significant if the infection occurs postpubertally. After age 11, unilateral orchitis occurs in 30% of mumps infections and bilateral orchitis in 10%. Mumps orchitis is thought to cause pressure necrosis of testis tissue from viral edema. Marked testis atrophy is usually obvious later in life. Cryptorchidism is also associated with decreased sperm production. This is true for both unilateral and bilateral cases. Longitudinal studies of affected boys have shown that abnormally low sperm counts can be found in 30% of men with unilateral cryptorchidism and 50% of men with bilateral undescended testes. Differences in fertility have not been as easy to demonstrate, but it appears that boys with unilateral cryptorchidism have a slightly higher risk of infer-

Table 42–4. Components of the infertility history.

Medical history
  Fevers
  Systemic illness—diabetes, cancer, infection
  Genetic diseases—cystic fibrosis, Klinefelter syndrome
Surgical history
  Orchidopexy, cryptorchidism
  Herniorraphy
  Trauma, torsion
  Pelvic, bladder, or retroperitoneal surgery
  Transurethral resection for prostatism
  Pubertal onset
Fertility history
  Previous pregnancies (present and with other partners)
  Duration of infertility
  Previous infertility treatments
  Female evaluation
Sexual history
  Erections
  Timing and frequency
  Lubricants
Family history
  Cryptorchidism
  Midline defects (Kartagener syndrome)
  Hypospadias
  Exposure to diethylstilbestrol
  Other rare syndromes—prune belly, etc.
Medication history
  Nitrofurantoin
  Cimetidine
  Sulfasalazine
  Spironolactone
  Alpha blockers
Social history
  Ethanol
  Smoking/tobacco
  Cocaine
  Anabolic steroids
Occupational history
  Exposure to ionizing radiation
  Chronic heat exposure (saunas)
  Aniline dyes
  Pesticides
  Heavy metals (lead)

tility. However, only 50% of men with a history of bilateral undescended testes are fertile. It is important to remember that orchidopexy performed for this problem does not improve semen quality later in life.

Exposure and medication histories are very relevant to fertility. Decreased sperm counts have been demonstrated in workers exposed to specific pesticides, thought to result from a shift in the normal testosterone/estrogen hormonal balance. Ionizing radiation is also a well-described exposure risk, with temporary reductions in sperm production seen at doses as low as 10 cGy. Several medications (Table 42–5) and ingestants such as tobacco, cocaine, and marijuana have all been implicated as gonadotoxins. The effects of these agents are usually reversible on withdrawal. Androgenic steroids, often taken by bodybuilders to increase muscle mass and development, act as contraceptives with respect to fertility. Excess testosterone inhibits the pituitary-gonadal hormone axis. The routine use of hot tubs or saunas should be discouraged, as these activities can elevate intratesticular temperature and impair sperm production. In general, a healthy body is the best reproductive body.

The family and developmental histories may also provide clues about infertility. A family history of cystic fibrosis (CF), a condition associated with congenital absence of the vas deferens (CAVD), or intersex conditions is important. The existence of siblings with fertility problems may suggest that a Y chromosome microdeletion or a cytogenetic (karyotype) abnormality is present in the family. A history of delayed onset of puberty could suggest Kallmann or Klinefelter syndrome. A history of recurrent respiratory tract infections may suggest a ciliary defect characteristic of the immotile cilia syndromes. It is important to remember that reproductive technologies enable most men afflicted with such conditions to become fathers and therefore allow for the perpetuation of genetic abnormalities that may not be normally sustained.

PHYSICAL EXAMINATION

A complete examination of the infertile male is important to identify general health issues associated with infertility. For example, the patient should be adequately virilized; signs of decreased body hair or gynecomastia may suggest androgen deficiency.

The scrotal contents should be carefully palpated with the patient standing. As it is often psychologically un-

Table 42–5. Medications associated with impaired ejaculation.

Antihypertensive agents
Alpha-adrenergic blockers (Prazosin, Phentolamine)
  Thiazides
Antipsychotic agents
  Mellaril (thioridazine)
  Haldol (haloperidol)
  Librium
Antidepressants
  Imipramine
  Amitriptyline

comfortable for young men to be examined, one helpful hint is to make the examination as efficient and as matter of fact as possible. Two features should be noted about the testis: size and consistency. Size is assessed by measuring the long axis and width; as an alternative, an orchidometer can be placed next to the testis for volume determination (Figure 42–5). Standard values of testis size have been reported for normal men and include a mean testis length of 4.6 cm (range 3.6–5.5 cm), a mean width of 2.6 cm (range 2.1–3.2 cm), and a mean volume of 18.6 mL (± 4.6 mL) (Figure 42–6). Consistency is more difficult to assess but can be described as firm (normal) or soft (abnormal). A smaller or softer than normal testis usually indicates impaired spermatogenesis.

The peritesticular area should also be examined. Irregularities of the epididymis, located posterior-lateral to the testis, include induration, tenderness, or cysts. The presence or absence of the scrotal vas deferens is critical to observe, as 2% of infertile men may present with CAVD. Engorgement of the pampiniform plexus of veins in the scrotum is indicative of a varicocele. Asymmetry of the spermatic cords is the usual initial observation, followed by the feeling of an "impulse" with increased intra-abdominal pressure associated with a Valsalva maneuver. Varicoceles are usually found on the left side (90%) and are commonly associated with atrophy of the left testis. A discrepancy in testis size between the right and left sides should alert the clinician to the possibility of varicocele.

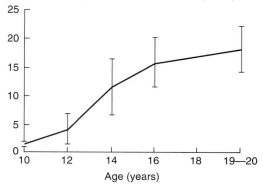

Normal ranges for testicular volume (mean)

Figure 42–6. Normal values for testicular volume in relation to age. (Redrawn and reproduced, with permission, from Zachman M et al: Testicular volume during adolescence: Cross-sectional and longitudinal studies. Helv Paediatr Acta 1974;29:61, and McClure RD: Endocrine investigation and therapy. Urol Clin North Am 1987;14:471.)

Prostate or penile abnormalities should also be noted. Penile abnormalities such as hypospadias, abnormal curvature, or phimosis could result in inadequate delivery of semen to the upper vaginal vault during intercourse. Prostatic infection may be detected by the finding of a boggy, tender prostate on rectal examination. Prostate cancer, often suspected with unusual firmness or a nodule within the prostate, can occasionally be diagnosed in infertile men. Enlarged seminal vesicles, indicative of ejaculatory duct obstruction, may also be palpable on rectal examination.

LABORATORY

Laboratory testing is an important part of the male infertility evaluation.

Urinalysis

A urinalysis is a simple test that can be performed during the initial office visit. It may indicate the presence of infection, hematuria, glucosuria, or renal disease, and as such may suggest anatomic or medical problems within the urinary tract.

Semen Analysis

A carefully performed semen analysis is the primary source of information on sperm production and reproductive tract patency. However, it is not a measure of

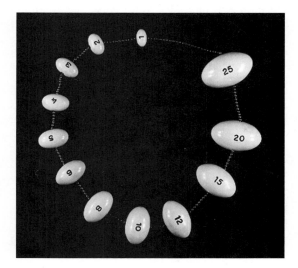

Figure 42–5. Prader orchidometer for measuring testicular volume. (Reproduced, with permission, from McClure RD: Endocrine investigation and therapy. Urol Clin North Am 1987;14:471.)

fertility. An abnormal semen analysis simply suggests the likelihood of decreased fertility. Studies have established that there are certain limits of adequacy below which it may be difficult to initiate a pregnancy. These semen analysis values were identified by the World Health Organization (1992) and are considered the minimum criteria for "normal" semen quality (Table 42–6). It is statistically more difficult to achieve a pregnancy if a semen parameter falls below any of those listed. Of these semen variables, the count and motility appear to correlate best with fertility.

A. SEMEN COLLECTION

Semen quality can vary widely in a normal individual from day to day, and semen analysis results are very dependent on collection technique. For example, the period of sexual abstinence before sample collection is a large source of variability. With each day of abstinence (up to 1 week), semen volume can rise by up to 0.4 mL, and sperm concentration can increase by 10–15 million/mL. Sperm motility tends to fall when the abstinence period is longer than 7 days. For this reason, it is recommended that semen be collected after 48–72 h of sexual abstinence.

To establish a baseline of semen quality, at least 2 semen samples are needed. Semen should be collected by self-stimulation, by coitus interruptus (less ideal), or with a special, nonspermicidal condom into a wide-mouthed, clean (not necessarily sterile) glass or plastic container. Because sperm motility decreases after ejaculation, it is important to have the specimen analyzed within 1 h of procurement. During transit, the specimen should be kept at body temperature.

B. PHYSICAL CHARACTERISTICS AND MEASURED VARIABLES

Fresh semen is a coagulum that liquefies 5–30 min after ejaculation. After liquefaction, semen viscosity is measured and should not show any stranding. Ejaculate volume should be at least 1.5 mL, as smaller volumes may not sufficiently buffer against vaginal acidity. Low ejaculate volume may indicate retrograde ejaculation,

Table 42–6. Semen analysis—minimal standards of adequacy.

Ejaculate volume	1.5–5.5 mL
Sperm concentration	$> 20 \times 10^6$ sperm/mL
Motility	> 50%
Forward progression	2 (scale 1–4)
Morphology	> 30% WHO normal forms (> 4% Kruger normal forms)

No agglutination (clumping), white cells, or increased viscosity.

ejaculatory duct obstruction, incomplete collection, or androgen deficiency. Sperm concentration should be > 20 million sperm/mL. Sperm motility is assessed in 2 ways: the fraction or percentage of all sperm that are moving and the quality of sperm movement (how fast, how straight they swim). A normal value for sperm motility is 50–60% motile and quality or progression score of at least 2 (on a scale of 0 [no movement] to 4 [excellent progression]).

Sperm cytology or morphology is another measure of semen quality. By assessing the exact dimensions and shape characteristics of the sperm head, midpiece, and tail, sperm can be classified as "normal" or not. In the strictest classification system (Kruger morphology), only 14% of sperm in the entire ejaculate are truly normal looking. In fact, this number correlates with the success of egg fertilization in vitro and thus is ascribed real clinical significance. In addition, it is accepted that sperm morphology is a sensitive indicator of overall testicular health, because the sperm morphologic characteristics are determined during spermatogenesis. The role of sperm morphology assessment in the male infertility evaluation is to complement other information and to better estimate the chances of fertility.

C. COMPUTER-ASSISTED SEMEN ANALYSIS (CASA)

In an effort to remove the subjective variables inherent in the manual semen analysis, there have been attempts to quantify sperm motility, concentration, and morphology with computers. Computer-aided semen analyses couple video technology with digitalization and microchip processing to categorize sperm features by algorithms. Most commonly, CASA systems report sperm concentration, motilities, and velocities (curvilinear, straight-line) and can be used to analyze sperm shape by examination of nuclear features. Although the technology is promising, when manual semen analysis findings are compared with those from CASA on identical specimens, CASA can overestimate sperm counts by 30% in the presence of high levels of contaminating cells such as immature sperm or leukocytes. In addition, at high sperm concentrations, motility can be underestimated with CASA. At this point, CASA has accepted value in the research setting and is gaining further clinical acceptance.

D. SEMINAL FRUCTOSE AND POSTEJACULATE URINALYSIS

Fructose is a carbohydrate derived from the seminal vesicles and is normally present in the ejaculate. If absent, the condition of seminal vesicle agenesis or obstruction may exist. Seminal fructose testing is indicated in men with low ejaculate volumes and no sperm. A postejaculate urinalysis is a microscopic inspection of the first voided urine after ejaculation for sperm. If sperm are found in the voided urine, then retrograde ejaculation is diagnosed. Such an analysis is indicated in diabetic patients with low semen volume and sperm counts; patients with a history of pelvic, bladder, or retroperitoneal surgery; and patients receiving medical therapy for prostatic enlargement. In general, the semen analyses of infertile men have patterns that may suggest a diagnosis (Table 42–7).

Hormone Assessment

An evaluation of the pituitary-gonadal axis can provide valuable information on the state of sperm production. In turn, it can reveal problems with the pituitary axis that can cause infertility (hyperprolactinemia, gonadotropin deficiency, congenital adrenal hyperplasia). It is recommended that FSH and testosterone levels be measured in infertile men with sperm densities of $< 10 \times 10^6$ sperm/mL. Testosterone is a measure of overall endocrine balance. FSH reflects more on the state of sperm production rather than endocrine balance. This combination of tests will detect virtually all (99%) endocrine abnormalities (Sigman and Jarow, 1997). Serum LH and prolactin levels may be obtained if testosterone and FSH are abnormal, to help pinpoint the endocrine defect. Thyroid hormone, liver function, and other organ-specific tests should be obtained if there is clinical evidence of active disease, as uncontrolled systemic illnesses can affect sperm production. The common patterns of hormonal disorders observed in infertility are given in Table 42–8.

With relatively normal spermatogenesis, low levels of plasma LH and FSH have no clinical meaning; likewise, an isolated low LH with normal testosterone is not significant. The measurement of plasma estradiol should be reserved for those men who appear underandrogenized or have gynecomastia in association with low, normal, or elevated testosterone levels.

A large retrospective study on 1035 infertility patients examined the prevalence of endocrine disorders (Sigman and Jarow, 1997). On initial testing, 20% of infertile men had an abnormal hormone level, but only 9.6% of men harbored a true endocrinopathy on repeat testing. If FSH elevations are excluded, the incidence of clinically significant endocrinopathies in infertile men is 1.7%.

In summary, the indications for hormonal evaluation of the infertile male are:

1. Sperm density of $< 10 \times 10^6$ sperm/mL on semen analysis
2. Evidence of impaired sexual function (impotence, low libido)
3. Findings suggestive of a specific endocrinopathy (eg, thyroid)

ADJUNCTIVE TESTS

Many adjunctive tests are available to help evaluate male-factor infertility if the initial evaluation fails to lead to a diagnosis. One guiding principle in this era of cost-containment is to order tests only if they will change patient management.

Semen Leukocyte Analysis

White blood cells (leukocytes) are present in all ejaculates and may play important roles in immune surveillance and clearance of abnormal sperm. Leukocytospermia or pyospermia, an increase in leukocytes in the ejaculate, is defined as $> 1 \times 10^6$ leukocytes/mL semen and is a significant cause of male subfertility. The prevalence of pyospermia ranges from 2.8% to 23% of infertile men. In general, neutrophils predominate among inflammatory cells (Table 42–9). This condition is detected by a variety of diagnostic assays, including differential stains (eg, Papanicolaou), peroxidase stain that detects the peroxidase enzyme in neutrophils, and immunocytology.

The reason for the immune cell infiltrate in pyospermia is poorly understood, although some proposed causes include an inflammatory response associated with infection, sensitization of the immune system to sperm antigens, or a reaction to low-grade toxins like cigarette smoke or alcohol.

Antisperm Antibody Test

The testis is a curious organ in that it is an immunologically privileged site, probably owing to the blood-testis barrier. Autoimmune infertility may occur when the blood-testis barrier is broken and the body is exposed to sperm antigens. Trauma to the testis and vasectomy are 2 common ways in which this occurs, giving rise to antisperm antibodies (ASA). ASA may be associated with impaired sperm transport through the reproductive

Table 42–7. Frequency of semen analysis findings in infertile men.

	Percent
All normal	55
Isolated abnormal	37
Low motility	26
Low count	8
Volume	2
Morphology	1
No sperm	8

Table 42–8. Characteristic endocrine profiles in infertile men.

Condition	T	FSH	LH	PRL
Normal	NL	NL	NL	NL
Primary testis failure	Low	High	NL/High	NL
Hypogonadotropic hypogonadism	Low	Low	Low	NL
Hyperprolactinemia	Low	Low/NL	Low	High
Androgen resistance	High	High	High	NL

T, testosterone; FSH, follicle-stimulating hormone; LH, luteinizing hormone; PRL, prolactin; NL, normal.

tract or impairment in egg fertilization. An assay for ASA should be obtained when:

1. The semen analysis shows sperm agglutination or clumping.
2. Low sperm motility exists with history of testis injury or surgery.
3. There is confirmation that increased round cells are leukocytes.
4. There is unexplained infertility.

Antisperm antibodies can be found in 3 locations: serum, seminal plasma, and sperm-bound. Among these, sperm-bound antibodies are the most relevant. The antibody classes that appear to be clinically relevant include IgG and IgA. IgG antibody is derived from local production and from transudation from the bloodstream (1%). IgA is thought to be purely locally derived.

Hypoosmotic Swelling Test

The most clinically useful measure of sperm viability is cell motility. However, a lack of motility does not necessarily signify absent viability. Indeed, there are clinical conditions, such as immotile-cilia syndrome and extracted testicular sperm, in which there may be immotile but otherwise presumably healthy sperm. Such sperm can now be used clinically for micromanipula-

Table 42–9. Cells involved in leukocytospermia.

Cell Type	Relative Abundance
Neutrophils	++++
Monocyte/macrophage	+
T-helper lymphocytes	+
T-suppressor lymphocytes	++
B lymphocytes	+

tion and in vitro fertilization (IVF). Cell viability can be evaluated noninvasively by using the physiologic principle of hypoosmotic swelling. Conceptually, viable cells with functional membranes should swell when placed in a hypoosmotic environment (25 mM citrate and 75 mM fructose). Since sperm have tails, the swelling response is very obvious in that tail coiling accompanies head swelling. This sperm test is indicated in cases of complete absence of sperm motility.

Sperm Penetration Assay (SPA)

It is possible to measure the ability of human sperm to penetrate a specially prepared hamster egg in a laboratory setting. The hamster egg allows interspecies fertilization but no further development. This form of bioassay can give important information about the ability of sperm to undergo the capacitation process as well as penetrate and fertilize the egg. Infertile sperm would be expected to penetrate and fertilize a lower fraction of eggs than normal sperm. The indications for the diagnostic SPA are limited to situations in which functional information about sperm are needed, that is, to further evaluate couples with unexplained infertility and to help couples decide whether intrauterine insemination (IUI) (good SPA result) or IVF and micromanipulation (poor SPA result) is the appropriate next treatment.

Sperm–Cervical Mucus Interaction

Infertility can be caused by impaired sperm transport in the female reproductive tract. An evaluation of interaction between sperm and cervical mucus is one way to assess the quality of the transport process. One way to examine sperm-mucus interaction is by measuring the rate of sperm movement through a pool of cervical mucus on a microscope slide or within a capillary tube. This assay involves controls, in which sperm are placed in seminal fluid instead of cervical mucus. An abnormal cervical mucus–sperm interaction may suggest infertility treatment in which sperm are placed beyond the cervix into the uterus (IUI).

Chromosomal Studies

Subtle genetic abnormalities can present as male infertility. It is estimated that between 2% and 15% of infertile men with azoospermia (no sperm count) or severe oligospermia (low sperm counts) will harbor a chromosomal abnormality on either the sex chromosomes or autosomes. A blood test for cytogenetic analysis (karyotype) can determine if such a genetic anomaly is present. Patients at risk for abnormal cytogenetic findings include men with small, atrophic testes, elevated FSH values, and azoospermia. Klinefelter syndrome (XXY) is the most frequently detected sex chromosomal abnormality among infertile men (Figure 42–7).

Figure 42–7. Klinefelter syndrome. **Left:** Note the eunuchoid habitus, female escutcheon, gynecomastia, and lack of temporal blading. **Right:** Characteristic firm, small testes. (Reproduced, with permission, from McClure RD: Endocrine investigation and therapy. Urol Clin North Am 1987;14:471.)

Cystic Fibrosis Mutation Testing

A blood test is indicated for infertile men who present with cystic fibrosis (CF) or the much more subtle condition, CAVD. Similar genetic mutations are found in both patients, although the former group is generally considered to have an atypical form of CF, in which the scrotal vas deferens is nonpalpable. Approximately 80% of men without palpable vasa will harbor a CF gene mutation. Recent data also indicate that azoospermic men with idiopathic obstruction and men with a clinical triad of chronic sinusitis, bronchiectasis, and obstructive azoospermia (Young syndrome) may be at higher risk for CF gene mutations.

Y Chromosome Microdeletion Analysis

As many as 7% of men with oligospermia and 15% of azoospermic men have small, underlying deletions in one or more gene regions on the long arm of the Y chromosome (Yq). Several regions of the Y chromosome have been implicated in spermatogenic failure, identified as *AZFa, b,* and *c* (Figure 42–8). Deletion of the *DAZ* (deleted in azoospermia) gene in the *AZFc* region is the most commonly observed microdeletion in infertile men. Fertility is possible in men with these

deletions with IVF and micromanipulation of sperm. A polymerase chain reaction–based blood test can examine the Y chromosome from peripheral leukocytes for these gene deletions and is recommended for men with low or no sperm counts and small, atrophic testes.

Radiologic Testing

A. SCROTAL ULTRASOUND

High-frequency (7.5–10 mHz) ultrasound of the scrotum has become a mainstay in the evaluation of testicular and scrotal lesions. In men who have a hydrocele within the tunica vaginalis space, the testis may be nonpalpable and should undergo ultrasound to confirm that it is normal. Any abnormality of the peritesticular region should also undergo a scrotal ultrasound to determine its characteristics or origin.

Recently, scrotal color Doppler ultrasonography has been used to investigate varicoceles (Figure 42–9). By combining measurements of blood-flow patterns and vein size, both physiologic and anatomic information can be obtained for more accurate assessment. The diagnostic criteria that define a varicocele vary from study to study, but in general, a pampiniform venous diameter of > 2–3 mm is considered abnormal. Retrograde blood flow through the veins with a Valsalva maneuver is also an important radiologic feature of a varicocele.

B. VENOGRAPHY

Venography is generally accepted as the most accurate way to diagnose varicoceles. Although found by palpation in approximately 30–40% of subfertile men, varicoceles can be detected by venography in 70% of pa-

Figure 42–8. Regions of the Y chromosome that have been associated with male infertility include azoospermia factor (AZF) regions *a, b,* and *c*. The *AZFc* region contains the *DAZ* gene, one of the few true infertility genes isolated to date. TDF, testis-determining factor.

Figure 42–9. Scrotal ultrasound. Varicoceles are imaged as tubular echo-free structures. (Reproduced, with permission, from McClure RD, Hricak H: Scrotal ultrasound in the infertile male. Detection of subclinical unilateral and bilateral varicoceles. J Urol 1986;135:711.)

tients. Renal and spermatic venography is fairly invasive and is usually performed through percutaneous cannulization of the internal jugular vein or common femoral vein. Venographically, a varicocele is defined by a Valsalva-induced, retrograde flow of contrast material from the renal vein into the scrotal pampiniform plexus. This test is expensive and technician-dependent; at present its main indications are to guide simultaneous percutaneous treatment of varicoceles or for the diagnosis of varicocele recurrence after prior treatment.

C. Transrectal Ultrasound (TRUS)

High-frequency (5–7 mHz) TRUS offers superb imaging of the prostate, seminal vesicles, and ejaculatory ducts. Transrectal ultrasound has virtually replaced surgical vasography in the diagnosis of obstructive lesions that cause infertility. Demonstration by TRUS of dilated seminal vesicles (> 1.5 cm in width) or dilated ejaculatory ducts (> 2.3 mm) in association with a cyst, calcification, or stones along the duct is highly suggestive of ejaculatory duct obstruction (Figure 42–10). In addition, prostatic abnormalities such as tumors and congenital anomalies of the vas, seminal vesicle, or ejaculatory ducts are easily defined. The indications for TRUS in infertility include low ejaculate volumes in association with azoospermia or severe oligospermia and decreased motility.

D. Computed Tomography Scan or Magnetic Resonance Imaging of the Pelvis

The imaging techniques of CT and MRI can help define reproductive tract anatomy. However, since the ad-

Figure 42–10. Transrectal ultrasonography (sagittal view) in a man with low ejaculate volume and low sperm counts and motility. Ejaculatory duct cyst (white arrow); urethra (double white arrows); bladder (asterisk).

vent of TRUS, these studies have relatively few indications. They include evaluation of a patient with a solitary right varicocele, a condition often associated with retroperitoneal pathology, and evaluation of the non-palpable testis.

Testis Biopsy & Vasography

The testis biopsy is a useful adjunct in the infertility evaluation because it provides a more precise clinical diagnosis for several infertility disorders. Most commonly, the technique involves a small, open incision in the scrotal wall and testis tunica albuginea under local anesthesia. A small wedge of testis tissue is removed and examined histologically. Abnormalities of seminiferous tubule architecture and cellular composition can be assessed and categorized into several patterns. A testis biopsy is most useful in the azoospermic patient. It is often difficult to distinguish between a failure of sperm production and obstruction within the reproductive tract ducts in such patients. A testis biopsy allows delineation between these 2 conditions. In obstruction, formal investigation of the reproductive tract is warranted, beginning with a vasogram. A vasogram involves the injection of dye or contrast media into the vas deferens toward the bladder from the scrotum (Figure 42–11). In plain film radiographs, contrast material can delineate the proximal vas deferens, seminal vesicle, and ejaculatory duct anatomy and determine whether obstruction is present. Sampling of vasal fluid during the same procedure can also determine whether sperm exist within the scrotal vas deferens. Vasal sperm presence implies that there is no obstruction in the testis or epididymis. With this information, the site of obstruction can be accurately determined.

Whether a biopsy is indicated for oligospermia is controversial. Rare cases of partial reproductive tract obstruction may be diagnosed by biopsy, but the incidence of these disorders is low. While unilateral testis biopsies are usually sufficient, the finding of 2 asymmetric testes may warrant bilateral testis biopsies. This situation may reflect a unilateral unobstructed failing testis paired with a normal obstructed testis. Testis biopsies may also be indicated to identify patients at high risk for intratubular germ cell neoplasia. This premalignant condition exists in 5.5% of men with a contralateral germ cell tumor of the testis and is more prevalent in infertile than fertile men.

A relatively new indication for the testis biopsy is to determine whether men with atrophic, failing testes and elevated FSH levels actually have mature sperm that may be used for IVF and intracytoplasmic sperm injection (ICSI). A single testis biopsy can detect the presence of sperm in 30% of men with azoospermia, elevated FSH levels, and atrophic testes. Testicular sperm

Figure 42–11. Vasography demonstrating (**upper left**) normal vas and seminal vesicles and (**upper right**) normal reflux into the bladder, confirming duct patency. Epididymal imaging showing extravasation (**lower left**) that demonstrates the difficulty of vasal dye injection toward the testis. **Lower right:** Azoospermia from a midline ejaculatory duct cyst is shown with contrast material filling the cyst (arrow). (Reproduced, with permission, from McClure RD: Evaluation of the infertile male. In: deVere White R [editor]: *Problems in Urology.* Lippincott, 1987.)

that are harvested by biopsy are now routinely used to help men with severe male-factor infertility to achieve fatherhood.

Fine-Needle Aspiration "Mapping" of Testes (Figure 42–12)

Although testicular sperm is used with IVF and ICSI to achieve pregnancies, there is a failure to obtain sperm in 25–50% of men with testis failure. When testis biopsies fail to retrieve sperm, IVF cycles are canceled at great emotional and financial cost. To minimize the chance of failed sperm retrieval, percutaneous fine-needle aspiration and "mapping" of the testis has been described. This technique can detect sperm in 60% of men with nonobstructed azoospermia and has confirmed that

spermatogenesis can vary geographically in the failing testis such that "pockets" of sperm can exist.

Like a testis biopsy, fine-needle aspiration procedure is performed under local anesthesia. Percutaneously aspirated seminiferous tubules from various locations in the testis (5–10 mg) are smeared on a slide, fixed, stained, and read by a cytologist for the presence or absence of sperm. The information gained from this technique can fully inform patients of their chances of subsequent sperm retrieval for IVF and ICSI.

Semen Culture

Seminal fluid that passes through the urethra is routinely contaminated with bacteria. This can make the interpretation of semen culture difficult. Thus, semen

Figure 42–12. Technique of percutaneous fine-needle aspiration "mapping" for sperm in the testis. Cytologic samples are taken from various systematically sampled areas of the testis, guided by marks on the scrotum. (Reproduced, with permission, from Turek PJ, Cha I, Ljung B-M: Systematic fine needle aspiration of the testis: Correlation to biopsy and the results of organ "mapping" for mature sperm in azoospermic men. Urology 1997;49:743.)

cultures should not be obtained at random, but only in selected situations, given that 83% of all infertile men will have positive semen cultures and that the relationship between bacterial cultures and infertility is at best inconclusive. Semen cultures should be obtained when there are features suggestive of infection, including (1) a history of genital tract infection, (2) abnormal expressed prostatic secretion, (3) the presence of more than 1000 pathogenic bacteria per milliliter of semen, and (4) the presence of $> 1 \times 10^6$ leukocytes per milliliter of semen (pyospermia).

The agents most commonly responsible for male genital tract infections are listed in Table 42–10. Gonorrhea is the most common infection. Ten percent to 25% of chlamydial infections may be asymptomatic.

Table 42–10. Most common organisms in male genital infection.

Neisseria gonorrhoeae	Cytomegalovirus
Chlamydia trachomatis	Herpes simplex II
Trichomonas vaginalis	Human papilloma virus
Ureaplasma urealyticum	Epstein-Barr virus
Escherichia coli (other gram-negative bacilli)	Hepatits B virus
Mycoplasma hominis	Human immunodeficiency virus

Trichomonas vaginalis is a protozoan parasite responsible for 1–5% of nongonococcal infections; it is usually symptomatic. *Ureaplasma urealyticum* is a common inhabitant of the urethra in sexually active men (30–50% of normal men) and is responsible for one-fourth of all cases of nongonococcal infections. *Escherichia coli* infections are relatively uncommon in young men and are usually symptomatic. Mycoplasmas are aerobic bacteria that are known to colonize the male reproductive tract. Rarer but possible causes of infection include anaerobic bacteria and tuberculosis.

■ CAUSES OF MALE INFERTILITY

The causes underlying male infertility are numerous but are conveniently grouped by effects at one or more of the following levels: pretesticular, testicular, and posttesticular.

PRETESTICULAR

Conditions that cause infertility that act at the pretesticular level tend to be hormonal in nature (Table 42–11).

Table 42–11. Pretesticular causes of infertility.

Hypothalamic disease
  Gonadotropin deficiency (Kallmann syndrome)
  Isolated LH deficiency ("fertile eunuch")
  Isolated FSH deficiency
  Congenital hypogonadotropic syndromes
Pituitary disease
  Pituitary insufficiency (tumors, infiltrative processes, oper-
    ation, radiation, deposits)
  Hyperprolactinemia
  Exogenous hormones (estrogen-androgen excess,
    glucocorticoid excess, hyper- and hypothyroidism)
  Growth hormone deficiency

Hypothalamic Disease

A. GONADOTROPIN DEFICIENCY (KALLMANN SYNDROME)

Kallmann syndrome is a rare (1:50,000 persons), genetically heterogeneous disorder that occurs in familial and sporadic forms. The X-linked form of the disease is a consequence of a single gene deletion (Xp22.3 region, termed KALIG-1). It may also be autosomally transmitted with sex limitation to males. In either case, there is a disturbance of neuron migration from the olfactory placode during development. This neural region contains precursors not only for the olfactory nerves but also the LH-releasing cells of the hypothalamus, which explains the 2 most common clinical deficits in the disorder: anosmia and absence of GnRH. Pituitary function is normal. The clinical features include anosmia, facial asymmetry, color blindness, renal anomalies, microphallus, and cryptorchidism. The hallmark of the syndrome is a delay in pubertal development. The differential diagnosis includes delayed puberty. Patients have severely atrophic testes(< 2 cm) with biopsies showing germ cell arrest and Leydig cell hypoplasia. Hormone evaluation reveals low testosterone, low LH, and low FSH levels. Men can be fertile when given FSH and LH to stimulate sperm production. Virilization can be obtained with testosterone or human chorionic gonadotropin (hCG).

B. ISOLATED LH DEFICIENCY ("FERTILE EUNUCH")

This very rare condition is due to partial gonadotropin deficiency in which there is enough LH produced to stimulate intratesticular testosterone production and spermatogenesis but insufficient testosterone to promote virilization. Affected individuals have eunuchoid body proportions, variable virilization, and often gynecomastia. These men characteristically have normal testis size, but the ejaculate contains reduced numbers of sperm. Plasma FSH levels are normal, but serum LH and testosterone levels are low-normal.

C. ISOLATED FSH DEFICIENCY

In this extremely rare condition, there is insufficient FSH production by the pituitary. Patients are normally virilized, as LH is present. Testicular size is normal, and LH and testosterone levels are normal. FSH levels are uniformly low and do not respond to stimulation with GnRH. Sperm counts range from azoospermia to severely low numbers (oligospermia).

D. CONGENITAL HYPOGONADOTROPIC SYNDROMES

Several syndromes are associated with secondary hypogonadism. Prader-Willi syndrome (1:20,000 persons) is characterized by genetic obesity, retardation, small hands and feet, and hypogonadism and is caused by a deficiency of hypothalamic GnRH. The single gene deletion associated with this condition is found on chromosome 15. Similar to Kallmann syndrome, spermatogenesis can be induced with exogenous FSH and LH. Bardet-Biedl syndrome is another rare, autosomal recessive form of hypogonadotropic hypogonadism that results from GnRH deficiency. It is characterized by retardation, retinitis pigmentosa, polydactyly, and hypogonadism. The presentation is similar to Kallmann syndrome except it includes genetic obesity. The hypogonadism can be treated with FSH and LH. Cerebellar ataxia can be associated with hypogonadotropic hypogonadism. This rare condition can result from consanguineous unions. Cerebellar involvement includes abnormalities of speech and gait. These patients can be eunuchoid-looking with atrophic testes. Hypothalamic-pituitary dysfunction due to pathologic changes in cerebral white matter is thought to be the reason for infertility.

Pituitary Disease

A. PITUITARY INSUFFICIENCY

Pituitary insufficiency may result from tumors, infarcts, surgery, radiation, or infiltrative and granulomatous processes. In sickle cell anemia, pituitary and testicular microinfarcts from sickling of red blood cells are suspected of causing infertility. Men with sickle cell anemia have decreased testosterone and variable LH and FSH levels. β-Thalassemia patients have mutations in the β-globin gene that lead to an imbalance in α and β globin composition of hemoglobin; these patients are mainly of Mediterranean or African origin. Infertility is also believed to result from the deposition of iron in the pituitary gland and testes. Similarly, hemochromatosis results in iron deposition within the liver, testis, and pituitary and is associated with testicular dysfunction in 80% of cases.

B. Hyperprolactinemia

Another form of hypogonadotropic hypogonadism is due to elevated circulating prolactin. If hyperprolactinemia occurs, secondary causes such as stress during the blood draw, systemic diseases, and medications should be ruled out. With these causes excluded, the most common and important cause of hyperprolactinemia is a prolactin-secreting pituitary adenoma. High-resolution CT scanning or MRI of the sella turcica has classically been used to distinguish between microadenoma (< 10 mm) and macroadenoma (> 10 mm) forms of tumor. Stratification of disease based on radiologic diagnosis alone is misleading, as surgery for hyperprolactinemia almost always reveals a pituitary tumor. Elevated prolactin usually results in decreased FSH, LH, and testosterone levels and causes infertility. Associated symptoms include loss of libido, impotence, galactorrhea, and gynecomastia. Signs and symptoms of other pituitary hormone derangements (adrenocorticotropic hormone, thyroid-stimulating hormone) should also be investigated.

C. Exogenous or Endogenous Hormones

1. Estrogens—An excess of sex steroids, either estrogens or androgens, can cause male infertility due to an imbalance in the testosterone-estrogen ratio. Hepatic cirrhosis increases endogenous estrogens because of augmented aromatase activity within the diseased liver. Likewise, excessive obesity may be associated with testosterone-estrogen imbalance owing to increased peripheral aromatase activity. Less commonly, adrenocortical tumors, Sertoli cell tumors, and interstitial testis tumors may produce estrogens. Excess estrogens mediate infertility by decreasing pituitary gonadotropin secretion and inducing secondary testis failure. Exposure to exogenous estrogens has been implicated as a reason for the controversial finding of decreased sperm concentrations in men over the last 50 years. Supporters of this claim suggest that men are overexposed to estrogenic compounds during fetal life, which results in compromised semen quality later (Carlsen et al, 1992). Postulated sources of exposure include anabolic estrogens in livestock, consumed plant estrogens, and environmental estrogenic chemicals like pesticides. This xenoestrogen exposure theory, however, remains unproved as a cause of impaired sperm quality.

2. Androgens—An excess of androgens can suppress pituitary gonadotropin secretion and lead to secondary testis failure. The use of exogenous androgenic steroids (anabolic steroids) by as many as 15% of high school athletes, 30% of college athletes, and 70% of professional athletes may result in temporary sterility due to this effect. Initial treatment is to discontinue the steroids and reevaluate semen quality every 3–6 months until spermatogenesis returns. The most common reason for excess endogenous androgens is congenital adrenal hyperplasia, in which the enzyme 21-hydroxylase is most commonly deficient. As a result, there is defective cortisol synthesis and excessive adrenocorticotropic hormone production, leading to abnormally high production of androgenic steroids by the adrenal cortex. High androgen levels in prepubertal boys results in precocious puberty, with premature development of secondary sex characteristics and abnormal enlargement of the phallus. The testes are characteristically small because of central gonadotropin inhibition by androgens. In young girls, virilization and clitoral enlargement may be obvious. In cases of the classic 21-hydroxylase-deficient congenital adrenal hyperplasia that presents in childhood, normal sperm counts and fertility have been reported, even without glucocorticoid treatment. This disorder is one of the few intersex conditions associated with fertility. Other sources of endogenous androgens include hormonally active adrenocortical tumors or Leydig cell tumors of the testis.

3. Glucocorticoids—Exposure to excess glucocorticoids either endogenously or exogenously can result in decreased spermatogenesis. Elevated plasma cortisone levels depress LH secretion and induce secondary testis failure. Sources of exogenous glucocorticoids include chronic therapy for ulcerative colitis, asthma, or rheumatoid arthritis. Cushing syndrome is a common reason for excess endogenous glucocorticoids. Correction of the problem usually improves spermatogenesis.

4. Hyper- and hypothyroidism—Abnormally high or low levels of serum thyroid hormone affect spermatogenesis at the level of both the pituitary and testis. Thyroid balance is important for normal hypothalamic hormone secretion and for normal sex hormone-binding protein levels that govern the testosterone-estrogen ratio. Thyroid abnormalities are a rare cause (0.5%) of male infertility.

5. Growth hormone—There is emerging evidence that growth hormone may play a role in male infertility. Some infertile men have deficient responses to growth hormone challenge tests and may respond to growth hormone treatment with improvements in semen quality. Growth hormone is an anterior pituitary hormone that has receptors in the testis. It induces insulin-like growth factor-1, a growth factor important for spermatogenesis. The routine measurement of serum growth hormone is presently not indicated in the infertility evaluation.

TESTICULAR

Conditions that cause infertility that act at the testicular level are listed in Table 42–12. Unlike most pretes-

Table 42–12. Testicular causes of infertility.

Chromosomal (Klinefelter syndrome [XXY], XX sex reversal, XYY syndrome)
Noonan syndrome (male Turner syndrome)
Myotonic dystrophy
Vanishing testis syndrome (bilateral anorchia)
Sertoli-cell-only syndrome (germ cell aplasia)
Y chromosome microdeletions (*DAZ*)
Gonadotoxins (radiation, drugs)
Systemic disease (renal failure, liver failure, sickle cell anemia)
Defective androgen activity
Testis injury (orchitis, torsion, trauma)
Cryptorchidism
Varicocele
Idiopathic

ticular conditions, which are treatable with hormone manipulation, testicular effects are, at present, largely irreversible. If sperm are observed, however, assisted reproductive technology can provide biological children for affected men.

Chromosomal Causes

Abnormalities in chromosomal constitution are well-recognized causes of male infertility. In a study of 1263 infertile couples, a 6.2% overall incidence of chromosomal abnormalities was detected. Among men whose sperm count was < 10 million/mL, the incidence was 11%. In azoospermic men, 21% had significant chromosomal abnormalities. For this reason, cytogenetic analysis (karyotype) of autosomal and sex chromosomal anomalies should be considered in men with severe oligospermia and azoospermia.

A. KLINEFELTER SYNDROME (FIGURE 42–7)

Klinefelter syndrome is the most common genetic reason for azoospermia, accounting for 14% of cases (overall incidence 1:500 males). It has a classic triad: small, firm testes; gynecomastia; and azoospermia. This syndrome may present with delayed sexual maturation, increased height, decreased intelligence, varicosities, obesity, diabetes, leukemia, increased likelihood of extragonadal germ cell tumors, and breast cancer (20-fold higher than in normal males). In this abnormality of chromosomal number, 90% of men carry an extra X chromosome (47,XXY) and 10% are mosaic, with a combination of XXY/XY chromosomes. Paternity with this syndrome is rare but more likely in the mosaic or milder form of the disease. The testes are usually < 2.0 cm in length and always < 3.5 cm; biopsies show sclerosis and hyalinization of the seminiferous tubules with normal numbers of Leydig cells. Hormones usually demonstrate decreased testosterone and frankly elevated LH and FSH levels. Serum estradiol levels are commonly elevated. Since testosterone tends to decrease with age, these men will require androgen replacement therapy both for virilization and for normal sexual function.

B. XX MALE SYNDROME

XX male syndrome is a structural and numerical chromosomal condition, a variant of Klinefelter syndrome, that presents as gynecomastia at puberty or as azoospermia in adults. Average height is below normal, and hypospadias is common. Male external and internal genitalia are otherwise normal. The incidence of mental deficiency is not increased. Hormone evaluation shows elevated FSH and LH and low or normal testosterone levels. Testis biopsy reveals absent spermatogenesis with fibrosis and Leydig cell clumping. The most obvious explanation is that SRY, or the testis-determining region, is translocated from the Y to the X chromosome. Thus, testis differentiation is present; however, the genes that control spermatogenesis on the Y chromosome are not similarly translocated, resulting in azoospermia.

C. XYY SYNDROME

The incidence of XYY syndrome is similar to that of Klinefelter, but the clinical presentation is more variable. Typically, men with 47,XYY are tall, and 2% exhibit aggressive or antisocial behavior. Hormone evaluation reveals elevated FSH and normal testosterone and LH levels. Semen analyses show either oligospermia or azoospermia. Testis biopsies vary but usually demonstrate arrest of maturation or Sertoli-cell-only syndrome.

Other Syndromes

A. NOONAN SYNDROME

Also called male Turner syndrome, Noonan syndrome is associated with clinical features similar to Turner syndrome (45,X). However, the karyotype is either normal (46,XY) or mosaic (X/XY). Typically, patients have dysmorphic features like webbed neck, short stature, low-set ears, wide-set eyes, and cardiovascular abnormalities. At birth, 75% have cryptorchidism that limits fertility in adulthood. If testes are fully descended, then fertility is possible and likely. Associated FSH and LH levels depend on the degree of testicular function.

B. MYOTONIC DYSTROPHY

Myotonic dystrophy is the most common reason for adult-onset muscular dystrophy. In addition to having myotonia, or delayed relaxation after muscle contraction, patients usually present with cataracts, muscle atrophy, and various endocrinopathies. Most men have testis atrophy, but fertility has been reported. Infertile men may have elevated FSH and LH with low or normal testosterone, and testis biopsies show seminiferous tubule damage in 75% of cases. Pubertal development is normal; testis damage seems to occur later in life.

C. Vanishing Testis Syndrome

Also called bilateral anorchia, vanishing testis syndrome is rare, occurring in 1:20,000 males. Patients present with bilateral nonpalpable testes and sexual immaturity due to the lack of testicular androgens. The testes are lost due to fetal torsion, trauma, vascular injury, or infection. In general, functioning testis tissue must have been present during weeks 14–16 of fetal life, since wolffian duct growth and müllerian duct inhibition occur along with appropriate growth of male external genitalia. Patients have eunuchoid body proportions but no gynecomastia. The karyotype is normal. Serum LH and FSH levels are elevated, and serum testosterone levels are extremely low. There is no treatment for this form of infertility; patients receive lifelong testosterone for normal virilization and sexual function.

D. Sertoli-Cell-Only Syndrome

Also referred to as germ cell aplasia, the hallmarks of Sertoli-cell-only syndrome are an azoospermic male with testes biopsies that show the presence of all testis cell types except for germinal epithelium. Several causes have been proposed, including genetic defects, congenital absence of germ cells, and androgen resistance. Clinically, these men have normal virilization with small testes of normal consistency. There is no gynecomastia. Testosterone and LH levels are normal, but FSH levels are usually (90%) elevated. The use of the word "syndrome" implies that no recognized insult has occurred, since gonadotoxins like ionizing radiation, chemotherapy, and mumps orchitis can also render the testes aplastic of germ cells. There is no known treatment for this condition. In some patients, extensive testis sampling with fine-needle aspiration mapping or multiple biopsies can reveal sperm that can be used for pregnancy with assisted reproductive technologies.

E. Y Chromosome Microdeletions

Approximately 7% of men with low sperm counts and 13% with azoospermia have a structural alteration in the long arm of the Y chromosome (Yq). The testis-determining region genes that control testis differentiation are intact, but there may be gross deletions in other regions that may lead to defective spermatogenesis. The recent explosion in molecular genetics technology has allowed for sophisticated analysis of the Y chromosome.

At present, 3 gene sites are being investigated as putative AZF (azoospermia factor) candidates: *AZFa, b,* and *c.* The most promising site is *AZFc,* which contains the *DAZ* gene region. The gene, of which there are at least 7 copies in this region, appears to encode an RNA-binding protein that regulates the meiotic pathway during germ cell production. Homologs of the *DAZ* gene are found in many other animals, including mouse and *Drosophila.* A quantitative polymerase chain reaction–based assay is used to test blood for these deletions. In the future, sperm DNA may also be tested as part of a semen analysis. Since men with these microdeletions can have sperm in the ejaculate, they are likely to pass them on to offspring if assisted reproductive technology is used.

Gonadotoxins

A. Radiation

The effects of radiotherapy on sperm production are well described. They are derived mainly from a series of remarkable experiments performed during the "atomic age" but only recently published. In a study of healthy prisoners in Oregon and Washington in the 1960s, Clifton and Bremner (1983) examined the effects of ionizing irradiation on semen quality and spermatogenesis. Before a vasectomy, each of 111 volunteers was exposed to different levels of radiation, from 7.5 to 600 cGy. Sperm counts were analyzed weekly and each prisoner served as his own control. There was a distinct dose-dependent, inverse relationship between irradiation and sperm count. A significant reduction in sperm count was observed at 15 cGy, and sperm counts were temporarily abolished at 50 cGy. Azoospermia was induced at 400 cGy in 4 of 5 patients; this persisted for at least 40 weeks. Despite these profound effects, sperm counts rebounded to preirradiation levels in most patients during recovery.

From examination of testis tissue after irradiation, it was concluded that spermatogonia are the germ cells most sensitive to irradiation. Given the dramatic sensitivity of testis tissue to irradiation, subsequent studies have focused on the "scatter" to testes of men undergoing radiation therapy for cancer. In patients subjected to abdominal radiation with gonadal shielding, the estimated mean unintended gonadal exposure was approximately 75 cGy. There does not appear to be an increase in congenital birth defects in offspring of irradiated men.

B. Drugs

Medications are usually tested extensively for their potential as reproductive hazards before marketing. Despite this, it is wise to discontinue unnecessary medications that can be safely stopped during attempts to conceive. A list of gonadotoxic medications can be found in Table 42–13. These can result in infertility by various mechanisms. Ketoconazole, spironolactone, and alcohol inhibit testosterone synthesis, whereas cimetidine is an androgen antagonist. Recreational drugs such as marijuana, heroin, and methadone are associated with lower testosterone levels. Certain pesticides, like dibromochloropropane, are likely to have estrogen-like activity.

Cancer chemotherapy is designed to kill rapidly dividing cells; an undesired outcome is the cytotoxic effect on normal proliferating tissues. Differentiating spermatogonia appear to be the germinal cells most sensitive to cytotoxic chemotherapy. Alkylating agents such as cyclophosphamide, chlorambucil, and nitrogen mustard are the most toxic agents. The toxic effects of chemotherapeutic drugs vary according to dose and duration of treatment, type and stage of disease, age and health of the patient, and baseline testis function. Despite this toxicity, the mutagenic effects of chemotherapy agents does not appear to be significant enough to increase the chance of congenital defects or genetically linked diseases among offspring of treated men. However, patients should wait at least 6 months after chemotherapy ends before attempting to conceive.

Systemic Disease

A. Renal Failure

Uremia is associated with infertility, decreased libido, erectile dysfunction, and gynecomastia. The cause of hypogonadism is controversial and probably multifactorial. Testosterone levels are decreased, and FSH and LH levels can be elevated. Serum prolactin levels are elevated in 25% of patients. It is likely that estrogen excess plays a role in hormone axis derangement. Medications and uremic neuropathy may play a role in uremic-related impotence and changes in libido. After successful renal transplantation, the hypogonadism usually improves.

B. Liver Cirrhosis

Hypogonadism related to liver failure may have various contributing factors. The reason for organ failure is im-

portant. Hepatitis is associated with viremia, and fevers can affect spermatogenesis. Excessive alcohol intake inhibits testicular testosterone synthesis, independent of its liver effects. Liver failure and cirrhosis are associated with testicular atrophy, impotence, and gynecomastia. Levels of testosterone and its metabolic clearance are decreased; estrogen levels are increased owing to augmented conversion of androgens to estrogens by aromatases. Decreased testosterone levels are not accompanied by proportionate elevations in LH and FSH levels, suggesting that a central inhibition of the HPG axis may accompany liver failure.

C. Sickle Cell Disease

As mentioned earlier, sickle cell disease can cause pituitary dysfunction, likely due to the sludging of erythrocytes and associated microinfarcts. This same mechanism may also occur in testis tissue and contribute to primary hypogonadism. As a result, spermatogenesis is decreased, accompanied by lower serum testosterone levels.

Defective Androgen Activity

Peripheral resistance to androgens occurs with 2 basic defects: (1) a deficiency of androgen production through the absence of 5α-reductase or (2) a deficiency in the androgen receptor. In general, these conditions are a consequence of single gene deletions. Figure 42–13 shows the algorithm of normal male development. Androgen insensitivity syndromes stem from aberrations in this pathway.

Table 42–13. Medications associated with infertility.

Calcium channel blockers	Allopurinol
Cimetidine	Alpha blockers
Sulfasalazine	Nitrofurantoin
Valproic acid	Lithium
Spironolactone	Tricyclic antidepressants
Colchicine	Antipsychotics

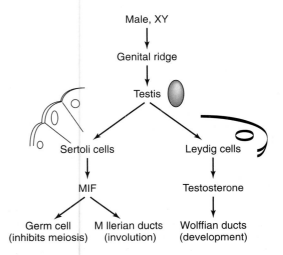

Figure 42–13. Differentiation pathway for the male. Aberrations in the pathway result in androgen insensitivity syndromes. MIF, müllerian inhibiting factor.

A. 5α-Reductase Deficiency

5α-Reductase deficiency results in normal development of the testes and wolffian duct structures (internal genitalia) but ambiguous external genitalia. The ambiguity results from an inborn deficiency of the 5α-reductase enzyme that converts testosterone to DHT in androgen-sensitive tissues like the prostate, seminal vesicle, and external genitalia. Thus far, 29 mutations have been described in the culprit enzyme. The diagnosis is made by measuring the ratio of testosterone metabolites in urine and confirmed by finding decreased 5α-reductase in genital skin fibroblasts. Spermatogenesis has been described in descended testes; however, fertility has not been reported in these patients. The lack of fertility may be due largely to functional abnormalities of the external genitalia.

B. Androgen Receptor Deficiency

Androgen receptor deficiency is an X-linked genetic condition marked by resistance to androgens. The androgen receptor, a nuclear protein, is absent or functionally altered such that testosterone or DHT cannot bind to it and activate target cell genes. Since androgens have no effect on tissues, both internal and external genitalia are affected. Fertility effects depend on the specific receptor abnormality. Some patients are 46,XY males with complete end-organ resistance to androgens. They have female external genitalia with intra-abdominal testes. Testes show immature tubules and the risk of testis cancer is elevated: Tumors will develop in 10–30% of patients without orchiectomy. Fertility is absent. Patients with mild receptor defects may present as normal-appearing infertile men. Spermatogenesis may be present, although impaired. It is unclear exactly how common this occurs in infertile men.

Testis Injury

A. Orchitis

Inflammation of testis tissue is most commonly due to bacterial infection, termed epididymo-orchitis. Viral infections also occur in the testis in the form of mumps orchitis. Orchitis is observed in approximately 30% of postpubertal males who contract parotitis. Testis atrophy is a significant and frequent result of viral orchitis but is less common with bacterial infections.

B. Torsion

Ischemic injury to the testis secondary to twisting of the testis on the spermatic cord pedicle is not uncommon in prepubertal and early postpubertal boys. When diagnosed and corrected surgically within 6 h of occurrence, the testis can usually be saved. Torsion may result in inoculation of the immune system with testis antigens that may predispose to later immunological infertility.

It recognized that the "normal" contralateral mate of a torsed testis could also exhibit histologic abnormalities. It has not been clearly demonstrated whether this is related to the actual torsion or to an underlying abnormality in testes predisposed to torsion.

C. Trauma

Because of the peculiar immunologic status of the testis in the body (ie, it is an immunologically privileged site), trauma to the testis can invoke an abnormal immune response in addition to atrophy resulting from injury. Both may contribute to infertility. Trauma to the testis that results in fracture of the testis tunica albugineal layer should be surgically explored and repaired to minimize exposure of testis tissue to the body.

Cryptorchidism

The undescended testis is a very common urologic problem, observed in 0.8% of boys at 1 year of age. It is considered a developmental defect and places the affected testis at higher risk of developing cancer. Although the newborn undescended testis is morphologically fairly normal, deterioration in early germ cell numbers is often seen by 2 years of age. The contralateral, normally descended testis is also at increased risk of harboring germ cell abnormalities. Thus, males with either unilaterally or bilaterally undescended testes are at risk for infertility later in life. Prophylactic orchidopexy is generally performed by 2 years of age to allow the testis to be palpated for cancer detection. It is unclear whether orchidopexy alters fertility potential in cryptorchidism.

Varicocele

A varicocele is defined as dilated and tortuous veins within the pampiniform plexus of scrotal veins. It is the most surgically correctable cause of male subfertility. The varicocele is a disease of puberty and is only rarely detected in boys under 10 years of age. A left-sided varicocele is found in 15% of healthy young men. In contrast, the incidence of a left varicocele in subfertile men approaches 40%. Bilateral varicoceles are uncommon in healthy men (< 10%) but are palpated in up to 20% of subfertile men. In general, varicoceles do not spontaneously regress. The cornerstone of varicocele diagnosis rests on an accurate physical examination.

Several anatomic features contribute to the predominance of left-sided varicoceles. The left internal spermatic vein is longer than the right; in addition, it usually joins the left renal vein at right angles. The right internal spermatic vein has a more oblique insertion into the inferior vena cava. This particular anatomy in the standing man may cause higher venous pressures to be transmitted to the left scrotal veins and result in retrograde reflux of blood into the pampiniform plexus.

Varicoceles are associated with testicular atrophy. It has also been demonstrated that varicocele correction can reverse atrophy in adolescents. There is indisputable evidence that the varicocele affects semen quality. In fact, based on the work of MacLeod and Gold (1951), a classic semen analysis pattern has been attributed to varicoceles in which low sperm count and motility is found in conjunction with abnormal sperm shapes. The finding of semen abnormalities constitutes the main indication for varicocele surgery in infertile men.

Precisely how a varicocele exerts an effect on the testicle remains unclear. Several theories have been postulated; it is likely that a combination of effects results in infertility. Pituitary-gonadal hormonal dysfunction, internal spermatic vein reflux of renal or adrenal metabolites, and an increase in hydrostatic pressure associated with venous reflux are also postulated effects of a varicocele. The most intriguing theory of how varicoceles affect testis function invokes an inhibition of spermatogenesis through the reflux of warm corporeal blood around the testis, with disruption of the normal countercurrent heat exchange balance and elevation of intratesticular temperature.

Idiopathic

It has been estimated that at least 25%–50% of male infertility has no identifiable cause. As our knowledge expands, it is likely that genetic and environmental factors will explain many of these cases.

POSTTESTICULAR (TABLE 42–14)

Reproductive Tract Obstruction

The posttesticular portion of the reproductive tract includes the epididymis, vas deferens, seminal vesicles, and associated ejaculatory apparatus.

A. Congenital Blockages

1. Cystic fibrosis—Cystic fibrosis (CF) is the most common autosomal recessive genetic disorder in the United States and is fatal. It is associated with fluid and electrolyte abnormalities (abnormal chloride-sweat test) and presents with chronic lung obstruction and infections, pancreatic insufficiency, and infertility. Interestingly, 98% of men with CF are missing parts of the epididymis. In addition, the vas deferens, seminal vesicles, and ejaculatory ducts are usually atrophic, or completely absent, causing obstruction. Spermatogenesis is usually normal. Congenital absence of the vas deferens (CAVD) accounts for 1–2% of infertility cases. On

Table 42–14. Posttesticular causes of infertility.

Reproductive tract obstruction
  Congenital blockages
    Congenital absence of the vas deferens (CAVD)
    Young syndrome
    Idiopathic epididymal obstruction
    Polycystic kidney disease
    Ejaculatory duct obstruction
  Acquired blockages
    Vasectomy
    Groin surgery
    Infection
  Functional blockages
    Sympathetic nerve injury
    Pharmacologic
Disorders of sperm function or motility
    Immotile cilia syndromes
    Maturation defects
    Immunologic infertility
    Infection
Disorders of coitus
    Impotence
    Hypospadias
    Timing and frequency

physical examination, no palpable vas deferens is observed on one or both sides. As in CF, the rest of the reproductive tract ducts may also be abnormal and unreconstructable. This disease is related to CF. Even though most of these men demonstrate no symptoms of CF, up to 65% of patients will harbor a detectable CF mutation. In addition, 15% of these men will have renal malformations, most commonly unilateral agenesis.

2. Young syndrome—Young syndrome presents with a triad of chronic sinusitis, bronchiectasis, and obstructive azoospermia. The obstruction is in the epididymis. The pathophysiology of the condition is unclear but may involve abnormal ciliary function or abnormal mucus quality. Although spermatogenesis is usually normal, reconstructive surgery is associated with lower success rates than that observed with other obstructed conditions.

3. Idiopathic epididymal obstruction—Idiopathic epididymal obstruction is a relatively uncommon condition found in otherwise healthy men. There is recent evidence linking this condition to CF in that one-third of men so obstructed may harbor CF gene mutations.

4. Adult polycystic kidney disease—Adult polycystic kidney disease is an autosomal dominant disorder associated with numerous cysts of the kidney, liver, spleen, pancreas, epididymis, seminal vesicle, and testis. Disease onset usually occurs in the twenties or thirties with symptoms of abdominal pain, hypertension, and renal failure. Infertility with this disease is usually secondary to obstructing cysts in the epididymis or seminal vesicle.

5. Blockage of the ejaculatory ducts—Blockage of the ejaculatory ducts, the delicate, paired, collagenous tubes that connect the vas deferens and seminal vesicles to the urethra, is termed ejaculatory duct obstruction. It is the cause of infertility in 5% of azoospermic men. Obstruction can be congenital and result from müllerian duct (utricular) cysts, wolffian duct (diverticular) cysts, or congenital atresia or is acquired from seminal vesicle calculi or postsurgical or inflammatory scar tissue. It presents as hematospermia, painful ejaculation, or infertility. The diagnosis is confirmed by finding a low-volume ejaculate and TRUS showing dilated seminal vesicles or dilated ejaculatory ducts.

B. Acquired Blockages

1. Vasectomy—Vasectomy is performed on 750,000 men per year in the United States for contraception. Subsequently, approximately 5% of these men have the vasectomy reversed, most commonly because of remarriage.

2. Groin and hernia surgery—Groin and hernia surgery can result in inguinal vas deferens obstruction in 1% of cases. There has been concern that Marlex mesh used for hernia repairs may add to perivasal inflammation and increase the likelihood of vasal obstruction.

3. Bacterial infections—Bacterial infections (*E coli* in men age > 35) or *Chlamydia trachomatis* in young men) may involve the epididymis, with scarring and obstruction.

C. Functional Blockages

Besides physical obstruction, functional obstruction of the seminal vesicles may exist. Functional blockages may result from nerve injury or medications that impair the contractility of seminal vesicle or vasal musculature. A classic example of nerve injury affecting ejaculation is after retroperitoneal lymph node dissection for testis cancer. This can cause either retrograde ejaculation or true anejaculation, depending on the degree of injury to postganglionic sympathetic fibers arising from the thoracolumbar spinal cord. These autonomic nerves overlie the inferior aorta and coalesce as the hypogastric plexus within the pelvis and control seminal emission. Multiple sclerosis and diabetes are other conditions that result in disordered ejaculation.

Evidence from animal models indicates that the seminal vesicles, lined by smooth muscle, possess contractile properties similar to those of the urinary bladder, making it conceivable that seminal vesicle organ

dysfunction may underlie some cases of ejaculatory duct "obstruction." Medications implicated in this functional problem are those classically associated with ejaculatory impairment. Table 42–5 lists these medications.

Disorders of Sperm Function or Motility

A. Immotile Cilia Syndromes

Immotile cilia syndromes are a heterogeneous group of disorders (1:20,000 males) in which sperm motility is reduced or absent. The sperm defects are due to abnormalities in the motor apparatus or axoneme of sperm and other ciliated cells. Normally, 9 pairs of microtubules are organized around a central pair within the sperm tail and are connected by dynein arms (ATPase) that regulate microtubule and therefore sperm tail motion. Various defects in the dynein arms cause deficits in ciliary and sperm activity. Kartagener syndrome is a subset of this disorder (1:40,000 males) that presents with the triad of chronic sinusitis, bronchiectasis, and situs inversus. Most immotile cilia cases are diagnosed in childhood with respiratory and sinus difficulties. Cilia present in the retina and ear may also be defective and lead to retinitis pigmentosa and deafness in Usher syndrome. Men with immotile cilia characteristically have nonmotile but viable sperm in normal numbers. Sperm nuclear material is thought to be unaffected. The diagnosis is made with electron microscopy of sperm.

B. Maturation Defects

After vasectomy reversal, normal sperm counts but low motility is often observed. This is thought to be due to elevated epididymal intratubular pressure and epididymal dysfunction, a consequence of time after vasectomy-induced blockage. As a result, sperm may not gain the usual maturation and motility capacities during transit through the epididymis.

C. Immunologic Infertility

Autoimmune infertility has been implicated as a cause of infertility in 10% of infertile couples. The testis is a curious organ in that sperm are highly antigenic, yet normally coexist within the host; it is an immunologically privileged site, probably owing to the blood-testis barrier, which consists of Sertoli cell tight junctions and locally downregulated cellular immunity. Autoimmune infertility may result from an abnormal exposure to sperm antigens after, for example, vasectomy, testis torsion, or biopsy, which then incites a pathologic immune response.

Clinically, antisperm antibodies (ASA) are found in 3–12% of men who undergo infertility evaluation. Antibodies may disturb sperm transport or disrupt normal sperm-egg interaction. Antibodies may cause clumping or agglutination of sperm, which inhibits passage, or may block normal sperm binding to the oocyte. Many assays are available to detect ASA. In the most widely used assay, polyacrylamide beads are coated with antihuman antibody and then exposed to motile sperm. Attachment of beads to sperm indicates antibody presence.

D. Infection

The agents most commonly responsible for male genital tract infections are listed in Table 42–10. Various products of activated leukocytes can exist in infected semen. A significant correlation has been demonstrated between leukocytes in semen and the generation of superoxide anions, hydrogen peroxide, and hydroxyl radicals (reactive oxygen species), all of which can damage sperm membranes. Sperm are highly susceptible to the effects of oxidative stress because they possess little cytoplasm and therefore little antioxidant activity. Damage to sperm from oxidative stress has been correlated to loss of function. Although genital tract infection has been linked to infertility in epidemiologic studies, the correlation between individual organisms and infertility is unclear. Uncontrolled studies suggest that pregnancy rates may improve after treatment, but controlled studies do not confirm these findings. It is important to remember that seminal fluid that passes through the urethra is routinely contaminated with bacteria.

Disorders of Coitus

A. Impotence

Sexual dysfunction stemming from low libido or impotence is a frequent cause of infertility. The male hormonal evaluation can detect organic reasons for such problems. Most cases of situational impotence, in which the stress of attempting to conceive results in poor erections, are treated with sexual counseling.

B. Hypospadias

Anatomic problems like hypospadias can cause inappropriate placement of the seminal coagulum too distant from the cervix and result in infertility.

C. Timing and Frequency

Simple problems of coital timing and frequency can be corrected by a review of the couple's sexual habits. An appropriate frequency of intercourse is every 2 days, performed within the periovulatory period, the window of time surrounding ovulation when egg fertilization is possible. Charting of basal body temperature by the female partner allows for the calculation of that period for the next ovulatory cycle. Home kits that detect the LH surge in the urine before ovulation are also helpful. Couples should be counseled to avoid lubricants if at all possible. It is also wise to discontinue any unnecessary medications during attempts to conceive. Other coital toxins include heat exposure from regular saunas, hot tubs, or Jacuzzis and the use of cigarettes, cocaine, marijuana, and excessive alcohol.

■ TREATMENT OF MALE INFERTILITY

SURGICAL TREATMENTS

The role of surgery in the treatment of male infertility is well established and cost-effective when compared to high-technology approaches. Surgery also attempts to reverse specific pathophysiologic effects and may allow for conception at home rather than in the laboratory.

Microsurgery in Urology

The rise of microsurgery as a surgical discipline followed 3 advances. The first was refinements in optical magnification; the second, the development of more precise microsuture and microneedles; and the third, the ability to manufacture smaller and more refined surgical instruments. In urology, microsurgical techniques were first applied to renal transplantation and vasectomy reversal. Microsurgical techniques evolved quickly from humble beginnings using borrowed forceps from the local jewelry store (the "jeweler's forceps") and human hair for fine suture material to its current highly refined state.

Even with these advances, microsurgery in urology is one of the most challenging disciplines in the field.

Varicocele

Although most men with varicoceles are fertile, the association of varicoceles with infertility is well established by observational, retrospective, and prospective studies. Several treatment modalities, both surgical and nonsurgical, are available for varicoceles. These include incisional ligation of the veins through the retroperitoneal, inguinal, or subinguinal approaches; percutaneous embolization; and laparoscopy. The common goal of all treatments is to eliminate the retrograde reflux of venous blood through the internal spermatic veins. Treatments can be compared in terms of expected success rates (semen improvement and pregnancy), cost, and outcomes (pain pills, return to work or other activity), and their relative merits can be analyzed. A basic comparison of 3 treatment options is outlined in Table 42–15. Remember that if watchful

Table 42–15. Varicocele treatments: Comparison of outcomes.

Outcome Parameter	Treatment		
	Incisional	**Laparoscopic**	**Radiologic**
Semen improvement	66%	50–70%	60%
Pregnancy rate	35%	12–32%	10–50%
Recurrence	0–15%	5–25%	0–10%
Technical failure	Negligible	Small	10–15%
Pain pills	9.4	11	Minimal
Days to work	5.0	5.3	1

waiting is chosen, a pregnancy rate of 16% can be expected. If IVF is chosen, a pregnancy rate of 35% can be expected. An overall complication rate of 1% is associated with the incisional approach, compared with a 4% complication rate for laparoscopy and 10–15% for radiologic occlusion. A significant component of the complications with the radiologic approach is technical failure, meaning the inability to access and occlude the spermatic vein.

Vasovasostomy

About 35,000 men per year undergo vasectomy reversal in the United States. The most common reason is remarriage and the desire for more children. Occasionally, an unfortunate individual will have lost a child and desire another. Infection, deformities, trauma, and previous surgery are less frequent indications for vasovasostomy or epididymovasostomy. A problem with duct obstruction is suspected in men with normal hormones and normal testis size and no sperm in the ejaculate.

There are several methods for performing a vasovasostomy. None has been proved superior to any other, except that magnification with an operating microscope has been shown to result in better success rates. Generally, either a single-layer anastomosis or a strict, two-layer anastomosis is performed (Figure 42–14). Although these procedures are technically different, the experience of the surgeon is the most important factor for success. Depending on these factors, 95% or more of patients may have a return of sperm after a vasovasostomy. If the vas fluid contains no sperm below the vasectomy site, a second problem may exist in the delicate tubules of the epididymis. The longer the time since vasectomy, the greater the "back-pressure" behind the blocked vas deferens. This may cause a blowout at some point in the single, 18-foot-long epididymal tubule, the weakest point in the system. A blowout results in blockage of the tubule as it heals. In this case, the vas must be connected to the epididymis above the blowout to allow sperm to travel through the reproductive tract. This is called an epididymovasostomy. After epididymovasostomy, approximately 60–65% of men will have sperm in the ejaculate. These rates, however, have improved remarkably during the last several years, with the evolution of surgical techniques and equipment.

The achievement of sperm in the ejaculate after vasovasostomy depends on the surgeon and the patient, but pregnancy after surgery obviously involves a third party. It is rare that more than 67% of men who have normal sperm counts after vasectomy reversal will impregnate a woman. Therefore, it is critical to delve into the reproductive health of the female partner before embarking on the procedure. Other reasons that reproductive tract microsurgery fails are (1) the quality of preblockage semen may not have been normal; (2) ASAs develop in roughly 30% of men who have had vasectomies (high antibody levels may impair fertility); (3) postsurgical scar tissue can develop at the anastomotic site, causing another blockage; (4) when the vas deferens has been blocked for a long time, the epididymis is adversely affected and sperm maturation may be compromised.

Ejaculatory Duct Obstruction

For over 20 years, transurethral resection of the ejaculatory ducts (TURED) has been used to relieve pain due to ejaculatory duct obstruction. More recently, it has become obvious that ejaculatory duct obstruction causes infertility in 5% of azoospermic men. Ejaculatory duct obstruction is suspected when the ejaculate volume is < 2.0 mL and no sperm or fructose is present. Clinical suspicion can be confirmed by TRUS demonstration of dilated seminal vesicles or dilated ejaculatory ducts. Patients with ejaculatory duct obstruction sufficient to cause coital discomfort, recurrent hematospermia, or infertility should be considered for treatment.

Transurethral resection of the ejaculatory ducts is performed cystoscopically (Figure 42–15). A small resectoscope and electrocautery loop are inserted, and the

Figure 42–14. Two-layer microsurgical vasovasostomy. **A:** Mucosal stitches of 10-0 nylon are placed in the "back wall" of the vas lumen, incorporating mucosa and a small amount of submucosal tissue. **B:** The "front wall" mucosal sutures are then placed. **C:** Finally, serosal sutures of 9-0 nylon are placed in the outside wall of the vas deferens to complete the anastomosis. (Reproduced, with permission, from McClure RD: Microsurgery of the male reproductive system. World J Urol 1986;4:105.)

verumontanum is resected in the midline. Since the area of resection is at the prostatic apex, near the external urethral sphincter and the rectum, careful positioning of the resectoscope is essential. Long-term relief of postcoital pain after TURED can be expected in 60% of patients. Hematospermia has also been effectively treated with TURED, but this literature is anecdotal. There is convincing evidence from several large studies of patients treated for infertility that 65–70% of men show significant improvement in semen quality after TURED and that a 20–30% pregnancy rate can be expected. The complication rate from TURED is approximately 20%. Most complications are self-limited and include hematospermia, hematuria, urinary tract infection, epididymitis, and a watery ejaculate. Rarely reported complications include retrograde ejaculation, rectal perforation, and urinary incontinence.

Electroejaculation

A complete failure of emission and ejaculation occurs most commonly from spinal cord injury (10,000 cases/year in the United States) and as a result of deep pelvic or retroperitoneal surgery that injures the pelvic sympathetic nerves. With rectal probe electroejaculation, the pelvic sympathetic nerves undergo controlled stimulation, with contraction of the vas deferens, seminal vesicle, and prostate, such that a reflex ejaculation is induced. The semen is collected from the penis and the bladder, as retrograde ejaculation is often associated with electroejaculation. Semen acquired in this way generally requires assisted reproductive technology for success.

In men with anejaculation after retroperitoneal surgery or spinal trauma, successful recovery of sperm with electroejaculation is possible in the vast majority of patients. Sperm motility tends to be lower than normal when obtained in this way, an effect independent of electrical or heat effects inherent to the procedure. In men with spinal cord injuries above the T5 level, it is often possible to induce a reflex ejaculation with high-frequency penile vibration, termed vibratory stimulation. With the use of handheld vibrators set to a frequency of 100 cycles/s at an amplitude of 2–3 mm, patients may be taught to perform the procedure and attempt to conceive at home with cervical insemination.

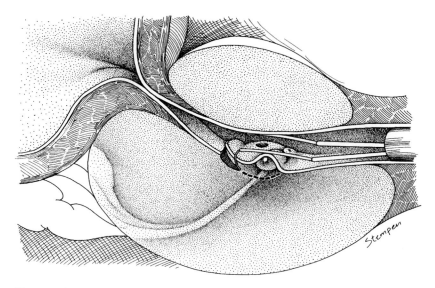

Figure 42–15. Transurethral resection of the ejaculatory ducts. A cystoscope with a resecting loop is used to remove the verumontanum and unroof an associated obstructing cyst that has compressed and obstructed the ejaculatory ducts. (Reproduced, with permission, from Turek PJ: Seminal vesicle and ejaculatory duct surgery. In: Graham SD [editor]: *Glenn's Urologic Surgery,* 5th ed. Lippincott, 1998.)

Sperm Aspiration

Sperm aspiration techniques are indicated for men in whom the transport of sperm is not possible because the ductal system is absent or surgically unreconstructable. An example of this is vasal agenesis. Acquired forms of obstruction may also exist, the most common of which is failed vasectomy reversal. Aspiration procedures can involve microsurgery to collect sperm from the sperm reservoirs within the genital tract. At present, sperm are routinely aspirated from the vas deferens, epididymis, or testicle. It is important to realize that IVF is required to achieve a pregnancy with these procedures. Thus, success rates are intimately tied to a complex program of assisted reproduction for both partners (Table 42–16). In cases of sperm aspiration from the testicle and epididymis, IVF along with ICSI is required. An obvious prerequisite for these procedures is ongoing sperm production. Although evaluated indirectly by hormone levels and testis volume, the most direct way to verify sperm production is with a testis biopsy.

A. VASAL ASPIRATION

After a scrotal incision and with an operating microscope, a vasotomy is made, and leaking sperm are aspirated into culture medium. Once enough sperm are obtained (> 10–20 million), the vasotomy is closed with microscopic sutures. Vasal aspiration provides the most

Table 42–16. Sources of aspirated sperm and associated reproductive technologies.

Procedure	Source	IVF	Micromanipulation
Vasal aspiration	Vas deferens	Usually	No
Epididymal aspiration	Epididymis	Yes	Yes
Testis biopsy	Testicle	Yes	Yes

IVF, in vitro fertilization.

mature or fertilizable sperm, as they have already passed through the epididymis, where sperm maturation is completed.

B. Epididymal Sperm Aspiration

Epididymal sperm aspiration is performed when the vas is not present or is scarred and unusable. Sperm are directly collected from a single, isolated epididymal tubule (Figure 42–16). After sperm are obtained, the epididymal tubule is closed with microscopic suture, and the sperm are processed. Epididymal sperm are not as mature as vasal sperm; as a consequence, epididymal sperm require ICSI to fertilize the egg. Egg fertilization rates of 65% and pregnancy rates of 50% are possible with epididymal sperm, but results vary among individuals because of differences in sperm and egg quality.

C. Testis Sperm Retrieval

The most recently developed aspiration technique is testicular sperm retrieval, begun in 1995. It is a breakthrough in that it demonstrates that sperm do not have to pass through the epididymis to fertilize the egg. Testicular sperm extraction is indicated for patients in whom there is an unreconstructable blockage in the epididymis, or in cases of severe testis failure, in which so few sperm are produced that they cannot reach the ejaculate. In this procedure, a small piece of testis tissue

Figure 42–16. Microscopic epididymal sperm aspiration. A small "window" incision is made in the scrotum and held open with a small retractor. Under 20 × magnification, the epididymis is dissected, and a single epididymal tubule is incised with microscissors. Fluid containing sperm is aspirated for use with in vitro fertilization.

is taken in a manner similar to that of a regular testis biopsy. The testis tissue is specially treated in the laboratory to separate sperm from other cells. High egg fertilization rates (50–65%) and pregnancy rates (40–50%) are possible with testis sperm.

Orchidopexy

An undescended testis occurs in 0.8% of male infants at 1 year of age. Spontaneous descent into the scrotum is unlikely after 1 year. Although the most important reason for orchidopexy is to make testicles with a higher risk of cancer palpable, preservation of fertility is another, more debatable reason. Histologic studies of undescended testis show that significant decreases in spermatogonial numbers occur between birth and 2 years of age. Orchidopexy has been recommended within 2 years of age with the idea that some of this germ cell degeneration might be prevented, although proof of this is lacking. Given that sperm can be retrieved from even the smallest failing testis and used for biologic pregnancies, orchidopexy and not orchiectomy should be the primary goal in these cases.

Torsion of the testis is a urologic emergency. There are significant data from animal (but not human) studies to suggest that the unaffected, contralateral testis can become infertile after torsion of its mate. This has been termed sympathetic orchidopathia and is assumed to be immunologic in nature. It is the basis for the recommendation that the nonviable torsed testicle be removed at diagnosis. However, given the advances in assisted reproductive technologies, such recommendations should be reconsidered.

Pituitary Ablation

Elevated serum prolactin levels stemming from a pituitary adenoma can be treated medically and surgically. If the adenoma is radiologically visible (macroadenoma), then transphenoidal surgical ablation of the lesion is possible. If the adenoma is not visible (microadenoma), then medical therapy with the dopamine agonist bromocriptine or a derivative is indicated.

NONSURGICAL TREATMENTS

Specific Therapy

Specific therapy seeks to reverse known pathophysiologic effects to improve fertility. For the most part, they are cost-effective treatments.

A. Pyospermia

The presence of elevated numbers of leukocytes in semen is termed pyospermia and has been associated with (1) subclinical genital tract infection, (2) elevated reactive oxygen species, and (3) poor sperm function and infertility. Sperm are highly susceptible to the effects of oxidative stress induced by leukocytes or infection because they possess little cytoplasm and therefore little antioxidant activity. The treatment of pyospermia is controversial in the absence of overt bacteriologic infection. It is important to evaluate the patient for sexually transmitted diseases, penile discharge, prostatitis, or epididymitis. An expressed prostatic secretion is examined for leukocytes, and urethral cultures are obtained for chlamydia and mycoplasma. The use of broad-spectrum antibiotics such as doxycycline and trimethoprim-sulfamethoxazole has been shown to reduce seminal leukocyte concentrations, improve sperm function, and increase conception. Generally, the female partner is also treated.

In pyospermia with a documented prostatic source (> 20 leukocytes per high-power field in expressed prostatic secretion), frequent ejaculation (more than every 3 days) and doxycycline may result in a more durable resolution of pyospermia (55% of treated men) than either treatment alone (5–17% resolution) (Branigan and Muller, 1994). There is increasing evidence that the antioxidant vitamins (A, C, and E) as well as glutathione and other antioxidants may help scavenge reactive oxygen species within semen and improve sperm motility in pyospermic men (Baker et al, 1996).

B. COITAL THERAPY

Simple counseling on issues of coital timing, frequency, and gonadotoxin avoidance can improve fertility. It is important to review the essentials of basal body temperature charting or home kits that detect the LH surge in the urine immediately (< 24 h) before ovulation. Since sperm reside in the cervical mucus for 48 h and are released continuously, it is not necessary that coitus and ovulation occur at the exact same time, a fact that can reduce the stress associated with infertility. Coitus every other day around ovulation is the best recommendation. Coital lubricants should be avoided if possible. If necessary, vegetable oils, olive oil, and petroleum jelly are the safest.

Retrograde ejaculation results from a failure of the bladder neck to close during ejaculation. Diagnosed by the finding of sperm within the postejaculate bladder urine, it can be treated with a trial of sympathomimetic medications. Approximately 30% of men will respond to treatment with some degree of antegrade ejaculation. Begun several days before ejaculation, imipramine (25–50 mg twice a day), Nasal-D (twice a day), Ornade (twice a day), or Sudafed Plus (60 mg 4 times a day) have all been used with success. The side effects associated with these medications usually limit the efficacy of this therapy. For medication failure, sperm harvesting techniques can be used with IUI to achieve a pregnancy. Premature ejaculation occurs when men ejaculate before the partner is ready. Sexual counseling combined with tricyclic antidepressants, Prozac, or other serotoninergic uptake inhibitors can be very effective.

C. IMMUNOLOGIC INFERTILITY

Antisperm antibodies are a complex problem underlying male infertility. Available treatment options include corticosteroid suppression (Table 42–17), sperm washing, IUI, IVF, and ICSI. Steroid suppression is based on the concept that an overactive immune system can be weakened to reduce antibodies on sperm. Intrauterine insemination places more sperm nearer the ovulated egg to optimize the sperm-egg environment. Pregnancy rates with this technique generally fall in the 10–15% range. Assisted reproductive technology with IVF and ICSI is very effective in this scenario. In general, if > 50% of sperm are bound with antibodies, then treatment should be offered. In addition, head-directed or midpiece-directed sperm antibodies appear more relevant than tail-directed antibodies. Since the presence of ASA is associated with obstruction in the genital tract, these lesions should be sought and corrected. There is renewed interest in the causes and possible treatments of this interesting problem, as several animal models exist that mimic the condition in humans.

Table 42–17. Corticosteroid therapy for immunologic infertility.

Year	Investigator	Control	Daily Dose	No. of Patients	% Pregnant
1983	Alexander	Yes	60 mg pred.	19	45
1986	Hendry	No	40/80 mg predl.	76	33
1987	Hass	Yes	96 mg methylpred.	20	15
1988	Smarr	No	15 mg pred.	60	43
1990	Hendry	Yes	20/5 mg predl.	29	31
1990	Hendry		Placebo	21	9

pred., prednisone; methylpred., methylprednisolone; predl., prednisolone.

D. MEDICAL THERAPY

Effective hormonal therapy can be offered to patients with diseases that predispose to infertility. Hormone therapy is effective when it is used as specific and not empiric treatment. Specific replacement therapy seeks to reverse well-established, pathophysiologic states. Empiric treatments attempt to overcome pathologic conditions that are ill-defined or have no proven treatment.

1. Hyperprolactinemia—Normal levels of prolactin in men help sustain high intratesticular testosterone levels and affect the growth and secretions of the accessory sex glands. Hyperprolactinemia abolishes gonadotropin pulsatility by interfering with episodic GnRH release. Visible lesions are generally treated with transphenoidal surgery, and nonvisible lesions are treated with bromocriptine, 5–10 mg daily, to restore normal pituitary balance.

2. Hypothyroidism—Both elevated and depressed levels of thyroid hormone alter spermatogenesis. States of thyroid dysfunction account for 0.5% of infertility cases but are very treatable. Replacement or removal of low or excessive thyroid hormone is effective treatment for infertility. As these diseases are clinically very evident, routine thyroid screening is not recommended for infertility patients.

3. Congenital adrenal hyperplasia—Most commonly, the 21-hydroxylase enzyme is deficient, and defective cortisol production results. The testes fail to mature because of gonadotropin inhibition due to excessive androgens. The diagnosis is rare and classically presents as precocious puberty; careful laboratory evaluation is essential. In both sexes, the condition and the infertility associated with it are treated with corticosteroids.

4. Testosterone excess/deficiency—Patients with Kallmann syndrome lack GnRH that stimulates normal pituitary function. Infertility associated with this condition can be very effectively treated with hCG, 1000–2000 U 3 times weekly, and recombinant FSH 75 U twice weekly, to replace LH and FSH. It is also possible to give GnRH replacement in a pulsatile manner, 25–50 ng/kg every 2 h, by a portable infusion pump. Pituitary diseases associated with testis failure are not amenable to GnRH treatment but respond well to hCG and human menopausal gonadotropin therapy. Individuals with fertile eunuch syndrome or isolated LH deficiency respond well to hCG therapy alone. One can expect to find sperm in the ejaculate beginning 9–12 months after therapy is started. Since injectable drug regimens are long, complex, and costly, it is good practice for men to cryopreserve motile sperm once achieved in the ejaculate. Anabolic steroids are a common and underdiagnosed reason for testicular failure in which excess exogenous testosterone and metabolites depress the pituitary-gonadal axis and spermatogenesis. Initially, the patient should discontinue the offending hormones to allow the return of normal homeostatic balance. Second-line therapy generally consists of "jump-starting" the testis with hCG and FSH as with Kallmann syndrome.

Empiric Medical Therapy

In at least 25% of infertile men, no identifiable cause can be attributed to the problem. Because the pathophysiology is ill-defined, this is termed idiopathic infertility. There is a second group of men in whom a cause of infertility may be identified but no specific therapy is available. Both groups of men are candidates for empiric medical therapy. This form of therapy seeks to overcome pathologic conditions that are ill-defined or have no proven treatment. As a rule, it is important to establish a timeline of therapy and decide with the patient when empiric treatment is to be discontinued and other avenues pursued.

A. CLOMIPHENE CITRATE

Clomiphene citrate is a synthetic nonsteroidal drug that acts as an antiestrogen and competitively binds to estrogen receptors in the hypothalamus and pituitary. This blocks the action of the normally low levels of estrogen on the male hormone axis and results in increased secretion of GnRH, FSH, and LH. The enhanced output of these hormones increases testosterone production and sperm production. Clomiphene therapy is given for idiopathic low sperm count. It is less effective as a treatment for low motility. The dose is 12.5–50 mg/d either continuously or with a 5-day rest period each month. Serum gonadotropins and testosterone should be monitored at 2–4 weeks and the dose adjusted to keep the testosterone level within the normal range. Higher than normal testosterone levels may result in a decrease in semen quality. Therapy should be discontinued if no semen quality response is observed in 6 months. Although there have been over 30 published trials on clomiphene since 1964, only a few include control arms. In general, there are as many trials showing that clomiphene is equivalent to placebo as there are showing that it improves sperm density and pregnancy rates. Decreased sperm densities have also been observed on this therapy.

B. TAMOXIFEN

Tamoxifen is commonly used for the treatment of metastatic breast cancer in women. It is also an antiestrogen that works in a manner similar to clomiphene citrate. It may have less estrogenic activity than clomiphene, however. Also indicated for idiopathic oligospermia, the dose of tamoxifen is 10–15 mg twice daily for 3–6 months. Serum testosterone, LH, and FSH should be measured 2–4 weeks after initiating therapy. Semen analyses are taken at 3 months and regularly thereafter.

C. KALLIKREINS

The kallikrein-kinin system is involved with tissue proliferation, the coagulation cascade, and the complement system. Components of this system are also present in male reproductive tract secretions. They may be involved in induction of sperm motility and stimulation of spermatogenesis. Kallikrein is a pancreatic enzyme that acts on kininogens to release kinins. It has been used for idiopathic oligospermia with the idea that it may enhance sperm metabolism, increase testis blood flow, and stimulate accessory sex gland secretions. For the treatment of low sperm motility, oral porcine pancreatic kallikrein is used in Europe at a dose of 600 IU/d. A recent placebo-controlled clinical trial with 90 subjects showed significant improvements in sperm density, motility, and forward progression in treated men. Pregnancy rates were 38% in the treatment arm and 16% in the placebo arm.

D. ANTIOXIDANT THERAPY

There is evidence that up to 40% of infertile men have increased levels of reactive oxygen species in the reproductive tract. These species (OH, O_2 radicals, and hydrogen peroxide) can cause lipid peroxidation damage to sperm membranes. Treatment with scavengers of these radicals may protect sperm from oxidative damage: glutathione, 600 mg daily for 3–6 months, or vitamin E, 400–1200 U/d. These agents may be useful in a subgroup of infertile men with elevated levels of seminal reactive oxygen species.

E. GROWTH HORMONE

There is emerging evidence that growth hormone–induced insulin-like growth factor-1 may be important for spermatogenesis. In recent European trials of growth hormone in infertile men, individuals with maturation arrest and azoospermia developed sperm counts. The use of growth hormone or its releasing factor may become a new and effective treatment for oligospermia.

ASSISTED REPRODUCTIVE TECHNOLOGIES

If neither surgery nor medical therapy is appropriate for male infertility treatment, assisted reproductive techniques can be used to achieve a pregnancy.

Intrauterine Insemination

Intrauterine insemination (IUI) involves the placement of a washed pellet of ejaculated sperm within the female uterus, beyond the cervical barrier. The principal indication for IUI is for a cervical factor; if the cervix is bypassed, then pregnancies may ensue. IUI is also used for low sperm quality, for immunologic infertility, and in men with mechanical problems of sperm delivery (eg, hypospadias). There should be at least 5–40 million motile sperm in the ejaculate (volume × concentration × motility) to make this procedure worthwhile. Success rates vary widely and are directly related to female reproductive potential; given this, pregnancy rates of 8–16% per cycle have been reported with IUI as a treatment for male infertility. Success rates are improved if ultrasound is used to document that follicles are enlarging and if urine testing is used to predict ovulation precisely.

In Vitro Fertilization and ICSI (Figure 42–17)

In vitro fertilization is a more complex technique than IUI and removes even more of the formidable obstacles to sperm in the female reproductive tract. It involves controlled ovarian stimulation and ultrasound-guided transvaginal egg retrieval from the ovaries before normal ovulation. Eggs are then fertilized in petri dishes with anywhere from 500,000 to 5 million motile sperm. This is excellent technology with which to bypass moderate to severe forms of male infertility in which low numbers of motile sperm are present. Most recently, a revolutionary addition to IVF has been described that is referred to as sperm micromanipulation, or ICSI. The sperm requirement for egg fertilization has dropped from hundreds of thousands for IVF to 1 viable sperm for ICSI. This has led to the development of aggressive new surgical techniques to provide sperm for egg fertilization from men with apparent azoospermia (no ejaculated sperm). The availability of these techniques has pushed urologists to look beyond the ejaculate and into the male reproductive tract to find sperm for biologic pregnancies. At present, sources of sperm include the vas deferens, epididymis, and testicle. Two notes of concern are the following: (1) Since IVF and ICSI may eliminate many natural selection barriers that exist during natural fertilization, genetic defects that caused the infertility are expected to be passed on to offspring unabated. This has large ethical implications, especially with respect to X-linked diseases like Klinefelter syndrome that might be expected to resurface again in grandchildren of the affected but treatable infertile male. (2) Recent data show that offspring born to infertile couples with this technique have a 4-fold

Figure 42–17. The intracytoplasmic sperm injection procedure. (**Top**) A mature oocyte (left) is readied for injection with a sperm (arrow) in a micropipet under the microscope. (**Bottom**) The micropipet is placed directly into the oocyte, and the sperm is deposited into the cytoplasm.

higher incidence of sex chromosomal anomalies than do children who are naturally conceived.

Preimplantation Genetic Diagnosis

Preimplantation genetic diagnosis is a highly specialized technique that enables the laboratory to precisely define the genetic normality of embryos. In patients with heritable, possibly life-threatening diseases, it is possible that offspring conceived with IVF and ICSI may have these diseases transmitted to them. This complex technique involves the removal of single cells from the early embryo while it is grown in petri dishes before transfer to the uterus. The genetic material from these "biopsied" cells can then be examined to determine whether the embryo carries an abnormal chromosome or gene. Through preimplantation genetic diagnosis, early human embryos that result from IVF and ICSI can be individually examined as they develop for the presence or absence of suspected genetic traits. Because of the real-time nature of the technique, decisions regarding embryo transfer are made within 24 h and help ensure that lethal diseases are not transmitted to offspring. Remarkably, the removal of a few cells from the embryo is not detrimental to the survival and normal development of most embryos.

REFERENCES

Male Reproductive Physiology

Aitken RJ, West K, Buckingham D: Leukocytic infiltration into the human ejaculate and its association with semen quality, oxidative stress, and sperm function. J Androl 1994;15:343.

Amann RP, Howards SS: Daily spermatozoal production and epididymal spermatozoal reserves of the human male. J Urol 1980;124:211.

Hess RA et al: A role for estrogens in the male reproductive system. Nature 1997;390:509.

Mather JP, Woodruff TK, Krummen LA: Paracrine regulation of reproductive function by inhibin and activin. Proc Soc Exp Biol Med 1992;20:1.

Turek PJ: Immunopathology and infertility. In: Lipshultz LI, Howards SS (editors): *Infertility in the Male,* 3rd ed. Mosby Year Book, 1997.

Turek PJ et al: Observations on seminal vesicle dynamics in an in vivo rat model. J Urol 1998;159:1731.

Von Eckardstein S et al: Serum inhibin B in combination with FSH is a more sensitive marker than FSH alone for impaired spermatogenesis in men, but cannot predict the presence of sperm in testicular tissue samples. J Clin Endocrinol Metab 1999;2496.

Whitmore WF, Kars L, Gittes RF: The role of germinal epithelium and spermatogenesis in the privileged survival of intratesticular grafts. J Urol 1985;134:782.

Diagnosis Of Male Infertility

Aitken R et al: Analysis of the relationship between defective sperm function and the generation of reactive oxygen species in cases of oligozoospermia. J Androl 1989;10:214.

Carlsen E et al: Evidence for decreasing quality of semen during the past 50 years. Br Med J 1992;105:609.

Cayan S et al: Response to varicocelectomy in oligospermic infertile men with and without coexisting genetic infertility. Urology 2001;57:530.

Clarke GN, Elliot PJ, Smaila C: Detection of sperm antibodies in semen using the immunobead test: A survey of 813 consecutive patients. Am J Reprod Immunol Microbiol 1985;7:118.

Clifton DK, Bremner WJ: The effect of testicular X-irradiation on spermatogenesis in man. J Androl 1983;4:387.

Davis RO, Katz DF: Computer-aided sperm analysis: Technology at a crossroads. Fertil Steril 1993;59:953.

Guzick DS et al: Sperm morphology, motility and concentration in fertile and infertile men. N Engl J Med 2001;345:1388.

Kruger TF et al: Predictive value of abnormal sperm morphology in in vitro fertilization. Fertil Steril 1988;49:112.

Liu DY, Baker WHG: Tests of human sperm function and fertilization in vitro. Fertil Steril 1992;58:465.

MacLeod J, Gold RZ: The male factor in fertility and infertility: Spermatozoan counts in 1000 men of known fertility and in 1000 cases of infertile marriage. J Urol 1951;66:436.

MacLeod J, Hitchkiss RS: The effects of hyperpyrexia on spermatozoa counts in men. Endocrinology 1941;28:780.

McClure RD, Hricak H: Scrotal ultrasound in the infertile man: Detection of subclinical unilateral and bilateral varicoceles. J Urol 1986;135:711.

Meacham RB, Hellerstein DK, Lipshultz LI: Evaluation and treatment of ejaculatory duct obstruction in the infertile male. Fertil Steril 1993;59:393.

Meinertz H et al: Antisperm antibodies and fertility after vasovasostomy: A follow-up study of 216 men. Fertil Steril 1990; 54:315.

Meng MV et al: Impaired spermatogenesis in men with congenital absence of the vas deferens. Hum Reprod 2001;16:529.

Petros JA et al: Correlation of testicular color Doppler ultrasonography, physical examination and venography in the detection of left varicoceles in men with infertility. J Urol 1991;145:785.

Rodriguez-Rigau LJ, Smith KD, Steinberger E: Varicocele and the morphology of spermatozoa. Fertil Steril 1981;35:54.

Schlegel PN, Chang TSK, Marshall FF: Antibiotics: Potential hazards to male fertility. Fertil Steril 1991;55:235.

Sigman M, Jarow JP: Medical evaluation of infertile men. Urology 1997;50:659.

Sigman M, Lipshultz LI, Howards SS: Evaluation of the subfertile male. In: Lipshultz LI, Howards SS (editors): *Infertility in the Male*, 3rd ed. Mosby Year Book, 1997.

Turek PJ et al: Diagnostic findings from testis fine needle aspiration mapping in obstructed and non-obstructed azoospermic men. J Urol 2000;163:1709.

Urban MD, Lee PA, Migeon CJ: Adult height and fertility in men with congenital virilizing adrenal hyperplasia. N Engl J Med 1978;299:1392.

Weintraub MP, De Mouy E, Hellstrom WJG: Newer modalities in the diagnosis and treatment of ejaculatory duct obstruction. J Urol 1993;150:1150.

World Health Organization: *WHO Laboratory Manual for the Examination of Human Semen and Sperm-Cervical Mucus Interaction*, 3rd ed. Cambridge Univ Press, 1992.

Zamboni L: The ultrastructural pathology of the spermatozoa as a cause of infertility: The role of electron microscopy in the evaluation of semen quality. Fertil Steril 1987;48:711.

Causes of Male Infertility—Pretesticular

Aiman J et al: Androgen insensitivity as a cause of infertility in otherwise normal men. N Engl J Med 1979;300:223.

Carter JN et al: Prolactin-secreting tumors and hypogonadism in 22 men. N Engl J Med 1978;299:847.

Fairman C et al: The "fertile eunuch" syndrome: Demonstration of isolated luteinizing hormone deficiency by radioimmunoassay technique. Mayo Clin Proc 1968;43:661.

Griffin JE: Androgen resistance: The clinical and molecular spectrum. N Engl J Med 1992;326:611.

Lieblich JM et al: Syndrome of anosmia with hypogonadotropic hypogonadism (Kallmann syndrome): Clinical and laboratory studies in 23 cases. Am J Med 1982;73:506.

Mozaffarian GA, Higley M, Paulsen CA: Clinical studies in an adult male patient with "isolated follicle stimulating hormone (FSH) deficiency." J Androl 1983;4:393.

Causes of Male Infertility—Testicular

Aiman J, Griffin JE: The frequency of androgen receptor deficiency in infertile men. J Clin Endocrinol Metab 1982;54:725.

Aynsley-Green A et al: Congenital bilateral anorchia in childhood: A clinical, endocrine and therapeutic evaluation of twenty-one cases. Clin Endocrinol 1976;5:381.

Coburn M, Wheeler TM, Lipshultz LI: Testicular biopsy: Its uses and limitations. Urol Clin North Am 1987;14:551.

Gorelick J, Goldstein M: Loss of fertility in men with varicocele. Fertil Steril 1993;59:613.

Kass EJ, Belman B: Reversal of testicular growth failure by varicocele ligation. J Urol 1987;137:475.

Kjessler B: Chromosomal constitution and male reproductive failure. In: Mancini RE, Martini L (editors): *Male Fertility and Sterility*. Academic Press, 1974.

Kostiner DR, Turek PJ, Reijo RA: Male infertility: Analysis of the markers and genes on the human Y chromosome. Hum Reprod 1998;13:3032.

Lipshultz LI et al: Testicular function after orchiopexy for unilaterally undescended testis. N Engl J Med 1976;295:15.

Okuyama M et al: Surgical repair of varicocele at puberty: Preventive treatment for fertility improvement. J Urol 1988; 139:562.

Turek PJ, Lowther DN, Carroll PA: Fertility issues and their management in men with testis cancer. Urol Clin North Am 1998;25:517.

Turek PJ et al: The reversibility of anabolic-induced azoospermia. J Urol 1995;153:1628.

World Health Organization: The influence of varicocele on parameters of fertility in a large group of men presenting to infertility clinics. Fertil Steril 1992;57:1289.

Causes of Male Infertility—Posttesticular

Afzelius BA, Mossberg B: The immotile-cilia syndrome including Kartagener's syndrome. In: Stanbury JB et al (editor): *The Metabolic Basis of Inherited Disease*, 5th ed. McGraw-Hill, 1983.

Chillon M et al: Mutations in the cystic fibrosis gene in patients with congenital absence of the vas deferens. N Engl J Med 1995;332:1475.

Handelsman DJ et al: Young's syndrome: Obstructive azoospermia and chronic sinopulmonary infections. N Engl J Med 1984; 310:3.

Jaffe T, Oates RD: Genetic abnormalities and reproductive failure. Urol Clin North Am 1994;21:389.

Matsuda T, Horii Y, Yoshida O: Obstructive azoospermia of unknown origin: Sites of obstruction and surgical outcomes. J Urol 1994;151:1543.

Matsumiya K et al: Clinical study of azoospermia. Int J Androl 1994;17:140.

Nagler HM, Deitch AD, deVere White R: Testicular torsion: Temporal considerations. Fertil Steril 1984;42:257.

Turek PJ: Immunopathology and infertility. In: Lipshultz LI, Howards SS (editors): *Infertility in the Male,* 3rd ed. Mosby Year Book, 1997.

Genetic Causes of Male Infertility

Kent-First MG et al: Infertility in intracytoplasmic-sperm-injection-derived sons. Lancet 1996;348:332.

Kuroda-Kawaguchi T et al: The AZFc region of the Y chromosome features massive palindromes and uniform recurrent deletions in infertile men. Nat Genet 2001;29:279.

Mak V, Jarvi K: The genetics of male infertility. J Urol 1996; 156:1245.

Mulhall JP et al: Azoospermic men with deletion of the DAZ gene cluster are capable of completing spermatogenesis: Fertilization, normal embryonic development and pregnancy occur when retrieved testicular spermatozoa are used for intracytoplasmic sperm injection. Hum Reprod 1997;12:503.

Nudell D et al: Increased frequency of mutations in DNA from infertile men with meiotic arrest. Hum Reprod 2000;15:1289.

Pryor JL et al: Microdeletions in the Y chromosome of infertile men. N Engl J Med 1997;336:534.

Reijo R et al: Diverse spermatogenic defects in humans caused by Y chromosome deletions encompassing a novel RNA-binding protein gene. Nat Genet 1995;10:383.

Reijo R et al: Severe oligospermia resulting from deletions of the Azoospermia Factor gene on the Y chromosome. Lancet 1996;347:1290.

Tiepolo L, Zuffardi O: Localization of factors controlling spermatogenesis in the nonfluorescent portion of the human Y chromosome long arm. Hum Genet 1976;34:119.

Xu EY, Moore FL, Reijo Pera RA: A gene family required for human germ cell development evolved from an ancient meiotic gene conserved in metazoans. Proc Nat Acad Sci (USA) 2001;98:7414.

Treatment of Male Infertility

Anguiano A et al: Congenital bilateral absence of the vas deferens: A primarily genital form of cystic fibrosis. JAMA 1992; 267:1794.

Baker WHG et al: Protective effect of antioxidants on the impairment of semen motility by activated polymorphonuclear leukocytes. Fertil Steril 1996;65:411.

Belker AM et al: Results of 1,469 microsurgical vasectomy reversals by the vasovasostomy study group. J Urol 1991;145:505.

Bennett CJ et al: Sexual dysfunction and electroejaculation in men with spinal cord injury: Review. J Urol 1988;139:453.

Branigan EF, Muller CH: Efficacy of treatment and recurrence rate of leukocytospermia in infertile men with prostatitis. Fertil Steril 1994;62:580.

Burris AS et al: A low sperm concentration does not preclude fertility in men with isolated hypogonadotropic hypogonadism after gonadotropin therapy. Fertil Steril 1988;50:343.

Cohen J et al: In vitro fertilization: A treatment for male infertility. Fertil Steril 1985;43:422.

Damani MN et al: Post-chemotherapy ejaculatory azoospermia: Fatherhood with sperm from testis tissue using intracytoplasmic sperm injection. J Clin Oncology 2002;20:930.

Devroey P et al: Pregnancies after testicular sperm extraction and intracytoplasmic sperm injection in non-obstructive azoospermia. Hum Reprod 1995;10:1457.

Enquist E, Stein BS, Sigman M: Laparoscopic versus subinguinal varicocelectomy: A comparative study. Fertil Steril 1994; 61:1092.

Goldstein M: *The Surgery of Male Infertility.* Saunders, 1995.

Goldstein M et al: Microsurgical inguinal varicocelectomy with delivery of the testis: An artery and lymphatic sparing technique. J Urol 1992;148:1808.

Haas GG Jr, Manganiello P: A double-blind, placebo-controlled study of the use of methylprednisolone in infertile men with sperm-associated immunoglobulins. Fertil Steril 1987; 47:295.

Hendry WF et al: Comparison of prednisolone and placebo in subfertile men with antibodies to spermatozoa. Lancet 1990; 335:85.

Kadioglu A et al: Does response to treatment of ejaculatory duct obstruction in infertile men vary with pathology? Fertil Steril 2001;76:138.

Madgar I et al: Controlled trial of high spermatic vein ligation for varicocele in infertile men. Fertil Steril 1995;63:120.

Matthews GJ, Schlegel PN, Goldstein M: Patency following microsurgical vasoepididymostomy and vasovasostomy: Temporal considerations. J Urol 1993;154:2070.

Nudell DM et al: The mini-MESA for sperm retrieval: A study of urological outcomes. Hum Reprod 1998;13:1260.

Ovesen P et al: Growth hormone treatment of subfertile males. Fertil Steril 1996;66:292.

Royle MG, Hendry WF: Why does vasectomy reversal fail? Br J Urol 1988;57:780.

Schoysman R et al: Pregnancy after fertilisation with human testicular spermatozoa. (Letter.) Lancet 1993;342:1237.

Sharlip ID: What is the best pregnancy rate that may be expected from vasectomy reversal? J Urol 1993;149:1469.

Steckel J, Dicker AP, Goldstein M: Relationship between varicocele size and response to varicocelectomy. J Urol 1993;149:769.

Tournaye H et al: Are there predictive factors for successful testicular sperm recovery in azoospermic patients? Hum Reprod 1997;12:80.

Turek PJ, Magana JO, Lipshultz LI: Semen parameters before and after transurethral surgery for ejaculatory duct obstruction. J Urol 1996;155:1291.

Van Steirteghem AC et al: High fertilization and implantation rates after intracytoplasmic sperm injection. Hum Reprod 1993; 8:1061.

Renovascular Hypertension

R. Ernest Sosa, MD, & E. Darracott Vaughan, Jr, MD

Renovascular disease is one of the most common causes of secondary hypertension. Renovascular hypertension is underdiagnosed in clinical practice. Although emphasis has been placed on developing accurate tests to identify the 5% of hypertensive patients who have renovascular hypertension, there are no perfect screening tests for its detection. Improved detection is possible because of a better understanding of clinical clues and pathophysiology of renovascular hypertension (Table 43–1). The diagnosing of renovascular hypertension is important for several reasons: (1) Renovascular hypertension can be difficult to manage medically. (2) Many renal artery lesions are progressive and may result in complete renal artery occlusion despite adequate medical management. Renovascular disease is a major cause of end-stage renal disease, especially in elderly patients. (3) High-renin hypertension is associated with an increased rate of cerebrovascular and cardiovascular complications. (4) Renal revascularization by surgical correction or angioplasty can potentially cure or better control the hypertension and reverse renal insufficiency. Renal parenchymal diseases can also cause hypertension (Table 43–2). In many cases the hypertension is correctable if properly diagnosed and treated.

Etiology

Renal disease in association with hypertension has been recognized since the early nineteenth century. In 1898, Tigerstadt and Bergman demonstrated that a water-soluble substance—extracted from the renal cortex of a healthy rabbit and termed **renin**—produced marked and sustained hypertension when injected intravenously into a second healthy rabbit.

In 1934 Goldblatt described 2 models of experimental hypertension. In a 2-kidney animal, clipping of one renal artery results in sustained hypertension. Removal of the clip or of the ischemic kidney returns the blood pressure to normal. This model is analogous to unilateral renal artery stenosis in humans: The hypertension is renin-dependent. In humans, as in the Goldblatt 2-kidney, 1-clip model of hypertension, unilateral renal ischemia has been shown to produce high-renin, angiotensin-dependent hypertension that can be cured by reconstruction of the renal artery, percutaneous balloon catheter dilation of the stenosed artery, or nephrectomy (Figure 43–1). In the second model—1 clip, 1 kidney—the hypertension is sodium volume–dependent. Blockade of the renin-angiotensin system has little effect on blood pressure, unless the animal is sodium-depleted. This model is analogous to renal artery stenosis in a solitary kidney. It may also resemble bilateral renal artery stenosis.

Natural History

Atheromatous renal arterial disease predominantly occurs in the proximal third of the renal artery and is often part of diffuse atherosclerosis, affecting many other vascular beds (eg, coronary, carotid, and pudendal arteries). In many cases, a plaque in the wall of the aorta may encroach on the ostium of the renal artery. Atheromatous disease of the renal artery most commonly afflicts older men. The disease is often bilateral (40%) and progressive (44%), resulting in total occlusion (16%) despite medical treatment of the hypertension.

Fibromuscular dysplasia of the renal arteries is the most common cause of renovascular hypertension in younger patients. It is diagnosed in one-third of patients with renovascular hypertension. These lesions can be progressive in up to 33% of cases but rarely result in total arterial occlusion. There are 4 different pathologic types of fibromuscular dysplasia. Medial fibroplasia is the most common and accounts for 70% of cases. The angiographic appearance is that of a string of beads owing to thickening of the media interspersed with areas of aneurysmal dilation. These lesions are rare in children.

In a study of potential renal donors, 27% of the normotensive patients with incidentally found fibromuscular dysplasia subsequently became hypertensive over the ensuing 7.5 years.

Thus, renal arterial lesions are often progressive. This fact provides strong support for angioplasty or surgical revascularization to maintain renal function and correct hypertension.

Pathogenesis

The renin-angiotensin-aldosterone system is an integrated hormonal cascade that simultaneously controls blood pressure and sodium and potassium balance, and influences regional blood flow. Renin is a proteolytic

Table 43–1. Causes of renovascular hypertension.

Common causes
Atherosclerosis (66%)
Fibromuscular dysplasia (33%)
Intimal fibroplasia (about 5%)
Fibromuscular hyperplasia (about 2%)
Medial fibroplasia (about 80%)
Perimedial fibroplasia (about 15%)
Rare causes
Polyarteritis nodosa
Takayasu's arteritis
Arteriovenous fistula
Aortic aneurysm
Coarctation of the aorta
Middle aortic syndrome
Radiation arteritis
Cholesterol emboli

enzyme produced in the juxtaglomerular cells of the afferent arterioles. It acts on renin substrate (angiotensinogen), an alpha-2 globulin produced in the liver, to form the decapeptide angiotensin I. Converting enzyme cleaves 2 amino acids from angiotensin I to form the octapeptide angiotensin II, a potent arterial vasoconstrictor. Angiotensin II also stimulates the zona glomerulosa of the adrenal gland to secrete aldosterone. Elevation of blood pressure and restoration of sodium balance inhibit further renin secretion.

The mechanisms responsible for renin secretion include an afferent arteriolar baroreceptor responding to

Table 43–2. Nonvascular causes of renal hypertension in unilateral renal parenchymal disease.

Surgery indicated
Renal cell carcinoma
Wilms tumor
Reninoma
Obstructive uropathy
Nonfunctioning atrophic kidney
Surgery only upon proved indications
Chronic pyelonephritis associated with vesicoureteral reflux
Polycystic kidney
Radiation nephritis
Perinephric scarring (Page kidney)
Segmental hypoplasia (Ask-Upmark kidney)
Renal tuberculosis

decreased renal perfusion pressure, a sensor at the macula densa responding to decreased delivery of sodium and chloride to the distal tubule, and increased activity of the sympathetic nervous system, mediated by beta-1-adrenergic receptors. Frequent causes of hypersecretion of renin include sodium depletion, hemorrhage, shock, congestive heart failure, and renal artery stenosis.

Plasma renin activity is closely related to the patient's sodium intake and urinary sodium excretion, that is, sodium balance. Figure 43–2 illustrates how the plasma renin activity varies with the sodium balance, which is determined by measuring the urinary excretion of sodium in a 24-h specimen.

Pathology

Stenosis of the renal artery (and, therefore, renovascular hypertension) is most commonly caused by arteriosclerotic plaques or fibromuscular dysplasia (Table 43–1). Not all renal artery stenoses are physiologically significant and cause hypertension, however. A lesion must produce a reduction in luminal diameter of at least 70% before renal plasma flow is reduced to the point that clinically significant ischemia results. The clinical significance of an anatomic stenosis noted on angiography or magnetic resonance angiography is assessed by renin assays, as discussed subsequently.

Other urologic lesions that may cause renin-dependent hypertension include obstructive uropathy, benign and malignant renal masses, and chronic pyelonephritis, the latter most commonly associated with vesicoureteral reflux (Table 43–2). However, hypertension due to renal parenchymal disease usually is not curable by surgical means. Most patients require medical management to control blood pressure.

History & Physical Examination

A. History

A complete and thorough medical history and physical examination provide important information about the patient's current general health, past medical history, and family medical history. Clinical clues and other factors suggestive of renovascular hypertension are set forth in Table 43–3. The patient's age and circumstances at onset of hypertension, recorded blood pressure ranges, previous treatment, results of therapy, and history of end-organ damage are noted. The past history is investigated for evidence of diseases (eg, glomerulonephritis, chronic pyelonephritis with or without vesicoureteral reflux, hydronephrosis, urolithiasis) or other factors (eg, renal trauma, radiation therapy to the abdomen) that could contribute to the development of hypertension.

Figure 43–1. **Left:** Characteristics of the early phase of 2-kidney, 1-clip Goldblatt hypertension in the rat. **Right:** The criteria derived from the animal model that serves to identify patients with correctable renal hypertension. Roman numerals relate left and right parts of figure. (Modified and reproduced, with permission, from Vaughan ED Jr et al: Clinical evaluation of renovascular hypertension and therapeutic decisions. Urol Clin North Am 1984;11:393.)

Hypertension may have an abrupt onset and progress rapidly in children with Wilms tumor, in young adults with fibromuscular dysplasia, and in older patients with arteriosclerotic occlusion of the renal artery. However, the absence of symptoms is not sufficient to rule out a diagnosis of curable hypertension.

Pulmonary edema is relatively frequent in patients with advanced renovascular hypertension with bilateral disease and azotemia.

B. PHYSICAL EXAMINATION

Physical examination should include serial measurements of the patient's blood pressure to establish the degree of hypertension. Measurements are taken in each arm with an appropriate-sized cuff while the patient is standing, sitting, and lying down. If 3 measurements are higher than 140/90 mm Hg in an adult, further evaluation is warranted. A funduscopic examination should be performed to look for hemorrhage, exudates, and papilledema. The physician should palpate all peripheral pulses. Diminution of pulses and decreased blood pressure in the lower extremities in a young patient may signify coarctation of the aorta; an intrascapular murmur is another characteristic sign. In patients with renal artery stenosis, a continuous abdom-

inal bruit may be heard on either side of the midline immediately above the umbilicus.

Laboratory Evaluation

A. RENOVASCULAR HYPERTENSION

The low prevalence of renovascular hypertension among hypertensive patients, together with the cost and less than perfect accuracy of screening tests for renovascular hypertension, makes screening for this disease impractical. Pickering and colleagues have suggested that for patients with a low index of suspected disease, only basic evaluation is needed (Table 43–3) (Figure 43–3). These include patients with borderline, mild, or moderate hypertension in the absence of clinical clues, and patients with low renin hypertension. For patients with a moderate index of suspected disease, noninvasive tests should be performed as described below. For this group the prevalence of renovascular hypertension is between 5% and 15%. For patients with a high index of suspected disease, for example, those with severe hypertension (diastolic > 120 mm Hg) refractory to aggressive medical treatment or with an increase in creatinine, or patients with malignant hypertension (type III or IV retinopathy), arteriography or magnetic resonance

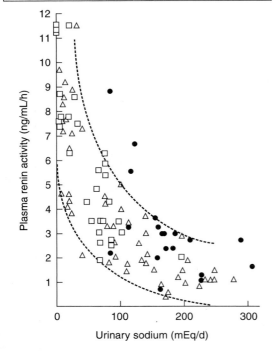

	No. of subjects	No. of assays
△ Balanced diet – Outpatient	19	53
☐ Balanced diet – Metabolic ward	14	31
● Random sample	20	20

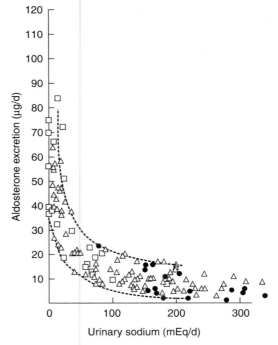

	No. of subjects	No. of assays
△ Balanced diet – Outpatient	19	88
☐ Balanced diet – Metabolic ward	12	24
● Random sample	18	18

Figure 43–2. Plasma renin activity levels obtained at noon (**left**) and 24-h urinary aldosterone excretion levels (**right**) in relation to daily urinary sodium excretion levels in normal subjects. In such subjects, plasma renin activity and excretion of aldosterone describe similar hyperbolic curves in relation to sodium excretion. The fact that a random sampling of nonhospitalized subjects consuming uncontrolled diets yielded similar results enhances the validity of this nomogram for use in studies of outpatients or subjects not consuming a constant diet. (Reproduced, with permission, from Laragh JH: *Hypertension Manual.* York Medical Books, 1973.)

angiography is indicated. These patients are likely to have deterioration in renal function when treated with converting-enzyme inhibitors and are at high risk for ischemic nephropathy.

1. Basic tests—Laboratory examination of patients with suspected renovascular hypertension (Figure 43–3) should begin with basic tests that assess the patient's general health: complete blood count, serum electrolytes and fasting blood glucose determinations, blood urea nitrogen and serum creatinine measurements, urinalysis and urine culture, and an electrocardiogram.

2. Plasma renin activity profile—In patients in whom the diagnosis of hypertension has been definitively established, evaluation with a plasma renin activ-

ity profile (plasma renin activity must be plotted against 24-h urinary sodium excretion) is performed. These measurements should be obtained while the patient is on a diet containing normal amounts of sodium; antihypertensive medication must be withheld for 2 weeks before sampling. The blood sample for the renin determination is drawn at the end of the 24-h period in which the urine is collected and after 4 h of ambulatory activity. This test will reveal elevated plasma renin activity levels in about 80% of patients with renovascular hypertension (Figure 43–4, left). However, 15% of patients with essential hypertension also have high renin, which lowers the predictive value of the test.

3. Captopril challenge test—Peripheral plasma renin activity is measured before and 1 h after administration

Table 43–3. Testing for renovascular hypertension: Clinical index of suspicion as a guide to selecting patients for workup.

Low (should not be tested)
   Borderline, mild, or moderate hypertension, in the absence of clinical clues
Moderate (noninvasive tests recommended)
   Severe hypertension (diastolic blood pressure > 120 mm Hg)
   Hypertension refractory to standard therapy
   Abrupt onset of sustained moderate to severe hypertension at age < 20 or > 50 years
   Hypertension with a suggestive abdominal bruit (long, high-pitched, and localized to the region of the renal artery)
   Moderate hypertension (diastolic blood pressure exceeding 105 mm Hg) in a smoker, a patient with evidence of occlusive vascular disease (cerebrovascular, coronary, peripheral vascular), or a patient with unexplained but stable elevation of serum creatinine
   Normalization of blood pressure by an angiotensin-converting enzyme inhibitor in a patient with moderate or severe hypertension (particularly in a smoker or patient with recent onset of hypertension)
High (may consider proceeding directly to arteriography)
   Severe hypertension (diastolic blood pressure greater than 120 mm Hg) with either progressive renal insufficiency of refractoriness to aggressive treatment (particularly in a patient who has been a smoker or has other evidence of occlusive arterial disease)
   Accelerated or malignant hypertension (grade III or IV retinopathy)
   Hypertension with recent elevation of serum creatinine, either unexplained or reversibly induced by an angiotensin-converting enzyme inhibitor
   Moderate to severe hypertension with incidentally detected asymmetry of renal size

---

of captopril (a converting-enzyme inhibitor), 25 mg orally. In renin-dependent hypertension, inhibition of the converting enzyme occurs. If the 3 criteria found by Muller (Table 43–4) are present in a patient with normal renal function who is not taking diuretics, renovascular hypertension can be distinguished from essential hypertension. Other investigators confirmed the value of the captopril test, although they found it less reliable than first reported. The overall sensitivity is approximately 61%, and specificity is 86%. Previous sodium depletion due to use of diuretics, dietary restrictions, and chronic treatment with captopril increases plasma renin activity and causes the captopril challenge test to be nonspecific. Patients taking beta blockers remain responsive to the test as described previously, unless the baseline plasma renin activity is less than 2.5 ng/mL/h, in which case the test may be unreliable.

Most studies have found the test to be less reliable in azotemic patients, and it does not discriminate between unilateral and bilateral disease. Moreover, the test may be less reliable in black patients than in white patients.

4. Captopril renography—An addition to the captopril test is the comparison of ^{131}I-hippurate and ^{99m}Tc-diethylenetriaminepentaacetic acid (^{99m}Tc-DTPA) or ^{99m}Tc mercaptoacetyltriglycine (MAG3) renography before and after single-dose captopril. Patients with renal artery stenosis show a fall in glomerular filtration confined to the affected kidney and thus a selective fall in ^{99m}Tc-DTPA uptake with preservation or even an increase in ^{131}I-hippurate and ^{99m}Tc-DTPA uptake to the normal side. Captopril renography has been found to have 90–92% sensitivity and 86–93% sensitivity in various studies. It has become one of the most popular noninvasive tests for renovascular hypertension. Captopril renography may be less reliable in patients with impaired renal function or in patients with severe renal artery stenosis.

5. Ultrasound scans—Renal Doppler ultrasound scanning is gaining widespread use for the evaluation of renovascular disease. Doppler ultrasound scanning can record velocity profiles of blood flow from the renal arteries and parenchyma. Several criteria have been used to identify a stenosis. One is to take the ratio of the peak systolic velocity between the aorta and the renal artery. A renal-aortic ratio of 3.5 or more and peak systolic velocity of more than 200 cm/s are considered indicative of a significant stenosis. Another is the "tardus-parvus" pattern, which occurs distal to a stenosis and is characterized by a smaller and more rounded waveform.

Doppler exam of the main renal arteries may fail technically in up to 40% of patients. An alternative strategy is to use the flow profile from the interlobar arteries. This can be quantified as the renal resistive index, which is defined as the peak systolic flow velocity peak end-diastolic flow velocity/peak systolic flow velocity × 100. A difference of resistive index between the 2 kidneys of more than 5% has been used as an indication of renal artery stenosis. Also, the absence of flow in the artery and a low-amplitude parenchymal signal is diagnostic of occlusion of the renal artery.

The advantages of duplex scanning are that it is noninvasive and free of adverse effects. For the patient with an elevated serum creatinine in whom the physician wants to determine, with a high degree of likelihood, whether significant renal artery disease is contributing to the azotemia, duplex scanning is useful. It can also be used for following up patients after percutaneous transluminal renal angioplasty, renal artery stents, or bypass surgery.

Figure 43–3. Suggested workup for renovascular hypertension.

An interesting development has been to use the hemodynamic effects of captopril to improve the diagnostic accuracy of Doppler scanning. Rene et al (1995) found that the pulsus tardus pattern was more likely to be seen after captopril in stenotic renal arteries; 68% of stenoses could be diagnosed before captopril, and 100% could be diagnosed after captopril. Another technique is to compare the resistive index of the ischemic and nonischemic kidneys before and after captopril.

6. Magnetic resonance angiography (MRA)—Magnetic resonance angiography is a technique that has the ability (Figure 43–5) to visualize arteries noninvasively without contrast material. Using phase contrast imaging, the gadolinium-enhanced MRA with 3-dimensional reconstruction of the images, sensitivities, and specificities has been reported to be > 90% when compared with conventional angiography. MRA is much better at detecting proximal than peripheral lesions. The low false-negative rate for detecting major atherosclerotic lesions means that a normal MRA obviates the need for traditional angiography in high-risk patients. Its expense and the high degree of expertise required to obtain and correctly interpret good images precludes its use as a general screening test.

7. Helical (spiral) computed tomography—Computed tomography (CT) can be used to visualize arteries as well as solid tissues. Spiral CT differs from conventional CT in that it incorporates a rapidly rotating gantry, which enables acquisition of images with sufficient rapidity to visualize arteries as the contrast material passes through. The resolution compares very favorably with that of MRA, although both techniques have limited ability to detect accessory renal arteries. The main appeal of spiral CT is that it enables construction of 3-dimensional images of the aorta, renal arteries, and kidneys all at the same time, using one of 2 procedures (maximal intensity projection or surface shaded display). Both are time-consuming to construct and re-

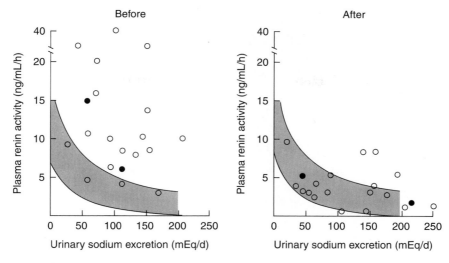

Figure 43–4. Effect of angioplasty on peripheral plasma renin activity level plotted against 24-h urinary sodium excretion. **Left:** Before angioplasty. **Right:** Six months after angioplasty. Hatched area shows normal range. o = Cured or improved, • = Failed to improve. (Reproduced, with permission, from Pickering TG et al: Predictive value and changes of renin secretion in hypertensive patients with unilateral renovascular disease undergoing successful renal angioplasty. Am J Med 1984;76:398).

quire a highly skilled radiologist or technician. The sensitivity and specificity of spiral CT for detecting renal artery stenoses have been reported to be in the region of 95%. Unlike MRA, it can be used to examine the patency of renal arteries with intravascular stents. The chief disadvantages are the cost and the much greater volume of contrast agents needed to obtain adequate images (about 150 mL, compared with 15 mL for conventional digital subtraction angiography). This greatly limits its use in patients with impaired renal function.

Table 43–4. Single-dose captopril test. Criteria distinguishing patients with renovascular hypertension from those with essential hypertension.

Stimulated plasma renin activity of 12 ng/mL/h or more **and**
Absolute increase in plasma renin activity of 10 ng/mL/h **or** more **and**
Percent increase in plasma renin activity of 150% or more **or** of 400% if the baseline plasma renin activity is less than 3 ng/mL/h.

Source: Reproduced, with permission, from Muller FB et al: The captopril test for identifying renovascular disease in hypertensive patients. Am J Med 1986;80:633.

8. Renal vein renin sampling—Patients with high peripheral plasma renin activity levels or those in whom the captopril challenge test is positive may undergo further evaluation with renal vein sampling for renin. Samples are collected from each renal vein (V1 and V2) and from the distal inferior vena cava before and after administration of captopril, 25 mg orally.

According to criteria established by Vaughan et al, potentially reversible hypertension is characterized by ipsilateral hypersecretion of renin ([V1 − A] divided by A ≤ 0.50), contralateral suppression of renin secretion ([V2 − A] divided by A = 0), and an increase in the peripheral plasma renin activity level. In patients with stenoses of both renal arteries, the pattern of renal vein renins often shows the same degree of asymmetry as in unilateral stenosis, lateralizing to the kidney with the greater degree of stenosis. The most marked asymmetry is seen in patients who have complete occlusion of one renal artery.

Renal vein renins are performed less widely today, in part because of high cost and the noninvasive tests described above, but also owing to the high false-negative rate that tends to exclude patients from the benefit of renal revascularization.

B. RENAL PARENCHYMAL DISEASE

In patients with suspected renal parenchymal disease, preoperative evaluation of plasma renin activity is

Figure 43–5. Three-dimensional, gadolinium-enhanced magnetic resonance angiography showing a thrombosis of the left renal artery (**A**) and severe stenosis of the left renal artery (**B**). (From Grenier N, Trillaud H: BJU International 2000;86(Suppl):84.)

similar to that described for patients with renovascular hypertension. The captopril challenge test is recommended in these patients to elicit evidence of a reactive rise in plasma renin activity and a fall in blood pressure. Hypertension due to renal parenchymal disease is less frequently curable by surgical treatment than is renovascular hypertension. Nephrectomy should be avoided if the blood pressure can be controlled with antihyper-

tensive medication and if the glomerular filtration rate in the involved kidney is sufficient to ensure the patient's survival if removal of the contralateral kidney ever becomes necessary.

Treatment

Patients with known or suspected hypertension must be methodically evaluated to identify those with renin-dependent hypertension and to plan individualized treatment.

There are 3 principal modes of treatment for renovascular hypertension: medical, surgical, and angioplasty with and without stents. Because renal artery stenoses impair renal function and cause hypertension, renal revascularization is preferred over medical management.

A. MEDICAL MEASURES

Medical management of patients was difficult before the advent of modern antihypertensive therapy, and survival has improved with angioplasty or surgical treatment. Currently, blood pressure can be controlled effectively but renal function may deteriorate, especially in patients with atherosclerotic disease. Converting-enzyme inhibitors are the most powerful drugs for patients with renovascular hypertension. However, the inhibition of angiotensin II constriction of the efferent glomerular arteriole may lead to decreased glomerular filtration rate and even renal failure in patients with bilateral renal arterial disease. In patients with bilateral renal artery stenosis or stenosis of a renal artery in a solitary kidney, use of converting-enzyme inhibitors may increase creatinine and blood urea nitrogen. Moreover, renal artery stenosis is progressive, with 15% of patients having complete occlusion despite adequate blood pressure control. Calcium channel blockers vasodilate the afferent arteriole and have been shown to lower blood pressure with less impairment of function than converting-enzyme inhibitors. In summary, medical management is limited to patients who are not candidates for intervention or in whom revascularization has failed. In these patients both blood pressure and renal function must be monitored carefully.

B. TRANSLUMINAL ANGIOPLASTY

Patients who meet the criteria for reversible renovascular hypertension can now be treated with percutaneous transluminal balloon dilation of the stenotic renal artery (transluminal angioplasty; see Chapter 8). In successful cases, angiograms obtained after transluminal angioplasty show enlargement of the diameter of the renal artery (Figure 43–6), and measurements show that the renin activity returns to normal levels and the

Figure 43–6. Aortograms showing unilateral right renal artery stenosis before (**left**) and after (**right**) successful percutaneous transluminal angioplasty. (Reproduced, with permission, from Vaughan ED Jr: Renal artery stenosis. In: Brenner BM, Stein JH [editors]: *Hypertension,* vol. 8 of *Contemporary Issues in Nephrology.* Churchill Livingstone, 1981.)

blood pressure likewise returns to normal or near-normal levels (Figures 43–4 and 43–7). Angioplasty is now the initial treatment of choice in all patients with fibromuscular hyperplasia and in patients with atherosclerotic disease, excluding those with osteal lesions and total occlusion. Successful dilation in more than 80% of these patients precludes the need for major surgery and can lower blood pressure while preserving or improving renal function. The results in patients with fibromuscular dysplasia are good. There is an overall benefit of 93% (58% cured, 35% improved, and 7% failed). Restenosis is uncommon in these patients. In patients with renal artery stenosis due to atheroma, the benefit is about 80% (22% cured, 58% improved, and 20% failed). The restenosis in patients with atheromatous disease is 19% after 9 months. It has been shown that failed angioplasty does not reduce the success rate of subsequent surgical renal revascularization.

C. Renal Artery Stents

Renal artery stents can be placed to maintain patency of the renal artery following angioplasty. The indications for stent placement include renal ostial stenoses that have a high restenosis rate following angioplasty. Other atheromatous lesions that were dilated unsuccessfully or have restenosed can be stented as well. The restenosis rate for these high-risk patients is less than that for angioplasty alone. The availability of stenting has changed treatment of patients with atheromatous lesions dramatically. Angioplasty with stenting is now the treatment of choice unless there is diffuse aortic disease with involvement of other intra-abdominal arteries.

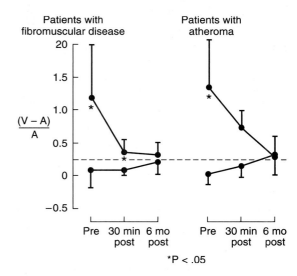

Figure 43–7. Effect of angioplasty on renal vein renin levels. Blood samples were drawn immediately before, 30 min after, and 6 months after angioplasty. The higher values are for the ischemic kidney; the lower ones, for the contralateral kidney. The asterisks indicate a significant difference between the 2 kidneys, and the dashed line represents the normal level of $(V - A)$ divided by A (0.24). (Reproduced, with permission, from Pickering TG et al: Predictive value and changes of renin secretion in hypertensive patients with unilateral renovascular disease undergoing successful renal angioplasty. Am J Med 1984;76:398.)

D. SURGICAL MEASURES

Surgery is indicated for patients with total renal artery occlusion and preservation of function, osteal lesions, and complex lesions, and those in whom percutaneous transluminal dilation is not successful. The first surgical cure of hypertension was achieved by unilateral nephrectomy. However, unilateral nephrectomy has benefited only 26–37% of the large group of unselected patients with hypertension who have been so treated. Unilateral nephrectomy is now reserved for treatment of 2 groups of patients with hypertension: (1) those who have poor or absent renal function in the involved kidney but normal function in the contralateral kidney and in whom attempts at revascularization have failed, and (2) those at such high risk that the loss of functioning nephrons is offset by the elimination of the cause of significant excess renin secretion. Partial nephrectomy may be performed if the kidney has multiple renal arteries and only one is stenotic.

Today, surgical treatment emphasizes preservation of renal function. Accordingly, various methods may be used to attempt to revascularize an ischemic kidney; these include endarterectomy, aortorenal bypass graft using the saphenous vein or hypogastric artery, and hepatorenal and splenorenal bypass procedures for patients with severely diseased aortas. Hypertension has been cured or improved in more than 90% of the carefully selected patients treated surgically by experienced operating teams; the mortality rate has been about 2%. Renal revascularization for preservation of renal function in azotemic patients with renal arterial disease is gaining wider acceptance irrespective of blood pressure or renin values. Long-term improvement or stabilization of renal function has been reported in about 70% of patients. All azotemic patients without a clear cause of renal failure should be evaluated for renal arterial disease.

REFERENCES

Darling CR et al: Outcome of renal artery reconstruction analysis of 687 procedures. Ann Surg 1999;230:524.

Dorros G et al: Four-year follow-up of Palmz-Schatz stent revascularization as treatment for atherosclerotic renal artery stenosis. Circulation 1998:98;642.

Johansson M et al: Evaluation of duplex ultrasound and captopril renography for detection of renovascular hypertension. Kidney Int 2000;58:774.

Novick AC, Fergany A: Renovascular hypertension and ischemic nephropathy. In: Walsh PC et al (editors): *Campbell's Urology,* 8th ed, Chapter 7, p. 229. Saunders, 2002.

Pedersen EB: New tools in diagnosing renal artery stenosis. Kidney Int 2000;57:2657.

Pickering TG, Blumenfeld JD: Renovascular hypertension and ischemic nephropathy. In: Brenner BM (editor): *The Kidney,* p. 2007. Saunders, 2000.

Pickering TG, Mann SJ: Renovascular hypertension: Medical evaluation and nonsurgical treatment. In: Laragh JH, Brenner BM (editors): *Hypertension: Pathophysiology, Diagnosis and Management,* 2nd ed, Chapter 120, p. 2039. Raven Press, 1995.

Ramos F et al: Renal function and outcome of PTRA and stenting for atherosclerotic renal artery stenosis. Kidney Int 2003; 63:276.

Snidow JJ et al: Three-dimensional gadolinium-enhanced MR angiography for aortoiliac in-flow assessment plus renal artery screening in a single breath hold. Radiology 1996;198:725.

Vaughan ED Jr, Sosa RE: Renovascular hypertension and ischemic nephropathy. In: Gillenwater JY et al (editors): *Adult and Pediatric Urology,* ed 4, Chapter 23, p. 972. Lippincott Williams & Wilkins, 2002.

Appendix: Normal Laboratory Values*

Marcus A. Krupp, AB, MD

Values may vary with method of measurement and population.

HEMATOLOGY

Antithrombin III: [P] 86–120%.

Bleeding time: Template method, 3–9 min (180–540 s).

Cellular measurements of red blood cells (erythrocytes):

Average diameter = 7.3 μm (5.5–8.8 μm).

Mean corpuscular volume (MCV): Men, 80–94 fL; women, 81–99 fL (by Coulter counter).

Mean corpuscular hemoglobin (MCH): 27–32 pg.

Mean corpuscular hemoglobin concentration (MCHC): 32–36 g/dL erythrocytes (32–36%).

Color, saturation, and volume indices: 1 (0.9–1.1).

Clot retraction: Begins in 1–3 h; complete in 6–24 h. No clot lysis in 24 h.

Fibrin D-dimer: [P] 0–250 ng/mL.

Fibrinogen split products: < 10 μg.

Fragility of erythrocytes: Begins at 0.45–0.38% NaCl; complete at 0.36–0.3% NaCl.

Glucose-6-phosphate dehydrogenase (G6-PD): [B] 4–8 μg/g Hb.

Hematocrit (PCV): Men, 40–52%; women, 37–47%.

Hemoglobin: [B] Men, 14–18 g/dL (2.09–2.79 mmol/L as Hb tetramer); women, 12–16 g/dL (1.86–2.48 mmol/L). [S] 2–3 mg/dL.

Partial thromboplastin time: Activated, 25–37 s.

Platelets: 150,000–400,000/mL (0.15–0.4 × 10^{12}/L).

Prothrombin: INR, 1–1.4.

Erythrocyte count: Men, 4.5–6.2 million/μL (4.5–6.2 × 10^{12}/L); women, 4–5.5 million/μL (4–5.5 × 10^{12}/L).

Reticulocytes: 0.6–1.8% of erythrocytes.

Sedimentation rate: Less than 20 mm/h (Westergren).

White blood count (leukocytes) and differential: 5000–10,000/μL (5–10 × 10^9/L).

Segmented neutrophils	40–70%
Myelocytes	0%
Juvenile neutrophils	0%
Band neutrophils	0–15%
Lymphocytes	15–45%
Eosinophils	1–3%
Basophils	0–5%
Monocytes	0–7%

Lymphocytes: Total, 1500–4000/μL	
B cell	5–25%
T cell	60–88%
Suppressor	10–43%
Helper	32–66%
H:S	> 1

BLOOD, PLASMA, OR SERUM CHEMICAL CONSTITUENTS (Values vary with method used.)

Acetone and acetoacetate: [S] 0.3–2 mg/dL (3–20 mg/L).

Aldolase: [S] Values vary with method used.

α-Amino acid nitrogen: [S, fasting] 3–5.5 mg/dL (2.2–3.9 mmol/L).

Aminotransferases:

Aspartate aminotransferase (AST; SGOT): [S] 15–55 IU/L.

Alanine aminotransferase (ALT; SGPT): [S] 10–70 IU/L. Values vary with method used.

Ammonia: [B] 9–33 μmol/L.

Amylase: [S] 80–180 units/dL (Somogyi). Values vary with method used.

α₁-Antitrypsin: [S] > 180 mg/dL.

Ascorbic acid: [P] 0.4–1.5 mg/dL (23–85 33 μmol/L).

Base, total serum: [S] 145–160 mEq/L (145–160 mmol/L).

Bicarbonate: [S] 24–28 mEq/L (24–28 mmol/L).

Bilirubin: [S] Total, 0.2–1.2 mg/dL (3.5–20.5 μmol/L). Direct conjugated, 0.1–0.4 mg/dL (< 7 μmol/L). Indirect, 0.2–0.7 mg/dL (< 12 μmol/L).

Calcium: [S] 8.5–10.3 mg/dL (2.1–2.6 mmol/L). Values vary with albumin concentration.

Calcium, ionized: [S] 4.25–5.25 mg/dL; 2.1–2.6 mEq/L (1.05–1.3 mmol/L).

β-Carotene: [S, fasting] 50–300 μg/dL (0.9–5.58 μmol/L).

---

*Blood [B], Plasma [P], Serum [S], Urine [U].

Ceruloplasmin: [S] 25–43 mg/dL (1.7–2.9 μmol/L).

Chloride: [S or P] 96–106 mEq/L (96–106 mmol/L).

Cholesterol: [S or P] 150–240 mg/dL (3.9–6.2 mmol/L). (See Lipid fractions.) Values vary with age.

Cholesteryl esters: [S] 65–75% of total cholesterol.

CO$_2$ content: [S or P] 24–29 mEq/L (24–29 mmol/L).

Complement: [S] C3 (b1C), 90–250 mg/dL. C4 ($β_{1E}$), 10–60 mg/dL. Total (CH$_{50}$), 75–160 mg/dL.

Copper: [S or P] 100–200 μg/dL (16–31 μmol/L).

Cortisol: [P] 8:00 AM, 5–25 μg/dL (138–690 nmol/L); 8:00 PM, < 14 μg/dL (385 nmol/L).

Creatine kinase (CK): [S] 10–50 IU/L at 30 °C. Values vary with method used.

Creatine kinase MB fraction: [S] < 4% total CK.

Creatinine: [S or P] 0.7–1.5 mg/dL (62–132 μmol/L).

Cyanocobalamin: [S] 200 pg/mL (148 pmol/L).

Epinephrine: [P] Supine, < 0.1 μg/L (< 0.55 nmol/L).

Erythropoietin: [S] 5–20% IU/L.

Ferritin: [S] Adult women, 20–120 ng/mL; men, 30–300 ng/mL. Child to 15 years, 7–140 ng/mL.

α-Fetoprotein: [S] 0–8.5 ng/mL.

Folic acid: [S] 2–20 ng/mL (4.5–45 nmol/L). [Erythrocytes] > 100 ng/mL (> 318 nmol/L).

Glucose: [S or P] 65–110 mg/dL (3.6–6.1 mmol/L).

α-Glutamyl transpeptidase: [S] 8–78 IU/L.

Glycosylated hemoglobin (HbA$_{10}$): [B] 4–7%.

Haptoglobin: [S] 40–200 mg of hemoglobin-binding capacity.

Iron: [S] 40–175 μg/dL (9–31.3 μmol/L).

Iron-binding capacity: [S] Total, 250–410 μg/dL (44.7–73.4 μmol/L). Percent saturation, 20–55%.

Lactate: [B, special handling] Venous, 4–16 mg/dL (0.44–1.8 mmol/L).

Lactate dehydrogenase (LDH): [S] 55–140 IU/L. Values vary with method used.

Lipase: [S] 0.2–1.5 units.

Lipid fractions: [S or P] Desirable levels: HDL cholesterol, > 40 mg/dL; LDL cholesterol, < 150 mg/dL; VLDL cholesterol, < 40 mg/dL. (To convert to mmol/L, multiply by 0.026.)

Lipids, total: [S] 450–1000 mg/dL (4.5–10 g/L).

Magnesium: [S or P] 1.8–3 mg/dL (0.75–1.25 mmol/L).

Myoglobin: [P] 15–100 ng/mL.

Norepinephrine: [P] Supine, < 0.5 μg/L (< 3 nmol/L).

Osmolality: [S] 280–296 mOsm/kg water.

Oxygen:

Capacity: [B] 16–24 vol%. Values vary with hemoglobin concentration.

Arterial content: [B] 15–23 vol%. Values vary with hemoglobin concentration.

Arterial % saturation: 94–100% of capacity.

Arterial P$_{O_2}$ (Pao$_2$): 80–100 mm Hg (10.67–13.33 kPa) (sea level). Values vary with age.

PaCO$_2$: [B, arterial] 35–45 mm Hg (4.7–6 kPa).

pH (reaction): [B, arterial] 7.35–7.45 (H$^+$ 44.7–45.5 nmol/L).

Phosphatase, acid: [S] 1–5 units (King-Armstrong), 0.1–0.63 units (Bessey-Lowry).

Phosphatase, alkaline: [S] 38–126 IU/L.

Phospholipid: [S] 145–200 mg/dL (1.45–2 g/L).

Phosphorus, inorganic: [S, fasting] 3–4.5 mg/dL (1–1.5 mmol/L).

Potassium: [S or P] 3.5–5 mEq/L (3.5–5 mmol/L).

Prostate-specific antigen (PSA): [S] 0–4 ng/mL.

Protein:

Total: [S] 6–8 g/dL (60–80 g/L).

Albumin: [S] 3.5–5.5 g/dL (35–55 g/L).

Globulin: [S] 2–3.6 g/dL (20–36 g/L).

Immunoglobulin: [S] IgA 78–400 mg/dL. IgG 690–1400 mg/dL. IgM 35–240 mg/dL.

Fibrinogen: [P] 0.2–0.6 g/dL (2–6 g/L).

Prothrombin clotting time: [P] By control. INR, 1–1.4.

Pyruvate: [B] 0.6–1 mg/dL (70–114 mmol/L).

Serotonin: [B] 0.05–0.2 μg/mL (0.28–1.14 μmol/L).

Sodium: [S or P] 136–145 mEq/L (136–145 mmol/L).

Specific gravity: [B] 1.056 (varies with hemoglobin and protein concentration). [S] 1.0254–1.0288 (varies with protein concentration).

Sulfate: [S or P] As sulfur, 0.5–1.5 mg/dL (156–468 μmol/L).

Transferrin: [S] 200–400 mg/dL (23–45 μmol/L).

Triglycerides: [S] < 165 mg/dL (1.9 mmol/L). (See Lipid fractions.)

Troponin: [S] < 0.5 ng/mL.

Urea nitrogen: [S or P] 8–25 mg/dL (2.9–8.9 mmol/L). Do not use anticoagulant containing ammonium oxalate.

Uric acid: [S or P] Men, 3–9 mg/dL (0.18–0.54 mmol/L); women, 2.5–7.5 mg/dL (0.15–0.45 mmol/L).

Vitamin A: [S] 15–60 μg/dL (0.53–2.1 μmol/L).

Vitamin B$_{12}$: [S] > 200 pg/mL (> 148 pmol/L).

Vitamin D: [S] Cholecalciferol (D$_3$): 25-Hydroxycholecalciferol, 8–55 ng/mL (19.4–137 nmol/L); 1,25-dihydroxycholecalciferol, 26–65 pg/mL (62–155 pmol/L); 24,25-dihydroxycholecalciferol, 1–5 ng/mL (2.4–12 nmol/L).

Volume, blood (Evans blue dye method): Adults, 2990–6980 mL. Women, 46.3–85.5 mL/kg; men, 66.2–97.7 mL/kg.

Zinc: [S] 50–150 μg/dL (7.65–22.95 μmol/L).

HORMONES, SERUM, OR PLASMA

Adrenal:

Aldosterone: [P] Supine, normal salt intake, 2–9 ng/dL (56–250 pmol/L); increased when upright.

Cortisol: [S] 8:00 AM, < 5–20 μg/dL (0.14–0.55 μmol/L); 8:00 PM, < 10 μg/dL (0.28 μmol/L).

Deoxycortisol: [S] After metyrapone, > 7 μg/dL (> 0.2 μmol/L).

Dopamine: [P] < 135 pg/mL.

Epinephrine: [P] < 0.1 ng/mL (< 0.55 nmol/L).

Norepinephrine: [P] < 0.5 μg/L (< 3 nmol/L). See also Miscellaneous Normal Values.

Gonad:

Testosterone, free: [S] Men, 10–30 ng/dL; women, 0.3–2 ng/dL. (1 ng/dL = 0.035 nmol/L).

Testosterone, total: [S] Prepubertal, < 100 ng/dL; adult men, 300–1000 ng/dL; adult women, 20–80 ng/dL; luteal phase, up to 120 ng/dL.

Estradiol (E2): [S, special handling] Men, 12–34 pg/mL; women, menstrual cycle 1–10 days, 24–68 pg/mL; 11–20 days, 50–300 pg/mL; 21–30 days, 73–149 pg/mL (by radioimmunoassay [RIA]). (1 pg/mL = 3.6 pmol/L.)

Progesterone: [S] Follicular phase, 0.2–1.5 ng/mL; luteal phase, 6–32 ng/mL; pregnancy, > 24 ng/mL; men, < 1 ng/mL (by RIA). (1 ng/mL = 3.2 nmol/L.)

Islets:

Insulin: [S] 4–25 μU/mL (29–181 pmol/L).

C-peptide: [S] 0.9–4.2 ng/mL.

Glucagon: [S, fasting] 20–100 pg/mL.

Kidney:

Renin activity: [P, special handling] Normal sodium intake: Supine, 1–3 ng/mL/h; standing, 3–6 ng/mL/h. Sodium depleted: Supine, 2–6 ng/mL/h; standing, 3–20 ng/mL/h.

Parathyroid: Parathyroid hormone levels vary with method and antibody. Correlate with serum calcium.

Pituitary:

Growth hormone (GH): [S] Adults, 1–10 ng/mL (46–465 pmol/L) (by RIA).

Thyroid-stimulating hormone (TSH): [S] < 10 μU/mL.

Follicle-stimulating hormone (FSH): [S] Prepubertal, 2–12 mIU/mL; adult men, 1–15 mIU/mL; adult women, 1–30 mIU/mL; castrate or postmenopausal, 30–200 mIU/mL (by RIA).

Luteinizing hormone (LH): [S] Prepubertal, 2–12 mIU/mL; adult men, 1–15 mIU/mL; adult women, < 30 mIU/mL; castrate or postmenopausal, > 30 mIU/mL.

Corticotropin (ACTH): [P] 8:00–10:00 AM, up to 100 pg/mL (22 pmol/L).

Prolactin: [S] 1–25 ng/mL (0.4–10 nmol/L).

Somatomedin C: [P] 0.4–2 U/mL.

Antidiuretic hormone (ADH; vasopressin): [P] Serum osmolality 285 mOsm/kg, 0–2 pg/mL; > 290 mOsm/kg, 2–12+ pg/mL.

Placenta:

Estriol (E_3): [S] Men and nonpregnant women, < 0.2 μg/dL (< 7 nmol/L) (by RIA).

Chorionic gonadotropin: [S] Beta subunit: Men, < 9 mIU/mL; pregnant women after implantation, > 10 mIU/mL.

Stomach:

Gastrin: [S, special handling] Up to 100 pg/mL (47 pmol/L). Elevated, > 200 pg/mL.

Pepsinogen I: [S] 25–100 ng/mL.

Thyroid:

Thyroxine, free (FT_4): [S] 0.8–2.4 ng/dL (10–30 pmol/L).

Thyroxine, total (TT_4): [S] 5–12 μg/dL (65–156 nmol/L) (by RIA).

Thyroxine-binding globulin capacity (T_4): [S] 12–28 μg/dL (150–360 nmol/L).

Triiodothyronine (T_3): [S] 80–220 ng/dL (1.2–3.3 nmol/L). Reverse triiodothyronine (rT_3): [S] 30–80 ng/dL (0.45–1.2 nmol/L).

Triiodothyronine uptake (rT_3U): [S] 25–36%; as TBG assessment (rT_3U ratio), 0.85–1.15.

Calcitonin: [S] < 100 pg/mL (< 29.2 pmol/L).

NORMAL CEREBROSPINAL FLUID VALUES

Appearance: Clear and colorless.

Cells: Adults, 0–5 mononuclear cells/μL; infants, 0–20 mononuclear cells/μL.

Glucose: 50–85 mg/dL (2.8–4.7 mmol/L). (Draw serum glucose at same time.)

Pressure (reclining): Newborns, 30–88 mm water; children, 50–100 mm water; adults, 70–200 mm water (avg = 125).

Proteins: Total, 20–45 mg/dL (200–450 mg/L) in lumbar cerebrospinal fluid. IgG, 2–4 mg/dL (0.02–0.04 g/L).

Specific gravity: 1.003–1.008.

RENAL FUNCTION TESTS

ρ-Aminohippurate (PAH) clearance (RPF): Men, 560–830 mL/min; women, 490–700 mL/min.

Creatinine clearance: calculation from serum creatinine:

$$\text{Men: } \frac{(140 - \text{age}) \times (\text{wt in kg})}{72 \times \text{serum creatinine mg / dL}} = \frac{\text{creatinine clearance}}{\text{mL / min}}$$

Women: calculated value × 0.85

Creatinine clearance, endogenous (GFR): Approximates inulin clearance (see below).

Inulin clearance (GFR): Men, 110–150 mL/min; women, 105–132 mL/min (corrected to 1.73 m² surface area).

Maximal glucose reabsorptive capacity (Tm$_G$): Men, 300–450 mg/min; women, 250–350 mg/min.

Maximal PAH excretory capacity (Tm$_{PAH}$): 80–90 mg/min.

Osmolality: On normal diet and fluid intake: Range 500–850 mOsm/kg water. Achievable range, normal kidney: Dilution 40–80 mOsm; concentration (dehydration) up to 1400 mOsm/kg water (at least 3–4 times plasma osmolality).

Specific gravity of urine: 1.003–1.030.

MISCELLANEOUS NORMAL VALUES

Adrenal hormones and metabolites:

Aldosterone: [U] 2–26 µg/24 h (5.5–72 nmol). Values vary with sodium and potassium intake.

Catecholamines: [U] Total, < 100 µg/24 h. Epinephrine, < 10 µg/24 h (< 55 nmol); norepinephrine, < 100 µg/24 h (< 591 nmol). Values vary with method used.

Cortisol, free: [U] 20–100 µg/24 h (0.55–2.76 mmol).

11,17-Hydroxycorticoids: [U] Men, 4–12 mg/24 h; women, 4–8 mg/24 h. Values vary with method used.

17-Ketosteroids: [U] Under 8 years, 0–2 mg/24 h; adolescents, 2–20 mg/24 h. Men, 10–20 mg/24 h; women, 5–15 mg/24 h. Values vary with method used. (1 mg = 3.5 mmol.)

Metanephrine: [U] < 1.3 mg/24 h (< 6.6 µmol) or < 2.2 µg/mg creatinine. Values vary with method used.

Vanillylmandelic acid (VMA): [U] Up to 7 mg/24 h (< 35 µmol).

Fecal fat: Less than 30% dry weight.

Lead: [U] < 80 µg/24 h (< 0.4 µmol/d).

Porphyrins:

Delta-aminolevulinic acid: [U] 1.5–7.5 mg/24 h (11.4–57.2 µmol).

Coproporphyrin: [U] < 230 µg/24 h (< 345 nmol).

Uroporphyrin: [U] < 50 µg/24 h (< 60 nmol).

Porphobilinogen: [U] < 2 mg/24 h (< 8.8 µmol).

Urobilinogen: [U] 0–2.5 mg/24 h (< 4.23 µmol).

Urobilinogen, fecal: 40–280 mg/24 h (68–474 µmol).

Index

Note: Page numbers in bold face type indicate a major discussion. A t following a page number indicates tabular material and an f following a page number indicates a figure. Drugs are listed under their generic names. When a drug trade name is listed, the reader is referred to the generic name.